The Papers of George Catlett Marshall

I think we can look forward to the time when we will have world peace. . . . That's what General Marshall has spent the best part of his life working for ever since he was Chief of Staff and I think General Marshall will go down in history as the man of the age.

—Harry S. Truman
November 3, 1953

Published under the auspices of
The George C. Marshall Foundation

To Larry I. Bland (1940–2007)
Founding Editor of the Marshall Papers

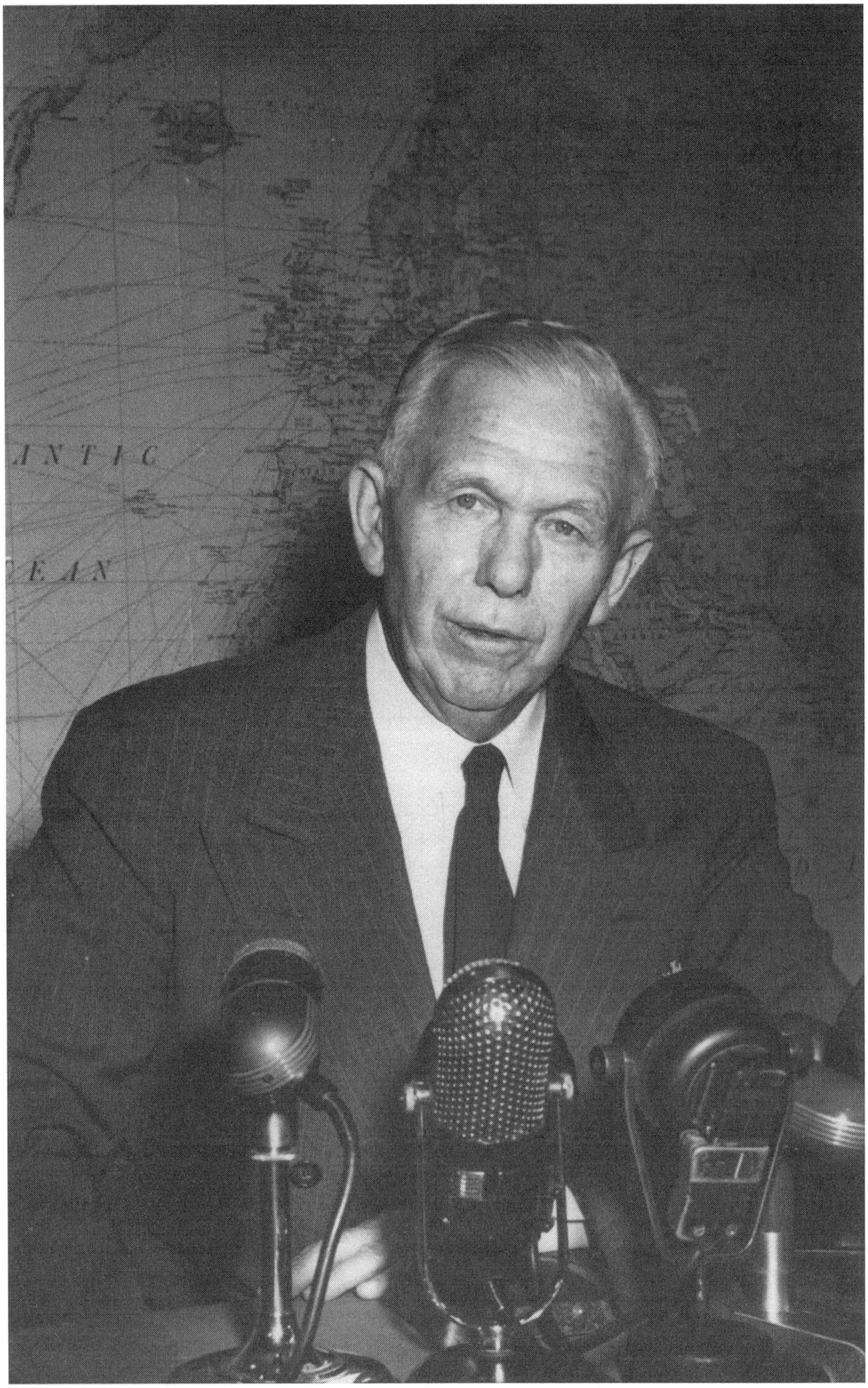
ANTIC
EAN

The Papers of George Catlett Marshall

Volume 7

"THE MAN OF THE AGE"

OCTOBER 1, 1949 – OCTOBER 16, 1959

Mark A. Stoler, Editor

Daniel D. Holt, Managing Editor

Anne S. Wells and Mame Warren, Senior Assistant Editors

Gregory C. Franke, Assistant Editor

Joanne D. Hartog, Research Assistant

THE JOHNS HOPKINS UNIVERSITY PRESS
Baltimore
2016

Printed in the United States of America on acid-free paper.

The Johns Hopkins University Press
2715 North Charles Street
Baltimore, Maryland 21218-4363
www.press.jhu.edu

Library of Congress Cataloging-in-Publication Data
(Revised for volume 7)
Marshall, George C. (George Catlett), 1880–1959.
The papers of George Catlett Marshall.
Includes index.
Contents: v. 1. "The soldierly spirit," December 1880–June 1939.
v. 2. "We cannot delay," July 1, 1939–December 6, 1941.
v. 3. "The right man for the job," December 7, 1941–May 31, 1943.
v. 4 "Aggressive and determined leadership," June 1, 1943–December 31, 1944.
v. 5. "The finest soldier," January 1, 1945–January 7, 1947.
v. 6. "The whole world hangs in the balance," January 8, 1947–September 30, 1949.
v. 7. "The man of the age," October 1, 1949–October 16, 1959.
1. Marshall, George C. (George Catlett), 1880–1959.
2. United States—History, Military—20th century—Sources.
3. Generals—United States—Correspondence.
4. United States—History, Diplomatic—20th century—Sources.

I. Stoler, Mark A. II. Holt, Daniel D. III. Title

E745.M37 1981 973.918′092′4 81-47593

ISBN 0-8018-2552-0 (v. 1)
ISBN 0-8018-2553-9 (v. 2)
ISBN 0-8018-2967-4 (v. 3)
ISBN 0-8018-5368-0 (v. 4)
ISBN 0-8018-7871-3 (v. 5)
ISBN 10: 1-4214-0792-2 (v. 6)
ISBN 13: 978-1-4214-0792-0 (v. 6)
ISBN 10: 1-4214-1962-9 (v. 7)
ISBN 13: 978-1-4214-1962-6 (v. 7)

A catalog record for this book is available from the British Library.

The preparation and publication of this volume was made possible in part by grants from the National Historical Publications and Records Commission and the National Endowment for the Humanities, independent agencies of the United States government; the Carnegie Corporation of New York; Furthermore Grants, a program of the J. R. Kaplan Fund; the Ambrose Monell Foundation; the Dr. Scholl Foundation; FedEx Corporation; the Miller Family Fund; and Mark Baruch and the Baruch Family Foundation.

Contents

Preface

The Marshall Papers

The George C. Marshall Research Library is the repository for Marshall's personal papers. Since 1956 this collection has been supplemented by contributions of documents by his friends, associates, and admirers and by the Marshall Foundation's program of copying relevant documents in other repositories, primarily the US National Archives.

This seventh and final volume of Marshall's papers, which includes 626 documents from the Marshall material available to the editors, differs in some significant ways from most of the previous volumes. Whereas the first five volumes focused largely on Marshall's extensive army career and his work as army chief of staff during World War II and the sixth volume concerned his two-year tenure as secretary of state, this volume concentrates on his civilian work as head of the American Red Cross from October 1949 to December 1950, as secretary of defense from September 1950 to September 1951, and as longtime chairman of the American Battle Monuments Commission, as well as the eight years of his retirement until his death in October 1959. As head of the US Army General Staff from 1939 to 1945 and as secretary of state from 1947 to 1949, Marshall signed numerous documents that he did not draft. He continued to do so as head of the US Department of Defense from September 1950 to September 1951, when Defense Department civilians and military officers drafted many documents bearing his signature. Scholars are often less concerned with who actually drafted a document than with who authorized or signed it. Thus, the secondary literature for the period covered in this volume has citations to important documents emanating from Marshall's office and bearing his name that have not been included here. This volume does not seek to publish the papers of the secretary of defense's office but only those created or edited by Marshall himself.

Regardless of their importance, many staff-written documents are thus not included except as noted in the annotations. With a few exceptions as explained below, Marshall wrote, dictated, spoke, and/or edited all of the documents that are included. As with staff-originated documents produced for his signature as army chief of staff and secretary of state, however, Marshall as secretary of defense continued to carefully oversee the contents of such documents. He frequently edited and modified the drafts of his subordinates so extensively that the editors have considered the final products to be Marshall documents.

Marshall was sixty-nine years old when appointed secretary of defense and turned seventy that winter. While he was still vigorous and mentally alert, he clearly did not possess the strength and stamina of his earlier years. Consequently, he relegated a great deal of work to his deputy secretary, Robert Lovett, who would succeed him as defense secretary in September 1951. He also relied much more heavily than in the past on staff members to draft or dictate to secretaries his letters, memoranda, and speeches—most notably his executive officer Marshall Carter and his aide C. J. George. During the retirement years, George and Mary Louise Spilman, the secretary in Marshall's Pentagon office, became even more important in drafting Marshall's correspondence. It is obvious, however, from the style as well as the contents of these documents—many of which contain personal information and memories Carter, George, and Spilman could not have known in advance—that Marshall told them what he wanted to be included. He also continued to heavily edit material they and other staff members had drafted. Consequently, the editors have chosen to include these letters as well.

Volume seven also contains more documents relating to Marshall's personal life than previous volumes. This is primarily due to the recent acquisition and use of a new collection of Marshall documents that Katherine Marshall retained after the death of her husband and the establishment of the George C. Marshall Research Library. This material remained in the family's possession until 2013, when her grandson James J. Winn Jr. donated it to the Marshall Library. Officially entitled the George Catlett Marshall and Katherine Marshall Collection, it is cited in this volume as the Marshall-Winn Collection. Marshall also wrote particularly personal letters to his goddaughter Rose Page Wilson and close friend Frank McCarthy as well as to family members and former colleagues, especially in his retirement years, many of which the editors have included in this volume and most of which are available in the collections of the George C. Marshall Research Library.

When Marshall resigned as secretary of defense in September 1951, he maintained a Pentagon office but spent most of his time at his home in Leesburg, Virginia, and his winter residence in Pinehurst, North Carolina, where he had very limited secretarial help. He frequently communicated with his office at the Pentagon, often dictating over the telephone or sending letters and speeches drafted by hand for M. L. Spilman or C. J. George to type. He also mailed many handwritten letters. Marshall's spelling was notoriously poor, and when the editors have transcribed such handwritten letters they have retained the spelling errors in the original. Secretarial errors in typing, however, have been corrected (see *Silent Corrections* in the Guide to Editorial Policies).

Given the number of years covered in this volume as well as the ancillary materials described above, a significant number of documents originally selected could not be included. Typescripts of these selected documents, together with unedited annotations, will be placed on the Marshall Foundation's website in the future as a supplement to the published volume.

Marshall's shift in position to secretary of defense led to a different focus on sources, with many of the documents included in this volume coming from Department of Defense records in Record Group 330 of the National Archives as well as the Secretary of Defense subgroup in the Marshall Papers. A detailed description of this subgroup exists in John N. Jacob, *George C. Marshall Papers, 1932–1960: A Guide* (Lexington, VA: George C. Marshall Foundation, 1987). A scanned version of this collection guide is available at www.marshallfoundation.org.

Considering the large number of extensive meetings Marshall attended as secretary of defense, the editors decided to provide very brief summaries of many of them, along with citations to the official minutes of these meetings available in the above-cited sources and the 1950 and 1951 volumes of the State Department's documentary series, *Foreign Relations of the United States*. They have also provided summaries of and excerpts from some of Marshall's speeches and congressional appearances during that year, as well as a listing of his published testimonies during this time period.

During Marshall's final year, when he was no longer able to communicate, Katherine Marshall, C. J. George, and M. L. Spilman sent important messages to family, friends, and former colleagues describing the final months of Marshall's life. A summary of this correspondence is included in the *Afterword*. Most of this material has not been published previously; extracts with citations are provided to complete the story. The details of Marshall's funeral and burial are readily available in several sources and are not included in this volume. (In particular, see B. D. Mossman and M. W. Stark, *The Last Salute: Civil and Military Funerals, 1921–69* [Washington: Department of the Army, 1971], 158–67.)

This seventh and final volume of the Marshall Papers differs in one other way from previous volumes. As explained in the preface to volume six, on November 27, 2007, Dr. Larry I. Bland, editor of and project director for the Marshall Papers for thirty years, suddenly and unexpectedly died (see *Papers of GCM*, 6: x–xi). The Marshall Foundation decided that work on the last two volumes of the papers would continue and appointed a team to finish the series composed of University of Vermont emeritus professor of history Mark A. Stoler as editor and Eisenhower Library former director Daniel D. Holt as managing editor and project director, with Sharon Ritenour Stevens, who had been with the project since its inception as associate editor, retaining that position. Anne S. Wells of the staff of the *Journal of Military History* served as a part-time assistant editor. Stevens became seriously ill and incapacitated in 2011, however, and was unable to complete volume six or work on any of volume seven beyond chapter one. Mame Warren, formerly director of Hopkins History Enterprises at the Johns Hopkins University, joined the team in April

2011 as assistant editor. Stevens died on August 9, 2013. With her passing, the project lost both an experienced documentary editor and, in effect, its historical memory; she has been sorely missed. After her death, Warren and Wells became senior assistant editors and Gregory C. Franke, who was the principal research assistant on volume six, became assistant editor, while Joanne Hartog joined the team as a research assistant.

ACKNOWLEDGMENTS

Given the change in both Marshall's position and the sources used in volumes six and seven, two highly distinguished senior diplomatic historians were added to the advisory board to review drafts and advise the editorial team on these two volumes: Robert L. Beisner, emeritus professor of history at American University; and George C. Herring, emeritus professor of history at the University of Kentucky. They joined eminent senior military historian Edward M. Coffman, emeritus professor at the University of Wisconsin–Madison; and Edwin A. Thompson, former director of the Records Declassification Division, National Archives, both of whom had advised on previous volumes. When Thompson died in April 2013, Allan Millett, a distinguished senior military historian and professor emeritus at the Ohio State University, agreed to serve as the fourth member of the advisory committee. The editors are deeply grateful for both their commitment and comments. We are also indebted to Dr. Daun van Ee, a former editor of the Eisenhower Papers who served as an essential editorial consultant, for his thoughtful insights.

Marshall Foundation executive assistants Alice Lee and Debbie Barron cheerfully and dependably supported the editors in countless ways. Marshall Library staff Jeffrey Kozak, Paul Barron, and Cara Sonnier shared their expertise. Joellen Bland, Katie Kain, and Gregory Franke keyed the documents for this volume. Robert S. Keefe patiently and meticulously composed the volume camera-ready for the printer. Marilyn Holt attentively compiled the index. Donelle DeWitt produced all the maps and set the charts in the volume. Evan Haberman (VMI, 1976) painstakingly proofread every document in this volume and provided important observations that improved our efforts.

The National Historical Publications and Records Commission and its staff have given the editors vital moral and financial support since the beginning of the Marshall Papers. Without this support, the project very likely could not have been completed. The editors also express gratitude to the National Endowment for the Humanities for its continuing financial support.

The George C. Marshall Foundation acknowledges with deep appreciation the financial support of the Carnegie Corporation of New York, Furthermore Grants (a program of the J. M. Kaplan Fund), the Ambrose Monell Foundation, the Dr. Scholl Foundation, the FedEx Corporation, the Miller Family Fund, and Mark Baruch and the Baruch Family Foundation.

Robert J. Brugger of the Johns Hopkins University Press has nurtured this project for years; the editors appreciate his dedication and wish him well in his retirement. Without the assistance of historians and archivists, no undertaking such as this would be possible. The editors acknowledge their indebtedness to the following persons: Timothy Nenninger and Tab Lewis at the National Archives; Conrad Crane at the Army Military History Institute; Timothy Rives and Christopher Abraham at the Dwight D. Eisenhower Presidential Library; William Baehr at the Franklin D. Roosevelt Library; Craig G. Wright at the Herbert Hoover Presidential Library; Randy Sowell at the Harry S. Truman Presidential Library; Jill Severn of the Richard B. Russell Library, University of Georgia; Rosalba Varallo Recchia at the Seeley G. Mudd Manuscript Library, Princeton University; Alissa Link at the Arthur and Elizabeth Schlesinger Library, Harvard University; Bill Massa, Dika Goloweiko-Nussberg, and Robert Klingernberger at Sterling Memorial Library, Yale University; Allen Packwood, Emily Morris, Katharine Thomson, and Francesca Alves at the Churchill Archives Centre, Churchill College, Cambridge; Anne S. Turkos at the University of Maryland; Lynn Conway at Georgetown University; Tonya Moore, Diane Jacob, and Mary Laura Kludy of Preston Library, Virginia Military Institute; Elizabeth Teaff and Tom Camden at the Leyburn Library, Washington and Lee University; Amy Fitch at the Rockefeller Center Archives; Dieter Ullrich, LaDonna Hamontree, and Cynthia Barnes at the Forrest C. Pogue Library, Murray State University; Jennifer Kirmer and Miranda Rectenwald at the Washington University Archives; and Laura J. Kissel at the Byrd Polar Research Center Archival Program, University Libraries, the Ohio State University. We would also like to give special thanks to Richard Langworth, editor of *Finest Hour*; and Frank Costigliola, editor of the George F. Kennan diaries.

The editors gratefully acknowledge the permission of the following individuals, publishers, and institutions to reproduce materials: Daniel J. Linke at Princeton University for permission to extract from the George F. Kennan diaries; Robert Faurot of Chicago for permission to quote from his grandfather William Spencer's correspondence with Marshall; the Radcliffe Institute at Harvard University for permission to quote from the Anna Rosenberg Papers; Hege Puntervill of NTB scanpix for permission to publish a photograph of the 1953 Nobel Peace Prize ceremony; and Lori Birdsong of Wright's Media for permission to publish a 1951 *U.S. News and World Report* interview with Secretary Marshall.

Guide to Editorial Policies

STYLE

Document texts and quotations in the annotation follow the writer's style, except as noted below. The editors' style generally conforms to that suggested by *The Chicago Manual of Style*, 15th ed. (Chicago: University of Chicago Press, 2003).

TEXTUAL CHANGES AND INSERTIONS

Document Heading. The organization, sequence, and sometimes the content of the document heading have been supplied by the editors. Heading information is taken from the source documents when available; however, if research indicates an error in the original date or place, a correction has been made using brackets and italics (see *Brackets* below). The heading consists of between three and seven elements: addressee, date, originator, place of origin, message designation, security classification, and title.

The addressee for letters, telegrams, and radio messages is always in the form TO HARRY S. TRUMAN. Civil titles (e.g., Senator, Dr., The Honorable, Judge, etc.) are not included in the document heading. If the recipient was a married woman, Marshall usually used "Mrs." with her husband's name if he knew it (e.g., Mrs. James J. Winn rather than Molly B. Winn). The editors have used the form Marshall indicated. For military personnel, including retired professionals, the rank used is that correct as of the date of the document. No distinction is made between permanent and temporary ranks in the annotation.

The addressee for memoranda is usually in the form MEMORANDUM FOR _________. With a few exceptions, the form of address used by Marshall is followed, but abbreviations (e.g., ACS, Col., etc.) have been spelled out. If the memorandum is to an addressee's title only and that individual (excepting the president) has not been previously identified, the editors have supplied the name in the heading or an endnote.

The security classification in a document's heading is given in italic type beneath the sender-recipient line. (See *Radio, Telegraph, and Cable Messages.*)

Salutation and Complimentary Close. When present, these elements have been printed with the first and last lines respectively of the document text rather than on separate lines as they appear in the original. Marshall usually addressed male recipients by their last names with a few exceptions. The capitalization and punctuation of the original have been retained.

Signature. Most documents in this volume have been reproduced from file (carbon) copies in the Marshall Papers or in various Defense Department and other official records. A name (or initials) at the end of a document published herein usually indicates that the editors have used a signed copy as the source text. During Marshall's term as secretary of defense and his retirement years, he often dictated messages and on occasion approved correspondence drafted by others. (See also *Preface.*) After Marshall retired in 1951, he often dictated letters over the telephone to Mary Louise Spilman, the secretary in his Pentagon office. Research indicates that no correspondence was sent without his approval even if his signature is missing on the copy of the original document. These are considered to be Marshall documents.

Silent Corrections. In making silent corrections, the editors have distinguished between documents physically produced by the author and those produced by a clerk or secretary from dictation or handwritten drafts. No silent changes have been introduced into author-produced documents unless misspellings in the originals cause confusion or change the meaning of the document. (See also *Brackets.*) Misspellings are common in Marshall's handwritten letters. (See also *Preface.*) In documents typed by a clerk or secretary, the original capitalization and punctuation have been retained, but the occasional spelling errors have been silently corrected. Marshall sometimes made minor corrections to documents prior to having them sent; these changes are accepted as the final version of the source text. If corrections were made by Marshall with strikeovers, strikeovers are left in place.

Brackets. All information within brackets in document texts has been supplied by the editors unless otherwise stated. If the bracketed material is in italic type, it is to be read in place of the preceding word or letter (e.g., "Last week I did 7500 miles and 14 [*fifteen*] cities." If the bracketed material is in roman type, it indicates additional rather than substitute information (e.g., "Wednesday afternoon [August 3] President Truman").

Italics to Emphasize and Differentiate. Except where used in brackets, italic type appears in the text of a document or in a quotation if the emphasis was in the original—indicated on the source text by underlining.

Merged Correspondence. During Marshall's term as secretary of defense and particularly in his retirement, he occasionally wrote his responses on the incoming correspondence by hand rather than create a new document. The response was then drafted by staff using Marshall's handwritten comments. When a correspondent posed specific questions Marshall chose to answer, the questions are inserted into Marshall's response in italic type within brackets (e.g., see pp. 709–11).

Speeches. As secretary of defense and during his retirement years, Marshall often departed from the prepared text. Consequently, in order to provide an accurate text of speeches as delivered by Marshall, transcripts and recordings of the speeches—rather than reading copies—have been used as the source documents when available.

Cross-references. References to documents within this volume are to page numbers, and document numbers are specified only if more than one set of notes appears on the cross-referenced page. Citations to previous volumes in this series are usually given as: see *Papers of GCM*, 5: 186; citations to *The Papers of Dwight David Eisenhower*, 21 volumes (Baltimore: Johns Hopkins University Press, 1970–2001) are usually given as: see *Papers of DDE*, 11: 1014. All previous volumes of *The Papers of George Catlett Marshall* are online in searchable format (www.marshallfoundation.org).

Radio, Telegraph, and Cable Messages. The term "Radio" is used to designate messages sent by radio, telegraph line, submarine cable, or some combination of these. When Marshall addresses a message to an agency, office, official, or specific person for transmission to a designated addressee, the ultimate recipient is normally given in the document heading, and the sender's message number is included if known (e.g., "To Robert A. Lovett, Radio No. _____. *Secret* Personal Eyes Only from Marshall"). Depending on the version used as a source text, radio messages may be in standard form (i.e., upper and lowercase letters with punctuation marks) or in all capitals with spelled-out punctuation and numerals. In the latter case, the editors have silently converted the text to standard form, including converting spelled-out numbers, dates, and names (e.g., C-54 instead of C HYPHEN FIVE FOUR).

Document Source Citations

Source Line. At the end of each document and prior to any endnotes, the source of the text is given in the following format: Repository/Collection (Main entry, Subentry, Sub-subentry)—e.g., GCMRL/G. C. Marshall Papers (American Red Cross, Categorical, Memoranda). Multiple copies may exist of certain documents, and these may be found in different repositories or collections. The version used by the editors as the source text is the one cited. Abbreviations used in the source citations are listed in the glossary.

Manuscript Notation. Most of the source texts for documents printed in this volume were typewritten by a clerk or secretary from dictation, notes, or a draft. Marshall's handwritten documents are designated by an "H."

Annotation

The editors use two types of annotation within the section of the volume containing documentary material:

Document Endnotes. Printed in small type at the end of documents.

Editorial Notes. General explanatory material referring to one or more subsequent documents; printed in document-size type. To distinguish these visually from documents, such notes have no heading, begin with a large dropped capital letter, and end with a star.

Editors' Summaries of Selected Meeting Texts, Speeches, and Testimo-

nies. Summaries of the minutes or transcripts of lengthy meetings in which Marshall is a key participant (e.g., see p. 14). To distinguish these visually from documents, such summaries have a centered heading, begin with a large dropped capital letter, and end with a star.

In the endnotes and editorial notes, the editors have attempted to explain all potentially obscure references, provide cross-references to important related material, and summarize the key parts of incoming or outgoing documents of relevance. Graduates of the federal service academies and the Virginia Military Institute have been identified by school and year of graduation (e.g., VMI, 1901) the first time that person is cited in this volume. Personal identifications normally include only the status, rank, or role at the time of the citation. Members of Congress's state and party affiliations are identified in prose or parentheses (D-VT) the first time they are mentioned. Later citations give changes that had occurred since the previous citation. Indexes to the various volumes of *The Papers of George Catlett Marshall* will enable the reader to follow a particular individual's development or relationship to Marshall. For acronyms, abbreviations, and code names, please consult the glossary.

The editors have not cited individual uses of certain reference works such as the *Army Register*, the Civil Service Commission's *Official Register*, *Cullum's Biographical Register of the Officers and Graduates of the U.S. Military Academy*, the *Congressional Directory*, and *Who's Who in America*. The editors frequently consulted Marshall's engagement calendars and logs to verify dates and places.

The editors have sought to minimize the use of secondary sources in the annotation. Whenever appropriate and feasible, quotations from Marshall documents not selected for publication, or from other primary sources, have been used. The editors have provided citations to the unpublished referenced documents. The Marshall Papers project is intended to provide a cohesive, intelligible story of Marshall in his own words, not to provide a detailed discussion of every facet of his life and times or to examine numerous questions not mentioned in Marshall's documents.

Illustrations

The following are the sources for the illustrations used in this volume.

frontispiece

Secretary of Defense George C. Marshall comments on Korean War armistice negotiations during a press conference, July 24, 1951. US Army photo; GCMRL/Photographs (1094).

following p. 538

1. General Marshall sits at his desk at American Red Cross headquarters in Washington, DC, September 13, 1950. Harris & Ewing photo; GCMRL/Photographs (950).
2. General Marshall visits with Red Cross staff and volunteers at Fort Bragg, North Carolina, c.1949–50. US Army photo; GCMRL/Photographs (371).
3. General Marshall speaks on the second anniversary of the enactment of the European Cooperation Act in Washington, DC, April 3, 1950. GCMRL/Photographs (161).
4. Marshall takes the oath of office as secretary of defense at the Pentagon, September 21, 1950. US Army photo; GCMRL/Photographs (272).
5. Secretary Marshall addresses the NATO defense ministers meeting at the Pentagon, October 28, 1950. US Army photo; GCMRL/Photographs (783).
6. Anna Rosenberg takes the oath of office as assistant secretary of defense at the Pentagon, November 15, 1950. Department of Defense photo; GCMRL/Photographs (789).
7. Secretary Marshall, General Eisenhower, President Truman, and Secretary Acheson shake hands in Washington, DC, January 6, 1951. GCMRL/Photographs (283).
8. Secretary Marshall administers the oath of loyalty to Civil Defense volunteers in New York City, February 27, 1951. Acme photo 963116; GCMRL/Photographs (792).
9. Secretary Marshall sits behind General MacArthur, April 19, 1951. US Army photo; GCMRL/Photographs (849).
10. Secretary Marshall smiles at the press following testimony on General MacArthur's relief, May 11, 1951. Associated Press photo; GCMRL/Photographs (1103).

11. Secretary Marshall speaks at the dedication of the Marshall Arch in the VMI barracks in Lexington, Virginia, May 15, 1951. GCMRL/Photographs (300).
12. Secretary Marshall and Generals Ridgway, Almond, and Van Fleet prepare to leave for X Corps headquarters in Hongchon, Korea, June 8, 1951. US Army photo; GCMRL/Photographs (2460A).
13. Secretary Marshall inspects the honor guard at X Corps headquarters in Hongchon, Korea, June 8, 1951. US Army photo; GCMRL/Photographs (870).
14. General Ridgway, Colonel Carter, and Secretary Marshall disembark Ridgway's plane in Seoul, Korea, June 8, 1951. US Air Force photo; GCMRL/Photographs (4028).
15. General Marshall and Assistant Secretary Rosenberg lead the members of the Defense Advisory Committee on Women in the Services up the steps of the Pentagon, September 17, 1951. Department of Defense photo; GCMRL/Photographs (305).
16. President and Margaret Truman visit the Marshalls in Leesburg, Virginia, c.1952. Photo by William J. Heffner. GCMRL/William J. Heffner Collection (Photographs/Prints).
17. General and Mrs. Marshall tend to their garden in Leesburg, Virginia, September 15, 1951. GCMRL/© Marshall-Winn Collection (Retirement, Photographs).
18. Generals Omar N. Bradley and Emmett O'Donnell, President Eisenhower, Undersecretary Walter Bedell Smith, and General Marshall pose with their godsons, at Fort Myer, Virginia, April 6, 1953. GCMRL/Photographs (7966).
19. General Marshall sits aboard the SS *Andrea Doria* en route to Naples, Italy, December 1953. Provided by Elizabeth Stetson Barry; GCMRL/Photographs (1321).
20. General Marshall receives the Nobel Peace Prize in Oslo, Norway, December 10, 1953. Credit: NTBscanpix.
21. General Marshall cuts the cake on his seventy-fifth birthday in Pinehurst, North Carolina, December 31, 1955. GCMRL/© Marshall-Winn Collection (Retirement, Photographs).
22. General and Mrs. Marshall watch a golf tournament in Pinehurst, North Carolina, n.d. GCMRL/Photographs (2043).
23. General and Mrs. Marshall chat with Frank McCarthy in Leesburg, Virginia, July 1956. Photo by William J. Heffner. GCMRL/© Marshall-Winn Collection (Retirement, Photographs).

Chronology

October 1, 1949–October 20, 1959

The following is a selective list of important events of General Marshall's life (in roman) and of influences on him (in italic type) during the period covered by this volume. Unless otherwise noted, events involving Marshall took place in Washington, DC, or in the Pentagon. All times are local.

During the last ten years of his life, the Marshalls alternated between two homes: Dodona Manor in Leesburg, Virginia, where they usually lived from late spring to late fall; and Liscombe Lodge in Pinehurst, North Carolina, where they spent the rest of their time. They also rented a small apartment in Washington, DC, during part of the year he served as secretary of defense.

Most of the appointment records for Marshall's presidency of the American Red Cross (October 1949–December 1950) are available in GCMRL/G. C. Marshall Papers (American Red Cross, Travel Schedules and Appointment Diary). The latter part of 1949 is also covered in GCMRL/G. C. Marshall Papers (Pentagon Office, Engagement and Visitor Records). The last months of Marshall's Red Cross presidency, as well as his term as secretary of defense (September 1950–September 1951), are documented in the detailed appointment records in GCMRL/G. C. Marshall Papers (Secretary of Defense, Engagement, Visitor, and Correspondent Records). The appointment records for his retirement (September 1951–October 1959), which are much less inclusive, are available in GCMRL/G. C. Marshall Papers (Retirement, Engagements and Correspondent Records).

For Marshall's year as secretary of defense, this chronology includes meetings with the president, the cabinet, and the National Security Council, but omits meetings with other officials he saw frequently, such as Robert A. Lovett, Dean Acheson, W. Averell Harriman, and the Joint Chiefs of Staff, except when the president was involved. It also excludes many of his appointments with the Armed Forces Policy Council, the Business Advisory Council, and foreign officials as well as numerous social engagements and many of his meetings with the Pan American Airways Board of Directors while head of the American Red Cross.

October 1949

1 President Truman's appointment of Marshall as ARC president takes effect.

3 Meeting with President Truman and Basil O'Connor, outgoing ARC president, 11:30 a.m.

6–8 State Department roundtable discussion on US policy toward China; ARC Board of Governors Executive Committee on the 8th, 11:00 a.m.
18 Receives award at New York Board of Trade dinner, New York City, 8:00 p.m.
19 New York Red Cross chapter luncheon and meetings, 12:30 p.m.
20 National Geographic Society Board of Trustees meeting, 4:30 p.m.
21 Testifies before House Armed Services Committee on unification of the national defense program, 10:00 a.m.
24–30 Six-day tour of Red Cross chapters and meetings with chapter and community representatives as well as press, traveling from Washington to Pittsburgh, PA; Cleveland, OH; Chicago, IL; Minneapolis, MN; Bismarck, ND; Seattle, WA; Portland, OR; San Francisco, CA; Los Angeles, CA; Phoenix, AZ; Kansas City, MO; St. Louis, MO; Memphis, TN; New Orleans, LA; and Atlanta, GA; returns to Washington overnight.

November 1949
2 Edward R. Stettinius Jr. funeral, New York City, 10:00 a.m.
4 VMI Board of Visitors meeting, Lexington, VA, 8:00 p.m.; VMI football game on the 5th.
9 ABMC meeting, 10:00 a.m.
10–14 ARC meetings; addresses meeting of ARC Large City Chapters on the 10th.
17–19 Speaks to students and faculty at Princeton University and attends Princeton-Dartmouth football game on the 19th, Princeton, NJ.
25 Receives United States Conference of Mayors award for distinguished public service from President Truman at the White House, 12:30 p.m.
29 Speaks at United Negro College Fund Forum at Hunter College, New York City, 8:30 p.m.

December 1949
2 Meeting with Baltimore Red Cross chapter, Baltimore, MD, 4:00 p.m.
5–6 Advisory Committee on Blood meeting, Washington, 9:30 a.m.; travels to New York City for afternoon meeting at International House and dinner with John D. Rockefeller Jr.; then luncheon on the 6th with radio and television executives followed by Pan American Airways Board of Directors meeting, 2:30 p.m.
7 National Geographic Society Board of Trustees meeting, Washington, 4:30 p.m.
13 Addresses ARC staff, 4:00 p.m.
14 Lectures at the National War College, 8:45 a.m.
27 Travels from Pinehurst to Hobcaw Manor, Bernard Baruch's home near Georgetown, SC, returning to Pinehurst on January 3.

January 1950
16 Begins second tour of Red Cross chapters in preparation for 1950 fund campaign with visit and address in Boston, followed by luncheon hosted by American Legion; press conference; dedication of Massachusetts Regional Blood Center; travel to Providence, RI, for meetings with area chapter representatives; address to patients at Veterans Administration Hospital; and press conference.

19 Attends General Henry H. Arnold's funeral, Washington National Cathedral; serves as honorary pallbearer at burial, Arlington National Cemetery, 3:00 p.m.

22–27 Resumes Red Cross tour with meetings, speeches, and press conferences in Jacksonville and Tampa, FL; Montgomery and Birmingham, AL; Houston and Dallas, TX; Oklahoma City, OK; Wichita, KS; Nashville, TN; and Louisville, KY; returns to Pinehurst on the 28th.

February 1950

6–7 Departs Pinehurst for meetings in New York City and continues Red Cross tour with visits to Rochester and Buffalo, NY.

8–25 Continues Red Cross tour with meetings, press conferences, and speeches in Buffalo, NY; Detroit, MI; Toledo, OH; Indianapolis, IN; and Cincinnati, OH; returns to Pinehurst February 10–14; then resumes tour with visits to Philadelphia, PA; New York, NY; Newark, NJ; New Orleans, LA; Los Angeles, CA; Honolulu, HI; and San Francisco, CA.

27 Speaks at Voice of Democracy program, Colonial Williamsburg, VA, 2:00 p.m.

28 Records remarks for Voice of America, and introduces the president in a radio broadcast opening the 1950 Red Cross Drive, White House, 10:30 p.m.

March 1950

5 Makes radio broadcast about ARC during the United States Steel Corporation's *Theatre Guild on the Air*, New York City, 8:10 p.m.

6–7 Continues Red Cross tour with visits to Pittsburgh and Erie, PA; Akron and Youngstown, OH.

11 Review of the 82d Airborne Division and luncheon, Fort Bragg, NC, 11:00 a.m.

27 Attends ARC Board of Governors meeting; promotes the ARC fund campaign on Arthur Godfrey's radio and television programs, 8:45 p.m., and on the *Lux Radio Theatre*, 9:55 p.m.

29 ABMC meeting, 10:00 a.m.

April 1950

3 Speaks to ECA employees at the program's mid-point anniversary, 11:15 a.m.

4 Speaks at International House luncheon and attends Pan American Airways Board of Directors meeting, New York City.

May 1950

5 ARC Blood Committee luncheon, 1:00 p.m.

8 Meeting with Secretary of the Army Frank Pace, followed by lunch with General Omar Bradley, 1:15 p.m.

10 Speaks to annual convention of military chaplains, noon.

16 Speaks at International House dinner, New York City, 8:00 p.m.

17 Speaks to National Boys Club Executive Association meeting and then at the presentation of *The Papers of Thomas Jefferson*, volume 1, to President Truman and Marshall, the Library of Congress, 3:30 p.m.

30 Delivers Memorial Day address at Arlington National Cemetery, 1:00 p.m.
31 Speaks at dinner for Red Cross chapter representatives, Denver, CO, 5:30 p.m.

June 1950

1 Speaks at luncheon in Fort Leavenworth, KS.
7 Testifies first before House Foreign Affairs Committee and then in executive session before Senate Foreign Relations and Armed Services Committee on Mutual Defense Assistance Program, 10:30 a.m.
12 Delivers commencement address at Pennsylvania College for Women, which awards Mrs. Marshall an honorary degree, Pittsburgh, PA; attends VMI dinner, Lexington, VA, 7:00 p.m., and delivers address at VMI graduation on the 13th.
14 Lunch with the president and BAC meetings; meeting with Pace at the Pentagon on the 15th, 3:00 p.m.
25 *North Korean Army invades South Korea.*
24–29 In Detroit for ARC convention; delivers keynote address at first plenary session on the 26th and closing remarks on the 29th.

July 1950

1 Meeting with Acheson, Charles E. Bohlen, W. Averell Harriman, and George F. Kennan in Leesburg, 1:00 p.m.
4 Meeting with President Truman in Leesburg.
5 Testifies before a subcommittee of the Senate Foreign Relations Committee on educational activities to combat communism; meeting with Pace; luncheon meeting with the president, Generals Dwight D. Eisenhower and Bradley, and Admiral Forrest P. Sherman, Blair House, 1:00 p.m.
11 Meeting with Red Cross Blood Program committees, 10:00 a.m., and speech on the ARC National Blood Program, Boston, MA, 7:00 p.m.
28 Records statement for Lockheed Aircraft Corporation in support of the ARC National Blood Program, 10:45 a.m., to air on August 11.

August 1950

2 Travels to Huron Mountain Camp, MI, for vacation.
26 *President Truman calls Marshall in Michigan.*

September 1950

2 Leaves Huron Mountain Camp and arrives Washington, 6:00 p.m.
6 Meetings with Bradley, 9:00 a.m.; the president, noon; and Pace.
7 Hosts Averell Harriman for lunch, Leesburg.
10–11 ARC meetings, Washington and Leesburg.
12 *President Truman accepts Louis Johnson's resignation as secretary of defense and appoints Marshall to succeed him.*
15 *UN forces launch a successful amphibious assault at the port of Inchon in Korea, and on the following day open an offensive against North Korean forces from the Pusan Perimeter; in Washington, US Senate passes a waiver making Marshall eligible to become secretary of defense.*

18–19 Checkup in Walter Reed Army Hospital. *President Truman signs H.R. 9646, making Marshall eligible to serve as secretary of defense.*
19–20 Testifies before Senate Armed Services Committee on his nomination to be secretary of defense and is confirmed by Senate.
21 Sworn in as secretary of defense, 9:47 a.m.; speaks at testimonial dinner for Congressman James W. Wadsworth, Rochester, NY, 6:30 p.m.
22–23 Attends meetings of US, British, and French foreign and defense ministers, New York City.
26 Meeting with the president, 12:30 p.m.; cabinet meeting, 4:00 p.m.
27 Speaks at ARC Volunteer Services meeting in Cleveland, OH, 8:00 p.m.
29 *Restoration of the Republic of Korea government in Seoul announced.* Cabinet meeting, 10:00 a.m.; luncheon with the president and Acheson, 12:45 p.m.; NSC meeting, 3:00 p.m.

October 1950

4 *Robert A. Lovett is sworn in as deputy secretary of defense.*
6 Speaks to Conference of Mayors, noon.
10 Meeting with the president, 12:30 p.m.; addresses Community Chest Federation, 1:15 p.m.
12 NSC meeting, 3:00 p.m.
13 Meetings with Acheson and French defense and finance ministers.
15 *President Truman meets with MacArthur on Wake Island.*
16 Meeting with French defense minister, 12:15 p.m.
19 Receives award from Disabled American Veterans, noon.
20 Morning cabinet meeting; records remarks for *Time for Defense* radio program and United Nations Day program (both to be broadcast on the 24th), 2:12 p.m.
23 Attends Henry Stimson's funeral, Highhold, NY, 2:30 p.m.
24 ABMC meeting, 10:00 a.m.; addresses National Guard Association Conference, 3:00 p.m.
25 National Geographic Society Board of Trustees meeting, 4:30 p.m.
27 Cabinet meeting, 10:00 a.m.; meeting with the president and others about the food situation in Yugoslavia, 10:30 a.m.
28–30 Welcomes NATO defense ministers and attends their meetings.
31 Meetings with NATO defense ministers, the president, and the cabinet.

November 1950

1 Speaks at unveiling of memorial to Sir John Dill, Arlington National Cemetery, 3:00 p.m.
2 NSC meeting, 3:00 p.m. *President Truman names E. Roland Harriman to succeed Marshall as president of ARC, effective December 4.*
3–5 BAC meetings, Sea Island, GA; speaks at BAC dinner on the 4th.
7 Meeting with the president, 3:00 p.m.
9 Opening remarks to consultants to Research and Development Board, 9:30 a.m.; NSC meeting, 3:00 p.m. *Appointment of Anna Rosenberg as assistant secretary of defense for manpower and personnel is announced.*
10 ARC meetings, 9:30 a.m.; statement to press on Rosenberg appointment, 3:55 p.m.

11 Speaks at the gravesite of General John J. Pershing and attends Armistice Day ceremonies, Arlington National Cemetery.
13 Addresses Army War College students and faculty, 8:20 a.m.
14 Attends Carnegie Corporation annual meeting in New York City, 11:24 a.m.; returns to Washington, and attends presidential dinner at Blair House, 8:00 p.m.
15 *Anna Rosenberg is sworn in as assistant secretary of defense, 11:00 a.m.*
16–19 Travels to Chicago to attend ARC meetings.
21 Meeting with the president, 12:30 p.m.; cabinet meeting, 4:00 p.m.
22 NSC meeting, 3:00 p.m.
24 *United Nations Command offensive begins in Korea.* Speaks at event and at dinner honoring American Legion national commander Erle Cocke, Dawson and Fort Benning, GA, 9:00 p.m.
25 *In northern Korea, Chinese Communist forces attack UN forces in strength.* Returns to Washington, 11:50 a.m.
27 *Congress reconvenes.* Testifies off the record before House Appropriations Committee, 3:30 p.m.
28 Meeting with the president, 12:30 p.m.; addresses Women's Press Club, 1:00 p.m.; NSC meeting, 3:00 p.m.; cabinet meeting, 4:00 p.m.
29 Addresses dinner honoring Israeli President Chaim Weizmann, New York City, 8:00 p.m.
30 Addresses National Preparedness Orientation Conference, 10:05 a.m. *President Truman in a press conference does not rule out use of the atomic bomb in Korea; British Prime Minister Clement Attlee decides to travel to Washington to confer with Truman.*

December 1950

1 Cabinet meeting, 10:00 a.m.; presidential meeting on Korea, 11:00 a.m.; testifies before Special Subcommittee on National Defense Appropriations of the House Appropriations Committee on second supplemental appropriations bill for 1951, 2:00 p.m.
2 Attends Army-Navy football game in Philadelphia but returns to Washington earlier than planned, 2:37 p.m.; meeting with the president, Acheson, and Bradley, 8:00 p.m.
3 Meeting with the president, 12:20 p.m.
4 Addresses ARC staff and turns over ARC presidency to E. Roland Harriman, 8:30 a.m.; attends first talks between the president and British Prime Minister Attlee, 4:00–5:35 p.m.
5 Meeting with the president, 12:30 p.m.; luncheon for Attlee on the presidential yacht, 1:00 p.m.; Truman-Attlee talks, 2:45–4:45 p.m.; cabinet meeting, 5:00 p.m. *Truman orders military and diplomatic officials overseas to clear "all but routine" public statements before release.*
6 Truman-Attlee talks, 11:30 a.m.–12:30 p.m. and 3:30–4:35 p.m; reception for Attlee, 6:30 p.m.; dinner at British embassy; post-dinner talks with Truman, Attlee, Acheson, and others, 9:30 p.m.–midnight.
7 Hosts luncheon for Attlee, which the president attends, 12:45 p.m.; Truman-Attlee talks, 3:45–5:10 p.m.
8 Cabinet meeting, 10:00 a.m.; speaks in New York City at ARC luncheon honoring Roland Harriman and Marshall, 1:00 p.m., and at annu-

al dinner of the Congress of American Industry of the National Association of Manufacturers, 9:00 p.m. *Truman-Attlee talks in Washington conclude.*

9 Testifies in executive session before Senate Appropriations Committee on the second supplemental appropriation bill, 10:00 a.m.

11 Testifies before Senate Appropriations Committee on the second supplemental appropriation bill, 2:00 p.m.; NSC meeting, 3:30 p.m.

11–24 *X Corps withdraws to Hungnam in eastern North Korea and evacuates by sea to South Korea.*

12 Cabinet meeting, 10:00 a.m.

13 Presidential meeting with congressional leaders to discuss national emergency, 10:00 a.m.

14 Addresses National Chamber of Commerce and National Association of Broadcasters Advisory Council; NSC meeting, 3:00 p.m.; meeting with Eisenhower, 5:07 p.m.

15 Cabinet meeting, 10:00 a.m. *President Truman declares a national emergency during a radio address, 10:30 p.m.*

18 Briefs Democratic congressional leaders at White House, 10:00 a.m.

19 Meeting with the president, 12:30 p.m.; cabinet meeting, 4:00 p.m. *President Truman announces the designation of General Eisenhower as SACEUR.*

20 National Geographic Society luncheon meeting, 12:20 p.m.; records message for United Defense Fund, 3:35 p.m., to be broadcast on the 30th. *"Great Debate" over Truman administration's focus on Europe and plans to send US troops to NATO begins.*

21 NSC meeting, 3:00 p.m.

22 Cabinet meeting, 10:00 a.m.

23 *Lieutenant General Walton H. Walker dies in Korea and is succeeded as US Eighth Army commander by Lieutenant General Matthew B. Ridgway.*

26 Dinner conference with the president, 7:30 p.m.

29 Meeting with the president, 9:30 a.m.; cabinet meeting, 10:00 a.m.; records message at 11:55 a.m. for CBS to broadcast on the 31st.

January 1951

2 Meeting with the president, 12:30 p.m.; Walker's funeral, Arlington National Cemetery, 1:45 p.m.; cabinet meeting, 4:00 p.m.

3 Meeting with Eisenhower, 12:32 p.m.

4 Briefs press, 10:15 a.m.; NSC meeting, 3:00 p.m.

5 Cabinet meeting, 10:00 a.m.; manpower conference, 11:31 a.m.

9 Meeting with the president, 12:30 p.m.; cabinet meeting, 4:00 p.m.

10 Testifies before the Preparedness Subcommittee of the Senate Armed Services Committee on UMT, 10:30 a.m.; NSC meeting, 3:30 p.m.

11 Speaks to National Advertising Council, 10:00 a.m.

12 Cabinet meeting, 10:00 a.m.; presidential meeting about Korea, 10:30 a.m.

15 VMI Board of Visitors meeting in Richmond, VA, 10:00 a.m.

16 Speaks to International Development Advisory Board, 9:05 a.m.; meeting with the president, 12:30 p.m.

17 NSC meeting, 3:30 p.m.
18 Makes opening remarks to BAC and attends BAC luncheon.
19 Cabinet meeting, 10:00 a.m.
20 Briefs press, 10:03 a.m.
21 Speaks at memorial service for Henry Stimson, 5:00 p.m.
22 Records ARC statement, 11:47 a.m.; cabinet meeting, 4:00 p.m.
23 Testifies before House Armed Services Committee on UMT, 10:00 a.m.; meeting with the president, 12:30 p.m.
24 Speaks at Armed Forces Staff College graduation, Norfolk, VA, 11:00 a.m.; NSC meeting, 3:30 p.m.
25 Records *Time for Defense* program, 3:30 p.m.; addresses Women's Patriotic Conference on National Defense, 9:00 p.m.
26 Cabinet meeting, 10:00 a.m.; US Chamber of Commerce dinner, 7:00 p.m.
28 Speaks at dedication of Washington Post Building, 3:00 p.m.
29–30 Conferences with visiting French Prime Minister René Pleven.
31 Cabinet meeting, 2:30 p.m.; addresses General Federation of Women's Clubs, 4:05 p.m.

February 1951

5 Cabinet meeting, 4:00 p.m.
6 Meeting with the president, 12:30 p.m.
8 Testifies in executive session before the Preparedness Subcommittee of the Senate Armed Services Committee on UMT, 2:30 p.m.
9 Cabinet meeting, 10:00 a.m.
12 Cabinet meeting, 4:00 p.m.
14 Greets magazine editors and book publishers, 10:05 a.m.; NSC meeting, 3:30 p.m.
15 Testifies before Senate Foreign Relations and Armed Services Committees concerning the assignment of US ground forces to Europe, 10:00 a.m.; greets Veterans of Foreign Wars, 1:59 p.m.
16 Cabinet meeting, 10:00 a.m.
19 Addresses American Association of School Administrators convention, Atlantic City, NJ.
20 Meeting with the president, 12:30 p.m.
21 Masonic breakfast honoring President Truman, 7:45 a.m.; departs for his Washington apartment because of illness, 9:30 a.m. *John D. Small reads Marshall's prepared statement about the St. Lawrence Seaway to the House Public Works Committee, 10:05 a.m.*
22–26 At home because of illness.
27 Swears in civil defense volunteers, New York City, 5:00 p.m.; speaks at opening of Red Cross 1951 fund campaign, Madison Square Garden, New York City, 8:45 p.m.

March 1951

1 Testifies before House Armed Services Committee on UMT, 10:00 a.m.
2 Cabinet meeting, 10:00 a.m.
5 Speaks at Columbia University, New York City, 8:30 p.m.
7 NSC meeting, 3:30 p.m.

21 Records television broadcast for United Service Organizations, 10:40 a.m.; NSC meeting, 3:30 p.m.
23 Meeting with the president, 11:00 a.m.
27 Meeting with the president, 12:30 p.m.; press conference, 3:00 p.m.
30 Cabinet meeting, 10:00 a.m.

April 1951

2 Records statement for third ECA anniversary, 8:45 a.m.; Armed Forces Day Proclamation signing, White House, 12:15 p.m.; cabinet meeting, 4:00 p.m.
3 Meeting with the president, 12:30 p.m.; records statement for Armed Forces Day (May 19), 3:45 p.m.
4 Speaks to selected judge advocates and legal officers, 10:59 a.m. *Senate approves sending additional US troops to Europe.*
5 *Representative Joseph W. Martin (R-MA) releases a letter from General MacArthur dated March 20, criticizing administration policy.*
6–8 Series of meetings with cabinet, the president, Acheson, Averell Harriman, and Bradley regarding MacArthur.
9 Welcoming address to Joint Civilian Orientation Conference, 9:04 a.m.; cabinet meeting, 11:00 a.m.; meeting with the president, Vice President Alben Barkley, Acheson, Harriman, and Bradley regarding MacArthur; ARC Board of Governors luncheon, noon; meeting with Belgian Prime Minister Joseph Pholien, 3:00 p.m.
10 Briefs press on plan for military manpower, 12:11 p.m.; meetings with the president, Acheson, Harriman, and Bradley regarding MacArthur, 12:30–4:20 p.m.
11 *White House spokesman announces that President Truman has relieved MacArthur of his commands and named Ridgway as his successor, 1:00 a.m.; Lieutenant General James A. Van Fleet succeeds Ridgway as commander of Eighth Army.* NSC meeting, 3:30 p.m. *President Truman makes national broadcast regarding MacArthur and Korea, 10:30 p.m.*
12–16 Cabinet meetings on 13th and 16th, 11:00 a.m.
17 Meetings with the president, 12:30 p.m. and 4:30 p.m.
18 NSC meeting, 3:30 p.m.
19 *MacArthur addresses Congress, 12:15 p.m.* Attends MacArthur Day ceremonies, 1:36–2:58 p.m.
20 Briefs American Society of Newspaper Editors, 9:15 a.m.; cabinet meeting, 11:00 a.m.
21 Speaks at Hood College convocation, Frederick, MD, 10:30 a.m.
23 Cabinet meeting, 11:00 a.m.
24 Meeting with the president, 12:30 p.m.
30 Addresses National Newspaper Promotion Managers luncheon, 12:02 p.m.

May 1951

1 Meeting with the president, 12:30 p.m.
2 NSC meeting, 3:30 p.m.; US Chamber of Commerce annual dinner, 7:15 p.m.
3 Departs for Winchester, VA, 1:00 p.m., for the Apple Blossom Festival.

3–5 *General MacArthur testifies before the Senate Armed Services and Foreign Relations Committees in the MSFE hearings.*
4 Meeting with Israeli Prime Minister David Ben-Gurion, 10:00 a.m.; cabinet meeting, 11:00 a.m.
7 Welcomes Women's Advisory Council, 10:13 a.m.; testifies in MSFE hearings, 10:30 a.m.
8–12 Testifies daily in MSFE hearings.
14 Concludes his testimony in MSFE hearings.
15 Speaks at VMI's Marshall Day, Lexington, VA.
18 Cabinet meeting, 11:00 a.m.; addresses second National Armed Forces Day banquet, 7:30 p.m.
19 Reviews Armed Forces Day Parade, 9:50 a.m.
22 Meeting with the president, 12:30 p.m.
23 NSC meeting, 3:30 p.m.
24 Records message about ARC Blood Bank for *Pint Parade*, 3:10 p.m., to be broadcast at midnight on the 30th.
25 Speaks at Industrial Public Relations Orientation Conference, 9:35 a.m.; cabinet meeting, 11:00 a.m.
28 Cabinet meeting, 11:00 a.m.
29 Meeting with the president, 12:30 p.m.; testifies before Senate Banking and Currency Committee about the Defense Production Act, 2:30 p.m.

June 1951

1 Speaks at graduation exercises, US Naval Academy, Annapolis, MD, 11:00 a.m.
4 Meeting with the president, 10:45 a.m.; cabinet meeting, 11:00 a.m.
5 Speaks at graduation exercises, US Military Academy, West Point, NY, 10:00 a.m.
6–7 Speaks at graduation exercises, Washington University, St. Louis; flies to Japan with stops in Washington state and Aleutian Islands, AK. *Congress passes UMTS legislation.*
8 Arrives Yokota Air Force Base, Japan, 9:00 a.m.; departs Yokota, 9:15 a.m.; arrives Korea, 1:30 p.m.; flies in liaison planes around front, 2:00–6:00 p.m.; holds informal press conference; departs Taegu, Korea, 7:30 p.m.; arrives Tokyo, 11:30 p.m., where he stays with the Ridgways until the 11th.
11–12 Press conference; departs Tokyo with stops in Naknek and Anchorage, AK, arriving in Washington on the 12th, 11:33 a.m.; meeting with the president, 12:30 p.m.; press conference, 3:00 p.m.
13 NSC meeting, 3:30 p.m.
14 Testifies in executive session before House Banking and Currency Committee regarding the Defense Production Act, 10:00 a.m. *Senator Joseph McCarthy (R-WI) attacks Marshall in a speech on the Senate floor.*
18 Cabinet meeting, 11:00 a.m.
19 Speaks at graduation exercises, National War College, 10:00 a.m.; witnesses signing of the UMTS law, White House, 12:15 p.m.; meeting with the president, 12:30 p.m.; records statement on passage of UMTS law, 3:03 p.m.

21 Meeting with the president, 12:30 p.m.
22 Cabinet meeting, 11:00 a.m.
23 Meeting with the president, 11:00 a.m. *Soviet UN representative Jacob Malik proposes talks regarding a cease-fire in Korea.*
24 Hosts President Truman and Supreme Court Justice and Mrs. Fred M. Vinson in Leesburg, where Bernard Baruch is also visiting.
25 Welcomes Joint Civilian Orientation Conference, 9:00 a.m.; dinner with the president, Acheson, Treasury Secretary John M. Snyder, and ECA Administrator William C. Foster, 7:00 p.m. *MSFE hearings end.*
27 NSC meeting, 3:30 p.m.
29 Testifies before House Foreign Affairs Committee on Mutual Security Program, 10:00 a.m.; dinner on the presidential yacht with the president, Acheson, Lovett, Bradley, and Dean Rusk, 7:00 p.m.

July 1951

2 Testifies before House Foreign Affairs Committee on the Mutual Security Program, 10:00 a.m.
3 Meeting with the president, 12:30 p.m.; speaks at the play *The Common Glory*, Williamsburg, VA, 8:15 p.m.
4 Broadcasts remarks for Independence Day program from Arthur Godfrey's studio, Leesburg, 10:15 p.m.
6 Meeting with the president, 10:50–10:55 a.m.; cabinet meeting, 11:00 a.m.
9 Cabinet meeting, 11:00 a.m.
10 Meeting with the president, 12:30 p.m. *Formal armistice talks begin in Kaesong, Korea.*
11 Receives gift of a Norwegian elkhound, 10:00 a.m.; NSC meeting, 3:30 p.m.; meeting with the president, Acheson, Bradley, and Sherman, 3:40 p.m.
13 Cabinet meeting, 11:00 a.m.
18 Testifies before House Appropriations Committee's Subcommittee on Department of Defense Appropriations, 3:00 p.m.
19 Meeting with the president, 10:45 a.m.
20 Cabinet meeting, 11:00 a.m.
24 Meeting with the president, 12:30 p.m.; press conference, 3:05 p.m.
26 Speaks at Air Staff Orientation Course, 11:40 a.m.
27 Testifies before Senate Foreign Relations and Armed Services Committees on the Mutual Security Program, 10:30 a.m.; funeral of Admiral Sherman, Arlington National Cemetery, 3:00 p.m.
28–30 Begins vacation by flying to Mitchel Field, NY, and Camp Edwards, MA; drives to Waquoit, MA, for vacation until August 24.

August 1951

10–12 Spends weekend on Naushon Island, MA.
24 Travels to Toronto, Canada; speaks at Canadian National Exhibition luncheon, 12:15 p.m., and formal opening, 2:30 p.m.; attends evening ceremonies, 8:30 p.m.
25 Attends exhibition functions; travels to Ottawa and stays in US embassy, returning to Washington on the 26th, 6:00 p.m.

28 Meeting with the president, 12:30 p.m.; records remarks for the ARC Blood Campaign program, 5:55 p.m.; hosts dinner for Admiral William Fechteler, the new chief of naval operations, which is attended by the president, 7:30 p.m.
29 Meeting with the president, 3:25 p.m.; NSC meeting, 3:30 p.m.
30 Witnesses signing of US-Philippines Mutual Defense Treaty, 12:00 p.m.; presidential luncheon for Philippine President H. E. Quirino, Blair House, 12:30 p.m.
31 Cabinet meeting, 11:00 a.m.

September 1951

1 *Australia–New Zealand–United States Security Treaty is signed, San Francisco, CA.*
8 *Japanese Peace Treaty and US-Japan Security Treaty are signed in San Francisco, CA.*
11 Meeting with the president, during which he accepts Marshall's resignation as secretary of defense effective the 12th, 12:30 p.m.
12 Staff meeting, 10:10 a.m.; briefs press, 10:19 a.m. *White House announces Marshall's resignation and the appointment of Lovett to succeed him, 11:00 a.m.* NSC meeting, 3:00 p.m.; meeting with the president and Lovett, 3:30 p.m.
14 *Senate unanimously confirms Lovett's appointment as secretary of defense.*
17 Addresses Defense Advisory Committee on Women in the Services, 9:05 a.m.; swearing-in of Lovett as secretary of defense.
18 Attends meeting of the VMI Board of Visitors, Lexington, VA.

October 1951

1 Speaks at National Governors' Conference, Gatlinburg, TN.
5–8 Travels to New York City; speaks at Freedom House dinner honoring Paul G. Hoffman on the 7th.
19 Cabinet meeting, at which Truman gives Marshall the chair he used as secretary of state and defense, 11:00 a.m.
24 Speaks at dedication of new ARC building, 12:30 p.m.; speaks at Washington Board of Trade dinner for UN veterans, 8:25 p.m.
30 Speaks at Drexel Institute's sixtieth anniversary convocation, Philadelphia, PA.

November 1951

11 Speaks at Armistice Day ceremonies, Valley Forge Military Academy, Wayne, PA.

December 1951

3 Speaks at Council for World Affairs meeting in Cleveland, OH.

January 1952

8 VMI Board of Visitors meeting, Richmond, VA.
9–10 Meetings with Anna Rosenberg and BAC.
17 Lunch at British embassy with Prime Minister Winston Churchill following his address to Congress.

February 1952

5 Meeting with the president, 9:45 a.m.

9 Vacations in Cuernavaca, Mexico, through March 4.

March 1952

12–13 Speaks at Lawrenceville School, Lawrenceville, NJ, and Wellesley College, Wellesley, MA.

14 Speaks at Four Freedoms Foundation dinner after receiving its award, New York City, 8:00 p.m.

May 1952

11 *Clifton S. Brown, Marshall's stepson, dies of lung cancer at Walter Reed and is buried in Arlington National Cemetery on the 13th.*

June 1952

3 Records remarks for the Congress of European-American Associations.

6 Addresses bicentennial luncheon at National Guard Armory in Winchester, VA.

7 Gives commencement address at Woodberry Forest School, Woodberry Forest, VA; VMI Foundation meeting, Lexington, VA.

8 Hosts President Truman in Leesburg.

18 National Geographic Society Board of Trustees meeting.

25 James Wadsworth's funeral, Washington National Cathedral.

August 1952

2 Flies to Santa Barbara, CA, and stays with Mrs. George Bolling Lee and her daughter, Mary, Clifton Brown's fiancée.

September 1952

1–2 Returns from Santa Barbara.

4–5 Departs Leesburg for New York City; sails with Mrs. Marshall and Mary Lee aboard SS *United States* on ABMC trip to inspect US military cemeteries in Western Europe, Africa, and England.

10 Lands in Le Havre, France, and drives to Normandy cemeteries; spends night in Caen, France.

11–16 In Paris; meets with French President Vincent Auriol; presides at dedication of US war memorial in Suresnes.

16–25 Travels to the Netherlands; Luxembourg; Nancy, France; Venice, Florence, Rome, Anzio, and Capri, Italy.

October 1952

4–8 Travels from Capri to Naples, Italy; Carthage, Tunisia; Nice, France; Cambridge and London, England; on the 8th, lunch with Anthony Eden and dinner with Winston Churchill.

9–14 Departs London for Southampton; return trip on SS *United States.*

22 National Geographic Society Board of Trustees meeting, 3:00 p.m.

November 1952

4 *Eisenhower is elected president of the US.*

27–28 VMI football game in Roanoke, VA, and VMI Board of Visitors meeting, Lexington, VA.

December 1952

4 Dinner honoring past and present Truman cabinet members, White House, 8:00 p.m.
5 ABMC meeting, 10:00 a.m.

January 1953

8 Dinner with Winston Churchill at the British embassy, Washington.
14 VMI Board of Visitors meeting in Richmond, VA, 10:00 a.m.; BAC meeting, Washington, 1:00 p.m.
20 Attends Eisenhower inauguration.

February 1953

17 Briefs JCS about the ABMC, 2:00 p.m.
18 Speaks at Milton Academy, Milton, MA.
19 *Secretary of Defense Charles E. Wilson names Marshall senior military consultant to the Rockefeller Committee on the Organization of the Defense Department.*
24–28 Hunts with James Bruce on Pinckney Island, SC.

March 1953

2 First meeting of the Rockefeller Committee.
3 Meeting with Secretary of Defense Wilson at the Pentagon, 9:00 a.m.; luncheon honoring General Van Fleet, White House, 12:45 p.m.
6 *President Eisenhower announces that Marshall will lead the US delegation to the coronation of Queen Elizabeth II, June 2, 1953.*
20–21,
26–31 Rockefeller Committee meetings.

April 1953

3–7 Rockefeller Committee meetings.

May 1953

1–2 Attends installation of new VMI superintendent, Lexington, VA.
13–14 Lecture and meetings with students and trustees, University of Louisville, KY.
19 Interview by Edward R. Murrow for *See It Now* television program for broadcast on the 24th, Leesburg.
22–23 Flies from Washington to New York City and sails with Mrs. Marshall on the SS *America* for Le Havre, France, en route to London for coronation of Queen Elizabeth II.
30 Flies from Le Havre to London and begins series of coronation events and visits.

June 1953

2 Represents the US at the coronation of Queen Elizabeth II at Westminster Abbey, 9:00 a.m.; attends queen's lunch at Westminster School, 1:30 p.m.
3–10 Coronation-related events and private visits in England.
11 Leaves London for Southampton and sails for New York on SS *United States*, arriving on the 16th and flying to Washington.
22 ARC dinner, Washington.

23 Dinner honoring the Trumans, 7:30 p.m.

August 1953

3 Travels to Binghamton, NY, to start vacation in Adirondacks; stays with Margaret Emerson at Sagamore Camp, Raquette Lake, August 4–15, and Ambassador and Mrs. Joseph E. Davies at Topridge, Upper Saint Regis Lake, August 20–29; returns to Leesburg on September 1.

September 1953

3 ABMC meeting, 10:00 a.m.

8 General Jonathan M. Wainwright's funeral, Arlington National Cemetery, 11:00 a.m.

19–22 Visits sister Marie Singer in Greensburg, PA; attends events in Fort Necessity and Uniontown, PA.

23 Becomes ill with influenza.

October 1953

30–31 Wins Nobel Peace Prize; holds press conference in his Pinehurst living room.

November 1953

1–16 At Walter Reed for treatment of influenza.

27–28 Flies from Pinehurst to Newark, NJ, and spends night in New York City; holds press conference onboard SS *Andrea Doria* and sails with C. J. George for Naples, Italy, en route to Oslo, Norway, for Nobel Peace Prize ceremonies.

December 1953

6–9 Arrives Naples at noon; flies to Paris and stays with General Alfred M. Gruenther; flies to Oslo on the 9th and holds press conference, 4:00 p.m.

10 Meets with Norwegian King Haakon VII, 11:00 a.m.; accepts Peace Prize in ceremony beginning at 1:00 p.m.; speaks briefly at the Nobel dinner.

11 Luncheon, Oslo City Hall, 1:00 p.m.; delivers Nobel lecture at Oslo University Festival Hall, 7:00 p.m.

12–17 Flies from Oslo to Heidelberg, Germany, and stays with General Thomas Handy; returns to Paris on the 15th and stays with General Gruenther; returns to Washington by air with Defense Secretary Wilson and then to Pinehurst on the 17th.

January 1954

18 VMI Board of Visitors meeting in Richmond, VA.

March 1954

17–18 BAC and ABMC meetings.

May 1954

5 National Geographic Society Board of Trustees meeting.

10 Dinner at Achesons' home with the Trumans, 8:00 p.m.

June 1954

4 Dutch ambassador's presentation to President Eisenhower and Marshall in appreciation for US aid to the Netherlands since the war, White House, noon.
11–12 VMI Board of Visitors meeting in Lexington, VA.
23–24 BAC meetings.
25 Dinner for Winston Churchill, White House, 8:00 p.m.

July 1954

3 Speaks at 200th anniversary of the Battle at Fort Necessity near Uniontown, PA.

October 1954

5 International House Board of Trustees meeting, New York City.

December 1954

2 *US Senate votes to condemn Senator Joseph McCarthy.*
8–10 ABMC and BAC meetings; receives award at AMVETS banquet on the 10th.

February 1955

17 General Brehon B. Somervell's funeral at Fort Myer Chapel, 2:00 p.m.
20–27 Hunts with James Bruce on Pinckney Island, SC.

May 1955

12 ABMC meetings, 4:00 p.m.
17 General Charles P. Summerall's funeral, 2:30 p.m.; meeting with Clarence Streit concerning the Atlantic Union, 3:15 p.m.

June 1955

16 Luncheon honoring Marshall, where he receives the first copy of Harry B. Price's *The Marshall Plan and Its Meaning*, 12:30 p.m.; records comments for a CBS television special on the tenth anniversary of the United Nations.
22 Ridgways' reception at Fort Myer, 6:00 p.m.; BAC dinner, 7:30 p.m.

August 1955

1–31 Vacation in Eagles Mere, PA.

September 1955

9 National Geographic Society Board of Trustees meeting, 4:00 p.m.

December 1955

14–17 At Walter Reed.

January 1956

26 At Walter Reed until February 7.

May 1956

23–24 Luncheon at Pentagon for Rockefeller Committee members; meeting with Admiral Thomas C. Kinkaid, ABMC.

June 1956

12 Speaks at VMI graduation, Lexington, VA.

29 Fleet Admiral Ernest J. King's funeral, Washington National Cathedral.

July 1956

31 At Walter Reed with bronchitis.

October 1956

25 Receives the Woodrow Wilson Foundation's Distinguished Service Award, 2:00 p.m.

November 1956

6 *Eisenhower is reelected president.*

December 1956

17–24 At Walter Reed.

18 ABMC meeting.

May 1957

6–12 At Walter Reed.

June 1957

5 Receives a medal from the Organization for European Economic Cooperation, Blair House.

1958

In hospital at Fort Bragg, NC., late March; and at Walter Reed, May 11–24, August 4–23, and September 23–October 16; visit from Queen Frederica at Pinehurst, October 25.

January–May 1959

Suffers first stroke on January 18 and is admitted to Womack Army Hospital at Fort Bragg, NC, where he survives a second stroke on February 17; flown to Walter Reed on March 11, where he is visited by Eisenhower on March 13 and May 18, Truman on May 3, and Eisenhower together with Churchill on May 5.

October 1959

16 Dies at Walter Reed.

19–20 Marshall's body lies in Bethlehem Chapel, Washington National Cathedral, from noon on the 19th until noon on the 20th; President Eisenhower and former President Truman attend funeral in Fort Myer Chapel, 2:30 p.m.; burial in Arlington National Cemetery.

30,000 Miles and 30,000 Interviews

October 1, 1949–June 26, 1950

I just came in at midnight last night from my final Red Cross trips to a total of somewhere near 30,000 miles and it seemed to me 30,000 press interviews with never a question about the Red Cross if they could avoid it. . . . And if anybody invites me to do anything in the next few months it is at personal peril.

—Marshall to Lieutenant General Richard J. Marshall
March 8, 1950

MARSHALL recalled in 1950 that President Harry S. Truman had first mentioned the possibility of heading the American Red Cross (ARC) "several weeks" before his November 1945 retirement as army chief of staff. "I did not feel then that I could undertake a job of that magnitude before gaining some rest," he wrote, though he and his wife Katherine did discuss the matter "frequently and at some length." Marshall's retirement was immediately followed by his mission to China, however, and then by his tenure as secretary of state. In March of 1949, after his January retirement, Truman again raised the subject. "I told the President that I appreciated the compliment he was paying me and that Mrs. Marshall and I would talk the matter over as we had done four years before. I had promised her that I would undertake no further public tasks without her approval." (George C. Marshall, "My New Job," published in the *Washington Post* [February 16, 1950, p. B1] and the *Red Cross Courier* [March 1950, pp. 4–9].) Still recuperating from his December 1948 surgery, Marshall informed Truman on March 15 that "I have been thinking about the Red Cross business and talking it over with Mrs. Marshall. I feel that I will be honored and ready to accept about May 1st or whatever later date meets your convenience. . . . I appreciate so much your desire to have me in that position, and particularly what I sense to be the real fact, that you wish to provide me with a dignified post that, at the same time, would not be too demanding for my health and peace of mind." (*Papers of GCM*, 6: 673.) On July 28, Marshall confided in his goddaughter, Rose Page Wilson, that he would "probably be appointed President of the American Red Cross on Sept. 15th." On September 22, Truman informed Marshall of his appointment, to be effective October 1 (ibid., 739, 748). Marshall met with Truman and outgoing Red Cross President Basil O'Connor on October 3, and on October 24, he began an extraordinary air tour of Red Cross chapters across the country (see pp. 19–21). In the intervening three weeks he attended numerous Red Cross meetings as well as a series of meetings at the State Department regarding China, where Mao Tse-tung's Communists were defeating Chiang Kai-shek's Nationalists and had just proclaimed the People's Republic of China. (See pp. 5–14.) Marshall also testified before the House Armed Services Committee on unification of the armed services while simultaneously continuing his extensive correspondence. ★

1

TO LADY MARY BURGHLEY[1]

October 6, 1949
Washington, DC

Dear Mary: I am sending you today a rather dilapidated-looking book "The Kentucky Cardinal and the Aftermath" by James Lane Allen, a famous Kentucky writer of some years ago.[2] The reason for the appearance of the book is because it has been read so often and I have neglected to have it rebound. I wanted to send it to you for many reasons but did not find it until the other day when I was cleaning out my books to make room for newer ones. I apologize for its appearance.

To me it is a very sweet story and I think you will find it that. Also, it gives a rather delightful impression of Kentucky in those early American days.

As you can see from the stationery, I am at my new job which I find already very interesting but, at least for the time being, rather exacting.

I had the good pleasure the other day at East Hampton to meet at a dinner of Trippes' (Pan American Airways) the Episcopal Bishop from the Diocese of Pittsburgh, Pennsylvania, who I found was an intimate friend of yours and a delightful person. I also confessed to him that it was in the same Diocese in a small Episcopal Church that I was fired from my job of pumping the organ for becoming too engaged in a little light literature.[3] Mrs. Trippe is the sister of my dear friend, Ed Stettinius, one time Secretary of State.[4] Affectionately,

GCMRL/G. C. Marshall Papers (American Red Cross, General)

1. Mary Theresa Scott, Lady Burghley, was the ex-wife of David Cecil, Lord Burghley. Marshall had visited Bermuda while Lord Burghley was its governor in 1944. He had corresponded frequently with Lord and Lady Burghley in subsequent years, sending her the songs from *Oklahoma!* as well as whooping-cough shots for her children shortly after his visit; see *Papers of GCM*, 4: 370, 379.

2. Marshall had previously attempted to send Allen's *A Kentucky Cardinal* and *Aftermath* to her; see *Papers of GCM*, 4: 378–79. Writing from England in February 1947, Lady Burghley had remarked that she missed "the 'Bluebirds' & 'Cardinals' of Bermuda." (Burghley to Marshall, February 7, 1947, GCMRL/G. C. Marshall Papers [Pentagon Office, Selected].)

3. The Marshalls had been guests of Juan and Elizabeth (Stettinius) Trippe from August 1 to 3 during a board of directors meeting for Pan American Airways, of which Trippe was president, in New York. Marshall had accepted Trippe's invitation to join the board on May 11; Trippe's July 21 telegram had informed Marshall that the stockholders had elected him with the "largest vote in company's history." (Marshall to Trippe, May 11, 1949, GCMRL/© Marshall-Winn Collection [Marshall Correspondence Collection, Personal]; Trippe to Marshall, telegram, July 21, 1949, ibid.; *Papers of GCM*, 6: 739–40n1.)

Harry Austin Pardue Jr. was bishop of the Pittsburgh Episcopal Diocese. Marshall recalled the days of his youth and pumping the organ at Saint Peter's Episcopal Church in Uniontown, Pennsylvania, in *Papers of GCM*, 1: 6. "The pumping was not difficult except you had to be there," Marshall later recalled. "But there was a long period of wait during the sermon. One of these mornings, I was occupying this period of waiting by reading a five-cent novel of that day about Nick Carter. Just in the most exciting portion, and it was very much like Jesse James, my attention was called to the organ by the thump, thump, which the organist, Miss Fanny Howe, could make from the keyboard. And I realized that she had started to play at the end of the sermon and no music was coming out. So I pumped the organ very hurriedly. Of course, she was not only displeased but rather outraged." (*George C. Marshall Interviews and Reminiscences for Forrest C. Pogue*, 3rd ed. [Lexington, VA: George C. Marshall Research Foundation, 1996], 54–55.)

4. "I am *so* delighted," Burghley replied, "to have that delightful book *and* I am more than glad that you have neglected to have it rebound for I like it all the more for being like what it is. . . . It made me laugh to think of you being fired from the job of organ-pumping! The Bishop of Pittsburgh spent a weekend here and very nobly preached in our village Church, which was very good of him considering that all the 'grand' places were *clamouring* for him. He is a remarkable personality." (Burghley to Marshall, November 1949, GCMRL/G. C. Marshall Papers [Pentagon Office, Selected].)

2

Remarks at the State Department Roundtable Discussion on American Policy toward China[1]
Confidential

October 8, 1949
Washington, DC

General Marshall. I am not speaking formally when I tell you I have derived a great deal of information and satisfaction from listening to the discussion here. I should explain to you gentlemen that since last December I have been obtaining my information from the press and a white book and have not been briefed by the State Department, so my reactions, I would assume, would be very much the same as yours.[2] There may be many things of which I am not aware between our Government and the Chinese Kuomintang Government, and between MacArthur and Japan and the State Department, and Indochina even and the Indonesian affair, with which I am familiar, the British and French particularly, and also with Australia and New Zealand.[3] All those things come into the picture and are vitally concerned with what you are called upon to discuss here—for the State Department decision.

I was wondering driving in this morning just what would be the best line for me to take. I am a little embarrassed by reason of the fact that I have been debating intangibles both over there and over here. Dr. Fairbank and myself perspired together in Chungking; at least, he gave encouragement from time to time. I had a great deal to do with him in missionary fields; he and I picked up one of our greatest missionaries, I think, Dr. Stuart, over there.[4]

(Discussion off the record.)

General Marshall. I was involved very heavily at the start, of course, with getting the Japanese out of the country; I had to get 3,000,000 out. I have been in Japan quite a little bit, before the war, just as I have been in the Philippines—as a matter of fact, I was in the tail end of the insurrections, the beginning of a building up of a basis for democratic government.[5]

Now, the ordinary term, the "complexity" of the problem has been overused, but I have never known any problem that had so much complexity involved in it—because, you might say, the simplest part of it is the Chinese people themselves and the immediate situation in China—when you take the conditions in Japan; you take the situation in Indonesia; you take the situation in Indochina; you take the situation in India; then you introduce Pakistan just to help out a little bit; and then the British former economic, almost, domination in China, and the labor of the Labor Government to maintain itself and the reaction of the Conservatives against it, which affects what you are getting into; and the French with relation to Indochina; and then the Dutch in the western European compact, and then over in Indonesia in a sense doing something else; then Australia, very difficult, particularly difficult with respect to some special aspects which I won't name here.

I might say, not in the spirit of levity, the first week I was the Secretary of State, I was introduced to what was being made an international incident over one whaler going to the Antarctic—the Australian Ambassador came to see me three times in 4 days. To get a little off the center in this, I will say the issue was, MacArthur sent it down there to get some of the oils and fats they needed so much in Japan for various production purposes, and it was being resisted—the Japanese were defended before the war in their handling of their whaling industry—because no Japanese trade was to be permitted if it could be stopped. But there was no offer to pay what we were paying in Japan to keep the show going. So the variety of influences involved in this thing are just fantastic when you try to arrive at a sound basic decision.

Then, of course, you have your immediate action and then the longer view, and it is much easier to approach the longer view than the immediate action. In relation to the immediate action, I think we have to take this into consideration. I am going to ask you to pardon me for making military references because I am more familiar with them and when they furnish a parallel they are useful to me at the risk of boring you. But, at least to me, one of the great struggles of conducting the strategy in a large war is the political necessity for action as compared to the military necessity of making haste slowly. When you have a situation, to use as an example, like our channel crossing, we were over a year and a half getting ready for that. The great question was what did you do during the year and a half to keep the public quiet—the political leaders had to have some action. The dangerous factor was if you started action anywhere you immediately began with assurances of a minimum and ended up with a maximum, and something this and something that, and delayed your whole operation. I have been through all the agonies of that.[6]

Now you have been confronted with that—the State Department has been—with the Chinese; they want action and they want it today, the political action. That is the way a democracy goes and you cannot get away from it. There is no use in wrangling about it, that is a fact.

Now, at the same time, I must add that time is of vast importance in this affair; then, again, that goes to extremes. There is great danger of making the very serious error that I often think government departments make—I used to think the War Department made in the past—waiting until the situation built up against you and then you are on the defensive, and then move in. That is fatal. I always want to move in first. On the other hand, it is equally dangerous that the first doesn't get you in before it is the proper time to get in. So timing is a vital consideration in this.

Another thought that occurred to me, listening to your discussion, is the thought Governor Stassen made reference to, but I suggested the reference so I will take credit for it. A good many of the things I have heard proposed here, in my opinion, could not possibly be handled by our Congress.

Now, at the risk of appearing immodest, although I don't think it is anything to brag about, certainly up until recently I had the unenviable reputation of having been before more committees more times and more hours than any other person in America. [Laughter.] As a soldier, I speak not only of political but military and sociological considerations, and especially more recently of economic considerations. When I was turning over in my mind what I might say that would be helpful, and I have to be very careful because of my past responsibilities in connection with this matter—I am trying in a sense to get away from that—I arrived at what may seem to you a half-baked conclusion, that the best way would be to decide what is the idealistic solution.

Now, what is the idealistic solution to this business? After you have decided on that, we will mold that, trim it down and put it on a practical basis; there would be many amendments, many modifications, and some introductions. You have got to keep the idealistic in mind, there is the spiritual involved in this thing.

I have been tremendously impressed in our dealings with Turkey and Teheran, particularly in Turkey, with the effects of our missionary efforts and Robert College in Turkey.[7] That just meant everything to us in the associations we had with them in connection with the Soviet Union. I was very much interested in the resumption by the Methodist mission, I will call it the Methodist mission, for the reestablishment of schools around Teheran which the Government had taken over because that was erecting a barrier of a kind that is acceptable to the world and has great strength in the root it establishes. Of course, that takes a long time; you cannot put it up tomorrow and have it effective the day after tomorrow, but those considerations must be taken into account.

You have an immediate situation in China that is closely related to the current situation in Japan because of the economic factors involved. I am going to turn over to Japan for a minute because I think it is very much concerned in our relationship to China. Japan is costing us a great deal of money; that cannot go on indefinitely. We have established this operation in Western Europe and we have done it on the basis of its reaching a termination in 1952.[8] I am speaking purely for myself, and without the intimate knowledge of what has occurred behind the scenes in the last 10 months, but it ought to be terminated in 1952. Part of the reason why they imply it cannot be terminated then comes from the opponents of the present appropriations, and part comes from the foreign fellows who naturally would like to see it prolonged beyond 1952, but you have got to stop somewhere. It is a very serious matter, not political generalization, that this Government remain strong, so there has to be a very definite limit. You get the man to a certain point and then he has to do, and he has to know he has to do.

When you come to this Japanese affair, you have a very serious affair on your hands which has to do with the question of trade between Japan and China—trade with the Communist government—and when we have General MacArthur out there, in a sense as head of the Japanese Government, certainly dominating the Japanese Government, I feel that we just cannot go on putting out large sums of money indefinitely into Japan. You have got this much smaller area into which we have poured many more Japanese; in other words, we have greatly increased the density of the population there. There has been taken away from them Manchuria, with all of its rich contributions to the economy of the country, Korea, Formosa, and the general trade with China. We have increased the population very decidedly, reduced the area, and even involved their fishing rights in the

Kurile Islands because of Russian problems of interference there, and that poses an economic problem of which I would not attempt to predict the outcome.[9] But I do know this—with the opposition we find further south in Australia, and possibly so long as the Dutch have a certain control in Indonesia, and the feeling is well understood with the Filipinos with regard to the Japanese—there has to be some outlet and some import-export, particularly import in raw materials and export of finished goods, in relation to Japan because that, I don't think, can go on indefinitely.

What we have to be so on our guard against is that we don't weaken ourselves economically so that the whole structure collapses. I am just as much opposed to sitting still and letting the world revolve around us; I am opposed naturally to that, but at the same time I am equally opposed to going along and dripping and dripping, it isn't dripping, it is bucketfuls and we find our own economic position in danger.

Now you are all pretty familiar, I guess, with these factors. When you come back to the question of Chinese-Japanese trade, I certainly think it should be permitted. Mr. Herod commented that if you leave the businessman alone he probably will promote the business if you don't get in his way—I don't know what that does to the conceptions of the State Department, it is just my kind of thinking. Something of that kind has to be done.

I might say when I was talking about putting whatever policies were decided upon on a practical basis, I didn't mean that you submit to the practice of just not doing anything, we will say, or a good thing, because you think the other fellow is going to oppose it. Of course you will have opposition, opposition to practically everything that is put up, but I think we must be very careful that we don't produce a "must" situation unless it is a "must."

For example, to go back into the experiences I have had with Congress, take the war situation, the extension of the draft.[10] Well, that was termed by the political leaders all around, by all parties, as being an absolute impossibility but it was a must. It could not be anything else, it was a must. We couldn't have everything we had dissolving in face of the world as it was. How did you go about to meet it? You have to do that, but you have to be careful. If it is a must, make clear to everybody it is a must and not a question of this judgment or that judgment. I don't think you can call the Japanese-Chinese trade exactly a must but it comes pretty close to being that. We are not going to go on forever providing the goods, the foods, and the money that has been necessary to keep Japan afloat, unless we are going to have a condition of riot, starvation, and things the American Government cannot tolerate within its control areas.

I have sort of indicated my thoughts at the moment, regarding the government proclaimed by the Chinese Communists, in saying there is a great question of timing involved in this thing on one side or the other—it is kind of a fine balance with the political pressures that are coming on. Also involved in that is the British attitude and the French attitude. I don't know what they are, I have not been in the conferences. I don't know how the pressures go, one way or another, and I am glad I don't know, but we have got to proceed very carefully and not be plunged by political momentary pressures into action that we may find later was highly inadvisable.

I will just interject for a moment some of my reactions at the time I was in China regarding these fellows that are at the head of the Chinese Communist government—Mao Tze-tung and Chou En-lai—and everybody, but those two I knew better than any of the rest.[11] I had officers pretty much all over north China, along the Yangtze and in Manchuria, and I always felt that the reports I got were far better than those the Generalissimo received. He was being fooled time and again because the fellow would defend himself, if he withdrew in an ignominious fashion, he always made it a great battle with Russian tanks and Russian soldiers. The only thing they did not introduce was the Russian paratroops; they had everything else. I would find out from my people it was a patrol encounter, and that went on all the time. Always I was trying to find out anything you could put your finger on that was authentic as to the Soviet influence or Soviet help in all this; I never got anything except the influence of what I would call the spiritual, or something akin to that.

They had Soviet advisers in Yenan—I think they gave me the citizenship of Yenan once; I am not quite certain—but we had them too.[12] But they were more closely in contact than our people. They made no pretense about being aloof from the Soviet Union; they had Stalin's picture and Lenin's picture over the theater there when they entertained me with a very finished performance of about 3 or 4 hours. (Discussion off the record.)

General MARSHALL. I never could get my hands on the thing. As I say, they had no reservation at all; they were Marxist Communists and totally resented implications that they were agrarian Communists of the new stripe. They were Marxist Communists. I remember Chou En-lai startled my wife—we had no place to go and had lunch with him—and he was telling her just what he was and that was it, and she had never heard anything like that before. They appealed to me to stop the procedure of dragging Stalin's painting through the street in the mud. They did not make any pretense of their association with the Communists of Russia; that was rather natural. They were Communists; they were Marxists, and that was the seat of all that development.

When it came to Soviet assistance at all, I never could get my hands on it. I was given all sorts of schedules but, in the opinion of all my advisers and Intelligence, they were not supporting them. Sometimes they were records of little conferences, but you could change a single sentence and change the whole impression of that particular affair. What did worry me more seriously than anything else was it seemed apparent to me that the Soviets were leaning over backward, except as to Dairen, in their attitude out there.[13] Now, they were not supporting their treaty obligations, but there is a great difference between actually supporting the thing and just remaining quiescent. Well, they were remaining quiescent with their treaty agreement to support the Generalissimo's Government, but they went much farther than that. In connection with the railroad in Manchuria, where they had a right to 50 percent of the employees and the Kuomintang government was obligated to protect the railroad, it did not protect the railroad, and the Russians withdrew all of their railroad personnel. Well, as far as I could see, what they were preparing themselves for was a case before the United Nations, where they could appear as clean as the driven snow and we would have our hands muddied by every bit of propaganda they could put on it. I would probably be the particular lump of mud they would throw on it, and that worried me.

Now, I am not talking about the ravaging of Mukden. That was a booty transaction under their claim, just the same as we had it in parts of Europe, in the enemy countries.[14] I am talking about the procedure that followed under the treaty. I was always concerned, and I think it is still going to show up here when they get to this, that they will make a case that they sat back and gave the Generalissimo a wide sweep of opportunity and look at what has happened—the United States interfered and brought about this catastrophe. They could accomplish almost all their purposes by negative action. All they had to do was to abandon the dumps, leave them to fall into the hands of the other fellows. All they had to do was to make it impossible for the Nationalist Government to use the railroad, and yet not introduce any complications about the movements of Communist troops that were moving in and getting set up in Manchuria, we will say, for later action. But that worried me a great deal, and I think that is a consideration you have to have in mind here because I think you will hear from it later.

As to Formosa, I heard that discussed here at the table, and I am not in a position to discuss that. I would have to talk with the Department and find out what has happened, what is the precise situation, and what are the relationships we have had with the British, and so forth. I think that is a dangerous situation, in one sense, because Formosa lies in the general direction from Japan to the Philippines, and if it were taken over by infiltration, as it well might be, it might be very serious. I don't know what we will do about it.

I will say right now in connection with that, though I have been in accord with most of the comments that I have heard around the table as to the futility of military support at the present time, and the great importance of immediate economic considerations dominating part of the thing, as well as the sociological and the spiritual, that leads me to this thought: I don't know at all what the Department thinks about this. Certainly, they would have a very much more reasoned-out opinion; but it seemed to me, when I was listening to Governor Stassen's talk about establishing an American center in Bangkok, that the psychological focus for the United States in approaching this area, if it did through any such procedure, is the Philippines. I may be entirely wrong about this because I don't know enough of what is happening in the Philippines, or other aspects, and about Bangkok, too, for that matter, but all of the Far East looks on the Philippines as a manifestation of the square deal. We certainly went through with it there.

There was a great deal of propaganda about all the reservations, we put into it, in the way of bases and things of that sort—and we ended up, I think, with practically keeping none of them. I don't know who did that. I think we overdid that vastly in requirements, but meanwhile matters changed just as they did in the far southwest Pacific, the Admiralty Islands, and things of that sort, where ideas got boiled down to the practicality of peacetime.

But the Filipinos, of course, realize that their dependence for security rests very heavily on us. They, of themselves, would have a terrible time. But I am quite certain that if the people, say the have-nots, of Indonesia, ask us for independence—the spirit of nationalism has been rapidly developing and all those people look to America as it relates to their action in the Philippines—it might be turned the other way: that we have come there and that we have got the Philippine Government under our domination.

I don't know, but I think there is great significance to our action in the Philippines which affects all those people. I have talked to some of the Philippine leaders and they have emphasized that pretty much to me. I am on dangerous ground now because I have not been fully enough informed, but that is my own reaction.

When I was thinking of Bangkok, I was thinking, just as I left as Secretary of State, the Soviets had established an embassy there with, I think, 50 persons in their little spot. So, they have a command post, as we say in the Army, already established in Bangkok. How wise it is for us to establish a post across the street, I don't know; but, with the data on hand, the State Department could tell you much more about that.

It is difficult for me to get into the general Asian picture because I don't know enough at the moment about the progression of events in Indonesia. Apparently right now it is headed along toward a desirable settlement, or it seems so from what I have read in the papers. If we can untwist that, with the Philippines right above it, and get Japan reasonably established so it does not burden us to death, you are beginning to get a front.

Now you turn over to Indochina. To be honest with you, my principal concern about Indochina after I got out of China—well, I will give you a little color. The very instant the war terminated in the Pacific and our Chinese divisions, that we had been responsible for training, got into Indochina, we had a strenuous demand from the French to get the American officers out of there. So, the first thing that happened the first week was to get every American officer, that had been advising these divisions, away from them. We had to do that and, moreover, there we were getting it from the French, and up north we were getting it from the Communists. It was twisted all over the place. One of our generals said "good morning" to somebody and that was reflected in all the papers as a hideous example of our duplicity. I am exaggerating a little bit. But he is an old friend of mine and I sympathize with him. So we began with that.

Then my next intimate contact with the affair—of course, I had heard quite a bit about China—was when we reached the problem of increasing the security of Western Europe. I found all the French troops of any quality were all out in Indochina, and I found the Dutch troops of any quality were out in Indonesia, and the one place they were not was in Western Europe. So, it left us in an extraordinarily weak position there because we just did not have anything there to make a front to the threats, the bluffing—I hope we can call it that—of the Soviet Union.

I don't know enough about the Indonesian question to comment on what I have heard here, and I might be very misleading if I did comment; so, I will refrain from that.

The general picture indicates to me what would seem to be more desirable is the slow build-up in the actions we take, not big things but many little things. Your greatest difficulty is keeping that out of the debates. The debates are essential to democracy, but they certainly can make you lots of trouble when you try to skate along this thin ice. You have the perimeter of the various affected countries with all the involvements, economic and sociological.

In that respect I would like to add it has seemed to me for quite a long time that we are in the midst of a world revolution and you cannot confine it to what you are thinking about in the Pacific. You have got to come back and think very carefully about Latin America, and when you talk about the absence of the middle class you put your finger right on Latin America, and that is much closer to home. That can affect us in the Far East because there is no doubt in my mind that there is a great sort of world revolution, and, I think someone said here that the communistic factor was more or less of an incident but it was riding on that flood. Well, the actions we take, I think, have to be adapted somewhat to the fact that is the temper of people all over the world, of the have-nots as has been characterized here, and we cannot ignore that.

Thinking hurriedly of what I have said, I don't think I have contributed anything in the way of a definite recommendation, but it is a very difficult thing to do unless you are pretty sure of all of your factors. I have learned through dealing with big organizations that about the time I decide this must be done they come in and prove to me it just cannot possibly be done because I didn't understand this and I didn't understand that, and I find out it is so time after time; so, I have gotten rather sensitive about declaring myself. Maybe if I were political I would be a little bit more free-handed. [Laughter.] Without having the various factors—and there are so many in this—I believe in the end it is a fairly sensible selection to figure out what is your ideal, and then trim that down to its practical application, and with amendments it is pretty hard to recognize, but our Constitution was so established and it has done pretty well. I am sorry I have talked so long.

US Senate, Institute of Pacific Relations, *Hearings before the Subcommittee to Investigate the Administration of the Internal Security Act and Other Internal Security Laws of the Committee on the Judiciary*, 82d Cong., 1st sess. (Washington: GPO, 1951), 5: 1651–56.

1. On September 16, 1949, Secretary of State Dean Acheson had invited Marshall to join "a few persons interested in American foreign policy toward China" at an October 6–8 "confidential consultative meeting" for the purpose of providing "an exchange of views valuable to the department in development of American foreign policy in this area." (Acheson to Marshall, telegram, September 16, 1950, GCMRL/G. C. Marshall Papers [Pentagon Office, Selected].) Marshall agreed and on October 6 joined twenty-four scholars, businessmen, and political and diplomatic figures for a three-day roundtable discussion. The meeting was chaired by Ambassador-at-Large Philip Jessup, and included briefings by such high level officials as State Department Policy Planning Staff head George F. Kennan and Assistant Secretary of State for Far Eastern Affairs W. Walton Butterworth. Marshall knew these individuals as well as some of the roundtable participants as a result

not only of his 1947–49 tenure as secretary of state (see *Papers of GCM*, 6), but also his preceding mission to China. For further information on that mission see *Papers of GCM*, 5: 369–776 and *George C. Marshall's Mediation Mission to China: December 1945–January 1947* (Lexington, VA: George C. Marshall Foundation, 1998).

While much of the discussion at the October 6–8 roundtable centered on whether or not to recognize Mao's newly declared government in China, the participants also dealt with future US policy in the rest of Asia and the western Pacific. Marshall was present on all three days but did not make any statements or ask any questions until the third and final day, when he opened the morning session with the comments that follow.

Two years later, Harold Stassen, president of the University of Pennsylvania and former Republican governor of Minnesota, would charge in sworn testimony before a senate subcommittee that the dominant group at the roundtable had favored recognition of Mao's government and that Jessup had agreed with them. Responding to congressional and press demands, the State Department released its confidential transcript of the roundtable on October 11, 1951. On the following day Francis H. Russell, director of the State Department's Office of Public Affairs, sent Marshall a copy of the transcript. That copy is in the Marshall Papers, Secretary of Defense files, but it does not contain all the comments by Marshall and others as released by the department on October 11, perhaps because the version sent to Marshall included "only those portions of the discussion of particular interest to Department officers." The version of Marshall's comments reproduced here has consequently been taken from the fuller version released by the department and published as an appendix to the hearings of the subcommittee of the Senate Judiciary Committee.

2. Marshall is probably referring to the State Department's so-called "China White Paper," published as *United States Relations with China: With Special Reference to the Period 1944–1949* (State Department Publication 3573, Far Eastern Series 30).

3. General of the Army Douglas MacArthur (USMA, 1903) was at this time supreme commander for the Allied Powers in Japan (SCAP).

4. Fairbank had headed the US Information Service in Chungking at the beginning of Marshall's 1945–46 mission to China. John Leighton Stuart had been a Presbyterian missionary in China as well as the president of Yenching University and had been appointed US ambassador to China in July 1946.

5. See *Papers of GCM*, 1: 23–28.

6. Marshall had first proposed what would become the Normandy invasion in the spring of 1942 (see *Papers of GCM*, 2: 157–59), but it was delayed by the decision to invade North Africa in 1942 and Sicily/Italy in 1943 and was not launched until June of 1944.

7. Robert College in Istanbul, Turkey, was an American institution founded in 1863.

8. Marshall is referring here to the European Recovery Program.

9. The Soviet Union had obtained the Kurile Islands from Japan at the end of World War II.

10. Marshall is referring here to the effort to extend the term of service for those drafted in the Selective Service Act of 1940, an extension that the House of Representatives passed in August of 1941 by only one vote.

11. Chou En-lai had been the chief Communist negotiator during the Marshall mission to China and had recently been appointed premier and foreign minister of the new Communist government.

12. Yenan was the Communist capital during the Chinese Civil War.

13. Dairen had been internationalized at the end of World War II with recognition of preeminent Soviet interests in the port.

14. Marshall is referring here to the Soviet military occupation of Mukden at the end of World War II.

3

EXCHANGE FOLLOWING REMARKS AT STATE DEPARTMENT ROUNDTABLE ON AMERICAN FOREIGN POLICY TOWARD CHINA
October 8, 1949 Washington, DC

IN THE question and answer session that followed Marshall's comments, he was asked whether Mao and Chou "would accept Moscow or Kremlin dictation when it went against their own size-up of their advantage or the advantage of their own group?" Warning that his response "would just be the wildest guess on that," Marshall said that "it would depend on how seriously the decision affected their own thinking." There would not be the "same domination" as the Soviets exercised in Eastern Europe, "but I would say that with a great many qualifications." Chou En-lai, he had found during his 1945–46 mission to be a serious as well as "a very able" negotiator, but for a while it looked like he would be relieved because "They thought he compromised too much." Mao "I could not penetrate. There is a real iron curtain when you get there," and he reminded Marshall of Soviet Foreign Minister Vyacheslav Molotov at times. (US Senate, Institute of Pacific Relations, *Hearings before the Subcommittee to Investigate the Administration of the Internal Security Act and Other Internal Security Laws of the Committee on the Judiciary*, 82d Cong., 1st sess., 5: 1656–58.)

Marshall also stated in response to questions that Mao had never proposed Russian participation in the mediation effort and that American aid to Japan should continue "as long as it seems necessary," but not "indefinitely. It just cannot be done. It cannot be done politically, for one thing, and it cannot be done economically, I think, for another." When asked to comment "on what the abandonment of Chiang Kai-shek is going to mean, what its significance may mean politically," Marshall responded with a lengthy explanation of the problems Chiang had faced in terms of his "tenuous control" over subordinates who "had become corroded by long tenure of office without any opposition whatsoever" and who were unwilling to give up their power. He concluded by apologizing for "running off" and left for an 11:00 a.m. meeting of the Red Cross Board of Governors' Executive Committee. (Ibid.) ★

4

TO HAROLD S. VANCE[1]

October 11, 1949
Washington, DC

My dear Mr. Vance: Hoffman called me up this morning to tell me that your company was generously ordering me a new Studebaker car. He didn't say whether he'd read my recent note to him to you but I assume that he did.[2]

Mr. Johnson and Mr. Engelmann have just been in to notify me of this gift and get my choice of a color for the car.[3] I appreciate this very much both personally and for the Red Cross and I know it will give me a very comfortable means of transportation here and about Washington. Please accept my thanks.

I think I remember you as an assistant to Mr. Knudson in the old pre-war days along the fall of 1940 over in the Public Health Building. In any event, I hope I may have the pleasure of thanking you personally in the near future.[4] Faithfully yours,

GCMRL/G. C. Marshall Papers (American Red Cross, General)

1. Harold S. Vance, a member of the board of directors of the South Bend, Indiana, chapter of the American Red Cross, was chairman of the board and president of the Studebaker Corporation. Vance had been chairman of Studebaker since 1935 and had succeeded Paul G. Hoffman as its president when Hoffman resigned in 1948 to direct the Economic Cooperation Administration (ECA).

2. "I find on taking over this new job of mine that the automobile assigned for my use is your famous Studebaker," Marshall had written to Paul Hoffman. "They are begging me for photographs though I've had a million taken. I think I will have them do me with my hand resting on this latest model!" (Marshall to Hoffman, October 6, 1949, GCMRL/G. C. Marshall Papers [American Red Cross, General].)

3. Courtney Johnson, assistant to the president of Studebaker Corporation, and George E. Engelmann, manager of Studebaker's Washington office, met with Marshall at 2:30 p.m. on October 11. Engelmann sent Marshall literature on the 1950 model Studebaker Land Cruiser. (Engelmann to Marshall, October 11, 1949, ibid.)

4. William S. Knudsen, president of General Motors from 1937 to 1940, had served on the National Defense Advisory Commission and as principal administrator of the Office of Production Management during World War II. Marshall is referring to Harold Vance and Knudsen reviewing American factory and machine tools production capability to manufacture guns for Britain during October 1940. (See *Papers of GCM*, 2: 334–35.)

George Engelmann delivered the new Studebaker Land Cruiser for the American National Red Cross to Marshall on November 30; Vance was not able to attend the presentation. "It is a beautiful car," Marshall wrote to Vance the next day, "and already I'm deriving much pleasure from it." (Marshall to Vance, December 1, 1949, GCMRL/G. C. Marshall Papers [American Red Cross, General].)

5

To Arthur H. Vandenberg — October 17, 1949
Washington, DC

Dear Arthur: I was so pleased as was Katherine to read in the newspaper that you had returned home and also to see a very cheerful looking photograph of you taken at the time of your leaving the hospital.[1] I do hope the whole business has been successful and that you are entirely out of the woods.

Katherine wrote to Hazel, I think about two days ago and I had written her the day before you went into the hospital.[2]

I was much worried about you because I thought that you probably delayed longer than you should have, in the interest of the country, going into the hospital. My delay was only a matter of about three months but yours amounted to at least a year.

I have dieted down to the point where I can get my clothes on comfortably and wear all of my wardrobe again. The diet was imposed by me because of clothes and not by the doctor in the interest of good health.

My love to both of you.[3] Affectionately,

GCMRL/G. C. Marshall Papers (Pentagon Office, General)

1. Arthur H. Vandenberg, Republican senator from Michigan, had been chairman of the Senate Committee on Foreign Relations during the 80th Congress and had worked closely with Marshall on numerous foreign policy issues in 1947 and 1948; see the index to volume six of *Papers of GCM.* He had half of his left lung removed during surgery on October 3 at the University of Michigan Hospital. The October 16 *New York Times* featured a photograph of Vandenberg smiling as he was released from the hospital to recuperate at home. ("Senator Vandenberg 'Doing Fine' after Operation of Five Hours on Left Lung," *New York Times*, October 4, 1949, p. 29 and "On the Recovery List," October 16, 1949, p. 43.) See pp. 315 and 490–91.

2. Katherine Marshall, General Marshall's second and current wife, had written to Senator Vandenberg's wife, Hazel.

3. "Thanks for your last letter—and all your precious messages," Vandenberg replied. "Like you, I probably put off 'my operation' longer than was wise. But, also like you, I am officially promised 'complete success.' I am told that every vestige of the lung lesion is removed. I am also emphatically told that I am '*on the shelf*' for 90 hermit-days while Nature completes the 'cruel and unusual punishment' which is supposed to be *unconstitutional* (everywhere except in hospitals). At the moment I seem to be of a frame of mind to prefer even Vishinsky to some Doctors with whom I am on much too familiar terms. But I expect to bless them in the end—despite their 50 stitches and their maddening appeals to 'patience' (of which I have little left after surviving the Senate Foreign Relations Committee and the White House the last few years)." Vandenberg concluded, "Thanks again for your stimulating messages. Your friendship has a top priority in my heart." (Vandenberg to Marshall, October 26, 1949, GCMRL/G. C. Marshall Papers [Pentagon Office, General].) Andrey Vyshinsky was Soviet deputy foreign minister throughout Marshall's tenure as secretary of state and had a reputation for making personal attacks; see the index to volume six of *Papers of GCM.* He became the Soviet foreign minister in March 1949.

6

To Frank McCarthy

October 17, 1949
Washington, DC

Dear Frank: I received your note at Leesburg on Saturday and we were both very glad to hear from you.[1]

I asked them to invite you during my quick passage through Los Angeles because I wanted very much to see you. However, it is not possible for me to delay my departure because I can only give each place about two and a half hours as I am making the entire circuit including Kansas City, St. Louis and then down to New Orleans, in six days.

I am leaving for New York in the morning to be there two days—part business, part pressure engagements and a little pleasure (South Pacific).[2] Incidentally, if you have any big theatrical connection in New York, give them my name if they can facilitate my getting tickets from time to time.[3] Hastily and affectionately,

GCMRL/G. C. Marshall Papers (Pentagon Office, General)

1. McCarthy (VMI, 1933), Marshall's former aide then employed by the Twentieth Century–Fox Film Corporation in Beverly Hills, California, had written to report that the chairman of the local Red Cross chapter, Clarence Beesmyer, had informed him that Marshall would be coming soon to California on Red Cross business. Beesmyer had invited

McCarthy to join him and Marshall at dinner on October 27. "Beesmyer also told me of your hurried schedule, with arrival in the afternoon and departure after dinner," wrote McCarthy. "This sounds like the old days. Wouldn't it be possible for you to bring Mrs. Marshall along and have two or three days here? I could arrange anything you like, inside or outside the studios, or at Palm Springs. This is one of the most beautiful times of the year on the edge of the desert, and I think you would find real relaxation there. There are so many people who would like to see you." (McCarthy to Marshall, October 13, 1949, GCMRL/G. C. Marshall Papers [Pentagon Office, Selected].) See p. 34n1.

2. Marshall's visit to New York included a meeting of the Pan American Airways Board of Directors and a banquet hosted by the New York Board of Trade, at which he received an award, on October 18. See p. 4n3. The following day Marshall attended a Red Cross luncheon, toured the Manhattan Red Cross blood center, and met with the New York Chapter staff and volunteers; he capped off the evening by attending the Broadway musical *South Pacific* at the Majestic Theatre.

3. McCarthy replied that he talked with Joseph Moskowitz, vice president for Twentieth Century–Fox with headquarters in New York, whose office would be pleased to handle Marshall's theater tickets. "I told him you would let him know, when you first had occasion to approach him on the subject, whether you objected to having your name used in connection with securing tickets. This would help, but it is not necessary in view of the prestige of his office in the theater and in view of the fact that all producers are glad to assist the motion picture companies in any way they can. I also made it clear to Mr. Moskowitz that you would want to pay for the tickets on each occasion." (McCarthy to Marshall, October 19, 1949, ibid.)

7

Testimony on the National Defense Program before the House Committee on Armed Services
October 21, 1949 Washington, DC

MARSHALL began by stating that he had been "notified of the desire to have me appear before the committee while I was in New York, from where I returned yesterday evening." Consequently he had "no prepared statement" and had "not discussed the immediate issues with anybody. I can only bring to you my point of view as it was formed through my experience before and during the war and therafter while I was Secretary of State.

"From the very first time I came to Washington in 1919, in the fall," Marshall informed the committee, "I became convinced that something had to be done in order better to insure a respectable posture of national defense." The key problem had been lack of money in peacetime, and he noted the post–World War I US Army's "downgrade to almost extinction. . . . Later I inherited the problem which had resulted from those years of attrition and had a great deal of time in which to mull the matter over in my own mind." Congress acted on the army without asking its opinions, and the General Staff then had to make spending decisions that irritated many representatives. "So I became a firm advocate of some form of unification." Furthermore, "it became more and more evident to me that something should be done in the interest of national security, and, to put it more politely, in the interest of the taxpayer, to produce a more unified procedure which was calculated to give us the most for whatever number of dollars the Congress felt that it could appropriate for the national defense." (US House of Representatives Committee on Armed Services, *The National Defense Program—Unification and Strategy*, 81st Cong., 1st sess., October 21, 1949 [Washington: GPO, 1949], 597–99.)

The World War II Joint Chiefs of Staff (JCS) organization had been an informal one, Marshall reminded the committee members, and "was not calculated to work as smoothly as would be highly desirable in the dangerous days we were then confronting." For example, the army air forces had remained subordinate to him as army chief of staff, even though he had granted the air chief, General Henry H. "Hap" Arnold (USMA, 1907), virtual autonomy and arranged for him to be a member of the JCS. Marshall also noted that he had had to overcome President Franklin D. Roosevelt's reluctance to improve the military's organization at the top by appointing Admiral William D. Leahy (USNA, 1897) as chief of staff to the commander in chief. Wartime emergency measures, however, were likely to be inadequate in times of peace when budget requests were significantly reduced. "I felt all along there hadn't been enough emphasis given to that phase of the matter," Marshall continued. "I felt particularly here in the past 2 or 3 years that we have been misled as to the workability of what we are doing in some respects by the fact that we have a great stimulant toward military appropriations which I hope in due time will be completely lacking—that is our feelings regarding the Soviet Union. When that lapses and we do get to a better accord, then, immediately the military forces are in great difficulties to maintain themselves at a reasonable state of efficiency and a reasonable state to provide for prompt expansion." (Ibid., 599–600.)

Marshall made clear, however, that he was not a proponent of excessive military spending in peacetime. He recalled that during the second half of 1945, military planning was being based on budget projections that he believed entirely unattainable; consequently, he "was in disagreement with almost everything that was being proposed." He believed that the military services needed a better method of doing business, one that avoided both the disastrous effects of excessive postwar funding cuts and "a financial effect on our economy which would be as disastrous to us as a war might well be. Now, my associates who differed with me did so, I felt, largely on the ground that they thought America had learned its lesson. When it comes to appropriations in piping times of peace, I don't think America will ever learn its lesson, because the political pressures are tremendous." (Ibid., 601.)

The military services had to "find more economical ways of doing some of these things that must be done." Spending had to be done "with great discretion." Marshall contended that "unity is absolutely mandatory," and he had hoped it "would have been smoothly worked out long ere this time." (Ibid., 602.)

To give the Congress some basis upon which to evaluate the military's funding requests, Marshall had long advocated that the Joint Chiefs of Staff be required by law to produce an annual report giving their views on the requirements for the national defense. This would avoid the situation that he recalled in the early 1920s:

"I saw Pershing in the position where his views didn't count at all. He never could get them up for consideration. And yet he was a man of great prestige in this country. But the cuts, and cuts and cuts came despite what he felt. The main reason for this was that he had no opportunity to give public expression without being in the position of disloyalty. Of course, he never would have done that." (Ibid., 604.) General of the Armies John J. Pershing (USMA, 1886) had been commander of the American Expeditionary Forces (AEF) during World War I from 1917 to 1918 and army chief of staff from 1921 to 1924; Marshall had served as his aide in Washington from September 1919 to June 1924.

"I want to congratulate you, General," committee chair Carl Vinson (D-GA) concluded in thanking Marshall for his testimony. "While I wasn't a unification convert at first, I became a Saul of Tarsus after many days and much tribulation. I am an advocate of it now. I am going to use everything in my power as long as I am in Congress to see that the spirit of it works and see that it works as it should—as a team, instead of for the advancement or the aggrandizement of any particular service." (Ibid., 605.) ★

8

American Red Cross Press Release — October 24, 1949
Army Message Center Radio. — Washington, DC

General George C. Marshall, new ARC President, is going to find out for himself how Organization operates by making flying tour Red Cross chapters across country. Going by air will cover 6,000 miles in 6 days, talk to Red Cross leaders at 12 stopping points. At each stop he will talk with leaders from many chapters in that area.

In reply to New York newspaperman's request for comment on the importance of the Red Cross to the Armed Forces during peacetime, General Marshall said, "I am sure you all know this—it is very important to the fellows overseas to have Red Cross services, as well as those in hospitals in this country. During the war there was quite a discussion as to whether the Red Cross should be at the docks and railway stations when the men left for overseas. It was a matter of balancing secrecy and morale. The question came to me for decision. I took the responsibility of deciding that the Red Cross should be there to preserve morale and they did a wonderful job throughout the war during the hot summer months and the cold winter days and nights."[1]

Referring to forthcoming tour, General Marshall declared, "It is my business now to find out from the Red Cross leaders about the inside workings of the Organization. At the end of the tour I should know a great deal more about the activities of the Red Cross and particularly what its workers are thinking. I know that as in any large Organization there are many points of view and that there are many things about morale and program which I should know."

General Marshall will not be a figurehead. He made this clear to newspapermen in New York, pointing out he had come into Red Cross only short while before it will be necessary for him to preside at meetings of large city chapters, Board of Governors, and Subcommittees of Board. He asserted, "I have come in at an active period of the Red Cross year and have to work very rapidly in order to acquaint myself with the services so that I will not be a figurehead."

General Marshall inspected New York Chapter Blood Center October 19. Later held First Press Conference. Announced there his air tour. Cities to be covered October 24 through October 30: Pittsburgh, Cleveland, Chicago, Minneapolis, Seattle, Portland, San Francisco, Los Angeles, Kansas City, St. Louis, New Orleans and Atlanta.

GCMRL/G. C. Marshall Papers (American Red Cross, Categorical, Memoranda)

1. Marshall defended using American Red Cross services during troop embarkations in a memorandum for the British Chiefs of Staff; see *Papers of GCM*, 4: 81–82.

ACCOMPANIED by Red Cross Executive Vice President and General Manager James T. Nicholson and Ramone S. Eaton, vice president and assistant general manager, Marshall between October 24 and October 29 actually traveled seventy-five hundred miles and visited fifteen cities—not the six thousand miles and twelve cities as announced in the Red Cross press release—in a Pan American Airways converted B-26 Martin Bomber. (The three additional stop-over cities were Bismarck, Phoenix, and Memphis.) His route took him from Washington, DC, to Pittsburgh, Cleveland, and Chicago on October 24; Minneapolis and Bismarck on October 25; Seattle, Portland, and San Francisco on October 26; Los Angeles and Phoenix on October 27; Kansas City, St. Louis, and Memphis on October 28; and New Orleans and Atlanta on October 29. He attended luncheon or dinner meetings in twelve of these cities, met the chairmen of 158 chapters and numerous other local Red Cross officials, inspected chapter houses, and held a press conference at each stop. "I'm not going to discuss war," he told the New Orleans press during one of those conferences; "I've been talking war for 10 years and I'm fed up. I'm talking Red Cross." (George Korson, "General Marshall's Flying Trip," *Red Cross Courier* 29 [December 1949]: 4–6, quote on 6.) See photo #2.

Marshall's healthy appearance, fast pace, and ability to maintain such a grueling schedule surprised many who thought that his kidney operation had left him permanently impaired. The *Portland Journal* quipped that Marshall "captured" the city "in a lightning maneuver that left local Red Cross personnel and civic leaders spinning in their tracks. . . . For a man who only a few months ago was believed to be seriously ill, Marshall's performance was amazing." (Ibid., 5–6.) His schedule each day illustrates why. On the first day of the trip he left Washington at 9:45 a.m.; was met at the Pittsburgh airport at 10:45 a.m. by Red Cross chapter leaders and the press; met with chapter representatives and community leaders at the Duquesne Club in Pittsburgh at noon; left Pittsburgh for Cleveland at 2:30 p.m.; arrived in Cleveland at 3:15 p.m.; met with chapter chairs and the press at a Hotel Statler reception in his honor at 5:00 p.m.; had a dinner meeting at the Union Club with chapter representatives and community leaders at 5:30 p.m.;

departed Cleveland at 8:00 p.m.; landed in Chicago at 8:45 p.m.; and then rode with chapter representatives to the Blackstone Hotel. His day in Portland that so impressed the *Journal* was equally if not more filled. It began with an 8:00 a.m. flight of over a thousand miles from Bismarck, North Dakota, to Seattle, where at 12:30 p.m. he was met by chapter officials and the press. That was followed by a 1:00 p.m. luncheon meeting at the New Washington Hotel with chapter and community representatives and a 3:30 p.m. flight to Portland. Arriving at 4:15 p.m., he was met by chapter representatives and the press, and at 5:00 p.m. he toured the Portland chapter headquarters. That was followed by a dinner meeting with chapter and community representatives at the Multnomah Hotel and then a 7:30 p.m. flight to San Francisco, where at 10:30 p.m. he was again met by chapter officers and the press and then driven with chapter representatives to the Saint Francis Hotel.

As amazing as this schedule was, Marshall was only late once during the entire trip—in New Orleans—for a total of twelve minutes. "I could take that delay," he later quipped; "it was at Antoine's," a famous restaurant in the French Quarter. Although official Red Cross business obviously dominated this trip, Marshall received a silver key in Portland to the old house he had occupied when in command of Vancouver Barracks (1936–38), and in San Francisco he had breakfast with Hap Arnold. He returned to Washington from Atlanta by train on October 30. (Ibid., 10–11). ★

9

TO LIEUTENANT GENERAL WALTER BEDELL SMITH — November 3, 1949, Washington, DC

Dear Smith: I was sorry not to see you when I was in New York Tuesday but I did not arrive until 2 p.m. and went directly to the Chrysler Building—thanks to your transportation.[1] Then I had to see David Rockefeller and ended up by going to bed at 8 o'clock at the Club. The next morning was devoted to Ed Stettinius' funeral from which I proceeded directly to the station.[2]

When I was in New York the other day I did not call you up at all because I feel it a great imposition to be continually making demands on your services and the Board of Trade people turned a car over to me for my use.[3]

Last week I did 7500 miles and 14 [*fifteen*] cities in six days and, while I am not traveling this week, I will be just as busy. I do have to go to a Board of Visitors meeting at V.M.I. on Saturday night and am compelled to motor down because of no rail transportation and no nearby airfield.[4]

Give my love to Mary.[5] Again, my thanks for the car. Faithfully yours,

GCMRL/G. C. Marshall Papers (American Red Cross, General)

1. Marshall attended the luncheon meeting of the Board of Directors of Pan American Airways on Tuesday, November 1, held in the Chrysler Building's Cloud Club. General Smith had served as US ambassador to the Soviet Union from March 1946 to March 1949, at which point he took over command of the First Army at Governors Island, New York.

General Smith had arranged for a car to meet Marshall, as he had done in September. See *Papers of GCM*, 6: 747.

2. The funeral service for former Secretary of State Edward R. Stettinius Jr. was held at Saint James Episcopal Church in New York City on November 2, 1949.

3. Marshall had received an award from the New York Board of Trade on October 18. (See p. 17n2.)

4. Marshall had been a member of the Virginia Military Institute's Board of Visitors since 1946. (See *Papers of GCM*, 5: 493, 576.)

5. Mary Eleanor Smith was Walter Bedell Smith's wife.

10

To Thomas J. Watson

November 9, 1949
Washington, DC

Dear Tom: Katherine and I greatly appreciate the compliment Mrs. Watson and you desire to pay us, and also in giving us such a wide choice of dates.[1] I am very sorry that I do not see our way clear to accepting at this time.

I will be in New York December fifth and sixth for a business meeting and for two dinners—International House and the Masaryk Memorial affair of which I am United States Chairman.[2] I am due to talk the next day at the War College.[3] Therefore, December eighth would be too soon for me to attempt another trip to New York because I really have to be careful of my energy now because the Red Cross demands are pretty heavy at the present time.

The thirteenth and fourteenth I am involved in one Red Cross date and the Business Advisory Council meeting. The fact that I missed the Hot Springs meeting makes it more desirable that I should not miss this meeting, besides I have something I want to say to them pertaining to the Red Cross. The fact is I am much overloaded for November, December and I am trying to see what I can do to lighten the burden. Last week I flew some 7,500 miles and visited fourteen [*fifteen*] cities in six days. That was a pretty heavy tax and this week is equally bad for I have five continuous days of Red Cross Chapter and Board of Governors meetings.

I hope you and Mrs. Watson understand because we are very appreciative of your desire to convey this honor.[4] Faithfully yours,

GCMRL/G. C. Marshall Papers (American Red Cross, General)

1. Watson, president of International Business Machines (IBM), had written Marshall inviting him to a dinner in his honor recognizing his acceptance of the presidency of the Red Cross. Watson was anticipating inviting "a number of representative people of the Red Cross along with a group of your friends from different parts of the country." He offered Marshall five dates in December upon which the dinner could be held. (Watson to Marshall, November 5, 1949, GCMRL/G. C. Marshall Papers [American Red Cross, General].)

2. On December 5, Marshall was the guest of philanthropist John D. Rockefeller Jr., and he visited International House, a residence and club in New York City where Marshall served as chairman of the board of trustees, before dining with his host that evening. (Rockefeller's son David was chairman of the Executive Committee of International House.) On December 6, he attended the Pan American Airways board meeting in the Chrysler Building. Marshall served as chairman of the US Masaryk Memorial Fund, a project dedicated to perpetuating the memory of Jan Masaryk through a physical memorial and

scholarship fund. Masaryk had been the foreign minister of Czechoslovakia whose death in 1948, ruled suicide by the authorities, was widely suspected to be a murder perpetrated by Czech Communists. ("Marshall Heads Drive," *New York Times*, September 14, 1949, p. 27.)

3. Marshall delivered an off-the-record address to the National War College in Washington, DC, on December 14 discussing "The Role of the Military in Foreign Policy." Commandant Lieutenant General Harold R. Bull (USMA, 1914) wrote, "Your splendid talk was a moving experience to each of us. Students and staff, I know, are deeply grateful for and proud of the direct and forthright manner in which you shared with us the wealth of your experience." (Bull to Marshall, December 16, 1949, GCMRL/G. C. Marshall Papers [American Red Cross, Categorical, Invitations, Accepted].)

4. "You can rest assured that Jeannette and I understand fully your situation," Watson replied. "We want you to know that your room is always ready at our house any time you would like to use it. It is understood that you will be guests with the same independence and freedom that you would have if you were in a hotel. I know that I am speaking for all your friends when I say do not over-tax your health—you mean too much to your family, your friends, your country and the world." (Watson to Marshall, November 11, 1949, GCMRL/G. C. Marshall Papers [Pentagon Office, General].)

11

TO HAROLD W. DODDS — November 10, 1949
[Washington, DC]

Dear Dodds: I am sorry I am causing you so much of a complication both with the long delay as to the subject of my talk and now as to publicity concerning it.[1] In all probability I will talk off hand though I have been endeavoring to formulate what line of discussion I might best take. Confidentially, I have had more difficulty in settling this matter than any other talk I think I've ever made, for the reason that I have to be so very careful these days not to intrude in matters in which the State Department is critically engaged and regarding which an unfortunate phrasing of mine or sense divorced from the context might lead to considerable newspaper publicity or columnistic discussion.

This situation has left us bereft of much that would be very interesting to your people but I have not the time and I would not care to take the risk of engaging in anything but very vague generalities regarding the present international situation.

I assume your astonishment of the subject I have selected but it happens to have been of great interest to me and something regarding which I was personally and officially heavily involved. My dilemma has been how to carry such coals to New Castle, meaning a talk in the presence of your faculty. However, I'll do the best I can.[2]

With apologies again for causing you so many complications,[3] Faithfully yours,

GCMRL/G. C. Marshall Papers (American Red Cross, Categorical, Invitations, Accepted)

1. Harold Dodds, president of Princeton University, and Marshall had been attempting to set up an acceptable date for Marshall to deliver a lecture to the university community; see *Papers of GCM*, 6: 718. Marshall wished his speech to be off the record, but Dodds had mistakenly forwarded a request from the university's public relations department for

an advance copy of the speech. While apologizing for the oversight, Dodds cautioned, "[Y]ou are not an obscure individual who can come to a university campus without arousing the curiosity of the public. For this reason it is an inescapable assumption that whatever you say is bound to get into the papers in some form or other. . . . It is the price that a man pays for eminence in public life, but as one humble American citizen I am most happy that you have been willing to pay the price of public service, for the nation has had great need of you." (Dodds to Marshall, November 9, 1949, GCMRL/G. C. Marshall Papers [American Red Cross, Categorical, Invitations, Accepted].)

2. Marshall planned to talk about educational technique in his speech at Princeton; see pp. 25–33.

3. "I can quite sympathize," Dodds replied, "with the position in which you find yourself in respect to a subject for your address here Thursday evening [November 17], because I have so often found myself in the same position. Anything you say will arise from experience and will, therefore, be particularly valuable to an academic audience. Please don't have our faculty in mind at all. The audience will be composed of undergraduates, plus men and women of the University community." (Dodds to Marshall, November 14, 1949, ibid.)

12

To Arthur H. Vandenberg — November 17, 1949, Washington, DC

Dear Arthur: I had a note from Hazel this morning along with a formal letter from her endorsing a Red Cross invitation. In her note she said that you were having some discomfort from an arthritic condition which was painful. She used the expression "in such pain at times" that it suggested to me that this reaction of yours was identical with mine.[1]

The first three days after my operation I apparently stood No. 1 on the list of quick recoveries and excited much "favorable comment" but the fourth day the trouble began. They didn't call it arthritic but said it was nerve pains that often follow an operation, in my case particularly because it related to the big nerve (No. 12, I believe—they seem to deal them out in sizes) which fanned out like the Delta of the Mississippi across my abdomen. For almost three weeks I was barely able to move without setting up a terrifically painful reaction—the worst pain I had ever suffered. Even to gulp when I drank would produce it; to turn my head on the pillow sometimes started it and my worst attack came when the nurse was fixing the sheets and tickled the sole of my foot. This lasted about two hours and was most painful.

Maybe you are suffering the same trouble with No. 12. However, when that wears off you find yourself in top shape and soon forget it ever happened. The point is that the nerve pain seemingly has no relation to the wound recovery. The other thing in my case was that ten months later when the small nerves began to heal, or rather make their junction, I became very sensitive where I previously had been numb. And with all of these suggestions and services, for which I charge nothing, I send you my profound sympathy.

Lovett and I were talking about you in New York the other day and incidentally I have to dictate a short statement that Roland Harriman (head of Lovett's firm) wishes to include in an introduction of Lovett at some dinner tonight. I am sorry I can't also quote from you.[2]

My love to you both.[3] Affectionately,

GCMRL/G. C. Marshall Papers (Pentagon Office, General)

1. Hazel Vandenberg had written to Marshall in his capacity as president of the Red Cross to pass on a request from "a very up-and-coming Chapter Chairman, Mr. O. B. Snow," who had asked her to ask Marshall to open the Red Cross national campaign in Grand Rapids, Michigan. "He has many logical reasons for this very unusual procedure but I told him that it was unprecedented to open the National Red Cross Campaign any place but in Washington." (Vandenberg to Marshall, November 12, 1949, GCMRL/G. C. Marshall Papers [Pentagon Office, General].)

She also included a more personal note that "Arthur is not 'coming back' from his operation as quickly as we hoped he would. Everything in connection with the operation is entirely satisfactory but he has developed an arthritic condition which is very painful and makes him want to stay in bed most of the time. His morale is down as a result of all this and I don't mind telling you it has affected mine. There is so little to be done for him apparently and he seems in such pain at times that it is simply maddening." (Vandenberg to Katherine and George Marshall, November 12, 1949, ibid.)

2. Robert A. Lovett had served as Marshall's undersecretary of state from July 1947 to January 1949. E. Roland Harriman (W. Averell Harriman's brother and a colleague of Lovett's at Brown Brothers Harriman and Company) read Marshall's tribute to introduce Lovett as the guest of honor and speaker at the dinner meeting of the Newcomen Society for the History of Engineering and Technology that evening. "I doubt if there is really anybody outside of those in top positions in the State Department," read Marshall's statement, "who vaguely realize the great service rendered by Bob Lovett as under-secretary of state. As a matter of fact, he had the very difficult role of being acting secretary of state almost one year and during a most critical period. The job would have been much easier for him had he actually been secretary instead of acting in my absence. He combined several characteristics that are of the greatest importance in public office and particularly in a position which involved world-wide considerations; integrity of the highest order, complete loyalty and great wisdom along with a selfless dedication of all his efforts to represent the government and those serving me." (Dictated to Mr. Hera [Roland Harriman's secretary], November 17, 1949; Harriman to Marshall, November 18, 1949, GCMRL/G. C. Marshall Papers [American Red Cross, General].)

3. Mrs. Vandenberg replied that Marshall's letter had buoyed her husband's spirits. She wrote to Katherine Marshall, "I think George's letter about the aftermath of his operation was a real tonic to Arthur because he has gotten terribly impatient over the constant pain in his side over the area where the rib was taken out." (Vandenberg to Katherine Marshall, November 29, 1949, GCMRL/G. C. Marshall Papers [Pentagon Office, General].)

13

Speech Delivered at Princeton University — November 17, 1949, Princeton, New Jersey

Educational Technique[1]

Considering the title of this talk, most of you, and certainly the members of the faculty, will wonder just why I come to Princeton to discuss a subject so far out of my normal line of activity—and to discuss it before many here who are the experts in the educational field. I ask you please to have in mind while I'm talking that I am not considering those phases of education which relate primarily to the training of the mind or to the development of the basic cultures, but rather to several elementary phases of education which lean towards the vocational and to another focused on the lessons of history. I have never been accused of being an educator—in fact, the most recent accusation applied to me in some European propaganda, "the Shylock of Wall Street," is one I have little hope of attaining and one that intrigues Mrs. Marshall, who handles our bank book. At this point, I add with some feeling that it is a relief to be discussing matters which are not directly involved in critical international relations after the long endurance trial which occupied all of my energies during the past few years.

If I seem to make too frequent reference to the military, it is only because the examples I refer to have come for the most part out of my military life and problems. When I entered the service 47 years ago it was a tradition, especially accented in popular fiction relating to Army life on the plains which absorbed most of the troops in those days, to stress the silent soldier, that officer of forbidding mien who spoke only to order, and that with terse finality. Now that may have been all right for a purely professional force not ever to be subjected to vast expansions, but it did not meet the requirements of the situation in which I found myself in 1939 as head of an Army of 179,000 men, air and ground, with more than 8 million yet to go. America's security, America's interest in the world and America's democracy could only be defended as a last resort by recourse to the citizen-soldier numbering in the millions, and the more rapidly he and especially his officers could be trained—that is, instructed—the more secure we would be.

Obviously, highly expeditious as well as effective educational methods are necessary to any such astronomical expansion. Professional soldiers must not only know; they must be experts in imparting that "know how" in the most expeditious manner. And please remember that *all* of the students or recipients must absorb and understand the instruction—not merely those favorably disposed. Nor could we drop the poor or indifferent student and send him back home. I am not talking about prospective Rhodes scholars, born scientists or natural students. I am thinking more of our young people who may have completed the last two years of grade school or perhaps up to the first two years of high school, where the maximum numbers of fairly developed minds of our democracy can be reached.

Understand me, I am not referring merely to purely military matters—infantry tactics, artillery fire, armored forces, air combat and bombing. I am referring, rather, to topographical engineering, electrical communications, motor and tank maintenance, matters logistical which mushroom in wartime into colossal problems of supply, transportation, shelter, maintenance and hundreds of related items. No business or trust, monopoly or industry in the world can compare even remotely with the vastness of the Army logistical requirement. And I might remark parenthetically that the maintenance of a modern bomber seemingly involves every complication of electronics, gas engines, radar and compressed air! There were also important matters pertaining to morale, the psychological reactions of soldiers in camp, at work and in battle. In some respects I found my war problems relating to organization and strategy were simple in comparison with all that went to create, maintain, transport, supply and insure the leadership and fighting qualities of the Army.

It was at once apparent that our main emphasis must be placed on the teaching technique of simplicity. Not just plain simple unadulterated simplicity—rather a virile, above-board, convincing simplicity. The kind of simplicity that makes the student realize his own unlimited capabilities, and instills in him the desire or enthusiasm necessary for full development of those capabilities. And out of this studied simplicity automatically develops personal incentive. Let me mention a few small incidents from my own early experiences—experiences which helped immeasurably in setting the pattern of training we followed in the last war. During the rainy season in the Philippines 37 years ago, I found myself suddenly confronted with the problem of teaching my NCOs [noncommissioned officers] topographical sketching before a certain inspection date. It was the season when heavy rains and deep mud made outside work almost impossible. Those old-time regulars dreaded this particular task. Hands like hams—with little knowledge of any of the mathematical or graphical bases for topographical engineering, they were bluffed at the start. Working in the mess hall and by my careful avoidance of every technical term, they made good preliminary progress. Outdoors on the roads between rain storms, their field of operations was extended, still avoiding technical terms such as intersections, resections, back sights, contours, etc. I speeded up their work, simplified their pencil recordings and moved up to the Philippine Department's annual garrison inspection. My group started out on the assigned task at 8 o'clock and was back by 1 o'clock. The groups from other companies drifted in—mostly with incompleted work—at dusk. Meanwhile I was being questioned, or rather investigated, by the Department's inspecting officer and my own Colonel, who thought there must be some skulduggery in the business. The Colonel commented that the sketches of my men were better than he had seen most of the officers do. I am not telling this as a personal triumph, but to illustrate my initial plea for simplicity in the business of teaching or instructing.

Somewhat later with my Philippine group, I grew tired of hearing fine old non-commissioned officers murder the King's English. "I 'seen' him when he 'done' it" was a commonplace, and the murders were unrestricted. On an unexpected rainy day, I discussed this problem, laying stress on the point that, however much they had to sell in the civilian market of integrity, courage, dependability, and knowledge along certain lines, they would usually destroy their chances of employment suitable to their special capabilities because of the devastating impression their grammatical errors would make on the prospective employer. I listed on the blackboard the most glaring of their errors and also the correct form of the same expressions or sentences. Then I emphasized the errors to see if they did not offend the men's ears—and they didn't! That was the entire course of instruction, about a half-hour in all. The First Sergeant asked me later if they could not leave on the blackboard the sentences I had written, so the Company Clerk made mimeographed copies for general distribution. But the impressive reaction to me was an inquiry from the YMCA [Young Men's Christian Association] secretary for some suggestions, as most of the men had gone to him in an appeal for instruction. His only solution was to volunteer the use of an old English grammar that somehow had found its way into the YMCA library. The point I wish to make is that by a few rather simple, obvious remarks, a real incentive to learn had been established in the minds of a hard bitten group of professional soldiers.

And that incident leads me to a third which I believe points up the importance of both simplicity and incentive.

The teaching of languages, considered on a percentage basis, is, in my opinion, nearly a total failure in this country. It seems to me that the fault is largely with the teaching and not with the limited opportunity for the use of foreign languages. The grammatical fence is usually placed as the first hurdle and few ever progress beyond that Becher's Brook.[2] Yet in China in 1927 the officers of my regiment and a large selected group of the men acquired real facility in speaking and understanding Chinese.[3] It is true that there is not much of grammar to the Chinese language, but those men were taught to speak and understand Chinese in from nine to twelve months with only sessions of an hour four or five times a week. The niceties of the so-called grammatical rules could, and I think should, come later.[4]

I experimented with the Chinese language teaching method by instructing my Chinese teacher in speaking and writing English in order that he could pass the examination qualifying for employment in the postal service. He did not apparently know ten words of English yet he was able, after four months, to pass the examination which, incidentally, was given by foreigners. Of course he worked hard, presumably many hours a day, but the fact was that he passed his examination and yet knew little or nothing of the grammatical rules governing the English language. I am not proposing the abolishment of the teaching of grammar but I am criticizing the failure of American schools to give their students a working, talking basis of the languages on which they put in so many hours usually to no profitable purpose.

Finally, before I demobilize my old regiment at least for this evening, I wish to make one more point related to what I term vocational training. It has always seemed to me that the habit of observation is of vital importance in any line of work, in any career. I mean a really personal, critical type of observation designed to retain in the memory those important aspects of any occurrence—to provide an ever-expanding reservoir of personal knowledge and experience upon which subsequent judgments can reflect before decision, or action, is taken. Someone once said, "Experience is the best teacher" or a paraphrase meaning roughly the same thing. What I am concerned with here is the procedure by which we teach our youth that while experience is a wonderful thing acquired only through the passage of time and involving in varying progressive degree such reactions as harassment, dismay, complacency, delight, and I am told even ecstasy, the experience itself is worthless unless we retain permanently in our minds those major aspects of value for future reference.

Of course we don't want to overdo the pedagogical approach to this technique. It would certainly be a dismal world if we were to embark on every experience wondering what, if anything, we were going to get out of it. And I refer here to any sort of possible experience you might be thinking of at this moment! But there are a number of ways in which the habit of observation can be taught to our youth, to get them started on the right track toward developing that retentive memory that will serve them so well in the future. One such method I used with considerable success, again in the Philippines.

I found myself one morning again barred from a planned outdoor training procedure by heavy rain. Somewhat at a loss as to what of interest I might manage indoors for these hardened old regulars, I suddenly hit on the idea of having them make a memory sketch in 30 minutes of the 6-mile route of the street car line connecting the post with the city of Manila. They were to include the terrain and other features within 300 yards of the track, which ran across an open, hilly countryside.

Now those men had taken that trip probably once a week during the past three years, yet they literally could produce nothing conveying any definite impression of the route and bordering country. After they turned in their work I did the sketch, explaining the procedure as I worked. Later they compared this with an accurate map on their own initiative. I made no further reference to the business until during a ten-minute rest period several months later on a practice march I called on the same group for a sketch of the route we had followed during the past hour. A few did a fair job but the majority bogged down again. They challenged me to try them again on the car line, but I replied that the principle I was endeavoring to impress on them applied to any country any time. As soldiers especially they must form the habit of observing, consciously or unconsciously. To be brief, those men developed really astonishing capability thereafter, entirely on their own. Very occasionally, possibly at intervals of several months or more, I would unexpectedly test them on a rapid piece of memory sketching, ten or fifteen minutes for the work, and it always resulted in a betting contest as to whose work I deemed the best. No real teaching was required. It was purely a question of pointing out the lack of observing, and establishing the incentive for self-improvement in this important attribute.

In later years I tried the same test on several hundred officers, men who understood the simple procedure of accurate instrumental mapmaking, and I found most of them at first entirely lacking in the ability which depends on a definite development of the power or art of observation.

I have cited these examples because for me they illustrate the fact that much of schooling fails to interest the pupil because of routine, cut and dried methods, when so little actual instruction is required if the interest is aroused. And once interest is aroused—once a firm incentive is established—there seems to be no barrier insurmountable to the enthusiastic student, regardless of age.

These illustrations also conveniently point out that much of past history can be capitalized on for guidance in the present. I drew on my own experiences—history of a sort, at least to me—to help solve certain critical problems of my more recent past. Let me see what I can now make out of that analogy.

It has become evident to me through the years that *no* national policy could be thoroughly realistic and *continuing* without a better understanding of the lessons of history along similar lines on the part of the average voter and especially the average legislator. In other words a fair, if not a thorough, understanding is necessary of the significance of the cause and effect of great events on world history—of the fall of Greece, the growth and decline of Roman power, the development and decline of power in European nations and, for example, the lessons of our experience in our own wars.

I am not stressing a study of wars, but rather of the reasons for the rise and fall of nations which usually have grown out of wars. However small your interest in wars as such, you must recognize that our gigantic debt today, a result of war, heavily burdens our economy on which our prosperity, our strength and our influence, and also to some extent the peace of the world, depend. How could this situation possibly have been avoided? We tried one method after the First World War and evidently it did not work. Study the situations and actions in Europe prior to the last war. Could that war have been avoided? War is the great evil of our civilization and I think that it can be avoided or, at the very least, contained and/or shortened. But I am convinced that the corrective measures or policies can never be secured through the necessary political action unless our people and legislators acquire a better understanding and knowledge of the lessons of history.

And now to the procedure most interesting to me in the teaching of history. As our recent great war Army was in the process of development, it became apparent that, despite the carefully prepared material placed at their disposal, the company officers had little success in interesting or instructing their men in the background of European and Japanese events of the preceding ten years which had resulted in the debacle of war and which were illustrative of the reasons for the stand our people eventually took in the matter. The officers were more successful in putting their tired soldiers to sleep than they were in depicting the situation in all of its important ramifications. Such a condition would not do for an army, especially with the diverse or distant points of view of those on the East Coast from others in the Mississippi Valley, in the Rocky Mountain region, the Southwest or the Pacific Slope. Something had to be done to give unity to the individual thinking or purposes of the millions of men who made up our Army.

In this dilemma I turned to the motion picture and the skill of a great director, Frank Capra, with the assistance of other equally distinguished experts. A series of moving pictures were produced, the first covering the period from the Limitation of Arms Conference in 1921 to [German Chancellor Adolf] Hitler's movement into Austria in 1936 [*1938*].[5] The Mukden incident and the rape of Ethiopia were of course included in the review of events.[6] The speeches, the regimentation of the children in Japan, Germany and Italy, and all the important procedure and propaganda leading up to the final tragedy were presented with a background of music and other methods of holding interest in which the great directors are experts. The picture ran about one hour and every soldier was supposed to have seen it. But the most interesting reaction to me was its effect on people who had been leading participants, some members of Lord Lytton's Commission to Manchuria, Mr. Stimson, our great Secretary of State in those prewar days, and others equally prominent.[7] They could hardly believe their eyes and ears as the full drama was placed before them. It seemed inconceivable that our people could have lived through such a period with the wealth of information poured out by our press, radio and screen without more quickly having reacted positively to the awful threat that was now made so glaringly apparent on the screen. Mark you, the picture was not propaganda in the sense that it was representing events with prejudice or perversion. The pictures were actual movies of that period assembled in proper sequence and glued together on a background of music and explanation.

From then on we progressed through a series of movies recording the development of the war, and finally presented movies explaining our Allies to the American soldier. "Know Your Ally, Britain" was the most successful of these and, in effect, was an outline history of why for many reasons the British are as they are, what brought about the development of the British Empire, etc. This picture was so effective from the British point of view that Mr. [British Prime Minister Winston] Churchill had it shown in all the English theatres. Our producers barred it because its length interfered with their feature pictures.

Out of this experience I reached the belief that in our school system much of history could be presented by film during the review periods for example, in such a manner that the grammar school or high school student would carry away with him a lasting impression of, say, the reasons behind the fall of Greece, the governmental experiments or experience common to Roman history and similar studies of governmental developments and failures in Europe after the dark ages. The critical phases of the early struggles in America during the Colonial period and the later development of the new Republic could be depicted. This would mean not only a comprehensive impression registered through the eye and ear but the carrying to the student of what would amount to illustrated lectures by the most noted historians, the voices and the picture of events being the work of experts of the stage and screen. I think in this way we would greatly encourage in the casual student a genuine interest in the cause and effect of historical events. Eventually this might also limit the proposals, frequently legislative, to enter into governmental experiments that had been tried and failed hundreds or even thousands of years ago.

In the introduction to these remarks I made reference to the fact that I was not discussing certain fundamental phases in the field of education. I wish to emphasize again that my remarks have been directed not to college or university students, not primarily even to the young people in the senior years of high school, but rather to that larger number out of which comes a reasonably informed public opinion—the last two years in grade school and the first two years in high school. It is that source which provides, in my opinion, a very important group of voters that influences the legislator in his home district.

I have gone through many struggles with this phase of public opinion during the war years, and afterwards during the struggle for a settled peace. I feel that it is of great importance that the level of teaching in our town or country grade and high schools be raised by all means available and I have suggested one definite method to that end.

I ask indulgence of the members of the faculty in considering some of the ideas I have expressed. Only an intense interest in the matter had provoked me to take the risk of entering into such discussion before this particular audience. While I may find no agreement with much of what I have said, at least I have brought the subject before you from my point of view.

And to you young men I would say that I am aware of the great traditions of Princeton dating from the earliest Colonial days; I am aware of the great services that have been rendered by the graduates of Princeton and particularly by representatives of the faculties of our universities, notably Princeton, who were so widely used in the major effort of the Government during the most critical years of the past decade.

I am now engaged in work with the American Red Cross. No doubt you will agree that the Red Cross makes an important contribution to the field of human welfare and that now or later you will probably make your contribution to such work either by gift or personal labor. I do not wish to sound bromidic, but I do feel that you who enjoy the advantages of this institution and others similarly placed could render a *greater* service to the country by exerting your influence toward the education of young America to the full meaning of democracy and our place, and opportunities, and obligations in the world today.[8]

GCMRL/G. C. Marshall Papers (American Red Cross, Speeches and Statements)

1. See pp. 23–24. Marshall edited several drafts of this lecture (initially titled "The Lessons of History") until he shifted focus in a handwritten draft to educational techniques, reducing his previous discourse on history to an abbreviated discussion of the role history plays in educating the public regarding foreign policy in a democracy. The drafts are located in GCMRL/G. C. Marshall Papers (American Red Cross, Speeches and Statements).

2. Becher's Brook was a notoriously difficult fence to be jumped in the course of the Grand National horse race near Liverpool, England; it is a term used proverbially to indicate a significant obstacle to achieving a goal.

3. Marshall's immersion in Mandarin Chinese helped him acquire the language. He remarked in 1925 that he spoke Chinese to his English-speaking valet just for practice, saying, "Now I can carry on a casual conversation in Chinese with far, far less difficulty than I ever could manage in French. And I can understand even the wranglings and squabbles of the coolies and rickshaw men." (See *Papers of GCM*, 1: 281.)

4. See p. 532.

5. The seven films in Frank Capra's "Why We Fight," series were *Prelude to War*, *The Nazis Strike*, *Divide and Conquer*, *The Battle of Britain*, *The Battle of Russia*, *The Battle of China*, and *War Comes to America.*

The Limitation of Arms Conference to which Marshall is referring took place in Washington, DC, from November 12, 1921, through February 6, 1922, and produced a series of treaties relating to naval arms limitation and maintenance of the peace in Asia and the Pacific. Signed by Great Britain, France, Italy, Japan, and the United States, the Five Power Treaty halted a looming naval arms race by dismantling numerous existing capital ships, establishing a ten-year moratorium on the construction of new capital ships and limits as well as ratios on the tonnage of future ships, limiting naval gun sizes, and prohibiting new fortifications in the Pacific. The Four Power Treaty among Great Britain, France, Japan, and the United States abolished the 1902 Anglo-Japanese Alliance and obligated the four powers to respect each other's Pacific possessions. In the Nine Power Treaty the five previously mentioned powers as well as Belgium, China, the Netherlands, and Portugal endorsed the American Open Door Policy calling for equal trade opportunity in China and preservation of its administrative and territorial integrity.

Hitler's movement into Austria refers to his March 1938 military seizure and annexation of Austria in direct violation of the Treaty of Versailles that had ended World War I and prohibited such annexation.

6. In the Mukden Incident of September 18, 1931, officers in the Japanese Kwantung Army accused the Chinese of blowing up a section of the Japanese-run South Manchurian Railway and used the incident, which they had fabricated, as a pretext for a military takeover of Manchuria in violation of the Washington Treaties and other international agreements, followed by the establishment of the puppet state Manchukuo in March of 1932. In 1935 Italy invaded and annexed the previously independent African kingdom of Ethiopia.

7. The Lytton Commission was a fact-finding mission chaired by the British Earl of Lytton and established under the auspices of the League of Nations. Its investigation of the Mukden Incident in Manchuria led to a resolution in the League condemning Japanese aggression—a move that sparked a walkout of Japanese representatives and the subsequent withdrawal of Japan from the League. Although the United States was not a member of the League, then Secretary of State Henry L. Stimson announced, in what became known as the Stimson Doctrine, a policy of nonrecognition of any territorial changes achieved by force or in violation of international agreements.

8. Marshall requested that Princeton University divide his thousand-dollar honorarium for the Stafford Little Lecture equally between Saint James Episcopal Church and the Loudon County Hospital, both in Leesburg, Virginia. (Dodds to Marshall, November 30, 1949, GCMRL/G. C. Marshall Papers [Pentagon Office, General].)

14

TO HENRY L. STIMSON

November 26, 1949
Leesburg, Virginia[1]

My dear Mr. Stimson: The tale of your vacations arrived last evening and I had read it before I went to sleep. Before I got up this morning I gave it a partial review, particularly the chapter relating to "Highhold."[2]

It is a delightful book and a fascinating account of a very remarkable life in your lighter moments. I wish I had read it before I visited Colorado and Glacier Park with you. I recalled the old guide at the Park and the site of your Camp on Lake St. Marys.[3]

Thank you for remembering me in the distribution. Katherine has now taken the book and will have the great pleasure of reading a remarkable account of a remarkable life.

I have been very busy taking over my responsibilities in the Red Cross. Three weeks ago I did 7,500 miles and fourteen [*fifteen*] city meetings in 6 days. Flew into Seattle and Portland with all commercial aviation grounded—the old problem of rain and fog in the north west.

With affectionate regards to Mrs. Stimson and you, and my thanks again,

G. C. Marshall

Yale/H. L. Stimson Papers (General Correspondence); H

1. The Marshalls owned a home, Dodona Manor, in Leesburg, Virginia.

2. Stimson's self-published book, released in 1949 and entitled *My Vacations*, was a personal memoir and travelogue. "Since the publication of 'On Active Service in Peace and War,'" wrote Stimson, "several of my younger relatives and friends have suggested that I should record some of the activities and interests of my youth, which were mainly outdoor diversions and which could not properly be included in that book—devoted as it was almost exclusively to official matters." Harper & Brothers published Stimson's *On Active Service in Peace and War*, co-authored with McGeorge Bundy, in 1948.

My Vacations' final chapter, entitled "Highhold," describes Stimson's Long Island estate, given the name Highhold for its views of the Long Island Sound to the north and the Atlantic Ocean in the distant south. Stimson purchased Highhold in 1903, after the demands of his career made it impossible to continue with his frequent vacations. Highhold, for Stimson and his wife Mabel, was an escape from the storm and stress of New York living. "We had aimed to establish a country home," wrote Stimson, "not a city home in the country, and we did it." (Henry L. Stimson, *My Vacations*, vi, 168.)

3. During an inspection trip in August 1941 in the west, Chief of Staff Marshall and Secretary of War Stimson spent a few days fishing at Glacier National Park in northern Montana. They also visited Rocky Mountain National Park in Colorado. See *Papers of GCM*, 2: 575, 591, 604, 692.

15

Remarks at Meeting, Hunter College — November 29, 1949, New York, New York

RE: "AMERICA'S STAKE IN THE EDUCATION OF THE NEGRO"[1]

I think I should explain in the introduction to my remarks this evening my reasons for accepting this invitation. Since my retirement I have endeavored to avoid occasions requiring me to make public addresses and the only exceptions have been when I was duty bound to speak in accepting some generous or complimentary award. Therefore I would have declined the invitation for this evening, but for two very special reasons I decided to accept.

I am intensely interested in the whole educational problem because of its dominant importance in the sound development of a great democracy, especially at a time when a generous knowledge of the world of affairs, of peoples and their traditions and reactions, of the history of nations as regards the why and wherefore of their rise and fall, and above all of the slow and difficult development of the freedoms we enjoy in this country and accept as a matter of course.

Then there was another reason for my acceptance and a more personally compelling one. The invitation was delivered to me by Doctor Patterson, the head of Tuskegee Institute. During the war years I was brought into frequent contact with Doctor Patterson and formed a very high regard for him.[2] What was more important, he was of great assistance to me in meeting many of the complications involved in raising our great war Army. He was wise and objective, unselfish and courageous, and I felt when he called on me to speak tonight that I owed him my acceptance.

As I have already said, I am intensely interested in all that pertains to education in its broadest sense. Success in the American world of today demands educational preparation that was not so vitally necessary in the past. The poorly educated man has a poor chance in this particular world of ours today. I am talking now of the mass of the people and I am thinking of the opportunities for the individual. But my personal interest goes far beyond that. Largely as a result of experience in raising and training a democratic citizen-soldiery and later on in experiencing the lack of public understanding in meeting the problems of international relations, I am concerned with the development of a sound basis for public opinion in such worldly matters.

With America by common consent the leading nation of the world, comes a vast responsibility which only an understanding public can enable our political and governmental leaders successfully to discharge. The decisions of the heads of our government, particularly in matters pertaining to foreign affairs, and the speeches and actions of our legislators in Congress are in essence but a reflection of informed public opinion. And that so-called "informed public opinion" cannot reflect sound judgments unless it has a basis of sound education. I also believe that that requirement is accentuated by the conflicting mass of opinions, representations and urgings of the commentator and columnist on the radio and in the press. Therefore my interest is focused on the educational problem.

But that is but one aspect of the matter which pertains largely to the grade schools and to the high schools. There is the problem of the college phase of education. Everyone must realize that this is necessary to the higher development of brains, and of leadership in government, business, the professions and the sciences. The consideration of university and post graduate education go a little further than I wish to discuss this evening.

Now what is the situation in regard to these matters I have just referred to? I'll try to put most of it, from my point of view, in the proverbial nut shell: We have a long way to go in improving the teaching and facilities in our grade and high schools, particularly those in the small towns and country districts. We are lamentably weak in teaching staffs and teaching qualifications. We are weaker still in many regions in the provision of the most ordinary facilities. The most serious weakness, I think, relates to quality and to type.

The immediately foregoing, it seems to me, is one of the most serious of America's problems. Incidentally, I think it ranks with and also is inter-related with the general economic problem. I have previously referred to its importance in connection with our present position of world leadership. Now how does this relate to the subject of the meeting tonight, "America's Stake in the Educated Negro"?

I have not had the benefit of a personal examination of the actual situation as to schools and teaching, except by way of occasional opportunities in various parts of the country, and from what I have read on the subject from time to time. With that as the basis of my thinking, it appears evident to me that possibly the most serious failure of this country in relation to the Negro problem, as it is commonly referred to, has been with regard to the lack of reasonably good educational facilities and opportunities for members of the Negro race. This failure has been both grossly unfair to the members of that race and seemingly indifferent to its importance in the development of a stable, a dependable democracy. The issues are usually confused by partisan debates and oratory, but I think the facts are reasonably clear. A phase of the problem that it seems to me has been seriously obscured in the acrimonious political battles has been the undoubted fact that public opinion in this country, public opinion Negro and White, today requires, or rather demands, a much sounder basis of understanding of the problems involved, which can only flow from an improved educational preparation or background. A healthy, safe development of our democracy imposes this demand and I feel that momentum is slowly being gathered to this end.

As to the Negro colleges and their very modest necessities, I think any fair-minded American will agree that these colleges should be generously supported until their product is sufficiently numerous and the improvement in general educational opportunities for the race has been similarly productive to permit the support of these institutions largely through the efforts of the successful graduates, whatever other educational opportunities may be made available.

I have made frequent reference to the urgent need for a better informed public opinion as to world affairs, or, as we regard them in these uneasy days, world problems. That necessity should be evident to all and the place of the Negro in the problems is two-fold. He forms a part of the body of American opinion that in the end determines our policies. Then also he is a special subject of frequent propaganda broadcasts directed against the state of health of our democracy. This even finds its way into debates in the halls of the United Nations.

We are very generously and aggressively interested in the preservation of the liberties of the democracies of Western Europe. The European Recovery Plan is directed to that end. Its first two years, according to my information, have been successful beyond our initial hopes—that is mine and those with whom I was associated in the launching of the undertaking. Personally, knowing the state of affairs in Western Europe in the late spring of 1947, the desperate, hopeless feeling of the people and their abject poverty and consequent state of hunger, the same scene two years later is bright beyond belief, however great the present problems and dangers.

I have always regretted that we could not have proceeded on the Recovery Plan on a Europe-wide basis as was originally suggested, regretted that suspicions for which there was no basis—or Communistic intentions, as seems to have been the case, caused the gauntlet to be flung down by others along the line of the iron curtain.

It might interest you to know that the foreign minister of one of these satellite states once remarked to me: "Everything would have been all right if only you had first consulted [Soviet Foreign Minister Vyacheslav] Molotov as you did [French Foreign Minister Georges] Bidault and [British Foreign Minister Ernst] Bevin." It was impossible for me to convince him of the complete truth of my statement to him that no foreigner was consulted and less than a dozen Americans. The last precaution was felt to be necessary in order to avoid a premature debate on this side of the Atlantic.

We are now entering the third year of the program and, in my opinion, it involves by far the toughest problems because two factors of great importance to sovereign powers dominate the field; they are currency and trade barriers. A solution to these two problems would be difficult at best as they involve national concessions which affect the business, banking and industrial interests, and the labor situation, of each country involved, and therefore the political interests or the political life of every government.

However, the necessity for a solution is so urgent and apparent that I am hoping that the influential group interests can be brought to support their respective governments in meeting the plain requirements of the situation, if American support is to continue. The difficulty to a public understanding of the problem will be materially increased by the onslaught of hostile propaganda which can be expected and which will be calculated to confuse the issue and distort the actions of the several governments. We must therefore guard against irritations and impatience and keep in mind that the problem of these Western European democracies is immensely difficult politically and otherwise.

In all of this we stand before the world somewhat as a model for all that individual freedom really means. We must be careful to remove the motes from our own eyes as we seek to clear the eyes of the world.

GCMRL/G. C. Marshall Papers (American Red Cross, Speeches and Statements)

1. Marshall prepared a handwritten draft of this speech, which he presented during the United Negro College Fund Forum on Higher Education.

2. Frederick D. Patterson had been president of the Tuskegee Institute since 1935. Marshall had worked with him in the years preceding World War II to support an army air corps training program at Tuskegee; see *Papers of GCM*, 2: 518–19, 525–27. Marshall further corresponded with Patterson during the war when the latter had requested small contributions on the order of fifty cents to a dollar from friends of the Institute. Marshall donated fifty dollars; see *Papers of GCM*, 4: 153–54. Marshall and Patterson were also involved in the postwar controversy relating to further use of the Tuskegee airfield—a move African-American leaders objected to because of the facility's location in the segregated South; see *Papers of GCM*, 5: 330–31.

Patterson had asked Marshall to speak at this forum and had presented him in early October with a draft for his consideration. Marshall apparently did not use this draft in preparing his remarks, though he did mention some of the key points that the Fund had desired. (Stebman to Patterson, October 1, 1949, and Stebman to Bonham, November 1, 1949, GCMRL/G. C. Marshall Papers [American Red Cross, Speeches and Statements].) See pp. 215–16 and 474–75.

16

To Robert A. Lovett — December 2, 1949
Washington, DC

Dear Lovett: I want to thank you particularly for your contribution to my day in New York Monday [*Tuesday*] and apologize again for keeping you waiting so long. I realize you are being very helpful to me behind the scenes in this Red Cross business and I want you to know that I am grateful.[1]

If I can bull through the next three months with reasonable success, I think I can get the whole business under control to my own satisfaction rather than merely compromising with other people's attitudes and policies.

Give my love to Adele and keep a fair share for yourself.[2] Faithfully yours,

GCMRL/G. C. Marshall Papers (American Red Cross, General)

1. Marshall traveled to New York on Tuesday, November 29; he had a one o'clock luncheon with Lovett and E. Roland Harriman at the Links Club on the Upper East Side.

On October 5, Lovett had written to congratulate Marshall on his new leadership of the Red Cross. "The problem of morale was rapidly becoming bad in this area and in several other cities," wrote Lovett. "One of my Partners, Roland Harriman, (Averell's younger brother) has been active on the top committees and devotes a good deal of his time to the Red Cross. He was getting very fed up with certain aspects of the determination of policies under the O'Connor regime." (Lovett to Marshall, October 5, 1949, GCMRL/G. C. Marshall Papers [American Red Cross, General].) "Since I still instinctively feel as though I were a member of your invisible staff," Lovett had written on November 3, "I ventured yesterday to suggest to Roland that he draw on his experience as Chairman of last year's Fund and prepare a brief outline of the principal sources of income, the principal expenses, peculiar problems, tested solutions of them, etc." While living in Washington, Lovett had heard complaints from chapter representatives attending the national meetings that their point of view was "lost sight of by Mr. O'Connor's tendency to let the 'professional group' make excessively long-winded 'reports', thus dragging out the proceedings with a consequent choking off of suggestions and discussions by the spokesmen for the various Chapters." (Lovett to Marshall, November 3, 1949, ibid.)

Roland Harriman gives his account of his family's work with the Red Cross and his appointment by Basil O'Connor in 1946 to chair a committee to reorganize the governing body in his autobiography, *I Reminisce* (Garden City, NY: Doubleday and Company, 1975), 185–99. His wife, Gladys, had been an active volunteer since 1920. Harriman served as vice chairman of the American Red Cross Board of Governors during Marshall's tenure.

2. Adele Lovett was Robert Lovett's wife.

17

TO LIEUTENANT SAM S. WALKER

December 7, 1949
Washington, DC

Dear Sam: Your momentous news reached me this morning.[1] Everything about it seems so strange to me—and yet so natural—addressing a "lieutenant", a husband and a father. It's hard to realize that I am so old that that amusing young boy has worked this great transformation in the world.

My congratulations to your wife first, and then to you and then to your mother and father. I am happy for you and for them.

I have been doing almost as much running around recently as in the war years. Three weeks ago 7,500 miles in 6 days and meetings in 14 [*fifteen*] cities—all Red Cross. In between times are a lot of short trips. I got back from New York last night.[2]

We leave for our place at Pinehurst the 16th, moving into town the 12th, closing the house here.[3] Then I hope to get four weeks complete rest.

Mrs. Marshall joins me in warmest congratulations. She is a very busy grandmother herself these days—5 grandchildren.[4] Affectionately,

G. C. Marshall

GCMRL/G. C. Marshall Collection (S. Walker)

1. Marshall is referring to the birth of Sam Walker's son, Walton Harris Walker II, born on November 6, 1949. Lieutenant Walker (USMA, 1946) was stationed in Japan; see *Papers of GCM*, 6: 518–19. Marshall had known the Walker family since 1939 when Sam Walker's father, Lieutenant General Walton H. Walker (USMA, 1912), had served as post executive officer at Vancouver Barracks in Washington State (see *Papers of GCM*, 1: 573).

2. See pp. 20–21.

3. The Marshalls owned a second home, Liscombe Lodge, in Pinehurst, North Carolina.

4. The grandchildren were her daughter, Molly, and James Winn's children: Jimmy (b. 1941), Kitty (b. 1943), and Ellene (b. 1948); her son Allen and Madge Brown's son, Tupper (b. 1941); and her son Clifton and Em Bowles Brown's newborn daughter, Carter (b. November 15, 1949).

18

Memorandum for Major General Orlando Ward[1] December 12, 1949
[Washington, DC]

I finally reviewed the volume on the Army Command Post—History of OPD. (I have forgotten the exact title and do not have the papers with me at this moment.)[2] I have no comments to make except with regard to two subjects:

CASABLANCA CONFERENCE[3]

I think the initial comments regarding the great advantage the British had over the American members from the point of view of British organization, numbers, experience, etc. and the fact that this in effect gave them the initiative are important. What is not mentioned are three very pertinent factors in the matter—

a. The insistence of the President on a very small staff for the trip. He would frequently refer to the small staff of the Marshal Foch when he was Allied Commander-in-Chief.[4] I think the eventual number was almost double the original prescribed.
b. The extreme difficulty of attaining Army and Navy smooth cooperation which made a united front, particularly in the preparation of papers, very difficult. I recall one paper Cook[e] hastily prepared and we, the Army and Air members were considering only to find that Admiral King was objecting emphatically to the entire paper.[5]
c. The British advantage which they enjoyed by reason of the movement of their staff to Casablanca by a "Command Ship" which gave them ample office accommodations, communications, as well as space for the party.

The repeated reference to this matter, particularly with decided implication that we were defeated apparently in everything, is both unwise and not wholly correct. Great as were our difficulties, we succeeded in imposing a condition for the transfer from the Mediterranean of 7 divisions to England, which eventually was carried out after the occupation of Sicily and before the further advance into Italy. This represented a very reluctant agreement on the part of the British and was a very definite commitment for the concentration of troops for Overlord.[6]

What I am really questioning is the continued reference to the matter with the resulting over-emphasis.

AIR CORPS

With reference to the freedom of actions accorded General Arnold and his air corps, which was much to be desired, I had to see that matters in the JCS did not degenerate from a two-sided situation (Army-Navy) to a three-sided or triangular argument which would have presented an almost impossible situation.

There are no records, I believe, on the following and therefore I do not think it wise to feature it: There was great difficulty in building up the conception of three Chiefs of Staff for our JCS to meet the British three Chiefs of Staff. This flowed from reluctance on the part of the Navy to have the Army Air so represented and not the Navy Air and at the same time *apparently* the Navy unwillingness to give their Air prominent position. I finally succeeded in establishing the three Chiefs of Staff basis, as I recall the matter, by getting Harry Hopkins to include in a Presidential message to Congress, or it may have been a public statement—but I think the former—a reference to the Chiefs of Staff by name: Marshall, King and Arnold. That settled the matter.[7]

G. C. Marshall

NA/RG 319 (Records of the Army Staff, Historian Background File, "Washington Command Post," Comments on OPD Manuscript, Entry p. 27, Box 19)

1. Major General Orlando Ward (USMA, 1914) was chief of the Department of the Army's historical division.

2. *Washington Command Post: The Operations Division* by Ray S. Cline was published by the Office of the Chief of Military History, Department of the Army, in 1951.

3. From January 14 to 24, 1943, Marshall along with the other wartime US chiefs of staff met in Casablanca, Morocco, with their British counterparts as well as Roosevelt and Churchill.

4. Marshal Ferdinand Foch, who commanded French troops throughout World War I, was named supreme commander of the Allied Armies in early 1918.

5. During World War II, Rear Admiral Charles M. Cooke (USNA, 1910) was navy assistant chief of staff for plans and Admiral Ernest J. King (USNA, 1901) was chief of naval operations and commander in chief of the US Fleet.

6. The agreement to transfer these divisions was actually reached at the May 1943 TRIDENT Conference in Washington, DC, not the January 1943 Casablanca Conference, and it took place after the September invasion of the Italian mainland as well as the July invasion of Sicily, not between the two events.

7. Harry L. Hopkins was Roosevelt's closest adviser during World War II.

19

To Mrs. Anna M. Rosenberg[1] — December 15, 1949, Washington, DC

Dear Anna: I don't want to allow this Christmas period to go by without expressing to you my appreciation for the friendly influence I find you have exerted in my behalf from time to time and to repeat my thanks to you for the daily reminder I have of you in the dispatch case that you procured for me at Bedell Smith's request. Every time I open it I think of you.

I'm going to add this bit of information which does not mean very much now and never did come to a head:

I had in mind constantly while I was in the State Department locating you, if you proved agreeable, in some place in Europe where I thought your influence might prove very helpful. The first choice was Moscow, but Smith's health held out and I did not have to find a replacement for him.

I turned over the question of representation in several satellite countries but I did not have the heart to propose such a mission, though I think probably you could have done more to correct matters than any other individual I had in mind. This is all water over the dam but I thought you might like to know what was in my mind.

With my greetings to you for the Christmas season and all my best wishes for you in the new year, believe me[2] Faithfully yours,

GCMRL/G. C. Marshall Papers (American Red Cross, General)

1. Anna M. Rosenberg, an expert on labor mediation and social services, was an adviser to Presidents Franklin Roosevelt and Truman and had served on the War Manpower Commission and Office of Defense Health and Welfare Services during World War II. She advised the War Mobilization and Reconversion Advisory Board during the postwar years.

2. "I don't know of any letter that I have ever received that gave me such pleasure as did your most kind and generous note of December 15th," Anna Rosenberg replied. "In this cynical age you are one of the few people who are held in reverence by all citizens in the nation individually and collectively. No one, therefore, can earn a greater personal tribute than to have your confidence and respect. It means a great deal to me." (Rosenberg to Marshall, January 4, 1950, GCMRL/G. C. Marshall Papers [American Red Cross, General].)

20

To Queen Frederica of the Hellenes — December 23, 1949
Pinehurst, North Carolina

Your Majesty, I have been long in replying to your last letter, but not idle.[1] After Acheson's return from France, I showed him your letter and talked things pertaining to Greece over with him. I saw the various State Department officials concerned with Greece and talked to various political leaders.[2]

As you know far better than I do, the atmosphere has cleared remarkably in your country. The United Nations action has been decided and firm, quite in contrast to my day. The Congress, I feel sure, will act favorably on your affairs and [Paul G.] Hoffman tells me the E.C.A. program indicates material contributions. The State Department informed me that your people were in agreement as to the 1950 program; I hope this was sincere. But what is I think most important, they predict favorable consideration of all phases of the proposed program by Congress.

You and His Majesty have had a hard struggle but the sun now seems to shine again and the future appears definitely hopeful. I pray that this may be so.

Mrs. Marshall has been having a hard time with an attack of that strange nerve affliction "shingles" in her eyes. We are down here at Pinehurst in our winter home and will be here until April. However, I will be traveling almost continuously from January 15 to March 7 on Red Cross business, some 20,000 miles in all. I have done 9,000 miles in the same cause since taking on this new responsibility in October.

I trust that both you and His Majesty are well and that the children are thriving. Mrs. Marshall charged me particularly to inquire about them. May you be enjoying a happy Christmas together.

With great respect, and admiration.[3] Faithfully yours,

GCMRL/G. C. Marshall Papers (Pentagon Office, Selected); H

1. Queen Frederica had written to Marshall on August 29 that recent military victories had chased Communist guerrillas across the Albanian border but "unless effective pressure is brought to bear upon Albania by the Western Allies, we shall be forced to keep a large army on that frontier to prevent the bandits from returning and reestablishing themselves. . . . The successes in Greece should be followed up relentlessly, and be considered only as a minor battle won within a great war." Greece also had to deal with the resettlement of seven hundred thousand refugees who might turn into "a power of unrest and unhappiness, which would be the feeding ground for a new communist danger." (Frederica to Marshall, August 29, 1949, HSTL/Dean Acheson Papers, Box 35 [George C. Marshall].) See the index to volume six of *Papers of GCM.*

On a more positive note, she had written about the successful efforts of her husband King Paul's "re-educational schools on the Dodecanese Island of Laeros for young bandits between the ages of 15 and 23" to reintroduce them as useful members of the community after completing "technical, agricultural and psychological education." The queen concluded, "Greece of to-day is a great human experiment. If given the chance, we shall succeed not only within our own frontiers, but also carry a ray of hope to those people who are still behind the iron curtain." (Ibid.)

2. Marshall had forwarded the queen's letter to the State Department and discussed how he might reply with John D. Jernegan, chief of the Division of Greek, Turkish, and Iranian Affairs. (Jernegan to Acheson, November 28, 1949, ibid.)

3. Queen Frederica replied on January 28 by extensively reviewing the political situation in Greece that had led King Paul to dissolve parliament and call new elections as the governing coalition crumbled. Aside from political troubles, she was optimistic that the people of Greece would rebuild "in spite of all the superhuman hardships they have gone through." Citizens had contributed money to rebuild schools in the destroyed villages. "We want to start a nation-wide drive amongst all those who have houses to adopt a family that has its home destroyed and to help them with all they need to restore their home life in the villages. Our slogan will be 'No more refugee winter in Greece.' " (Frederica to Marshall, January 28, 1950, GCMRL/G. C. Marshall Papers [Pentagon Office, Selected].)

As with Frederica's previous letter of August 29, 1949, Marshall forwarded this letter to the State Department. "The Queen is a remarkable personality," Acheson replied, "but it seems to us that she displays a tendency to overlook the danger of compromising the Crown by excessive involvement in the operation of parliamentary democracy in her country." (Acheson to Marshall, March 6, 1950, ibid.) See also an unsigned and undated memorandum reporting comments by Deputy Undersecretary of State Dean Rusk and Officer in Charge for Greek Affairs Leonard J. Cromie with attached memorandum, "Greek Refugee Children." (Ibid.) See pp. 132–34 and 304–6.

21

To Mrs. John White Pendleton[1]

December 25, 1949
Pinehurst, North Carolina

Dear Madge: Thanks for the tie. Your taste is mine and therefore perfect. Also please thank Tupper for his handy work, the book binding.

I hope your Xmas was a happy one. It should have been.

We leave for Baruch's place near Georgetown So. Carolina on the 27th, returning the 3d.[2] I am off on almost continuous travel on Jan. 15th lasting until the first week in March.

Much love— Affectionately,

G. C. M.

GCMRL/Xerox 2237 (GCM Family, Personal Letters); H

1. The widow of Marshall's stepson Allen Brown, Madge had married John White Pendleton (VMI, 1928) on June 3, 1949. Mr. Pendleton's father, Colonel Hunter Pendleton, had been a chemistry professor at VMI and a close friend with Marshall and his first wife, Elizabeth Carter Coles (known as Lily), in Lexington, Virginia. (See *Papers of GCM*, 6: 698.) During World War II John W. Pendleton served with the rank of major in US Army Air intelligence in Africa and Italy. After the war he was associated with the Central Intelligence Agency (CIA) as a foreign affairs analyst for the Middle East.

2. The Marshalls had visited previously with their longtime friend Bernard M. Baruch, a financier and political consultant who advised numerous presidents, at Hobcaw Manor, his home near Georgetown, South Carolina. See pp. 44n4, 743, and *Papers of GCM*, 6: 307, 627–28, and 667.

22

To Colonel Harris F. Scherer[1]

December 31, 1949
Georgetown, South Carolina

Dear Scherer: "Leisure—How Do You Use It?", should make a very interesting subject for the discussion and I would have liked very much in the past ten years to have enjoyed a little of it, but I am sorry to say that during that period I almost forgot the meaning of the word.

In response to your request I might say that when the opportunity occurs I usually occupy myself by reading, particularly history and biographies, more of the former because so many of us are reluctant to think of its importance and its effect on the rapid occurring events of today, and also because so many of us are weak on the subject. During the spring and summer most of my free time is spent in the garden attempting to produce sufficient vegetables and fruit for our own table. When time, weather and distance are in my favor I like to partake in the pleasures of hunting and fishing.

At this very moment I am hunting the country side near Georgetown, South Carolina and the results so far have exceeded my expectations.

I have no objection for direct quotation of any or part of the above.

With best wishes to you, the staff and members of the school for a happy New Year. Faithfully yours,

GCMRL/G. C. Marshall Papers (American Red Cross, Categorical, Requests)

1. Scherer (USMA, 1919), commandant of the Adjutant General's School at Camp Lee, Virginia, had written that leisure time was to be the subject of discussion for his students, faculty, and staff. "Sports, travel, hobbies, study, social activities, and just 'doing nothing', consume millions of spare hours in our country today. For the average man who embarks on an army career this means that during his thirty years he will have 112,400 hours, exclusive of the normal forty-hour duty week, to use for himself. The way in which he uses this time can very easily determine the success or failure of any individual." Concluding that it would be valuable "to teach a wise expenditure of leisure time," Scherer asked Marshall to "advise us how you occupy yourself outside normal duty hours." (Scherer to Marshall, December 22, 1949, GCMRL/G. C. Marshall Papers [American Red Cross, Categorical, Requests].)

23

To General of the Air Force Henry H. Arnold — December 31, 1949
Georgetown, South Carolina

Dear Arnold: I appreciate very much the birthday telegram from you and Bee, but what I especially appreciate is your remembering me at this time.[1]

Katherine and I are enjoying a visit with Baruch at his place in South Carolina.[2] I have been doing some hunting with excellent results while Katherine is resting and relaxing in an effort to rid herself of a disturbing case of shingles of the eyes.

I do hope that the excitement of Christmas hasn't set you back and that you are one of the inactive members of that select group of "Cardiac Valley".[3]

With best wishes for health, happiness and a fruitful New Year from both of us to you. Faithfully yours,

G. C. Marshall

[P.S.] Got my limit (15) two days out of four hunting about 2 hours a day.[4]

GCMRL/G. C. Marshall Collection (Arnold)

1. Bee was Arnold's wife, Eleanor. Their birthday telegram is not in the Marshall Papers.
2. See p. 43n2.
3. Arnold had a long history of heart problems.
4. Marshall added this handwritten postscript. A week later he reported to General of the Army Dwight D. Eisenhower (USMA, 1915), then president of Columbia University in New York City, "Katherine and I have just returned to Pinehurst after spending a few delightful days in South Carolina where there was some fine quail shooting. In five afternoons of two hours each I got sixty birds." (Marshall to Eisenhower, January 7, 1950, DDEL/D. D. Eisenhower Papers [Pre-Presidential, Principal Files, Box 80].)

24

To Gordon Gray — January 6, 1950
Pinehurst, North Carolina

My dear Mr. Secretary: I have delayed too long, I fear, in replying to your letter of December sixteenth regarding the Hoover Board recommendation as to the transfer of Corps of Engineer civil duties—River and Harbor and Flood Control to the Bureau of Reclamation.[1] I have been away and also I desired to consult some of my Engineer associates.[2]

Very pertinent arguments can be put forward convincingly regarding the admirable record in civil work by the Engineer Corps, and considerable doubts can find some justification as to the ability of the Bureau of Reclamation to take over the vast increase of responsibility proposed. However, that is beside the point of your question as to the effect that the Hoover proposal "might have on our overall military capabilities in peace and in war."

I think the efficiency, the capacity of the Corps of Engineers to undertake its inevitable wartime problems would undoubtedly suffer materially through lack of the experience now gained through River and Harbor and Flood Control work. Such experience cannot well be secured otherwise in time of peace.

The argument that only 200 Engineer officers are involved in the work of some 4,000 (I think it is) civilian assistants indicates a limited performance and achievement by the Engineers; that argument is fallacious. It is just that directorship ability which is required in war to implement the work of hundreds of thousands of citizen-soldier engineers.

I think some adjustment is demanded but I am not qualified at this time to indicate just what it should be—possibly the withdrawal from Flood Control.

I am sorry not to be more helpful. Faithfully yours,

GCMRL/G. C. Marshall Papers (American Red Cross, General)

1. Secretary of the Army Gray had written to Marshall on December 16 to ask for his views on the Hoover Commission on Organization of the Executive Branch of the Government's proposal to transfer the civil works functions of the Army Corps of Engineers to the Department of the Interior. He asked specifically for "any comments you may have on the effect that the subject proposal might have on our overall military capabilities in peace and war." (Gray to Marshall, December 16, 1949, GCMRL/G. C. Marshall Papers [American Red Cross, General].) Former President Herbert C. Hoover's commission had issued its final report to Congress, recommending organizational changes to promote economy, efficiency, and improved service, the previous May.

2. Marshall had asked Brehon B. Somervell (USMA, 1914), a retired general who had commanded the Army Service Forces during World War II, to offer his opinion on the matter. Somervell, president of the Pittsburgh-based coal company Koppers, responded directly to Secretary Gray and sent a copy of the letter to Marshall. Somervell warned Gray against transferring the civil works of the Corps of Engineers to the Interior Department's Bureau of Reclamation, saying it would result in work performed "less efficiently" and "more influenced by political considerations." (Somervell to Marshall, December 28, 1949, and Somervell to Secretary of the Army, December 28, 1949, ibid.)

25

TO MRS. NANCY DILL

January 10, 1950
Pinehurst, North Carolina

Dear Nancy: Katherine and I appreciate very much your good wishes to us for Christmas and the New Year.[1] I am happy to report that we spent a delightful

Christmas at Pinehurst and on the 27th motored down to Georgetown, South Carolina, where we enjoyed a week's visit with Mr. Baruch. While there I celebrated my birthday and the coming of the New Year.[2]

It is good to know that the Heseltine statue of Jack is such a fine likeness and I too hope the casting will be successful. I hear frequently from Bliss and I know that he will tell me when the job is done and when it is expected in Washington.[3]

You do me great honor in asking me to unveil the statue and I accept with great humility. Katherine and I are looking forward to welcoming you and Sonia.[4] Katherine has been having a hard time with "shingles" in her eyes.

Give my love to Sonia. Affectionately,

GCMRL/G. C. Marshall Papers (American Red Cross, Subject, Field Marshal Sir John Dill Memorial Committee)

1. Nancy Dill, widow of Field Marshal Sir John Dill, had written to wish the Marshalls "a very happy Christmas" and "peaceful New Year." She had seen the equestrian statue of her late husband by sculptor Herbert Haseltine that was slated for placement in Arlington National Cemetery. "It is a remarkable likeness of him, and a very good horse, and I do earnestly hope the casting will be successful, and no further delays." She asked Marshall to let her know when the statue would be unveiled so that she and her daughter, Sonia, might attend. She concluded, "May I ask you to unveil it, George? You were his friend, and it is through you that he is buried in Arlington. Such a great honour for an Englishman." (Dill to Marshall, December 12, 1949, GCMRL/G. C. Marshall Papers [American Red Cross, Subject, Field Marshal Sir John Dill Memorial Committee].) See pp. 127–28, 143–44n2, 151–52, 159–60, and 222–24.

2. See pp. 43n2, 44n4.

3. Robert Woods Bliss, former US ambassador to Argentina, chaired the committee in charge of raising money for the John Dill memorial at Arlington.

4. Sonia Furlong was the late field marshal's stepdaughter.

26

To Brigadier General Claude M. Adams — January 14, 1950
Pinehurst, North Carolina

Dear Flap: I was most interested in your report on the bird shooting in your part of the country.[1] After returning to Pinehurst I went out in the early morning to see if I could bag some doves and the only thing I caught was a cold.

I plan to be in Nashville on January 27th only four hours and in looking over my engagements while there I find that I have been booked so solid that I doubt very much the possibility of our getting together for a chat. I am asking the Chapter Chairman to extend to you and Ruth an invitation to the Red Cross luncheon and if you care to come I shall see you there.

Mrs. Marshall will not accompany me on this trip. She joins me in warm regards to you and Ruth. Faithfully yours,

GCMRL/G. C. Marshall Papers (American Red Cross, General)

1. Marshall's former assistant and longtime friend retired Brigadier General Claude "Flap" Adams had written with a quail-hunting report from Humboldt, Tennessee, that

"pickings here have been rather slim. We have lots of birds but the shooting is poor." (Adams to Marshall, January 10, 1950, GCMRL/G. C. Marshall Papers [American Red Cross, General].) Adams was an old friend of Marshall who had served as his executive officer at Vancouver Barracks in 1937–38. During that time he and his wife Ruth had joined the Marshalls on weekend hunting and fishing trips (*Papers of GCM*, 1: 551; Forrest C. Pogue, *George C. Marshall*, vol. 1, *Education of a General, 1880–1939* [New York: Viking, 1963], 311–12).

27

To Mrs. Henry H. Arnold — January 15, 1950
Telegram. — Washington, DC

I arrived in Washington tonight to learn of Arnold's death.[1] Mr. Truman telephoned me about him and expressed great affection and sorrow. You have all of my sympathy. I am so glad we had breakfast together last October.[2] I will treasure that last contact with an old and dear friend.[3]

GCMRL/G. C. Marshall Papers (American Red Cross, General)

1. General Arnold died following a heart attack on January 15, 1950, at Sonoma, California.

2. Marshall and Arnold had breakfast together at the Saint Francis Hotel on October 27, 1949, during Marshall's Red Cross trip to San Francisco, California. (George to Arnold, October 24, 1949, GCMRL/G. C. Marshall Papers [Pentagon Office, Selected].)

3. "Your telegram which arrived so soon after Hap's passing was a great comfort to me and the children," Eleanor Arnold wrote to Marshall in February. "Hap's long association with you meant a great deal to him and he enjoyed the breakfast with you at the St. Francis that morning more than anything that happened to him during the past year. . . . Thank you so much for your telegram, and also for weathering the stormy day at Arlington together with so many of our dear friends." (Arnold to Marshall, February 3, 1950, GCMRL/G. C. Marshall Papers [American Red Cross, General].) Marshall had served as an honorary pallbearer at the funeral services for Arnold held at Arlington National Cemetery on January 19 during sleet and snow. ("Arnold's Body Lies in State, Burial Today," *Washington Post*, January 19, 1950, p. 1; "General Arnold Buried at Arlington as All Services Pay Him Honor," January 20, 1950, pp. 1, 5.)

FROM mid-January through early March, Marshall undertook a second extensive tour of Red Cross chapters throughout the country in preparation for the 1950 Fund campaign (see pp. 19–21 for the first tour in October), with a return to Washington for General Arnold's funeral on January 19 (see previous document) and three stops for rest in Pinehurst. This time he covered thirty thousand miles, visited forty-one cities, and addressed more than thirty thousand people. Most of them were Red Cross volunteers, but tens of thousands more gathered for parades held in his honor. Fifty thousand people lined the streets for the parade through downtown Boston on January 16, during which he rode in an open car. During another parade in Youngstown, Ohio, on March 7, he left a closed car and walked because "All these people came here to see me." A local newspaper editorialized the next day, "The words were characteristic of the man. . . . The people expected their famous guest to be riding in pomp and splendor. They didn't look for him to be walking, like an ordinary man. General Marshall doesn't try to look different from other men. The difference is in what he does." ("General Marshall Winds up Speaking Tour," *Red Cross Courier* 29 [April 1950]: 13; "General Marshall Urges Campaign Workers to 'Finish the Job,'" ibid., 10–12; John Larner, "Boston Welcomes General Marshall," ibid. [February 1950]: 6–9.)

Once again Marshall kept up an extraordinary pace on the tour. His speed "almost bowled you over," wrote Gertrude Samuels of the *New York Times* after accompanying Marshall on part of the trip. "After just three days of flying, entraining, motoring, running and walking up and down stairs and in and out of rooms with flying squads of people led by a general still obviously on some maneuvers, after untold official breakfasts, luncheons, dinners with thousands of people, after official and unofficial press and radio conferences (and small-fry stolen ones), veterans' interviews and industry and labor meetings, all of them done on the double—all I can say is that any report of General Marshall's retirement appears to be greatly exaggerated." Marshall's tempo, she noted, "leaves workers with the distinct feeling of being alerted to battle call." Once again his ability to stay on schedule astounded those who witnessed it. During one forty-two–hour period "of plane, trains, motor trip, dinners, rallies and press and radio conferences, we lost four minutes," Samuels wrote, two of them "waiting for the General's baggage to show up on a plane. He couldn't understand that. 'Minutes lost,' he kept muttering. 'Golden minutes of time wasted.'" While it was "clear that the whole world is still his major interest," Marshall emphasized, "'I am now concerned solely with the Red Cross. I have no other plans for the future, and I assume that this will be my last public effort.'" (Gertrude Samuels, "Touring with Marshall of the Red Cross," *New York Times Magazine*, February 26, 1950, pp. 7, 27–28, 30.) ★

28

SPEECH TO THE AMERICAN LEGION[1]

January 16, 1950
Boston, Massachusetts

I am very glad that I found it possible to be here today. We have shared a great many experiences, some of them bitter, some of them tragic and many of them triumphant. But all of them have been part and parcel of our common determination to protect, defend and strengthen our country. We speak the same language.

Some of you, like myself, have fought and lived through two world wars. We have learned many things. One of them is the elementary truth that there is no security in weaknesses; but I think you will agree with me that the strength of a people is not measured solely in terms of armaments and wealth. Of equal importance are the things of the spirit, the principles to which we hold fast, and the health and welfare of the American people.

In our several ways, and according to our abilities, we are all devoting ourselves to activities that improve the welfare of the American people and, thus, strengthen the nation.

As you probably know, I have a new job. If I ever had the comfortable feeling that my appointment to the American Red Cross would be a restful, easy assignment, I have been thoroughly disabused of that notion. My initiation has been a strenuous one, including a trip of some 7,500 miles around the country, more meetings and conferences than I can recall, and a course of orientation which has obliged me to cram much basic knowledge into little more than three months.

There is a great deal to learn about the Red Cross because it reaches deep into American life and into every community. Many of its activities are so deeply embedded in our social structure and so familiar that we take them for granted without pausing to consider the enormous amount of effort and the great financial expenditures that are required to carry them on.

I am still studying the Red Cross and learning new things about it every day. I wish all of you had the opportunity to do likewise. One thing I promise you: the better you know it, the better you like it.

This trip to Boston, which has given me the added pleasure of being with you today, is a further step in my Red Cross education. Specifically, I am here to assist in the ceremonies dedicating the new Boston Regional Blood Center which opens its doors today.[2]

I know that the Red Cross National Blood Program is of particular interest to you. The men of the Legion who fought in World War II have first hand knowledge of the benefits to be derived from blood. They know how many of their comrades were spared because blood donated by the American people thru the Red Cross was flown to all the fighting fronts of the world. The exact figure, I believe, is that 97% of our casualties survived—largely because blood was available wherever and whenever needed.

Legionnaires all over the country are cooperating with the Red Cross to make a success of this program, and I am sure that this is true in Boston.

When the Red Cross launched this program a little more than two years ago it made, in effect, a commitment to the American people. Simply stated, this was that the Red Cross had accepted the responsibility for organizing, perfecting, and expanding a program which would eventually provide blood and blood products to all the American people, except in those communities where the need for blood was being adequately met by local resources. We are standing by that commitment and will continue to stand by it until it is fully met.

Let's take a look at the record and see if it substantiates this claim. In the past two years the Red Cross has opened 30 regional blood centers which, with the mobile units attached to them, have collected over 500,000 pints of blood and supplied them to 1550 hospitals and clinics for the sick and injured. The center which opens here today makes the 31st link in the national chain, and it is expected that ten more will open their doors in the current year.

This is substantial progress. The record shows that we are moving forward to the attainment of our objective. It is essential that we do attain it because the demand for blood increases with each discovery of new properties of blood and of improved techniques for its use. Surgical operations that would have been impossible a few years ago can now be performed with the aid of blood therapy. Children whose births are attended by complications of the RH factor can be saved in the majority of cases by replacing their entire blood stream with blood of the right type.[3] Victims of fire and explosion whose lives would have been despaired of five or ten years ago, now have hope of survival through the use of the blood fractions—those products derived by the breaking down of blood into its component parts. The medical profession believes that, in time, new fractions will be discovered and that these may be of use in treating specific ills of the human race.

All of this proves that there is a tremendous field of usefulness for the Blood Program as an aid to every day medical practice.

I think we should emphasize to the American people that only a national program with regional centers distributed throughout the country can give them the protection they need against the hazards of sickness and injury and the possible havoc of great disaster or national emergency.

It has been estimated that a national military emergency might require more blood in one week than all our requirements during one year of World War II.

The generosity of the American people is not open to doubt and it is certain that in the event of a great national calamity hundreds of thousands of blood donors would volunteer immediately, but without the machinery and technicians to receive them, vital time would be lost while centers for blood were hastily organized and staffed.

It has been pointed out frequently that the Blood Program is a program *for* the people. It is an inescapable corollary that it is a program *by* the people as well. It cannot be successfully brought to full growth without the support of the people. The Red Cross can provide leadership, but it cannot create blood. That can come only from people.

And so, we have to tell the American people frankly that the Red Cross needs three things from them if it is to continue honoring this commitment: It needs blood donors; it needs volunteers to help staff the centers; it needs the financial resources to bring the program to full maturity.

That is a big order, perhaps, but I do not think it is too big for the people of America.

Many of you know the Red Cross best through its work with the Armed Forces and with veterans. You saw it in action at home and overseas. You remember the clubmobiles and the clubs, and the coffee and doughnuts—Someone has said that the doughnut almost became a regimental insignia for the Club service—You remember the Red Cross office or tent or Quonset hut where your comrades unburdened themselves of trying personal problems or sought assistance in family emergencies.

I said a moment ago that many Red Cross activities come to be taken for granted. I think that was true to a great extent during the war. You saw the Red Cross nearly everywhere, doing a wide variety of things. It seemed to be an integral part of the whole wartime landscape. Many servicemen took the things it did for granted without stopping to consider the enormous effort in supply, staffing and financing that brought them about.

One thing we all do know: nothing is easy in war.

That applies to the Red Cross war effort as well as to the campaigns of the Army, Navy and Air Force.

I suppose being taken for granted is a compliment in a way, but it has its dangers, too. When the fighting ceased, the Red Cross was subjected to a good deal of undeserved criticism—largely directed at the charges that were made in the overseas clubs.

I assure you that complaints of this nature are wholly unjustified because the charges were made at the request of the War Department, although the Red Cross would have much preferred doing everything on a "gift" basis in line with usual Red Cross policy.

The charges were nominal and came nowhere near covering the actual expenses incurred in operating the club service. Actually, it cost the Red Cross more than $78,000,000 over and above what was taken in.

Another complaint concerns the alleged sale of free or donated cigarettes by Red Cross representatives. There is only one such case on record, and what happened to the guilty man is exactly what would have happened to an officer or soldier guilty of such an irregularity. He was court-martialed.

What did happen, unfortunately, was that on a number of occasions Red Cross supplies were mixed up with Army supplies. Cigarettes meant for the Post Exchanges went to the Red Cross, and cigarettes bearing the Red Cross symbol found their way into post exchanges where they were sold. Errors of this kind are an inevitable result of the vast upheaval and confusion of war.

Perhaps the most annoying complaint—because it is the most illogical—is the charge that Red Cross girls were "Brass Happy," by which is meant that they were usually unavailable for personal social engagements with enlisted men. There were several good reasons for this but the best one is a simple matter of logistics—that's a favorite word with military men, you know.

Overseas there was an average of *one* Red Cross girl for every *fifteen thousand* servicemen. Being reasonable men, I am sure you will see at once what a slight chance any serviceman had of a personal social engagement with a Red Cross girl. The only solution would have been to have one girl for every man—and that obviously was impossible.

I have nothing but admiration for the thousands of Red Cross girls who worked in the rain and mud and snow alongside the troops, wherever they were assigned.

I am not trying to persuade you that no mistakes were made. It is almost certain that there were errors of judgment and human frailty in an operation as extensive as the Red Cross war effort. I *am* saying that the overall job was magnificent, and that the continuing service of the Red Cross to the armed forces is too important to the welfare of the enlisted man and his family to be impaired by unthinking criticism.

I hope that all of you will do your utmost to correct misconceptions and misinterpretations of the Red Cross when they come your way. The American Legion is an influential factor in American life. We look to you to use your influence wisely and fairly.

We hear occasionally the suggestion that it is time for the Red Cross to get back to a peacetime basis. By this, I suppose, is meant a return to the status of the late nineteen thirties. I wonder if anyone would be so bold as to make that suggestion to the Army and the Air Force and the Navy—or to the American Legion?

If I remember correctly, in the nineteen thirties we had a total military establishment of about 300,000 men. What would you think of attempting to carry out the nation's responsibilities in 1950 with a force of that size?

A reduction to the status of the nineteen thirties is equally unrealistic when applied to the Red Cross, because it ignores the framework in which the Red Cross carries on a large part of its program.

In serving the Armed Forces it is obliged to go where our servicemen go; it is obliged to relate the size of its staff and the extent of its activities to the size of the military establishment. And this is indisputable: no matter how extensive the Red Cross job may be, it cannot permit any deterioration in the *quality* of the service.

The Secretary of National Defense [Louis A. Johnson], the Joint Chiefs of Staff and Commanding Officers in every theatre of operations have emphatically reaffirmed the importance of Red Cross Services to the Armed Forces. It is their determination to have a military establishment that is not only the best trained and the best equipped, but also girded and strengthened by the highest morale of any force in the world. The Red Cross has a traditional role to play in this and will continue to play it.

It is a natural sequence to think of the veteran in any discussion of Red Cross activities with the military, and, of course, the welfare of our veterans is the great concern of the American Legion. It is, also, a primary consideration of the American Red Cross. So long as the nation maintains a large armed force, the veteran population will increase proportionately; and so long as we have wars that cause vast numbers of men and women to sacrifice their best years, their health, and in some cases their lives, we must have organizations to serve them and their dependents. Government can't do the total job. Far from doing too much for these men and women, for *some* of them we do not yet do enough. I am thinking particularly of the hospitalized veterans.

Perhaps you were as shocked as I was some weeks ago to read in the newspapers of the shameful neglect of many mentally disturbed veterans by their families and friends.[4] According to officials of the Veterans Administration, some of these men have not been visited or communicated with for months and years—except by workers and volunteers of the Red Cross, the American Legion and other service organizations. The Veterans Administration doctors have said that in many cases friendly solicitude and normal contact with the outside world might be the determining factors in restoring mental balance, while the lack of them might cause the lengthening of mental shadows into total darkness.

Here is a field in which the Red Cross can and should do much, much more. I know that our volunteers are working strenuously to this end, and that they are not confining their efforts to the psychiatric veterans hospitals, but are extending their assistance to many civilian mental hospitals as well.

I cannot think of work that is more worthwhile. I cannot think of a personal satisfaction greater than to know that one has helped to restore a normal adjustment to life to a mind that has been disordered and tortured.

There is a great deal that still remains to be done for many of our people—unfinished business for both the Legion and the Red Cross.

The American Legion can count on the continued cooperation of the Red Cross in assisting our veterans to a secure place in civilian life. The Red Cross looks to the American Legion for support and leadership in bringing the National Blood Program up to full strength and usefulness.

If we work together and lead the way, the things that need doing will be done. The American people have never lost sight of human values. They have seldom failed to recognize the necessity of meeting human needs.

On the larger front of world affairs also, there is much that requires unity of purpose and action. The United States stands committed to peace, yet resolved to resist aggression; committed to the role of good neighbor on a global scale, yet obliged to expend enormous energy and resources for preparedness and unpredictable moves on the international chessboard.

Let us continue to demonstrate, in this tense and exacting time, the unity that is so essential to our nation in carrying out its heavy responsibilities.

GCMRL/G. C. Marshall Papers (American Red Cross, Speeches and Statements)

1. Marshall had traveled to Boston by overnight train, where he was met by Red Cross officials at 8:10 a.m. That morning he had attended meetings about the national blood program with prominent Red Cross contributors, as well as several hundred "key personnel of the fund campaign organization" at the Federal Reserve Bank. (Boston itinerary, January 16, 1950, GCMRL/G. C. Marshall Papers [American Red Cross, Speeches and Statements].)

Daniel G. Holland, chairman of the Boston blood program, also served as commander of the local American Legion Post and had arranged for Marshall to speak to "over a thousand of the leading citizens of Boston" at a luncheon at the Copley Plaza Hotel at 12:15 p.m. (Eaton to Marshall, January 11, 1950, ibid.)

2. The American Red Cross established its first regional blood center in Rochester, New York, on January 11, 1948. By the beginning of 1950, the organization had opened thirty of these regional free blood banks, which supplied 1,550 hospitals and their surrounding communities. ("Blood Bank Network Now Covers Nation," *New York Times*, January 12, 1950, p. 34.)

3. The Rh, or rhesus, factor refers to a series of antigens, which can either be present (Rh-positive) or absent (Rh-negative) on the surface of red blood cells.

4. Both the *New York Times* and *Washington Post* had published articles documenting the lack of attention given to veterans under treatment for mental conditions. One article noted that over seventeen thousand mental patients in veterans' hospitals had yet to receive a visit from either friends or relatives. The Veterans Administration made a plea to friends and families to visit the nation's "forgotten men" because such visits had a demonstrated benefit on the patient's health. ("Kin Shun Veterans in Mental Wards," *New York Times*, December 28, 1949, p. 26; "Forgotten Men," *Washington Post*, December 29, 1949, p. 10.)

29

To Charles R. Brannan

January 19, 1950
Washington, DC

My dear Mr. Secretary: I received your letter of January sixth with its invitation to be Fund Chairman of the Battle Monuments Commission for the 1950 Red Cross Campaign.[1]

I wish it were possible for me to do as you ask but in my present position as President of Red Cross I will be traveling around the country the rest of this month, all of February and the first week of March, doing what you have already started to do in the Government Unit. I have already traveled 9,000 miles visiting Red Cross chapters and will, in all probability, cover 25,000 miles before it is over.

If it is convenient, I would like to designate Brigadier General Thomas North, Secretary of the Battle Monuments Commission, in my stead.

With my best wishes to you for a successful campaign, Faithfully yours,

GCMRL/G. C. Marshall Papers (American Red Cross, Subject, American Battle Monuments Commission)

1. Marshall had been elected chairman of the American Battle Monuments Commission (ABMC) on January 26, 1949. Secretary of Agriculture Brannan, fundraising chairman for the government unit of the 1950 Red Cross Fund, had written to Marshall as chairman of the ABMC to ask him to serve as fundraising chairman for the commission. (Brannan to Marshall, January 6, 1950, GCMRL/G. C. Marshall Papers [American Red Cross, Subject, American Battle Monuments Commission].)

30

To Richard C. Wing

February 1, 1950
Pinehurst, North Carolina

Dear Wing: Mrs. Marshall and I were so glad to learn that you are leaving the sanatorium and are planning to re-enter college.[1] I feel confident that entering school right away will give you an entirely different perspective and you will find that you are not "branded" as you say but that your friends will welcome your return.

Since taking over my duties with Red Cross I have been doing much traveling in connection with the coming campaign. Last week I was in Florida, Alabama, Texas, Oklahoma, Kansas, Tennessee and Kentucky and have just returned to Pinehurst for a breather before starting out Sunday night for another swing of the country. I find the work very interesting and despite the amount of travel I am feeling fine. Unfortunately Mrs. Marshall has been suffering this winter with "shingles" in the eyes but is slowly improving.

We spent several days during the Christmas holidays with the Baruchs' at Hobcaw where there was fine quail shooting, and in five afternoons of two hours each I got 60 birds.[2]

Anna is here in Pinehurst with us and frequently speaks of you and wishes to be remembered to you.[3]

With best wishes and warm regards in which Mrs. Marshall joins me, Faithfully yours,

G. C. Marshall

GCMRL/R. C. Wing Collection

1. Wing, Marshall's former cook and orderly, had written that he was preparing to leave the Pottenger Sanatorium in California after a fourteen-month stay for tuberculosis. Planning to return to college, Wing wrote of his concern that "it won't be easy to adjust myself with that unwelcomed and hideous TB sign branded on me." Yet, despite his illness, the stay had been restful and provided an opportunity to read books, listen to music, and cultivate "some good points for myself." He concluded, "And sir, if I may say so, because I once served you, consequently I have gained much respect from others because of you. And too, sir, I have gained much confidence in myself which help me seek for the better things in life." (Wing to Marshall, January 23, 1950, GCMRL/G. C. Marshall Papers [American Red Cross, General].)

2. See p. 44n4.

3. Wong Renxian (Anna Wong) had worked for the Marshalls since April 1946, when General Marshall hired the Shanghai native to be Mrs. Marshall's maid. She came to the US with them in January 1947 and continued to work for them until 1951.

31

TO CLARKE W. COSTIKYAN — February 6, 1950
Pinehurst, North Carolina

My dear Mr. Costikyan: Thanks for your invitation to be present at the presentation by the Montclair Golf Club of the Montclair Yale Bowl for 1950 to Bob Lovett.[1] I am genuinely sorry that I cannot manage to be present as I shall be in Hawaii at that time.

May I compliment the Club members on their choice for I consider that Lovett made one of the great contributions to his country, first in the development of our mighty wartime Air Corps, but even more importantly during his service as Under Secretary of State.[2] During the entire period of his latter service the problems of our foreign relations were almost without precedent in American history in difficulty, complexity and critical importance. During the major portion of this service he was Acting Secretary of State and carried a truly vast responsibility for his countrymen.

You are right in honoring him and I am particularly glad that you do so because his fine services are so little realized by the people of this country. Faithfully yours,

GCMRL/G. C. Marshall Papers (American Red Cross, General)

1. Costikyan, an expert on antique rugs and fine carpeting in New York City, had written as president of the Yale Club of Montclair, New Jersey, that their Yale Bowl was given annually to an alumnus "who through his own efforts has reached the top of his profession, so to speak and thereby has won his 'Y' in life." Requesting Marshall's attendance at the presentation ceremony to Robert A. Lovett on February 24 at the Montclair Golf Club,

Costikyan wrote, "I imagine this may be difficult because of the great amount of work that you must have at this time. I was wondering, however, if you could not attend, whether you would be willing to send us a letter to read that evening to the alumni that are there. It would be quite appropriate in view of the long services Mr. Lovett had with you, and I know it would be appreciated by everyone. Of course, if you could attend, so much the better, and I will promise you 'no speeches.'" (Costikyan to Marshall, February 2, 1950, GCMRL/G. C. Marshall Papers [American Red Cross, General].)

2. Robert A. Lovett was assistant secretary for air in the War Department during World War II.

32

To John D. Rockefeller III[1] February 9, 1950
Pinehurst, North Carolina

My dear Rockefeller: I have just received an itinerary of the Hawaiian trip and if this schedule is maintained, I will be in Williamsburg on the 27th for the "Voice of Democracy" program.[2]

Mrs. Marshall and I appreciate the kind invitation we received from you and your wife and we accept with much pleasure. At this time we plan to arrive at Fort Monroe the afternoon of the 26th. My wife's daughter and her family are there and we will pay them a visit.

I will ask the Army to motor us over to Williamsburg the morning of the 27th, joining you and Mrs. Rockefeller wherever you say.

With our thanks and best wishes,[3] Faithfully yours,

GCMRL/G. C. Marshall Papers (American Red Cross, Categorical, Invitations, Accepted)

1. "Understand you have received invitation from 'Voice of Democracy' to speak in Williamsburg in late February," Rockefeller had cabled on January 4. "This wire is just to tell you how much I hope it will be possible for you to accept. Mrs. Rockefeller and I would be so happy to welcome you and Mrs. Marshall to Williamsburg." (Rockefeller to Marshall, January 4, 1950, GCMRL/G. C. Marshall Papers [American Red Cross, Categorical, Invitations, Accepted].)

2. The Voice of Democracy program invited high school students from across the country to deliver addresses on the subject of democracy. That year's finalists were invited to spend a day in Colonial Williamsburg touring the reconstructed and restored buildings of the colonial era Virginia capital. The Rockefeller family had largely financed the historic site's restoration in the 1930s, and John D. Rockefeller III served as chairman of its board of trustees.

3. Rockefeller replied that he and Mrs. Rockefeller welcomed the Marshalls' visit at their home in Williamsburg, Bassett Hall. The luncheon would be held at the Williamsburg Inn, and the program and Marshall's speech would be at the colonial House of Burgesses. (Rockefeller to Marshall, February 15, 1950, ibid.) See pp. 57–60.

33

To Louis R. Marick February 15, 1950
Washington, DC

My dear Louis: I have just returned to my office from an extended trip around the country visiting Red Cross chapters and found your letter and book.[1]

I complied with your request and the book is now on its way back to you. You did a good job in compiling the articles and pictures and I can readily understand why the teacher gave you an "A".

History is a very important subject and we should all try to learn as much of it as we can. Many of our young men and women of today will be the leaders of our Government in the future and it is important that they have a good background in history, for it invariably affects the thinking of those confronted with world problems. Faithfully yours,

GCMRL/G. C. Marshall Papers (Secretary of Defense, Number Indexed, M203-1-18)

1. Marick had written from Michigan, "When I was in the ninth grade at Grosse Pointe Highschool our Civics teacher had us follow the Moscow Meeting which you attended. This book is a daily report about the Moscow Meeting and is composed of all newspaper articles. I wondered if you will please autograph this book which I am sending to you. The main reason I kept this book was that our Civics teacher told us that in years to come it will be an important historical document." (Marick to Marshall, January 22, 1950, GCMRL/G. C. Marshall Papers [Secretary of Defense, Number Indexed, M203-1-18].)

34

Speech for Meeting in the House of Burgesses[1] — February 27, 1950, Williamsburg, Virginia

Just two [*three*] years ago last Wednesday, before a Washington's birthday audience at Princeton University, I made the following comment:

> "I am therefore greatly concerned that the young men and women of this country . . . students in every university, college and high school in the United States, shall acquire a genuine understanding of lessons of history as they relate to governments and the characteristics of nations and peoples . . ."[2]

Here today, in this program, we have the evidence of youthful interest in this matter. We find four high school students whose addresses on the subject of democracy have won for them national acclaim;[3] and we find them in the historic House of Burgesses in Williamsburg, a restored edifice of democracy which stands on ground that is hallowed in our nation's struggle for freedom.

The echoes of the past in Williamsburg are the sounds of men whose hearts and spirits cried out against oppression; whose determination was such that they dared death and endured painful hardship to attain their goals; and whose hope for all mankind inspired them to set down in our Constitution the principles by which we live today.

Democracy to them, and to us, was not a new formula for peaceful pursuit among mankind. As a system, it was the best that had emerged from dark ages of a long struggle. It is not more than that today, although refined by experience and improved by wider understanding. Democracy still is an old idea, and its pursuit is even now a race to be won only by the courageous and the determined.

Would you remember who spoke these immortal words:

"The administration of our Constitution favors the many and not the few—that is why we are called a democracy. Our laws provide equal justice for all. Socially, advancement is based on ability and merit, without regard to considerations of class or financial status. If a man is able to serve the state, he is not to be held back by the obscurity of his position or condition . . .

"And the freedom we enjoy in our government extends also to ordinary life. Each of us goes about his business without encroachment from the other; nor do we cast jealous eyes at a neighbor for doing as he pleases.

"We place our trust less in a rigid system or a rigid policy than we do in the feelings and the native spirit of our citizens.

"Instead of regarding public discussion as a stumbling block to effective action, we regard it as an indispensable preliminary to any wise action at all."

Those words were spoken by Pericles five hundred years before the birth of Christ.[4] You can find in them little that differs from our concept of democracy today. And so, when I just said that democracy was still an old idea, that word "old" covered a period of at least 2500 years.

In March of 1947, during a meeting of the foreign ministers in Moscow, I gave this as my explanation of American democracy, to quote: "I realize that the word 'democracy' is given many interpretations. To the American government and citizen, it has a basic meaning. We believe that human beings have certain inalienable rights—that is, rights which may not be given or taken away. They include the right of every individual to develop his mind and his soul in ways of his own choice free of fear or coercion—provided only he does not interfere with the like right of others. To us, a society is not democratic if men who respect the rights of their fellowmen are not free to express their own beliefs and convictions without fear that they may be snatched away from their home and family. To us, a society is not free if law-abiding citizens live in fear of being denied the right to work or deprived of life, liberty and the pursuit of happiness."[5]

The free expression of opinion today perhaps becomes even a stronger implement for forging world peace and understanding than in the day of Pericles. Five hundred years before the birth of Christ, Pericles could only be heard within the range of his voice; nor did there exist methods for wide distribution of his written words.

Today the words we speak, as on this occasion today, are heard by millions not only in our own country, but throughout the world. The great lines of communications, offering as they do the avenues for spreading understanding represent, I believe, a first line of defense against another world conflict.

It is imperative that the implications of this fact be understood thoroughly by all peoples the world over. It is through communications that we distribute the information upon which the people base their own decisions. This is as true in a demagogic nation as in a free democracy. The only difference between the two lies in the kind of information that is made available to the people.

We must not permit ourselves to forget so quickly that one nation, within the last two decades, militarized its people to launch a world war by controlling and coloring the knowledge it distributed through government-controlled channels of communication.

If the youth of today, upon whose shoulders must fall the responsibility for tomorrow's world, have one duty that looms larger than all the others, it is this: to defend to the uttermost the right of men to speak freely. That is the essence of democracy. When it is understood in all parts of the world—when it is practiced in every nation—there should be little fear of war. For the people will know the truth.

Young men and women must show an eagerness to learn—not only the circumstances which make our lives so complicated today, but the historic happenings which have led to these circumstances.

Learning the causes of world strife which, in almost every generation, has suppressed the hopes of men for peace, should be, I think, an elective subject of every young person today. He can look for those causes in our history books and in the history of other nations. He will not find them easily, and in the course of his search, he may become confused and rebellious. But as years add wisdom, he will discover one dominant factor which has contributed to conflict in the past. And that is misunderstanding. Sometimes, less softly, it is called ignorance.

We must understand people and their motives, and we must learn to be tolerant of their ideas when they differ from ours.

If the geographical radius of your activities is about six miles, as it was mine when I was a youngster, or if it is six thousand miles, your understanding should encompass the universe. Threats to peace know no particular climate nor place nor people. The threats to peace are found in the compulsions of history which bring nations to certain determined courses.

Youth's consideration of the lessons of history should not be confused by the pressure of day-to-day crises, even though these are very important. One hundred years from now, an hour's crises of 1950 will represent less than a second in the history of the world's development. We need perspective, then, in a world sense; we need to discover not only the nature of our relationship to the men and women in our own neighborhood, but that relationship to the neighborhood of everywhere.

There is a pitfall along the way to permanent peace. History demonstrates that people cannot live happily when they are afraid. Fear can grow swiftly, like a weed, and smother everything good that grew before it took root. In times such as these in which we are living, in the age of the atom if you will, we must not let fear stand before us in our search for world amity.

Justice Black put it well the other day in a speech when he said: ". . . There is no country in the world that provides more opportunities for people's happiness than does the United States. So long as we remain at peace with the world and cling with unshakable finality to the right of the people to think, speak and write as their consciences may dictate and so long as the people of our generation retain the same courage which gave this free government to the world, Americans have no reason to fear."[6]

In a world which offers us so many opportunities, many of them the products of man's progress in science, our responsibilities do become larger. Particularly do they become large in this field of free expression. By reason of the very fact that our voices can be heard by millions today where audiences were measured in scores before, we should never speak hastily. Idle words can easily become evil words.

Therefore, young people must first learn to search for the facts pertaining to a given situation before they offer comment. Once they have weighed them carefully, once they have arrived at their own best decisions, the sincerity of their purpose cannot well be questioned. But first of all they must be certain of the facts.

We should all strive to be good citizens, of course, and that means participating in the government of our nation through observing its laws and through electing its officials. We must be willing, as Pericles said so many years ago, to serve it in any capacity, and no such capacity should be considered menial.

And since there are many lies abroad today in the world, and there always have been, we must speak the truth—forcefully and repeatedly, but only if we have made sure of the facts. Democracy is a truth. Do not accept it complacently; we must take it as the true belief, and live it throughout our lives.

Certainly the fact that one million high school students this year took the time to write and speak for democracy is an indication that the subject is not dormant, as some would have us believe.

The sermon of its rightness is recorded in the journals of man's progress and inscribed on the sacrifices and shields of fallen millions.

GCMRL/G. C. Marshall Papers (American Red Cross, Speeches and Statements)

1. Marshall delivered this speech in the House of Burgesses at Colonial Williamsburg during a radio broadcast over the Columbia Broadcasting System (CBS) in honor of the four winners of the Voice of Democracy contest, a program that invited high school students to record five-minute addresses on the subject "I Speak For Democracy." Robert K. Richards, chair of the Voice of Democracy Committee, had prepared a draft for Marshall "by putting together in one format words you had uttered before." (Richards to Marshall March 1, 1950, GCMRL/G. C. Marshall Papers [American Red Cross, Categorical, Invitations, Accepted].) Marshall edited the draft and delivered it as amended.

John D. Rockefeller III, who presented introductory remarks, had personally encouraged Marshall to accept the invitation of the National Association of Broadcasters (NAB), one of the sponsors of the contest, to deliver the address; see p. 56. A report of the contest, including texts of addresses, was published by the NAB in "The Voice of Democracy: 1949–1950," *Station Management,* March 6, 1950, pp. 13–21.

2. The ellipses are in the copy text. For the full speech given at Princeton on February 22, 1947, see *Papers of GCM,* 6: 47–50.

3. The four winners were Richard L. Chapman of South Dakota, Anne Pinkney of Colorado, Robert Shanks of Indiana, and Gloria Chomiak of Delaware, who delivered her script during the broadcast.

4. Marshall quoted from Pericles' funeral oration. (Thucydides, *The History of the Peloponnesian War*, trans. Richard Crawley [New York: E. P. Dutton and Company, 1910], 119–28.)

5. See *Papers of GCM*, 6: 77–79.

6. Supreme Court Justice Hugo L. Black had spoken these words in his speech on January 21, 1950, at the forty-third annual meeting of the American Jewish Committee at the Plaza Hotel in New York. ("Black says Fear Obscures Reason," *New York Times*, January 22, 1950, p. 44.)

35

To Harold W. Dodds

February 27 [*28*], 1950
Washington, DC

Dear Dodds: Thank you very much for your letter of February fourteenth inviting me to attend and speak at the meeting on May ninth at the Library of Congress.[1]

I appreciate the compliment of your invitation and am delighted at the opportunity of adding Thomas Jefferson's writing to my library collection. But what I appreciate most of all is your generous expressions and gracious thought of me in writing as you did. I shall be honored to do as you ask.

Mrs. Marshall and I have just returned from a trip to Hawaii and en route out stopped in New Orleans for the Mardi Gras ball, then spent a day in Los Angeles where I spoke on behalf of Red Cross, and on our return from Honolulu made a stop in San Francisco for a day. After arriving back in New York we flew to Williamsburg where I participated in the Voice of Democracy program.[2] Now I am back at my desk trying to catch up on accumulated correspondence. Tomorrow we are flying down to Pinehurst for a little rest and relaxation. While we both are a little tired, we thoroughly enjoyed the trip.

Mrs. Marshall has asked to be remembered to you and Mrs. Dodds and with kindest regards to you both, I am Faithfully yours,

GCMRL/G. C. Marshall Papers (American Red Cross, Categorical, Invitations, Accepted)

1. Dodds had written to invite Marshall to an event at the Library of Congress "to celebrate the publication of the first volume (fifty-one are to follow) of the complete writings of Thomas Jefferson, under the auspices of Princeton University and the Princeton University Press, with a grant of $200,000 from the *New York Times*." Asking Marshall to join President Truman, himself, and historian Douglas Southall Freeman, chairman of the documentary edition's advisory committee, as speakers for the event, Dodds added, "We hope that you will agree to accept a second copy of the first volume. I ought to add perhaps that the succeeding volumes will be supplied you, with less formality however than the first. There are a good many reasons which make this invitation appropriate. One is that your life and thoughts have been in the Jeffersonian tradition. To me personally, however, the chief reason is that in my private book you are America's number one citizen measured by standards of wise and self-denying public service." (Dodds to Marshall, February 14, 1950, GCMRL/G. C. Marshall Papers [American Red Cross, Categorical, Invitations, Accepted].) Due to a scheduling conflict with a presidential trip, Marshall later accepted the revised date for the event, May 17. (Marshall to Dodds, March 24, 1950, ibid.) See pp. 89–91.

2. See previous document.

36

To Major General Frank R. McCoy

March 1, 1950
Washington, DC

Dear Frank: Sergeant George has just reminded me that you were going to give us a treat and arrive at Pinehurst on the fourth to stay over with us.[1]

This notice is to tell you that Katherine went into the hospital yesterday for her "shingles" and a bad cold—the Walter Reed. We arrived here yesterday morning on the completion of a trip to New York, New Orleans, Los Angeles, Hawaii, San Francisco and return to New York and then to Williamsburg for a broadcast and back to Washington. She did finely until the final flight from San Francisco to New York when the altitude affected her shingles and besides that, she apparently picked up a cold at the transfer from New York to Fort Monroe. So when we arrived in Washington yesterday morning she went directly to Walter Reed to consult the doctors about her shingles and they put her to bed. She will be there until the eighth when I come through on the finish of my last trip and fly her to Pinehurst. As I am leaving Pinehurst on the fourth I will not be there either. Allene and Sterling were planning to come up to the hotel in Pinehurst on the third.[2] I am going to telephone them tomorrow to see if they will change their plans and come up immediately and stay with me.

This is a very hasty note as I am leaving in a few minutes.

With love to you both.

GCMRL/G. C. Marshall Papers (American Red Cross, General)

1. Sergeant C. J. George had been Marshall's aide since January 21, 1947, the day Marshall was sworn in as secretary of state. Marshall's longtime friends Frank and Frances McCoy were vacationing in Charleston, South Carolina, and had planned to visit with the Marshalls in Pinehurst March 4–6. For more on General McCoy's career, see pp. 869–71.

2. Allene Lacy, Katherine Marshall's sister, and her husband, Sterling, who also lived in Leesburg, were vacationing at a hotel in Daytona Beach, Florida. See next document.

37

To Mrs. Sterling Lacy[1]

March 1, 1950
Washington, DC

Dear Allene: Katherine and I arrived in New York from Hawaii and San Francisco Sunday morning at 9 and left within 15 minutes in my plane for Langley Field—15 minutes from Fort Monroe. Katherine had had a bad night because the altitude of thirteen thousand feet affected her badly, particularly as she did not begin to take oxygen until she had developed the bad effects.

However, the next morning she made the shift and we arrived at Fort Monroe and the Chamberlin in fair shape and slept most of the afternoon, as Molly did not arrive until 5 o'clock from Pinehurst.[2] Jim and Molly [Winn] came over for dinner and Katherine had a good night.

The next day it was mostly grandchildren, but it was evident that Katherine was developing a cold although she claimed it was sinus. She insisted on going for dinner that night and then passed a miserable night, sneezing almost constantly. The next morning we flew up to Washington—I had wanted her to stay in Fort Monroe. She went directly to the hospital to have her eyes looked at. Once there the doctors insisted she go to bed, which fortunately she agreed to do and did so immediately as George had her baggage with her.[3] She is now at Walter Reed

Hospital and, while she was feeling badly yesterday afternoon when I saw her, the night nurse told me she was sleeping and in better spirits. She had X-rays, cardiographs, blood tests and more particularly she had had injections of the new rare remedy for shingles and that made her feel badly because it is painful for a time.

I just telephoned the hospital and they said she had had a very good night—one sleeping pill, and only complained of a dull feeling in the back of her head this morning and she is now taking another nap.

I am leaving for Pinehurst in about a half hour. I'll be there until Saturday, maybe until Sunday morning. I propose to telephone you late this afternoon to see if you and Sterling wish to change your plans and come and stay at the cottage; as I will be there alone, you can have two bedrooms, or no one will be there until the late afternoon of the 8th when Katherine and I should arrive.

This is a hasty note to amplify a telephone message yet to be made. Affectionately,

GCMRL/G. C. Marshall Papers (American Red Cross, General)

1. See previous document n2.
2. The Chamberlin was a waterfront hotel in Hampton, Virginia.
3. Marshall is referring to C. J. George.

38

To Harry S. Truman

March 2, 1950
Pinehurst, North Carolina

Dear Mr. President: Your very gracious and thoughtful note reached me here this morning. Thank you for your thoughtfulness and kindly interest. As you have seen me you know that I am still going on all cylinders.[1] Also, it may reassure you to know that I have just gotten up *at ten A.M.* to a bright sun and a beautiful day, and that I went to bed at ten last night. I do know how to relax.[2]

They telephone[d] me this morning that Mrs. Marshall is much better, the pain from the "shingles" in her eyes is gone, her cold much better, eats well and had a good night. Thank goodness she is in bed and can't mix up with the hospital house keeping.

With great respect, Faithfully yours,

G. C. Marshall

HSTL/A. Robert Ginsburgh Papers; H

1. "Of course, as always I am interested in what you are doing. As usual you are doing a thorough job," President Truman had written to Marshall referencing an article in the *New York Times* profiling Marshall's Red Cross travels. (Truman to Marshall, February 26, 1950, GCMRL/G. C. Marshall Papers [American Red Cross, General].) The author had noted that "the 'retired' General sets the pace of a young lieutenant on maneuvers." (Gertrude Samuels, "Touring With Marshall of the Red Cross," *New York Times Magazine*, February 26, 1950, p. SM4.)

2. "Please be careful of your health and physical well being," Truman cautioned. "I want you to be alive and fit when I quit here so we can do some things that need to be done

in this great republic of ours. You have made the greatest of contributions toward saving it. I've tried to make a small contribution.

"There is much to be done," the president continued. "I want you as a living partner to finish the job. Please take care of yourself. Don't make me responsible for your demise. I have enough to answer for without that!" (Truman to Marshall, February 26, 1950, GCMRL/G. C. Marshall Papers [American Red Cross, General].)

39

United States Steel Corporation
Theatre Guild on the Air Broadcast[1]

March 5, 1950
New York, New York

My fellow Americans—

The troubled times in which we live call urgently for the qualities of the human spirit—unselfishness, tolerance, compassion for others. Because the work of the Red Cross is a genuine expression of these ideals, it offers the great medium for the individual to make his personal contribution to the world.

Faced with the misgivings and misunderstandings that fill our thoughts today, it is important for all of us to build up in every way we can a renewed feeling of good faith and good will which are essential to a peaceful world.

People search constantly for an answer to the question: "What can I do as an individual to make this a better—a more secure world?"

In the long perspective of history it has been proved time and again that high ideals and humanitarian causes, when supported by vast numbers of people, do have great impact on the course of civilization. But these vast numbers have been but the combined expression of the multitude of individuals. The men and women of the Red Cross, who devote themselves to the welfare of their communities and of the nation, are making their individual contribution to a better world.

In my short experience as the head of the Red Cross—I assumed office only last October—I have been deeply impressed by the scope of the tremendous volunteer effort that is being given to our people all over America. I have visited chapters both great and small. I have talked with community leaders and with the man in the street. I have learned at first hand what the Red Cross does for the victims of disaster—how it considers no disaster job completed until the needs of the homeless and injured have been met; I have seen what Red Cross volunteers are doing in hospitals and community agencies across the nation. I have learned that the National Blood Program has saved lives and hastened the recovery of the injured or sick; and I know that this program is essential to preparedness for any great disaster. I have always known, of course, how important the work of the Red Cross is to the men and women of the armed forces and to the veterans—a million and a half of the one and twenty million of the other. I have had my belief in its importance confirmed.

The Red Cross has great spiritual significance because it symbolizes love for humanity and the impulse to give generously from the heart to those in need of help. That is what is most needed in the world today.

That spirit will make a stronger America and a better world.

GCMRL/G. C. Marshall Papers (American Red Cross, Speeches and Statements)

1. Marshall delivered this address after the second act of the radio broadcast of *Lady in the Dark*, the March 5 presentation on the popular Sunday evening *Theatre Guild on the Air*, starring Gertrude Lawrence and Macdonald Carey. The weekly program, sponsored by the United States Steel Corporation, presented both current and classic drama. This particular Sunday evening program was dedicated to the American Red Cross Fund Drive.

40

TO REGINALD H. HALL

March 8, 1950
Washington, DC

My dear Mr. Hall: I have just returned to Washington from my final Red Cross tour to find your letter of February 21 regarding my reference to veterans of the A.E.F., to a short war, to 40 days of combat, etc.[1]

I think you have misinterpreted what I was endeavoring to do through the reference referred to. In the first place, I too am a veteran of that war. I arrived on the first transport and left on the last. I was present at the first raid, saw the first dead on the ground and wrote the order terminating the fighting of the First American Army November 11, 1918. So I am not apt to depreciate the services of the veterans of that war.

I was answering the criticism made by many businessmen and others that the Red Cross today had not demobilized, and that compared the budget and obligations of 1938 with those of 1950. In my comparison of an armed force of 265,000 men in 1938 with one today of 1,600,000 scattered through 69 countries, and a comparison of something over 3½ million veterans in 1938 as against almost 20 million today, I added to the last comparison a further explanation of the difficulties in effect of a short war in healthy countries as compared to a long war in jungles, in mountains, the Arctic Circle, the Greenland Cap, Iceland, and the heart of Africa with jungle rot, malaria and terrible diseases that produced today psychoneurotic cases to the extent of 60% of the 110,000 in the hospitals.

In further explanation of the difficulties, I referred to the fact that the First World War was a short war; that only 2 million went abroad and 1 million only for the last five months and of those most had not more than 40 days of combat—this is accurate and is no reflection whatever. Faithfully yours,

GCMRL/G. C. Marshall Papers (American Red Cross, General)

1. Hall, a World War I disabled veteran who had served as a runner with Company H of the 168th Infantry, had listened to Marshall's broadcast for the American Red Cross from Los Angeles on February 20. "Listening to your remarks I heard you mention, three million from first World War. Two million were overseas, and then something about five months followed by—the majority or most off saw no more than forty days combat service.

"To me this remark was unkind, it seemed to have a tenor to minimize. A natural reaction publicly would be 'that war could not have been so hot, forty days'. . . . The more I thought about your remark the more I gripped inside. I thought of the lads with my Co four months in Lorraine (which was no picnic) Champaigne, Mihiel, Chateau Thierry, and twice in the Argonne, from Feb to Nov. without a letup except to fill up and catch a breath, to go through all that and then get theirs a few days before the end 'I wonder what they would think of that forty days?'" (Hall to Marshall, February 21, 1950, GCMRL/G. C. Marshall Papers [American Red Cross, General].)

41

To George R. Pattullo — March 8, 1950, Washington, DC

Dear George: I found your letter of February twenty-seventh on reporting in here from my final Red Cross trip.[1] I have traveled somewhere near thirty thousand miles, mostly since January, and now I am through for the time being and I will never attempt it again. But I now know something of the Red Cross as I have seen some thousand chapter chairmen and twenty-five to thirty thousand principal workers.

Incidentally, the Chapter Chairman in Phoenix is owner of the Westward Ho Hotel. He gave me a delightful suite when I was there in October and then I had to attend a breakfast party in the suite at seven thirty in the morning before I took off for Kansas City.

I was so glad to learn something about you and I take it you are in good health but not in good temper.[2] I shall certainly call you up and try to see you when both of us are in New York. I have to go up quite frequently to attend meetings with the directors of Pan American Airways. I usually stay at the Metropolitan Club but I'm seldom there for more than a night and not always that. We make our home from the middle of December until the latter part of April at Pinehurst where we have a nice bungalow. The rest of the year we are located in Leesburg where we have too much of a house, too much antiquity (1780) and too many rooms.[3] If you ever get near Washington telephone or telegraph me so that we can arrange to have you come down (and Mrs. Pattullo if she is with you) and stay with us. I have so much to talk over with you.[4]

As to the horse, I'll talk about that when I see you. I have had no time for riding for the past three years but I'm starting the day after tomorrow. I leave for Pinehurst in the morning to settle down a bit and there is delightful riding there.[5]

With warmest regards, Faithfully yours,

GCMRL/G. C. Marshall Papers (American Red Cross, General)

1. Pattullo, writer of Western stories and a correspondent for the *Saturday Evening Post* during World War I, was a resident of New York City but had written from Phoenix, Arizona, to ask "when you plan to quit? It strikes me that after winning a war as Chief of Staff, then a tough China mission and a term as Secretary of State, you had earned rest. Another case of the willing horse. Speaking of horses, how're you off for a good saddle-horse? By that I mean a real one—Kentucky thoroughbred, or Virginia. I fain would make you a birthday present of one before I kick off, or grow too work-worn for the saddle. Please let me know about this matter, as I have had the inclination for some years but waited until you retired from public office." (Pattullo to Marshall, February 27, 1950, GCMRL/G. C. Marshall Papers [American Red Cross, General].) For previous correspondence with Pattullo, see *Papers of GCM*, 3: 496–97.

2. "As for my own fortunes," wrote Pattullo, "I can't describe them better than by my reply to a Washington telegram in 1944 as to whether I wished to reacquire my yacht Done Gone under Act So-and-so and the Amendment So-and-So, which boat had been taken over for coastguard duty after Pearl Harbor. I wired back from Palm Beach: 'No, I do not wish to reacquire yacht Done Gone, because Henry Morgenthau has whittled me down to rowboat size and I'll have to do the rowing myself.' A big income, but Uncle Sam, he takes. However, I've given up my daily ravings against Washington, as it has achieved nothing except high blood pressure for me. Besides, I've long since come to the conviction that Washington is afflicted with tinnitus, which the dictionary defines as a baffling disease of noises in the head." (Ibid.) Henry Morgenthau Jr. had served as secretary of the treasury from January 1934 until July 1945.

3. See pp. 39n3 and 908.

4. Pattullo was married to the former Lucile Wilson of Dallas, Texas.

5. "Your letter gave me a lift, because the mood you spotted in mine still holds," replied Pattullo. "We're in an era of little men and they give me gooseflesh. . . . About that horse—please do me a favor, General. . . . Do take a look-see around and pick out a Kentucky or Virginia thoroughbred in which you will find not only comfort, but pride. Then have the breeder send me the bill. You'll be doing me a kindness, because this has been close to my heart for years and I only waited until you became a private citizen." He concluded, "I get around the country a lot; and often I wonder whether you realize the place you hold in the respect and affection of your countrymen?" (Pattullo to Marshall, March 19, 1950, ibid.)

42

To Lieutenant General Richard J. Marshall — March 8, 1950, Washington, DC

Dear Marshall: Sergeant George tells me he communicated with you regarding lodging for my driver on the night of June 12th.[1]

I found myself in a jam through a confusion of dates. A few years ago I became involved and obligated to appear at this ancient female academy (the academy not the females) across the river from Pittsburgh. Mrs. Marshall was to make an address there at their one hundredth anniversary, I think, and she developed pneumonia or something of that sort and couldn't appear and I agreed to square the deal.[2] The previous communication indicated June 15 but it was not until about a week ago I discovered it was actually June 12 at 10:30 in the morning, so I am inflicted with the necessity of motoring up there and then flying that afternoon to Roanoke or Lynchburg, whichever you think is the better point from which to motor to Lexington. I am sorry I will not be present at the meetings of the Board of Visitors prior to my arrival but it couldn't be helped. I told Sergeant George to tell you that I would stay over at the new quarters for the Board. I merely wanted to secure lodging for my driver who will have to meet me down there.[3]

I just came in at midnight last night from my final Red Cross trips to a total of somewhere near 30,000 miles and it seemed to me 30,000 press interviews with never a question about the Red Cross if they could avoid it.[4]

Mrs. Marshall is now in the Walter Reed having treatment for shingles in her eyes and a severe cold.[5] She has recovered sufficiently for me to fly her down to Pinehurst tomorrow morning. And if anybody invites me to do anything in the next few months it is at personal peril. Faithfully yours,

GCMRL/G. C. Marshall Papers (American Red Cross, Categorical, Invitations, Accepted)

1. General R. J. Marshall (VMI, 1915), superintendent of George Marshall's alma mater, the Virginia Military Institute, had written on February 10 to invite Marshall to deliver the commencement speech to the Class of 1950-B on June 13. "This is the first regular postwar class to graduate," he added. (R. J. Marshall to Marshall, February 10, 1950, GCMRL/G. C. Marshall Papers [American Red Cross, Categorical, Invitations, Accepted].) "I am more pleased and grateful than I can say that you have accepted the invitation," the superintendent wrote on February 16. (R. J. Marshall to Marshall, February 16, 1950, ibid.) See pp. 108–10.

2. Jocelyn Griffith, vice president of the senior class at the Pennsylvania College for Women, had written to Marshall on June 26, 1949, to invite him to be their commencement speaker. (Griffith to Marshall, June 26, 1949, ibid.) "As a result of my new job I was forced to regret invitations which had been on the books for some time, so you can see it is difficult for me to predict just what I will be doing or where I will be come next June," Marshall wrote to Griffith after she repeated her request. (Marshall to Griffith, October 6, 1949, ibid.) "Mrs. Marshall was in the office when your second letter arrived. She is a strong supporter of your cause and is most anxious that I make the date if possible." (Ibid.) "I will be able to accept your invitation to speak at the commencement exercises on June 12 at 10:30 a.m.," Marshall confirmed on February 28, 1950. (Marshall to Griffith, February 28, 1950, ibid.) See pp. 102–8.

3. R. J. Marshall recommended Roanoke since "the Army maintains a detachment" there. (R. J. Marshall to Marshall, March 10, 1950, ibid.) He also confirmed that a reservation was in place for Marshall's driver, Sergeant William J. Heffner, at the Colonial Inn in Lexington, and for Marshall in the new quarters for the board of visitors. (Ibid.)

4. See pp. 47–48. "I am appalled by the amount of traveling you are doing," Superintendent Marshall had written to Marshall on February 16. (R. J. Marshall to Marshall, February 16, 1950, ibid.) "Notwithstanding your having refused to answer most of the 30,000 interviewers," the superintendent responded, "I have thought that the publicity was splendid." (R. J. Marshall to Marshall, March 10, 1950, ibid.)

5. See pp. 62–63.

43

To Robert H. Ruby[1]

March 11, 1950
Pinehurst, North Carolina

My dear Doctor Ruby: Reference your letter of March 2 which I just found on my return to Pinehurst, the "little people" I was referring to are not in this country but in India, Africa, the Orient and like places (especially in Latin America).[2] They work but know no five-day week, they are usually on the edge of starvation or dying of starvation. They have no luxuries and only a limited number of what we consider necessities.

You and I are thinking of quite different groups. Faithfully yours,

GCMRL/G. C. Marshall Papers (American Red Cross, General)

1. Robert H. Ruby was completing his residency in pathology and surgery at St. Louis County Hospital in St. Louis, Missouri.

2. "An AP [Associated Press] release dated Honolulu, Feb. 25 refers to statements attributed to you," wrote Ruby. "One statement is quoted as, 'The revolution I'm talking about is that of the little people all over the world. They're beginning to learn what there is

in life, and what they're missing.' This is all of your statement. No other statements with explanations are given. So this letter is not to take exception to your statements because no one could without those qualifications necessary. The purpose of this letter is to ask what is there in life that little people are missing? . . . Limiting these to the peoples of the United States how could they possibly want more economic security than they have now. I as a young physician could discontinue my residency training now and draw any number of pensions or benefits if I should lose my desire for work and study and such. . . . People today work less than ever before, draw more money and have time left for more play." (Ruby to Marshall, March 2, 1950, GCMRL/G. C. Marshall Papers [American Red Cross, General].)

44

To Sharlene Adams[1]

March 16, 1950
Pinehurst, North Carolina

Dear Miss Adams: I have your letter of March 3 with its request to write you a letter for inclusion in the Randolph Junior High School's Treasure Chest.

I seriously doubt that my boyhood habits and ideals differed from those of the majority of children of today. However, sincerity, integrity and tolerance are, to my mind, the first of many requirements to a fine, strong character. Faithfully yours,

GCMRL/G. C. Marshall Papers (American Red Cross, Categorical, Requests, Statements, Comments, and Advice)

1. Adams, a seventh-grade student from Randolph, Vermont, had written, "The boys and girls of Randolph Junior High School . . . are building a Treasure Chest. We are going to fill it with Good Habits, High Ideals and Right Attitudes. Perhaps when you were in junior high school you started developing habits that helped to make you the successful person you are today. Would you write me a letter stating any habits, ideals, or attitudes that we would be wise to follow in order to be better citizens of our community?" (Adams to Marshall, March 3, 1950, GCMRL/G. C. Marshall Papers [American Red Cross, Categorical, Requests, Statements, Comments, and Advice].)

Marshall had received a similar request in February from Peter R. DuPont, a student at the Brooks School in North Andover, Massachusetts, and secretary of *The Next Voter*, a political science magazine published by him and sixteen classmates. He had written, "we are so very anxious . . . to publish the reply by fifteen of America's most distinguished citizens to the following question: 'What, in your opinion, is the most valuable and useful advice—in one word, one sentence, one paragraph or more—that you would like to give to any American boy on his graduation from School?'" Marshall's response to DuPont was virtually identical to his answer here. (DuPont to Marshall, February 15, 1950, ibid.)

45

To Philip C. Jessup

March 17, 1950
Pinehurst, North Carolina

My dear Jessup: I am shocked and distressed by the attack on your integrity as a public servant.[1] Throughout your intimate service with me when I was Secretary of State you were clearly outstanding as a representative of the government both as to your masterful presentations and the firmness of your opposition to all Soviet or Communistic attacks or pressures. This was conspicuously the case during your handling, on the Security Council, of the Berlin Blockade issue.

Both the Under Secretary, Mr. Lovett, and I counted you as a great source of strength to the State Department during those critical days.[2] Faithfully yours,

G. C. Marshall

LC/P. C. Jessup Papers; H

1. Jessup had recently come under attack by Wisconsin Republican Senator Joseph R. McCarthy for having "an unusual affinity for Communist causes." Recalled from his post as ambassador-at-large in the Far East to address these accusations, Jessup produced this letter and another from Dwight D. Eisenhower decrying the charges at a Senate investigatory hearing on March 20, 1950. (William S. White, "Jessup Denounces M'Carthy Charges as Danger to U.S.," *New York Times*, March 21, 1950, p. 1.) "Your long and distinguished record as a scholar and a public servant has won for you the respect of your colleagues and of the American people," Eisenhower, then president of Columbia University, had written to Jessup, who was also a professor of international law at Columbia. "No one who has known you can for a moment question the depth or sincerity of your devotion to the principles of Americanism. Your University associates and I are confident that any impression to the contrary will be quickly dispelled as the facts become known." For Eisenhower's full letter, see Alfred D. Chandler et al., eds., *Papers of Dwight David Eisenhower*, 21 vols. (Baltimore: Johns Hopkins University Press, 1970–2001), 11: 1014; hereinafter volumes of the *Eisenhower Papers* are referred to as *Papers of DDE*.

2. Alfred Kohlberg, chairman of the American China Policy Association and a leading figure in the pro–Chiang Kai-shek "China Lobby," wrote to ask Marshall whether his letter endorsing Jessup was meant to be taken literally. Marshall replied with an emphatic yes; see pp. 80–81.

46

To John Seabrook — March 27, 1950, Washington, DC

My dear Seabrook: On returning to my office from the Red Cross Board meeting today I found your interesting letter of March seventeenth.[1]

While I was not prepared to hear of General Arnold's death, I was not too surprised. My first trip for Red Cross—that was in October—took me to the West Coast and I had the opportunity to have breakfast with him at my hotel. I thought he looked very badly at that time. I attended his funeral at Arlington Cemetery and the only snow of any consequence this winter fell on that day. This made a sad occasion even more depressing. He was a loyal and good friend and I miss him very much.[2]

I find my job with Red Cross very interesting and stimulating. As a matter of fact, since joining the organization on October first, I have traveled some thirty thousand miles in connection with its activities. Fortunately I am able to get some time off to spend at my winter home in Pinehurst where I can do a little horseback riding.

My health has been good although Mrs. Marshall has been troubled during the fall and winter with "shingles" in the eyes. The condition seems to be clearing up but slowly.

The photograph you request has been sent to you under separate cover. I feel honored that it will hang beside that of Sir John Dill.

Mrs. Marshall joins me in warm regards to you and your family. Faithfully yours,

GCMRL/G. C. Marshall Papers (American Red Cross, General)

1. Seabrook, a New Zealand Air Force attaché in Washington during World War II, had written to Marshall that he was "shocked to learn of the passing of General Arnold recently. . . . He was always so kind and helpful to me personally during the time I was stationed in Washington, and he had a happy way of making us feel that we were welcome and part of his own Forces. In mentioning this I feel that I should also tell you how much we loved and respected the late Vice Admiral J. S. McCain, U.S.N. [United States Navy], who also took a special interest in our New Zealand combat aircraft requirements in the South Pacific. He was a staunch friend to we New Zealanders. If you could spare me a photograph of yourself, Sir, to put in my den at home, alongside the one I have of Sir John Dill, I would appreciate it very greatly." (Seabrook to Marshall, March 17, 1950, GCMRL/G. C. Marshall Papers [American Red Cross, General].) Admiral John S. McCain Sr. (USNA, 1906) had been a naval aviator, taking command of the Air Forces for the Western Sea Frontier and South Pacific Force at the outbreak of World War II. In August 1943 he became the deputy chief of naval operations (air) and returned to lead the Fast Carrier Task Force in the Pacific theater in 1944. He died in September 1945.

2. See p. 47.

47

REMARKS DURING THE *LUX RADIO THEATRE* PROGRAM[1] — March 27, 1950, Washington, DC

I have just finished an extensive tour of the country, some thirty thousand miles, and I am tremendously impressed by the leadership and work of our 3700 Red Cross chapters and by the large numbers of public-spirited men and women who have volunteered their services as campaign workers.

The American people believe in the Red Cross.

They judge the Red Cross by its works. Year in and year out they have seen it mobilize its resources to aid the victims of disaster with both emergency relief and long-range rehabilitation. Last year it helped in 330 disasters, the greatest number in a single year.—And here's an interesting point—April is the month of greatest disaster frequency. So we must anticipate more Red Cross assistance in the next thirty days. In recent weeks we had thousands of volunteer Red Cross workers in the field on flood relief, and we were caring for—that is, feeding, sheltering and sometimes clothing as many as 23,000 families. Nearly two millions of Red Cross funds were or are involved.

The Red Cross goes right on day in and day out serving the men and women in the armed forces—a million and a half of them—in this country and overseas. Our workers daily bring comfort to those in military and veterans hospitals; the National Blood Program supplies blood to the hundreds of thousands of sick and injured; and our volunteers stand trained and ready to assist in these and other Red Cross services.

To do the things that the American people expect, the Red Cross is appealing this year for sixty-seven million dollars. Last year the public subscribed over sixty-eight million. Four hundred and thirty-eight of our 3700 chapters have reached their quotas. To meet our minimum needs the other chapters must reach their goals.

I urge our campaign workers to increase their efforts. I am confident that the people will respond if it is properly presented to them.

In these days of misunderstandings and misgivings, the beneficent arms of the Red Cross reach out to recreate that feeling of good faith and good will which is essential to the world if we are to have peace.

GCMRL/G. C. Marshall Papers (American Red Cross, Speeches and Statements)

1. The *Lux Radio Theatre* was a weekly, hour-long program that adapted films to the radio. ("William Keighley Dies at 94; Theater and Movie Director," *New York Times*, June 26, 1984, p. B8.) Marshall spoke during the evening radio program that featured an adaptation of *The Man Who Came to Dinner* with Lucille Ball and Clifton Webb. ("Today's Greater Washington Radio Programs," *Washington Post,* March 27, 1950, p. B9.)

48

To Louis A. Johnson[1]

March 29, 1950
Washington, DC

My dear Mr. Secretary: Beginning during World War I and with the approval of the military authorities, the American Red Cross has developed and maintained an extensive program of service in military hospitals which has included medical and psychiatric social service and organized recreation directed by trained professional workers.

These activities have been maintained in addition to the communication and welfare services that are available to all members of the armed forces, including able-bodied and hospitalized personnel, and the varied and extensive activities of trained Red Cross volunteers serving in military hospitals.

During this thirty-two year period, there has been increasing recognition of the essential contribution of medical social workers to the medical treatment of the sick and injured. The Red Cross has made a significant contribution to this advance by the maintenance in military hospitals of social services supported by the voluntary contributions of the American people at a time when these services had not received such general recognition as could provide the basis for their maintenance by the expenditure of funds available to the military establishment. The Red Cross effort in this particular field has therefore been in the nature of a demonstration which now has reached a point at which plans for an orderly conclusion should be considered and agreed upon.

At its meeting March 27, 1950, the Board of Governors of the American National Red Cross directed that plans be made to discontinue the medical and psychiatric social work service in military hospitals and requested the staff to work out a program to accomplish this by July 1, 1951.

The action to be taken in compliance with this resolution will of course be carefully considered with your office and with the Surgeons General of the respective services. I am sure that the interests of all concerned with this matter will be served by an early discussion and I shall greatly appreciate your cooperation in naming representatives to work with us in developing the procedures and the timing to accomplish this policy decision of the Board of Governors.

I wish you to know that the American Red Cross will continue its military welfare services to the men in the armed forces, and to their families, and that the thousands of volunteers who are now working in the military hospitals will be urged to continue and to increase their numbers and activities.[2] Faithfully yours,

G. C. Marshall

NA/RG 330, SD 080 (American National Red Cross)

1. Undersecretary of war from 1937 to 1940, Louis A. Johnson had been secretary of defense since March 28, 1949.

2. "Thank you kindly for your recent letter telling of plans to discontinue medical and psychiatric social work service in military hospitals," Johnson replied. "In many ways I am sorry to hear of it, since innumerable outstanding contributions have been made by the Red Cross in this field. Both from an individual as well as on a service wide basis, this work has earned our deepest appreciation. However, while its necessity is regretted, your action is entirely understandable under the circumstances. . . . May I take this opportunity also to express my appreciation for the many splendid services being performed daily for the Armed Forces by your devoted staff. They are our friends indeed." (Johnson to Marshall, April 5, 1950, NA/RG 330, SD 080 [American National Red Cross].)

49

To General J. Lawton Collins[1]

March 29, 1950
Washington, DC

My dear Collins: I hoped that I would find an opportunity to see you while I was in Washington on this trip but I have been so completely engaged with the three-day meeting of the Board of Governors of the Red Cross that I have not had an opportunity to get over to the Pentagon. I am meeting with the Battle Monuments Commission this morning and leave immediately thereafter for Pinehurst. I will be back for a half a day on the third, en route to New York, but I think this letter will serve my purpose.

I find we are in difficulties in the Battle Monuments Commission over the fact that we have not been able to get the guidance necessary for the historical appreciation of various battles or campaigns that is included in each cemetery memorial and is really the most interest compelling phase of these very artistic structures. General [Thomas] North tells me the trouble is that he cannot get the detail of an officer, who knows enough about the matter to work out the details, to guide the artist. We are going to have to hire a civilian for the purpose if we cannot secure any army officer but I think this would be an unfortunate way to proceed.

North tells me he tried to make progress through General [Orlando] Ward's section but that has not been satisfactory and I am appealing to you direct.

This is a very important consideration in our cemeterial set-up and the time has arrived where we must get immediate action because the mosaics, carvings and other matters involved have to be decided upon and gotten under way.

If I have not made the matter clear, and North is not here with me to guide me at the moment, I would suggest that you give him an opportunity to state the case in detail. I will only add that the army's interest in this is, in my opinion, deserving of more than routine consideration.[2] Faithfully yours,

GCMRL/G. C. Marshall Papers (American Red Cross, Subject, American Battle Monuments Commission, 1949–1950)

1. J. Lawton Collins (USMA, April 1917) had been army chief of staff since August 16, 1949.

2. Vice Army Chief of Staff General Wade H. Haislip (USMA, 1912) informed Marshall on March 31 that Deputy Chief of Staff Lieutenant General Matthew B. Ridgway (USMA, 1917) and General North had agreed to appoint Lieutenant Colonel Joseph B. Mitchell (USMA, 1937) to provide the ABMC with historical background for the battles or campaigns included in each cemetery memorial. (Haislip to Marshall, March 31, 1950, NA/RG 319 [Records of the Chief of Staff, Secretary, General Staff, Security Classified General Correspondence, 1950, 166.040 ABMC].)

50

Speech Delivered at the Mid-Point Anniversary of ECA

April 3, 1950
Washington, DC

I am very glad to participate in this gathering today because it celebrates a momentous occasion, the half-way point of the ECA.[1] I never consider the European Recovery Program without recapturing in my mind the tragic state of Western Europe in the late spring of 1947. The situation appeared almost hopeless and every plan we made seemed to be thwarted in advance by a vicious circle of conditions which were the product of war.

Frankly, in those days I thought of the rehabilitation of Europe more in terms of material reconstruction—harbors, buildings, communications and similar matters. But slowly I learned that the most serious phase of rehabilitation was related to other considerations—political, moral, spiritual. These were less tangible, but far more difficult to deal with. Not only had the trade and business relations of hundreds of years been completely obliterated, but with them had gone the faith and confidence in many of the key institutions of modern civilization. It was the rehabilitation of these that was by far the most difficult task, and one in which we are still engaged. It is in the meeting of these problems that I feel the European Recovery Program is making its greatest contribution to the world.

The debates on the question of continuing the program, it seems to me, are confused by a variety of motives. An appraisement of the requirements of the day is befogged by a failure to realize that we are now engaged in a great struggle. You here may not be in the same sort of physical danger as troops on the battlefield, but you are engaged in a contest with a foe who has designs no less deadly than those we have ever faced. Make no mistake about it, the chips are down. Winning this struggle is as vital to the peace and prosperity of the world as any military campaign in history. I think it is important these critical days to have constantly in mind the fact that the original suggestion for the European Recovery Program applied to all of Europe. The present division between the East and the West was drawn by Mr. Molotov for the Kremlin. Indeed, unless we achieve victory our great military and financial sacrifices may have been largely in vain, I fear.

The nature of this struggle should be clearly understood. It seemed to me during the time I served as Secretary of State that at each meeting of the Foreign Ministers, assaults against the enactment of progress of the recovery program were timed to confuse the understanding of the negotiations in the minds of the public. They were directed at weakening the program by forcing expenditure of funds beyond our calculations and appropriations.

The opposition has not been confined to strikes and purely political manifestations. It has followed through in every conceivable manner, even to the point where I found myself within an hour of the event, publicly accused over the radio of being the major planner in the assassination of an important and popular public figure in Bogota.[2]

But despite these determined efforts to prevent the rehabilitation of Western Europe on a basis which would permit a healthy revival of democratic processes, the plan has succeeded, thanks to the financial endorsement of our Congress, the leadership of the President and the Secretary of State, Mr. Acheson, and the splendid work of you people of ECA here and abroad, under the able direction of Mr. Hoffman, Mr. Foster and Ambassador Harriman.[3]

But your job is only half done. I must emphasize the tremendous imprtance of carrying through on the scale planned. We must avoid proposals to emasculate and reduce ECA to a mere relief affair. At the same time, it seems clear to me that we cannot continue this sort of extraordinary aid indefinitely; therefore the termination date of June 30, 1952, should be adhered to. I feel that if this date is settled and clear it will spur the work of the European leaders and people to accomplish the extremely difficult task ahead of lifting themselves above the need for our financial assistance. There will always be in this generation of men a need for our moral and spiritual backing.

To those who assert that our targets cannot be reached within the short span of two more years, I would say that perfection of accomplishment cannot always be expected. But we have seen a close approach to that perfection in these past two years.

It is true that for Western Europe to get its economic house in such order that it can survive and prosper in this competitive modern world requires a tremendous final effort over the next two years. The erasing of old trade barriers and the construction of new channels, such as a clearing union for Europe's varied moneys, may require a miracle of cooperation.

But, looking again at the conditions prevalent in the spring of 1947, and again considering the situation at this moment, I can only feel that one near miracle has been accomplished. We must work for, and expect, another miracle.

Let me sum it up: We are engaged in a perilous struggle with an implacable foe: we must carry this battle to the finish; we must avoid the temptation to imperil the whole investment—and it is just that, an investment in saving all those precious articles of faith and ways of life we call democracy. It is an investment in preserving the freedoms of men in a clean and decent world.[4]

GCMRL/G. C. Marshall Papers (American Red Cross, Speeches and Statements)

1. Marshall delivered this speech at the Hotel Statler in Washington for a gathering of several hundred employees of the ECA to celebrate the second anniversary of congressional approval of the Economic Cooperation Act, which had established the ECA to administer the European Recovery Program (ERP). The program was scheduled to begin at approximately 11:15 a.m. and be broadcast on radio. (George to Marshall, March 31, 1950, GCMRL/G. C. Marshall Papers [American Red Cross, Subject, ECA].) Also in attendance were Dean Acheson, Paul G. Hoffman, Deputy ECA Administrator William C. Foster, and numerous ambassadors and senators from both parties. (Ferdinand Kuhn, "Reds Labeled No. 1 Peril in U.S. History," *Washington Post*, April 4, 1950, pp. 1 and 4). See photo #3.

2. Marshall had been in Bogotá for an Inter-American Conference when, on April 9, 1948, Colombian Liberal leader Jorge Eliécer Gaitán was assassinated. Rioting ensued, and rebel radio quickly accused Marshall of complicity in the assassination. ("Bogata Rebels Accused Marshall," *Washington Post*, April 23, 1948, p. 10.) See *Papers of GCM*, 6: 435–36.

3. W. Averell Harriman had served as secretary of commerce under President Truman from 1947 to 1948 and was US special representative to the European Recovery Program nations from 1948 to mid-1950.

4. Hoffman wrote on April 5 to thank Marshall for the speech, adding that during the town hall program in Richmond, Virginia, the previous evening, he "found that the most effective lines in my speech were excerpts from your statement. Once again it is evident that a whisper from Marshall can do more to move the world than a shout from most of us." (Hoffman to Marshall, April 5, 1950, GCMRL/G. C. Marshall Papers [American Red Cross, General].)

51

Speech to International House Sponsors — April 4, 1950
New York, New York

I have asked you to meet with me today because of your known interest in international affairs. All of us earnestly desire world peace and security and we realize that it requires cooperation and good will among men and nations. But how are these things to be gained and made secure for our children, and for our children's children?

Since succeeding Colonel Stimson a year ago as Chairman of the Board of International House, I have become increasingly convinced that a part of the answer lies in the field of international education.[1]

International House was conceived as a means of bringing together under one roof a group of outstanding international graduate students. It began as an experiment in international living; and the question at that time was: "Would the difference of race, religion, and culture prove insurmountable barriers to friendship and understanding?"

Today there is an answer to that question. International House is no longer an "experiment." It has demonstrated on a large scale that it *is* possible for young men and women from all parts of the world to live, work, play and study together, and through their day by day experiences to learn to understand and appreciate each other.

The program of International House over the past 25 years has been a significant one, but the job ahead far surpasses that of the past, for a quarter of a century ago, the United States was just emerging as a first rate power in the world. It was in many respects provincial. Not many realize that in 1898 there was not one ambassador accredited to this government.

Today, the situation has completely changed. We are the leading power in the world of nations. Many of our institutions which served us well in the last 50 years are becoming inadequate to do the larger job required today. Among such is the New York International House.

What I mean is this: twenty-five years ago we had some 6,000 foreign students in the United States. Young people abroad preferred to go to England, France or Germany. Today almost all those students wish to study in this country . . . and the trickle of the past has grown to some 27,000 this year.

A large number of people seem to have the idea that anyone coming to this country will automatically become one of our admirers, regardless of what his life here may be like. Recent surveys have made it clear, however, that if we are to make friends of these students from abroad, we must see that they find adequate housing, good counsellors, and help in making friends and in becoming oriented to our way of life. International House is one of the few places which has been deliberately geared to meet these needs. And it is a measure of the value of the work of the House that if these young people understand and like the United States, they will serve as interpreters of the real America in their own countries—the kind of service which no propaganda machine can provide.

International House only does a small part of the job. But in the past it has done a large part of it directly, and has had an even wider influence indirectly. Over 20,000 students have enjoyed the happy, home-like atmosphere of International House. Some have gone home to fill positions of authority and trust. Others are now members of delegations to the United Nations, and of foreign embassies in Washington. They are doing their utmost to help create that spirit of international friendship and peace which was a part of their daily lives here in New York.

The purposes of International House have perhaps not been entirely clear to some of you, so I should like to point out one or two things which the House seeks to do, aside from providing a decent home-away-from-home.

First, it brings the students together in an international community which has a real life of its own, a place where each has the opportunity to learn at first hand and intimately the ways and problems of people from distant lands. There are really very few places in the world where young people may sit down for a cup of coffee and chat with a British Member of Parliament, a Buddhist priest, a United Nations delegate or a foreign ambassador. There are even fewer places where students from over 65 nations are in constant, daily association with each other. This kind of education for international understanding is one of the advantages International House offers both to our own students and to those from abroad.

Another primary purpose of the House is to see that foreign students are thoroughly exposed to American culture and life. One method the House has used with great success has been the "Living America" series. Last year the House brought together outstanding national leaders in their fields to meet foreign students and to give them a more complete picture of America. Those who spoke included a labor leader, Mr. James Carey; a successful businessman, John Orr Young, co-founder of the firm of Young and Rubicam; an outstanding writer, Bernard De Voto; and the President of the Farm Bureau Federation, Allan Kline, a mid-western farmer who knows how to raise corn and hogs on a large scale.[2] This year's "Living America" series has included a splendid set of documentary films. Any student who stays at International House is bound to go home with a broader understanding of American life than when he arrived.

There are a number of other reasons why the role of International House today can be especially significant. I have already mentioned America's enormously increased influence in world affairs. More than ever before, there is a great need for young Americans who have an understanding of other peoples. Take our Point Four program, for example.[3] We can't merely export the techniques we have found useful here. These techniques must be adapted to suit the particular country where they are to be used. And this job requires not only technical knowledge. Above all, it requires a feeling for the way other peoples think and react.

Take, for example, Indonesia, and the other countries of Southeast Asia and the Middle East. We need representatives in Indonesia, who know the country, because they have eaten many a meal with Indonesians, have discussed their customs, religion, ways and habits, either in public forums at the House, or in midnight bull-sessions upstairs in a dormitory room. If we are to prove competent to assume a leading role in the world's affairs, this kind of training is of greater importance than ever before.

These are some of the reasons why we ask your support today. An institution which so usefully serves to promote understanding among those who will be the leaders of tomorrow *must have* the support it needs to do the job.[4]

We appreciate your coming here today and I hope I have been able to give you a fairly clear outline of the work of International House and its value to the country today.[5]

GCMRL/G. C. Marshall Papers (American Red Cross, Speeches and Statements)

1. David Rockefeller, chairman of the executive committee of International House, had contacted Marshall in March 1949 to formally invite him to succeed Henry Stimson as chairman of the board of trustees of International House in New York. Upon receiving Rockefeller's invitation, Marshall replied: "I am most appreciative of the compliment paid to me by the Board of Trustees of International House in inviting me to succeed Mr.

Stimson as Chairman of the board and am honored in accepting the office." Writing to Marshall upon news of his acceptance, Stimson noted that the general would "find that the Board of Trustees contains some very fine, capable, and foresighted men and women, and that you will profit by your intercourse with them." (Rockefeller to Marshall, March 15, 1949, GCMRL/G. C. Marshall Papers [Pentagon Office, General]; Stimson to Marshall, May 6, 1949, GCMRL/G. C. Marshall Papers [Pentagon Office, Selected]; *Papers of GCM*, 6: 678, 705–6.)

2. James Carey had been the first president of the United Electrical, Radio, and Machine Workers of America from 1936 to 1941, a member of the National War Labor Board from 1941 to 1942, secretary-treasurer of the Congress of Industrial Organizations (CIO) in 1942, a member of the President's Committee on Civil Rights in 1946, and a member of the Trade Union Advisory Committee on International Affairs since 1947. John Orr Young and fellow advertising consultant Raymond Rubicam had started the highly successful advertising firm Young & Rubicam in 1923; Young retired in 1935. Bernard De Voto was an award-winning author, journalist, and historian. Allan Kline had been elected as president of the American Farm Bureau Federation in late 1947 and had testified before the House Foreign Affairs Committee in support of the Marshall Plan in early 1948.

3. Proposed by President Truman in early 1949 and approved by Congress and launched in 1950, the Point Four Program provided technical assistance to "underdeveloped areas" of the world.

4. George S. Franklin, who worked at the Council on Foreign Relations, had explained in a letter to Marshall that at the conclusion of the sponsors' group lunch, those in attendance would be presented with a list of possible contributors to International House and asked, if they were amenable, to indicate up to five names they would be willing to contact. Either Franklin or David Rockefeller would also make a brief statement regarding the financial needs of the House. Marshall's speech had been drafted with such need in mind, although focusing upon the broader purpose of the house rather than the need for funds. Marshall made numerous edits to the proposed draft. (Franklin to Marshall, March 27, 1950, GCMRL/G. C. Marshall Papers [American Red Cross, General].)

5. "It was pleasant having a glimpse of you at the International House luncheon and to hear you speak so effectively in its behalf, which was indicated by the way in which the guests got busy with their pencils checking off names on lists which were circulated," Roland Harriman wrote Marshall two days later. (Harriman to Marshall, April 6, 1950, ibid.) See p. 82.

52

TO CLIFTON S. BROWN

April 5, 1950
Washington, DC

Dear Clifton, I am so sorry you had such hard luck and was sorry that it has not been possible for me to get down to see you.[1] I got in at 9 o'clock last night from New York and we are leaving at 10 o'clock this morning for Pinehurst.

We will keep in touch with you through Allene and Sergeant George. He telephones me daily and he will call Allene first to find out how you are getting along.

Sergeant Heffner will stay down at the house so you need not concern yourself about there being nobody there.[2] Also, I will tell him to drop by the hospital to find out what you may want done for you at the house or in the town.

Try to have patience with this tribulation and not go out of the house without your hat on! Affectionately,

P.S. Madge called up yesterday and when she learned about you said she is planning to go down and see you.

GCMRL/G. C. Marshall Papers (American Red Cross, General)

1. Clifton Brown, Marshall's stepson, had been hospitalized at the Loudoun County Hospital in Leesburg with a stomach illness. See p. 81.
2. Sergeant William J. Heffner, who had served in the army since 1932, was Marshall's chauffeur and orderly.

53

To William D. Pawley — April 5, 1950, Washington, DC

Dear Pawley: I have not heard of you or from you for a long time.[1] What are you and Edna doing?

I came into Washington the third and left almost immediately for New York. Got back from there late last night and we are leaving at 10 o'clock this morning for Pinehurst.

Mrs. Marshall came up with me to see the Walter Reed about her eyes—shingles. She is on her fifth month of this tribulation, but otherwise she is feeling very well.

I am going bass fishing tomorrow morning and riding this afternoon. The rest of the schedule is open but it will probably be about the same thing. We are coming up to Leesburg the end of the month.

My affectionate regards to Edna and to you.[2] Faithfully yours,

GCMRL/G. C. Marshall Papers (American Red Cross, General)

1. Former US Ambassador to Brazil Pawley had written to Marshall most recently on October 3, 1949.
2. A typed note at the end of this document indicates that Marshall dictated the letter but "got away before he could sign it."

54

To Alfred Kohlberg — April 6, 1950, Pinehurst, North Carolina

My dear Mr. Kohlberg: I believe it necessary for you to re-read the text of my letter to Ambassador Jessup as I think it can be interpreted but one way.[1]

As to the contention of some of your directors that it was a meaningless statement, I assure you that was not the case. I wrote the letter because I was responsible for his selection and assignment, because he rendered me in his official capacity a great service and because I admire him and have complete confidence in his integrity. Very truly yours,

GCMRL/G. C. Marshall Papers (Pentagon Office, General)

1. Philip C. Jessup had recently been accused by Senator Joseph McCarthy of having Communist sympathies. Marshall and Eisenhower had both written letters defending Jessup's service that Jessup produced in the course of his Senate hearings; see pp. 69–70.

Alfred Kohlberg wrote in the aftermath of these letters being published in the press, "In discussing with some of the Directors of our Association the meaning of your letters of endorsement given to Ambassador Philip C. Jessup, I contended that these letters were meant to be an endorsement by both of you of Ambassador Jessup's record, including his affiliation with Communist fronts, his long and close association with Communist and Fellow-Travelers, and even his public appearance as a character witness for Alger Hiss in both Hiss trials. Some of our Directors contended that your letters were not to be taken literally. They said they should only be considered as a formal and meaningless statement very similar to the statements of recommendation commonly given by business firms to unsatisfactory employees who have been let out. I would greatly appreciate hearing from you . . . as to which interpretation should be put on your letters." (Kohlberg to Marshall, April 3, 1950, GCMRL/G. C. Marshall Papers [Pentagon Office, General].) Hiss had served in various positions in the Roosevelt administration and attended the Yalta Conference in February 1945 as a member of the US delegation. In 1948, he was accused of transmitting classified State Department papers to members of the Communist Party in the United States prior to World War II. He was found guilty of perjury on January 26, 1950, sentenced to five years in prison, and released in 1954.

55

To Oveta Culp Hobby — April 11, 1950
Georgetown, South Carolina

Dear Mrs. Hobby: Thanks for sending me the tear sheets of some of the Red Cross fund articles and even more for the support your paper has given Red Cross.[1] I was much interested and gratified to learn that Houston had already exceeded its quota and I'm sure that *The Houston Post* played a large part in getting them over the top.

I am writing you from Hobcaw where I am getting some relaxation for a week. Mrs. Marshall is in Leesburg where she can be near her son who is hospitalized for a diagnosis of a stomach condition.[2]

With warm regards to you both, Faithfully yours,

GCMRL/G. C. Marshall Papers (American Red Cross, General)

1. Oveta Culp Hobby, wartime head of the Women's Army Auxiliary Corps (later the Women's Army Corps), was the executive vice president of the *Houston Post*. Marshall had stayed with her and her husband William P. Hobby, the former Democratic governor of Texas from 1917 to 1921, during his visit to Houston, Texas. (Hobby to Marshall, January 5, 1950, GCMRL/G. C. Marshall Papers [American Red Cross, Invitations, Accepted].) She sent three articles from her newspaper dealing with the Red Cross fundraising drive to Marshall: "The one from the first of March opened the drive—the other two are a closing appeal and the final figures for Houston." (Hobby to Marshall, April 7, 1950, GCMRL/G. C. Marshall Papers [American Red Cross, General].)

2. See pp. 79–80.

56

To David Rockefeller

April 11, 1950
Georgetown, South Carolina

Dear David: I have your letter of April seventh confirming Tuesday, May 16th as the date for the dinner.[1] I agree that it should be a very worthwhile evening considering that Mr. Dulles will be the principal speaker and that we shall have the opportunity to hear a few words from your father.[2]

My Pan American luncheon and meeting gets under way at one o'clock on the 16th but we should adjourn in time for me to make the 5:30 meeting at International House.[3]

I appreciate very much Peggy's and your invitation to spend the night.[4] I accept with much pleasure as I should enjoy seeing her and the children again. I'm afraid at this time that I cannot say whether Mrs. Marshall will accompany me but as soon as I find out definitely I will let you know. It will be necessary for me to fly back to Washington the morning of the 17th as I have an engagement to speak before the Boys' Club of America Executive Association luncheon at 12:30 p.m.

Mrs. Marshall joins me in warm regards to you both and love to the children.
Faithfully yours,

GCMRL/G. C. Marshall Papers (American Red Cross, General)

1. On April 5, Marshall had written to Rockefeller concerning plans for the twenty-fifth anniversary of International House, "As to the dinner, would Tuesday, May 16th be a possible date? The week of the 9th does not fit very well into my plans." (Marshall to Rockefeller, April 5, 1950, GCMRL/G. C. Marshall Papers [American Red Cross, General].) Rockefeller had replied on April 7, "May 16th, has now been cleared with all concerned and we have settled on it for the final dinner of the . . . celebration at which you have kindly agreed to be toastmaster. . . . We are indeed grateful to you for being willing to speak for us and to send out the invitations over your signature. There is no doubt at all but what the success of the luncheon is to be attributed to your cooperation." (Rockefeller to Marshall, April 7, 1950, ibid.) See pp. 76–79.

2. John Foster Dulles had attended several Council of Foreign Ministers conferences (see *Papers of GCM*, 6: 73, 121, 235, 270, 477) and served as a foreign policy adviser to Republican presidential candidate Thomas E. Dewey in 1948; he was appointed chairman of the United States delegation to the United Nations (UN) meeting in Paris when Secretary Marshall had to return to the United States in November 1948. President Truman had appointed him foreign affairs consultant to Secretary Acheson on April 6, 1950.

3. The editors have not been able to locate a copy of Marshall's remarks at the dinner.

4. Margaret "Peggy" McGrath Rockefeller was David Rockefeller's wife.

57

To Lieutenant General Willard S. Paul

April 17, 1950
Pinehurst, North Carolina

Dear Paul: George tells me that he had the pleasure of breaking bread with you the other day at the Canteen and that you spoke of your forthcoming move South. Time moves so rapidly that I hadn't realized that the date of your departure would soon be here.[1]

I understand that you were fortunate in finding a home with a lake at your front stoop. Knowing of your keen interest in fishing, these surroundings should provide plenty of pleasure and excitement—and house guests. Frankly, I think you made a wise decision in selecting a place which is not mid-way between Walter Reed and Arlington. Far too many retired service people hang around Washington instead of picking out a place in the country where life would be more pleasant.

I am sorry that I will not be in the office prior to your departure, but as you take your leave I wish to express my appreciation for the valuable services you have rendered Red Cross. As for me, my sincere thanks for your helpful assistance during the war years and since joining this fine organization.[2]

With warm regards to Mrs. Paul and to you, Faithfully yours,

GCMRL/G. C. Marshall Papers (American Red Cross, General)

1. Paul was retiring from his position as consultant and special adviser to the American Red Cross. He had previously served as both a division commander and deputy chief of staff at Supreme Headquarters Allied Expeditionary Force (SHAEF) during World War II, and as assistant chief of staff for personnel in the Army General Staff after the war.

2. "You were very kind to drop me such a pleasant note," Paul replied; "please understand that my 13 months of service here at Red Cross, much of which was spent in the field visiting chapters and installations, has been most helpful, constructive, and pleasant. I don't know of any group that I have enjoyed more. It may be that you will want some of the ideas I have picked up during the period I have been here. I have left with [James T.] Nicholson the study of reorganization, which I feel, if given the thought it should have, will do much to facilitate the activities and cut down expenses. Also he has separate papers on Volunteers, a new Hospital Service, and other matters. I would appreciate it if you would look those over." (Paul to Marshall, April 19, 1950, GCMRL/G. C. Marshall Papers [American Red Cross, General].)

58

To Millard E. Tydings[1]

April 24, 1950
Pinehurst, North Carolina

My dear Senator Tydings: I have received your letter of April 17 in which you refer to a recent statement, in connection with the hearings of the Subcommittee on Foreign Relations under S. Res. 231, that "Owen Lattimore is the principal architect of our Far Eastern policy". Your letter then asks the extent to which, in my opinion, "Lattimore was the principal architect of our Far Eastern policy" during the period in which I served as Secretary of State.[2]

The statement referred to above is completely without basis in fact. So far as I and my associates can recall, I never even met Mr. Lattimore.[3]

I take the liberty of commenting on the harmful effect on our foreign relations of such statements, charges or insinuations broadcast with so little regard for the truth. They undoubtedly confuse our friends abroad, undermine and weaken our position before the world and actually lend assistance to the powers that would destroy us.[4] Faithfully yours,

GCMRL/G. C. Marshall Papers (American Red Cross, Subject, State Department, 1949–1950)

1. On April 21, C. J. George had sent Marshall two drafts for this letter. One had been prepared by the State Department and "cleared by the China Affairs people," including Assistant Secretary of State for Far Eastern Affairs W. Walton Butterworth and his subordinate Philip Sprouse; the other was a revised version George had written because he "believed you would not want to do any name calling." (George to Marshall, April 21, 1950, GCMRL/G. C. Marshall Papers [American Red Cross, General].)

2. Chaired by Senator Tydings (D-MD), the subcommittee had been established in February 1950 to investigate charges by Senator Joseph McCarthy that known Communists were working in the State Department. Previously McCarthy had attacked Philip Jessup, resulting in Marshall's letters to Jessup and Alfred Kohlberg. (See pp. 69–70 and 80–81.) On March 21, McCarthy, in an executive session of the subcommittee, accused Owen Lattimore of being a top Communist spy. Lattimore was not a member of the State Department. He was a central Asian scholar, Johns Hopkins University professor, and former editor of the Institute of Pacific Relations' journal, *Pacific Affairs*, who during World War II had served as an adviser to the head of the Nationalist Government of China, Chiang Kai-shek; director of the Pacific Bureau of the Office of War Information; and member of Vice President Henry Wallace's 1944 mission to Siberia and China. McCarthy amended his charge and publicly asserted on March 30 the one cited in Marshall's and Tydings's letters. Tydings noted in his letter and request to Marshall that he was sending similar letters to Dean Acheson, Marshall's successor as secretary of state, and to Marshall's predecessors Cordell Hull and James Byrnes (Tydings to Marshall, April 17, 1950, GCMRL/G. C. Marshall Papers [American Red Cross, Subject, State Department, 1949–1950].)

On April 20, McCarthy had attacked Marshall directly for the first time, labeling him during a question-and-answer session following a speech before the American Society of Newspaper Editors as "completely unfit" to have been secretary of state and claiming he had "boned up" on China by reading Lattimore's work. ("M'Carthy Labels Marshall 'Unfit,'" *New York Times*, April 21, 1950, p. 3.)

On April 6, Francis H. Russell had written "purely on my own" to suggest that Marshall write to Tydings in response to McCarthy's attacks. Marshall had decided not to do so when Tydings's April 17 letter arrived. "This at once put a different face on the matter as the initiative was Tydings and the question was specific," Marshall informed Russell. "So I answered accordingly, including an expression of views regarding the effect of the present destructive and dangerous procedure on our foreign relations and our position in the world." (Russell to Marshall, April 6, 1950, GCMRL/G. C. Marshall Papers [American Red Cross, General]; Marshall to Russell, n.d., ibid.; H.)

3. "I don't remember the fellow at all," Marshall told George during a telephone conversation the morning of April 21. "Either General Hull or Jim Shepley can tell you more about that—they did all the conferring with the State Department. I was busy with the Pearl Harbor investigation then." (Transcript of Marshall's call to George, morning of April 21, 1950, GCMRL/G. C. Marshall Papers [American Red Cross, General].) For more on Marshall's testimony on Pearl Harbor, see *Papers of GCM*, 5: 377–83, 387–88, 520–21.) Lieutenant General John E. Hull had been chief of the Operations Division of the Army General Staff during the last year of World War II and had helped to draft the directive for Marshall's 1945–46 mission to China (Forrest C. Pogue, *George C. Marshall*, vol. 4, *Statesman, 1945–1959* [New York: Viking, 1987], 65); at this time he was deputy chief of staff for operations and administration in the Office of the Secretary of Defense (OSD). James R. Shepley was the Washington bureau chief for *Time* magazine who had worked on Marshall's 1943–45 report as army chief of staff and had assisted him in China in early 1946. For more on Marshall's final report see p. 879n4; for more on Shepley and Hull's part in Marshall's mission to China, see the index of *Papers of GCM*, 5.

Later on April 21, George reported that "As a result of our telephone conversation this afternoon, I first called General Hull—he was out of the city. I then called Jim Shepley and raised the questions we discussed. Shepley first said that he personally did not think that he had ever seen Lattimore unless it was at a time he didn't know about. He also confirmed that you had attended only one conference at the State Department and those present were [then Director of the Office of Far Eastern Affairs John Carter] Vincent, Byrnes, and Acheson. He said, 'Neither Hull nor I ever saw Lattimore anywhere, any time, any place.' He further stated that as a matter of independent recollection you never saw Lattimore and he doubts you ever heard of him." George also told Marshall that he had called Brigadier General Henry A. Byroade (USMA, 1937), former chief of the international affairs section of the Army General Staff who was then working in the State Department, who verified that "as far as he could recall you had never seen Lattimore and doubted that you had ever heard of him." Byroade added that "he himself had seen Lattimore but is positive that he did not participate in any of the conferences he attended and is sure without question that he was not present at the one conference you took part in." (George to Marshall, April 21, 1950, GCMRL/G. C. Marshall Papers [American Red Cross, General].)

Lattimore and Marshall had both participated in the State Department's roundtable discussions of October 6–8, 1949 (see pp. 5–14), but so had twenty-three other invited participants along with numerous State Department officials, and there is no record in the transcript of any verbal communication between the two men.

4. According to Marshall's American Red Cross secretary Alice McPherson, Marshall's letter was "dictated over the 'phone by General Marshall from Pinehurst" and delivered to Tydings's office on April 24, just in case the copy Marshall mailed from Pinehurst on a Sunday had not yet arrived. The same day Lattimore's brother-in-law Robert Armstrong Andrews wrote to Marshall that he and his wife "were very pleased this morning to hear over the radio the report of your 'NO COMMENT' to the ridiculous statement of Senator Joseph R. McCarthy. . . . We have been very disturbed by the McCarthy method, which is really trial by hearsay instead of trial by rules of evidence. Your attitude toward McCarthy is one we wish would become universal. He is beneath contempt." (McPherson to Tydings, and Andrews to Marshall, April 24, 1950, ibid.)

59

To Colonel Charles S. Roller Jr. — April 26, 1950
Pinehurst, North Carolina

Dear Chief: I read your interesting letter of the 17th which was addressed to Leesburg and just reached me here at Pinehurst. Mrs. Marshall and I are enjoying our winter quarters as the weather has been delightful and I have had fine sport—riding, fishing and on occasion hunting.

Your request for my views on R.O.T.C. is quite ethical, but I am entirely out of touch with matters of this nature and am avoiding intruding myself into military policies.[1]

I am scheduled to address the graduating class of the Pennsylvania Women's College in Pittsburgh the morning of June 12th.[2] I leave there by air for Roanoke, arriving late in the afternoon then motor over to Lexington and will have to leave before lunch the next morning. Mrs. Marshall will not accompany me and my itinerary denies me the pleasure of spending the night. Thanks anyway.[3] With warm regards, Faithfully yours,

GCMRL/G. C. Marshall Papers (American Red Cross, General)

1. Roller, a classmate of Marshall's in the VMI class of 1901 and the principal of Augusta Military Academy in Fort Defiance, Virginia, had written twice—on February 16

and again on April 17—to complain about an alteration in army regulations that had previously allowed students at junior Reserve Officer Training Corps (ROTC) schools to be commissioned as second lieutenants in the reserves upon graduation but now required two additional years of attendance at a senior college or university with an ROTC unit before commissioning. "If I am entirely ethical," he wrote to Marshall on April 17, "I would like your views." (Roller to Marshall, April 17, 1950, GCMRL/G. C. Marshall Papers [American Red Cross, General].) "I value your advice and judgment more than anyone in America today, so please write me with some constructive criticism for or against what I have written you." (Ibid.)

2. See pp. 102–8.

3. "It would give Janet and myself the greatest pleasure in the world to have you and Mrs. Marshall come some time and spend the night with us," Roller concluded, noting that Marshall was scheduled to give the commencement address at VMI in June. (Ibid.) See pp. 67–68 and 108–10. Roanoke, Virginia, is fifty-five miles south of Lexington; Fort Defiance is forty-five miles north of Lexington.

60

To F. Trubee Davison

April 28, 1950
Pinehurst, North Carolina

Dear Trubee: I have just read the excellent editorial in Thursday's edition of the New York Times on your retirement as President of the American Museum of Natural History and Mrs. Marshall and I hasten to add our tribute of "a job well done" to the many you will receive.[1] We doubt very seriously that you will actually retire to a life of rest and relaxation but will continue as you have in the past working for the benefit of your countrymen.

We close our place here on Monday next and move North to Leesburg. For the most part the winter was very pleasant and it afforded us the opportunity of spending many hours out of doors. I have had fine sport, riding most every day and frequent fishing and hunting excursions, but I should add that all these pleasures came between and after the trips I made in connection with the Red Cross campaign. Incidentally, my travels took me some 35,000 miles, with numerous meetings, speeches and the usual press conferences.

With our very best wishes and warm regards to you and the family,[2] Faithfully yours,

GCMRL/G. C. Marshall Papers (American Red Cross, General)

1. "The news that F. Trubee Davison will retire at the end of eighteen years in office as president of the American Museum of Natural History," the *New York Times* opined on April 27, "certainly calls for an expression of public gratitude for his services. . . . He has devoted himself continuously to an institution that gives pleasure and instruction to millions and carries on research of great value to mankind. . . . We gladly pay tribute to a man who has been useful to his city and his country." ("Mr. Davison's Service," *New York Times*, April 27, 1950, p. 28.)

2. "I appreciate tremendously your very nice letter about my retirement as president of the American Museum of Natural History," Davison replied. "I have no specific plan for the future, but will be on this job for another 18 months, so I will have plenty of time to talk myself into trouble by then. It was nice to know that you had such a plea[*sa*]nt winter in Pinehurst, in spite of the strenuous Red Cross campaigning which you had to do, and which

I heard about from many sources. It was a red letter day for the Davison family when you became president of the Red Cross." (Davison to Marshall, May 4, 1950, GCMRL/G. C. Marshall Papers [American Red Cross, General].) Davison's father, Henry Pomeroy Davison, had served as chairman of the War Council of the American Red Cross during World War I, had been instrumental in founding the international League of Red Cross Societies, and had served as its chairman until his death in 1922.

61

To W. Walton Butterworth

May 8, 1950
Washington, DC

My dear Butterworth: Thank you for your note of the fifth and Page A 3445 of the Congressional Record.[1] The Record these days does not occupy a position on my reading agenda and it is only through the thoughtfulness of people such as you that I have the opportunity to read something of what is being said on the Hill.

Mrs. Marshall and I are now back in Leesburg. I find that my job with Red Cross is quite demanding of my time and I will be making frequent visits to the office. Mrs. Marshall is still being harassed by shingles in the eyes and in an attempt to secure some relief has taken to drinking carrot juice. I certainly hope it has some curative powers.

With warm regards to you and the family, Faithfully yours,

G. C. Marshall

GCMRL/W. W. Butterworth Papers

1. "I suppose you do not feel it incumbent upon you to read the Congressional Record these days," wrote Butterworth, the assistant secretary of state for Far Eastern Affairs, on May 5. "I must say that I wish I could say the same. Nevertheless, I thought you would be interested to see the attached and take note of the Honorable Ralph W. Gwinn's name for future reference." (Butterworth to Marshall, May 5, 1950, GCMRL/G. C. Marshall Papers [American Red Cross, Subject, State Department, 1949–1950].) Representative Gwinn (R-NY) had spoken in defense of Alfred Kohlberg, one of Gwinn's constituents, on the floor of the House and had expanded his address to include attacks on Marshall and others, calling Marshall "a prisoner of the Communist cell in the Department who knew exactly how to feed him the right information and keep any doubters far from him." (*Congressional Record* 96, pt. 8, 81st Cong., 2d sess., A3258.) See pp. 80–81.

62

To Clyde Lewis[1]

May 10, 1950
Washington, DC

My dear Lewis: At the time of the death of Field Marshal Sir John Dill, the Congress passed a resolution regarding his contribution to our joint war effort with England (copy attached).[2] This action of the Congress was unique in that it had never been taken in connection with any other foreigner.

We of the American Chiefs of Staff, Admiral King, General Arnold and myself and our immediate associates, General [Brehon B.] Somervell, General [Muir S.] Fairchild and several others, were so keenly aware of the tremendous importance of Sir John's contribution to the necessary British-American accord involved in our world strategy that we thought it essential a memorial be erected so that his memory and the Resolution in Congress might be kept alive to impress future generations with the importance of an intimate understanding between our two countries.[3] Probably that is more evident now than it was even at the time of our joint effort in the war.

Dill was interred in Arlington Cemetery by authority of the Secretary of War, Mr. Stimson, and with the recognition of that procedure by the Congress.

In furtherance of our purpose a committee was formed and Mr. Robert Woods Bliss was asked to act as chairman. A list of the committee is attached.[4] We proceeded to raise the necessary funds for a suitable memorial which would fix the attention of the passer-by sufficiently to cause him to pause and read the resolution of the Congress, and also the citation of the President, Mr. Roosevelt. Arrangements were made with a sculptor for the execution of the memorial, a very fine statue of Sir John mounted. The area in the cemetery assigned by the Secretary of War is suitable, in fact was selected, for that purpose.

Having gone so far there then developed a resolution submitted by the Department of Virginia which eventually, I think, was called Resolution No. 510, proposing that Sir John's interment in Arlington Cemetery be terminated and, in effect, reflecting very seriously on the procedure contemplated. This was somewhat modified at a meeting of your national convention but its effect was to stir up hostile references in certain newspapers whose policy has been one of antagonism to most things British.

General Eisenhower, as Chief of Staff, brought the matter to the attention of the Judge Advocate General who confirmed the procedure contemplated.[5] Now as the time draws near for the erection of the statue another article appears provoked by the visit of Sir Basil Brooke, Prime Minister of Northern Ireland, who incidentally is the nephew of Field Marshal [Alan] Brooke, wartime Chief of the Imperial General Staff and Chairman of the British Chiefs of Staff.

I am addressing you directly to learn if your organization is contemplating any action regarding this project which would tend to defeat its purpose. I regard this matter as very serious because, in my opinion at least, at no time has it been so important that the United States preserve as much of an accord as practical with the leading nation of Western Europe.

I would appreciate your treating this matter, for the time being at least, as confidential between you and myself.[6] Faithfully yours.

GCMRL/G. C. Marshall Papers (American Red Cross, Subject. Subject, Field Marshal Sir John Dill Memorial Committee)

1. Clyde A. Lewis was the national commander of the Veterans of Foreign Wars (VFW).
2. The resolution, which had been approved by Congress on December 20, 1944, read: "WHEREAS the Congress having been informed of the death of Field Marshal Sir John Dill, in Washington, District of Columbia, on November 4, 1944; and WHEREAS the Arlington National Cemetery has been chosen as the final resting place of this distinguished soldier; and WHEREAS as the Senior British representative on the Combined Chiefs of Staff, Field Marshal Sir John Dill, by his wisdom and devotion to the vital cause

of British-American military cooperation, rendered a great service to the United Nations: Now, therefore, be it Resolved by the Senate and the House of Representatives of the United States of America in Congress assembled, that the outstanding service rendered to the United Nations by Field Marshal Sir John Dill be, and it hereby is, recognized by the American people and the Congress of the United States." (Public Law 516, 78th Cong., 2d sess.) See *Papers of GCM*, 4: 694–95 and 5: 5–6.

3. Major General Muir S. Fairchild had been director of military requirements for the army air forces.

4. In addition to Marshall, members of the Field Marshal Sir John Dill Memorial Committee were Admiral King, Vice Chief of Naval Operations Admiral Frederick J. Horne (USNA, 1899), General Brehon Somervell, Deputy Commander in Chief of the United States Fleet and Deputy Chief of Naval Operations Admiral Richard S. Edwards (USNA, 1907), Deputy Chief of Staff of the United States Fleet Rear Admiral Bernhard H. Bieri (USNA, 1911), Chairman of the Board of Chase National Bank Winthrop Aldrich, President of International General Electric Clark H. Minor, and Robert Woods Bliss. General Arnold had served on the committee until his death in January; General Fairchild, who had died on March 17, 1950, had also been on the committee.

5. Eisenhower was army chief of staff from November 19, 1945, to February 6, 1948.

6. Lewis replied that there was presently no resolution pending but that one "might be offered" at the Virginia State Encampment. He had been assured by state officers that if the national staff was opposed, "every effort will be made to discourage its adoption should it come up for consideration." While there was "some sentiment" in the state against "unusual honors to a foreign soldier" in Arlington, he continued, the national staff took "a dim view of such an elaborate memorial" as the one being proposed. "The principal bone of contention is the fact that such an unusually large plot of ground had been set aside" for the memorial. The staff would have "no objection" to Dill's remains staying in Arlington or to a small statue, but felt it "unreasonable to set aside approximately one acre of ground in the Cemetery for this memorial. . . . I sincerely believe that if the memorial to Sir John Dill could be limited to a small plot of ground not in excess of that which has been allocated to some of our own great Americans, that we could oppose any resolutions calling for the removal of the remains of Sir John Dill or objecting to the erection of a memorial statue." Lewis concluded that the staff had "the greatest esteem and affection for you as our wartime leader and as a distinguished American and that we will go as far as possible in trying to accede to your wishes." (Lewis to Marshall, May 22, 1950, GCMRL/G. C. Marshall Papers [American Red Cross, Subject, Field Marshal Sir John Dill Memorial Committee].)

63

Remarks at the Library of Congress[1] — May 17, 1950, Washington, DC

In the presence of this distinguished company and associated here this afternoon with great authorities on the life and contributions to American history of Thomas Jefferson, it would be presumptuous, to put it more plainly, it would be foolish of me to offer any comments of mine on the subject of Thomas Jefferson. However, I think it permissible to take the liberty of expressing a thought regarding him and his associates that has been in my mind for some time, and it is this:

What has impressed me most regarding Thomas Jefferson and his time was his age when he made his first great contribution in drafting the Declaration of Independence and the fact of the extreme youth of his immediate associates who played such a great part in the struggle for our freedom and independence and an even greater part in the drafting of the Constitution of the United States. I refer, of course, to Alexander Hamilton, James Madison and James Monroe. The average age of these three men in 1776 was 20 years.[2] Jefferson was 33. That is astonishing when one considers the tremendous part they were to play while still very young men in the birth of this government. But what is more impressive to me was the breadth and depth of their research into the lessons of history and the recorded philosophy of the great thinkers of the past on the subject of the rights of men. I admit to a feeling of humiliation when I realized how profound had been their studies when so very young and how sketchy and superficial mine have been over a long period of years.

These four men of course reached manhood in the most critical period of the Colonies, when every man's mind was focused on the limitations and restrictions imposed on his local government and on himself personally by the rulers of the mother country. They had little to distract them from consideration of the issues involved. The Bill of Rights was born and then came the Declaration of Independence, recognized the world over, I think, as a great milestone in the history of man. And after that there followed the long years of bitter endurance until the Revolutionary War was brought to a conclusion. There was much time for sober thinking and prolonged discussions. Finally came the victory and with the victory, as seems usually to be the case, came the greatest dilemma of all.

These young men were now to pass through a post graduate course, as it were, on the futility of a national government based on a loose confederation. They arrived at last, after this prolonged period of self-education and remarkable experience, at the hour for drafting the great concluding chapter of this extraordinary period— the Constitution of the United States of America. I must remark on the fact that their youth was tempered by the calm poise of a Washington and the profound wisdom of one of the greatest philosophers and realists in history, Benjamin Franklin.

What interests me particularly in this matter is a comparison with the situation today, a comparison relative to the principal actors. I see no group of young men, such as these four I have been referring to, exercising a dominating, at the very least a strong immediate influence on the development of our country. On the contrary I see an educational system which confines most young men to the proposition of education in the abstract until they are well into their middle 20s and in some cases approaching their 30s. In other words, the present system seems to retard the active participation of young men during that virile period when the sap is running to the full.

I think I am correct in saying that Thomas Jefferson was an American pioneer in the field of education, but I doubt if he foresaw the course of its development in this highly complicated and technical age.[3]

GCMRL/G. C. Marshall Papers (American Red Cross, Speeches and Statements)

1. Princeton University President Harold Dodds had invited Marshall to speak at the ceremony marking the publication of the first volume of the writings of Thomas Jefferson. See p. 61.

2. Alexander Hamilton was born on January 11, 1757; James Madison was born on March 16, 1751; James Monroe was born on April 28, 1758.

3. On May 19, Dodds wrote Marshall to "confirm my oral thanks to you for your part in the celebration of the publication of the first volume of the Jefferson Papers held at the Library of Congress Wednesday. It was a tremendous personal pleasure to me to have you there and be able to hand you a suitably bound copy of the first volume." (Dodds to Marshall, May 19, 1950, GCMRL/G. C. Marshall Papers [American Red Cross, General].)

64

To John Seabrook

May 17, 1950
Washington, DC

My dear Seabrook: It was good to receive your letter of May eighth and learn of your close association with the Auckland Center of the New Zealand Red Cross.[1]

A number of our publications are being sent to you under separate cover. I feel that Dr. MacCormick will be particularly interested in the material on fund raising and hope he will find it useful as plans for Auckland's forthcoming fund campaign are developed.

We recently moved north to Leesburg and are devoting a good number of hours of our day to the garden. While Mrs. Marshall's eyes are improving with the aid of carrot juice, she still suffers some discomfort. I am happy to report that my health is good.

With my heavy schedule of Red Cross work together with commencement speeches I have agreed to make, I expect to be constantly on the go for the next few months. I thoroughly enjoy all of this activity but arrange it so I will have time for relaxation.

With warm regards, Faithfully yours,

GCMRL/G. C. Marshall Papers (American Red Cross, General)

1. Seabrook had written Marshall on May 8 in reply to an earlier letter (see pp. 70–71). Seabrook's friend, Dr. Kenneth MacCormick, had recently been appointed president of the New Zealand Red Cross, and Seabrook had forwarded him information on Marshall's Red Cross activities for use on his "recently-launched campaign to put Red Cross in this part of New Zealand on its feet." He continued, "Dr. MacCormick is organizing a Red Cross drive for increased membership and funds, and I am sure he will meet with the success he deserves. In this work my wife and I shall do all we can to assist him. It would be greatly appreciated if you could arrange for one of your staff to post me some booklets or descriptive matter outlining the activities of American Red Cross, because I am sure that this material will be of great assistance and value here." (Seabrook to Marshall, May 8, 1950, GCMRL/G. C. Marshall Papers [American Red Cross, General].)

65

To Madame Chiang Kai-shek[1]

May 29, 1950
Washington, DC

Dear Madame: Katherine has wanted to write you a long newsy letter but she is still suffering quite a bit from her shingles, now seemingly confined to her right eye. So I am going to give you all the news that might be of interest to you and she will complete the letter in her own long-hand.

She tells me she wrote to you from Hawaii where we were for four days on combination Pan-American Airlines business and Red Cross affairs. She stood the trip around and back to San Francisco in fine shape but flying East from there, in a plane like the "Sacred Cow"—which as you know has no pressure cabin—she suffered from altitude sickness because they had to fly rather high and she did not tell anyone she was feeling badly and therefore did not take oxygen in time.[2] However, on arrival in New York we took off in fifteen minutes for Fort Monroe where Molly is and got down there without any inconvenience.[3] But there it was quite cold and she proceeded to take cold. So when we left thirty-six hours later she was in rather bad shape and on arrival in Washington went straight to the hospital and was confined there for a week and, incidentally, was herself very weak. As a matter of fact, I was relieved to have her there because I was on a Red Cross schedule which required me to be on the road for just a week. On checking in at Washington I picked her up and flew her down to Pinehurst where, with the lovely weather and the early spring flowers, she got back to normal in a very short time, except for the shingles.

I, incidentally, was away most of January, February and early March. As a matter of fact, my Red Cross activities kept me on the road for some thirty thousand miles and averaged about two cities a day.

We found Molly and the children all well and nicely located, though the apartment was rather small. Kitty in particular inquired about you and, of course, Molly and Colonel Winn.

We did not see Clifton and his wife in New York because we were only there fifteen minutes and that at the airport early in the morning. However, later I took Katherine to New York with me on a Red Cross trip and she saw them there. Their baby is a lovely little boy—apparently a good looking fine specimen.[4]

Allene and her husband spent part of the winter in Florida and then three weeks at Pinehurst at a hotel quite near our place. They did not come to the cottage because they did not want to impose any burden on Katherine until she fully recovered. They preceded us to Leesburg by about a month.[5] We came up May 3 and found everything shipshape and the tulips that you planted were in beautiful bloom. The whole place looked better this year than ever before and now is a riot of blooming peonies, poppies and other early flowers. The dogwood and azaleas were very lovely this spring.

We had a large dinner to celebrate Allene's wedding anniversary and I think we go to a dinner in a few nights celebrating Sterling Lacy's birthday.

Katherine and I left Dodona at 7:15 this morning and drove in to town.[6] She immediately went shopping. She meets me for a luncheon that I am giving the President of the International Red Cross Committee from Switzerland.[7] Tomorrow we come up in town for me to make the Memorial Day address at the amphitheater in Arlington Cemetery, and then to a lunch for this same official at the Swiss Legation. The next day I leave for Denver at 11 a.m., arriving there in time for a dinner meeting and leave the next morning at 7:30 for a talk I am to give at the Staff College at Fort Leavenworth. Katherine will not be with me.

On the 12th of June she receives a degree (Humane Letters) from the Pittsburgh Women's College, an old institution in Pittsburgh, Pennsylvania. From there we fly down to Lexington, Virginia, where I deliver the graduation address and attend a meeting of the Board of Visitors of which I am a member.[8] Then we turn to a motor car and drive over to Charlottesville for the night and visit some of the relatives of the first Mrs. Marshall, but I am due here in Washington for a meeting of the Business Advisory Council for luncheon and the remainder of the afternoon.[9]

The end of the month Katherine will be with me for four or five days in Detroit for the National Convention of the Red Cross, some four thousand representatives.[10]

We have not made up our minds where to go this summer. Margaret Emerson wishes us to pay her a visit but I doubt if we do this.[11] And we have been considering South America, Canada and several mountain resorts in this country.

We have seen quite a bit of Margaret Emerson who, incidentally, spent a week end with us at Pinehurst. She is a very cheerful person.

We have had you in mind almost daily, knowing how difficult and troubled your life must be. Occasionally we see some reports of you direct and have heard that you have been in the newsreels although we missed the showings. Generalissimo, in spite of all the strain he must be undergoing, appears to be in good shape. Just how he manages to do so is hard to understand.

I have learned this morning that Hollington Tong is in town and wishes to see me.[12] I'll arrange to see him a little later in the week when I am back.

I gave your wonderful luggage a good bit of travel this winter as my mileage indicates and I also used that coat you gave me throughout, reinforcing it with an interlining when I struck very cold weather. I have been in good shape this winter and have gotten back to the point where I can do fairly heavy physical work down at Leesburg without undue fatigue providing I confine it to half-day efforts.

Katherine and I are learning to play Canasta but she cannot last out an entire game because of her eye. And now, Madame, I'll turn you over to Katherine for a more intimate report. I send you my most affectionate regards and please make my compliments to the Generalissimo.

GCMRL/G. C. Marshall Papers (Pentagon Office, Selected)

1. Madame Chiang Kai-shek (Soong Mei-ling) was the wife of Generalissimo Chiang Kai-shek.

2. The *Sacred Cow* had been President Franklin Roosevelt's personal airplane. See *Papers of GCM*, 6: 194.

3. Molly Brown Winn was Katherine Marshall's daughter. For other family members mentioned in this letter, see p. 39n4.

4. Clifton Brown's wife, Em Bowles Locker, gave birth to a daughter, Carter Boardman Brown, on November 15, 1949.

5. See p. 62n2.

6. See p. 34n1.

7. Paul Ruegger was the president of the International Committee of the Red Cross.

8. Marshall was scheduled to deliver the commencement address at the Pennsylvania College for Women on June 12 as well as at VMI on June 13. See pp. 102–10.

9. See p. 110n4.

10. See pp. 113–22.

11. Emerson was a friend of Katherine Marshall. See *Papers of GCM*, 6: 744–45.

12. Hollington Tong was a Chinese Nationalist diplomat and scholar.

66

Remarks Memorial Day Services at Arlington Cemetery[1]

May 30, 1950
Arlington, Virginia

This is Memorial Day—a day dedicated some 80 years ago to the stirring of our memories of those who fell in the Country's battles, many of whom surround us here in Arlington Cemetery. There have been many Memorial Day addresses here and there will be many more but, as for me, my memories go back to a certain day where in an olive grove on the scene of a fierce battle which had just terminated in a great allied victory, I joined with troops resting from the ordeal of battle on that field. They observed their Memorial Day on the ground they had just fought for and where their fallen comrades had but a few days previously been laid to rest.[2] There we were not talking of the remote past—our thoughts were centered on the scenes of fury and devastation around us and the certainty of greater struggles soon to follow. Many of the men in that particular regiment, an unusually large percentage as a matter of fact, fell in the further fighting, and it was evident that each man was thinking of the sacrifice he very probably would too soon be called upon to make. The setting that evening, the expressions on the faces of those men, and the prospects of the immediate future made a profound impression upon me which I would re-create in your minds today, if it were possible for me to translate the emotions of that hour. Those men quite evidently looked to us to redeem the sacrifices their comrades had already made and that they felt they were soon to make, as so many did. The situation was concrete and very much of the present, and not a retrospect of the past as is largely ours today.

As Chairman of the Battle Monuments Commission I am concerned with plots of ground all over the world where our men lie buried, young men brought to a sudden ending of life in the fight to maintain our way of life. Our great responsibility to them is to protect their loved ones and their friends from the agonies and miseries of war. Their living comrades, the veterans of today, alone know what war really is—that there is nothing to be said in favor of war except that it *is* the lesser of two evils. For it *is* better than appeasement of aggression because appeasement encourages the very aggression it seeks to prevent. And it *is* far better than submission to tyranny and oppression, because without freedom and respect for human dignity life would not be worth living.

Unless we are faced with the choice of these terrible alternatives, I think we should concentrate on finding peaceful solutions to the world's problems. Peace should be a dynamic force and not a negative condition that is merely the absence of armed hostilities. We should support to the full every existing instrument to the building of a more stable world. *So long* as there is a forum for open discussion of international disputes, the United States should be a participant. *So long* as there remains a conference table around which the nations can gather, the United States should be the first to attend and the last to retire. Only thus can we earn the right to stand here in the presence of the graves of these many men who were cut off in their youth from the life we enjoy and say in good conscience, "We are doing our best to justify your sacrifice."

A most terrible aspect of war is the toll it takes of the youth of the country. The average age of the men of the armed forces in the last war was about 26 years. The average age of those who perished would probably be less since the older men in service were not generally employed in combat.

And so, we lost almost Three Hundred Thousand of the nation's youth.

Repeated depletion of vigorous and productive manpower has been the undoing of many civilizations. We have been relatively fortunate in that our wars have not resulted for us in wholesale destruction. But we cannot be certain of the future.

It would be unwise, it seems to me, to console ourselves with the thought that we would ultimately win if hostilities should break out again, because I fear that the victorious power in another war will stand amidst its own ruins with little strength left to re-establish itself or to offer assistance to its neighbors. It will only enjoy the empty triumph of inheriting the responsibility for a shattered and impoverished world.

To one who follows the current trend of thought among the Western European Powers it is evident that they are well aware of this. They realize that whoever wins another war, their generation will lose it; they know that peace is a condition necessary to their survival and they look to this country not only for material and military strength to offset the probability of war, but, more importantly, I am sure that they look to us for a clear restatement of the moral principles we feel are essential to a peaceful international society.

Some have suggested that the United States should take the lead in dissolving the United Nations and in setting up a new organization composed only of like-minded nations. Personally I think it would be unfortunate for the peace of the world deliberately to upset the precarious equilibrium that now exists. The United Nations symbolizes one of mankind's highest aspirations—an international house of democracy, a true brotherhood of the nations. We should not, it seems to me, deliberately turn away from that symbol, else we would weaken our moral position before the world and surrender at least a part of our leadership in the fight for peace.

One of the things for which our comrades gave their lives was to bring fellowship closer to reality. We have not realized that dream. Admittedly the United Nations is an imperfect organization. But remember it does provide a forum where words can be used instead of bullets. And so long as this forum remains open there are cracks in the iron curtain through which some of our ideas will penetrate.

Those who have lost faith in the organization profess alarm because the Eastern Powers use it as a platform for the dissemination of communist propaganda. But we also have the privilege of telling our story through the same medium. And in any contest of ideas, I think honesty will finally win in the long run for truth must prevail, and I'll wager my money on American principles of freedom and equality under law, and tolerance and justice for all men.

Then too, we have much the better story if we tell it well and tell it affirmatively. We have taken the offensive regarding communism. But we should constantly remind all people that no nation has ever embraced any form of totalitarian rule through exercise of the popular will.

However, the ferment that is stirring around the world today is not all communist inspired. A large part of it, I believe, results from an upsurge of peoples who have long suffered in poverty and misrule. And the millions who live under such sub-normal conditions are entitled to a fair share of the God-given rights of human beings. It is a challenge to the more favored nations to lend assistance in bettering their lot.

Furthermore, self-interest demands that we give close attention to these peoples for their situation is the seedbed for either one of two ways of life—democracy or communism. If we act with wisdom we can guide this yearning to the better things of life through democratic channels.

We must present democracy as a force holding within itself the seeds of unlimited progress for the human race. We should make clear that it is a means to a better way of life within nations and to a better understanding among nations. Tyranny inevitably must fall back before the tremendous moral strength of the gospel of freedom and self respect for the individual.

But we must have in mind that these democratic principles do not flourish on empty stomachs. And that people turn to the false promises of dictators because they are hopeless and anything promises better than the miserable existence they endure.

However, I am certain that material assistance alone is not sufficient. The most important thing for the world today, in my opinion, is a spiritual regeneration which would restore a feeling of good faith and good will among men generally. Discouraged people are sorely in need of the inspiration of great principles. Such leadership can be the rallying point against intolerance, against distrust and against that fatal insecurity that leads to war. I hope that we will provide that leadership. But we will have to get back to first principles if we are to speak with a voice that will kindle the imagination and rouse the spirit.

We have made much of America's strength and material prosperity. We have talked a great deal about the American way of life. But our material prosperity may or may not be exportable. A dynamic philosophy, on the other hand, knows no restrictions of time or space. And we *do* have an American creed that comes to us from the deep roots of the past. It springs from the convictions and hopes of men and women from many lands who founded this nation and made it great. You will find that creed, that heritage in the Declaration of Independence and the Constitution with its Bill of Rights.

Although it may have been without a clear realization, those were the things for which our men fought and died; those are the ideals which we can offer to the world with the certainty that they have the power to inspire people and to impel them to action.

I do not mean that we should try to persuade other people to accept our form of government, but rather the great fundamentals on which it is based. I mean that the basic principles on which our government was founded are timeless and have validity for all mankind.

But it must be remembered that raising our voice to the world imposes upon us a most serious obligation. We cannot convince others unless we are true to ourselves. We must be satisfied in our own hearts that we give more than lip service to these principles we profess.

When we call for our great individual freedoms, we must be sure that no infringement of these rights is permitted or tolerated because of emotions of the moment.

In some such spirit let us devote ourselves to a generous service to our fellow men just as these dead about us dedicated their lives to that service. I believe that our lost comrades would want it exactly that way.

We have before us the greatest task ever faced by any generation of men in the fight to preserve peace. War, I say again, is no longer just an evil. In this age it seems intolerable.

Our greatest tribute to our dead will be a devotion to the resolve that war must not happen again. But we must not—I emphasize, we must not, as we invariably have done in the past, render ourselves impotent, an invitation to the ruthless aggressor. Also, we should not place complete dependence on military and material power. It is a difficult road we have to follow but we have a wealth of lessons from the past and with clear heads and with genuine willingness to support our efforts, I think we can lead the world into a better life than now seems apparent.

"With malice toward none; with charity for all; . . . let us strive on to finish the work we are in; . . . to care for him who shall have borne the battle, and for his widow, and his orphan—to do all which may achieve and cherish a just and lasting peace among ourselves, and with all nations."[3]

GCMRL/G. C. Marshall Papers (American Red Cross, Speeches and Statements)

1. Lee R. Pennington, president of the Grand Army of the Republic Memorial Day Corporation, had written Marshall on April 14 that the corporation's officers and directors "would deem it a signal honor to have you as our speaker at the Memorial Day Services at the Arlington Amphitheater" on May 30, 1950. "I appreciate the compliment of your invitation," Marshall replied on April 20, "and accept with pleasure." (Pennington to Marshall,

April 14, 1950, and Marshall to Pennington, April 20, 1950, GCMRL/G. C. Marshall Papers [American Red Cross, Categorical, Invitations, Accepted].)

2. The event took place in Tunisia in May 1943. See *Marshall Interviews*, 323–25.

3. This is an abbreviated quotation from the final paragraph of Abraham Lincoln's second inaugural address, delivered in Washington on March 4, 1865. "I thought your Memorial Day address was a masterpiece," President Truman wrote to Marshall on June 7, (Truman to Marshall, June 7, 1950, GCMRL/G. C. Marshall Collection [Truman].)

67

TO ARTHUR H. VANDENBERG

June 6, 1950
Washington, DC

Dear Arthur: I feel especially complimented by your comments regarding my address at Arlington.[1] As usual you are very generous in your expressions and I am duly appreciative.

Katherine and I were glad to see the picture of you in the paper the other day for it indicates that you have weathered well your struggles and are on the road back to good health.[2]

We had the Hoffmans' down for early supper on Saturday and I found him to be quite an expert on the problems of gardening.[3] Between us we devised a plan to combat the persistent bugs and beetles.

We pray that your Hazel is on the mend as we do hope to have you both down here in the country soon. Affectionately,

GCMRL/G. C. Marshall Papers (American Red Cross, Subject, Memorial Day Speech Comments)

1. Vanderberg had written "to say that I should have been very proud to have made the speech you made at Arlington on Memorial Day. It was a brilliant, vital, moving address which greatly needed to be made and which could best be made by you." (Vandenberg to Marshall, June 2, 1950, GCMRL/G. C. Marshall Papers [American Red Cross, Subject, Memorial Day Speech Comments].) See previous document.

2. See "Text of Acheson's Statement on Foreign Arms Aid Program," *New York Times*, June 3, 1950, p. 2.

3. Marshall is referring to ECA Director Paul Hoffman and his wife, Dorothy.

68

TO JAMES R. SHEPLEY

June 6, 1950
Washington, DC

Dear Shepley: Many thanks for your comments on my Memorial Day speech.[1] So far the reaction to my talk has been very satisfying.

Mrs. Marshall and I ran into Frank McCarthy as we were leaving the amphitheater and we asked him down to Leesburg for dinner and the night, which he accepted.[2] He appeared to be in fine shape and quite enthusiastic about his work.

I will have George telephone you and arrange for our getting together. It might be that we can have lunch on Wednesday next, however I will let you know.[3]

Faithfully yours,

GCMRL/G. C. Marshall Papers (Secretary of Defense, Selected)

1.Shepley had written to compliment Marshall on his Memorial Day speech at Arlington (see pp. 94–98) and to comment on Marshall's statement that "there is nothing to be said in favor of war except that it is the lesser of two evils. For it is better than appeasement of aggression. . . . And it is far better than submission to tyranny and oppression, because without freedom and respect for human dignity life would not be worth living." Shepley remarked that "I wish this statement could be added to the American Constitution. Then, of course, we would not only have a Bill of Rights, but a Bill of Obligations." (Shepley to Marshall, May 31, 1950, GCMRL/G. C. Marshall Papers [Secretary of Defense, Selected].)

2. Shepley had written, "I chanced on Frank McCarthy shortly after his arrival in town this week and his first question to me was of you." (Ibid.)

3. "If you have free time on one of the occasions you are next in Washington on Red Cross business," Shepley had added, "I would appreciate very much an opportunity to come by and spend a few minutes with you. Perhaps, if your schedule is not too rigid, we could have lunch somewhere." (Ibid.) Shepley and Marshall had lunch in Washington on Wednesday, June 7.

69

Testimony on the Mutual Defense Assistance Program
June 7, 1950 Washington, DC

House Foreign Affairs Committee, 10:30 a.m.–12:20 p.m.

HE HAD not thought it "a very wise business" to attempt to be briefed by the State Department and the Pentagon prior to his appearance before the committee, Marshall said, so he would confine himself "to the fundamentals involved." He repeated what he had told the House Armed Services Committee in October (see pp. 17–19) about the initial concentration of US funding on economic recovery in 1947–48, and only subsequently on the need for rearmament in Western Europe. "There was no thought at the time of becoming involved in any armament program. However, as time went on, it became glaringly apparent" that the morale of the West Europeans "was very materially affected, not only by their fear of the military power of the Soviets, but particularly of their own weakness, which at that time was very marked. . . . They felt quite helpless. And as their fear grew their feeling of helplessness grew with it, so it became apparent to many of us close to the program that something had to be done to bolster up their morale, in addition to the economic rehabilitation on which we had initially engaged. The only method that appeared practical at the time to accomplish this was the armament program." Marshall had first discussed the program at length with European representatives during the fall 1948 UN meeting in Paris (see *Papers of GCM*, 6: 551–626). He believed it had definitely helped to restore Western Europe's morale and should be continued, albeit not indefinitely. (US House of Representatives, Committee on Foreign Affairs, *To Amend the Mutual Defense Assistance Act of 1949: Hearings . . .* , 81st Cong., 2d sess. [Washington: GPO, 1950], 85–86.) The act sought $1 billion for the program's second year.

"To sit impotent is the most dangerous thing you can do," Marshall said in response to questions by Committee Chair John Kee (D-WV) and Charles A. Eaton (R-NJ). Soviet leaders were coldly calculating realists, so there was a greater possibility of reconciliation between the USSR and the West when the Soviets found themselves "up against an implacable determination on our part not to submit to the police-state procedure." Soviet leaders had their own troubles, "which I think will grow with time—I hope a short time—but certainly their growth will be encouraged by the fertilizing we are giving to western Europe." (Ibid., 88–89.)

Asked if he believed that another world war could be avoided only by being militarily strong, Marshall noted "that it is a matter of very fine judgment to what extent we go in our military restrengthening in relation to the necessary strength of our economy. That is one of the most difficult things to decide. You can wreck the economy of a country in a military effort, and you can have it wrecked because of your military impotency." (Ibid., 93.)

As he usually did whenever Marshall testified before the House Foreign Affairs Committee, Minnesota Republican Walter Judd, a perennial supporter of Nationalist China, raised the issue of the failure of the United States to support Chiang Kai-shek's regime to the extent it did European governments, particularly that of Greece. Judd asserted that the US government offered China only moral lectures and public criticisms rather than encouragement against the Communists. "I was there on the ground," Marshall replied, "and I think we did" offer more. Recognizing that he and Judd "have a complete difference of opinion" on this matter, Marshall emphasized the substantial aid, similar to the aid for the Europeans, that had been sent to China but that had "proved to be utterly futile." Why did we not send someone to China of the caliber of General James A. Van Fleet (USMA, 1915, head of the Joint US Military Advisory Group in Greece), Judd asked. "There was only one Van Fleet," Marshall asserted. "We sent him to Greece. . . . We sent [to China] what we thought were good men." (Ibid., 95–96. See also 104–8.)

Asked more than once by committee members to comment on the proposition that any attempt to build up Western Europe's military strength would precipitate a Soviet attack there to prevent the balance of power from shifting against it, Marshall dismissed the idea that a rearmed Western Europe would be an "aggressor force" as "a military absurdity" and said that the alternative idea to rearming the Europeans—that the United States could arm "to the teeth here" while "leaving Europe impotent"—was "psychologically wrong and militarily wrong, and just generally wrong. That procedure also assumes the policy that when Europe is overwhelmed we can go about our business in the usual way, which we could not in my opinion. We will be curbed and restricted in many ways aside from the direct threat to our own peace. We would have the whole world in the other camp." But could rearmament increase Soviet suspicions, Rep. John M. Vorys (R-OH) asked, thereby building "toward a fight?" Quite the opposite would be the case, Marshall thought. The Soviet leaders "are military men and they have developed a real military staff out of their great war experiences, and leaders, who would know full well that this western Europe set-up could not carry out an aggressive policy." (Ibid., 88–91, 100–101.)The US defense budget would need to be more than doubled should it decide to arm itself vigorously while not arming Western Europe, Marshall asserted, and given that the United States' greatest strength was its economy, cold calculation required that the economy be protected from excessive burdens by having Western Europe do its part. (Ibid., 102.)

Senate Committee on Foreign Relations and Committee on the Armed Services, 2:00–2:45 p.m.

Unlike the morning's public meeting, this one was held in executive session. Marshall repeated many of the points he had made to the House committee: e.g., that he had not been briefed and thus could only talk about "fundamentals"; that the original recovery program had been "purely economic" and included all of Europe; that the Soviets bore responsibility for the ensuing division of the continent; that military as well as economic aid had been "very regrettable" but "very necessary" to restore Western Europe's morale in the face of the Soviet threat; and that "it would be a grave error to withdraw into our shell right now and not go ahead with this program." Continuing the efforts of America's intelligence services was vital, he added in response to a question from Committee Chair Tom Connally (D-TX), but Americans "talked too much about it. That sort of thing has to be done in the dark." (US Senate, Committee on Foreign Relations, *Executive Sessions of the Senate Foreign Relations Committee* [*Historical Series*], vol. 2, 81st Cong., 1st and 2d sess., 1949–1950 [Washington: GPO, 1976], 426–28.)

It would be far less wasteful of scarce resources if the Dutch, Belgians, and French concentrated on providing ground forces and the United States on naval and air forces. Marshall described some of his previous efforts to convince European leaders of this proposition. (Ibid., 429–31.) Command and control of European military forces should be under a European, Marshall thought; in the event of a general war, however, "eventually we would have to take over the entire command." As secretary of state, "I was in favor of [British General Bernard Law] Montgomery" as Supreme Commander in Europe. "He is hard to get along with, but if he is on top he gets along pretty well with the fellow that is under him. I thought you needed a pretty tough actor. . . . I didn't see anyone there who could control Montgomery. I thought he had a better chance of control than any other fellow." (Ibid., 433.) ★

70

To Harry S. Truman

June 12, 1950
Washington, DC

My dear Mr. President: I have received your communication of June 5, notifying me of my reappointment as a Governor of The American National Red Cross for a term of three years from June 12, 1950, and designating me to act as the principal officer of the corporation during that period.[1]

I am highly honored by your confidence in me and will discharge my responsibilities to the best of my ability.

With great respect, Faithfully yours,

GCMRL/G. C. Marshall Papers (American Red Cross, General)

1. "Pursuant to the provision of Section 5, as amended, of the Act to incorporate the American National Red Cross," Truman had written, "I hereby reappoint you a Governor of the Corporation to serve on its Board of Governors for a term of three years from June 12, 1950. I also designate you to act as the Principal Officer of the Corporation, with such title and such functions as may from time to time be prescribed in the bylaws of said Corporation." (Truman to Marshall, June 5, 1950, GCMRL/G. C. Marshall Papers [American Red Cross, General].)

71

COMMENCEMENT ADDRESS AT THE PENNSYLVANIA COLLEGE FOR WOMEN[1]

June 12, 1950
Pittsburgh, Pennsylvania

I have been somewhat puzzled as to what I best might talk about to you young ladies this morning. I must not bore you with innocuous pleasantries or presumptuous advice. Just what I can find to talk about between those two poles is difficult to determine. However, I can say this, that I have been deeply interested all of my life, and more so as I grew older, in young people and their interests, their reactions and their possibilities.

In my business of soldiering I have had constantly to do with young men in large numbers and in a good many cases been responsible for the assignment of very young men to vast responsibilities and saw them discharged in a truly remarkable manner.

With regard to the very young, I want to tell you of an experience of mine with seven men of nine years each—professional Cub Scouts, who called on me in the State Department three years ago. Their chairman wrote to me requesting an opportunity to present their report on a so-called Junior Marshall Plan.[2] He was referring to the European Recovery Plan. I agreed to receive them, despite the fact that I was unusually busy. They arrived in my office one morning, spotless in their freshly pressed uniforms, each boy apparently having just had a haircut and all had scrubbed or been scrubbed until they shone. With them came, of course, the State Department press correspondents and a battery of photographers.

I seated the boys at a table and took the eighth seat myself.

When I called on the chairman to explain their visit he delivered himself of the complete information in one sentence. And while I was thanking him for his expressions and congratulating him on the brevity of his speech, it occurred to me what a complete contrast their action was to the days of my youth, what a perfect illustration it was of the tremendous change in America during the period of my own lifetime—a change which seems now not to be realized by the many debating or discussing the Recovery Program.

I am going to take the liberty of reading to you what I said to those boys on the spur of the moment that day, because it seemed then and seems now to me a pretty good illustration of the rapid development of this country as concerns its relations with the rest of the world. I said this, in speaking to those seven young men:

"I think what you are planning is a very fine thing. When I was a boy, I do not believe it would have been possible.

"As a matter of fact, in those days, about all we knew of the world was through our histories and geographies. We learned something of Europe, something of Africa, something of Asia. We knew, for instance, that they had kangaroos in Australia, and hot springs in New Zealand, but not much else.

"As I recall, 10 to 15 miles was nearly our limit of action because that meant a 20 to 30-mile drive or ride before you got home. When the bicycle came in, our radius of action was extended a bit.

"We knew little about the world—as a matter of fact, we knew very little about the United States except for those fortunate few who could afford railroad travel. Now, of course, that is all changed.

"Just recently I returned from London in a single night. I returned from Rio de Janeiro in Brazil, well south of the Equator, in a night and part of a morning the other day. I went out to attend a dinner in Salt Lake City and did not leave Washington until noon and I was back in Washington in time for breakfast the next morning.

"Now, Salt Lake City in my young days was a far-off place where there were Mormons. I thought probably I would never live to see it. But the other day it was merely a destination for a dinner engagement.

"I remember the first time I was aware of Manila and of the Philippines. It was when Admiral Dewey sailed from Hongkong at the opening of the Spanish-American War in 1898.[3] I knew about Manila rope and that was all I knew of the Philippines. And the high officials of the government knew little more, as the records show.

"Since then I have spent five years in the Philippines and more recently I was involved with a great operation to recover the Philippines from the hands of the Japanese.

"But the greatest change of all, I think, is our place in the world, from being little known and almost ignored when I was your age, until today, when in the short period of my lifetime we are now recognized as the most powerful of nations and the acknowledged leader in the world. In my youth there was not a foreign ambassador accredited to Washington—we only ranked foreign ministers.

"All this is why I think it is so impressive for a group of boys of your age to undertake to provide food for a year for a number of starving children in Europe. It is a generous and fine action on your part for those children who are in dire need of such help. And it is of real international importance to this government in establishing a basis of friendship and good will and trust that is so important to our people, and to the world and to peace.

"Therefore, I am very glad to welcome you here and I congratulate you in taking the lead in what you are setting out to do.

"I wish very much that I could have had something like this in my record as a boy."

That little meeting was of considerable importance to me as Secretary of State because a photograph of this intriguing little group and a print of my comments made the first page of a large number of the most important papers in this country.[4] I received many letters from people, almost all of whom expressed astonishment to learn how inconspicuous and unimportant this country was before the world in 1898 and they seemed for the first time to understand something of the necessity for radical changes in our attitude today and the critical importance of how we carried ourselves in our present position of vast responsibility.

In referring to the great changes that have occurred in this country since the early 90's, I think it would be pertinent to these remarks to mention the fact that the change regarding the status of women has been even more rapid and much greater. I don't know whether you realize it or not, but as late as 1890 about the only opportunities offered women in this country, aside from marriage and raising a family or finding a relative who would provide a home, were nursing and teaching. You are, I assume, familiar with the world of opportunity for women today. But it is only since August 1920 that our Constitution was so amended as to give women the vote.

In that brief period since 1890 not only has the whole position of this country been altered before the world, but the women in that short span of time, speaking historically, have arrived at the point where they are conspicuous, and admirably so, in the Senate and in the House of Representatives of the United States. They have been governors of states, mayors of cities, principal officials of great corporations, and a tremendous force in the molding of public opinion.

That men are still dubious or reluctant about this tremendous change is both natural and at times still plainly evident, as I found when I proposed the necessary legislation during the war to authorize the Women's Army Corps, better known as the WAC's. I not only found male resistance in the process of obtaining the legislation but even more markedly in the process of integrating the WAC's into the Army. Many of the older officers thought the world was being turned upside down and it fell to me, as one of my duties, to modernize that view.

However, I want to pay tribute here to the tremendously effective influence of women in supporting the war effort. Time after time when I found myself opposed by very stubborn reluctance to this or that war measure, I turned to the women's organizations and to committees of women and in every case they backed me solidly and very effectively. Later when I became Secretary of State and was in the midst of the Congressional debate as to whether or not there should be a European Recovery Program, I again turned to the women, the Federation of Women's Clubs, and they gave me tremendously effective support.[5]

It might interest you to know, in connection with the WAC organization, that when the group was first organized I took a lieutenant into my office as receptionist, purely because I thought it was important that I should show some evidence of confidence in the prospective efficiency of the organization. Later the Secretary of the General Staff came to me for permission to utilize this lieutenant in briefing for me the studies and recommendations of various sections of the General Staff. I agreed, though personally I had never even seen the lady at that time. Later this same officer requested my approval of her appointment as an assistant secretary of the General Staff, to which I agreed.

To give you some idea of the importance of this appointment of a woman to this particular post in the military hierarchy, I should explain that the work was being done by a number of Assistant Secretaries and the importance of it can best be illustrated by telling you that among those assistants during the early period of my service as Chief of Staff were the present head of the Chiefs of Staff, General [Omar N.] Bradley, the present Chief of Staff of the Army, General [J. Lawton] Collins, the former Ambassador to Russia and Chief of Staff to General Eisenhower, [Walter] Bedell Smith, and other officers who later became lieutenant generals and army corps commanders and made outstanding reputations as combat leaders.[6] So the young lady was to join a rather distinguished company.

Later on when it became apparent that I must have a secretary who could devote his entire time to the documents, studies and proposals of the United States Chiefs of Staff and the Combined British-American Chiefs of Staff, this particular WAC, now a major, was recommended for the job. So, for the remainder of the war, before attending any meeting of the Chiefs of Staff, she would brief me on the various problems on the agenda. She not only briefed but also advised me, and was called on to perform similar services for the head of the Air Forces, General Arnold, and the head of the vast services of supply, General Somervell, now president of Koppers Company here in Pittsburgh. She ultimately became a lieutenant colonel and when the legislature of her home state passed a resolution to set aside a day for celebration in her honor, she declined the honor feeling it was not appropriate for war time. I am referring to Florence Newsome of Providence, Rhode Island.[7]

As President of the Red Cross I come in contact with many young people. There are 19 million in the Junior Red Cross, and a great many young women volunteer workers.

There is a tremendous amount of work that must be done every day of the week by volunteers of the Red Cross. I am certain you do not vaguely realize how much has to be done—the Motor Corps, the Gray Ladies, those who provide some diversion and entertainment for the hospitalized, of whom we now have 110 thousand in the veterans hospitals alone. I have been happy to learn that your College program has included some fine work for the veterans in Aspinwall Hospital. Then they do outstanding work in time of emergency—in flood disasters and where the cyclone strikes. It might interest you to know that there were 225 emergencies during the past 12 months, for which the Red Cross has expended about 6 million dollars.

Now I have the feeling that the time has arrived when every young woman should be definitely trained to give some service as a citizen. Home nursing is one of the simplest examples and a tremendously important matter, as we find when there is a disaster or an epidemic or trouble generally in the field of activity of the Red Cross. But there are many other specialties suited to young women which would make them much more valuable as citizens. And I think it would be a fine thing if the graduates of all the colleges in these troubled days would entertain that feeling and do something about it.

I think it is very important, and it is an actual obligation now that you have the vote, that young women should know more about the practical aspects of politics. I am using the term in the sense of government rather than in the frequently accepted meaning of some form of skulduggery.

We have a two-party system plus practical politics. If you citizens make the political procedures right you make government right.

A friend of mine told me of a test he had recently made in his home town. He prepared a list of questions, such as: Are you a registered voter? Who represents you and your party in your town? Who is the chairman of that committee? Who is your state committee representative? Who is the vice-chairman of your state committee? Who is your national committee chairman? Who is your national committee-woman? Who represents you in the State Legislature? And who represents you in the United States Houses of Congress? He asked these questions of those to whom the people of the community looked for leadership—the principals of the two public schools, the headmasters of the two private schools, the presidents of the two banks, the presidents of the two country clubs. Then he addressed them to those who looked to the others for leadership—the merchants, the bartender, the gardener on his estate, the bootblacks. It is hard to believe, but he told me that the bootblack group could answer 86% of the questions and—I mention this in fear and trepidation—the teacher group could only answer 2%.

Now let me ask you something; how can we make democracy work if the leaders of the community know less about local government than the persons who look to them for guidance?

The wise voice of old Ben Franklin on the sidewalks of Philadelphia a century and a half ago, tired and weary after a long session of the Constitutional Convention, when questioned as to the kind of government the Convention proposed to give them, replied, "We are giving you the greatest form of government—a republic, *if* you can keep it."

Never was there a time in history when this form of government was in so much danger or was so important to the salvation of mankind.

Speaking of Franklin, I am tempted to tell you a little story of a school boy who was called upon to give an outline of Franklin's life. The young man said, "Franklin as a boy started walking in Boston and ended up in Philadelphia. There he met a young lady on the sidewalk with a loaf of bread under her arm. He married her and discovered electricity." Whatever else he did, Franklin gave us one of the great examples of practical realistic philosophy regarding the affairs of men and the government of countries.

I have been especially pleased to participate in this occasion this morning because of the honor that is to be done Mrs. Marshall for that, of course, is the quickest way to my heart.

When she told me the other day of having received a telephone message from your President, Dr. Anderson, to the effect that the Board of Trustees had voted her a degree, I naturally asked her what degree. She replied it was for "Humane Letters" and in a very serious vein I suggested it might be more appropriate if there were added to it the words "phonetically or otherwise" because though she is a charming speller, quite a unique speller, I must confide in you that she could never win a spelling bee—nor could I, incidentally. I was frequently embarrassed while Secretary of State by having my question as to how to spell this or that word treated as a joke, though my trouble was very real; I didn't know how to spell the word.

It has been a very real pleasure for me to talk to you today and I hope I have not confused your thinking or bored you with my personal reactions. I wish for you every success, a very happy life, and lots of children.[8]

GCMRL/G. C. Marshall Papers (American Red Cross, Speeches and Statements)

1. See p. 68n2 (Document 42). Marshall wrote on the final copy of the speech that it had been "Delivered as written with a few interpolations."
2. See *Papers of GCM*, 6: 354–56.
3. Admiral George Dewey (USNA, 1858) had commanded American naval forces in a decisive victory over the Spanish in the Battle of Manila Bay on May 1, 1898.
4. See "'ERP' of Cub Scouts Pleases Marshall," *New York Times*, February 11, 1948, p. 3.
5. See *Papers of GCM*, 6: 465–69.
6. Former Army Chief of Staff Bradley (USMA, 1915) had been appointed chairman of the Joint Chiefs of Staff (JCS) in August 1949.
7. In February 1944, the Rhode Island legislature had passed a joint resolution to commend Lieutenant Colonel Newsome as the state's first WAC officer and the only female member of the Army General Staff and to express "the assurance of the pride of all Rhode Islanders in her distinguished service." Newsome also received a March 1944 invitation by William G. Lind, mayor of Cranston, Rhode Island, to attend a May 7 rally for the WAC as the guest of honor. She declined for several reasons that she expressed to Frank McCarthy: "I loathe publicity and prefer not to be in the spotlight. Also, I have been unusually fortunate in the Army venture and would prefer that some other WAC could share some of the glory. . . . After all, the enlisted women are the ones to be honored—their careers in the Army often entail great personal sacrifice. . . . Frankly the bestowing of honors on an individual who has done nothing but render the required service at no cost just doesn't seem right to me." McCarthy replied to Mayor Lind on Newsome's behalf that due to her duties in early May, she would be unable to attend the rally. ("R.I. Woman in War's Highest Councils," [Providence, Rhode Island] *Evening Bulletin*, July 5, 1944, p. 12; Lind to Marshall, March 24, 1944, GCMRL/G. C. Marshall Papers [Pentagon Office, General]; Newsome to McCarthy, March 30, 1944, ibid.; and McCarthy to Lind, March 31, 1944, ibid.)

Marshall had awarded Newsome the Legion of Merit in October 1945, and by the time he delivered this speech at the Pennsylvania College for Women, Newsome had become the widow of Dr. Charles Johnson of Providence, Rhode Island. Marshall sent her a copy of his speech on June 14 because of his reference to her, and he commented that it "doesn't sound normal" to address her as Mrs. Johnson. Johnson, then employed by the CIA, replied on June 19 to thank Marshall for the copy of the speech and for his "complimentary remarks about my wartime work for you." ("Rhode Island's Ace WAC Receives Legion of Merit,"

Evening Bulletin, October 30, 1945; "Dr. C. E. Johnson Dies at Age of 52," *Providence Journal*, March 21, 1950; Marshall to Johnson, June 14, 1950, and Johnson to Marshall, June 19, 1950, GCMRL/G. C. Marshall Papers [American Red Cross, General].)

For Marshall's wartime promotion of and comments on Newsome, see Mattie E. Treadwell, *The Women's Army Corps,* in *United States Army in World War II* (Washington: Office of the Chief of Military History, Department of the Army, 1954), 575–76, 761.

8. "I want you to know how real the honor was to have both you and Mrs. Marshall here for our commencement," Pennsylvania College for Women President Paul R. Anderson wrote on June 23. "We were happy to hear from you, and particularly so because you spoke to the students directly. They appreciated this more than I can say." The letter included a check for three hundred dollars "to express our appreciation and that of others to Mrs. Marshall for her devoted and creative life." Marshall responded, "Mrs. Marshall wishes to thank you for writing of her as you did, as do I," and noted that the honorarium "surprised me, but I would prefer to return it to you for such use, for an individual or in general, as you feel most desirable." (Anderson to Marshall, June 23, 1950, and Marshall to Anderson, July 5, 1950, GCMRL/G. C. Marshall Papers [American Red Cross, Categorical, Invitations, Accepted].)

72

VIRGINIA MILITARY INSTITUTE GRADUATION SPEECH[1] — June 13, 1950, Lexington, Virginia

It is a great pleasure for me, and I count it also as an honor, to be invited to talk to you men of the graduating class this morning and to the corps of cadets in the final ceremony of the year.[2] From my own experience, almost fifty years ago, I realize it is pretty hard to capture the attention of you young gentlemen at this particular hour. You have too many other wonderful things to think about, and a good many of them are here in the gallery.

When I was turning over in my mind what I might talk about this morning, I looked up my records to see what I had said here under similar circumstances on the day Paris fell before the terrific German onslaught in June 1940.[3] I know you could never read what I said, and I doubt if any member of the faculty today who was present on that occasion has any recollection of the incident. So I will take the liberty of reading a paragraph or two of my comments on that fateful day in the history of the world. But before doing so, I might explain that just before I came to the platform I received a message from the President, Mr. Roosevelt, to return to Washington at once and I left immediately on the conclusion of my remarks without having the opportunity of seeing the graduates of that day receive their diplomas.

What I said then I find very accurately expresses my feelings today, these many years later. Now if you will bear with me a few moments, I will read an extract from those remarks.

"This is a day of high emotions to you men of the graduating class; it is the culmination of your period of preparation for life. You step off this morning on your own, to make your way in the world.

"To me, for the moment, this morning recaptures my day of graduation. I think I can clearly recall my thoughts and plans. They were very personal, of course.

I was struggling for an appointment in the Army, to get into the campaign then in progress in the Philippines; and I was intent on getting married. I am not quite clear as to whether or not the Army career was incidental to the marriage problem, a necessary corollary with its impressive salary of the $116.67 a month of those days. But beyond those two compelling desires I apparently was indifferent to all other important issues of life.

"The point is that about six months later I *did* succeed in securing a commission in the Army, I *did* manage to marry and I *was* on my way to the closing phase of the Philippine Insurrection.[4]

"I have been attempting to recall this morning just when I first became conscious of the important influence of my cadet days on my career. In dealing with the men of my first company I did have the super-confidence of a recent cadet officer. I knew my drill, though I was a little vague about other matters. . . . The sword I carried at company formations was the same sword I had carried as a cadet officer, but the colt revolver on my hip as we filed along narrow mountain trails provided an entirely new reaction. It was very reassuring. I think there came to me very gradually, day by day, in my contact with the other officers, all senior to me, especially with those who showed the debilitating or sometimes demoralizing effect of several years of tropical campaigning, an appreciation of what the VMI had given me through its traditions and by its standards of conduct and responsibility.

"At retreat formation in some isolated garrison in the Philippines, my thoughts would go back to evening parade with the background of the Brushy Hills and the sunset over House Mountain and there would occur to me a thought of what the Corps, what the Institute expected of a cadet officer in the performance of his duty.

"I spoke of this day as being one of high emotions. It is your graduation day, but it may also be one of the most fateful days in the history of the world. No man can predict the outcome of the tragic struggle in Europe. No American can foresee the eventual effect on the Americas. The world we have known may be revolutionized; the peaceful liberties we have accepted so casually may be a hazard in this ghastly game abroad."

Much water has gone over the dam since then—a torrent—really a veritable flood of great and often terrible events, and all the world still seems poised in the balance of critical uncertainties. The peoples of the world and the leaders of the Western world are puzzling, and hoping, and praying for ways and means to maintain the peace. In America this summer there seems to be an abounding prosperity but even so there persists a feeling of uncertainty as to its duration, and that uncertainty, of course, is largely explained by the temper of the world these days.

Now I've seldom found myself in a position of importance concerning world affairs in war or in peace for which I could not find some historical parallel. Certainly it has become evident to all that you only win a war to find yourself confronted by a much more difficult and even greater problem consolidating the peace, both economically and politically. I think this was particularly true after the British-allied triumph at Waterloo to overthrow Bonaparte and bring to an end the 22 years of Napoleonic wars. When one reads the history of England for the succeeding decade or two, it is clearly evident what tremendous problems follow for the victors in a great war. However, the saying that "These are the times that try men's souls,"[5] while true in the application to the present, should not divert us from the realization that it is times like these that require men *of* great soul *and* great courage.

That is the world into which you are stepping forth this morning on your own for the first time in your lives. You have a wonderful heritage drawn from your years here, which will be far more important in your life than you can possibly realize today. Probably the most important requirement for success in life among men is a reputation for integrity. In addition to the influence for good you have received in your home life you leave here with a solid foundation for integrity of responsibility and of action drawn from the teachings, the associations and the traditions of the Virginia Military Institute.

Good luck to you—may God be good to you.[6]

GCMRL/G. C. Marshall Papers (American Red Cross, Speeches and Statements)

1. Marshall wrote on the top of the copy text that the speech had been "Delivered as written with a few interpolations."

2. See pp. 67–68.

3. See *Papers of GCM*, 2: 244–45.

4. Marshall married Elizabeth Carter "Lily" Coles of Lexington, Virginia, on February 11, 1902, eight days after receiving his commission as a second lieutenant. (The first Mrs. Marshall died in 1927.) He arrived in Manila in May, at the end of the Philippine Insurrection. On July 4, 1902, President Theodore Roosevelt announced an end to the fighting. (Pogue, *Education*, 67–69; *Papers of GCM*, 1: 23–25.)

5. This is the famous first line of Thomas Paine's Revolutionary War pamphlet entitled *The American Crisis*.

6. The next day Superintendent Marshall wrote to thank Marshall "for taking time out of your busy life to come down here and make the graduation address yesterday. I thought that your comparison of now and ten years ago was most appropriate and a pointed reminder to the members of our graduating class." (R. J. Marshall to Marshall, June 14, 1950, GCMRL/G. C. Marshall Papers [American Red Cross, Categorical, Invitations, Accepted].)

73

To J. Manly Cobb — June 14, 1950, Washington, DC

Dear Reverend Cobb: It is easy for me to understand how you feel about leaving St. James and Leesburg.[1] Many times during my Army career I had that same feeling, but at my new station I would meet old friends, make new acquaintances and of course find new problems. However, the past has always provided me with memories that will always be cherished.

I am especially complimented by your generous comments regarding my Memorial Day speech.[2] I have received a number of requests for copies; in this morning's mail I had one from Spokane and another from Los Angeles.

I appreciate your making available to me the book CHAPTERS IN CHURCH HISTORY and I will read it with much interest.[3]

My wife joins me in warm regards to you both. Good luck! Faithfully yours,

G. C. Marshall

GCMRL/G. C. Marshall Collection (J. Manly Cobb)

1. J. Manly Cobb, the rector of Saint James Episcopal Church in Leesburg, was moving to a church near Roanoke, Virginia. He had written to Marshall, "I wish I could put in words what the opportunity of having the privilege of knowing you and Mrs. Marshall has meant to me personally and in my ministry. As in all the deep experiences in life, this cannot be expressed in words, but it is there and I count it one of the greatest blessings in my life." (Cobb to Marshall, June 6, 1950, GCMRL/G. C. Marshall Papers [American Red Cross, General].)

2. Cobb had complimented Marshall on his recent speech at Arlington National Cemetery (see pp. 94–98), saying that it "should go down as one of the greatest utterances in history." (Ibid.)

3. Along with his letter, Cobb included a copy of this recent book by Powel Mills Dawley, *Chapters in Church History* (New York: National Council, 1950).

74

To Colonel Marshall S. Carter[1]

June 14, 1950
Washington, DC

Dear Carter: Mrs. Marshall and I enjoyed reading your interesting and informative letter of the 8th.[2] We would like to have you and the family come down to Leesburg the first Saturday or Sunday in July for lunch, say at 12:00 EST or an early supper at 4:30 EST.[3] I suggest you telephone George and let him know if you can make it or not.[4]

I was happy to hear of your arrangements for Sun Valley. I can now see your three ladies on the ice while you and the boy are out looking for a productive fishing hole. It was about two years ago at this time that the trout at Shadyside Farm took a fancy to a dry fly. Perhaps you can hitch a ride down there for a day of fishing with our whisky distributing friend.[5]

I hope to get over to Pawley's before I leave for the convention on the 23rd.[6] I went out the other day to Goose Creek but the best I could do was a six-inch bass, weight not determinable.

Troop duty in my opinion is the happiest period of one's service and I think the Army made a wise decision in getting you away from a desk job. Having the assignment on your record will have much to do with the furtherance of your career.

We are delighted with the jeep.[7] I hope you get as much pleasure from yours as we hope to have from ours.

With our very best to you and the family, Faithfully yours,

GCMRL/G. C. Marshall Papers (American Red Cross, General)

1. Colonel Marshall S. Carter (USMA, 1931) had been Secretary Marshall's aide at the State Department. See p. 604.

2. Carter, then completing his studies at the National War College, had written to update Marshall as he prepared to depart for a new assignment in Japan. "Dept. of Army," he wrote, "has directed that I have a troop command, and the latest information is that I will command the anti-aircraft group that is deployed around Tokyo. It consists of two white gun battalions, two negro automatic weapons battalions, and a negro band, plus assorted miscellaneous hdqtrs. and sections. . . . My directed command is good for only one year, but I hope to be able to keep the regiment for my entire tour. It will certainly be a new and most revealing experience for me, because my largest command to date has been a twenty-five man school detachment with 90 attached students! And that was back in 1941." (Carter to Marshall, June 8, 1950, GCMRL/G. C. Marshall Papers [American Red Cross, General].)

3. Leesburg, Virginia, remained on Eastern Standard Time while Washington, DC, had switched to Daylight Savings Time.

4. "We were disappointed not to be able to come to Dodona last Saturday," Carter had written, "and hope that a raincheck is still available." (Ibid.)

5. The "whisky distributing friend" was most likely Hy Berkowitz, who maintained a residence at Sand Springs Ranch in Wendell, Idaho.

6. Carter had written that "Bill Pawley telephoned me Sunday to come down and do some fishing." (Ibid.) In 1944, Pawley had purchased the Belvoir farm in Fairfax County, Virginia.

7. Carter had written, "We have ordered a gray Jeep Stationwagon . . . it is exactly like your new one, which I have heard about but not yet seen." (Ibid.) The Marshalls owned a 1950 Willys-Overland Jeep stationwagon. (Marshall to Roberts, April 5, 1951, GCMRL/G. C. Marshall Papers [Secretary of Defense, Number Indexed, M200-11-41].)

75

To Arthur Krock — June 15, 1950
Washington, DC

Dear Krock: I have your letter of June 13 with the invitation to join you to discuss the possible publication of several incidents of the past in which I figured.[1]

I would be glad to talk to you on a date convenient to us both. I must tell you in advance that I shall have nothing to say for publication, by quotation, implication or inference. If on this basis you still want to talk to me, I will be glad to see you, but I would prefer doing so here at the office. Faithfully yours,

GCMRL/G. C. Marshall Papers (American Red Cross, General)

1. Arthur Krock, "the dean of Washington newsmen," was the District's bureau chief for the *New York Times*. He had written to ask Marshall for an interview to discuss "several important incidents of the past in which you figured prominently, the publication of products—if any—to be determined by you. It seems to me that the time is about right for it." (Krock to Marshall, June 13, 1950, GCMRL/G. C. Marshall Papers [American Red Cross, General].)

76

AMERICAN RED CROSS ANNUAL CONVENTION KEYNOTE SPEECH

June 26, 1950
Detroit, Michigan

Mr. Robinson,[1] Your Honor, My fellow workers in Red Cross:

I must first express my deep appreciation, personal and official, for the reception that has been given to the Convention and its delegates by the city of Detroit and the Detroit Chapter. We owe to all those concerned, especially to His Honor the Mayor and to Mr. Ewald, the chapter chairman, and his workers, our very sincere thanks.[2]

As all of you are aware this is my first Red Cross convention. Fortunately for me I do not feel that I am a complete stranger because I have already had contact with many of you.

I think it will help me to explain my point of view regarding various Red Cross matters if I begin by giving you a brief outline of the experience I have already had as head of the organization.

When I was first appointed last October, it was necessary that I acquire very quickly some knowledge of the organization and its activities before the impending meeting of the Board of Governors which was to decide among other things the amount of the budget which would be the basis for the spring fund drive. It seemed imperative that I at least gather a superficial knowledge of the organization and its activities before that meeting. Therefore, in one week of October I traveled about 75 hundred miles visiting 15 cities and making contact with some 254 chapter chairmen. I not only came in contact with them but in most instances, after I got well started on the trip, I called on each one to express his views on operations and policies of the Red Cross.[3]

Following this came the meeting of the Board of Governors of 50 and while I could not at that time put forward any firm conclusions, I could at least listen intelligently and I was able to give the Board an outline of reactions of Red Cross workers in various parts of the country.

Later, in the middle of January, I started on a series of trips which were not completed until well into March. During this period in which I visited 29 cities within the continental limits and also a visit to Hawaii, I met nearly 800 chapter chairmen and saw about 25 to 30 thousand of the most active Red Cross workers. I sat with the Boards of Directors of many of the larger chapters and discussed Red Cross problems with the businessmen of a great many cities. From this trip I emerged with very definite views regarding a number of the most important problems of the Red Cross and, therefore, was prepared to discuss them at the meeting of the Board of Governors in March.[4]

There was one reaction, in particular, that I gathered from this travel that I think it well to mention at the start of my talk today, in order to give it the emphasis I think it deserves, and it is this: I was surprised to find how many of the most active workers in the organization had a very limited knowledge of the over-all operations and obligations of the whole organization. And, if this condition existed among the most active in the Red Cross, it is only fair to assume that such lack of knowledge was much greater in the lower echelons, and that the public with whom they came in direct contact must have gotten a very confused impression of what the organization is doing. Probably, in many cases, they acquired complete misconceptions. Therefore, I think it is of the utmost importance that a really determined effort be made to bring all the active Red Cross workers to a complete understanding of the general program of the Red Cross—just what it means and how it operates. To do this will require just as careful preparation as for the training in home nursing or first aid or for the other programs.

I have made reference to this situation a number of times in talking to Red Cross groups, but I do not think I have ever been able to make entirely clear my impression of how serious to us this weakness is and it might well be more serious later on.

The Red Cross is a publicly supported organization. This means that any member of the public feels that he has the right to criticize, and has the right to ask questions with the expectation of receiving full, authoritative answers. He naturally believes that any person closely associated with the Red Cross should be able to give him explicit information in answer to his questions, and when the answers are vague, inaccurate or misleading, the whole organization suffers.

It is up to you and to me—to everyone who has the interests of Red Cross at heart, to create a better public understanding of the organization's functions and limitations. Simply stated, the solution is this: Know your Red Cross.

Now, obviously, in an organization as vast as this it would not be humanly possible to make everyone connected with it a walking encyclopedia of detailed knowledge about everything we do. But there are certain elements in the broad, general picture with which we should all be familiar.

We should know the origin of the Red Cross and the world-wide significance of the Red Cross movement. We should know what relationship the American Red Cross bears to the International Red Cross Committee and to the League of Red Cross Societies. We should understand the national charter responsibilities the American Red Cross must fulfill in serving the armed forces and the victims of disaster. We should be very clear that these are definitely *national* and that they cannot be handled on any other basis. We should know *why* there is a need for a national blood program. We should know *how* the Red Cross proposes to meet that need.

If there were widespread public understanding of the responsibilities and limitations of the Red Cross, many of our problems would not arise.

So many of our present difficulties stem from misconceptions of what the Red Cross is and does that it would be well to review a few of the major misunderstandings with which I find I have to contend.

There is still a belief in some circles that the National Blood Program of the American Red Cross is a step in the direction of socialized medicine. While for the most part, the medical authorities of the country are solidly behind the Red Cross in its efforts to ensure a framework for an adequate blood supply for the nation, especially in great emergencies, yet in certain quarters the reproach, socialization, greets any mention of the Blood Program.

Actually, nothing could be very much further from socialization than the Red Cross approach. Socialization implies an activity required of the people by legislation or government decree. Asking the strong and healthy to donate their blood voluntarily for the relief of the sick and injured is the exact opposite of the socialized approach. Red Cross facilities serve merely as the channel through which generous impulses can be directed to the benefit of those in need of the great restorative powers of human blood.

Another criticism that is frequently heard implies that the Red Cross is trying to monopolize the blood resources of the nation and to close the doors of all existing blood banks. This is equally inaccurate. The Red Cross opens regional centers for the procurement and distribution of blood only where no facilities exist or where the existing facilities are inadequate to meet the need. And only upon the invitation of the local medical authorities.

And so, in connection with the Blood Program alone, there are two wide areas of misunderstanding in regard to Red Cross policies and practices.

To turn to another cause of misunderstandings, very few, even within the Red Cross organization, understand the difficulty that has been presented with the exhaustion of the surplus funds—reserves as they are usually called—that accumulated from the generous over-subscriptions during the war years. In brief, though our running expenses for the fiscal year just ending were to be almost 85 millions, yet the public was only asked to subscribe 60 millions because the difference was to be made up by the application of those reserve funds. Because these reserve funds are now close to exhaustion and despite the fact that in our budget estimates we have materially lowered the calculated expenses for the coming fiscal year to the extent of more than 6 million, we were compelled to ask the public to subscribe 7 million dollars more than last year, that is 67 million.

We have experienced recurrent waves of criticism and complaint having their origin in the services rendered by the Red Cross during World War II. The content of most of these is a compound of unreasonable expectations and misinformation.

How often have you heard:

"The Red Cross charged for food and lodging."

"The Red Cross wouldn't give me a loan."

"The Red Cross wouldn't get me home when my wife was ill."

"The Red Cross never did anything for me."

Complaints of this nature plainly indicate that the average serviceman did not understand the function of the Red Cross and the limitations imposed upon it by the military authorities and the exigencies of war.

Now let us be completely realistic and forget for a moment that we represent a great and widely respected welfare organization. Let me ask this question:

Could any business establishment long continue in operation if its representatives were unable to tell the public exactly what it had to offer and on what terms? Of course not. A good advertising program is, of course, essential, *but* when the customer comes to the shop it is the girl behind the counter and the man in the aisle who determine how much business the establishment will do.

That analogy is not far-fetched. The Red Cross has essential services to offer. Its relations with the public are generally good as evidenced by the fine support it has received year after year, but if we do not have well-informed and articulate workers that situation will change, and the problems that are now merely troublesome might grow great enough to present a serious dilemma.

Nowhere is this situation more crucial than in the matter of Red Cross fund raising policies. In my travels around the country, I have found that business and industrial leaders do not fully appreciate the national and international obligations of the Red Cross which make an independent fund campaign necessary.

Does chapter leadership have a responsibility here? Yes, I think it does. I think that in some quarters there has been a tendency to over-emphasize the community aspects of Red Cross at the expense of the great national and international functions of the organization which give the Red Cross symbol its greatest significance.

The national organization and the chapters are one and the same. Together they make up the American Red Cross. The national organization serves as the agent of the chapter in carrying out the national responsibilities which each chapter accepts under the charter which gives it the right to organize.

The money allocated to national in the fund campaigns is not taken away from chapters and spent without regard to local community needs. Actually, about 70% returns to the local community, or is spent in its behalf, through Services to the Armed Forces, through relief and rehabilitation to the victims of disaster, through the National Blood Program and in materials and services that implement the total Red Cross program.

We need to do much more in stressing this fact to the public and we must begin, as usual with *our own family* who, if they understand the matter thoroughly, can do much to help tell the story.

There is certainly an inadequate public realization of what is done, locally and nationally, with the funds allocated to serve the armed forces and the veterans. In certain respects there has not only been no demobilization since the war but actually a tremendous increase in our obligations. The number of veterans has increased from less than four million prior to World War II to nineteen million today.

The number of hospitalized veterans has risen to the unprecedented total of one hundred ten thousand with a steady increase inevitable for the next twenty-five to thirty years.

Compared with pre-war years, 1938 for example, we now have to meet the Red Cross needs of one and a half million members of the armed forces scattered throughout the world. Prior to 1938 this obligation pertained only to some two hundred sixty-five thousand men, most of whom were located in this country.

Serving the armed forces requires the closest partnership between the chapters and the national organization. Chapters provide the intimate contact with the American family which is the fundamental basis on which the Red Cross rests.

Chapters not only carry on the welfare program for the families of servicemen and veterans but, also, they are usually heavily engaged in making the necessary contacts in time of personal trouble between members of the armed forces and their families. Add to this the tremendous burden of daily work for veterans in the large hospitals adjacent to chapters and the work of serving nearby military installations, and it should be easy to understand that the chapter plays a major part in services to the armed forces.

Now all of this not only requires a well organized work program, largely staffed by volunteers, but it also requires money. The fund requirements frequently exceed the resources of the local chapter. This especially is the case where a small chapter lies in the vicinity of a large veteran's hospital or military installation. When chapter resources are inadequate additional funds must be provided by the national organization.

Another activity which is widely misunderstood both in respect to its operations and its financing is disaster relief and rehabilitation. Local chapters not only have a tremendous work problem on their hands in time of floods, hurricanes, great fires and similar misfortunes, but frequently, usually they must be heavily financed from the funds of the national organization.

Let me give you a few examples. During the past twelve months there have been some 225 emergencies for which the national organization has expended six million dollars. The disasters affected local communities, but the money came largely from the national organization. The floods and tornadoes that struck the midwest and south last Spring required allocations totaling nearly $1,300,000. They involved the support, that is, shelter, clothing and food, at one time of 23,000 families. Many other families were helped but those I have just mentioned were almost completely supported by the Red Cross. There were weeks when the Red Cross was carrying five to ten thousand of these families affected by the floods. Some 25,000 Red Cross volunteer workers were in the field; and I felt great pride, however brief my association with the Red Cross had been, in the fact that the work was done so quietly and efficiently that little of it made the headlines. This efficiency was due to the planning which we call disaster preparedness. Then, too, this was another illustration of a partnership between chapters and the national organization. Here the local chapters provided the manpower while the national organizations provided the necessary funds and also contributed the skills of trained staff officers.

It has been estimated that about 70% of every dollar allocated to each year's Disaster Budget is spent on post-disaster rehabilitation. It is easily demonstrable that this is money plowed back into the community by the national organization. And in many cases the sum spent on one disaster will far exceed national's fund campaign quota from the entire region in which the disaster occurred.

I found that in Texas the national organization has contributed more money in a single year than had been allocated by the state to the national organization in a period of three years. In the 1948 Fund Campaign the state of Texas raised $2,696,000 of which less than a million and a half was remitted to the national organization. In one disaster alone, the Fort Worth Flood of 1949, national returned to Texas nearly two million dollars.[5] There are numerous instances of a similar nature. They all illustrate that the Red Cross organization is, in a sense, more national than local.

It is true that chapters in certain areas relatively immune to disaster do not always receive a dollar for dollar return on the funds allocated to national from local campaigns. But one never knows when disaster may strike nor its nature, and it is the basic philosophy of the Red Cross to accept responsibility for the other fellow's welfare whether he be across the street or in the next county or in a distant state. If we begin now to question the soundness of that philosophy, then we are no longer the Red Cross, but some other organization.

Here again chapter leadership should take the initiative in spreading this philosophy in their communities.

The complaint that chapters are obliged to carry an inequitable share of the national budget also arises in connection with the National Blood Program because there are still many chapters that are neither part of nor adjacent to a regional blood center.

We have already proved that the Blood Program is potentially a service to every chapter—to every community in the United States. It was proved in Texas City three years ago when blood was flown to the injured from all over the United States.[6] It was demonstrated again in the South Amboy explosion this year when blood from adjacent communities reached that city within the hour following the disaster.[7]

In any major disaster or national emergency, blood centers now in operation and those in the planning stage would provide blood for any section of the country. More important, the development of this program has set a pattern. It has established a framework capable of rapid expansion in the event of a major national emergency. This is an essential element in the nation's plan for civil defense.

We need not depend upon disasters or a national emergency to bring the benefits of the Blood Program to the nation at large. Funds allocated to this purpose benefit every chapter directly or indirectly. Over three million dollars worth of the specific for measles, obtained from blood plasma, has been distributed by the national organization to the state health departments of every state in the Union. Almost seven hundred thousand dollars worth of a blood derivative has been distributed for the treatment of shock and kidney diseases. Neurologists have asked the Red Cross to distribute fibrin foam, another derivative which is used in delicate surgery, but at the present time we can only supply this product in limited quantities. But the fact of the matter is all of these valuable derivatives are going to your local communities.

Research, assisted by the Red Cross through provision of the blood products and the payment of laboratory charges is expected to develop new uses for additional blood products. They are being tested in two Red Cross pilot laboratories. When perfected and medically approved they will be of benefit to the entire nation.

My analysis of the American Red Cross convinces me that it is, predominantly, a *national* organization, that reaches into nearly every community in our land with services that are *both local and national.*

A weakening of the national status of the Red Cross would jeopardize its unique position in American life and would partly undermine its position as a strong link in the International Red Cross movement.

The logical deduction from this is, in my opinion, that the Red Cross cannot delegate its fund raising function. It must remain independent and flexible enough to meet emergencies on either the national or the international scene.

Because the Red Cross stands firmly by this point of view, many people assume that the organization is opposed to the idea of community chests. The Red Cross does not question the merits of joint campaigns where organizations with purely local objectives are banded together in their fund raising efforts. On the contrary, it is my belief that cooperative community arrangements leading to better local health and welfare programs should be encouraged.[8]

We do say—and we speak from experience—that for the Red Cross it will not work.

The two principal points to be considered in this matter are first, as I have already illustrated, that Red Cross requirements demand from time to time the expenditure of funds in a community far beyond the capacity of that community to provide. Yet these funds must be obtained every year because emergencies arise with dreadful regularity though fortunately not always in the same area. I think it would be quite impracticable to obtain the necessary amounts for issues that would seem at the time of a local drive remote from the interest of the local community. And always there are the Charter requirements that relate to the armed forces and veterans, and the treaty obligations of the Red Cross that relate to the entire world.

The second point of vital importance is the fact that unless there is a definite annual contact between the largest possible number of individuals and the Red Cross specifically, the organization would lose the special status and appeal which have been of such great importance to the nation throughout Red Cross history. I am therefore convinced that the separate fund raising policy of the organization is both wise and necessary.

The persistence of the debate on whether or not the Red Cross should participate in federated drives is harmful not only to the Red Cross but also to welfare organizations generally. Nothing is more certain to lower the morale of an army than to have its soldiers feeling sorry for themselves. During the war I found that public statements, and the mail from home inspired by such statements, caused a serious drop in morale directly affecting the striking power of an army. The same reaction has developed in our public today, and for much the same reasons.

At this point I might mention that not more than 2½% of the nation's income has ever been given to philanthropic causes. I will not try to present a contrast by estimating the huge sums that are spent each year for casual items of personal luxury by the great majority of our citizens. We are a very fortunate people and we have always been a correspondingly generous people. I hope we continue to be. The one should always be the corollary of the other.

The Red Cross has always emphasized the importance of individual effort—individual generosity—individual concern for the needs of the distressed. The volunteer is therefore the basis of the Red Cross effort.

As you already know, we are seriously short of volunteers. But what is of more importance to me is the fact, at least I think it is the fact, that the public is so little aware of the work the volunteers do every day of the week and what a severe reaction would be instantly set up if this volunteer effort was suspended or diminished.

For the veterans alone there are activities that must be carried out day by day, by volunteers. They require preliminary organization and precise arrangements, they require transportation facilities, they require the training of workers. These requirements grow daily as the veterans grow older and their ailments become more frequent and severe. This obligation will not dwindle with the years. Unfortunately it will steadily increase as the years go by. And if you can visualize the problem that we had in 1938 with the small numbers of hospitalized veterans of the First War, you may realize what a tremendous problem we have today. We are not only dealing with older and more feeble veterans of the First War but with more than 15 million additional veterans whose complaints in 60% of the cases are reported to be psychoneurotic.

I have worried a great deal about how to make the public more conscious of the fine work done largely by women volunteers and the necessity for more of them.[9] I have not yet found the solution, because the work is quietly done, therefore efficiently done, and that does not make the headlines.

Also we have to offset the sometime reaction that Red Cross activities pertain almost entirely to war times except in cases of disaster. This is a complete misconception because actually, in one sense, there is harder work to be done by the Red Cross in time of peace than in time of war. It is conceivable that we could get along without Red Cross services in time of war because volunteers spring from all sides at such times, though their efforts would be unorganized and therefore highly inefficient. But we would have these workers available as a result of the patriotic impulse of the times. Today we lack that impulse but we do have these tremendous tasks that do pertain to the last war, to the present situation of the armed forces, as well as to disasters and home service requirements.

I very much hope that we can build up a much stronger volunteer effort during the next twelve months. And to do so it is important that the volunteer be given important work, real responsibility and that she or he be made to feel that this effort is appreciated by the general public in the local communities.

There is another phase of the Red Cross effort that I little realized until recently. That is the Junior Red Cross which has an enrolled membership of some 19 million. I think that we have not made full use of this vast potential because there seems to be too great a loss of individuals in the transition between the Junior Red Cross and the senior organization.

I think it is important that young women—girls, as a matter of fact, should be encouraged to take advantage of certain excellent training opportunities that the Red Cross offers, the better to prepare themselves as citizens. I am thinking of the extensive health programs in home nursing, first aid, and food and nutrition. The position of women in the country is such that they are destined to take a large part in public affairs. Some preparation for the duty of citizenship is therefore an obligation for the young women of the nation.

We are looking into this phase of the matter but so far we have not produced a definite additional program. So I will merely express my own view that here is possibly the greatest potential for vigorous and enthusiastic action in the whole Red Cross scene if we only learn how to make better use of it.

Finally, I would like to speak to you about the possible influence of the Red Cross in these troubled times. Whatever may be considered the nature of the problem in our country's international relations, I think it should now be apparent to every thinking citizen that negotiatory agreements and treaty commitments can only be effective, that is, be depended upon, if they have a background of good faith and good will among the nations and people concerned. I have talked about this on numerous occasions but I think it very appropriate that I should mention it this morning because I am convinced that the future peace of the world depends on the re-establishment of these qualities that make for understanding among peoples and races and nations.

Now I know of no other organization with the facilities, the background and the reputation of the Red Cross for promoting the re-establishment of this desired state of affairs. All that we do is to help people, to help communities, to help regions. There is no maneuvering for power or for ulterior purposes. We work only for the welfare of human beings.

As members of the American Red Cross we should never forget that we are a part of the world-wide Red Cross movement. We are bound together with the peoples of 67 other countries. Basically their spiritual aspirations are the same as ours. They want to live in human dignity and peace. By our example of compassion for those in distress, whether in our local communities, across the nation or around the world, we can foster human welfare and promote world understanding.

So I think in these particular years that there is great good for all mankind that can be done by the Red Cross. It is not a task of a day, or a week, or even a year. We should never cease in our sincere and steady efforts to help others.

This expresses man's oldest and noblest impulse—which if released and realized to its full strength can become the most powerful force in the world for a lasting peace.

GCMRL/G. C. Marshall Papers (American Red Cross, Speeches and Statements)

1. Philip K. Robinson of Milwaukee served as chairman of the American Red Cross Convention from June 26 to June 29, 1950.

2. Republican Albert E. Cobo had been sworn in as mayor of Detroit earlier that year. ("CIO Defeat Widens Michigan Democratic Split," *Washington Post*, November 20, 1949, p. B3.) Henry T. Ewald was the chairman of the Detroit chapter of the American Red Cross.

3. See pp. 19–21.
4. See pp. 47–48, 72–73.
5. On May 17, 1949, twelve inches of rain fell on Fort Worth, Texas, causing the Trinity River to overflow its banks and flood the city. More than thirteen thousand people were left homeless, and City Manager W. O. Jones estimated that property damage would run "well over $6,000,000." ("Flood Hits Dallas; 8 Dead in Ft. Worth," *Washington Post*, May 19, 1949, p. 19.)
6. On April 17, 1947, a ship loaded with nitrates exploded in the harbor of Texas City, Texas. The Red Cross activated local chapters and transferred personnel working in tornado-ravaged Oklahoma to assist the Texas refugees. ("Ship Starts Havoc," *New York Times*, April 17, 1947, p. 1.)
7. On May 20, 1950, four munitions barges in the harbor of South Amboy, New Jersey, exploded. The Red Cross quickly declared the region a disaster area, mobilized workers, and sent blood supplies to aid the town. ("Town Designated as Disaster Area," *New York Times*, May 20, 1950, p. 3.)
8. See pp. 188–91.
9. See pp. 105–6.

Trembling on the Edge

June 27–November 27, 1950

I have been trembling on the edge of being called again into public service in this crisis, but I hope I get by unmolested, but when the President motors down and sits under our oaks and tells me of his difficulties, he has me at a disadvantage.

—Marshall to Rose Page Wilson
July 24, 1950

KOREA had been promised its independence from Japan in the 1943 Cairo Declaration. Following the Japanese surrender in 1945, it was occupied by US and Soviet troops, with the 38th parallel serving as a temporary dividing line. As the cold war developed and intensified that line became permanent, with each power establishing a rival government in its area before withdrawing its occupation forces: the Republic of Korea (ROK) under Syngman Rhee in the south and the Democratic People's Republic of Korea (DPRK) under Kim Il-sung in the north. Each sought to unify Korea under his own leadership.

On June 25, 1950, the North Korean Army crossed the 38th parallel and attempted to unify the peninsula by force. Perceiving this attack as a Soviet-inspired move, the Truman administration quickly decided to oppose it with force. General Douglas MacArthur in Tokyo was authorized to commit first US air and naval forces, and by June 30 US ground forces, to the peninsula. Simultaneously the administration requested and received UN Security Council resolutions condemning the North Korean attack as aggression and calling upon member states to support South Korea militarily, thereby sanctioning US military moves as a UN "police action." (The Soviet Union was at this time boycotting the Security Council for its refusal to seat Mao Tse-tung's People's Republic of China in place of Chiang Kai-shek's Nationalist government, which had retreated to Formosa, an island also known as Taiwan off the coast of mainland China.) Already supreme commander for the Allied Powers in Japan (SCAP) as well as commander in chief, Far East Command (CINCFEC) and commanding general of US Army Forces Far East (CGUSAFFE), MacArthur was now appointed commander in chief, United Nations Command (CINCUNC) as well. The administration also decided at this time to increase its military aid to the French in their war against the Communist Viet Minh in Indochina and to the Philippine government, and to send the Seventh Fleet into the straits of Taiwan to preclude any Communist effort to take the island or any move by Chiang back onto the mainland that would expand the war.

Marshall did not participate in and was not consulted on any of these decisions. During the first week of July, however, numerous government officials—including President Truman and Secretary of State Acheson—met with him both at his Leesburg home and in Washington (see pp. 128–31). While in Washington during that week he also testified before the Senate Foreign Relations Committee regarding the US Information and Education Program. ★

77

TESTIMONY ON EXPANDING THE INTERNATIONAL INFORMATION AND EDUCATION PROGRAM
July 5, 1950 Washington, DC

"I THINK it is very important that we meet the Soviet in what is sometimes called their 'conquest of the minds of the people,'" Marshall began. He understood that "propaganda" was technically the correct word, but he believed that it implied "that you are engaged in cunning practices to put over your bill of goods." It was important that the US government agencies "confine ourselves to the truth. . . . I think any propaganda machine is an unfortunate thing for a government like ours to have to set up, but I think a great military force is an unfortunate thing also, but sometimes you have to have it; and right now it seems most appropriate." (Senate Committee on Foreign Relations, *Expanded International Information and Education Program: Hearings . . . on S. Res. 243*, 81st Cong., 2d sess., 21.)

During his mission to China in 1946, Marshall noted, he faced propaganda "so outrageous that no sound man could be impressed by it. I discovered later that was not the case. I have seen it here. I have seen it carried to the point where it was quite evident that the Soviets knew from the instant they moved in a certain direction that we would know that it was the height of insincerity. Yet they could still do that and get a tremendous reaction publicly in this country, a very difficult thing for the State Department to endure." The United States had to meet the Soviet Union's skillful and determined propaganda attacks. As justification for this, Marshall cited a sentence from the Declaration of Independence—"A decent respect for the opinion of mankind impels us to explain why we are doing this"—but noted that "as a continuing Government function [such propaganda efforts] will not be a good thing. But I think it is now urgently necessary. . . . [T]he fundamental principle involved in this effort is that we confine ourselves to the truth. Just what particular truths, at what particular time, in what particular quantity, and how put out, is a technical question for experts." (Ibid., 22.)

Marshall reiterated these points in response to a question from Senator H. Alexander Smith (R-NJ), asserting that "the truth does prevail, maybe in a long time, too long a time, it seems, but it does prevail. . . . We are a little impatient about the prevailing truths, and I think it is most important for us to stick to the truth very accurately in any program such as this." Furthermore, whatever the US armed forces had accomplished by force, "to consolidate what they do requires a change of mind of the people of the world or it will not be lasting at all. That is what we are suffering from right now. We have had a conquest, a military conquest, but it is not lasting. There is a confusion of the mind. How you correct that, I do not know unless it is by some such method as this resolution proposes." As with the ECA, he responded to a question from Senator William Benton (D-CT), any program should be run outside the State Department "so long as we controlled the policy." (Ibid., 22–24.)

Senator Henry Cabot Lodge Jr. (R-MA) asked if, nevertheless, "the highest priority" should go to "the rebuilding of the military strength of the free world" since without military strength "none of our propaganda will be effective." Such rebuilding was "essential," Marshall responded, "because otherwise we will lose half that we have gained, if not all that we have gained, in the development particularly of western Europe. It is one of the unfortunate tragedies of the present situation that we have to proceed on that basis. But it is inevitable that we do, if we do not want to find ourselves in a hopeless position later on." (Ibid., 25–26.) ★

78

To Lewis W. Douglas July 5, 1950
Washington, DC

Dear Douglas: I have been delayed in acknowledging your letter in which you gave me a frank reaction regarding the question of my accepting the Freedom of the City.[1] I appreciate very much the care which you have taken in the matter and your views. But I think there is one phase of the question which concerns me most that I didn't make clear to you. I am not concerned personally in the matter at all as far as adverse reactions are concerned. My concern is the harm that might be done British and American relations and the honor we wish to pay Sir John Dill. As matters now stand I think I will hold to my earlier view that I should not accept and I am glad to have had you tell me that this will be completely understood.

I might tell you that I heard from Field Marshal Wilson, "Jumbo", who expressed the feeling of Nancy Dill, himself and Dill's friends that he thought it would be very bad to go ahead with the erection of the monument in Arlington because of the unpleasant reactions that might be stirred up in this country.[2] I don't agree with him on this but have consulted the British Ambassador to get his official reaction.[3] Informally, he agrees with me and we have gone ahead with instituting the final arrangements for setting up the monument in Arlington Cemetery.

I got your reference to the fishing and saw your letter to Carter (incidentally, he leaves tonight en route to Japan).

With affectionate regards to Mrs. Douglas and yourself and my very best to Sharman.[4] Faithfully yours,

GCMRL/G. C. Marshall Papers (American Red Cross, General)

1. Douglas, the US ambassador to Great Britain, had written to Marshall on May 2 regarding a proposal to give Marshall the Freedom of the City of London. Marshall replied on May 10 that he was "beginning to be a little doubtful of the wisdom of my considering this honor" because of its possible negative impact on congressional funding for the ECA and the ongoing opposition to the planned memorial to Sir John Dill in Arlington National Cemetery by "dyed-in-the-wool isolationists" who would "seize on this as just another opportunity to damn the British," as the *Chicago Tribune* and the other Patterson family–owned newspapers had been doing. Marshall had asked Douglas if declining the honor would embarrass him and the lord mayor of London, to which Douglas replied on June 2 that "you will be giving no offense whatsoever to anyone on this side of the water." (Douglas to Marshall, May 2 and June 2, 1950, and Marshall to Douglas, May 10, 1950, GCMRL/G. C. Marshall Papers [American Red Cross, General].) Marshall expressed similar reasons for declining the honor in a July 10 letter to Lady Mary Burghley. (Marshall to Lady Mary Burghley, July 10, 1950, ibid.)

2. Field Marshal Sir Henry "Jumbo" Maitland Wilson had headed the British Joint Staff Mission in Washington, DC, from Field Marshal Sir John Dill's death in late 1944 until April 1947. As such, he was a member of the Combined Policy Committee, which since late 1943 had been concerned with collaboration and exchange of information on atomic matters with the British and Canadian governments. Wilson was created Baron Wilson of Libya and Stowlangtoft in 1946.

3. See pp. 143–44.

4. "Your letter of July 5th is here," Douglas replied. "For purely personal reasons you know how much Mrs. Douglas and Sharman and I regret your decision. However, I can

understand the reasons thoroughly and sympathize with you." (Douglas to Marshall, July 14, 1950, ibid.) Sharman was Ambassador Douglas's daughter.

See also pp. 145–46.

79

To Arthur H. Vandenberg

July 7, 1950
[Washington, DC]

Dear Vandenberg: Katherine and I returned from a week in Detroit—the National Red Cross Convention—and the first thing we did was to find out if we might see you. However, we were told that visitors were not yet welcome.

I wanted to tell you that the Board of Governors passed a resolution regarding Hazel and stood in reverent silence to her memory.[1]

Katherine wanted me particularly to tell you how much impressed she was by the memoriam card. It was beautifully done and I know it will be treasured by all of Hazel's friends.

Confidentially, you might be interested to know that I have had a very active time the past few days. On about an hour's notice Acheson, Harriman, Bohlen, and Kennan showed up down at Leesburg and stayed for lunch.[2] You can imagine the character of the discussion.[3] At four o'clock Baruch flew into the little air field which is only a quarter of a mile from the house. He stayed until the following afternoon. Then the President telephoned he wanted me for lunch on Wednesday with Eisenhower and Bradley. The next morning before we had gotten up the President telephoned again and asked if he might come down which he did arriving at 9:30 our time with Margaret. They stayed until about noon.[4] While he was there a message came from Pace, Secretary of the Army, asking me to call at his office and be briefed on the situation there the *next* day.[5] I tried to catch up on my Red Cross business which had accumulated during my absence and then went up on the Hill at ten o'clock and had to wait until eleven to talk on Benton's resolution favoring an increased educational program by the United States in combating communism in foreign countries.[6] Tom Connally blew in and was photographed with me, or I with him and I got away at 11:30 and went to Pace's office and there I found mostly "brass." From there I arrived at the Blair House about two minutes late and lunched with the President, Eisenhower, and Bradley.[7]

Now, for a man who is trying to devote himself to Red Cross and keep out of governmental things, I certainly found myself up to the neck in this situation. It would have been a great relaxer to sit down and have a drink with you and Bob Lovett and decide just how we were going to manage the world and then have done it.

I suppose you saw that the President tried to get Lovett in service as American Deputy on the North Atlantic Treaty Council and he declined because of health reasons. Adele, his wife, who has always been very sturdy has been ill, I believe, for the first time in her life.

This is much too long a letter but some of the details may interest you.[8] Affectionately,

GCMRL/G. C. Marshall Papers (Pentagon Office, General)

1. Hazel Vandenberg, Arthur's wife, passed away on June 10, 1950, after a long illness. She had been a public relations officer for the Red Cross during World War II and was an active volunteer for the organization following the war.

2. Charles E. "Chip" Bohlen had served as a special adviser on Soviet affairs and counselor to Secretary of State Marshall and composed a first draft of the Marshall Plan speech delivered at Harvard University on June 5, 1947. (See *Papers of GCM*, 6: 142, 149–50.) In August 1949 President Truman named him minister of the US embassy in Paris. He was recalled to temporary duty in Washington upon the outbreak of the Korean War in late June 1950. Averell Harriman was simultaneously recalled to serve as special presidential assistant. ("Truman Shuffles State Department," *New York Times*, May 27, 1949, p. 11; "Diplomatic Problems Arise Over US Action in Korea," *New York Times*, July 21, 1950, p. 4; "Truman Appoints Harriman Special Foreign Affairs Aide," *New York Times*, June 17, 1950, p. 1.)

George F. Kennan had been director of the State Department's Policy Planning Staff from May 1947 until January 1950. President Truman appointed him Bohlen's successor as a special adviser and counselor to the secretary of state on Soviet affairs in August 1949. He had been poised to leave the State Department on July 1, 1950, but stayed on as counselor on Soviet affairs until late August because of the outbreak of the Korean War. ("Truman Shuffles State Department," *New York Times*, May 27, 1949, p. 11; "Kennan Maps Rest from US Duties," *New York Times*, December 11, 1949, p. 50; "Diplomatic Problems Arise Over US Action in Korea," *New York Times*, July 21, 1950, p. 4; "Kennan Steps Out as Guide on Soviet," *New York Times*, August 20, 1950, p. 48.)

3. Kennan in his diary reported a long and pessimistic intelligence briefing on the morning of July 1 regarding Korea, followed by a meeting with John Foster Dulles and Secretary of the Army Frank Pace. "Following that meeting," Kennan wrote, Acheson

> suggested that he, Averell Harriman, Chip Bohlen and myself go out to Leesburg and talk to General Marshall. A phone call was put through to the General, and it was arranged that we should come for lunch. We departed immediately and got out there soon after one o'clock. The General was in fine form. We sat on the lawn under the trees and had our business talk then and there, over our events of the week and the position in which we found ourselves today. The General listened very attentively and silently, as he always does when a problem is being exposed before him, and then gave us his views vigorously and without hesitation.
>
> Pointing out that all of his statements were based on the very scanty information which the Secretary had just been able to give him and not on any detailed background of fact, he said that there could be no doubt about the proper course for us to pursue. We had begun this thing; now we had to go through with it. His greatest worry had been that for the sake of Korea we might have risked an alienation of public opinion in Western Europe, which was the area of the greatest real strategic importance. What we had told him had relieved his fears on this point; but he was deeply disturbed over what he understood to be the attitudes in the Defense Establishment, particularly with their relation to the Department of State. He did not feel that we needed to send more in the way of military support to MacArthur. It was a common failing of commanders in the field to ask for more than they needed, and MacArthur was far from being an exception to this rule. He should be told to do this job with what he had. He could do it if he applied himself to it. The depletion of the forces on Japan was not dangerous. Any amphibious action against Japan would be a great undertaking, and a very risky one in the face of any sizeable air and naval defense. He was particularly concerned about the initial tendency of the Air Force to think that they could do this all alone. That, he said, was the same old thing. The Air Force and the Navy were full of ideas about how they could do things, and their

functions were indeed tremendously important; but when it came down to the last analysis, you could never get along without the "little fellow in the mud". Also, he felt that our people had made a mistake in the organization of the Korean Army. He had begged them to organize it along the lines of the Philippine scouts, using experienced older American non-commissioned officers and filling up the ranks with Koreans. Instead, they had insisted on trying to build up a new army from scratch, officers corps and all. Nevertheless, he was not discouraged, and he felt that this might turn out to be a good thing in many ways.

On the way back to Washington, we talked matters over and agreed that it was important that the General should have an opportunity to state his views to the President in the very near future. Mr. Harriman undertook to get into touch with the President and to make the suggestion, but we agreed that it would neither be fair to the General nor wise for any of us to try to relay the General's views to the President. (Kennan diary entry, July 1, 1950, Princeton/George F. Kennan Papers [box 232, folder 1]; Frank Costigliola, ed., *The Kennan Diaries* [New York: W. W. Norton & Co., 2014], 258–59.)

4. Truman's first telephone call to Marshall with its invitation to lunch on July 5 probably stemmed from the Acheson-Bohlen-Kennan-Harriman discussion on their drive back from Leesburg on July 1, described by Kennan in note 3 above. But his second telephone call and decision to visit Marshall in Leesburg on July 4 had an additional motive: the president had by this time decided to remove Secretary of Defense Johnson and wished to see if Marshall was able and willing to take the position.

Johnson had been attacking Acheson and the administration's China policy, meeting—according to Truman—with "enemy Senators of mine," and beginning "to show an inordinate egotistical desire to run the whole government. He offended every member of the cabinet," Truman recorded in his diary on September 14, 1950. "Finally in June 1950 I made up my mind he'd have to go. I made a trip to Leesburg with my daughter and talked to Gen. Marshall—about China, Formosa, Japan, MacArthur, Chiang Kai-shek and finally about the defense department. A most interesting morning." (Robert H. Ferrell, ed., *Off the Record: The Private Papers of Harry S. Truman* [New York: Harper & Row, 1980], 192.)

Marshall implied in a letter three weeks later that he and Truman had indeed discussed the Defense Department position on July 4 (see pp. 146–47). Perhaps for that reason the president took precautions to keep the visit secret: it is not in his appointments calendar for July 4 (which incorrectly places him in Blair House all day), and he had his daughter drive him to Leesburg. She reported the trip in her published diary entry for July 4. (Margaret Truman, *Souvenir* [New York: McGraw Hill, 1956], 275–76.)

5. Frank Pace Jr. had served as a special assistant to the US attorney general in 1946, executive assistant to the postmaster general from 1946 to 1948, and assistant director and director of the Bureau of the Budget from 1948 to April 12, 1950, when President Truman appointed him secretary of the army.

6. William Benton had served as an assistant secretary of state for public affairs from August 31, 1945, to September 30, 1947; he was appointed to the US Senate on December 17, 1949. He also served as chairman of the board and publisher of the *Encyclopedia Britannica* from 1943 to 1973. For Marshall's testimony see pp. 125–26.

7. Marshall had lunch with Truman, Eisenhower, and JCS Chairman General Bradley as well as Chief of Naval Operations (CNO) Admiral Forrest P. Sherman (USNA, 1917) on July 5, 1950. (Truman to Marshall, July 15, 1950, GCMRL/G. C. Marshall Papers [American Red Cross, General].) Admiral Sherman had served as deputy chief of staff to Admiral Chester W. Nimitz (USNA, 1905), Pacific Fleet commander, from November 1943 through the end of World War II. He had been CNO since October 1949 and represented Nimitz, who was on the West Coast at the time of this meeting. Connally had served in the US Senate since 1929. He was currently chairman of the Senate Committee on Foreign Relations.

Eisenhower noted in his diary that during the meeting he and Marshall "told the president that his decision of a week ago must be earnestly supported. Speed and strength, both are needed. We encountered good intentions but I'm not so sure we met full comprehension." (Robert H. Ferrell, ed., *The Eisenhower Diaries* [New York: W. W. Norton, 1981], 176.) Sherman informed Nimitz the next day that "We discussed the current situation and General Bradley went over the military situation in Korea at considerable length. In the discussion both General Marshall and General Eisenhower advocated that we do everything necessary to finish the Korean incident quickly and successfully, augmenting forces as necessary and practicable but avoiding general mobilization. . . . I got the impression," Sherman added, that Truman "wanted to talk the present situation over with his senior military advisers and that he would do so again from time to time as opportunity offers." (Sherman to Nimitz, July 6, 1950, NA/RG 330, CD 092 [Korea].) "The President said that Marshall and Eisenhower asked Bradley many penetrating questions about the military situation in Korea," presidential assistant George Elsey recorded on July 8, "and about the readiness of our military forces for action elsewhere. The President said that he found the questions and Bradley's answers highly illuminating." (Memorandum for the File, July 8, 1950, HSTL/George M. Elsey Papers [Subject File, Korea: July 1950].)

8. "I am deeply touched by the action of the Board of Governors of the American National Red Cross in passing its resolution and standing in reverent silence to her memory," Vandenberg replied. "I am tremendously interested in that portion of your letter which indicates your contacts with divers and sundry officers of the Government. It is comforting to me to know that they are pursuing you for advice because advice could come from no sounder, saner, solid source. I loved your reminiscence [about Lovett]. . . . Those were truly 'great days.' My part in them will always be my proudest record. Looking backward, it is really quite amazing how well we in the world got along together." (Vandenberg to Marshall, July 10, 1950, GCMRL/G. C. Marshall Papers [Pentagon Office, General].)

80

TO HARRY S. TRUMAN

July 10, 1950
Washington, DC

My dear Mr. President: I feel that I should add to your burden of correspondence by thanking you more formally for the two luncheons you have honored me with, and particularly for the visit you and Margaret paid us the other day.[1] Katherine and I really are deeply appreciative and she, like myself, is always hopeful that you will turn to our peace and quiet at Leesburg more frequently—some day even go so far as to let us bed you down for the night.[2]

With great respect. Faithfully yours,

G. C. Marshall

GCMRL/G. C. Marshall Collection (Harry S. Truman)

1. Truman visited Marshall at Dodona Manor with his daughter Margaret on July 4; see previous document.

2. "It was a very great pleasure to me to pay you a visit at Leesburg and it was also exceedingly helpful to have the opportunity of discussing the situation with you, General Eisenhower, General Bradley and Admiral Sherman. I had hoped to have Admiral Nimitz present but he had just landed in Berkeley and I didn't order him back," Truman responded. "We are pursuing direct policy in this present situation and trying to profit by the experience of 1941. I hope to have the opportunity of seeing you occasionally to discuss just what is going on. I'll either call on you at Leesburg or ask you to come up." (Truman to Marshall, July 15, 1950, GCMRL/G. C. Marshall Papers [American Red Cross, General].)

81

To Queen Frederica of the Hellenes July 10, 1950
Washington, DC

Your Majesty: In replying to your last letter I have been hoping to have some good news to give you regarding the tragic situation of the Greek children who were carried over the border to the Satellite states.[1] I am distressed that greater progress has not been made. Yugoslavia stated, I am told, more or less publicly that they intended to return the children but the situation appears rather discouraging on the part of the Cominform states although they are hoping that something may come at least from Yugoslavia.[2]

As head of the American Red Cross, I have been deeply interested in what this organization has done and is in the process of doing regarding your situation in Greece. I have found that something more than a half million dollars worth of wearing apparel was contributed in 1947 and that the most recent contribution consisting of one hundred thousand dollars worth of clothing and shoes for the children was made back in January 1949, the shipments occurring largely during the first six months of that year.

A recent report from the Greek Red Cross states that by February last, four-fifths of this children's clothing had been distributed to the villages in the north and those of Western Macedonia and the mountain area of Thessaly. Also, that the remaining items are still in process of being distributed. As you are the head of the Greek Red Cross I assume that you are familiar with these facts and in much greater detail than I am. I am told that the relationship between your Queens Fund and the Greek Red Cross is excellent and that the working members of the Ladies Committee of the Queens Fund are volunteers associated with the Greek Red Cross. My information is that supplies donated to the Greek Red Cross by our organization and other Red Cross societies has been turned over to the Queens Fund for the benefit of the refugee children.

As you probably know, acting on the initiative taken by the President of the International Committee of the Red Cross and the Chairman of the Board of Governors of the League of Red Cross Societies, the Secretary-General of the United Nations invited the Governments of Bulgaria, Czechoslovakia, Hungary, Roumania and Yugoslavia to designate representatives to meet him in Geneva on July 6th to discuss the problem of the return of the Greek children in accordance with the resolutions of the General Assembly of the United Nations. Because of the situation in Korea I understand this meeting has been postponed. I hope not indefinitely. However, I am assured that the International Red Cross is continuing its efforts to effect the repatriation of the Greek children.

I hesitate to outline these various facts because you are probably intimately familiar with them. However, I should comment on the fact that the combined mission of the International Committee of the Red Cross and the League of Red Cross Societies, recently returned from Greece and brought the necessary documents required by the Czechoslovak Red Cross and that Government for the repatriation of 122 of the 128 Greek children identified by the Czechoslovak Red Cross.

As you know on May 30th the American Delegate to the United Nations, Ambassador Warren R. Austin, transmitted a note from the United States to the Secretary-General of the United Nations expressing our formal regret that no Greek child so far has been returned to Greece and that even elementary indications, indispensable for the solution of the problem, have not been furnished by the Governments concerned.

Recently, the Bulgarian Government declared its willingness to cooperate in the repatriation of the children and visas, I am told, are now being awaited by the International Red Cross for the entry into Bulgaria by its mission. It is too bad that negotiations on the exchange of ministers with Yugoslavia broke down.[3]

Of course the present incident in Korea has tremendous possibilities either for good or bad and this Government will act with determination, I am sure, which I think is essential if we are to get a good result. The present fighting, of course, involves the usual disadvantage of democracy which cannot engage in secret mobilizations and arbitrary decisions for violent action. It will be some time before the United States Forces and other United Nations contingents have concentrated the necessary strength in Korea. But the process is under way at top speed though the distances are tremendous and the difficulties very great. The most heartening phase of the entire matter is the apparent unanimous attitude not only of the people of this country but of the democratic world.

I saw that my military selection, General Van Fleet, has been withdrawn.[4] I have not seen him but I hope he left with a spirit of good will and understanding with your officers.

Mrs. Marshall and I very frequently mention the possibility of that visit in our "private home" that I mentioned to you. I suppose protocol and secret service would introduce many complications but I think I am capable of making the satisfactory arrangements. Mrs. Marshall has been suffering for almost nine months with "shingles" in her eyes. She still finds it very difficult to read or write and suffers considerable reaction if she gets tired.

Your Majesty I must ask your pardon for dictating this note but it is a rather lengthy one and I thought it best to put it in that form.

With Mrs. Marshall's love to the children and our respectful regards and admiration to the King and yourself.[5] Faithfully yours,

GCMRL/G. C. Marshall Papers (Pentagon Office, Selected)

1. Frederica's July 2 letter to Katherine Marshall may have prompted the timing of Marshall's July 10 response. The Greek government had claimed that Communist guerrillas had abducted children from northern Greece and sent them to reeducation camps in the Balkan satellite states. "There is one thing which the world does not seem to have understood or taken to heart," Frederica had remonstrated. "28,000 Greek children have been carried across the frontiers and have disappeared behind the iron curtain. . . . I do not think there has ever been such a crime in history and there has never been such silence by the world over this crime against humanity." (Frederica to Katherine Marshall, July 2, 1950, GCMRL/© Marshall-Winn Collection.) In his March 6 letter to Marshall (see p.

42n3), Acheson had expressed his appreciation for the efforts of the American Red Cross, working through the International Committee of the Red Cross and the League of Red Cross Societies in Geneva, Switzerland, "to bring about the repatriation" of these children. "Progress has been discouragingly slow," he admitted, "but I feel that we must keep this humanitarian issue alive." (Acheson to Marshall, March 6, 1950, GCMRL/G. C. Marshall Papers [Pentagon Office, Selected].) For additional information on these Red Cross efforts, see an unsigned and undated memorandum reporting comments by Assistant Secretary of State for Far Eastern Affairs Dean Rusk and the officer in charge of Greek affairs in the State Department's Bureau of Near Eastern, South Asian, and African Affairs, Leonard J. Cromie, with attached memorandum, "Repatriation of Greek Children." (Ibid.)

2. The Cominform was the Soviet-dominated Communist Information Bureau that had been established in September 1947, from which Yugoslavia had been expelled in June 1948.

3. "Very little came of the efforts of the International Red Cross," Queen Frederica wrote in her memoir. "Of the thousands of children who were taken away a few hundred did come back and these were mostly from Yugoslavia. Shortly before our victory over the communists relations with Yugoslavia improved and some small groups came trickling home." (Queen Frederica of the Hellenes, *A Measure of Understanding* [London: Macmillan, 1971], 128.)

4. Major General James A. Van Fleet had been selected to command the Joint US Military Advisory Group in Greece (JUSMAG) in early 1948 to support the Greek government during the civil war there. See *Papers of GCM*, 6: 344–45, 353–54.

5. Queen Frederica sent Marshall a lengthy response commenting upon the political and military situation in Western Europe, remarking that "Western Germany is materially disarmed. France is spiritually disarmed. That is to say from a fighting spirit point of view only. Italy from an army point of view is always better to have as an enemy than as a friend." She encouraged the Allies, in the event of a third world war, to use Greece as "*The Bridgehead* for a *Spearhead attack* against the soft underbelly of the Russian Empire." Making the argument that Greece's army and national morale were in "good fighting spirit" and capable of "superhuman efforts," she recommended that the United States establish a series of forward operating military supply bases in Greece in preparation for a future war. She then outlined the current political situation in Greece, calling the Plastiras government "unspeakably awful." In closing, she remarked, "We have been very sad to see Van Fleet leave. He has been a first class friend. There was perfect cooperation between my husband, General Van Fleet and General Papagos. Van Fleet trusted us and we trusted him. He shared our hopes and fears and understood the Greek situation perfectly." (Frederica to Marshall, July 20, 1950, GCMRL/G. C. Marshall Papers [Pentagon Office, Selected].)

Greek military hero General Alexandros Papagos had been serving as the commander in chief of the Hellenic National Army at the recommendation of General Van Fleet since January 1949 and had been promoted to the rank of field marshal in October 1949. (Photini Tomai, ed., *Documentary History of Greece [1943–1951]: Truman Doctrine and Marshall Plan* [Athens: Ministry of Foreign Affairs of the Hellenic Republic, 2011], 433–34.) Nikolaos Plastiras had been serving as prime minister and head of the Foreign Ministry since April 1950. He had also been prime minister from December 1944 to April 1945. (Ibid., 436.) A State Department typist misspelled Plastiras's name while transcribing Queen Frederica's handwritten letter. See pp. 304–6.

82

TO MADAME CHIANG KAI-SHEK — July 10, 1950
Washington, DC

Dear Madame: I delayed in replying to your letter of May 23 until the return of Secretary Johnson from the Far East.[1] However, with his arrival came the Korean incident which nominates [*dominates*] all considerations at the present time. These recent events have considerably changed the situation you described and the arrival of American Naval vessels in Formosa waters has a very direct bearing on that situation.

At the present time as you of course know matters are in the train of rapid developments and it is too difficult to make any report of observations at the moment. However, there appears to be no question of unanimity of the people in this country that Western Europe is supporting the determined action on our part and I hope with more representation from other nations in the United Nations.

I brought Katherine in this morning. She's en route to the hospital for further treatment for her eyes and extraction of two teeth that should have come out long ago. She will undoubtedly spend the night there. I, meanwhile, am off for Boston in connection with scientific developments in the blood program of the Red Cross. We have just returned from a week in Detroit where we attended the National Convention of the Red Cross. Katherine got along very well there because I made very few engagements for her and she had considerable rest periods between events.[2]

However, we had a shocking accident in Leesburg Saturday when her brother-in-law, Sterling Lacy, driving his car with Allene in the seat with him, lost control and crashed into a tree. He was a little cut up and sustained a broken leg. Allene was thrown against the dashboard and the windshield breaking the latter and very badly cut her chin inside the mouth. She suffered a broken, really a shattered shoulder, and this morning—we dropped in the hospital at eight o'clock—was having a pretty difficult time. I think they are going to move her into Washington because the setting of her shoulder will require very skillful treatment.

All of this, of course, poured on Katherine who has spent most of her time since Saturday in the hospital from seven in the morning until late in the evening. She did not want to come in for her treatment today but I insisted.

I hope your health is built up and particularly during this summer heat that you are not suffering from your old trouble and hope that by being in the mountains you are escaping the heat. From the reports I get here, Generalissimo's health is good and he bears up under the strain. I was told this morning that General MacArthur is sending a member of his headquarters to Formosa to see what is needed to put it in a state of defense.

I am sorry for the delay in answering your letter but under the circumstances it seemed wise to do so. Katherine, I think, is writing you regarding the tea which just came two days ago. The hats have not yet shown up.

As usual I am traveling with your dressing gown—I mean mine but your gift and also your luggage. So far I have been well. I express myself regarding this rather cautiously because I do not want pride to go before a fall.

With affectionate regards to you and my compliments to the Generalissimo. Faithfully yours,

GCMRL/G. C. Marshall Papers (Pentagon Office, Selected)

1. Madame Chiang had written to relate to Marshall the details of a visit by several American journalists to Taipei. She also took the opportunity to press him on the subject of additional aid for the Nationalist government, remarking, "It is now undeniable, even on the part of the most skeptical, that Russian imperialism, clothed with communist fervor, has as a major, perhaps a primary objective, its complete and early establishment in the Western Pacific. The Russians are going all out to this end. Chinese observers, American civilian and military observers who have recently departed from the Chinese mainland, give complete confirmation of intelligence reports, that the Russians are moving into the China mainland by the thousands—Russian civilians, technicians, soldiers, many of them in uniform. Further, these Russians are reinforced by Japanese and German prisoners of war and by Koreans. . . . It seems to me obvious that the only possible way to check, possibly reverse, the growing strength of communism in Asia is to give life and strength to the tremendous opposition that is being generated on the mainland as well as in Formosa against communism, now that there is such vivid and desperate realization of what it means. . . . It all adds up that we immediately need military aid to match what Russia is pouring into Communist China. The flow of such supplies from the United States should be controlled by United States personnel, the flow being adjusted to the prospects of its efficient and effective use. This is the manner in which your ECA and JCRR [Joint Commission on Rural Reconstruction] aid is now coming into Formosa and accomplishing very fine results. We feel it is imperative that no one be in a position to say that United States resources are being wasted. We feel that we, as well as you, must make certain that every dollar is properly spent." (Madame Chiang to Marshall, May 23, 1950, GCMRL/G. C. Marshall Papers [Pentagon Office, Selected].)

She concluded by expressing her hope that a plan could be developed "so that the beacon light of freedom in Asia could be kept kindled to inspire the hundred millions of my poor countrymen who are reduced to desperation and starvation on the mainland. Their cries re-echo in my ears day and night, for there is so little that I personally can do to help them, but that little I am doing with all my might and main." (Ibid.)

2. For Marshall's speech in Boston, see the next document. For his speech at the Detroit Red Cross convention, see pp. 113–22.

83

Speech on the Red Cross National Blood Program[1]

July 11, 1950
Boston, Massachusetts

Mr. Bundy, ladies and gentlemen[2]:

I welcome the opportunity to talk to you about the Red Cross National Blood Program, for to me it is one of the most important services ever undertaken by the Red Cross or possibly any such organization, here or abroad.

I am a layman, so I will not presume to talk about the technical aspects of blood in medical practice, but I must refer to certain matters which are thoroughly familiar to the scientists here but may not be clear to some of you. I wish to speak of the problems which confront us in the development of a nationwide program, designed to help meet the demands for blood in civilian medical practice and to serve as a bulwark against a major disaster or national military emergency.

The National Blood Program was launched as a peacetime program. But who can think only of peace today? The possible need for blood for our military forces is no longer a vague, shadowy possibility. It is a concrete fact.

The fact of present danger and the possibility of its increasing must be met with dispatch but without hysteria. Those who are charged with the responsibility for safeguarding the nation's health and reinforcing its security must think in terms of both civilian and possible military needs.

A national military emergency would call for quantities of blood almost beyond estimate. There is only one source from which this blood can be obtained—that is from the veins of living, healthy American people. And it must come voluntarily. Not even the totalitarian states have ever been able to procure blood by government fiat. Certainly that would be unthinkable in America. It would also be unnecessary—for our people are always quick to respond to an emergency. The difficulty has been to make them recognize the emergency, until it is on us in full blast. If the Red Cross is again officially designated as the agency responsible for blood procurement for our military forces or our civil defense, we will need the cooperation of existing blood facilities and interested organizations, as well as the help of every individual qualified to give blood. It is for these reasons that this meeting is being held today.

People must be made to realize that the day by day needs for blood are great and constantly growing—that blood is as important to peacetime strength and health as to the treatment of the battle wounded. When all is said and done, the nation's strength depends upon a healthy people.

As some of you may be unfamiliar with all the factors underlying the establishment of the National Blood Program, it may not be amiss for me to sketch in a little historic background.

Because they were either patriotic donors or grateful recipients, millions of Americans know about the blood donor service operated by the Red Cross during the war. More than twelve million pints of blood were processed into dried plasma and other blood derivatives for use of our men overseas. Nearly four hundred thousand pints of whole blood were flown to battle fronts—being about equally divided between the Pacific and European theaters of war. This blood and plasma was a major factor in a brilliant medical record—the survival of more than 97% of all wounded American servicemen.

In view of the publicity given the wartime service, it is understandable that many people think of that blood program as the first Red Cross participation in blood procurement. That is not a fact.

Back in 1937 a Red Cross chapter in Augusta, Ga., commenced the enrollment of blood donors to supply blood to local hospitals. One after another, Red Cross chapters over the country started donor enrollment services. When war came and the Red Cross was officially designated as the blood procurement agency for the military forces, it already had a nucleus from which to develop the blood collection service. After the war many chapters continued their local participation in donor enrollment. In addition to the National Program, there are now more than 150 of these local services in operation.

The present Program was established only after many appeals from hospital authorities and medical leaders. Physicians who had seen the miracle working power of blood in treating the war wounded very naturally wished to avail themselves of this strong weapon against peacetime disease and death.

In 1947 a committee of private physicians surveyed the nation and discovered that only 20% of the country's hospitals had blood facilities of any kind. Many of these banks were inadequate to meet the needs of their own physicians. No one of them could possibly cope with a major disaster in the community. In view of the increased blood demands for medical practice, growing out of wartime knowledge and experience, this was an appalling unpreparedness for day after day needs, entirely aside from disaster. How to get enough blood became the major problem.

Against this background of need, the Board of Governors of the Red Cross voted to inaugurate a national blood program. The first regional center under this program was established in Rochester, New York, in January, 1948. Today there are 33 such regional centers serving more than 1,800 hospitals in 38 states. Already these centers have provided physicians and hospitals, without cost, more than 781,000 pints of blood. At least four more of these regional centers are planned for opening this year.

The National Program now in operation differs greatly from the wartime service. During the war Red Cross activities were confined to drawing blood from donors and turning it over to the military authorities for processing and shipment. Present regional centers collect blood, examine it for medical safety, mark it as to group and other pertinent technical data, refrigerate it and distribute it to hospitals and physicians in accord with need.

This complete blood operation demands highly skilled physicians, nurses and technicians. It also calls for extensive educational and promotional efforts directed toward securing donors.

In the face of world conditions today we recognize that blood procurement cannot be a purely independent Red Cross activity. Certain agencies of the government, as well as the medical profession and other private groups, also have a vital place in the development of our blood resources.

Facing this fact, we have recently made some basic changes in the organization pattern of the National Blood Program, through which we will be able to work in closer cooperation with government agencies and national medical and health groups.

Because of its growing importance to our national welfare and security, the Blood Program has been made a separate service of the Red Cross, reporting directly to its President.

Under the new pattern, the development of medical policies and procedures, as well as professional techniques and practices, will be the responsibility of a committee of five nationally known physicians. The chairman of this committee is Dr. Ross T. McIntire, wartime Surgeon General of the Navy, who has been national director of the program since its inception. Serving with him are such distinguished physicians as Dr. Charles A. Janeway of Harvard Medical School, Dr. I. S. Ravdin of the University of Pennsylvania, Dr. Charles A. Doan of Ohio State University School of Medicine and Dr. Carl Moore of Washington University, St. Louis.

Dr. Edwin J. Cohn has agreed to serve as special adviser and consultant to me and Dr. Louis K. Diamond, celebrated Boston Hematologist, will continue to serve as national medical director.

As President of the Red Cross, I have asked the Secretary of Defense, the chairman of the National Security Resources Board [NSRB] and the heads of other appropriate governmental agencies to name their chief medical officers as advisers in the planning and operation of the blood program.

I have also asked the American Medical Association and other medical groups, as well as the American Hospital Association and the American Pharmaceutical Association to designate representatives to cooperate with us.

These representatives, together with the medical committee I mentioned earlier, give us access, I feel, to the best knowledge and thinking on blood that is available in this country. There are here tonight representatives of these agencies and cooperating groups. The understanding support of these men assures the future success of this program.

In addition we have been assured by the National Research Council, which played such an important part in blood procurement during the last war, that it will continue close collaboration with the Red Cross in its efforts to build an effective national blood program.

It is obvious that in preparing to provide blood for a possible military emergency we must evolve a scheme by which all the blood collection facilities in the country can be linked to cooperate in time of need. I am happy to report that steps have been taken through which non-profit blood banks which now serve many communities will be drawn into blood procurement plans. We have been assured the support and help of the American Association of Blood Banks to this end.

This arrangement is essential if we are to realize the goal of a truly national program. And we must have a truly national program if we are to have a measure of safety—any community which suffered a major disaster would necessarily have to look outside for help.

A great deal of careful planning has gone into the establishment of our regional centers. Blood is too valuable a substance to risk waste—either of the blood itself or of blood collection facilities. Therefore, we have not attempted to establish regional blood centers in communities where needs were being met but, on the contrary, have tried to concentrate where blood supplies were non-existent or inadequate.

All our regional centers operate in close cooperation with local medical societies—they are supervised by a medical advisory committee selected by the medical society in the area served by the center.

While the majority of the physicians in the country have been solidly behind our efforts to ensure a national framework for an adequate supply of blood to meet any emergency, there has been resistance on the part of some.

They thought the program was a step in the direction of socialized medicine. Nothing, I think, could be further from the truth. Socialization implies an activity required of the people by their government. Red Cross blood centers serve merely as the channel through which the generous impulses of the healthy may be directed to the benefit of those in need of the restorative powers of human blood. The fact is that the National Blood Program is positive evidence of the values of a purely voluntary activity—voluntary gifts of blood as well as money make this blood service possible.

Others have suggested that the Red Cross was trying to monopolize the blood resources of the nation and close the doors of all existing blood banks. That, of course, was not true. There is no place in this country for monopoly of the people's impulse of compassion for the sick and injured—that is as true of the Red Cross as it is of any other agency or group. The health of our people is the business of every agency or group charged with the responsibility for the national welfare—whether we are at peace or at war.

While I have been talking to you about possible emergencies, I have not been unmindful of the every day needs of our people for blood; mothers suffering hemorrhage, babies born with the need for complete replacement of blood due to incompatible factors in their parents' blood, patients undergoing surgery, suffering severe burns, chronic anemia, leukemia, and accident victims. Accident victims undergoing amputations and those requiring medical treatment and surgery far outnumbered our war wounded during the period of conflict. The fearful record of the July 4th weekend is evidence of the accuracy of this statement. Many of these victims, possibly most of them, needed blood, plasma, and one or more of the several blood derivatives in common use today.[3]

In addition to whole blood there are certain blood derivatives which have become standard therapy. These derivatives must be supplied as well as whole blood. Moreover whole blood is unstable, it cannot now be preserved more than 21 days. Any stockpiling of transfusion materials against a future emergency must be in the form of these stable derivatives—plasma and albumin. But to stockpile these derivatives we must first have whole blood.

Most of the blood derivatives which have been used in this country during the last five years were processed from plasma returned to Red Cross by the armed forces at the end of the war. This surplus plasma is running low—it is about exhausted.

Of one derivative alone—immune serum globulin—the Red Cross has supplied more than two and a half million vials. This serum is used to combat measles. Many think of measles as a simple childhood ailment—physicians tell me it is not quite so simple. It brings with it serious complications—sometimes it brings death. Immune serum globulin has proven immeasurably valuable in keeping down complications and saving the lives of very young children and babies. . . . we cannot afford to see this help withdrawn from physicians who treat children.[4]

So we come back again to the great problem—procurement of blood. Not just enough blood to meet the daily needs of medical practice, and that need has never been adequately met, but enough more blood to give the surplus required for valuable blood fractions.

In addition—blood is essential to research. You have seen demonstrations today which have been very illuminating to me . . . You have seen the care which is taken to extract the last bit of value from every drop of blood.

This afternoon you have witnessed new developments in blood in the Harvard laboratory under the guidance of Dr. Cohn.

Does it surprise you to know that most of the research and discoveries leading to today's demonstration have been made under the guidance of the medical leaders here today? And that most of these demonstrations are the result of major developments in blood study during the past decade? Would any one of you be willing to accept a cessation of this work when you know how much it means to the welfare of our people? Of course not. Nor would any of our people, be willing if they were aware of the importance of these discoveries and the fact that all of them depend upon donated blood.

In view of these discussions today . . . it must be apparent to you that in spite of the phenomenal strides in research and knowledge during the war years, and since, only the top waters have been stirred. I would hazard the guess that not even these distinguished scientists who have been responsible for much of this knowledge would be willing to venture an opinion as to what may yet be expected. Though additional benefits may be just "around the corner," the doctors may still have a lot "up their sleeves", as it were, and will not pass this information along to us until it has undergone what in medical parlance is called "clinical investigation and proof." I am quite satisfied with that caution, as I am sure you will be.

In view of the knowledge we now have, thanks to gentlemen like these present tonight, and considering all the possibilities of the future, I am content. I would like to offer the assurance that the American Red Cross, not only because of its obligations but because it esteems it a great privilege, will lend every possible cooperation to our medical leaders in their search for new and better ways to make blood serve the needs of all our people. We will bend every effort toward increasing the availability of blood.

Under the guidance of the medical committee I mentioned earlier, four pilot plants will undertake to test and demonstrate new developments in blood usefulness as a medical agent. These plants will probably be located at Boston, Philadelphia, St. Louis and Columbus, Ohio. We will give to these scientists as they have given to us—the best of our cooperation . . . to the end that all of our people may benefit from our joint effort . . . to the end that no man, woman or child, no soldier, sailor nor civilian may die for lack of life saving blood or blood derivatives . . .[5]

GCMRL/G. C. Marshall Papers (American Red Cross, Speeches and Statements)

1. The 7:00 p.m. dinner took place at the Harvard Club following a demonstration at Harvard Medical School of what the *New York Times* called "Revolutionary methods for the collection and preservation of blood . . . that make possible for the first time the isolation of many new components that promise to serve as veritable 'elixirs of life.'" ("'Life Elixirs' Seen in Blood Advances," *New York Times*, July 12, 1950, p. 31.)

2. Harvey Bundy chaired the Boston Metropolitan Chapter of the Red Cross. From 1931 to 1933 Bundy had served as assistant secretary of state in charge of financial and economic questions under Henry L. Stimson. In 1941 then Secretary of War Stimson

named Bundy his special assistant on atomic matters. After the war he studied foreign activities of the US government for the Hoover Commission on Organization of the Executive Branch of the Government.

3. The holiday weekend of July 4, 1950, saw a dramatic increase in traffic accidents. On July 4, the *New York Times* reported that "traffic fatalities in the nation rose sharply yesterday to 336, an increase of ninety-six in twenty-four hours." ("Holiday Fatalities in Sharp Upswing," *New York Times*, July 4, 1950, p. 1.)

4. This and the following ellipses are in the original; nothing has been omitted.

5. Marshall recorded a statement on July 28 for the Lockheed Aircraft corporation to congratulate the company's employees on their "decision to give further support to the National Blood Program of the American Red Cross" and for "setting a fine example which other organizations may follow." (Recording for Lockheed Aircraft Corporation for use on August 11, 1950, recorded on July 28, 1950, GCMRL/G. C. Marshall Papers [American Red Cross, Speeches and Statements].)

84

To Harold W. Dodds — July 17, 1950
[Washington, DC]

Dear Dodds: While your note of July 14th did not call for a reply I can't help but express my appreciation of your gracious acknowledgment of my letter regarding the Red Cross Board of Governors.[1]

I was up at Cohasset the night of the tenth and at Manchester the night of the eleventh, first with Dr. Edwin Cohn of Harvard and his wife and then with Harvey Bundy of Boston and his wife—all for the purpose of a three-day meeting with all the government representatives concerned with the Blood Program, the civilian organizations and the Harvard scientists. It was a rather hectic three days and having your case in mind I'm a pretty good example of what can be done on one kidney.[2]

You will be very wise to go slow and as pleasantly as you can make out. If you do get to the city during the next five months take on nothing of a serious nature, conversation or otherwise, rather take a look at Gentlemen Prefer Blonds as it will brighten things up considerably for you whether or not Mrs. Dodds approves.[3] Faithfully yours,

GCMRL/G. C. Marshall Papers (American Red Cross, General)

1. Dodds, who was recovering from surgery, had written, "In reply to your gracious letter of July 5 . . . I am sorry that my letter arrived so late, but I confess to a measure of relief since I realize that after a kidney removal one does not get back to full strength at once. If when the next vacancy occurs among the members-at-large of the Board of Governors you still wish to submit my name I shall be happy to accept." (Dodds to Marshall, July 14, 1950, GCMRL/G. C. Marshall Papers [American Red Cross, General].)

2. See the previous document.

On December 7, 1948, surgeons had removed Marshall's enlarged right kidney on which they had previously found "a large mass" that turned out to be a "benign cyst." ("Final Summary, Abstract from Clinical Record of General George C. Marshall [Ret.]," n.d., GCMRL/G. C. Marshall Papers [Pentagon Office, Biographical Materials, Marshall, Katherine Tupper, 1939–1947]. See also *Papers of GCM*, 6: 491n1 and 637.) On July 7, 1950, Marshall had written to Paul Hoffman, who was recovering from surgery, that "One thing I can tell you now, aside from the differential in years between us, you're going to have a much longer time to regather your energies than now is probably your planning.

. . . I had no indication whatsoever of any trouble—the X-rays being the only indication of trouble—it took me all of eleven months to kick out of it. However, I had a very bad period of about six weeks with what they call a nerve pain which in one sense had nothing whatever to do with the operation but resulted from the disturbance of a painful nerve which lay over the kidney. The result was very much like an automobile rattle (that early Studebaker). The pain was all in one place while the cause was in quite another." (Marshall to Hoffman, July 7, 1950, GCMRL/G. C. Marshall Papers [American Red Cross, General].)

3. *Gentlemen Prefer Blondes* was a Broadway musical starring Carol Channing, and based on a 1925 novel by Anita Loos.

85

To Field Marshal Lord Wilson — July 17, 1950
[Washington, DC]

Dear Wilson: As you already know, since receipt of your letter, I saw Franks and he has just now sent me copy of his letter to you and your reply, which constitutes a complete answer to the question you raised with me.[1]

I am relieved that the matter is now being generally straightened out. All of the arrangements have been made at Arlington cemetery with the personal approval of the Secretary of the Army for the laying of the base of the monument. Bliss, the Chairman of the Committee, has done a yeoman's job in effecting the arrangements and is now on the West Coast for an operation but will be back, we hope, in good condition in the early fall.

We are planning the ceremony of the dedication in some detail. You will hear more about this later of course.[2]

With warm regards. Faithfully yours,

GCMRL/G. C. Marshall Papers (American Red Cross, Subject, Field Marshal Sir John Dill Memorial Committee, 1949–1950)

1. Wilson had handwritten to Marshall that he and other friends of Sir John Dill as well as Nancy Dill were "apprehensive that there may be opposition to placing the equestrian statue in Arlington Cemetery," and "rather than run the risk of public opposition to the site . . . being expressed publicly it would be better for the statue to be placed elsewhere in Washington." (Wilson to Marshall, June 5, 1950, GCMRL/G. C. Marshall Papers [American Red Cross, Subject, Field Marshal Sir John Dill Memorial Committee, 1949–1950].) For previous correspondence on this opposition, see pp. 127–28.

On June 22, the British ambassador to the United States, Sir Oliver Franks, had informed Wilson of a June 19 luncheon conversation during which Marshall had informed Franks of Wilson's letter and requested his advice. Marshall, according to Franks, asserted that the press criticism "was not at all representative of American feeling" and felt that maintaining the present plans to place the equestrian statue "in a very special site near the roadway in the Cemetery would be a standing reminder in decades to come of Anglo-American relations and their importance." Franks concluded in a July 13 letter to Marshall that he and Wilson were now "in complete agreement with your thoughts. . . . I hope therefore that you will feel happy, so far as the British are concerned, to carry out the full programme." (Franks to Wilson, June 22, 1950, and Franks to Marshall, July 13, 1950, ibid.)

2. On July 26, Marshall wrote to thank Franks for his "handling of the matter . . . and the attitude you took," and to inform him of Wilson's July 22 reply "expressing complete accord with what we are going to do. I hope we have nothing of a disagreeable nature," he concluded, "to mar what should be a lasting reminder of great importance of British-Amer-

ican accord and understanding." (Wilson to Marshall, July 22, 1950, and Marshall to Franks, July 26, 1950, ibid.) For more on the ceremony, see pp. 222–24.

86

To Henry L. Stimson

July 20, 1950
Washington, DC

My dear Mr. Stimson: I was so shocked to read in the paper that you had a fall and a bone break.[1] I hope it has not been too painful and inconvenient. Katherine joins me in deepest sympathy.

We have been visiting the hospital two or three times a day in Leesburg to see Katherine's sister and brother-in-law. They had an automobile accident and he is suffering with a broken leg and she with a crushed shoulder and various contusions and cuts.

Katherine is still struggling with "shingles" in her eyes but otherwise is in good condition.

I know how deeply you must be interested in the international developments in the past few days. Confidentially, Acheson, Harriman, Bohlen and Kennan came down to see me very unexpectedly at Leesburg and remained for lunch. Baruch flew in that evening and spent the night and the next day. The President came down the following morning on about an hour's notice, and had me for lunch with Eisenhower the following day. Pace, Secretary of the Army, got me over to his office to be briefed by the Deputy Chief of Staff and other military leaders. I also, during this hectic period of interviews, had to appear before a committee of Congress.[2]

Katherine and I are planning to go out on August 1st for the month to Huron Mountain Camp on the shores of Lake Superior in northern Michigan. We have a cottage but are eating at the lodge. It is a private set up. We considered Nantucket, declined an invitation to the Adirondacks and then turned to Jackson Hole in Wyoming, and ended up as I have indicated.

With our sympathy and affectionate regards to Mrs. Stimson and you.[3] Faithfully yours,

G. C. Marshall

Yale/H. L. Stimson Papers

1. The *Washington Post* reported on July 20 that Stimson "broke his leg when he fell Sunday night in his home." The article remarked that he was "resting comfortably" in the hospital. ("Stimson 'Comfortable,'" *Washington Post*, July 20, 1950, p. B15.)

2. See pp. 125–26 and 128–31.

3. "I cannot tell you how your letter of July 20th . . . has pleased me," Stimson replied. "I value tremendously the sympathy of you and Mrs. Marshall. I am glad to say I am getting along very well, and have been transported from the Hospital in New York, where I spent three weeks, to my bedroom in Highhold. . . . The crack was in the head of the femur, and it necessarily takes time to mend, but everything now indicates that I shall be around again pretty soon, after the final setting is beyond peradventure." (Stimson to Marshall, August 18, 1950, GCMRL/G. C. Marshall Papers [American Red Cross, General].)

87

To John J. McCloy[1]

July 20, 1950
Washington, DC

Dear McCloy: I recently decided that it would not be practicable for me to make a trip to Europe this fall and so must decline your gracious invitation of last spring.[2]

I might tell you most confidentially that last fall the Lord Mayor of London conveyed to me through Lew Douglas an invitation to accept in September or October of this year the highly regarded "Freedom of the City" award. This was a great honor that they wished to pay me but I was a little doubtful of the wisdom of my considering this honor. I arrived at this contention because of an article in the London Times which mentioned the possibility of my coming over, this was followed by several hints that I might receive invitations from Belgium and Holland in particular and I, of course, did not want to do anything which might have prolonged the battle for ECA funds which was then going on. There was no doubt in my mind that the opponents of the appropriation would have been very critical—even to the point of calling this award compensation for my part in the European Recovery Program.

I finally made the decision not to accept the honor when the erection of a monument in Arlington Cemetery to the memory of Sir John Dill was bitterly criticized by a Manassas Virginia newspaper and followed by a vicious column in the Patterson papers.[3] I am enclosing a clipping from the New York Daily News which will give you a clearer picture of the dispute. As I am a member of the Dill Memorial Committee and have worked closely on all the details I fear a visit by me to London would give rise to the nastiest of smear campaigns by the anti-British newspaper clique. My concern is the harm that might be done to British and American relations and the honor we wish to pay Sir John and not what might be said of me personally.

I originally intended to visit London first then come over to Germany, but in view of what I have written I know you will understand how unwise it would be for me to plan such a trip. Please express to Handy and Taylor my regrets on the basis of Red Cross commitments and the Korean situation.[4]

Mrs. Marshall joins me in affectionate regards to Ellen, the children and you of course.[5] Faithfully yours,

GCMRL/G. C. Marshall Papers (American Red Cross, General)

1. McCloy had been serving as the US High Commissioner for Germany (USHCG) since September 1949.

2. Major General Maxwell D. Taylor (USMA, 1922), US commander in Berlin, had written to Marshall on March 25 that "Mr. McCloy mentioned recently that he has invited you to come to Germany in the near future and hopes that you may be able to accept." He went on "to add my cordial invitation to include Berlin in any European itinerary" since "the economic future of this city depends largely upon funds provided under the plan which bears your name." Marshall had responded on April 3 that "I don't know whether or not it would be possible for me to visit Berlin but I shall certainly have it in mind. . . . I would

like so much to see you and Handy and others, and, of course, Jack McCloy." General Thomas T. Handy (VMI, 1914) had succeeded General Lucius D. Clay (USMA, 1918) as the commander in chief of US forces in Europe in September 1949. (Taylor to Marshall, March 25, 1950, and Marshall to Taylor, April 3, 1950, GCMRL/G. C. Marshall Papers [American Red Cross, General].)

3. For more on the Dill memorial, see pp. 87–89, 127–28, 143–44, 151–52, and 222–24.

4. For Marshall's regrets to Taylor on not having the opportunity to visit Europe in the fall, see pp. 150–51.

5. McCloy responded to Marshall that he was "sorry to learn that you are not coming to Europe this summer as a visit by you at this time to Germany would have, in my judgment, a very wholesome effect," and that he was "shocked by the thought that there should continue to be any criticism of the memorial to Dill." (McCloy to Marshall, August 18, 1950, ibid.) Ellen was McCloy's wife.

88

To Mrs. John B. Wilson[1]

July 24, 1950
Leesburg, Virginia

Dear Rose: I have just this moment opened the package with the leather frame and the two photographs of the boys. The container is attractive and the photographs of the boys charming—they have such interesting and really charming faces and expressions. You are good to remember me in this way and I will treasure the pictures—put them on my dresser with the one of you and me in 1924 that Celeste sent me several years ago.[2]

I saw Mayor Edwards in Detroit and he spoke of you. He has been made of governor of the National Red Cross. I spotted him last fall and was delighted to get him elected to the Board. He will go far, I think, in public life.[3]

We leave for New York the 31st and leave there the 2d for Huron Mountain Camp on Lake Superior in northern Michigan—have taken a cottage for the month. Most confidentially, I have been trembling on the edge of being called again into public service in this crisis, but I hope I get by unmolested, but when the President motors down and sits under our oaks and tells me of his difficulties, he has me at a disadvantage.[4]

With my love, and thanks, and my best to John and each of the boys, Affectionately,

G. C. M.

GCMRL/J. Page Wilson Collection; H

1. Marshall's goddaughter, Rose Page Wilson, had befriended Marshall in 1919, when he and his first wife had moved into an apartment building at 2400 Sixteenth Street NW, where the Page family lived. (Rose Page Wilson, *General Marshall Remembered* [Englewood Cliffs, NJ: Prentice-Hall, Inc., 1968], 1, 7.) See pp. 728–29.

2. Celeste Page Morgan was Rose Page Wilson's older sister.

3. Dan Edwards, then mayor of Durham, North Carolina, was a friend of Wilson. She replied to Marshall, "You mentioned seeing Dan Edwards in Detroit. Last night's paper announced his appointment to the Executive Committee of the Natl Red Cross. The other day he swam over to me in the pool addressing me formally as 'Hey Toots, I have a job for you.' Then he asked me to serve on the Board of Directors for the County Red Cross. I

said of course I would and dutifully attended the first meeting. Dan slipped one over on me and at the meeting it was announced that I was also to be Secretary of the Board. I think he meant this as a compliment to you and also he is a shrewd politician and my appointment might mean your personal appearance here sometime. I won't tell him but I'm afraid he has overestimated my drawing power. At any rate, imbued as I am with your enthusiasm for the Red Cross, I shall take my job seriously and try to make my appointment count for something." (Wilson to Marshall, July 26, 1950, GCMRL/G. C. Marshall Papers [American Red Cross, General].)

4. See pp. 128–31. "I supposed the President sits under your oaks in order to persuade you to become his Chief of Staff," Wilson remarked. "I wish he'd let you alone." (Ibid.)

Robert Lovett expressed his concern in a July 21 letter to Marshall Carter: "My Partner, Roland Harriman, tells me that he saw General Marshall last week and that he looked to be in fine shape. I hope to goodness he stays that way because if things really get rugged, this country is going to need him in a bad way." (Lovett to Carter, July 21, 1950, GCMRL/Marshall S. Carter Papers [Central File, Selected Correspondence].)

89

To Major General Orlando Ward — July 28, 1950
[Washington, DC]

Dear Ward: I have delayed unconscionably in giving you my reaction to the first three chapters of this book.[1] I find nothing in my more or less superficial examination which seems to be incorrect. However, my impression is that this particular history, at least the first three chapters, will create an unnecessary and unfortunate impression on the reader's mind.

There is so much of criticism and castigation of the Adjutant General's Department as to recruiting that one draws the conclusion that the WAC organization was a failure in the war, which it decidedly was not.

It is all very well to state things accurately from a historical viewpoint but this presentation goes far beyond that. I do not mean that it should not be made clear that there was a great reluctance of army officers generally, particularly those in high control, to the interjection of a female organization in the Army, and I see no reason for not making clear the early history of the failures to secure this organization at a much earlier date, but there is such an unnecessary concentration and repetition regarding the recruiting difficulties that one is left with the inevitable impression that the WAC organization was a failure.

I think the recruiting difficulties, failures to properly approach the question, and general reluctance in the matter can be plainly stated but much more briefly and much less repetitiously.

It would be tragic to leave an impression that the WACS were a failure as an organization. The fact that they triumphed over these difficulties was a grand thing and the greatest achievement of Mrs. Hobby, but one does not get that impression in these first three chapters.

I can speak very frankly here because I was anxious to have the WAC organization created and forced the issue behind the scenes, and usually not in writing, time after time.[2] There were great difficulties in even getting the bill from the Budget Bureau to Congress—difficulties that I do not care to put on paper but out of which grew my selection of Mrs. Hobby to engineer the passage of the draft through the Budget Bureau and lead off in its presentation before Congress. And, incidentally, I found to my combined consternation and amusement (this is most confidential) that the bitter opposition came from southern representatives, even intimate friends of Mrs. Hobby's father who had been known there as the parliamentarian of Texas legislation.[3] As Mrs. Marshall put it—they would kiss your hand and give you a corsage but they be damned if they would let you have any rank in the government, particularly in the military.

I was confronted at one state with opposition to any grade above major notwithstanding a prospective WAC population of one hundred thousand. The Army Nurses brought in very heavy influences either against certain WAC legislation or to ride with it to their desires which were being opposed by the Medical Department.[4] I mention these things to indicate that I was pretty familiar with the difficulties of the problem but I would not present them in a manner which damns the whole organization and, incidentally, only would leave the impression that men are slow to appreciate women in public office.[5]

GCMRL/G. C. Marshall Papers (American Red Cross, Subject, Army, Department of the, 1949–1950)

1. Ward was preparing a volume on the Women's Army Corps for the *United States Army in World War II* series. On April 24 he had sent the manuscript to Marshall with a request that he review it by June 1 "for inaccuracies of fact or interpretation. . . . To expedite your consideration, the author has marked the passages in the text in which actions and opinions are attributed to you, and has attached numbered tabs to such references." (Ward to Marshall, April 24, 1950, NA/RG 319, Records of the Army Staff, Office of the Chief of Military History, Historian Background Files, The Women's Army Corps, 330.14.)

2. For Marshall's support of women in the military, see *Papers of GCM*, 2: 641–42 and 3: 99, 135–37.

3. Oveta Culp Hobby's father, Isaac W. Culp, had served three nonconsecutive terms in the Texas legislature between 1899 and 1925.

4. For the complaints of the Army Nurse Corps, see *Papers of GCM*, 3: 540–41.

5. "I have been wading through the WAC manuscript myself and have come to the same conclusions that you did in reading it," Ward replied. "The point of view is not broad enough and it is written somewhat with a chip on the shoulder. I am sure that we can remedy the tone and make it into a very valuable history." (Ward to Marshall, August 2, 1950, GCMRL/G. C. Marshall Papers [American Red Cross, Subject, Army, Department of the, 1949–1950].) The Office of the Chief of Military History published the *United States Army in World War II* Special Studies: *The Women's Army Corps* by Mattie E. Treadwell in 1954.

90

To Major C. J. George[1] — August [7?] 1950

Huron Mountain Camp, Michigan

Dear George: First, date my letter as above and not merely "Huron Mt., Michigan." They tell me there will be confusion.[2]

Next, I enclose a letter from Queen Fredericka. Have it typed and hand to

Bradley's aid for Bradley's eye only. The estimate on Greek fighting characteristics is interesting.[3]

Now as to my god-child Page Wilson, 2815 Chelsea Circle, Durham, N.C.: I will have to send something to arrive by the 16th, something he can keep and therefore worded: "To Page Wilson from his god-father G.C.M." might do. You will have to make the choice. Spend up to $20.00, preferably about $15.00. Maybe one of the small sized photos in uniform in a silver frame—tho I don't think much of this. I have autographed a photo if you can't think of something better.[4]

We are having a really delightful time. There's good bass fishing but I have not done well as yet, but have hopes.

The mail, or telegrams, only leaves here once a day for Big Bay, about 9 a.m. It arrives here about 1 p.m. This letter, written at 2 p.m. will not get in the mail at Big Bay until about ten a.m. to-morrow.[5] Hastily, G.C.M.

GCMRL/G. C. Marshall Papers (Secretary of Defense, Selected); H

1. Marshall had Sergeant George recalled to active commissioned service in his reserve grade of major. See p. 157.

2. This undated letter is probably in response to one from George dated August 4, 1950, in which he reported to Marshall about various personal matters that had occurred since the Marshalls departed for Michigan on August 2. (George to Marshall, August 4, 1950, GCMRL/G. C. Marshall Papers [American Red Cross, General].)

3. Frederica had written to Marshall on July 20 in response to reading an article about Marshall in a recent issue of *Time*. There is no correspondence to or from Bradley regarding this letter in the Marshall Papers. For Marshall's response to Frederica's letter, see pp. 304–6.

4. The birthday of Marshall's godson Page Wilson was August 16. Marshall had asked Rose Wilson, Page's mother, for the address of the beach cottage where she was staying with her family so he could "remember Page on his birthday." Rose Wilson responded on August 4, "We will be back in Durham for Page's fifth birthday. We took the cottage for two weeks only so will have to get out on the fifteenth. Page's birthday is the sixteenth." (Marshall to Wilson, July 28, 1950, GCMRL/J. Page Wilson Collection; Wilson to Marshall, August 4, 1950, GCMRL/G. C. Marshall Papers [American Red Cross, General].) There is no evidence of what gift Marshall sent Page Wilson in the Marshall Papers.

5. "I would appreciate your letting me know how long it took for this pouch to arrive," George had written to Marshall. "We mailed it at 5 p.m. Friday evening." Marshall wrote "Monday noon" on George's letter. August 7, 1950, was a Monday. For more on Marshall's travel arrangements while in Michigan, see pp. 153–54.

91

To Major C. J. George — August 11 [*10*], 1950, Huron Mountain Camp, Michigan

Dear George: Heffner, I find, had a flat tire en route.[1] He must have run on it a bit before discovering the trouble, for the casing and tube are so far damaged that local repairs are inadequate.

So, I have no spare. Please express me one, or arrange for us to buy one in Marquette.

Weather here is cool, really brisk, 67°. We only have had one hot day. Fished yesterday without success, tho a fellow on another club lake caught a 4 3/4 lb bass and a 3 lb Lake trout.

I have order $16.50 of gear from L. L. Bean Inc. in Freeport, Maine. You will be getting the check.

Mrs. Marshall is off and on with her headaches. In good shape the past two days.

We have invited Erskine Wood of Portland, Ore. to visit us. I doubt if he accepts as he is convalescing at a sanitarium in Stockbridge, Mass.[2]

Thanks for looking after Molly.[3]

GCMRL/G. C. Marshall Papers (Secretary of Defense, Selected); H

1. Sergeant William Heffner had been Marshall's chauffeur since 1948. For more information on the spare tire, see pp. 153–54.

2. The Marshalls had spent time with Erskine Wood, a lawyer from Portland, Oregon, and his wife on a fishing trip along Oregon's Metoulis River in 1938 while Marshall was stationed at Vancouver Barracks. See *Papers of GCM*, 1: 564–65. Wood had written to Marshall on July 3 to thank him for his "kind and sympathetic letter" in the wake of the death of Wood's wife, Rebecca Baird Biddle Wood, on June 11. "All this has shaken me so, that next week I am going to the Austen Riggs Foundation at Stockbridge Massachusetts, to try to rebuild my shattered nerves. Again thank you for your invitation to visit you next winter at Pinehurst. We shall have to see what the future brings, but I shall remember it." Marshall's letter to which Wood replied on July 3 is not in the Marshall Papers. (Wood to Marshall, July 3, 1950, GCMRL/G. C. Marshall Papers [American Red Cross, General].)

Wood apparently did visit the Marshalls in Michigan, for he wrote again on September 5 that, "I hated to leave you, but it had to be. I can, however, still keep the memory of those happy days and hope I shall for some time. . . . I went from Chicago back to New York . . . and went up to Stockbridge for one night to say goodbye and get my things . . . I am back at work in the office and happier for being so." (Wood to the Marshalls, September 5, 1950, GCMRL/G. C. Marshall Collection [Erskine Wood].)

3. "Molly found it necessary to change her plans to arrive on Thursday as Col. Winn could not get free," George had written on August 4. "She and the children left Old Point Comfort on the Bay Line Thursday night and arrived this morning. I met them and drove them down to Leesburg." (George to Marshall, August 4, 1950, GCMRL/G. C. Marshall Papers [American Red Cross, General].)

92

To Major General Maxwell D. Taylor — August 11, 1950
Huron Mountain Camp, Michigan

Dear Taylor: Thank you for your letter of July 31 which reached me here in the woods of northern Michigan where Mrs. Marshall and I came to escape the heat of Washington and to enjoy a little rest and relaxation.[1] Mrs. Marshall has been troubled with shingles in the eyes for the past nine months and she feels, as do I, that being rid of all responsibilities—household and otherwise—will help measurably in her determination to regain normal health.

I appreciate your telling me about the ceremony and the generous references made to me. Incidentally, Reuter's cable didn't arrive until the evening of the 24th and by the time I learned of it and made the reply it was almost noon of the 25th.[2]

I have given up all hopes of visiting Europe this year. Meetings of the Board of Governors of Red Cross have been scheduled for September and November, and as this work is my primary responsibility I couldn't very well absent myself.[3]

With warm regards. Faithfully yours,

GCMRL/G. C. Marshall Papers (Secretary of Defense, Number Indexed, M200-2-41)

1. Taylor had written to tell Marshall of the "very impressive ceremony" on July 26 "at which the cornerstone was laid to the George C. Marshall Pavilion," a large hall that would be used to display the products of Berlin industry at the October German Industrial Exhibition. "The decision to name the hall after you was reached spontaneously by the Magistrat and was communicated, as you know, on rather short notice. . . . I tapped the first stone into place, after depositing your cable of reply and the preamble to the Marshall Aid Act of Congress into the foundation. There was the usual speech-making with many warm and genuine expressions of regard for you and for the importance of the plan which bears your name in the city of Berlin. We are still hoping that you will find it possible to come here sometime in the present year." (Taylor to Marshall, July 31, 1950, GCMRL/G. C. Marshall Papers [Secretary of Defense, Number Indexed, M200-2-41].)

2. Ernst Reuter, mayor of West Berlin, had cabled Marshall on July 22 of the desire to name the pavilion in his honor in light of his "services rendered to European reconstruction." Noting that on July 26 Taylor would be laying the "foundation stone of pavilion in which copy of U S Congress Act on ECA of 3 April 1948 will be walled in," Reuter added that he would "be very glad to add . . . message from you to Berlin people expressing your consent to the naming." Marshall accepted the honor on July 25. (Reuter to Marshall, radio, July 22, 1950, and Marshall to Taylor, cable no. WCL-34487, July 25, 1950, ibid.)

Reuter replied on August 4 to report that Marshall's message had been read at the cornerstone laying ceremony and had "met with the Berliners warmest thanks." He also invited Marshall to attend the opening of the exhibition on October 1. Marshall repeated on August 18 that he appreciated "the gracious thought which prompted this action" but declined Reuter's invitation due to Red Cross obligations. (Reuter to Marshall, August 4, 1950, and Marshall to Reuter, August 18, 1950, ibid.)

3. See pp. 247–51.

93

To Robert Woods Bliss — August 11, 1950, Huron Mountain Camp, Michigan

Dear Bliss: Your letter of August first and the print of the revised plan reached me here in the mountains where Katherine and I came to spend the month.[1] So far we have had a fine time amidst beautiful scenery and pleasant weather.

We were very glad to hear that your operation was successful and that you are making rapid progress towards normal good health, which you always seem to enjoy.

On checking the print I agree that the changing of the statue to a cater-corner position will not only provide a better view to the public but is also more geometrically attractive.

I didn't see Professor Earle's letter but Miss Snow suggested to Major George that it be sent on to you.[2]

Katherine joins me in warm regards to Mildred and yourself.[3] Faithfully yours,

GCMRL/G. C. Marshall Papers (American Red Cross, Subject, Field Marshal Sir John

Dill Memorial Committee, 1949–1950)

1. Bliss, the chairman of the fundraising drive to memorialize Sir John Dill at Arlington National Cemetery, had written after a meeting with various officials to inform Marshall of a decision to have the equestrian statue face diagonally rather than perpendicular to Roosevelt Drive as previously planned. He enclosed a print of the revised plan that also indicated the revised boundaries of the burial plot. "This is a greatly reduced area of the site originally set aside by Secretary Stimson," he noted. He also thanked Marshall for sending copies of the previous Franks-Wilson correspondence regarding this controversial issue. (Bliss to Marshall, August 1, 1950, GCMRL/G. C. Marshall Papers [American Red Cross, Subject, Field Marshal Sir John Dill Memorial Committee, 1949–1950].) For more on the Dill memorial, see pp. 87–89, 127–28, 143–44, and 222–24.

2. This letter, which Marshall never saw, was forwarded to Bliss, who had written at the end of his August 1 letter, "By this mail I am writing to Professor Edward Mead Earle, whose letter to you from the Institute for Advanced Studies at Princeton has been sent me by Miss McPherson." (Bliss to Marshall, August 1, 1950, ibid.) The letter from Professor Earle has not been found.

3. Mildred was Bliss's wife.

94

TO MAJOR GENERAL BRYANT E. MOORE — August 16, 1950
Huron Mountain Camp, Michigan

Dear Moore: Your letter of August 11 together with the photographs of the paintings of MacArthur and Eisenhower have been received here in the woods of northern Michigan where Mrs. Marshall and I are enjoying a most pleasant vacation.[1] I think the paintings are excellent likenesses.

I will sit for Stephens as you requested, but at this date it is not possible for me to arrange anything definite. I will be here until the first of September and after my return I am scheduled for a number of meetings and several visits to Red Cross chapters around the country. I do hope, however, to complete the task before Mrs. Marshall and I go down to Pinehurst for the winter and early spring. As it stands now, I would say October at the earliest.

To supplement whatever photographs you have of me, I am having sent to you several which have been taken over the past three years. I will write or telegraph you just as soon as the decks are cleared.[2]

With warm regards, Faithfully yours,

GCMRL/G. C. Marshall Papers (American Red Cross, Categorical, Portraits)

1. Moore (USMA, 1917), the superintendent of the US Military Academy, had first requested on May 25 that Marshall sit for a portrait to be painted by Thomas E. Stephens and placed in West Point's Grant Hall alongside portraits of the three other men holding the five-star rank of General of the Army at that time: Generals Arnold, Eisenhower, and MacArthur. Marshall replied on May 31 that he was honored that West Point would be "disposed to think of me, a non-graduate, so graciously," but he hesitated to agree "to take on the obligation of sitting for a portrait." He informed Moore that the only satisfactory portrait was painted by James Anthony Willis and had been created primarily from photographs. As such, Marshall asked if there was "any possibility of your commissioning Willis for the job," not to offend Stephens, "but rather to save me the time-consuming task of pos-

ing for hours." Moore replied on June 6 that West Point's Museum Board had reviewed one of Willis's portraits of Marshall but determined that it would not "be of the same character" as the ones painted by Stephens, and thus he requested that Marshall "sit for Stephens." If Marshall approved, Moore wrote further on August 11, "we shall take steps to provide Mr. Stephens with photographs, including any that you would be kind enough to send us, and he could then go to work on preliminary studies. Mr. Stephens is prepared to go anywhere at any time, and to suit your convenience absolutely as to time, place and any other conditions you may wish to set." (Moore to Marshall, May 25, June 16, and August 11, 1950; and Marshall to Moore, May 31, 1950, GCMRL/G. C. Marshall Papers [American Red Cross, Categorical, Portraits].)

2. On September 1, C. J. George sent eleven photographs of Marshall to General Moore for Stephen's reference. (George to Moore, September 1, 1950, ibid.) Marshall would sit for Stephens on three occasions in 1951: March 8 and 15, and May 5. Stephens completed the portrait later that year and it was placed in Grant Hall at West Point alongside portraits of Generals Arnold, Eisenhower, and MacArthur.

95

TO MAJOR C. J. GEORGE

August 27 [*28*], 1950
Huron Mountain Camp, Michigan

Dear George: I sent off a wire and a letter to you yesterday—Sunday, changing my time of departure from *noon* Sunday next to *noon* Saturday next. Mr. Truman got me into Big Bay at 10 o'clock Saturday night.[1] I only came in to dinner from fishing at 8-30, to find out when I was coming back, he wanted to talk things over with me. He agreed to my staying until Sunday but I think he wanted me earlier, tho he insisted that was soon enough for his purpose. Whether or not Matt Connelly knew of the conversation I do not know, but as the President asked me to telephone him as soon as he got back I sent word to you to tell Connelly of my ETA [estimated time of arrival] Saturday.[2]

I suppose Heffner told Munson why the landing at Houghton (where we did land) was most inconvenient—a 176 mile drive over a winding road a good bit of the way.[3] I think he should come into the Sawyer airport the evening before. Caution him to make no mention of my name and departure plans.

The tire came OK and has been put in "spare" condition. The car needs tuning up so Heffner had best have that done the first day some where.[4]

I got a few bass Saturday about 1½ lb. fellows. Rain and cold had limited the fishing. Better weather now seems on hand for this last week. F. yrs.

G. C. M.

GCMRL/G. C. Marshall Collection (C. J. George); H

1. For more on President Truman's call to Marshall, see Forrest C. Pogue, *George C. Marshall*, vol. 4, *Statesman, 1945–1959* (New York: Viking, 1987), 420; and Ferrell, *Off the Record*, 192. Big Bay, Michigan, was a popular destination for anglers.

2. Matthew J. Connelly was Truman's appointments secretary.

3. Colonel Homer C. Munson had been assigned to fly as personal pilot to General Marshall since June 1942. Marshall had been forced to land at Houghton, Michigan, due to bad weather and drive the distance to Huron Mountain Camp.

4. See pp. 149–50. "[W]hen Heffner comes up with Munson he will have in his hand

a canvas kit of spare parts," George had written to Marshall on August 22. "This will be some insurance against a possible breakdown of the Plymouth on the way back." (George to Marshall, August 22, 1950, GCMRL/G. C. Marshall Papers [American Red Cross, Categorical, Memoranda, George, C. J., 1949–1950].)

96

To Madame Chiang Kai-shek

September 5, 1950
Washington, DC

Dear Madame: Katherine and I have just returned from our month's vacation on Lake Superior. Your letter of August first reached me the day before I left Michigan.[1]

Naturally I was much interested in what you had to tell me about General MacArthur's visit but my special interest focused on the possibility of your being utilized to head up the Guerilla Movement on the mainland. I think this would be a terrible responsibility for you to take not only from the viewpoint of danger but also considering your uncertain state of health as you would be bound to suffer heavily from the hard living during such an enterprise.

Katherine told me she wrote you a letter shortly before we left Huron Mountain. She possibly told you most of the news. However, at a risk of repetition I will tell you something of what has been happening to us: We went up to New York on the 31st of July to attend a going away dinner for some friends of ours leaving for the Scandinavian Peninsula. The next day I had a Board meeting. We were staying in Margaret Emerson's apartment, she being in the Adirondacks. The following morning we took off by air for northern Michigan and arrived at our destination at two o'clock but could not land because of a low fog which came up at the last minute. The result was that we made a distant landing and had about a 176 mile drive that evening getting into camp at eleven o'clock. We had a perfectly delightful month except Katherine for a period of a week had a bad cold which affected her sinus and shingle complaint. However, she came through it very well. We were frequently out all day on the water. There were six lakes some three or four miles in extent. The fishing was fair. Katherine caught the largest bass on each occasion.

We left there Saturday morning and flew straight in to Washington arriving here at four o'clock. Molly and the children were still at Leesburg—and are leaving tonight for Fort Monroe. They all were well. Clifton was there also. Katherine is getting ready for a dinner of about fifty people on Sunday night—Red Cross governors. I am off to New York this morning but will fly back this evening if all goes well. Incidentally, it was 51 degrees when we left Michigan and 92 degrees when we hit Washington. This morning it is a little better—73 degrees. I do hope cool weather will reach you soon and I am so glad to know that you are established on high ground.

With affectionate regards and my best to the Generalissimo. Faithfully yours,

GCMRL/G. C. Marshall Papers (Pentagon Office, Selected)

1. Madame Chiang sent a lengthy letter detailing MacArthur's visit to Formosa in late July and his meetings with Nationalist military leaders. According to MacArthur, he went to Formosa "in order to determine its military capabilities for defense." (Douglas MacArthur, *Reminiscences* [New York: McGraw-Hill, 1964], 339.) The visit surprised the administration, however, and it led to consternation in Washington and fears that MacArthur's actions and statements violated administration policy on Formosa. It consequently led to sternly worded messages from the JCS and Secretary Johnson, on orders from Truman. (Dean Acheson, *Present at the Creation: My Years in the State Department* [New York: W. W. Norton & Co., 1969], 422; D. Clayton James, *The Years of MacArthur*, vol. 3, *Triumph and Disaster, 1945–1964* [Boston: Houghton Mifflin, 1985], 453–55.)

After reporting in detail on the conferences between the SCAP's staff and Nationalist military leaders, Madame Chiang remarked that "The Generalissimo also told General MacArthur that from various quarters, including the guerillas, there have come requests and suggestions that I head the Guerilla Movement on the mainland. He asked the General what he thought of the matter. The General replied that as far as the effectiveness of the work is concerned, he thought it would be fine. The person heading the movement should be some one the enemy would not suspect, and certainly I would be the last one the enemy would suspect. But that the sacrifice on my part would be tremendous because whoever heads the movement would be fraught with danger and subjected to torture worse than death if caught. . . . And therefore he felt the sacrifice would be too great on my part. His last words as we left the car at the field to me were, 'I would not like to see you in such danger.' I told him that I have long left personal considerations behind. My only objective is to serve my country in the best way possible." She concluded by asking if there was any way Marshall could "put in a word to facilitate our getting some radar sets." (Chiang to Marshall, August 1, 1950, GCMRL/G. C. Marshall Papers [Pentagon Office, Selected].)

PRESIDENT TRUMAN had first raised the possibility of Marshall's replacing Johnson as secretary of defense during his July 4 visit to Leesburg (see p. 130n4). Then in late August, while Marshall was still vacationing in northern Michigan, Truman had telephoned and asked him to visit upon his return. Marshall did so on September 6, whereupon Truman asked him to replace Johnson, who was being blamed for US military unpreparedness and whose behavior had become increasingly unacceptable. According to Acheson that behavior had by this time "passed beyond the peculiar to the impossible." (Acheson, *Present at the Creation*, 441.) Marshall agreed on condition that his tenure as secretary of defense would only last from six to twelve months. He also requested that Lovett be named his deputy secretary. (Pogue, *Statesman*, 420–22.) Marshall did add a warning: "I want you to think about the fact that my appointment may reflect negatively on you and your Administration. They are still charging me with the downfall of Chiang's government in China. I want to help not hurt you." "Can you think of anyone else saying that?," Truman wrote to his wife Bess on September 7. "I can't, and he's of the *great*." On that same day W. Averell Harriman had lunch with Marshall in Leesburg. "Wonder of Wonders," Truman told Bess, "Mrs. Marshall is for it! He could not possibly hurt me." (Ferrell, *Off the Record*, 189, 192–93.)

On Truman's instruction and at his insistence, Johnson on September 12 tendered his resignation and recommended that Marshall replace him. Naming "a man of such stature" would "promote national and international unity" and "be an inspiration to the people of the United States and to our allies." (Johnson to

Truman, September 12, 1950, NA/RG 330, SD 040 [Secretary of Defense, 1950].) On the same day, Truman accepted the resignation and nominated Marshall to become the third secretary of defense.

Marshall was actually ineligible for the position due to a clause in the 1947 National Security Act asserting that the secretary of defense must not have been on active duty within ten years of his appointment. Congress would have to amend that law prior to Marshall's appointment, which it quickly did. (See pp. 157–58n1 and 160–63.) ★

97

To Robert A. Lovett

September 16, 1950
[Washington, DC]

Dear Lovett: Just received your letter of the 14th acknowledging my birthday greetings and making generous reference to my acceptance of this new post.[1]

As always I am delighted to hear from you even though concerning such a sad matter as the advancing years. Incidentally, I have grown very much older in the past three or four days and whatever was sandy looking on my head will be an honest gray.

I hope Adele is back to her state of robust health and strength again.

Katherine joins me in affectionate regards to you both. Faithfully yours,

GCMRL/G. C. Marshall Papers (Secretary of Defense, Selected)

1. "It was thoughtful of you to remember my birthday," Lovett had written. "It was wonderful of you to respond to the President's call again in these grim times and it should give the country the leadership needed in the military establishment and remove much of the feuding that has been so disgraceful." (Lovett to Marshall, September 14, [1950], GCMRL/G. C. Marshall Papers [Secretary of Defense, Selected].)

See also the next document.

98

To Arthur H. Vandenberg[1]

September 16, 1950
[Washington, DC]

Dear Arthur: This letter is absolutely not to burden you with the necessity for replying. I merely want to tell you that I have just received yours of the thirteenth and appreciate very much your writing. Katherine was so much interested in hearing from you.

I just got off a note to Bob Lovett a moment ago thanking him for a nice letter.[2] I made no mention of what I really wanted out of him and I am still pondering the question as to whether or not I should embarrass him with the proposition—Under [*Deputy*] Secretary of Defense. The trouble is I am afraid he would accept because I asked him despite the fact he doesn't feel physically up to it or otherwise desire it. I have until the thirtieth to make a choice as Steve Early's time is not up until then.[3] I do hesitate to levy on Lovett again but he would be perfect for my dilemma.

You will be interested to know that Sergeant George is now Major George. I had him recalled to active commissioned service in his reserve grade. He is now looking very impressive as his tailor presented him with a complete outfit—aiguillette and all. This happened before the secretaryship was offered. George will cut quite a figure at the Pentagon.

Katherine charges me particularly to give you her love and to say how much she looks for an opportunity to see you again. Affectionately,

GCMRL/G. C. Marshall Papers (Secretary of Defense, Selected)

1. Vandenberg, who had cancer and had previously undergone surgery (see pp. 24–25), had written to update Marshall on his convalescence. He concluded, "I read in the morning papers that you have again responded to your country's call to duty. Knowing how you and Katherine have longed for relief from such responsibilities, I very humbly bow before your magnificent and unremitting loyalty. I wish you every success in your new task for which you are so superbly qualified." (Vandenberg to Marshall, September 13, 1950, GCMRL/G. C. Marshall Papers [Secretary of Defense, Selected].)

2. See previous document.

3. Stephen T. Early had been Franklin D. Roosevelt's White House press secretary from 1933 to 1945 and deputy secretary of defense since August of 1949; he resigned in September 1950.

Lovett would agree to become deputy secretary of defense on September 28 and would be sworn in on October 4, 1950. Marshall wrote to Adele Lovett to confess that he had "debated for quite a while as to whether or not to write to you most confidentially and get your reaction before I approached him. However, I let nature take its course, and I hope very much this does not impose too great a hardship, expense and inconvenience on your home life. It certainly raises hob with us." Adele Lovett assured Marshall that they could not be returning to Washington "under happier working conditions." (Marshall to Adele Lovett, October 2, 1950, and Adele Lovett to Marshall, October 3, 1950, GCMRL/G. C. Marshall Papers [Secretary of Defense, Number Indexed, M200-3-34].)

99

FROM HARRY S. TRUMAN — September 18, 1950
TO MRS. GEORGE C. MARSHALL — [Washington, DC]

Dear Mrs. Marshall: As you are the General's superior officer I send you a personal souvenir which you may wish to keep. Not attempting to settle the ancient question as to which is mightier, the pen or the sword—the General is facile in the use of both—I am forwarding the implement with which I had the pleasure of approving today H. R. 9646, "An Act to authorize the President to appoint General of the Army George C. Marshall to the office of Secretary of Defense."[1]

I wish for your sake and for the General's that this meant less instead of more work for him.[2] Cordially and sincerely,

HSTL/H. S. Truman Papers (Post-Presidential Files)

1. On Friday, September 15, the Senate passed a waiver in Marshall's case to the eligibility restriction in the National Security Act (see pp. 155–56), voting 47–21, with twenty Republicans and one Democrat opposed. ("Marshall Backed by Senate Group," *New York*

Times, September 20, 1950, pp. 1, 37.)

2. "What a thoughtful, wonderful person you are," Katherine Marshall responded. "In all your busy, pressing life—to send me the pen you signed George's appointment with. You know how much I shall treasure it and also your thought of me. I am praying that this appointment will bring some relief to you—and help to the country. With my affectionate regards to you, Mrs Truman and Margaret." (Katherine Marshall to Truman, September 19, 1950, GCMRL/G. C. Marshall Collection [Harry S. Truman].)

100

TO HENRY L. STIMSON

September 18, 1950
Washington, DC

Dear Mr. Stimson: I have just this moment read your letter of the thirteenth from "Highhold". It was good of you to write as you did and there is no one in the world whose opinion and support could mean so much to me as yours.[1]

I am in the midst of hard days and harder are ahead. However, that goes with democracy.

I do hope you are making a rapid recovery. Maybe I'd better return that sponge rubber cushion to you!

With most affectionate regards to you both. Faithfully yours,

G. C. Marshall

Yale/H. L. Stimson Papers

1. Stimson had written to congratulate Marshall on his recent appointment as secretary of defense. "My spirits gave a great leap of relief and happiness last night when I heard over the radio that you had been appointed Secretary of Defense. The President has at last taken the right step," wrote Stimson, "by placing the military preparation of our country on the right track for dealing with the world crisis with which we are faced, thank heaven. It is a great sacrifice that is asked of you, but thank God you are young enough and strong enough to deal with it. My heart goes with you in all the difficulties that you must face." (Stimson to Marshall, September 13, 1950, GCMRL/G. C. Marshall Papers [Secretary of Defense, Number Indexed, M205-4-10].)

101

TO DEAN G. ACHESON

September 18, 1950
Washington, DC

Dear Acheson: I appreciate very much your taking time from what must be a very hectic period to write me such a nice letter on my appointment.[1]

I thought I would escape a visit to the Hill, but just a few hours ago I received an invitation to appear before the Senate Armed Forces Committee tomorrow afternoon.[2] Perhaps after this I will be confirmed, then a short trip across the river where I am sure much hard work awaits me.

I read in the newspapers about your 72-hour confinement to your hotel and I suggest that you take a short respite from your duties for a walk through Central Park.[3]

Hoping to see you in the not too distant future and with warm regards, Faithfully yours,

GCMRL/G. C. Marshall Papers (Secretary of Defense, Selected)

1. Acheson wrote Marshall a note to congratulate him on his appointment as secretary of defense. "I am aware of the surge of relief and confidence that the whole country feels," he wrote, "and I know from the personal experience of our months together what a firm foundation the country's emotion has." (Acheson to Marshall, September 15, 1950, GCMRL/G. C. Marshall Papers [Secretary of Defense, Selected].) Acheson had been Marshall's undersecretary of state in 1947.

"No change could have been more welcome to me," Acheson later wrote, than the replacement of Johnson with Marshall. "It brought only one embarrassment. The General insisted, overruling every protest of mine, in meticulously observing the protocol involved in my being the senior Cabinet officer. Never would he go through a door before me, or walk anywhere but on my left; he would go around an automobile to enter it after me and sit on the left; in meetings he would insist on my speaking before him. To be treated so by a revered and beloved former chief was a harrowing experience. But the result in government was, I think, unique in the history of the Republic. For the first time and, perhaps, though I am not sure, the last, the Secretaries of State and Defense, with their top advisers, met with the Chiefs of Staff in their map room and discussed common problems together. At one of those meetings General Bradley and I made a treaty, thereafter scrupulously observed. The phrases 'from a military point of view' and 'from a political point of view' were excluded from our talks. No such dichotomy existed. Each of us had our tactical and strategic problems, but they were interconnected, not separate." (Acheson, *Present at the Creation*, 441.)

In sharp contrast with his predecessor, Marshall would establish a close working relationship with the State Department. In addition to his numerous conversations with Acheson, he would order the resumption of informal consultations between officials in both departments and institute weekly meetings between State Department representatives and the JCS, chaired by Dean Rusk. "Hence, proposed military actions with political implications were discussed with the State Department and cleared with the Secretary of State before being submitted to the President." (Walter G. Hermes, *United States Army in the Korean War*, vol. 2, *Truce Tent and Fighting Front* [Washington: Office of the Chief of Military History, US Army, 1966; repr. 2005], 55.) "I instituted the procedure of our meeting with the State Department officials in the Office of the Chiefs of Staff," Marshall would later inform a congressional committee, "and that has been paralleled by similar meetings of lower level officials of both the State Department and the Defense Department. . . . [O]ne thing I thought was important that was not going on at the time I took office was intimate discussions back and forth rather than exchange of memorandums." (Senate Committee on Armed Services and Committee on Foreign Relations, *Hearings to Conduct an Inquiry into the Military Situation in the Far East* [hereafter *MSFE*] . . . , 82d Cong., 1st sess., 379 and 523.)

2. See pp. 160–63.

3. "Secretary of State Dean Acheson has been so tied up with the Western defense conferences," the *New York Times* reported, "that he could not get out of the Waldorf-Astoria Hotel here for about seventy-five hours." ("Acheson Work Kept Him Within Hotel 75 Hours," *New York Times*, September 16, 1950, p. 8.)

102

To Lady Nancy Dill

September 19, 1950
Washington, DC

Dear Nancy: I would be most ungrateful if I neglected to reply to your very nice note of the fourteenth.[1] I appreciate having your and Sonia's reaction to my accepting the Defense post.

Katherine and I checked into the Walter Reed Hospital yesterday for some dental work and a general physical examination. I have been feeling extremely well but Katherine is still having difficulty with her eyes. I do hope that the work she is now having done will rid her of the eye shingles and neuritis which have been plaguing her for such a long time.

We look forward with anticipation to your and Sonia's forthcoming visit.

I had a note from Bliss this morning and he said that the statue is now on the high seas. Practically all of the arrangements for the unveiling have been made.[2] Faithfully yours,

GCMRL/G. C. Marshall Papers (Secretary of Defense, Selected)

1. Dill had written to thank Marshall for information on the date of the unveiling at Arlington Cemetery of the equestrian statue to her late husband as well as to offer her congratulations and those of her daughter, Sonia, on Marshall's appointment as secretary of defense. "Please don't answer this," she had added in parentheses at the end of her letter. (Nancy Dill to Marshall, September 14, 1950, GCMRL/G. C. Marshall Papers [Secretary of Defense, Selected].) See pp. 222–24

2. "Every sort of unexpected complication has combined," Robert Woods Bliss had informed Marshall on September 15, "not only to delay the completion of the statue but also to add greatly to the original estimated cost. But the statue is finished at last and is en route from Belgium where it has been cast." (Bliss to Marshall, September 15, 1950, ibid.)

103

Secretary Of Defense Confirmation Hearing
September 19, 1950 Washington, DC

ON JANUARY 8, 1947, the Senate had confirmed Marshall's appointment as secretary of state unanimously and without any hearings (see *Papers of GCM*, 6: 3–4). That would not be the case for his nomination as secretary of defense. At 2:15 p.m. on September 19, Marshall appeared before the Senate Armed Services Committee to answer questions. (Senate Committee on Armed Services, *Hearing on the Nomination of General of the Army George C. Marshall to be Secretary of Defense, September 19, 1950*, 81st Cong., 2d sess.)

Many of those questions during the ensuing fifty-five-minute session were asked by Senator William Knowland (R-CA). They involved such matters as withdrawing troops from Korea in 1948–49, arming West Germany, admitting Spain into NATO, and defending Formosa. Marshall consistently replied that he had not kept up with these issues since his January 1949 retirement as secretary of state and that he would need to discuss them with Secretary of State Acheson, President Truman, and the military before responding. Knowland also questioned Marshall regarding his previous views on service unification and civilian control of the military. Underlying these questions was the longstanding congressional fear of militarism. That fear had been expressed in the provision barring active or recently retired military officers from becoming secretary of defense, which had been revised four days earlier to make an exception for Marshall. (See pp. 155–56 and 157–58n1.)

Nevertheless Senator Harry P. Cain (R-WA) asserted that he would vote against Marshall's confirmation solely because he was "a professional military man." Others disagreed, with Senator Lyndon Johnson (D-TX) noting that "22 Presidents have appointed 38 men with military experience to the offices of Secretary of War and Secretary of the Navy." When Knowland asked Marshall about his "conception of the duties and the relationship of the Secretary of State and the Secretary of Defense," Marshall responded that the former was "the natural leader up to the President in the matter of our international relations" while the latter was "deeply concerned when these relationships, negotiations and treaties affect our defensive posture and our position in the world in a military sense." In case of disagreement, "then, of course, it would be for the President to decide the issue as he is the final determiner of foreign policy." Marshall also noted that he had opposed heavy military representation on the National Security Council (NSC), and that while as a second lieutenant he had stated "we would never get anywhere in the Army unless a soldier was Secretary of War," as he grew "a little older and served through some of our military history . . . , I came to the fixed conclusion that he should never be a soldier." (Ibid., 2–3, 7–8, 10.)

Although not a member of the committee, Senator William Jenner (R-IN), a fierce critic of Marshall and the Truman administration who attended the hearing, had submitted a series of hostile questions that committee chair Millard Tydings then asked Marshall after a majority of the committee voted to do so in open rather than executive session, with Marshall retaining the right to request executive session for any of his answers. (Ibid., 19–22.) In the congressional debate over modification of the National Security Act so as to allow Marshall to serve as secretary of defense, Jenner had attacked him as "not only willing," but "eager to play the role of a front man for traitors. The truth is this is no new role for him, for General George C. Marshall is a living lie." Jenner further labeled him an "errand boy, a front man, a stooge, or a conspirator" for an administration he defined as "a criminal crowd of traitors and Communist appeasers." ("Appointment of Gen. George C. Marshall to the Office of Secretary of Defense," *Congressional Record* 96, pt. 11, 81st Cong., 2d sess., 14913–17, quotes on 14914 and 14917.) His questions on September 19 continued the attack. Chairman Tydings read, "You use as an excuse for not writing your memoirs the fact that you did not wish to 'hurt' anyone. Whom are you protecting?" Marshall replied, "A great many people." When asked by Tydings if he wished to name them, Marshall said no. "Why did you permit the signing of the master lend-lease agreement with Russia which gave the Russians priority on our war material at the expense of the American fighting forces?" Tydings then asked. Marshall replied that he had not signed the agreement, but that "if I had done so, my answer would be the same. We had gone very carefully over all the proposals, we had pared them down, and we felt that was in the interest of the fighting, which was to defeat the Nazi forces." When asked why he had recommended "the appointment of Alger Hiss as executive secretary of the

American Secretariat" at the 1944 Dumbarton Oaks Conference, he replied that he did "not recall having made any such appointment." When asked why he had agreed to be the president's emissary to "force" Chiang Kai-shek "to take Communist China and its armies into the Nationalist Government," Marshall objected to the implication and replied that he accepted the assignment because President Truman "asked me to go," that "my job was to stop the fighting," and that he advised on "the demobilization of all the armies." (*Hearing*, 19–22.)

Tydings then read, "Why did you join in the suppression of the Wedemeyer report on China?" "I did not join in the suppression of the report," Marshall shot back; "I personally suppressed it." He then pointed out that Wedemeyer had called for putting Manchuria under trusteeship, that the Soviets would have been a partner to any such arrangement as would the UN, and that the United States was pressing the Greek issue in the UN at that time. Furthermore, "this was a report from a man I sent to find out something for me and not for a public speech," and Chiang had made clear to Marshall emphatically and "time after time that he would resign before he would accept any relationship in connection with China in which the Russians or the British had a part." The next question was why Marshall had approved "the suppression of the facts concerning the Bogotá Conference of April 1948." "I do not recall that I did approve it," Marshall responded. He then stated that he could not give a "'Yes' or 'No' answer" to whether he favored continuing Marshall Plan aid to nations "shipping war potential to Russia" because it was a "very involved question relating to the economics of Europe." When asked why he did not protest as army chief "the policies adopted at Tehran, Yalta, and Potsdam which handed half the world on a silver platter to Stalin," Marshall replied that he "did not think it would have been suitable to my position. I was very much engaged in a war at that time, and was engaged in the meetings with the Soviet commanders and staff," not with "political meetings with which I was not familiar" and which "took place at other places." (Ibid., 22–24.)

Marshall was then asked if he was "in favor of surrendering American sovereignty into the hands of an international superstate and the turning of American Armed Forces into a permanent foreign legion?" "That pretty well covers the water front," he replied. "No; I am not in favor of that." When asked if he was now sufficiently recovered physically from his surgery "to assume the arduous duties of Secretary of Defense," he offered "a very concrete answer"; he had come to the committee hearing directly from Walter Reed Hospital "and they say the machinery is all right." Tydings then asked the last Jenner question on his sheet: "Will you assure the American people unequivocally that as Secretary of Defense you will not be dominated by or carry out the policies of the Secretary of State Dean Acheson, who will not turn his back on Alger Hiss?" "I will not answer that question," Marshall replied. Two additional Jenner questions not on Tydings's sheet addressed Marshall's whereabouts and behavior immediately before the Pearl Harbor attack of December 7, 1941. (Ibid., 24–25.)

The committee then went into executive session and voted 9–2 to recommend confirmation, with Cain and Knowland opposed. The Senate approved by a vote of 57–11 with fifteen Republicans joining forty-two Democrats in the majority. Marshall was sworn in at the Pentagon on September 21. ★

104

To General Brehon B. Somervell

September 20, 1950
Washington, DC

Dear Somervell: I have just received your note of September fifteenth.[1] I did not have much choice in the matter and I realize that the going will be rough at least for a while.

I have been feeling extremely well, as a matter of fact I just checked out of Walter Reed where I had been for two days. I went in for a general check-up and the doctors reported that my machinery is in good working order.

With much appreciation for writing me as you did and with warm regards.

Faithfully yours,

G. C. Marshall

USAMHI/B. B. Somervell Papers (Correspondence)

1. Somervell wrote, "I want to congratulate the country on your appointment. You know I thought you should not have taken the last one but this is all to the good. *Do* take care of yourself. With every wish for the success that will be yours." (Somervell to Marshall, September 15, 1950, GCMRL/G. C. Marshall Papers [Secretary of Defense, Categorical, Congratulations re Appointment as Secretary of Defense].)

105

To Henry L. Stimson
Radio.

September 21, 1950
Washington, DC

Dear Mr. Stimson: In congratulating you on your birthday I want you to know that I took over your old chair at your old desk in your old room that you departed from with such high honor just five years ago today.[1] May you and Mrs. Stimson enjoy good health and plan to visit with me on this familiar ground and break bread with me in the room that was my office and now I find is a dining room.[2]

GCMRL/G. C. Marshall Papers (Secretary of Defense, Number Indexed, M200-1-1)

1. Marshall is referring to Stimson's Pentagon office that he occupied as secretary of war during World War II. Stimson retired from that position on September 21, 1945, and Marshall assumed the office of secretary of defense on September 21, 1950. That day also marked Stimson's eighty-third birthday. See photo #4.

2. Stimson replied, "Deeply cherish your birthday telegram and offer. I am planning to take you up on next 5 year anniversary." (Stimson to Marshall, September 22, 1950, GCMRL/G. C. Marshall Papers [Secretary of Defense, Number Indexed, M200-1-1].)

106

TESTIMONIAL DINNER FOR
JAMES W. WADSWORTH[1]

September 21, 1950
Rochester, New York

Many years ago, about 1908 as I remember, in studying the War Department reports on the conduct of the campaigns in the Philippine Islands, I found a reference to your guest of honor in a wire from the famous fighting General of those days, Lawton, to the Commanding General and Military Governor of the Philippines.[2] It seems young Wadsworth after graduating from Yale sought active service in the Philadelphia Battery in Puerto Rico. The quick peace denying him the service he desired, he succeeded in reaching the Islands in the heavy disguise of a commissary clerk and was pressing for opportunities to participate in the active fighting.

His was a mere name to me then, but I pondered over the fact that a top general in the heavy fighting of the moment should bother himself about a young fellow in such a humble position.

It was not until 11 years later when accompanying General Pershing to his first, and I believe his only, hearing before Congressional committees that I found that young commissary clerk was the very young Chairman of the Senate Military [Affairs] Committee.

In my work for General Pershing in connection with the proposed National Defense Act, I soon came to feel that Senator Wadsworth was probably the determining figure in whatever military legislation might be drafted. I was tremendously impressed then, and I have continued to be, with the evident integrity which formed the background of his every action. Succeeding events demonstrated that he was a shining example of that important factor for the success of a democracy, a man high in government position who acts only in the interest of his country as he sees it and utterly regardless of the effect on himself personally.

The events of that period are so instructive, I think that it might not be amiss to summarize what actually occurred.

Early in 1790 President Washington transmitted a plan for a complete national defense organization to the First Congress. It was based upon the principle that, in a self-governing republic, every able bodied young man should be trained to defend his country. Unfortunately, our forefathers did not accept this Washingtonian plan. If they had, we would have been prepared in the beginning for every military emergency in our subsequent history.

Now it is an interesting and arresting fact that in January 1920 after the First World War, James Wadsworth, Chairman of the Senate Military Affairs Committee, introduced a bill proposing a modern adaptation of the original Washingtonian defense plan. The result of this plan, if adopted, would have been to conserve the citizen army of World War I as a permanent national institution, ready for speedy mobilization at any time in the future. If Congress had passed the original Wadsworth Bill, I do not believe even a Hitler would have dared to provoke a second World War and, without the havoc of that war, there would be no present menace of a third world war.

After hearings involving all the leading actors in those war years, which were prolonged through the late spring, and summer into the fall of 1919, with the tragedy of the war and our appalling unpreparedness for that war fresh in everybody's mind, the Congress enacted a National Defense Act which received the approval of the President on June 4, 1920. The teeth or backbone of the Act had been emasculated by the refusal of the legislators to endorse universal military training [UMT], but otherwise the Act was a tremendous advance for the security of our national defense—though not to be compared with Senator Wadsworth's original proposal.

A standing Army of 280,000 was authorized. Personnel was provided for the efficient functioning of an elaborate ROTC system in the colleges and universities and general instruction and training of the National Guard. Personnel was also provided to make good with the troops the absenteeism of officers called for staff duty or student officers sent to our military educational institutions.

The point I wish to make is that after these long hearings, fresh on the conclusion of a terrible war, the most terrible the world had seen up to that time, reasonably sound action was taken by the Congress, except as to universal military training, and the Army for the first time was put on a basis which permitted it some opportunity to prepare in time of peace for what it might be called upon to do in time of war.

However, within nine months Congress, now confronted with the highly political problem of the national budget and an increase in taxes, took the first step to destroy the sensible action it had taken in the law approved June 4, 1920. By limiting appropriations, it necessitated the reduction of the Army from 280,000 men to 185,000. Eight months later the number had been reduced to 150,000 and for some years after June 30, 1922 the figure stood at 125,000. There was no reduction in the obligations of the Army's maintaining its services to the National Guard, the organized reserves, the ROTC, and for the personnel required as student officers in the highly important Army war college, staff college and the special service schools. It was the combat troops that must suffer.

First the war-strength units were reduced in strength. Then the third battalions were omitted from regimental units. The strength of the companies was materially reduced. Later the headquarters units of battalions, regiments and brigades were almost eliminated—those units that were responsible for the direction, control and supervision of the fighting elements. Finally it came to the point where half the bands were eliminated, and while a bandsman does not usually shoot, his music is of great importance to morale, particularly when the fighting men are deep in the mud or half-fed or half-frozen.

And then came a great movement towards the air and the Newton Baker Committee went into action and proposed very important things to be done for the Air Corps.[3] These Congress enacted into law but did not provide any of the personnel for the purpose. So again the infantry, the artillery and the tank units and all of their higher elements were levied upon for this purpose, until we reached the point in 1933 where there literally was no ground force worthy of the name in the Army.

During this emasculation I remember one instance where a regiment was ordered to move about 1200 miles in order to consolidate command and as there was no money for transportation, it marched with its dwindling companies. By the time it got half-way to its destination it lost several units which had to be eliminated and before it reached its new post the entire regiment was eliminated.

This was pretty much the picture of the ground forces of the Army when I came to Washington in 1938. The point I wish to emphasize is that despite what most people said, the Congress and the people had not learned a lesson from the First World War. And what is more important, again after 1945 and 46 we demonstrated that we still had not learned our lesson despite another catastrophic world war.

In later years your guest of honor took the lead in inducing Congress to pass the Selective Service Act.[4] He did everything in his power in the interests of the national security and international peace, and his actions were backed with great wisdom and a very special knowledge of the circumstances, requirements and the probable reactions of the Congress. I felt in those days immediately preceding our entry into the last war, as I did at the conclusion of the first war, and as I continued to feel through the long ordeal which lead to the final victory in 1945, that James Wadsworth had rendered a truly magnificent service to his country—quietly, unobtrusively but most effectively.

GCMRL/G. C. Marshall Papers (American Red Cross, Speeches and Statements)

1. Edward P. Curtis, an executive at Eastman Kodak, had written to Marshall in July 1950 asking him to give the opening remarks at the testimonial dinner for James W. Wadsworth (R-NY), who was retiring from Congress. As both a senator (1915–27) and a member of the House of Representatives (1933–51), Wadsworth had been deeply involved in military affairs. "While my schedule for September is very tight," Marshall replied, "I would like very much to attend this dinner and am going to try to arrange my schedule so that I can be in Rochester that evening." (Curtis to Marshall, July 10, 1950, and Marshall to Curtis, July 14, 1950, GCMRL/G. C. Marshall Papers [American Red Cross, General].) There are numerous mentions of Wadsworth in the first four volumes of the *Papers of GCM*. Please consult indexes.

2. Marshall is referring to Henry Lawton, a decorated officer who served in the Civil War, the Apache Wars, the Spanish-American War, and the Philippine-American War. Felled by a sharpshooter's bullet at the Battle of Paye on December 19, 1899, he is buried at Arlington National Cemetery. The commanding general and military governor of the Philippines at that time was Elwell S. Otis, who had taken over from Wesley Merritt (USMA, 1860) in August 1898 and was replaced by Arthur MacArthur in January 1900. (*Report of Major-General E. S. Otis, U. S. Volunteers, on Military Operations and Civil Affairs in the Philippine Islands. 1899* [Washington: GPO, 1899].)

3. Newton D. Baker, secretary of war from March 9, 1916, to March 4, 1921, chaired a committee in 1934 that concluded the army air corps was inadequate in strength and recommended greater autonomy via the creation of a General Headquarters Air Force, but rejected the calls of air advocates for a separate and independent air force. A General Headquarters Air Force to control operations was established on March 1, 1935.

4. Marshall is referring to the Selective Training and Service Act of 1940, also known as the Burke-Wadsworth Act. Nebraska Democrat Edgar R. Burke introduced the bill to the Senate on June 20, 1940, and Wadsworth introduced it to the House the next day. The bill passed and was signed by the president on September 16, 1940, thereby creating the first peacetime draft in US history.

MARSHALL'S first weeks in office were eventful and hectic. Only a day after his September 21 swearing in as secretary of defense, he joined Acheson in New York City at a meeting with the British and French foreign and defense ministers being held in conjunction with a full NATO (North Atlantic Treaty Organization) Council meeting. Simultaneously he had to deal with fast-moving events in Korea. On September 15, MacArthur had launched a bold and successful amphibious assault behind North Korean lines at the port of Inchon. A day later the US and South Korean forces that had established a defensive perimeter around the port of Pusan in the southeast corner of Korea (extending from the mouth of the Naktong River in the south to Taegu and on to Pohang on the east coast) launched their own successful offensive against the North Koreans, who began to withdraw on September 19. By September 23, they were in full retreat from the perimeter, with Allied forces in pursuit. On September 27, those forces linked up with those that had landed at Inchon two weeks earlier.

The North Korean invasion of South Korea in June had convinced the Big Three (Britain, France, and the United States) meeting in New York that, in Acheson's words, "the USSR was prepared to use force . . . to achieve political ends" and that a major expansion of NATO forces was therefore necessary. The United States was willing to increase its forces in Europe, provided the Europeans increased their forces and agreed to the rearming of West Germany within a NATO army—a proposal that Britain supported but France opposed. During a September 22 afternoon session Marshall warned of "a serious problem" with congressional appropriations if German rearmament did not occur, and on the morning of September 23, Acheson asked him to speak about the effect of French refusal on Congress and the public "and with regard to obtaining necessary appropriations." Marshall responded "that he would be immodest and say that no one in the history of the US had ever gotten as much money out of Congress as he. He said that he was thoroughly familiar with the difficulties of getting funds and mentioned the portion of our Congress which is isolationist, and another portion which is purely destructionist." The latter group "would try to kill the whole plan on the grounds that Germany was not participating." Such nonparticipation, he warned, would lead to "great difficulty" in obtaining the necessary appropriations. In response to a question by French Defense Minister Jules Moch as to whether the proposed German military units had to be of division size as opposed to smaller units, he said that he would have to study the matter, that the division "was the most efficient unit from a purely military standpoint" and would have to be adopted "sooner or later," but that "it might not be necessary to start with divisions." (*FRUS, 1950*, 3: 341, 1392–93).

According to Acheson, Marshall during the New York meetings was of "immense help in two ways. His great prestige and calm, compelling exposition left no doubt in any mind, including the French minds, that without Germany the defense of Europe was not possible. He also became convinced himself, and was able to persuade the Pentagon," that its previous insistence on a "rigid and brusque 'one package' proposal" that linked a united NATO command and increased US forces to German rearmament was counterproductive and "would not work." Acheson also noted that Marshall "did useful work in private talks with Moch by getting him off generalities and onto specifics, the matching of needs and resources." (Acheson, *Present at the Creation*, 444.)

Marshall returned to Washington late in the afternoon on Saturday, September 23, and went to Leesburg, where he spent Sunday. He spent much of the ensuing week dealing with how to proceed in Korea as the US/South Korean/UN forces approached the 38th parallel. ★

107

To Harry S. Truman

September 27, 1950
Washington, DC

Dear Mr. President: I am attaching, for your approval, a draft directive to the Commander of the United Nations' Forces in Korea implementing the primarily military aspects of NSC 81/1 which contains the agreed U.S. policy on future courses of action in Korea.[1]

The Secretary of State and I have concurred in this directive, which was prepared by the Joint Chiefs of Staff except for the final paragraph proposed by the Department of State.[2]

Your approval would permit the Commander of the United Nations' Forces in Korea to conduct the necessary military operations north of the 38° to destroy North Korean forces, subject to the conditions specified in paragraph 2 of the directive.[3]

With great respect, Faithfully yours,

NA/RG 330, CD 092 (Korea, 38th Parallel)

1. NSC 81/1 authorized military operations north of the 38th parallel, albeit with a series of provisos. The most important of these was that neither the Soviets nor the Communist Chinese had intervened or threatened intervention and that the president had authorized such operations in advance. President Truman approved NSC 81/1 on September 11. (NSC 81/1, "A Report to the President by the National Security Council on United States Courses of Action with Respect to Korea," September 9, 1950, NA/RG 273, P&O 091 [Korea]; Doris M. Condit, *History of the Office of the Secretary of Defense*, vol. 2, *The Test of War, 1950–1953* [Washington: Historical Office, OSD, 1988], 64–65.)

2. The JCS had on September 25 tentatively approved and forwarded the draft directive to Marshall, who on September 26 sent it to Acheson for State Department approval. Acheson approved it on September 27, subject to inclusion of an additional paragraph calling for restoration as soon as possible of the ROK government with Seoul as its capital but only in the South; the political future of the North would have to await UN action. (Bradley to Marshall, memorandum, September 25, 1950, Marshall to Acheson, September 26, 1950, Matthews to Marshall, September 27, 1950, NA/RG 330, CD 092 [Korea, 38th Parallel]; James F. Schnabel and Robert J. Watson, *The History of the Joint Chiefs of Staff: The Joint Chiefs of Staff and National Policy*, vol. 3, *The Korean War*, pt. 1 [Washington: Office of Joint History, Office of the Chairman of the Joint Chiefs of Staff, 1998], 98–99.)

3. Truman approved the directive on September 27 and the Joint Chiefs forwarded it to MacArthur on the same day. Paragraph 2 authorized military operations north of the 38th parallel to destroy the North Korean armed forces, with the proviso that "under no circum-

stances" were MacArthur's forces to cross or conduct any operations across the Chinese or Soviet borders and that "as a matter of policy, no non-Korean ground forces will be used in the northeast provinces bordering the Soviet Union or in the area along the Manchurian border." As per the State Department's final paragraph, MacArthur was also authorized to "facilitate the restoration" of the ROK government in Seoul, "but political questions such as the formal extension of sovereignty over North Korea should await action by the United Nations to complete the unification of the country." (Truman to Marshall, September 27, 1950, NA/RG 330, CD 092 [Korea, 38th Parallel]; Schnabel and Watson, *History of JCS*, 3, pt. 1: 99–100; James F. Schnabel, *United States Army in the Korean War*, vol. 3, *Policy and Direction: The First Year* [Washington: Office of the Chief of Military History, US Army, 1972], 181–83). For MacArthur's response, see p. 171n1.

On the same date, the Joint Chiefs informed Marshall that they and MacArthur had no objection to two State Department proposals regarding the termination of hostilities in Korea. (Bradley to Marshall, memorandum, September 27, 1950, NA/RG 330, CD 092 [Korea, 38th Parallel]; Schnabel and Watson, *History of JCS*, 3, pt. 1: 100.) On October 3, Marshall informed Acheson that the Defense Department had "no objection, from the military point of view, to those matters, in both of the letters, which are primarily within its purview" but he included a series of suggestions based on input from the three service secretaries. (Marshall to Acheson, October 3, 1950, and service secretaries to Marshall, memorandum, September 27, 1950, NA/RG 330, CD 092 [Korea, 38th Parallel]; *FRUS, 1950*, 7: 853–54. The two State Department letters are on 731–32 and 755–59.)

Direct correspondence with MacArthur went through the Joint Chiefs of Staff communication system but usually came from US Army Chief of Staff Collins or Army Secretary Pace via the dual chains of command then in existence. Furthermore, many of the telegrams MacArthur received actually came from Marshall, Acheson, and/or the JCS–State Department committee chaired by Dean Rusk that Marshall had initiated (see p. 159n1). While the JCS participated in the drafting of some of these, such as NSC 81/1, they merely put into military language many other directives emanating from civilians in the State and/or Defense Departments.

On September 27, Marshall also directed the service secretaries to appoint assistant secretaries or undersecretaries for fiscal management as well as departmental comptrollers and deputy comptrollers. Simultaneously he approved JCS recommendations regarding preparation of additional supplemental budget requests for fiscal years 1951 and 1952, including the assumption that "Combat operations in Korea will be concluded by 30 June 1951." (Condit, *Test of War*, 486; Marshall to service secretaries, memorandum, September 27, 1950, NA/RG 330 [OSD Index, 201–Marshall, George C.]; Marshall to service secretaries and JCS, memorandum and attachment, "Statement of General Assumptions," September 27, 1950, NA/RG 330, CD 111 [Gen.].)

108

TO MRS. JOHN W. PENDLETON

September 27, 1950
Washington, DC

Dear Madge: Congratulations. I was so relieved and delighted to get the news last night just before we went to bed. Katherine had just told me of her drive to town with you. It is splendid that all worked out so well, that you have a boy as Tupper desired and that now you can look forward to the wonderful part instead of the moment of suffering and uncertainty.[1] Devotedly,

G. C. M.

GCMRL/Xerox 2237 (GCM Family, Personal Letters); H

1. Madge Pendleton had given birth to a son, John W. Pendleton Jr., on September 26.

Tupper was her son from her marriage to Marshall's stepson Allen Brown. (See p. 43n1.) On September 30, she wrote to thank Marshall for his letter and reported that "Everything is going very well—John and Tupper carrying on at home, the baby flourishing & I am living the life of Riley here. When we send the baby home, I hope you can stop in and make a formal inspection of him." (Pendleton to Marshall, September 30, 1950, GCMRL/G. C. Marshall Papers [Secretary of Defense, Number Indexed, M200-2-43].)

109

To General Sir Hastings Ismay[1]

September 28, 1950
Washington, DC

Dear Ismay: I have just this moment read your note of September 20.[2] I can't begin to tell you how much I appreciate your warm expressions regarding this appointment I have just taken over. I wish I could feel that you and I were going to work closely again because my recollection of our associations is among the pleasantest of the war years—or my life, for that matter.

This new departure of mine is very hard on Mrs. Marshall, but she is game, though she was profoundly depressed when the papers reported her delighted with the matter. Unfortunately this means we will be separated most of the winter because she can't stand the Washington climate due to sinus trouble and will be at Pinehurst, N.C., and, of course, I have to be here.

With warmest regards from us both to Lady Ismay and yourself. Faithfully yours,

P.S. The old clan is gathering here. Bedell Smith comes to town for his new duties on October 1st.[3] Maybe (this is wholly off-the-cuff and confidential) Eisenhower will be about. Bob Lovett, Assistant Secretary for Air in the War Department during the war years, just telephoned me as I dictated this note to tell me that he informed the President he would accept the assignment as Deputy Secretary of Defense. I am in communication with Frank McCarthy, but I don't know if I can compete with the motion picture industry. He is in Germany now.[4]

GCMRL/G. C. Marshall Papers (Secretary of Defense, Selected)

1. Ismay had been Winston Churchill's chief of staff and representative on the British Chiefs of Staff Committee during World War II. See pp. 891–92.

2. "The news that you have again sacrificed yourself in the service of your country and of the world has been received here with the utmost admiration and gratitude," Ismay had written, "particularly by those of us who were fortunate enough to work with you and under you during World War II. We all feel that the United Nations have had a reinforcement amounting to several battleships, several divisions and several groups of aircraft: and we all wish you the very best of luck in your stupendous task." Ismay also noted that he recalled warning Marshall in November 1945 that he was "under an illusion if you imagined that your country could spare you for many many years. How right I was!" (Ismay to Marshall, September 20, 1950, GCMRL/G. C. Marshall Papers [Secretary of Defense, Selected].)

3. Smith became the fourth director of Central Intelligence on October 7, 1950.

4. McCarthy was in Bavaria working as an associate producer on the set of a Twenti-

eth Century–Fox war movie called *Decision Before Dawn*. ("Movie Realism Opens Old Wounds in Germany," *New York Times*, December 10, 1950, p. X9.) See also pp. 183–84.

110

To General of the Army Douglas MacArthur — September 29, 1950
Radio No. JCS-92985. *Top Secret* — Washington, DC

From JCS to PERSONAL FOR Genl of the Army Douglas MacArthur, SECDEF sends. FOR HIS EYES ONLY.

Reference present report of supposed announcement by Eighth Army that ROK Divisions would halt on 38th parallel for regrouping:[1] We want you to feel unhampered tactically and strategically to proceed north of 38th parallel. Announcement above is referring to may precipitate embarrassment in UN where evident desire is not to be confronted with necessity of a vote on passage of 38th parallel, rather to find you have found it militarily necessary to do so.[2]

NA/RG 218, Geographic File, CCS 383.21 (Korea, Sec. 34)

1. In response to the directive sent to him on September 27 (see pp. 168–69), MacArthur on September 28 had sent his plans for operations in North Korea. Sometime between October 15 and 30, the Eighth Army under Lieutenant General Walton H. Walker (USMA, 1912) would cross the 38th parallel in the West "with the objective of seizing Pyongyang," the North Korean capital, while the X Corps under Major General Edward M. Almond (VMI, 1915), which had landed at Inchon, would be sealifted to make an amphibious landing in the east at Wonsan and link up with the Eighth Army. Only South Korean forces would "conduct operation [north] of the line Chungjo-Yongwon-Hungnam." MacArthur concluded that there was "no indication at present of entry into North Korea by major Soviet or Chinese Communist forces." (MacArthur to DEPTAR [Department of the Army] for JCS, cable, September 28, 1950, NA/RG 330 CD 092 [Korea, 38th Parallel]; Schnabel and Watson, *History of JCS*, 3, pt. 1: 100–101, and map 4 illustrating MacArthur plan on 105.)

The JCS approved MacArthur's plans but before so informing him requested that Marshall obtain presidential approval "as soon as practicable since certain ROK Army forces may even now be crossing the 38th parallel." Marshall wrote on Bradley's memorandum that Truman and Acheson had approved these plans at a September 29 luncheon meeting at Blair House. (Bradley to Marshall, memorandum, September 29, 1950, NA/RG 330, CD 092 [Korea, 38th Parallel].)

At the same time that these events were taking place, however, Marshall received unconfirmed news reports that General Walker had informed reporters that his forces would halt at the 38th parallel to regroup and, according to the official army history of the Korean War, "ostensibly, to await permission to cross." These reports so disturbed Marshall that he sent MacArthur this personal message. (Schnabel, *Policy and Direction*, 183.) Acheson, however, concluded in his memoirs that "To me, the message seems directed toward soothing MacArthur's irritation at being required to submit his plan of operations. He was assured that Washington wanted him to feel unhampered in proceeding north, except as his orders confined him. His plan showed that he understood this perfectly." (Acheson, *Present at the Creation*, 453–54.)

2. The typescript of this message in NA/RG 218, CJCS File 091 (Korea [1950]) has an attached "handwritten note, signed N" and addressed to General Bradley's administrative assistant, Paul M. Kearney, stating that the original version of this document to General

MacArthur was written "in Gen Marshall's handwriting." The editors have been unable to locate Marshall's handwritten original. (See also Schnabel and Watson, *History of JCS*, 3, pt. 1: 103, 296n57.)

MacArthur responded the next day that he had received "no confirmation" of Walker's alleged announcement and doubted its authenticity. The 38th parallel, he continued "is not a factor in the mil[itary] employment of our forces. The logistical supply of our units is the main problem which limits our immediate advance. In exploiting the defeat of the enemy forces, our own troops may cross the parallel at any time in exploratory probing or exploiting local tactical conditions. My overall strategic plan for North Korea is known to you. Unless and until the enemy capitulated[*s*], I regard all of Korea open for our mil[itary] operations." (MacArthur to Marshall, cable, September 30, 1950, NA/RG 218, Geographic File, CCS 383.21 [Korea, Sec. 34]; Schnabel and Watson, *History of JCS*, 3, pt. 1: 103.)

111

To General of the Army Douglas MacArthur — September 30, 1950
Radio No. WCL-46338. — Washington, DC

From Secretary of Defense

Please accept my personal tribute to the courageous campaign you directed in Korea and the daring and perfect strategical operation which virtually terminated the struggle.[1] G C Marshall.

GCMRL/G. C. Marshall Papers (Pentagon Office, Selected)

1. MacArthur and South Korean President Syngman Rhee had on September 29 announced in Seoul, the recently recaptured South Korean capital, the restoration of the ROK government south of the 38th parallel. ROK troops would cross the parallel on October 1.

"Thanks, George, for your fine message," MacArthur replied on October 1. "It brings back vividly the memories of past wars and the complete coordination and perfect unity of cooperation which has always existed in our mutual relationships and martial endeavors. Again my deepest appreciation for your message and for your unfailing support." (MacArthur to Marshall, October 1, 1950, GCMRL/G. C. Marshall Papers [Pentagon Office, Selected].)

112

To Lieutenant General Richard J. Marshall — October 2, 1950
Washington, DC

Dear Marshall: I have just received your note of September 29, notifying me of my election as President of the Board of Visitors.[1] I hope my dubious view of this procedure will not be justified, but I am about to make a bad beginning.

The next meeting you scheduled for the evening of the 27th of October in Lexington. On that evening I am scheduled for a meeting with Defense Minister [Emanuel] Shinwell of Great Britain. What is more important, the following morning, the 28th, I am Chairman of a meeting of eleven defense ministers of the North Atlantic Treaty group, the meeting to last probably through Monday.[2] Under the circumstances, I cannot possibly be absent because matters of the most grave importance are to be discussed and I hope decided upon.

I am asking you now to read the foregoing portion of my letter to the Board of Visitors, that they may understand my situation.

I am certain we can get together on October 6, as you request, but I must explain now that I am involved with receiving for Mr. Truman (in his absence) the mayors from all over the United States, and I will be giving them a presentation here at the Pentagon about noon. At lunch, I am involved with Stuart Symington of NSRB and Anna Rosenberg. But, before the meeting of the mayors or after the lunch with Symington, I think we can manage a half hour.[3] Faithfully yours,

VMI Archives/Alumni Records (George C. Marshall File)

1. George Marshall had first been appointed to the VMI Board of Visitors in the spring of 1946. (See *Papers of GCM*, 5: 576.) He was elected its president on September 23, 1950. (R. J. Marshall to Marshall, September 29, 1950, GCMRL/G. C. Marshall Papers [Secretary of Defense, Number Indexed, M208-1-9].)

2. See pp. 218–20.

3. "There are several papers on which I want to get your signature," Superintendent Marshall had written, "and which I will bring to Washington on the 6th of October. If I am unable to see you then I will leave them with Major George. I have to be there on that date for a meeting of college presidents who are discussing the use of colleges in the event of a major mobilization. I suggest that rather than attempt to read the minutes that will come to you under separate cover I brief you on them verbally on October 6th." (Ibid.) The meeting took place on October 6 at 2:45 p.m., after Marshall had addressed the Conference of Mayors (see pp. 179–82) and had lunch with a group that included W. Stuart Symington, the first secretary of the air force from 1947 until becoming chairman of the National Security Resources Board on April 26, 1950, and Anna Rosenberg, Symington's consultant on mobilization policy.

While he agreed to serve as president of the VMI Board of Visitors, Marshall resigned from the board of directors of Pan American Airways, of which he had been a member since mid-1949, to be effective upon his confirmation as secretary of defense. Juan Trippe, president of the airline, accepted Marshall's resignation on September 21, 1950, and expressed the "keen disappointment" of the board's executive committee, "but also great relief that you soon were to head up the military establishment." (Trippe to Marshall, September 21, 1950, ibid., M200-3-30].)

113

To Millard E. Tydings[1] — October 2, 1950
Confidential — Washington, DC

Dear Senator: This note is primarily to tell you that your message to me the other day about Franklin arrived about six hours after the decision was made for the appointment of Lovett.[2] I was not free to comment on this at the time, which I know you will understand. Incidentally, the President told me that you had phoned him also.

Now to another matter, which I hope you will treat as exceedingly confidential. I am turning over in my mind the proposal to the President of a new head to the Munitions Board, and the thought has occurred to me that possibly Franklin is unusually well qualified for the job. What is your view in the matter—professionally, politically and otherwise?[3]

I must tell you that Sawyer is making inquiries without any reference to me whatever, in regard to Franklin.[4] Faithfully yours,

GCMRL/G. C. Marshall Papers (Secretary of Defense, Chronological, Secretaries, Ackerman)

1. In addition to heading the subcommittee to investigate Senator McCarthy's charges regarding the State Department (see p. 84n2), Tydings was chair of the Senate Armed Services Committee.

2. John M. Franklin was president of the United States Lines Company and a former major general who had served during World War II as assistant chief of transportation in the War Department.

3. Franklin on October 5 informed Tydings that he did not believe he was qualified for the position and requested that his name be withdrawn from further consideration. Tydings forwarded this letter to Marshall on the following day. (Tydings to Marshall, October 6, 1950, GCMRL/G. C. Marshall Papers [Secretary of Defense, Number Indexed, M200-3-31].)

4. Marshall is probably referrring to Secretary of Commerce Charles Sawyer, who was a member of the National Munitions Control Board.

114

NOTES BY BRIGADIER GENERAL A. ROBERT GINSBURGH ABOUT A CONFERENCE WITH GEORGE C. MARSHALL[1] — October 2, 1950, Washington, DC

The Secretary desired that I go over his book entitled, "Selected Speeches and Statements," and cut out all references that can be used in the current situation.[2]

He desired that the same thing be done with his final annual report.[3]

He also desired that his speeches be obtained from the State Department where he discussed or appeared on military programs.

It is evident from the conversations I had with him that trained manpower is what he is most vitally interested in and he looks upon UMT as the surest reservoir for a continual flow of men into the Guard, and trained men ready to volunteer in an emergency. He feels UMT will save billions. He apparently was not wholly pleased with the program that the services had drawn up but asked that I regard that as confidential, but that he certainly was going to work on training men and having adequate members.

It looks as though UMT is the big thing.[4]

HSTL/A. Robert Ginsburgh Papers (Diary, Office of the Secretary of Defense)

1. Ginsburgh, USAF, was the military assistant to the director of the Office of Public Information in the Defense Department. He met with Marshall at 11:35 a.m.

2. H. A. DeWeerd, ed., *Selected Speeches and Statements of General of the Army George C. Marshall* (Washington: Infantry Journal, 1945). See *Papers of GCM*, 4: 641.

3. *Biennial Report of the Chief of Staff of the United States Army, July 1, 1943, to June 30, 1945, to the Secretary of War* (Washington: GPO, 1945); and *General Marshall's Report: The Winning of the War in Europe and the Pacific: Biennial Report of the Chief of Staff of the United States Army, July 1, 1943 to June 30, 1945, to the Secretary of War* (New York: Simon and Schuster, 1945). For more on Marshall's final biennial report, see p. 879n4.

4. For more on Marshall's views on UMT and the differences between UMT and universal military service and training (UMST), see pp. 177–78.

President Truman was also a supporter of UMT and had attempted unsuccessfully to pass a program several times. Prior to Marshall's appointment as secretary of defense, Congress had instead reinstituted Selective Service in 1948. In 1950, it had been considering another iteration of a UMT bill that would train all men between eighteen and twenty for six months, followed by six months in the reserves. In late August, however, Truman asked the committees to stop hearings on the grounds that such a program could not possibly be implemented until the fighting in Korea had subsided. He did so, however, with the goal of taking additional action in January 1951. ("Universal Training Shelved in Senate," *New York Times*, August 31, 1950, p. 3.) Marshall's comments and directives to Ginsburgh appear to have been in preparation for this early 1951 effort. See pp. 325–29 and 338–47.

115

TO COLONEL MARSHALL S. CARTER — October 3, 1950, Washington, DC

Dear Carter: Commencing with Harriman and going down through quite a few others, I have many suggestions about bringing you back. My reaction has been that such procedure would be most unfair to you because if my tenure is short, you would be left adrift again on a staff raft. However, I would be curious to get your thought in view of your present situation and prospects in Japan or Korea.[1]

We were much distressed to learn of your father's death, and particularly the fact that both Preot's father's death and your father's should have come within such a short time. This is a tremendous shock for her as well as for you.[2]

George and I were delighted to learn that she had such a fine summer at Sun Valley. I think that probably did a great deal, both for her and her mother, and apparently the children were delighted. I will try to see them soon, but so far I have been up to my ears in tremendous problems in my first few days here.

Mrs. Marshall came to town yesterday with me and measured the rooms in the apartment she's leasing and decided on the decorations. We'll probably move into town about the 15th, closing Leesburg except for possible weekends. I am insisting that she go very promptly down to Pinehurst and I will try to weekend there. All this will depend on what happens in the world.[3]

With affectionate regards, Faithfully yours,

GCMRL/Marshall S. Carter Papers (Educational and Professional Papers, OSD 1950–1952)

1. For Carter's assignment in Japan, see p. 112n2.

2. Préot Nichols Carter was Marshall Carter's wife. Her father, Brigadier General William R. Nichols (VMI, 1906), had died on July 12, 1950. Marshall Carter's father, Brigadier General Clifton Carroll Carter (USMA, 1899), had died on the evening of September 19–20, 1950.

3. The Marshalls were renting apartment 505 at 3901 Connecticut Avenue in Washington.

Marshall later reported to Edmund Coles, brother of Marshall's first wife, Lily, that they would be moving "the bulk of our furniture" from Leesburg to this apartment on October 16 and that Katherine Marshall, who suffered from sinusitis while in Washington, would be leaving on November 15 to open their home in Pinehurst, North Carolina. (Marshall to Coles, October 12, 1950, GCMRL/G. C. Marshall Papers [Secretary of Defense, Number Indexed, M200-2-11].)

"Washington assignment preferable," Carter cabled on October 11. He also sent a letter on that date thanking Marshall "for your thoughts on Dad's death" and asserting that he had "not considered that I had ever been left adrift on a staff raft, and am not concerned about that possible angle. . . . I would prefer to return to Washington to work for you," he concluded, "under any conditions and for any period of time." (Carter to Marshall, October 11, 1950, GCMRL/Marshall S. Carter Papers [Educational and Professional Papers, OSD 1950–1952].)

"Unless you have important reason for holding Colonel M S Carter," Marshall cabled MacArthur on October 18, "please return him to Washington by air to report to the Office of the Secretary of Defense." (Marshall to CINCFE [MacArthur], telegram no. DEF-20176, October 18, 1950, GCMRL/G. C. Marshall Papers [Secretary of Defense, Selected].)

Marshall had Carter create in the Defense Department the equivalent of a general staff secretariat for central control of communications. Carter consequently organized the Executive Office of the Secretary (EXOS) and served as both its director and Marshall's executive officer. (Condit, *Test of War*, 483–88.) For additional detail on EXOS as well as information on Marshall's other administrative reforms in 1950 and early 1951, see pp. 371–74.

116

To Brigadier General John McAuley Palmer — October 4, 1950, Washington, DC

Dear John: When I get settled down in this new job I want to have you over some day for lunch, both for pleasure and to talk about your, and my favorite subject.[1] I can send a car for you, so that it will involve the minimum of effort, and they can bring you up here to my office in the elevator.

Katherine and I are taking a small apartment in town, very small, and we hope very hidden. I can't commute back and forth, so we will close that place about the 15th, I think.

The difficult time comes later on when she must go to Pinehurst on account of her sinus weakness, and naturally I have to be here except for weekends. This is a pretty poor prospect.[2]

My love to you both. Faithfully yours,

GCMRL/G. C. Marshall Papers (Secretary of Defense, Number Indexed, M200-3-13)

1. An old friend of Marshall, Palmer (USMA, 1892) had served as assistant chief of staff for operations for the AEF during World War I under General Pershing and was his aide-de-camp from 1921 to 1923. He was a major figure in the formulation of postwar US military policy and a strong proponent of a trained citizen-soldier army and UMST. Marshall recalled Palmer to active duty in 1941 as an adviser on military policy through the end of the war. (See the indexes of volumes 1–4 of *Papers of GCM.*) Palmer had lived in Washington since his retirement in 1946.

2. Palmer responded on October 8, "I have your note of October 4 and look forward to having lunch and a chat with you when you get settled in your new job." He was in the process of turning his papers over to the Library of Congress, but he expected "to close my study room at the Library of Congress and move my remaining papers to our apartment. . . . The bulk of my papers have already been transferred to the Manuscripts Division of the Library of Congress. There, they may enable some younger man to finish the job that I have had to leave unfinished." (Palmer to Marshall, October 8, 1950, GCMRL/G. C. Marshall Papers [Secretary of Defense, Number Indexed, M200-3-13].) For more information on the publication of Palmer's papers, see pp. 354–55.

117

STATEMENT TO THE AMERICAN LEGION CONVENTION[1]

October 5, 1950
Washington, DC

I regret that I am unable to be present in person to express to you the appreciation of the Department of Defense for the loyal support the Legion has always given to the preparedness measures and to urge your wholehearted efforts to give this country the strength it needs in the critical future we now face.

In the past, our military successes have invariably been received with an excess of optimism and an immediate reaction to reduce our armed forces or limit their further development. This was the case to a greater or lesser degree following almost every success we had in the last war, beginning with the victory in Tunisia.[2] The immediate reaction to the Korean campaign seems to indicate repetition of this unfortunate habit of ours. But this time, with your most active help, I hope, we must not give away to the heavy pressures to relax our vigilance or emasculate our strength.

In the world today, I am sorry to say, military strength seems the most essential factor in the support of our foreign policy and of difficult negotiations, and it seems for the moment to be the best means to prevent war—also the surest way to hasten victory if war should befall us.

To maintain a strong military posture through the years immediately ahead and at the same time not to wreck our economy, it is mandatory that we create and maintain a reservoir of trained manpower available for service. In other words, we must have some system of Universal Training. I will not go into the arguments in this message. You already know them well, I am sure, but, they never have been more impressive to me than they are today, and I am certain they will be tomorrow.

In March 1948, as Secretary of State, I said before the Armed Services Committee of the Senate:

"I see no possible way financially to maintain a reasonable military posture except on the foundation of universal military training. The consideration of this subject has been confused by discussion of amounts, requirements, administration and various conflicting beliefs. The clearcut issue is whether or not this country will stand before the world for at least the next five or ten years in a position appropriate to its leadership in furthering the perpetuation of free governments, and avoiding their transition into police states".[3]

In my final report as Chief of Staff in September 1945, I made a special and earnest plea for the immediate adoption of a system of Universal Military Training.[4] Last June we found ourselves of a sudden in a situation in Korea where the issue of trained manpower was of momentous importance. Now that that particular crisis seems moderated to some degree, I hope that the American people will recognize this urgent need and adopt it as a national policy. Just how we can best join the present imperative requirement for selective service action with the initiation of some system for Universal Military Training I am not now prepared to say. But one way or another, it must be done. Past proposals will undoubtedly have to be materially altered to meet the serious situation into which we have gotten ourselves by past failures to act in time. But I hope, with your help, that we can manage this time to overcome the vigorous opposition of small minorities that have dominated the decision in the past, and finally do what, in my opinion, is so much to the vital interest of the American people, not to mention the world at large.

GCMRL/G. C. Marshall Papers (Secretary of Defense, Speeches and Statements)

1. The American Legion convention took place in Los Angeles, California.
2. The Allied victory in Tunisia was completed on May 13, 1943, and resulted in the capture of over 238,000 German and Italian prisoners of war (POWs).
3. See *Papers of GCM*, 6: 408.
4. Marshall had concluded this final war report with an extensive section, entitled "For the Common Defense," regarding the need for a system of universal military training. In outlining his ideas for a system of universal military training, he made clear that "It is not universal military *service*—the actual induction of men into the combatant forces. Such forces would be composed during peacetime of volunteers. The trainees would be in separate organizations maintained for training purposes only. Once trained, young men would be freed from further connection with the Army unless they chose, as they now may, to enroll in the National Guard or an organized reserve unit, or to volunteer for service in the small professional army. When the Nation is in jeopardy they could be called, just as men are now called, by a committee of local neighbors, in an order of priority and under such conditions as directed at that time by the Congress." (*General Marshall's Report*, 117–23.)

Marshall had also used this statement as the basis for his testimony before the Senate Armed Services Committee on March 17, 1948, which was considering a program of UMT at that time. See *Papers of GCM*, 6: 407–10.

118

To Daniel A. Poling

October 6, 1950
Washington, DC

Dear Dr. Poling: I have your letter of September 12, requesting that I send a prayer to be included in the book, AN ARMED FORCES PRAYER BOOK, which you are editing.[1] The one I am submitting I composed and read at Sunrise Services in Arlington Amphitheater, April 9, 1944. Since that time Mrs. Marshall has used it in her book TOGETHER. Mrs. Marshall's book is copyrighted, so for your own protection you may want to contact her publishers Tupper & Love.

My prayer reads as follows:

"Almighty God:

"May those who have given their lives in the service of this nation rest in Thy care.

"May those who are wounded in body find spiritual comfort under Thy guidance in the knowledge that through their services a great cause has been served.

"May those who offer their lives in support of that cause, by land and sea and air, find strength in Thy divine guidance.

"May those of us who serve this nation in its great purpose to secure freedom for all peoples be sustained by Thy blessings.

"Give us strength, O Lord, that we may be pure in heart and in purpose to the end that there may be peace on earth and good will among men.

"May we be mindful this Easter morning 'still stands Thine ancient sacrifice, an humble and a contrite heart.' Amen."[2]

I appreciate your consideration in giving me an opportunity to repeat my supplication in the hope that it might, just as you express it, bring courage and comfort to others as it has to me.[3] Faithfully yours,

GCMRL/G. C. Marshall Papers (Secretary of Defense, Number Indexed, M200-3-28)

1. Dr. Daniel A. Poling was president and editor of the *Christian Herald* magazine and had been a member of the President's Advisory Commission on Universal Training in 1946 and 1947. "I have agreed to edit a book of prayers for the armed forces," he had informed Marshall on September 12. "In this connection I am writing men and women who have had experience in all the services either directly or through members of the family, requesting that they send me a prayer, a prayer that might be helpful to others. . . . I shall be most grateful if you will send me a prayer. I am eager to have the little volume appear at the earliest possible date." (Poling to Marshall, September 12, 1950, GCMRL/G. C. Marshall Papers [Secretary of Defense, Number Indexed, M200-3-28].)

2. See Katherine T. Marshall, *Together: Annals of an Army Wife* (New York: Tupper and Love, Inc., 1946), 190–91.

3. "I cannot tell you, sir, how grateful I am for your prompt response to my appeal for a prayer," Poling replied on October 10. "Your contribution is worthy and distinguished." (Poling to Marshall, October 10, 1950, GCMRL/G. C. Marshall Papers [Secretary of Defense, Number Indexed, M200-3-28].) The volume was published in the following year. (Daniel A. Poling, ed., *The Armed Forces Prayer Book* [New York: Prentice-Hall, 1951].) It included contributions from such individuals as Harry Truman, Dean Acheson, Dwight Eisenhower, Douglas MacArthur, Madame Chiang Kai-shek, and Eleanor Roosevelt, as well as Marshall, whose prayer was reproduced on page 52. Upon publication of the book, Poling reported to Marshall that its reception "has been unanimously excellent" and that he had asked the publisher to send Marshall a copy. Marshall replied on June 15 to thank Poling for the book and added: "We must not only never lose sight of God in our daily lives, but must turn to Him more and more for guidance in these difficult days. I know that the prayers in this book will be an inspiration to all who read them." (Poling to Marshall, n.d., and Marshall to Poling, June 15, 1951, ibid., M212-5-14].)

119

TRANSCRIPT OF REMARKS TO THE CONFERENCE OF MAYORS — October 6, 1950, Washington, DC

This has been a very brief presentation of the Korean operation. I think, though, it is sufficiently complete for you to get a pretty fair understanding.[1]

There are a great many lessons to be drawn from this experience. I will only take the time to mention a few which, I feel, it is important for you to have in your mind when you are discussing matters of this kind—matters of National Defense—with your friends and associates.

In the first place, considering the logistics involved in this operation, I mean the great movements which were required up to 9,000 miles distance, it should be evident to all of you that for our country to meet these unpredictable crises here and there which might arise, it is not a practical proposition to deploy troops in advance, because one never can know these days just where the next crisis will develop. We will have to depend on these logistical powers of ours to mobilize at the critical point what is needed at that time and place.

It also is impressive in another respect. When you look back to the heavy initial deployment of the North Korean Army, it is evident that a Democracy, by its very nature, will always get a late start. We are not in the business of launching surprise attacks on others, because that isn't in accordance with our conception of life and international relations. So we must usually start with the inevitable handicap of having the other man or men taking a decision without the deterring influence of the Press, without the influence of Legislators, without public opinion being permitted a voice. He or they decide to do something at a certain place at a certain time. We can't do that. We should never be able to do it. But it does present a very, very difficult proposition for your government and your Armed Forces, and in everything connected with the initial operations wherever they may be.

I can talk very frankly today because my appointment to the Defense Department only occurred since the collapse of the North Korean forces, so I knew nothing of the inner-workings here, the tremendous tasks that were performed until I became Secretary of Defense. So, as I say, I can talk frankly without your feeling that I am protecting the interests of the Defense Department.

Another very important lesson in this affair, from which to draw your own conclusions as to the legislative requirements that soon are going to arise, is the predicament in which we found ourselves because of the lack of trained men. It is a long, tedious, difficult road in procuring them, processing them, getting them into place, training them, moving them to where they are to go, allowing them to become acquainted with their new associates and to become real members of a team—that represents a long, long period of time. The country found itself without any such reserve and as you just heard we had to strip divisions in this country—take the trained soldiers out of them, take the critical leaders away from them—and rush them in any way we could, over to Korea. That must never happen again. Our situation was saved in Korea by the South Koreans, by the action of General MacArthur in inducting into our American units some 30,000 of them to fill our ranks and make good our complete lack of a reserve of trained personnel immediately available for duty.[2]

I am being rather emphatic about this, because I had a hard struggle during the last war, as Chief of Staff, with the manpower situation, with the political repercussions involved in it, with the various blocs of interest involved here and there, which I won't go into. But for a long time I couldn't get the men in sufficient numbers for the training of what we called "replacements." That term wasn't dramatic enough for the public but it was dramatic enough for the enemy. When we finally got the system well underway and our units were maintained at 100% strength by the following morning, no matter what the action was of today, and from that time on every division was always a sharp axe, high in morale, ready to strike.

Here we had this great struggle—by "we" I mean the staff here—to provide the men, and we could only do it by "robbing Peter to pay Paul," until we had virtually gutted our units in this country.

And yet that Korean affair was a very small campaign. A campaign in some respects fortuitous geographically because it was close to Japan where we did have some divisions and we did have a command set-up with all the necessary arrangements and communications and experience, and a wonderfully capable strategist and leader, in General MacArthur. Also we had sea power. We were dealing with a peninsula which we could surround on every side but one—the narrow northern strip; so too with our planes—the enemy had very few planes, and we had a great many eventually—so we had great advantages in those respects. But we had the gravest of disadvantages, not only in the tremendous distances involved in the support of the operation, but in the fact that we did not have immediately available a reserve of trained manpower.

You can't solve any military tactical problems by pushing a button; you must have men. And they must be trained men or a long period of time in preparation must first elapse.

The fact that we don't have adequate trained manpower is our greatest hazard, and is the reason for our involvement time after time in these tragic dilemmas which provoke terrific effort and great public interest on our part but only for a brief time; then there quickly follows a subsidence of interest. As a result we spend billions and billions and argue about these vast expenditures without getting at what is the real nubbin of the problem.

I appreciate very much your coming over. I am glad of this opportunity to have the Department of Defense present this picture to you. I was asked by the President to substitute for him in meeting you at the close of your conference. Well, I thought you wouldn't get much out of merely meeting me, but I do hope you may have gotten some meat out of hearing these gentlemen present the background of the Korean operation.

I would like Mayor Lawrence to have something to say.[3]

GCMRL/G. C. Marshall Papers (Secretary of Defense, Speeches and Statements)

1. Marshall spoke at noon in place of President Truman, who had to cancel his appearance. At Marshall's suggestion, the conference attendees heard briefings by several high-ranking officers, including General Bradley and Deputy Army Chief of Staff Ridgway, prior to his remarks. (Betters to Marshall and Marshall to Betters, October 2, 1950, GCMRL/G. C. Marshall Papers [Secretary of Defense, Number Indexed, M214-1-41].)

A revised and abridged version of Marshall's speech was published in the December 17, 1950, edition of *This Week* magazine entitled "A Warning to America."

2. General Ridgway had informed the mayors during his address that the army had been "compelled at once to make heavy inroads on our small General Reserve, robbing it of entire combat and service units, and ruthlessly stripping away trained specialists from it and every other source until we virtually had no Army General Reserve in the United States capable of responding to other emergencies elsewhere. So acute was the shortage of infantrymen and Artillerymen in the fighting units in KOREA that General MACARTHUR found it necessary to draw upon trained SOUTH KOREAN soldiers, and actually integrate some 30,000 into our Infantry and Artillery." (Transcript of Department of Defense Pre-

sentation to the Conference of Mayors, October 6, 1950, GCMRL/G. C. Marshall Papers [Secretary of Defense, Speeches and Statements].)

3. Mayor David L. Lawrence of Pittsburgh, president of the Conference of Mayors, thanked Marshall "and the others of his staff for this very, very interesting and profitable meeting here this morning." The American people were "very happy in the fact that you, once again, have sacrificed your own comfort and your own pleasure and your own opportunity for a well-deserved rest to come back again to the country when the country called upon you to fill this very important place at this particular time." They were also "very grateful to you and look upon you, in my opinion, as one of the greatest Americans of our time." (Ibid.)

Marshall then concluded the session by discussing the work of the Red Cross in civil defense, in connection with which "we have been given a tremendously large order and we have accepted it. It leads to 3 or 4 things: one, the blood program which we are in now a tremendous scale, and have been able to prove that we can increase rapidly enough to meet the situation. In fact, almost more rapidly than is required. That would be of very great concern to your civil defense.

"We are now setting the stage for meeting Mr. Symington's request for the training of some 20,000,000 in first aid, which is essential to civil defense, and it has to be done in a regularized manner or it would be quite ineffective. We are also getting ready to arrange for the training of some one-hundred thousand nurses' aides." (Ibid.)

120

To J. Clifford Folger[1]

October 9, 1950
Washington, DC

Dear Folger: I wish, through you, to express my thanks to the District Chapter for their prompt handling of the case of the Austrian DP [displaced person] couple I found stranded, wet and bedraggled the other day.[2] I am told this morning that your chapter has issued them sufficient provision to carry them through Tuesday, tomorrow, and, in the meantime, have contacted the pastor of St. Patrick's Church, who has access to DP records and is affiliated with the [National] Catholic Welfare Organization [*Council*].[3] Faithfully yours,

GCMRL/G. C. Marshall Papers (Secretary of Defense, Number Indexed, M200-3-38)

1. J. Clifford Folger had been chairman of the Washington, DC, chapter of the Red Cross since 1942.

2. A female Austrian displaced person had handed Marshall a note at Red Cross headquarters in Washington, DC, a few days previously. The editors have been unable to locate any further information about the contents of this note or the identity of this woman. (George to Marshall, memorandum, n.d., GCMRL/G. C. Marshall Papers [Secretary of Defense, Number Indexed, M200-3-38].)

3. Major George had also informed Marshall that the National Catholic Welfare Council had "arranged for the transportation and entry of this family into the United States, and they will handle the matter from here on out." (Ibid.)

121

TO FRANK MCCARTHY

October 9, 1950
Washington, DC

Dear Frank: Our radio interchanges have been rather unsatisfactory because I do not feel that I know your genuine reaction to the possibility of joining me here in the Pentagon.[1] You must reply to this letter with great frankness, and I would appreciate your giving a cryptic radio reply followed *immediately* by a letter to the extent of explanation necessary.

What Lovett and I want you for is Assistant Secretary of Defense. You would have a multitude of activities to coordinate, primarily a general control of administration of this department.

There is one Assistant Secretary who is Comptroller and works on all the financial and budgetary phases. There is another one who is Counselor and is involved in all the legal aspects of our business. What is left, which is the largest portion, would be yours.

Now as to timing. It would be necessary for you to take over early November. Your predecessor would drop out about the 30th of October, and it would be essential that you should be in the saddle before Congress reconvenes and before the Congressional committees get well under way with hearings. Just how this will affect your business commitments, I do not know and I would avoid at all cost embarrassing your future because I can get somebody else, but, of course, much prefer you.[2]

I am dictating this letter hastily in order to get an early reply. This time be certain the letter reply gets off because a radio is rather terse expression of one's innermost feelings and personal obligations.[3] Affectionately,

GCMRL/G. C. Marshall Papers (Secretary of Defense, Selected)

1. As early as July 21, McCarthy had informed Marshall from Germany that he was "eager to be of service to you on any notice, for any period, in any capacity, at any rank" should Marshall return to government service. Marshall responded on July 28 that while he appreciated the offer "tremendously" and that "there is nobody's services I would value quite so highly as yours if I took over a difficult and important job," he did not wish to disturb McCarthy's civilian career in the motion picture industry. (McCarthy to Marshall, July 21, 1950, and Marshall to McCarthy, July 28, 1950, GCMRL/G. C. Marshall Papers [Pentagon Office, Selected].) On September 14, McCarthy sent a telegram from Germany and repeated his "any place any time under any circumstances" offer. On the following day, Marshall asked when he would complete the picture on which he was working "and be free to return home." The second half of December, McCarthy cabled back on September 19. Assuming that Marshall intended to recall him to active duty, he added in a separate letter that he could come immediately if needed. (McCarthy to Marshall, September 14 and 19, 1950, Marshall to McCarthy, September 15, 1950, ibid.).

2. Paul Griffith, a native of Uniontown, Pennsylvania, was assistant secretary of defense for administrative and public affairs. For more on the changes to this position following Griffith's retirement, see pp. 206–7.

3. Marshall's letter reached McCarthy, who was on location in Mannheim rather than his Munich studio, by courier only on the evening of October 14. On the following day, he responded by both cable and lengthy letter. The one he had sent on September 19 stating he could resign and return immediately had "miscarried," and in the interim, shooting for

the film, *Decision Before Dawn*, had begun. Due to that fact and a series of "peculiar circumstances" relating to this particular film he could no longer resign. "I placed aside the possibility of asking for a postponement because it was clear, inherently in the situation as well as from your letter, that you must make the appointment immediately." He was "distressed for many reasons, the greatest of which is losing this opportunity to work again under your direction," and he would be "eagerly available" after the middle of December "to help in any way I can with the great burden." (McCarthy to Marshall, cable and letter, October 15, 1950, ibid.)

122

Conversation on European Defense
October 9, 1950 Washington, DC

DURING the September 22–23 meetings of the "Big Three" foreign and defense ministers in New York (see pp. 167–68), French Defense Minister Moch had made clear that American financial assistance as well as military equipment would be required to obtain any French agreement to expansion of their military forces and to West German rearmament. At an October 9 meeting of State, Defense, and Treasury Department officials held to discuss the feasibility of such financial assistance, Marshall stated that he had "serious reservations" about the Pentagon's "one package" approach to the French and that he favored a more gradual and piecemeal approach. He also concurred with the statement by Paul Nitze, head of the State Department's Policy Planning Staff, that "the successful defense of Europe was an integral part of the defense of the United States"; that if a beachhead on the European continent could not be maintained "a successful outcome of a global war would be hard to foresee"; and that "it would cost the United States less, both in terms of men and of money to cooperate with the Europeans in the development of a unified force for the defense of Europe than to increase the number of United States divisions stationed in Europe above those now contemplated." In this regard Marshall is referring to a forthcoming proposal by "a group of prominent educators" that compulsory military service be instituted so that the United States could station half a million men in Europe. While "not wholly in agreement," Marshall "thought that there was an element in their thinking which we should take seriously. In maintaining a large standing army, we would have problems not only with the Congress, but also with the soldiers themselves. We were even now running into problems in calling up reserve officers similar to those which we have always met in calling up men under the Selective Service Act. . . . It was of great importance that the European countries play their full part and a way be found to utilize German units. Perhaps as an initial step, we might contemplate incorporating German platoons in American divisions. In this way, our divisions could very rapidly be brought to an over-strength condition." (*FRUS, 1950*, 3: 364–66). For ensuing conversations with the French on these matters, see pp. 187–88 and 194–203. For more on the proposal by several US educators of compulsory military service, see p. 209n1. ★

123

MEMORANDUM FOR THE SECRETARY OF THE ARMY

October 10, 1950
Washington, DC

Subject: Calling Into Active Service of Officer Reserves

Senator Lucas telephoned me from Illinois to the following effect:[1]

"There is considerable feeling out here in regard to the procedure being followed in calling reserve officers to active duty. For example, to take specific illustrations, an officer with five children is called out and another officer with no children, living in the same small community, is left undisturbed, both in the same grade. In another instance, a man who has carefully built up a small farm on which he does a large portion of the work, has a wife and three children, and he has been called up, which means the forced sale of his farm in all probability, while other men in the same grade in the nearby community, without families or critical obligations, are not touched.

"Is there not some way to obviate this business? Please telegraph me c/o Stevens Hotel, Chicago".[2]

I realize that reserve officers are called out merely in their grade and the matter of family has heretofore not been considered. But in the present situation where a doubtful future is in prospect, it would seem that possibly some special considerations should enter into the selections. I had thought of talking to you sometime back about adopting a policy, for example, whereby an officer would be informed that his tour would not be beyond a year unless there was active war or a very grave emergency, *unless* he himself desired a longer tour. Unless there is some such policy, we are going to wreck the business careers of a large number of our reserve officer personnel because we are entering into a long pull, we hope, meaning that we are going to avoid war by being prepared for war.

Will you please look into this and telegraph Lucas what you think might be said to him there for his information or that he might use in meeting the problems of his constituency.[3]

GCMRL/G. C. Marshall Papers (Secretary of Defense, Chronological, Secretaries, Ackerman)

1. Scott W. Lucas (D-IL) was the Senate majority leader.
2. Complaints regarding the call-up of reserves for the Korean War had been numerous. See Condit, *Test of War*, 491–92, and Schnabel, *Policy and Direction*, 121–22.
3. On October 12, Army Secretary Pace responded that he had telegraphed Lucas and informed him that "definite criteria permitting delay because of hardship have been issued to all field agencies concerned" and that all reservists had the right to request delay to the chief of their military district and appeal decisions. He noted, however, that recall of officers was "based on military necessity" in particular branches, and that the cases Lucas had cited might have involved officers from different branches with different qualifications. Pace also informed Marshall that in the present recall of 20,000 officers, a system had been established for delays of not more than three months "to take care of all real hardship cases." The recall period was for twenty-one months, the legal maximum in the 1950 Selective Service Act, and all the services were presently "considering the problems

relating to the adoption of the policy which you have suggested." Six days later, Pace's office added that reservist officers could also request and be granted additional three-month delays "if the circumstances warrant." (Pace to Marshall, memorandum with attached telegram to Lucas, October 12, 1950, and Kreps to Marshall, October 18, 1950, NA/RG 330, SD 326.21.)

At the recommendation of the Defense Department's Civilian Components Policy Board, Marshall on October 23 directed that each service allow a reservist at least thirty days between call-up and the date he must report for active duty. The services were also directed to "determine and requisition their manpower requirements for six months in advance of recall" and then inform those reservists not selected that their possible future recall would be at least four months later "unless a material change in military requirements otherwise dictates." (Press release, October 23, 1950, GCMRL/G. C. Marshall Papers [Secretary of Defense, Number Indexed, M200-3-26].)

124

To General of the Army Douglas MacArthur — October 10, 1950
Radio No. DEF-93678. *Eyes Only Top Secret* — Washington, DC

The President urgently desires to meet with you in Honolulu Saturday morning, the fourteenth. He will be accompanied by General Bradley, Harriman and Rusk of State Department. The President realizes your difficulty with a new campaign starting or in progress. If Monday the sixteenth would be better for you than Saturday he will make that change. Furthermore if your presence in Japan or Korea is of critical importance the President would consider meeting you Saturday morning the fourteenth at Wake Island.[1] Please expedite reply because the President's plans must be firmed immediately.[2] G C Marshall

GCMRL/G. C. Marshall Papers (Pentagon Office, Selected)

1. Marshall stated during his Senate testimony regarding MacArthur's 1951 relief that "The original proposal to the President was that he [MacArthur] was to come to Hawaii, and I intervened with the President to say that I thought with conditions of affairs in Korea, that might be a very serious matter and would he have any objection if I also proposed Wake Island, and he said he had none, and I did it on that basis, but my purpose in doing it was to protect him [MacArthur] from a long trip and being absent at a critical moment." (*MSFE*, 439–40.)

2. Later on the same day, MacArthur responded with a preference for Wake Island, and Marshall replied, "your message received and the President agreeable. Since Wake Island is west of the date line the President's Saturday morning the fourteenth is your Sunday morning the fifteenth. He will arrive well after daylight but exact time will be given you later. In addition to those mentioned in previous message Secretary Pace of the Army and Jessup of State Department will also accompany him. President will discuss with you the rehabilitation of Korea for which the army will probably be designated the executive agent as well as other matters." (Marshall to MacArthur, cable, DEF-93763, October 10, 1950, GCMRL/G. C. Marshall Papers [Pentagon Office, Selected].)

Acheson reported on October 9 that Truman "raised with me once again the proposal made last week that he should meet General MacArthur either in Hawaii or on Wake. He said that he had been thinking this over and thought favorably of it. General Marshall had given his approval." Truman further informed Acheson that he wanted to review with MacArthur "the situation in Korea, the probable future developments and length of time necessary for the maintenance of American forces there. He would also like to appraise the possibilities of possible Chinese interference in Korea, which the President thought was not likely, and also possible Chinese interference in Indochina." (Acheson, "Meeting with the President, Subject: President's Proposed Trip to Hawaii," memorandum, October 9, 1950, HSTL/Dean G. Acheson Papers [Secretary of State File].)

Bradley had informed Marshall that the rehabilitation of Korea was "one of the subjects" Truman wished to discuss with MacArthur and that "the Army will probably be the executive agent." (Bradley to Marshall, memorandum, October 10, 1950, GCMRL/G. C. Marshall Papers [Pentagon Office, Selected].) Later that day Marshall cabled MacArthur again that "in view of the subjects to be discussed President feels it might be helpful for him if you bring Ambassador [to South Korea] John Muccio to Wake." (Marshall to MacArthur, cable, DEF-93805, October 10, 1950, ibid.)

On October 15, Truman, MacArthur, and their advisers met on Wake Island to discuss Korean operations. Marshall remained in Washington.

125

MEMORANDUM OF CONVERSATION — October 10, 1950
Top Secret — Washington, DC

SUBJECT: Visit of French Representative to the Standing Group with the Secretary of Defense[1]

General Ely came to pay his respects as French Representative to the Standing Group. He indicated his feeling of honor on the occasion of the call, especially in recognition of the great debt which France owes in its recovery efforts to General Marshall.

General Marshall inquired on the number of French divisions in Indo-China and the problem of maintaining their strength. General Ely replied that they averaged between five and six divisions and that there was a difficulty in maintaining the strength, since the shipment from France was mainly non-commissioned and commissioned officers, while those in basic training were limited to duty in France.

On General Marshall's inquiry General Ely stated that France maintained five divisions in Germany and France at this time, and planned to increase this number to ten during 1951 and to a total of twenty divisions available on D ≠ three by 1953–1954.

General Marshall reminisced with General Ely on leading French military figures he had known during World War II, particularly General Juin.[2]

The conversation then turned to an account by General Marshall of the occasion in 1931 while he was head of an Infantry school in Southern Georgia. The General had seen a copy of a French directive requiring the French Field Regulations to be modified as a result of reducing French military service from 24 to 18 months. The General directed four studies to be made separately on the methods of training in peacetime of France, Germany, the United Kingdom and Japan. The study on France was done by General Collins and the study on Germany was done by General Stillwell [*Stilwell*]. The study on the United Kingdom was conducted by an officer General Marshall did not mention by name, but identified as the Military Attache when Mr. Lindberg[*h*] received the invitation of Goering to inspect the German Air Force in 1937.[3]

General Marshall was particularly interested in the efforts of the French to extend military service from 12 to 18 months. He pointed out the difficulty that the United States forces had in the Korean campaign to maintain fighting strength. He also pointed out that arrangements, to which he was not a party, provided units but not replacements.

The meeting was intended to be a courtesy call and no matters of importance were discussed.

R. E. Beebe
Colonel, USAF
Office of Foreign Military Affairs

NA/RG 330, CD Memorandum of Conversation

1. The Standing Group of NATO's North Atlantic Military Committee was composed of permanent representatives of the British, French, and American chiefs of staff and maintained headquarters in Washington, DC.

Marshall met with Lieutenant General Paul Romauld Ely, French liaison officer to SHAEF during World War II and currently the French representative to the NATO Standing Group; Rear Admiral James. H. Foskett, director of the Standing Group; and Captain A. C. Murdaugh, assistant director of the office of foreign military affairs in the Defense Department, at 11:20 a.m. Colonel Royden E. Beebe, a member of the Office of Foreign Military Affairs and the son of Marshall's longtime friend, Brigadier General Royden E. Beebe (see pp. 241–42) took these minutes.

2. In World War II, General Alphonse Pierre Juin had commanded French land forces during the 1942–43 Tunisian campaign and the French Expeditionary Corps during the Italian campaign of 1943–44. In August 1944, he became chief of staff of the French Army. He visited the United States in late April and early May of 1945 and met with Marshall as well as other US officials. See *Papers of GCM*, 4: 452, 514, 719, and *Papers of GCM*, 5: 179–81. In April 1946, Marshall is referring to him as "a fine fellow, an old friend of mine, an outstanding commander of a French Corps in the American Fifth Army in Italy." (*Papers of GCM*, 5: 529.)

3. Marshall is referring to Generals J. Lawton Collins, an instructor at Fort Benning under Marshall as assistant commandant, and Joseph Stilwell (USMA, 1904), whom Marshall had appointed as head of the tactical section at Fort Benning. Then Major Truman Smith had been assistant military attaché in Germany from 1920 to 1924 and was an instructor at Fort Benning under Marshall from 1928 to 1932. Smith was the US military attaché in Germany from 1935 to 1939, during which time the famous aviator Charles Lindbergh received the invitation from German air chief Hermann Goering. For more on Smith, see pp. 884–85 and 919–20. See also *Papers of GCM*, 2: 162, 616–17, and 4: 161–62.

126

Remarks for the Community Chest Campaign Broadcast — October 10, 1950
Washington, DC

Mr. Parker, Mr. Duffield, Mr. Lyon and Members of the Community Chest Federation:[1]

During the past twelve months as President of the American Red Cross, I have traveled to all parts of the country and met with chapter leaders from over twelve hundred communities. At the same time in many cities I had occasion to discuss with Community Chest leaders the work of the agencies which comprise your organization. This has made evident to me the need for strengthening these community agencies, many of which work closely with the Red Cross.[2]

When I agreed to participate in this Community Chest Campaign I was merely President of the Red Cross and not an active member of the Government. Today I am Secretary of Defense, though still for the time being at the head of the Red Cross. Naturally when I talk of the importance of the Community Chest to the well being, the morale of our people, I am bound to think and talk of its effect on the morale of our armed forces in these difficult days and in relation to the growing military forces.

The National Defense is now gaining in its military phase. We are preparing to mobilize our resources on a tremendous scale to strengthen our combat potential and that of our associates. Much, in fact the most, remains to be done. And it will be done, I am sure.

There are special responsibilities locally in the country. That is your primary concern in undertaking the 1951 Community Chest Campaign. This fund campaign is a vital consideration not only to all our communities but also to those of us who are responsible for the defense of our nation. I look upon the success of your campaign locally and throughout the nation as a test of the moral strength of our people.

I know something of the despair and the suffering of those who become engulfed in tragedy. I know that our country has always been generous in its solicitude for the unfortunate of the world. That is something in which we can take pride. But regrettably we sometimes fail to recognize misfortune when we see it on our own doorstep. Poverty, disease and distress in our own communities are positive dangers both to national well being and to our security.

It is one of the great opportunities of the Community Chest and its agencies that they can do much to educate our people in this respect. Your Community Chest is more than a group of local charities. In serving children, the aged, the disabled; in providing healthful recreation; in furnishing guidance to youth; in relieving the anxiety of the distressed; it is a great educational medium in bringing about a better understanding of the needs of the unfortunate. In furthering this greater recognition of the total needs of the community, it is a very important unifying force in American life.

This life has undergone a radical change in the last one hundred years. A century ago the majority of our communities were based on a self-sufficient, largely agricultural economy. We now have an intricate industrial society residing in great metropolitan areas from which the old neighborly touch has gone. We turn to community services for the friendly assistance which used to be given by one neighbor to another.

We must remember that great changes have taken place in our social thinking in recent years. The modern concept of social welfare embraces a far greater range of services than those common to American life fifty years or more ago.

In those days welfare or charity as it was generally thought of—was, for the most part, concerned with doles to the poverty-stricken and shelter for orphaned children and the worn out aged who had become the flotsam and jetsam of society.

Today we have a broader understanding of the factors that create poverty, maladjustment and crime. Many of the Community Chest Agencies are directed to activities that will prevent social tensions rather than merely patch up sore spots in the social fabric.

Such activities as Family Service Agencies, Counseling Services and Youth Guidance Agencies are important because they help people to help themselves—a great principle for a democratic society.

This kind of social work does not coddle or pauperize. It helps its beneficiaries to become self-reliant citizens capable of playing a vigorous part in the stern times in which we live.

While the effort today must be community-wide we need in our personal lives a regeneration of the spirit of neighborliness that characterized the pioneer days of our expanding nation. If we are to keep the strength we have and gain increasing strength in the days to come we must match the determination of our men in uniform with a spirit of sacrifice on the part of everyone in the civilian population.

I have a particular reason as Secretary of Defense to ask your support. The community services rendered by the Chest Agencies are valuable in themselves because they benefit everybody. But, as an ever greater number of young men are called into military service, a greater proportion of our population will be families and dependents of servicemen. What you do to improve the welfare and security of our homes has a strong effect on military morale, and I know what morale means to a military organization.

In developing our modern fighting forces our military leaders are devoting more time to morale factors than ever before.

There is a special function of the Community Chest in relation to the Defense Establishment which I should like to commend. That is the obligation that has been assumed by various agencies of the Community Chest to provide recreation and welfare for the men and women on leave in communities near their stations.

During World War II there were few towns near our military and naval installations that did not boast at least one attractive Community Center extending hospitality to our servicemen. They were greatly needed and greatly appreciated. Now, many camps and training centers are being reactivated to handle the greatly increased forces we must have.

A sense of loneliness and confusion is often the first reaction of a young serviceman away from home. In providing him with wholesome recreation and entertainment in pleasant off-post surroundings, communities can make a tremendous contribution to his well being and to the development of the spirit that makes for a good soldier. This program is worthy of the immediate attention of every community where numbers of service personnel can be expected to spend their leaves.

I have said a good deal about the building of our national strength and the maintenance of morale, and the contribution that Community Chest Agencies can make to both. It is true that these things are essential. But your agencies go beyond the good of the mass and think and act in terms of the human being. In your philosophy the individual *does* count and must be assisted according to his needs.

So long as we in this nation keep our high regard for the sanctity and dignity of the individual, we can be sure that our democracy is a living institution that will stand up in the face of emergency or trial.

It is the privilege of Community Chests and their affiliated agencies to minister to the needs of the individual. Giving voluntarily to such a cause is a measure of our fitness as citizens of a great democracy.

Make no mistake. All over the world democracy is being forced to *prove* that it is the finest way of life.

The example we set here at home by our own sense of civic responsibility is the best way to demonstrate the virtues of democracy to the peoples of other lands. Let us prove that we here in this country know how to make good use of freedom by doing freely what others are compelled to do.

The Community Chest Campaign gives every American citizen an opportunity to strengthen the moral fibres of democracy at home.

This, in itself, will help to strengthen our hands abroad and bring us nearer to the world of peace and security we strive to attain.

GCMRL/G. C. Marshall Papers (American Red Cross, Speeches and Statements)

1. Chauncey G. Parker Jr., assistant US High Commissioner for Germany and director of administration of the International Bank for Reconstruction and Development, was president of the Washington, DC, Community Chest Federation. Hugh K. Duffield, general manager of Sears, Roebuck & Co. in the Washington, DC, area, had been appointed general chairman of the 1951 Community Chest fund campaign. Richard K. Lyon, a lawyer in the Washington area, was the chairman of the Business-Employees Unit of the Community Chest drive.

2. Community chests were regional organizations that coordinated fundraising and charitable services in a single unit. Some local Red Cross chapters worked with community chests in the 1920s and 1930s, but in 1936 national Red Cross leaders prohibited any additional local chapters from participating in joint fundraising with community chest campaigns. The Red Cross maintained its belief in the need for its own separate fund campaigns in spite of its postwar leadership reorganization until it loosened restrictions on local chapters from joining united fund drives in 1955. (Foster Rhea Dulles, *The American Red Cross: A History* [New York: Harper & Brothers, 1950], 332–33; Charles Hurd, *The Compact History of the American Red Cross* [New York: Hawthorn Books, Inc., 1959], 226, 251–55, 260; "United Fund Drive Backed by Red Cross," *Washington Post*, April 6, 1955, p. 1.)

127

To J. C. Bertrand

October 11, 1950
Washington, DC

Dear Bertrand: Both Mrs. Marshall and I appreciated very much your detailed letter of October 10 and all that you had already done for the place. The planting of the winter grass was done under the supervision of Colonel Hawes, who has handled this for us each year. He seems to have done it earlier this year than heretofore, and I hope that as a result it doesn't turn out too badly. However, it is kind of you to have done all you have already done to put the place in good shape.[1]

Mrs. Marshall was particularly touched by Mrs. Bertrand's offer to have two women step in and straighten the house up before her arrival. She will be very glad to take advantage of this and we will let you know in time. I was sorry to learn the other day that Mrs. Bertrand had called up the office during my absence and they had not obtained her telephone number. I tried to locate her in town but without success.[2]

We are still in the country at Leesburg but have started moving to a very small apartment in town. The decorators are still busy and not until Monday will we take over.

As you would anticipate, I am terribly busy now in connection with the North Atlantic Pact Meeting, of which I am the Chairman—the preliminary pick and shovel workers already being here—and the preparation for the presentation to Congress of the first of the budget of the new military program. This represents a tremendous amount of detail work and close attention. Also, of course, I am somewhat besieged by people who wish to see me.

As to Camp Chafee, I will look into the matter and see just what can be done. I do not know at the moment whether or not it is occupied or is to be occupied, but I will find out as soon as I have an opportunity, just what the situation is and what I might do. I would certainly enjoy very much getting a shoot out there, and I know Bradley would.[3]

With warm regards to you both. Faithfully yours,

GCMRL/G. C. Marshall Papers (Secretary of Defense, Selected)

1. Bertrand, a resident of Pinehurst, North Carolina, had written on August 31, 1950, to invite Marshall to go hunting with him and offered to send some of his workers to tidy up the Marshalls' home in preparation for their autumn return later. Though he declined the hunting invitation, Marshall on September 5 accepted "this generous offer" provided that Bertrand "would let me pay the men for the time occupied." (Bertrand to Marshall, August 31, 1950, and Marshall to Bertrand, September 5, 1950, GCMRL/G. C. Marshall Papers [American Red Cross, General].)

Bertrand reported on October 10, that his men had begun to clean the house three weeks prior but that someone else had already worked on the landscaping, which "looked pretty bad," so they had redone much of it. (Bertrand to Marshall, October 10, 1950, GCMRL/G. C. Marshall Papers [Secretary of Defense, Selected].)

Colonel George P. Hawes was a realtor in Pinehurst.

2. Bertrand had also offered to Katherine Marshall interior cleaning services under his wife's supervision. (Ibid.)

3. Bertrand included an invitation for Marshall and General Bradley to go quail hunting with him in Arkansas later in the autumn. Bertrand also asked Marshall if he could help to obtain permission for his trainer to train his dogs at Camp Chaffee in Arkansas and for Bertrand and his partner to hunt there as well. (Ibid.) Major George informed Marshall on October 12 that the camp had been activated. (George to Marshall, memorandum, October 12, 1950, GCMRL/G. C. Marshall Papers [Secretary of Defense, Number Indexed, M200-2-33].)

Bertrand died suddenly of an undetected heart condition on November 12 in Midland,

Texas. Marshall sent his condolences to Mrs. Bertrand on November 13, stating that he was "greatly shocked" by the news. (Marshall to Susan Bertrand, November 13, 1950, ibid.)

128

MEMORANDUM FOR THE RECORD October 11, 1950
Confidential Washington, DC

SUBJECT: Visit of Korean Foreign Minister to Secretary Marshall at 1400 on 11 October 1950[1]

The meeting was intended as a courtesy call, and matters of substance were not discussed. Mr. Limb opened the conversation by saying that he had long wished to meet General Marshall and was happy for this opportunity to pay his respects.

General Marshall welcomed Mr. Limb and his Korean colleagues and talked of his visit to Korea as a young officer in 1914.[2] There was some discussion of the change of geographic place names which had taken place.

Mr. Limb expressed the gratitude of his Government for the assistance of the U.S. in repelling the North Korean invasion.

Secretary Marshall expressed his admiration of the ROK soldiers, particularly those serving with U.S. forces. He mentioned his previous statement to this effect to the 200 Mayors.[3] Mr. Chang noted the widespread and favorable attention the statement had received in Korea.

General Marshall went on to discuss the method of integrating the individual ROK soldiers into the U.S. forces. He stated that, as Secretary of State, he had advocated, in the formation of the ROK Army, a method similar to that used in the Philippines and in Haiti, whereby there had been a gradual phasing out of U.S. troops and officers and a taking over by the country concerned until gradually control by the country of its own armed forces was complete. He described this in some detail and noted the importance of preserving standards of cohesion and discipline in the Army. Such an Army is a firm bulwark of stability to the government. He further noted that the experience of the campaign through which the Korean Army had just passed had now placed it beyond the training and taking-over stage.

Mr. Limb stated that they would require additional training help from the U.S. when hostilities were over. General Marshall, at some length, pointed out to him and his colleagues, as political leaders, the vital part they must play in the formation of the armed forces of the necessary character by selecting leaders on the basis of military merit, instead of friendship and political influence. He described the necessity, in a democracy, for complete loyalty on the part of the Army to President as Commander-in-Chief and to the Secretary of Defense, regardless of the incumbent of the office, and noted how ingrained this was in the U.S. forces. He cited examples from our past history and contrary examples from Latin American, Italian and Chinese history. In so doing, he also spoke of the influence of the West Point and Naval Academy graduates in promoting stability in the Philippine Constabulary. Mr. Chang asked whether U.S. law would permit Koreans to be trained at West Point. General Marshall continued the development of his main thesis. At the conclusion, Mr. Limb and Mr. Chang expressed their complete agreement with General Marshall's ideas, but hoped that, after the cessation of hostilities, U.S. military assistance, in the form of equipment and training, would be forthcoming in order to build up an army of the type described by General Marshall.

A. C. Murdaugh

NA/RG 330, CD Memorandum of Conversation

1. South Korean Foreign Minister Ben C. Limb was accompanied by Ambassador to the US John Myun Chang and Chang Taek-sang, the vice chairman of the ROK National Assembly. All of them had Western educations and spoke fluent English. The meeting took place from 2:00 p.m. to 2:29 p.m. Also present were Arthur B. Emmons of the State Department's Office of Northeast Asian Affairs; Escorting Officer Colonel R. L. Miller of the Foreign Liaison Branch of the Intelligence Division (G-2), Army General Staff; and Navy Captain Albert C. Murdaugh, assistant director of the Defense Department's Office of Foreign Military Affairs, who authored this memorandum. Colonel Miller also wrote a memorandum summarizing the meeting; it is located in the same file as this document.

The three Koreans were also scheduled to see President Truman at 11:45 a.m. and Secretary Acheson in the afternoon. For that 5:00 p.m. meeting, see *FRUS, 1950*, 7: 928–29.

2. During his second tour of duty in the Philippines in 1914, then First Lieutenant Marshall had visited Korea as well as Japan and Manchuria while on leave. See Forrest C. Pogue, *George C. Marshall*, vol. 1, *Education of a General, 1880–1939* (New York: Viking Press, 1963), 124–25; and *Papers of GCM*, 1: 85–92.

3. See pp. 179–82.

129

Memorandum of Conversation — October 13, 1950
Top Secret — Washington, DC

SUBJECT: Discussions on French Rearmament Program

(Note: This Conference was held at New State Department Building, Conference Room 5106, at 1100, Friday, 13 October. It was the initial meeting with the French Defense and Finance Ministers at which the French representatives presented the French Rearmament Program to representatives of the United States.)[1]

Mr. Moch presented the French plan for raising and rearming French forces. He stated that ten (10) divisions were to be raised by 1951, five (5) additional divisions by 1952, and five (5) more by 1953. Of these forces raised, ten will be at full battle strength and ten will be at 75% strength, but capable of being raised to full strength by D plus three days. All of these 20 divisions will be stationed in Germany or Metropolitan France.

At present, France has three (3) divisions in Germany at 75% strength and two (2) divisions in France at 50% strength, totalling about 90,000 men. The strength of these forces will be increased in 1951 to 185,000, in 1952 to 248,000 and in 1953 to 331,000. In addition to these forces, there will be other troops for logistical support, and for forces stationed in North Africa and in other overseas territories.

In 1950 the ground forces budget amounted to 111 billion francs. In 1951 it will require 287 billion francs for the ground forces alone. The 1950 armed forces budget for France is 282 billion francs, which will have to be increased to 610 billion francs to meet the 1951 program. To include the overseas defense requirements, 240 billion francs must be added, making a total defense budget of 850 billion francs for 1951. In figuring this budget of 610 billion francs, 1951 MDAP [Mutual Defense Assistance Program] deliveries have not been included as appreciable deliveries are not expected during calendar year 1951. The 1950 MDA Program, plus what France will produce under this program, should just about meet the 1951 requirement of 10 divisions. The fiscal year 1951 MDA Program, which is anticipated will be delivered during calendar year 1952, will be such that this force can be raised to 11 or 12 divisions. By 1953, deliveries under MDAP should be sufficient to permit the organization of 18 or 20 divisions.

It is necessary for the French to undertake an extensive production program because:

1. There are many items which they cannot get from the United States under MDAP;
2. It is necessary to use French industries to full capacity; and
3. Certain war materials can be produced cheaper in France than in the United States. The French are able to produce a new 12-ton tank, a light tank reconnaissance vehicle, a 50-ton tank, and a new Bazooka, all of which are now beyond the prototype stage.

It is intended to organize a new anti-tank division built around this new light tank which will have great mobility and fire power. It is very important to get these production programs under way at an early date, especially for the manufacture of the equipment for the new anti-tank division.

In order to organize and equip the forces which are proposed for 1951, it will be necessary to secure $770 million more than is now available to the French. If this financial problem is not solved, it will not be possible to raise the 10 divisions required in 1951. Of this deficit, only about 1/7 can be adequately covered by AMP [additional military production] projects.

Secretary Marshall in reply stated that the United States is giving top priority to the shipment of equipment to Indo-China; that the French program as presented appears to be very sound as regards to the forces to be raised in 1951.[2] There is no disagreement with the program. However, it is believed that possible economies may be effected without jeopardizing the plan. One area in which it appears that possible cuts may be made is in the Naval program. He made it clear that although the over-all program of 20 divisions had been presented, it was not to be confused with the over-all requirement which would be determined by the Military and Defense Committee later this month. He felt that before the French went too far into the financing of the entire 7 new anti-tank divisions, only one should be formed and tested before making a commitment to complete the others.

In regard to the request that Mr. Moch had previously made to Secretary Marshall for a light bomber group for Indo-China, he pointed out that the B-26 light bombers which were not readily available are needed for air operations in Korea and that it would be some time before others could be made available from the pipe line. He asked if the 40 F6Fs now en route to Indo-China would be a practicable substitute for the light bombers which were requested.[3]

Mr. Moch stated that the 40 F6Fs were to be used as replacements for the P-63's which were now worn out and wondered if B-25's could be made available in place of B-26's.

Secretary Marshall said that he would have the availability of B-25's investigated as a matter of priority.

General Lemnitzer then described the 1950 and 1951 regular and supplemental MDA Programs as they affected France and suggested that priority should be given to meeting equipment deficiencies of the combat forces which would be required for area defenses. He suggested that anti-submarine type aircraft instead of fighter type aircraft should be provided for the Naval forces, which would produce a substantial savings in the Naval program. He stated that the air program for air defense and tactical aircraft appear to be reasonable, but if any cuts were made it should be air defense aircraft rather than in tactical aircraft.

Mr. Moch presented the budget for Indo-China which required 154 billion francs for French forces, 46 billion francs for Viet Nam forces, and 7 billion francs for public works making a total of 208 billion francs. In addition, 31 billion francs are also required for other overseas territories. This represents an increase of 28 billion francs for Indo-China, which will provide 10 billion francs for pay increases, 11 billion francs for increases in native forces and 7 billion francs for increases for public works. This budget should provide for the organization of 18 additional Viet Nam battalions and equipment for 40,000 non-regulars. He pointed out that the equipment for the 18 new battalions and 40,000 non-regulars was in addition to equipment which had previously been requested. Secretary Marshall asked Mr. Moch if the United States had been meeting their requests for equipment in Indo-China. Mr. Moch replied that between March and September of this year they had prepared 16 lists according to priority. Of these lists the first three have been received, the second three are urgently required but have not been received, and that he is unable to provide any information on the ten remaining lists.

Secretary Marshall asked Mr. Moch if the United States had declined to provide anything for Indo-China. Mr. Moch replied that all requests had been approved except for two groups of 90mm/AA artillery which he agreed should not have been approved. Secretary Marshall then commented that the problem was to speed up deliveries. Mr. Moch agreed and said that it was urgent that lists D, E and F be delivered promptly.

Mr. Acheson commented that in view of the fact that the equipment for the 18 battalions and the 40,000 irregulars was not included in these initial requests there would have to be a revision of the entire Indo-China program as there was a financial limit as to what could be supplied.

Mr. Moch commented that the French High Command had informed him that as a matter of urgency six battalions, including one parachute battalion and 11,000 officers and NCO's, are being supplied to Indo-China immediately, that these 11,000 officers and NCO's are to supply cadres for native battalions and to improve the training of the native forces.

AFTERNOON SESSION

Mr. Acheson opened the afternoon session with a summation of the deliveries of equipment to Indo-China and stated that the French would have to provide additional lists in order that equipment may be programmed for the 18 battalions and the 40,000 irregulars.

Secretary Marshall stated that he would do what he could to see that the screening and delivery of the items were expedited. He further stated that in regard to the French request for light bombers for Indo-China he would give instructions that one squadron, plus 5 planes with spare parts and equipment, be taken from the pipe line and shipped to Indo-China as soon as possible. He believes that delivery would be made between 1–15 December and that the delivery of additional aircraft would be contingent upon the developments of the war in Korea. He pointed out that the French should very carefully screen the lists submitted by local commanders as it was essential that we all be realistic in our demands as the need for equipment was very great and it was necessary to confine demands to the bare essentials.

Mr. Moch expressed his appreciation for the offer of the light bomber squadron and reiterated that the equipment on the D, E, and F lists be supplied immediately.[4]

Mr. Petsche stated that every effort should be made to avoid waste and for that reason the French have requested a central procurement control and also a common budget. He stated that the immediate requirement was to finance the military program in order to get into production and in order to submit a military budget to the Assembly in January. He stated that the defense budget must be doubled and that it would amount to 15% of the national income of France. They have already decided to raise taxes by 200 billion francs and to decrease expenditures by 80 billion francs. He stated that home construction had been stopped and that even with loans of an inflationary nature there was still this deficiency of 270 billion francs. He pointed out that this deficiency must be met outside of France, otherwise French economy would be destroyed. He pointed out that France must be protected against inflation, which was the breeding ground of Communism, and would also upset the military program.

Mr. Snyder pointed out that our problems parallel those of France, that a threat of inflation also existed in this country, and that we had also tripled our expenditures since Korea. However, our people were willing to take chances and increase their taxes in order to provide for adequate defenses. He felt that each nation should do its utmost within its own means, and that our problem would be to supplement the French to the extent we are capable within our means.

Mr. Acheson asked if France could expend as much on military production as was budgeted for in the 1951 program. Mr. Moch replied that this represented only a small part of their production capacity and that they would be able to meet this increased production within existing capacity. However, with the provision of machine tools the rate of production could be increased. Mr. Moch pointed out that they proposed to manufacture the Vampire as a fighter type plane and also some 400 MD [Marcel Dassault] type, which was better than the Vampire; that they expected to produce land based anti-submarine aircraft by 1952; and that there are now four production lines in operation producing the tanks of which 135 are now on order. He stated that the French could start on production quicker than the United States but could not produce at as high a rate because of their need for modernizing their plants with new machine tools. Production has been started on 4,000 jeeps, 20,000 Bazookas, 254 Vampires, and 150 MD 400's.

In closing, Mr. Moch stated that the 1951 French Rearmament Program is a small part of the over-all program and provides for only 1/3 of the Army program, 1/2 of the Air program, and 1/3 of the Navy program. However, if they could get machine tools they could go beyond the 1951 program.

L. L. Lemnitzer
Major General, U.S. Army
Director, Office of Military Assistance

NA/RG 330, CD Memorandum of Conversation

1. These meetings took place from October 13 to 18, 1950. For background see pp. 167–68 and 184. See also the next document.

In attendance on October 13 were Marshall, Acheson, Treasury Secretary John W. Snyder, new ECA Administrator William C. Foster, and Ambassador to France David K. E. Bruce for the United States; Moch, Finance Minister Maurice Petsche, and Ambassador to the US Henri Lucien Bonnet for France; and numerous subordinates. These minutes were taken by Major General Lyman L. Lemnitzer (USMA, 1920), director of the Office of Military Assistance. A different set of minutes along with a complete list of those present is in *FRUS, 1950*, 3: 1396–1401.

Prior to this October 13 meeting, Marshall and Acheson had agreed that Marshall would "raise informally the German question" with Moch during an October 12 luncheon "and convince him of the firmness of the United States in its conviction that Germany must contribute to the defense of Western Europe." (Lemnitzer and Beebe for Lovett, memorandum, October 12, 1950, NA/RG 330, CD Briefings.)

2. The Korean War led to an expansion of US aid to the French in Indochina in their war against the Communist-led Viet Minh. In September and October, the French suffered defeats near the Chinese border, claimed they were no longer able to meet their military commitments to NATO and Indochina, and requested more military equipment but not US divisions "for the moment." (Condit, *Test of War*, 209.)

3. On October 12, Moch had handed Marshall a translated message from French Prime Minister René Pleven requesting these aircraft as well as other assistance. On that same day, the JCS were directed "as matter of priority" to consider this request and to provide Marshall with their recommendations so that he could give Moch a "definite reply" before October 15. On October 13, the chiefs informed Marshall that the aircraft would "not materially alleviate the situation in Indo-China" while their diversion to that area could "weaken our potentialities in north Korea or in Europe." Consequently they believed that "from a strictly military point of view" these bombers should not be sent to the French and that if "for politico-military reasons" they were sent, they should be given a priority that would enable them to be shipped by mid-December. (Lemnitzer to Kreps and Kreps to JCS, memoranda, October 12, 1950; and Davis to Marshall, memorandum, October 13, 1950, NA/RG 330, CD 091.3 [MDAP, Indochina].)

4. On October 17, the State Department announced in a press release that the United States would provide increased military aid to France and Indochina, with the latter

assigned "a particularly high priority." (*FRUS, 1950*, 3: 1427–28.) On October 18, the US minister in Saigon warned Acheson that Tonkin and perhaps Laos as well were in "grave danger" and that delivery of the light bombers earlier than the December 1–15 date Marshall had mentioned to Moch on October 13 was "imperative." Consequently he suggested having US crews fly them directly from operational or reserve squadrons in Korea or Japan. On the following day, Deputy Undersecretary of State H. Freeman Matthews made a similar recommendation to Acheson, asserting that the military situation in Indochina was "so grave as to require the very highest priority treatment" and suggesting that the secretary meet with Marshall to urge expedited deliveries from Korea. (*FRUS, 1950*, 6: 899–901.)

Marshall received a copy of Matthews's memorandum and asked Lovett who would be "the best man to put on the follow up on this job." Lovett replied "Gen Lemnitzer at present." (Marshall and Lovett handwritten comments on Matthews to Acheson, memorandum, October 19, 1950, NA/RG 330, CD 091.3 [MDAP, Indochina].) On October 20, Acheson had a brief discussion with Marshall before a cabinet meeting, during which Marshall told him that he had already called for a review of the bombers in order to speed up their delivery and that he was also trying to expedite shipment of other war material the French had requested. (*FRUS, 1950*, 6: 900.) Lemnitzer informed Marshall on the same date that the air force was "taking emergency action," that the aircraft would be ferried across the Pacific beginning November 5, and that the last should arrive in Saigon about November 25. On October 21, he informed Marshall that November 5 was "the earliest possible" date for deliveries to begin but that the 40 F6F fighter bombers already on their way to Indochina aboard a French aircraft carrier and due to arrive in Saigon the following week "should go a long way toward alleviating the present serious situation." On October 27, he informed Marshall that, weather permitting, the first set of B-26s designated for delivery to Indochina would begin its journey on October 31 and the last one on November 26. (Lemnitzer to Marshall, memoranda, October 20, 21, and 27, 1951, NA/RG 330, CD 091.3 [MDAP, Indochina].)

For additional information on Marshall's role in the high priority given to the dispatch of these aircraft, see pp. 320–22.

130

MEMORANDUM OF CONVERSATION — October 16, 1950
Top Secret — Washington, DC

SUBJECT: Visit of French Minister of Defense
with the Secretary of Defense[1]

Summation: M. Moch's basic points were: Russia would not take aggressive action but would push her "peace offensive"; Germany would, as always, side with the strongest force; German units could not be relied upon to defend the West; the mechanics of French politics is a 10 to 1 ratio against the rearmament of Germany; a defense line west of the Rhine is unacceptable to France; there is a need for delay and further study on the German issue. General Marshall's basic points were: We cannot afford to delay an agreement on German participation in European defenses; from the U. S. political point of view, we must reach a decision at the forthcoming October 28 Defense Committee meeting; the Russian threat is dual, either the long-range war of attrition or the always possible sudden move of military aggressive action; present indications are of a build up of Russian strength in all sectors. France must propose a practical alternative solution of the U. S. proposal is not accepted. The U. S. does not expect a simple yes or no answer but must take practical steps to include Germany in a defense plan.

1. The conversation opened by M. Moch questioning General Marshall on the idea of a meeting of the personal representatives of the Defense Ministers on October 18.[2] After an explanation by the General as to its possibility and suggesting that it was to the advantage of France to participate, M. Moch said he had obtained the services of Bonnet and Major General Vernoux as representatives.[3] It was agreed that French representatives would not be required to comment on the German issue unless they so desired. The General emphasized that in his previous experience the Defense Ministers would not be able to conclude their important duties in a short period of time unless these preliminary conversations were undertaken.

2. M. Moch indicated his interest in extending his technical visit, presently scheduled for October 31–November 2, to include demonstrations of rocket developments. The General indicated that this could be arranged. M. Moch said he would not be certain of his schedule until October 28 but it was agreed that tentative plans for this would be made.

3. M. Moch invited a group of American technicians to visit France to inspect military weapons, particularly in the field of bazookas, 12 and 50 ton tanks, field artillery, etc. General Marshall expressed his interest in this and said he would communicate with him further. He said that French technical developments are sometimes in advance of American efforts, particularly in the automotive field. The strength of the U. S. lies in her ability to mass produce weapons after they have passed the proto-type stage.

4. The General undertook to acquaint M. Moch with his personal estimate of the world-wide military situation. It was understood that the information was for M. Moch's personal use and was not intended to be officially conveyed to the French Government.

The continuing pressure by the USSR was discussed and the example of Korea analyzed. The General was concerned that the number of troops concentrated in Korea prior to hostilities with our full realization could be repeated elsewhere. The threat of Russian large-scale airborne operations was increasing and made the situation extremely difficult. It is possible for the USSR to move effectively in two or three directions at the same time. He expressed the belief that if the Russians were to continue a war of attrition, a war of nerves, that it would be to our advantage and not Russia's. On the other hand, a sudden decision for military action would be to our disadvantage.

The General expressed, very confidentially, the present thinking of the JCS and himself on the use of U. S. divisions, now in Korea, for duty in Europe and the measures to be taken if that was to be done. M. Moch agreed that the question of providing shelter in Europe for additional troops was a serious one. It was agreed that these problems were pressing and an approach to a solution should be begun at once.

The General reviewed the position of the French and British Governments in the present international circumstances. It was emphasized that unity of the North

Atlantic Treaty nations was essential although sometimes difficult of achievement. M. Moch interrupted to say that he well understood the major difficulty was on the question of the French viewpoint on Germany. The General went on to point out that all desired the main defensive line to be as far East as possible. How was this to be done? One of the great dangers, he pointed out, was the over-population of Germany and Japan. The strain on U. S. resources in this regard is large and must come to an end at the earliest possible time. M. Moch believed this was one of the prices of victory, but the General pointed out that the lack of resources in these countries and the present over-population may well drive them to a breaking point and force them to action. If Germany were to turn to the East this would indeed be bad for France. The U. S. cannot go on sending funds to Germany indefinitely. The wheels of progress have begun turning and the Schuman Plan should be of great assistance, nevertheless the situation was explosive.[4]

The General turned to plans for defense of Europe. How would it be possible to advance their defense line eastward without Germany? M. Moch asked the General's opinion of the total division strength required. He was informed that something on the order of 70 to 90 divisions throughout NATO might be required. M. Moch did not believe this feasible to maintain in peacetime and suggested that 50 divisions might be enough. The General replied how else other than the maintenance of a large number of divisions could we be prepared for conflict? He expressed the belief that 50 divisions could not advance on the defense line eastward but would in fact be west of the Rhine or further westward. M. Moch remarked that France could not accept such a defensive scheme and would prefer an understanding with the Soviets as an alternative.

After further discussion of the German rearmament problem M. Moch indicated that the problem of the French government was, as Ambassador Bruce put it, to say neither "yes" nor "no" in order not to say "no". The General sympathized with the French difficulties but pointed out our own problems. He felt that he must face Congress beginning November 20. The German question was on everybody's mind and unless practical steps had been taken it would be difficult to secure additional funds for European aid. There was complete agreement by both that the whole situation was extremely difficult. It was apparent that M. Moch dreaded the situation confronting him.

M. Moch analyzed the fighting capabilities of the Germans and their tendency to side with the force displaying the greatest military strength. He was very frank in his skepticism and went on to suggest that Germany would not remain loyal to the West if the military situation were in favor of the Russians.

M. Moch is to see Plevan [*Pleven*] immediately on his return to Paris. He believes, at the moment, that if the French are to say "yes" or "no" on the German question on October 28, the answer will be "no". He agrees that this is tragic but he believes that there is a 10 to 1 majority within the National Assembly in the decision against German rearmament.

General Marshall reiterated his insistence that the French must be consistent and logical. If the French Government were unable to agree with the majority of

NAT[O] nations on Germany, then some practical alternative must be reached. General Marshall was doubtful as to what future alternative courses might be. M. Moch expressed the belief that should hostilities be undertaken by the East German Police Force that West Germany would not fight their brothers. The General was in disagreement and pointed out that history would show differently—that the Germans were not much different than the Koreans.

In the final summing up of the conversation, M. Moch denied that his personal feelings toward the Germans influenced his governmental thinking.[5] The General did not believe that he or other Frenchmen could be entirely impartial in the matter of Germany. M. Moch expressed the belief that, disregarding the Communist problem, any political platform which was opposed to monetary aid to Catholic schools and the rearmament of Germany would receive 70% of the French votes. M. Moch further expressed his fear that any special general election prior to the scheduled 1951 general election would in itself constitute a victory for the Communist Party.

He asked if it would be possible to suspend the issue beyond October 28. The General made it quite clear that he did not believe this practical since he must face Congress and U. S. public opinion in November. M. Moch expressed the belief that it was always possible for the French government and French people to change their attitudes. M. Moch concluded that he thought it best if we should continue to study the German situation. Perhaps we could appoint the Supreme Commander at once and charge him with this study. The General said he favored the earliest appointment of the Supreme Commander but did not favor such a course of action.

R. E. Beebe
Colonel, USAF
Office of Foreign Military Affairs

NA/RG 330, CD Memorandum of Conversation

1. This meeting took place at 12:15 p.m. That morning Moch, Petsche, Bonnet, and other French officials had met with Acheson, Snyder, Bruce, and others to discuss French rearmament and requests for financial assistance. (Lemnitzer, memorandum, "Discussions on French Rearmament Program," October 16, 1950, NA/RG 330, CD Memorandum of Conversation.) Marshall did not attend this morning meeting.

2. A State Department briefing paper prepared for Marshall prior to his afternoon meeting with Moch asserted that the French defense minister was "apparently" calling on him to discuss French participation in this October 18 meeting and obtain assurance that Washington would not press at that time for a decision on German rearmament. "Such an assurance can be of course readily given," but Marshall was advised to "take advantage" of his meeting with Moch to have a "frank discussion" about this matter. "Moch is apparently becoming more and more bitter on this issue and determined to fight it even to the extent of resignation from the Cabinet. In working himself into this state of mind he has apparently become complacent about the Russian threat and espouses the real danger as being Germany." The briefing paper recommended that Marshall inform Moch of the safeguards that could presently be obtained regarding German rearmament, as well as present his views on "the present military situation in Europe, the danger of the Russian threat, and the possible limited time in which to prepare. The purpose of this approach would be to reassure Moch on the question of German units and at the same time, by laying the rather terrifying

military situation on the line *in a most forceful manner*, to convince him that the situation is such that he cannot, as Defense Minister, oppose available assistance in the defense of his country." ("Briefing Paper for Secretary Marshall," NA/RG 330, CD Briefings.) For the October 18 meeting, see *FRUS, 1950*, 3: 388–89.

3. General Raoul Vernoux was chief of staff of the Combined Staff, French Ministry of Defense.

4. Named for French Foreign Minister Robert Schuman and announced in May 1950, the Schuman Plan called for a single authority to control the production of coal and steel in France and Germany, with membership open to other European countries as well. It led to the formation of the European Coal and Steel Community in April 1951.

5. One journalist wrote at this time that Moch was "something of a fanatic about Germany because his son was tortured to death in a Nazi concentration camp." ("Moch Arrives for Talks on Rearmament," *Washington Post*, October 12, 1950, p. 1.)

131

To George M. Humphrey — October 16, 1950, Washington, DC

Dear Humphrey: I am enclosing a statement prepared for my information regarding the present status of the Munitions Board, which lacks a Chairman. I would appreciate very much your glancing through this in order to ascertain the contrast between the position of the old Munitions Board and the dominant authority of the present set-up. I believe I am not exaggerating when I say that the Munitions Board today can exercise a determining influence on American industry for good or bad during the next few years. It is the controlling agency in the relationship of government to industry and in the governing hand as it were over the materiel demands of the three Services.[1]

As I requested above, please read this over and then I would appreciate your telephoning me and giving me an opportunity to have a brief discussion regarding your possible relationship to this agency. Faithfully yours,

P.S. I am not unaware of Labrador.[2]

GCMRL/G. C. Marshall Papers (Secretary of Defense, Number Indexed, M200-3-42)

1. Humphrey had been the president of the M. A. Hanna Company, a leader in the iron and coal industries, based in Cleveland, Ohio, since 1929. In 1946, he had been chairman of the Department of Commerce's Business Advisory Council. ("George M. Humphrey Dies," *Washington Post*, January 21, 1970, p. C6.)

The statement Marshall enclosed summarized the organization, functions, and responsibilities of the Munitions Board, which had been established in the National Security Act of 1947 to coordinate Defense Department activities regarding industry, plan the industrial aspects of military mobilization, standardize specifications and technical equipment between the services, and streamline interservice agencies to promote industrial efficiency. ("National Security Act of 1947," Section 213, Public Law 253, 80th Cong., 1st sess., July 26, 1947.) It was the statutory successor to the Joint Army-Navy Munitions Board, which had been established in 1922 to coordinate procurement of munitions and supplies for the two services.

2. Humphrey had been elected president of the Iron Ore Company of Canada in January 1950 to "finance test drilling for iron ore in the Quebec-Labrador fields." ("Hear Iron Ore Concern," *New York Times*, January 5, 1950, p. 50.) For more on the Labrador iron ore fields, see pp. 398–400.

Humphrey responded on October 19 that he was honored by Marshall's offer but declined as he thought that "neither my training nor experience qualify me for its direction. . . . What this job requires is a high class director of purchases who has had experience in the detail of coordinating requirements and supplies for one of our larger manufacturing organizations." (Humphrey to Marshall, October 19, 1950, GCMRL/G. C. Marshall Papers [Secretary of Defense, Selected].) The position would eventually be filled by John D. Small (USNA, 1915), a New York businessman who had previously headed the Civilian Production Administration. (Condit, *Test of War*, 501–2.)

132

TO MAJOR GENERAL BRYANT E. MOORE

October 18, 1950
Washington, DC

Dear Moore: I have decided that I will take in the Army-Navy Game this year and I am writing you with regard to accommodations.[1]

In the first place, in view of my Army affiliations and connections, I was wondering if because of my present position it might be politic for me to sit on the Navy side. However, that seems rather odd,—at least it does to Mrs. Marshall, and I am turning to you for advice.

A solution, of course, is to cross over. I wish to avoid this because it is a procedure usually followed by the President, and another consideration is that President Truman is younger than I am,—and when I get wrapped up in two blankets I don't want to cross over, unless by some miracle you provide a sunshiny day.

However, please write me confidentially what you think.[2] Faithfully yours,

GCMRL/G. C. Marshall Papers (Secretary of Defense, Number Indexed, M214-2-23)

1. The annual Army-Navy football game was scheduled to be played on Saturday, December 2, in Municipal Stadium, in Philadelphia, Pennsylvania.

2. In his October 19 response, Moore informed Marshall that "The President sits in the same box each year. He does not cross over between the halves of the game. West Point and Annapolis alternate sides each year, the Academy sitting on the President's side acting as the host for the game and making all the arrangements. The Secretary of Defense sits on the side opposite the President. This will automatically put you on the Army side this year, a fact which I think will give Mrs. Marshall much pleasure, and I know will make us happy. The Secretary of Defense remains in his seat during the entire game, as does the President." Moore also informed Marshall that he would soon receive a formal invitation and twelve tickets. (Moore to Marshall, October 19, 1950, GCMRL/G. C. Marshall Papers [Secretary of Defense, Number Indexed, M214-2-23].) See pp. 225–26 and 279–80.

133

MEETINGS WITH THE BRITISH REPRESENTATIVE TO THE NATO STANDING GROUP, THE FRENCH FINANCE MINISTER, AND THE ISRAELI FOREIGN MINISTER

October 19, 1950 Washington, DC

ON OCTOBER 19, Marshall had separate meetings with three prominent officials from other nations: Marshal of the Royal Air Force Lord Arthur Tedder, deputy supreme commander of the Allied Expeditionary Force during World War II who was now serving as chairman of the British Joint Services Mission in Washington and British representative to the NATO Standing Group; French Finance Minister Maurice Petsche; and Israeli Foreign Minister Moshe Sharrett, formerly political adviser to the Jewish Agency for Palestine as Moshe Shertok.

The twenty-minute meeting with Tedder began at 11:45 a.m. with "an exchange of pleasantries and reminiscences on various military leaders" and then focused on the German rearmament issue. Tedder believed the French military was "in complete agreement" that German units had to be formed within NATO and that "This clearly demonstrated that the issue with the French is essentially a political one." Marshall believed that it "would have been wiser to approach the French on a more progressive basis and that it should have been done some time ago. As it was they were faced with a difficult question without preliminary considerations." As he previously had done with Moch (see pp. 199–203), Marshall also mentioned the possibility of attaching German battalions to American units, adding British units as well this time. (Memorandum of conversation, "Participation of Germany in European Defense Force," October 19, 1950, NA/RG 330, CD Memorandum of Conversation.)

The equally brief meeting with Petsche took place at the latter's request at 12:25 p.m. The chief concern of the French finance minister was that military rearmament could lead to "runaway inflation which could ultimately result in disaster for NATO nations" and "must be avoided at all costs." Addressing Marshall "as the author of the Marshall Plan" as well as secretary of defense, Petsche urged him to "exercise his great influence" to help solve "this vital problem." The Western nations "could win the peace and World War III if it is thrust upon us," but doing so would "require firm decisions and careful operation in the financial field if we are not to fall into financial traps that will defeat all of the objective we are seeking in the military field." Marshall responded that the United States was "keenly aware of the disastrous results which would result from inflation," that it "had a particularly difficult problem in this regard," and that he "would do everything possible to obtain a sound and workable solution." (Memorandum of conversation, "Conversation between Secretary of Defense and French Minister of Finance," October 19, 1950, ibid.)

The lengthier meeting with Sharrett took place from 2:30 to 3:30 p.m. Also in attendance were Israeli Ambassador Abba Eban and two US military officers. It consisted primarily of Sharret's disquisition on Israel's present situation, immigration policy, and ensuing military capacity. Marshall responded that he understood Sharrett had raised two questions, one regarding US willingness to provide military equipment and the other assistance in military training. Sharrett replied with "a third question of great importance. . . . what the United States plans were for the Middle East in the event of a war with Russia. Did the United States intend to defend the Middle East or to abandon it and re-enter at a later date? This was a matter of utmost importance to his country." The minutes contain no reply from Marshall to this question—or the previous ones for that matter. Sharrett then concluded that he would take these questions up "through the proper governmental channels between his Embassy and the State Department" and that he hoped Marshall, "being fully informed, would be able to give sympathetic consideration." Marshall replied by thanking Sharrett "for his very interesting and able presentation, which he found most enlightening and informative, and stated that he would give these questions his attention." (Memorandum for the record, "Meeting between the Secretary of Defense and Mr. Sharrett, Foreign Minister of Israel," October 24, 1950, ibid.) ★

134

MEMORANDUM FOR THE PRESIDENT

October 20, 1950
Washington, DC

My dear Mr. President: The attached is self explanatory.[1] If you approve how do you think we should proceed as to Eisenhower personally? Would you put the question to him or should I in your name?[2] G. C. Marshall

GCMRL/G. C. Marshall Collection (Harry S. Truman); H

1. Marshall attached to this note a memorandum that Bradley had sent him the same day officially confirming the October 13 oral recommendation of the JCS that General Eisenhower be designated as Supreme Allied Commander, Europe (SACEUR) of NATO forces.

2. A handwritten notation at the end of a typed Defense Department copy of this document states that "This matter was discussed by telephone with Gen Marshall by the President after paper's receipt. Conclusions not known." (NA/RG 330, CD 091.7 [Europe, 1950].) The editors have found no evidence that Marshall contacted Eisenhower on this matter, though Truman definitely did. The president later stated that on October 19 he had asked in a handwritten postscript to a letter that Eisenhower visit him the "First time you are in town." Eisenhower noted in his October 28 diary entry that Truman had called him on Monday, October 23, and said "that he would like me to come to Washington for a conversation, to talk in general terms about an assignment for me involving command of the Atlantic Pact Defensive Forces." That meeting took place on October 28. (Harry S. Truman, *Memoirs*, vol. 2, *Years of Trial and Hope* [Garden City, NY: Doubleday & Company, Inc., 1956], 257; *Papers of DDE*, 11: 1388–89.)

135

TO MRS. ANNA M. ROSENBERG

October 20, 1950
Washington, DC

Dear Anna: Will you consider an appointment as Assistant Secretary of Defense, at least until next June 30*th*?[1]

I enclose a brief of the present responsibilities of the office, in addition to which would be the coordination of man-power matters between the Munitions Board and the office of Personnel affairs here with me. Also the principal contact with the White House regarding political considerations, which Lovett is carrying at the present time. I can imagine something of the sacrifice this would impose on you. I won't attempt to debate the matter with you in the hope of over pursuading you. I have put the matter briefly but I hope clearly. Lovett and I hope so much you can see your way clear to do this.

I am writing this in long hand so that no one in my office will know of the proposal. I have not discussed it with the President. Faithfully yours,

G C Marshall

Harvard University, Radcliffe Institute, Schlesinger Library/Anna Rosenberg Hoffman Papers (Correspondence, Department of Defense, Assistant Secretary of Defense); H

1. On September 18, Rosenberg had written to congratulate Marshall on his appointment as secretary of defense and had added, "It is presumptuous, I think, to say if I can be of any help you have only to call on me, but I'm sure you know the spirit in which I mean it." Marshall had thanked her and then wrote at the bottom of the typed letter, "Please come in and see me when you are next in Washington." (Rosenberg to Marshall, September 18, 1950, and Marshall to Rosenberg, September 25, 1950, GCMRL/G. C. Marshall Papers [Secretary of Defense, Number Indexed, M205-1-12].) They saw each other at an October 6 lunch meeting of the Committee on Mobilization Policy, after which she informed Marshall that she would next be in Washington on October 17 and 18 for a meeting of the committee. (Rosenberg to Marshall, October 10, 1950, ibid., [M203-1-21].) They met on the morning of October 19, shortly after Marshall saw Paul Griffith.

In an unrecorded oral history interview for Marshall's biographer Forrest C. Pogue, Rosenberg said that while she was waiting in Marshall's outer office on October 19, "A man came out and I went in. The General said did you see that man. He is the tenth who has turned me down on a job I want to fill. He said he promised his wife he would go travelling. I told him there is a Mrs. Marshall and I promised her three times I would come home. And I haven't been able to do it. I said how can anyone refuse you General. There was a twinkle in his eye, but he didn't say anything." Two days later, she received this handwritten letter. Later she asked Marshall why he had not asked her during their October 19 meeting. "He said I was trying to get my courage up. He said I felt you couldn't turn me down after what you said." (GCMRL/Oral History Collection, Notes 71N, copy 2, interview with Rosenberg, December 30, 1957.) Pogue relates the story and ensuing events, adding that Marshall asked Baruch to help convince her to accept while warning her "that the people trying to get at him would attack her" and that she accepted but suggested that no announcement be made until after election day. (Pogue, *Statesman*, 430–31 and 578n19.) For Marshall's recommendation of Rosenberg to Truman and official announcement on November 10, see pp. 232–33.

136

To General of the Army Dwight D. Eisenhower October 23, 1950

[Washington, DC]

Dear Eisenhower: I have delayed answering your letter of October 18 until I had an opportunity to talk over the matter in some detail with Lovett and Bradley.[1] It is still too early for me to give you a very definite reply, as we are in the middle of working out an approach to the problem in connection with the preparation of the budget and the presentation before the Manpower Commission.[2]

In brief, my reaction and that of Lovett is that we can obtain the same result from an amendment to the Selective Service Act that we would obtain from the adoption of some form of universal military service. We both feel that in result the two procedures would be almost identical, but the former would avoid a tremendous political problem. We have a Selective Service Act which has been long debated and well understood.[3] It would be far easier to amend that to whatever extent is necessary than to come in with a new proposition which bears a title which is bound to produce a severe reaction from the American public.

Furthermore, we feel that the former procedure would lend itself better to the adoption of some system for building up trained reserves. We are therefore of the opinion—and we are still working on the practicability of the proposition, that there should be an immediate adoption of a law authorizing some form of Universal Military Training in such a fashion that it could be gradually initiated as the urgent need for the Selective Service action decreased. Whether that would be within six months, a year or two years, I am not prepared now to hazard an estimate, but I am completely convinced that unless we get started on this thing, get it into the law, and get the thinking headed towards it, we will inevitably be back in the same predicament we were six months ago.

The fact that the group in New York stood for such a drastic procedure, having in mind the distinguished position of most of the group, should be a great help to us in obtaining what we feel is necessary. But I am convinced, judging from my own experience, which has been rather terrific along these lines of changing public opinion, that unless we get into some system which does not involve so many men in uniform for prolonged service, we will find ourselves flat on our faces again as appropriations vanish. I have been through this too often—1921–1924, especially the summer of 1941, and finally the late summer and early fall of 1945—to feel that the American public has learned its lesson.[4] Taxes, the political importance of the budget, the reaction of restless young Americans and the tremendous influence of the family, would combine to wreck us again, however keenly we feel at the moment the necessity for taking drastic action.

In all this, I am not proposing cuts in the trained manpower requirements of the immediate future. I am thinking a great deal about the National Guard and its ineffectiveness for prompt service—the fact that we have 27 divisions and 22 separate regiments that might, backed by some form of Universal Military Training providing men for the ranks, be really a great force in the world and yet not on the daily payroll.

All this is confidential to you because I have not yet come forward with a complete statement of my views here in the Defense Department. Bradley and Collins know my general feelings only. Faithfully yours,

GCMRL/G. C. Marshall Papers (Secretary of Defense, Selected)

1. Eisenhower had written to inform Marshall of a statement he had made in support of universal military service at a September 28 meeting of prominent Americans at the Waldorf-Astoria Hotel in New York to discuss foreign affairs and defense policies. (The full letter is in *Papers of DDE*, 11: 1384–86.) Eisenhower advocated universal service rather than the universal military training that Marshall supported. (See ibid., 912–13, 1341–42, 1408–10.) For more on the differences between universal military service and universal military training, see pp. 177–78.

Upon Marshall's appointment as secretary of defense the previous month, Eisenhower had proposed postponing the meeting or cancelling his appearance. "In view of the close relationships that have existed between General Marshall and me for some years and of my great admiration of him as a military leader, organizer and thinker," Eisenhower wrote on

September 15, "I deem it my duty to confer with him in detail before appearing anywhere either publicly or semi-publicly to discuss these matters." Marshall suggested that Eisenhower and the program proceed as planned. (Ibid., 1318–19.)

In his October 18 letter, Eisenhower told Marshall that President James B. Conant of Harvard University supported universal service, as did the seven college presidents at the meeting. Indeed, none of the approximately fifty people present had expressed a dissenting opinion. "While these convictions are, I realize, at some variance with your own," Eisenhower noted, "I feel that an expression of them cannot damage whatever position you may personally choose to take in a program of so-called 'rearmament.' Nevertheless, I think you realize, without my saying it, that I certainly want to do nothing to embarrass you in your difficult task; consequently if you believe that repetition of my personal views would or could embarrass you, then I would like to hear from you as soon as possible, because I am called upon frequently to appear publicly." (Ibid., 1384–85.) For more on Marshall's appraisal of this plan, see p. 184.

2. The editors have not been able to determine to which commission he is referring. The reference may have been to the Defense Manpower Administration that had recently been established within the Department of Labor.

3. Marshall is referring to the Selective Service Act of 1948.

4. These episodes are covered in *Papers of GCM*, volumes 1, 2, and 5.

137

Transcript of Address before the Seventy-second General Conference of the National Guard Association — October 24, 1950, Washington, DC

General Walsh, and Gentlemen, I must explain to you first, not exactly by way of apology but because I haven't three or four different persons within myself, that up to the present moment I have not yet been able to go into the National Guard problem in the Defense Department thoroughly at all, hardly superficially. And what I am going to say will naturally apply largely to what I understood in the old days and the superficial knowledge I have as to the law regulating your organization at the present time, because I have never read it. I haven't had it discussed with me. I plunged into this job with several things of such momentous importance that I had to take them up because time was marching on and I had to meet the dates. Therefore, I am not prepared as I would like to be in talking to you here this afternoon.[1]

I am grateful to General Walsh for his generous comments in introducing me.[2] As he said, I have known him a long time. I have known these other gentlemen a long time. And there are a good many of you I have known a long time. And to those that I haven't known, those in particular who have come into the Guard largely during the last war and thereafter, I would like to say this: I began my Guard experience way back in 1907, with the Pennsylvania National Guard at Mt. Gretna; then in northern New York.[3] I remember arriving in a milk wagon up there; that was the only transportation I could get. And in Massachusetts, and in Florida, and with the National Guard of Utah and Wyoming, out in Pole Mountain Camp in Wyoming; some connection with the National Guard in California, though rather brief; and very intimately with the National Guards of the States of Washington, Idaho, and Oregon, and I believe Montana; and with the Michigan,

Illinois National Guard—Wisconsin National Guard.[4]

Now, I was with many of these at considerable length. So now I will make the very immodest assertion that up at least until last war I knew a little bit more about the National Guard than most of you did because I had served in more of your units.

Now, of course, I can't say that any longer. I have yet to make my experience in the light of the present situation and the present laws.

You have had various representatives of the Defense Department talking here—I believe Mr. Pace, the Secretary of the Army; General Collins, and I think they told me General Haislip is talking to you tomorrow. And I suppose you have had very concrete information upon what is worrying you a great deal at the present time in relation to service under the present conditions—its duration, probability, and matters of that character. There was a directive gotten out in the last few days which gives you some information. Beyond that at this time I will not go, because I would have to discuss it at great length with the Department of Defense that are concerned and with the personnel and manpower involvements.[5]

But, I would like to say this, though I am not prepared, really, to go into it in a very definite fashion. In contrast to what is your worry today, and it is a very real worry because it is an unusual situation, what is going to happen to you in relation to your families, in relation to your business, in this uncertain period before us?

You are a great agency of the defense organization of this Government. And we are confronted by a very serious situation. If things work out as we hope they will work out in the immediate future there will be no war; but there will be a great deal of service, unavoidably. The question is: how we do that?

We have never quite had this before. We had a period of the National Guard in 1940 and 1941, and if you recall, there was a great deal of talk about the National Guard in the Summer of 1941. And I had a very hard time to see that our Armies didn't disband at what eventually proved to be within a few months of our entry into a great war. The same applied of course to the Selective Service personnel.[6]

So this in a sense is an old story to me, but it is a very important consideration to you in your normal life. We all know if there was actual war, there is no question about what we would do and how we would do it. Now, we are confronted by a very serious situation, in which you are necessarily intimately involved. And how do we go about that, in relation to the complications that are set up? You are the largest strength connected in terms of organization with the National Defense of this Government. And naturally, this affects you very materially.

Now, I want to talk about something else. What I am interested in—and as I say I am not prepared to go into it in the most serious manner now as to details, probabilities of action at this time or some other time—but what I am interested in above all other things connected with you is how to make this National Guard a much stronger organization. We never can have a large standing Army.—I should say a *very* large standing Army. It isn't in keeping with our tradition and it isn't in keeping with our budget. But it is imperative, if we don't have a sufficient standing Army, particularly in days like this, that the quality of the National Guard be of such a nature that it will be far more readily available for service than I understand it can be under the present law today.

I remember telling General Reckord here when he was going out to a convention—I think it was in Chicago, wasn't it?

GENERAL RECKORD: Yes, sir.[7]

SECRETARY MARSHALL: We were talking at that time about Universal Military Training. I said, "Reckord, to me this is the great interest of the National Guard, above the Army, above any other organization in this Government, because that makes the National Guard, an effective, immediate weapon of power, and one that is within the reason of our financial budgets."

So I am deeply interested in the measures that might be taken to make your organization so strong that it is a great force for peace in the world.

Now, people use that expression a great deal, but I am using it very seriously now, that it is a great force for peace in the world. For example, I think you have twenty-seven divisions. Someone told me the other day, I think, you have twenty-two separate regiments. There are a great many other organizations. I will just mention those.

If that great force had availability, at the present time it would change the entire world picture. I don't mean by calling them all out; that is an impracticable, highly undesirable procedure. But we must in some way, I feel, bring the National Guard up to the point where it is much more readily available for service.

Now, how do you do it? I am not prepared to talk in detail now. You can surmise for yourself the general business end. But I think it is imperative that we find some way to make this great organization far, far more readily available for service on a time basis than it is at the present time.

Now, I am familiar with the training procedures of the National Guard, or I was familiar. I admit I am not familiar with them today, when almost all of the officer personnel, except possibly the very junior officers, have war experience. That is quite a different situation from what we had before this war, though we had a great many then in the Guard who had been in the First World War.

But I know from my intimate association, not only for a month or two, but right through the Winter, that to my mind it is almost impossible on the ordinary requirements of weekly training to produce the basic training that is essential for combat, short of a long period of service in getting ready again, which is a time-consuming and a time-losing procedure.

And I might say this, which has a little application to what I am talking about: During the war, I had what they called a sampling taken. I think Mr. Roper took most of the samplings. He wasn't getting election probabilities then. He was dealing with it in another way. I know it was quite a while before I could get it done without giving offense to commanding officers, because it isn't a very good thing to go around and inquire of the men how they liked this and how they liked that.[8]

When you set up the American mind to that, you pretty soon have not an army but a collection of individuals of all different points of view and being very free and handy with them. So it was tricky business. But they did it very well. And it was very carefully compiled and it was immensely informative.

In brief, we found this: In going into the things that were elements of the basic training, we found quite a number, quite a large number of items of that basic training that the men thought were either of no good purpose or there was far too much of them. Now, the interesting factor was that when we did the same thing abroad, we found almost invariably that the veteran of the combat said there was not enough of them and they were far too easy in the training period. In other words, he completely reversed himself the minute he came into the Combat Zone and the necessities of combat.

Well, I think you all who have had combat experience would recognize that. But it means that you are presented—I wouldn't say with an extraordinarily difficult situation—but an impossible situation to get under the ordinary training possibilities you have, that quality of basic training which you must have if you have a solid foundation that will stand up in the world today on the field of combat, without a long period of preparation after you come into the service. And that isn't so good, either, that long period of preparation, because there is so much pulling and hauling involved that that is a little bit unsatisfactory. And I had a long experience with that.

I might say that at the start, when the National Guard was called out in the War, it was seven weeks of basic training and we had to use the Guard, as you recall, to train the Selective Service people because we didn't have the weapons otherwise, nor did we have the instructors otherwise. I have received a great many formal recommendations, in some cases appeals to me, to reduce that seven weeks; there wasn't enough to do. Well, we ended up finding seventeen weeks hardly enough, when we did it under tremendously high pressure. So the misconception was very great and the necessities were even far more pressing than people realized.

So to summarize my thoughts at this time, it is that we must find some way to make our organization much stronger, *much* stronger, because it is bound to be the principal mass of defense for the ground fighting for this country and meaning for its influence on the world at large. How it is to be done, how long the procedure will be in doing it, and whether it will be done, of course, are matters to be debated. But I don't think we can go along any longer on the present basis and expect that we can at the same time be very moderate in what we require from the Regular Establishment.

Here we have a great opportunity to really have the sound, solid foundation of a great citizen army. We must make it just exactly that. And it can be done, I am quite certain. And much more simply done than under present struggles. I am not going into the air part of it so much. I found, however, in the period of 1934, we will say, up to 1938 or 1939, that the observation development in the National Guard worked on an easier basis and more efficient basis than in the Regular Establishment. That part alone was a much simpler business.

And when I came away from the National Guard contact and came to the other contact, I found it was very much the case. Of course, things have changed—the character of planes. And of course, each young fellow wants to have a jet fighter and project himself into the combat on that basis. And he will get his opportunity, no doubt.

I am sorry not to have a more concrete talk for you. I am sorry I do not know enough of the details of your problems today. I do realize your embarrassments today and I know full well you must realize ours.

Thank you very much.

(Standing applause)

Gentlemen, I am not running for office.[9]

GCMRL/G. C. Marshall Papers (Secretary of Defense, Speeches and Statements)

1. Major General Ellard A. Walsh was president of the National Guard Association of the United States. On September 29, he had invited Marshall to address the gathering on October 23, "either on or off the record as you desire" and "closed with no strangers admitted and no publicity of any kind in case you should so wish." Marshall had accepted tentatively on October 2, but the October 23 funeral for Henry Stimson, who had died on October 20 (see p. 337n1), forced him to push back the address to October 24. Although Marshall had originally requested executive session, his address, given at the Mayflower Hotel, was reported in the press. (Walsh to Marshall, September 29, 1950; Marshall to Walsh, October 2, 1950; and Foley to Marshall, memorandum, October 23, 1950, GCMRL/G. C. Marshall Papers [Secretary of Defense, Number Indexed, M214-1-31]; "Marshall Urges a Stronger Guard," *New York Times*, October 25, 1950, p. 12.)

2. Walsh had said "that one of the greatest state papers that was ever written was his [Marshall's] great state paper later embodied in War Department Circular 347." (Transcript of Marshall's Remarks to National Guard Association, October 24, 1950, GCMRL/G. C. Marshall Papers [Secretary of Defense, Speeches and Statements].)

War Department Circular 347, dated August 25, 1944, described, in part, Marshall's vision for the role of the military in the postwar world, including continued temporary US military presence in conquered Axis territory and a plan for UMT that would provide for a "professional peace establishment . . . to be reinforced in time of emergency by organized units drawn from a citizen army reserve." (Attachment to Transcript of Marshall's Remarks to National Guard Association, October 24, 1950, ibid.)

3. See *Papers of GCM*, 1: 38–45.

4. See ibid., 57–509 passim.

5. Other speakers at the conference included Secretary Frank Pace; chief of the army division of the National Guard Bureau, Major General Raymond H. Fleming; General J. Lawton Collins; Secretary of the Air Force Thomas K. Finletter; national director of the Selective Service System, General Lewis B. Hershey; and Senator Edward Martin (R-PA). ("Marshall Urges Stronger Guard," *New York Times*, October 25, 1950, p. 12.)

On October 23, Marshall had ordered the release of all reservists and members of the National Guard on involuntary active duty upon completion of their training and their replacement with draftees or volunteers. This order also required the armed forces to give reservists at least four months' notice before calling them for active duty and a thirty-day period between being called and reporting for duty. See also pp. 185–86. ("Reservists Freed from Forced Duty," *New York Times*, October 24, 1950, p. 20.)

6. Marshall is referring here to the 1941 debate over extending the term of service for draftees who had been inducted in the summer of 1940.

7. Major General Milton A. Reckord was serving as the adjutant general of the Maryland National Guard. During World War II, he had been the commander first of the Twenty-ninth Division and then of the Third Corps Area in Maryland, and after that theatre provost marshal in the European Theater of Operations until V-E Day.

8. Elmo B. Roper Jr. was a pollster who had worked with both the Office of Production

Management and the War Department during World War II to use opinion research to assist the war effort. (Marshall to Roper, May 3, 1941, GCMRL/G. C. Marshall Papers [Pentagon Office, General].) See also pp. 958–59.

9. "They are still your friends, General," Walsh added at this point. He then made clear that when Marshall had promulgated the policies in War Department Circular 347, "we thought it was right and the solution, and we think so still at this time, General Marshall. And I can assure the Secretary of Defense that we will never desist in our efforts to establish a system of Universal Military Training and Service." Marshall responded, "Thank you very much." (Transcript of Marshall's Remarks to National Guard Association, October 24, 1950, GCMRL/G. C. Marshall Papers [Secretary of Defense, Speeches and Statements].)

138

Statement for the United Nations Day Program[1] — October 24, 1950, Washington, DC

When the communists invaded the Republic of Korea, the United Nations acted immediately to uphold the rule of international law. It called upon its members to enforce its demand that the communists halt this unprovoked attack and withdraw from the country. When this notice was ignored, the United States moved instantly to enforce the demand, despite overwhelming odds.[2]

The highest moral principle dictated our action. We were moving to protect the freedom of a peaceful nation.

In this world so dwarfed by modern invention and so bound together by common interests, a blow at freedom anywhere is a blow at freedom everywhere.

I share the pride of all Americans in the courage and determination displayed by our armed forces in a desperately difficult situation. And I grieve with our people over the sacrifices that have been made in human life and suffering. But the unfriendly governments have been put on notice that force will be met with force and not by mere appeasement.

I am sure that the common people throughout the world are profoundly grateful to those who fought and still are fighting in Korea under the flag of the United Nations to make their world safe and secure against tyranny and evil.

GCMRL/G. C. Marshall Papers (Secretary of Defense, Speeches and Statements)

1. The United Nations General Assembly had declared October 24 United Nations Day, first celebrated in 1948, to commemorate the ratification of the treaty that established the organization in 1945. Marshall recorded this statement on October 20 for the October 24 broadcast by the Armed Forces Radio Service. For Marshall's recorded statement on the celebration of the first United Nations Day in 1948, see *Papers of GCM*, 6: 545–46.

2. Following the North Korean invasion of the South on June 25, 1950, the UN Security Council passed Resolution 82, which called for "the immediate cessation of hostilities" and called upon "the authorities in North Korea to withdraw forthwith their armed forces to the 38th parallel" as well as "all Member States to render every assistance to the United Nations in the execution of this resolution and to refrain from giving assistance to the North Korean authorities." (UN Security Council Resolution 82, June 25, 1950.)

The Security Council passed another resolution on June 27 in response to North Korea's failure to withdraw north of the 38th parallel, recommending "that the Members of the

United Nations furnish such assistance to the Republic of Korea as may be necessary to repel the armed attack and to restore international peace and security in the area." (UN Security Council Resolution 83, June 27, 1950.)

139

MEMORANDUM FOR ROBERT A. LOVETT

October 25, 1950
Washington, DC

The entire Defense Department congratulates you on the soundness of your great decision to remain in bed and conduct yourself—with restraint and ordinary wisdom.[1]

GCMRL/G. C. Marshall Papers (Secretary of Defense, Selected); H

1. Marshall had written to Lovett's wife, Adele, on October 17 to convey Mrs. Marshall's and his distress "to hear that you are sick-a-bed with bronchitis. We hope you will not rush matters and that you will not subject yourself to this damp Washington weather and humidity until you are free of this aggravating illness." Lovett may have become ill due to her bronchitis. (Marshall to Adele Lovett, October 17, 1950, GCMRL/G. C. Marshall Papers [Secretary of Defense, Number Indexed, M200-3-34].)

140

TO HARRY S. TRUMAN

October 25, 1950
Washington, DC

My dear Mr. President: Some time ago I was informed that Dr. Snazely [*Snavely*], Executive Director of the Association of American Colleges, had included the name of Dr. F. D. Patterson, President of Tuskegee University, for consideration as a member of the National Science Foundation, soon to be appointed. Dr. Patterson asked me if I would speak to you regarding his appointment.[1]

While I have carefully refrained from involving myself in such matters outside of my own department—War, State, or here—Dr. Patterson rendered such splendid service to me during the war and since with me as a director of the Red Cross that I feel I must make an exception in this case and warmly advocate his appointment. He is a very fine man and I found that, during the war, he had the courage to withstand very heavy pressures and endure resulting criticisms.[2]

With great respect, Faithfully yours,

GCMRL/G. C. Marshall Papers (Secretary of Defense, Selected)

1. President Truman had signed a bill into law on May 10, 1950, that established the National Science Foundation, run by a twenty-four-member board appointed by the president to grant funding for research, fellowships, and scholarships. Guy Snavely informed Patterson on May 15, 1950, that the Association of American Colleges, one of the organizations selected to nominate candidates for the board seats, would include him in its list of nominees. Patterson had written to Marshall on August 11 requesting his endorsement for this appointment. Marshall had responded from Huron Mountain Camp in Michigan on August 23 that he was "sending to the President my suggestion of you for this appointment. I hope it bears fruit." ("Truman Signs Bill to Set Up National Science Foundation," *New York Times*, May 11, 1950, p. 2; Snavely to Patterson, May 15, 1950; Patterson to Marshall,

August 11, 1950; and Marshall to Patterson, August 23, 1950, GCMRL/G. C. Marshall Papers [American Red Cross, General].)

2. "I certainly appreciated your letter about Dr. F. D. Patterson," Truman quickly responded. "I think very highly of him and I am more than happy that you have been able to try him out and know that he is a solid person." (Truman to Marshall, memorandum, October 27, 1950, GCMRL/G. C. Marshall Papers [Secretary of Defense, Selected].) For Marshall's previous work and relationship with Patterson, see pp. 34 and 37.

Truman announced his selections for the board on November 2, but Patterson was not chosen. ("Truman Names 24 to Science Board," *New York Times*, November 3, 1950, p. 37.)

141

To Admiral Lord Louis Mountbatten of Burma — October 25, 1950, Washington, DC

Dear Mountbatten: I received your letter of the 15th of October and a few minutes ago had a visit from Alan Moorehead, during which he posed your question as to the best method of securing a reasonably wide distribution of your report in this country. He will tell you what I had to say, which I hope may be helpful.[1]

Moorehead told me that he would send me a copy of the report and I look forward keenly to reading it.[2]

It has been a long time since I have heard from you, or about you directly, and my mind turns toward you at the moment because Monday we dedicate the Dill Memorial, and I am having Nancy Dill and her daughter, Major Dill and his wife, and the British Chiefs of Staff and also Mr. Shinwell, in here for lunch with me.[3] Incidentally, I find the lunch room for the Secretary of Defense is a very commodious and stylishly set up affair here in my old office, which, as you may remember, was next door to Mr. Stimson's office, in which I am now seated.

The Dill statue was received from Baltimore yesterday and was placed on the pedestal this morning; the bronze tablets for the gate posts showing the resolution of Congress and the citation by Mr. Roosevelt were flown in from Birmingham, England last week, so I think all will be ready for November 1, weather permitting, as you Britishers say.

With warm regards, Faithfully yours,

GCMRL/G. C. Marshall Papers (Secretary of Defense, Number Indexed, M200-4-12)

1. Mountbatten had been head of British Combined Operations and as such a de facto member of the British Chiefs of Staff Committee in 1942. In October 1943, he was appointed Supreme Allied Commander of the new South-East Asia Command, a position he held until June 1946. In December of that year, he was appointed viceroy of India and in August governor general of India, a position he held until June 1948, when British rule ended in India. On October 15, he had requested that Marshall meet briefly with Alan Moorehead, an award-winning British war correspondent and author then heading the public relations division of the British Ministry of Defense, to discuss how Mountbatten's "Report to the Combined Chief of Staff on South East Asia" could "best be presented to the American public." (Mountbatten to Marshall, October 15, 1950, GCMRL/G. C. Marshall Papers [Secretary of Defense, Number Indexed, M200-4-12].) Moorehead met with Marshall at 11:03 a.m. on October 25; no record of their conversation or ensuing correspondence is in the Marshall Papers.

2. Marshall received a copy of the report, which Mountbatten had inscribed: "Submitted to the great war time leader and Chief of Staff, U.S. Army, General of the Army George C Marshall with gratitude and deep appreciation for this unfailing support and friendship." Marshall thanked Mountbatten on February 12, 1951, for the report and the inscription "with so many superlatives for me." (Marshall to Mountbatten, February 12, 1951, ibid. For the inscribed copy, see Vice Admiral the Earl Mountbatten of Burma, *Report to the Combined Chiefs of Staff by the Supreme Allied Commander South-East Asia 1943–1945* [London: His Majesty's Stationery Office, 1951], inside front cover, GCMRL/Rare Books.)

3. Major John Dill, Field Marshal Dill's son, had married Heather Falkner in 1942. At 1:15 p.m. on November 1, 1950, Marshall ate lunch with members of the Dill Memorial Committee and other invited guests who attended the unveiling of the Dill statue at Arlington National Cemetery later that afternoon. See pp. 222–24.

142

STATEMENT FOR THE *HERALD-TRIBUNE* SPECIAL FORUM ISSUE[1] October 25, 1950
Washington, DC

In talking to Americans I feel free to go straight to the point in discussing the mobilization of our strength for world security.

Our armed forces know what is needed. Our citizens know that they want security. The time for endless debate and difference of opinion should shortly reach an end. We must settle on a firm foundation for our actions in the immediate future and then carry out our security program without hesitation or vacillation.

The mobilization of free men involves a long drawn out and intricately planned business and the longer the necessity continues, the more severe will be the test of the character of the men and nations involved. With each succeeding month, with each succeeding year, there will be heavier and more pressing demands on the moral and spiritual qualities and powers of our men and women.

The determined quest of security for the world, as we have come to learn, is a heavy burden to be carried along a steep and sometimes bloody road. Only strong nerves and firm resolution will suffice. But while we physically arm, we must keep clearly in mind that it is not the mere possession of weapons that will win the struggle. It will be more the spirit of the resolution to persist to the end that will achieve the ultimate victory, a stable peace.

Our thoughts are now dominated by what has been happening in Korea. But we must carry our thinking far ahead to other possibilities.

With regard to Korea I know of no other instance in the history of warfare in which our land, sea and air forces have pulled together so effectively. But what is far more important, I do not recall a similar situation in which free men of the world have combined in the field of action to right a great wrong and to put the unfriendly governments of the world on notice that force will now be met by force and there will be no appeasements in dealing with aggressors.

We must back our fighting men to the full. We must act now and in the future to prevent further sacrifices and terrible hazards due to failures here at home. The time for debates draws to a close. Americans must make their decision and stick to it for the years to come.

GCMRL/G. C. Marshall Papers (Secretary of Defense, Speeches and Statements)

1. Richard Weil Jr., president of R. H. Macy & Co., Inc., had written to Anna Rosenberg on October 10, asking her to pass along to Marshall a request for a statement for the 1950 *Herald-Tribune* Special Forum Issue, the theme of which was "Mobilizing America's Strength For World Security." Rosenberg forwarded this request to Marshall on October 13, reassuring him that "there is nothing commercial involved in this; it is merely a special issue which the Herald-Tribune likes to send out to its many thousands of participants. I think it would be wonderful if you could find it possible to do this." (Weil to Rosenberg, October 10, 1950, and Rosenberg to Marshall, October 13, 1950, GCMRL/G. C. Marshall Papers [Secretary of Defense, Number Indexed, M200-3-28].)

Major George informed Rosenberg on October 25 that Marshall's statement had been sent and that the proof, delivered on that date, was "in fine shape." The statement was published in the *New York Herald Tribune* on October 29, 1950. (George to Rosenberg, October 25, 1950, ibid.)

143

NATO Defense Ministers Meeting
October 28–31, 1950 Washington, DC

AT THEIR final "Big Three" defense ministers meeting on September 23, Marshall and his British and French counterparts had agreed to postpone the full NATO defense ministers meeting from October 16–20 to October 28–31 so as to give the French Parliament, scheduled to open on October 17, time to consider German rearmament within a NATO defense force. In the interim, Marshall continued to meet with French Defense Minister Moch and to correspond with British Defense Minister Shinwell. See pp. 167–68 and 194–203; Condit, *Test of War*, 322–23; and Marshall to Shinwell, October 20, 1950, NA/RG 330, SD 092 (NATO).

By the time the NATO defense ministers meeting opened on October 28, the French Parliament had overwhelmingly rejected direct German participation in NATO on a divisional level and had asserted its opposition to any German army or general staff. Instead French Premier René Pleven had proposed, in what became known as the "Pleven Plan," the immediate appointment of a NATO supreme commander and the creation of a new and experimental force, under a separate European defense minister, to be composed of French cadres and an equal number of French and German soldiers but no German units beyond the company or battalion level. (Condit, *Test of War*, 326.)

Acheson later stated that the Pleven Plan "caused us consternation and dismay" and that to him it was "hopeless, a view confirmed by General Marshall and concurred in by the President, and protracted discussion of it dangerous." (Acheson, *Present at the Creation*, 458–59.) Many of the NATO defense ministers who met with Marshall in the days preceding their conference voiced similarly negative views. Norwegian Defense Minister Jens Christian Hauge said there was "much in it that the Norwegians did not favor," while Portuguese Defense Minister Fernando dos Santos Costa told Marshall that his government found it "unacceptable, both militarily and politically." (Memorandum of conversation, "Visit of Defense Minister of Norway with Secretary of Defense," October 26, 1950; and memorandum of conversation, "Visit of Portuguese Minister to Secretary of Defense," October 27, 1950, NA/RG 330, CD Memorandum of Conversation.) During an October 27 meeting with Marshall, British Defense Minister Shinwell labeled the plan "military folly and political madness," as well as "disgusting and nauseous," and he warned that it could lead to British refusal to commit divisions to the European continent. Marshall responded that "we had been unable to penetrate the miasma of the French plan and discern any clear details; that we had hoped, on examination of the plan, to find some common ground between it and our proposal, but that the French proposal was so nebulous that no common ground could be said to exist." (Memorandum of conversation, "Visit of British Defense Minister Shinwell," October 27, 1950, ibid.) Immediately after this meeting with Shinwell, Marshall met with Moch, who reiterated France's opposition to any German army or general staff as well as German divisions, which he labeled "tantamount to a German army." Insistence on such divisions, he warned, would lead to the resignation of the French cabinet. (Memorandum of conversation, "Inclusion of Germany in an Integrated European Defense Force," October 27, 1950, ibid. The State Department summary of this meeting is in *FRUS, 1950*, 3: 410–12.)

In his welcoming remarks to the NATO defense ministers on October 28, Marshall as host and chair pressed for resolution of this conflict and the creation of a viable NATO defense force. "Economic recovery and increased military strength have given us greater courage to resist the communist challenge," he stated. "Victory in Korea is impressive evidence that the determined efforts of United Nations will have the backing of powerful military, naval and air forces to defend the peace of the world." Nevertheless, "the added confidence we now have gained must not be dissipated. We must not sink into an attitude of complacency or over-confidence, for the struggle may have only begun. . . . This is the time that we must complete a plan that will make it perfectly clear to all the peoples we represent, and also to any who plot against us, that we are organizing, training, and equipping forces that can successfully resist aggression in any form. We must adopt mutual defense plans that will exploit the full military potential that we possess among all of our twelve nations. . . . What has been done so far, good as it may be, is far from enough. The potential collective force of the United Nations was not enough to deter the aggressors in Korea. The actual collective forces of the North Atlantic States may not be enough to deter aggression in our North Atlantic area and definitely is not enough to resist attack without serious and critical initial losses. That gap in military strength we must now close as quickly as possible." (Remarks to NATO defense ministers, October 28, 1950, GCMRL/G. C. Marshall Papers [Secretary of Defense, Speeches and Statements].) See photo #5.

The gap could be closed, the United States maintained, only by German rearmament within a unified NATO military force and under a single commander.

With the French continuing to oppose German divisions, however, Marshall—despite his previous opposition to the Pentagon's "single package" approach and despite hints that Truman would agree to Eisenhower's immediate appointment as NATO military commander—proposed sending the issue of a unified NATO military force under a single commander back to the NATO Military Committee and the issue of German rearmament back to both the committee and the NATO Deputy Council, postponing action on both matters until the next meeting of the defense ministers in December. He suggested this on the grounds that it was not possible to give "final form" to the command and military structure of an integrated NATO military force until German participation in that force had been determined. (*FRUS, 1950*, 3: 415–26, quote on 423.) "The other Ministers received this," Marshall later informed the National Security Council, "as tantamount to the U.S. declining to send additional U.S. forces or staffs to Europe until agreement had been reached" on German rearmament. (Memorandum for the Executive Secretary of the National Security Council, "U.S. Position Regarding Strengthening the Defense of Europe and the Nature of Germany's Contribution Thereto," November 8, 1950, NA/RG 330, CD 091.7 [Europe].) Shinwell responded that Marshall's statement to the NATO defense ministers "only confirmed his worst fears" and that it "might mean UK reluctance [to] make additional contributions to Western Forces," but he and the other defense ministers had no choice save to agree to postponement. (*FRUS, 1950*, 3: 423–24.) "It may be inferred," the official history of the OSD noted, "that the postponement was intended to prod the alliance members, and particularly the French, to take positive action on German rearmament and a role in NATO." (Condit, *Test of War*, 327–28.)

Acheson, in a post-mortem on the conference, noted Marshall's "superb and impartial handling of Chairmanship," and blamed the failure to reach any agreement on the "quasi dictatorial" and "absolute intransigence of Moch." Continuation of this French attitude on German rearmament, he warned Paris, could preclude agreement on any militarily "sound plan" for the defense of Western Europe and endanger future US military assistance from Congress. (*FRUS, 1950*, 3: 426–32, quotes on 427, 428 and 431.)

For more on the December 1950 NATO defense ministers meeting, which Marshall did not attend, see pp. 303–4n1. ★

144

To E. Roland Harriman — November 1, 1950, Washington, DC

Dear Harriman: I have just read your letter of the 27th with your suggestion that I might possibly continue as the Head of the Red Cross on a "Chairman of the Board" basis with the necessary leave of absence during the continuation of my present occupation.[1] You are very thoughtful and very complimentary in making this suggestion. I am sorry that I do not feel free to go along with you.

From a number of points of view—not all personal—I think it is imperative that I resign from the Red Cross, to become effective the end of November. Most confidentially, when I found the pressure being exerted by many to fill my prospective vacancy, I became deeply concerned over what might happen. Therefore, I think it is important to get the matter conclusively settled. Now, also confidentially, and you probably know from what Kellstadt has told you, the President has favorably considered your name to be my successor.[2] I have been so occupied the past week, that I have had no time to think about Red Cross matters, though I think I did succeed last weekend in probably securing a three and a half million dollar contribution distributed over three years towards the maintenance of the pilot plants and the blood program. The Mellon Foundation people are very favorably impressed.[3] I have been uncertain as to when I should file my letter of resignation with the President, but I have now decided that I should do it within the next few days though it need not become public at that time.

Politically, I have had to consider the allegations to the effect that I had moved into the Defense Department only as a temporary political maneuver. So from that point of view, my actions should be positive in a way that cannot be misinterpreted.

I am intensely sorry to think of dropping out because my heart has been very much in the effort in the past year, but I am entirely convinced that it is the proper thing to do. Incidentally, I am not certain that I agree with you as to the amended set-up you suggest because I am inclined to feel that under the conditions the Red Cross must operate, the Head not only must take a very active part but must have a very *direct* responsibility or authority in connection with the routine operations which in any way affect public reactions. However, this is merely an opinion.[4]

With my love to Mrs. Harriman and my regrets to you in one sense and ~~respective~~ congratulations in another, Faithfully yours,

GCMRL/G. C. Marshall Papers (Secretary of Defense, Selected)

1. C. J. George recalled in September 1959 that upon Marshall's appointment as secretary of defense, President Truman "suggested that he go on terminal leave as head of the Red Cross with the thought, that, when he left the Pentagon, he could resume Red Cross duties. The General allowed this arrangement to continue for about two and a half months, but then decided that he could not do both and, more particularly, he felt that the Red Cross should have an active head." (George to Spencer, September 1, 1959, GCMRL/G. C. Marshall Papers [Retirement, General].) See also p. 650.

"I have Presidential agreement for going on in the Red Cross up to the November meeting in Chicago," Marshall had handwritten on an October 2 letter to Harriman. "Then I must drop out." (Marshall to Harriman, October 2, 1950, GCMRL/G. C. Marshall Papers [Secretary of Defense, Number Indexed, M200-3-49]. For the Chicago board of governors meeting, see pp. 247–51.) Harriman wrote to Marshall on October 16 and again on October 27 to ask that he reconsider. "If my information is correct and if I have correctly interpreted it," he noted in the second letter, "I understand that you will be asked to continue as head of Red Cross. With all the urgency at my command I beg that you give it favorable consideration, if not on the present basis then on a 'Chairman-of-the-Board' basis with the necessary leave of absence in that capacity. . . . My urgency stems from the realization of the imprint you have made in Red Cross life through your association with it the results of which it would be a tragedy to jeopardize at this serious juncture of national and world affairs." (Harriman to Marshall, October 16, 1950, ibid.; Harriman to Marshall, October 27, 1950, GCMRL/G. C. Marshall Papers [Secretary of Defense, Selected].)

2. On October 9, Marshall had met with Charles Kellstadt, vice president of Sears, Roebuck & Co. and first vice chairman of the American Red Cross, apparently to discuss proposing Harriman as his successor. He had then met with Harriman and written to Kellstadt that the two of them had concluded "the best procedure was for you to write a letter directly to the President, stating the case and suggesting a possible personal interview with the President in order for you to go into some of the important requirements of the Red Cross at this particular time." Marshall included a draft of this suggested letter but asked Kellstadt "not to interlard any reference to me because I think it would simply cloud the issue." Kellstadt forwarded a slightly revised version of this letter to President Truman on October 11, and he met with the president at 12:15 p.m. on October 26. (Marshall to Kellstadt, October 9, 1950, GCMRL/G. C. Marshall Papers [Secretary of Defense, Categorical, American National Red Cross, 1950–1951]; Kellstadt to Truman, October 11, 1950, and C. J. George to Kellstadt, October 19, 1950, GCMRL/G. C. Marshall Papers [Secretary of Defense, Number Indexed, M200-3-49].) Lovett met with Truman on October 11 and informed Marshall that the president "did not want to appoint another President, that apparently everybody in the country wanted the job but that he wanted you to continue to hold it, if necessary on the basis of a leave of absence." (Lovett to Marshall, memorandum, October 11, 1950, GCMRL/G. C. Marshall Papers [Secretary of Defense, Selected].)

3. Marshall had discussed this project in Leesburg with Donald D. Shepard of the A. W. Mellon Educational and Charitable Trust. A trust official notified Marshall on January 8, 1951, that the organization had declined to offer the funding upon learning that the project in question could not be centered in Pittsburgh, where the Mellon Trust was based. (Schmidt to Marshall, January 8, 1951, GCMRL/G. C. Marshall Papers [Secretary of Defense, Number Indexed, M200-8-16].)

4. In his October 27 letter to Marshall, Harriman had reported, "at the time of the reorganization of Red Cross serious thought was given to redefining the duties of the 'principal officer' (the Presidential appointee) and a newly created post of 'Chief Administrative Officer' to be elected by the Board of Governors. . . . I have been long convinced that for a variety of reasons, some of which I have discussed with you, in any event, such a set-up would be beneficial for all concerned regardless of personalities." (Harriman to Marshall, October 2, 1950, GCMRL/G. C. Marshall Papers [Secretary of Defense, Selected].) On November 2, Truman announced Harriman's selection to succeed Marshall as president of the American Red Cross, effective December 4. ("E. R. Harriman Gets Top Red Cross Post," *New York Times*, November 3, 1950, p. 24; "Red Cross Installs E. Roland Harriman," *New York Times*, December 5, 1950, p. 16.)

A month prior to this letter and Truman's November 2 announcement, Marshall had moved as head of both the Defense Department and the Red Cross to establish and clarify what he labeled "working relationships and liaison arrangement" between the two organizations. (Marshall to the service secretaries, memorandum, October 5, 1950, NA/RG 330, SD 080 [American National Red Cross].) In light of a March 25, 1950, Red Cross decision to discontinue medical and psychiatric social work service in military hospitals, Marshall on September 25 also authorized budget increases to allow for employment of qualified civil service personnel so that "this valuable service may be continued in military hospitals." (Marshall to the service secretaries, memorandum, September 25, 1950, ibid.)

145

Remarks at the Unveiling of the Sir John Dill Memorial

November 1, 1950
Arlington, Virginia

Here before us in Arlington Cemetery, among our hallowed dead lies buried a great Englishman, Field Marshal Sir John Dill. He was my friend, I am proud to say, and he was my intimate associate throughout most of the war years, commencing with the historic meeting at Argentia in Newfoundland, in August 1941.[1]

He gave his life in the service of his own country and of this country and for the hopes of all free peoples. On the morning following his death, President Roosevelt, in making a posthumous award of the Distinguished Service Medal, characterized his services in part, in these words, "Sir John Dill made an enduring contribution toward the victorious conclusion of the war and also to that harmony of purpose which is essential to our security in the years to come."[2] It was these last words referring to "that harmony of purpose which is essential to our security in the years to come" that moved a group of the American leaders in this war, Fleet Admiral Ernest J. King, General of the Army Henry H. Arnold, myself, and others to undertake the erection of a memorial to Sir John. But more especially we wished to commemorate down through the years and in a manner that would meet the eye of thousands of Americans, the vast importance of that harmony of purpose between Great Britain and the United States which is so essential to our security and the peace of the world in the years to come.

The Congress of the United States established a precedent in passing a joint resolution recognizing the burial of Sir John in this national cemetery and the outstanding services rendered by him to the United Nations.[3]

For those who did not have the good fortune to know Field Marshal Sir John Dill and for those who did not have the rare opportunity of working with him, I wish to say here today that in my opinion, and I know in the opinion of others intimately associated with the conduct of the war, his influence was greater than that of probably any other individual in welding together the military forces of our two countries. It was this complete accord that more than any other single factor gave us the victory in Europe.

I have never known a man whose high character shone so clearly in the honest directness of his every action. He was an inspiration to all of us in those trying days, and I think it is peculiarly fitting that this memorial to his memory should stand prominently at this crossroads where the avenues bearing the names of Roosevelt and Grant converge. It is especially fitting that the road to the Tomb of the Unknown Soldier should pass within a few feet of this statue, for it will enable the thousands upon thousands of Americans who annually visit this shrine to pause for a moment and read the resolution of the Congress and the citation of President Roosevelt in testimony of a great service rendered our two countries and its importance to us in the future.[4]

GCMRL/G. C. Marshall Papers (Secretary of Defense, Selected)

1. Then US Army chief of staff, Marshall first met Dill, his British counterpart as chief of the British Imperial General Staff, in August of 1941 when they both attended the meeting between Roosevelt and Churchill off the coast of Argentia, Newfoundland. See *Papers of GCM*, 2: 585–88. After US entry into the war, Dill headed the British Joint Staff Mission in Washington until his death on November 4, 1944. For his very close relationship with Marshall, see Alex Danchev, *Very Special Relationship: Field Marshal Sir John Dill and the Anglo-American Alliance, 1941–1944* (London: Brassey's Defence Publishers, 1986).

Marshall had been preceded in this ceremony by Angus Dun, the Episcopal bishop of Washington, DC, who delivered the invocation and who had also presided at Dill's memorial service on November 8, 1944. Dill Memorial Committee chair Robert Woods Bliss introduced each speaker.

2. Roosevelt awarded Dill the Distinguished Service Medal posthumously the evening of the British field marshal's death. On January 2, 1945, Marshall noted that Roosevelt had not yet presented the medal officially to his widow, Lady Nancy Dill; he did so on January 5. (*Papers of GCM*, 5: 5–6.)

3. House Joint Resolution 317, adopted on December 20, 1944, by the 78th Congress, recognized "the outstanding service rendered to the United Nations" by Dill due to his "wisdom and devotion to the vital cause of British-American military cooperation." (Public Law 516, 78th Cong., 2d sess., December 20, 1944.) Marshall was responsible for this joint resolution. He also arranged for Dill's burial in Arlington and the erection of the equestrian statue he was about to unveil, despite regulations against the burial of non-American soldiers and the creation of such memorials in that cemetery. (*Papers of GCM*, 4: 654; Forrest C. Pogue, *George C. Marshall*, vol. 3, *Organizer of Victory, 1943–1945* [New York: Viking, 1973], 482.) For Marshall's controversy with the Veterans of Foreign Wars regarding their objections to the statue, see pp. 87–89.

4. At Lady Dill's request, Marshall unveiled the statue following his remarks. (See pp. 45–46.) Remarks by British Ambassador to the United States Oliver Franks and President Truman followed the unveiling of the statue. Marshall had drafted those presidential remarks as well as a White House press release regarding this ceremony. (Marshall to Connelly, October 26, 1950, GCMRL/G. C. Marshall Papers [Secretary of Defense, Selected].)

Less than an hour prior to Truman's remarks, there had been an assassination attempt on him while he was resting in Blair House, an event that many of the attendees of the Dill statue unveiling did not know had transpired until a motorcyclist informed a photographer who passed the news along during Marshall's speech. ("President is Calm at Dill Dedication," *New York Times*, November 2, 1950, p. 1.)

146

To Tracy S. Voorhees — November 3, 1950
[Sea Island, Georgia[1]]

Dear Voorhees: Thanks for your letter of October 24th, jointly signed by your associates, on the project of organizing a citizens committee for strengthening public support of whatever stern measures may be necessary to achieve adequate Western European Defense.[2]

Your proposal is an undertaking of great importance.

I think it would be helpful if I could talk with you and as many of the group as can conveniently be present, in the near future, at your convenience. Such a meeting should assist us all in getting off on the right foot, particularly as to a possible public statement on the principles and purposes of the committee.[3]

I am sending identical letters to all the signers and ask you, if this proposal is agreeable to you, to make the arrangement with my office.[4] Faithfully yours,

NA/RG 330, SD 381 (European Defense)

1. Marshall was on Sea Island, Georgia, to attend a conference of the Business Advisory Council, called at the behest of Commerce Secretary Charles Sawyer, and gave an address on November 5. Marshall spoke in regard to a defense production program, then in preparation, of at least four years in duration. ("Marshall Reveals a Defense Program of 4 Years

or More," *New York Times*, November 6, 1950, p. 1.)

2. Voorhees had been undersecretary of the army from August 1949 to April 1950 and president of the Army Emergency Relief. He, along with ten others, had sent Marshall a letter stating that they were "gravely concerned by a realization of the problems which you and all of us face to achieve in time adequate Western European defense." The other signers of the letter included James Phinney Baxter III, president of Williams College; Vannevar Bush, wartime director of the Office of Scientific Research and Development and chairman of the National Military Establishment's Research and Development Board (RDB) from 1947 to 1948; Will Clayton, undersecretary of state for economic affairs under Marshall and a key drafter of the Marshall Plan; Harold Dodds, president of Princeton University; and Robert Patterson, undersecretary of war from 1940 to 1945 and secretary of war from 1945 to 1947. They believed "that a realistic defense must include not only a European army, but a hard core of American troops in Europe in strength adequate to raise the confidence and the morale of our allies to a level which will bring about their own full-scale effort to defend themselves." This plan would "probably require universal two-year service" in the military, and the signers assured Marshall they encouraged these steps "not because of a fatalistic acceptance of the inevitability of war, but because they together constitute the best and perhaps the only means of keeping the peace." They were contemplating "enlarging our group into a citizens committee wholly non-political in character, acting without partisan or other criticism of the past," to advance these proposals, which they listed in an enclosure. (Voorhees et al. to Marshall, October 24, 1950, NA/RG 330, SD 381 [European Defense].)

3. On November 20, Marshall met with the six individuals mentioned above in addition to six others. During and after that meeting Marshall made clear his appreciation of and respect for the group, whose members held subsequent meetings with Anna Rosenberg, by then assistant secretary of defense for manpower and personnel. (Marshall to Dodds, and Marshall to Wriston, December 14, 1950, ibid.)

4. Marshall Carter had noted in an October 31 memorandum for Marshall that "Mr. Lovett and Mr. Leva are enthusiastic about promoting the activities of such a citizens committee" but warned that the secretary was not "prepared to accept some of the statements contained in the group's proposed 'principles and purposes.'" He attached a reply that he had drafted, Lovett approved, and Marshall amended. (Carter to Marshall, memorandum, October 31, 1950, ibid.)

The *New York Times* reported on January 8, 1951, that thirty-three Americans had formed a Committee on the Present Danger that urged Americans to "help create the conditions necessary for the success of General Eisenhower's great mission" to lead the NATO forces in Europe. The eleven co-signers of the October 24, 1950, letter to Marshall and the additional individuals present for the November 20 meeting were all members of this new group. ("Civic Group Asks Aid to Eisenhower," *New York Times*, January 8, 1951, p. 1.)

147

To Margaret Emerson

November 6, 1950
Washington, DC

Dear Margaret: Katherine and I returned last evening from the Business Advisory Council Conference at Sea Island. We had a delightful weekend and a very easy trip to and from—about a two hour ten minute flight each way.[1]

When we returned to the apartment last night, we found the television set in place but not yet connected; I believe they do that at 10:00 this morning. It is most impressive and a most generous Christmas gift. You have provided me with a great deal of entertainment that I otherwise would have missed.

What I am dictating this note about is the Army-Navy Game. Katherine has decided she wishes to go and we have a private car for the trip. Would you care to join us? I might send your ticket to New York so that you could meet us at the box and then I thought possibly you might prefer to step over to the car with us, which will be on the siding, and come down to Washington with us, and spend the night here. We would get back about 7:30, I imagine. Katherine has asked Colonel Winn and Molly and I am about to ask Virginia Stettinius. All of them would stay in town that night and I thought I would get rooms for the whole party at the Lafayette which always puts out for me.[2]

Katherine is making this her wedding anniversary party, though it is a little late as far as dates are concerned. I do hope you will decide to join us, and I also hope that the weather will not be too disagreeable. It is almost certain to be cold and every now and then rain or snow adds to the pleasures. Affectionately,

GCMRL/G. C. Marshall Papers (Secretary of Defense, Number Indexed, M214-2-23)

1. See previous document, n1.

2. See p. 204. Marshall had also written to Molly Winn on October 23 to invite her and her husband, Jim, to attend the game, departing Washington around 9:00 a.m. and returning at 7:30 p.m. He had also invited Clifton Brown, Molly Winn's brother and Katherine Marshall's oldest child. Katherine Marshall hoped "very much that you can find some way to do this." (Marshall to Winn, October 23, 1950, GCMRL/G. C. Marshall Papers [Secretary of Defense, Number Indexed, M200-4-17].)

Emerson accepted the invitation on November 8, 1950, and Virginia Stettinius, the widow of former Secretary of State Edward R. Stettinius Jr., did the same within the following week. Marshall replied to Virginia Stettinius that Molly and James Winn might not go because "their boy Jimmy is being put in the hospital Saturday morning, here, for an operation, not serious, which will keep him in bed several weeks. She will stay at the apartment, so the gathering at the Lafayette we anticipated will not materialize." (Emerson to Marshall, November 8, 1950, and Marshall to Stettinius, November 14, 1950, ibid., [M214-2-23].) See pp. 239–40 and 279–80.

IN LATE October and early November, the nature of the Korean War changed dramatically as advancing Eighth Army and ROK forces began to face sharp and unexpected counterattacks by Communist Chinese forces that had entered Korea from Manchuria as well as Soviet aircraft based in that province. On November 5, General MacArthur informed the UN of the Chinese counterattacks and responded by ordering the initiation, on November 7, of an intensive bombing campaign north of UN front lines—including Sinuiju and the Korean side of the bridges over the Yalu River that marked the boundary between Korea and Manchuria. (*FRUS, 1950*, 7: 1046–47.) This campaign alarmed the administration. When Lovett informed Acheson and Rusk on the morning of November 6 of MacArthur's plans, they agreed that the bombing campaign should be postponed because it would violate a prior US commitment to consult the British before undertaking any action affecting Manchuria, because it might spill over into Chinese territory and trigger a Soviet intervention, and because Washington was about to request a UN resolution condemning the Chinese intervention and feared that the air campaign might alienate its UN allies. Lovett then telephoned Marshall, who agreed to the postponement—unless there was a threat to US troop security—until Truman, then in Kansas City, could be consulted. After that call, Lovett telephoned Air Force Secretary Finletter and instructed him to advise the Joint Chiefs of Staff of the situation and have them order postponement of the bombing until Truman could be contacted and his instructions received. Acheson then telephoned Truman, who concurred that the campaign should be postponed unless there was an "immediate and serious threat" to the security of US troops. (Memorandum of conversation between Acheson and Lovett, November 6, 1950, NA/RG 330, CD 092 [Korea]; *FRUS, 1950*, 7: 1055–58, quote on 1056. See also Schnabel and Watson, *History of JCS*, 3, pt. 1: 125–26; Condit, *Test of War*, 75–76; and Allan R. Millett, *The War for Korea*, vol. 2, *1950–1951: They Came from the North* [Lawrence: University Press of Kansas, 2010], 306–9.) The Joint Chiefs consequently ordered MacArthur to postpone any bombing within five miles of the border with Manchuria until he received further instructions. At presidential request they also asked him to explain why he had ordered the bombing campaign in the first place and to provide an estimate of the situation. (JCS to MacArthur, cable no. 95878, November 6, 1950, NA/RG 218, Geographic File, CCS 383.21 [Korea, Sec. 38].)

MacArthur strongly protested this JCS order, stating that Chinese soldiers and supplies were "pouring across all bridges over the Yalu from Manchuria. This movement not only jeopardizes but threatens the ultimate destruction of the forces under my command" and could be halted only by destroying the bridges. "Under the gravest protest that I can make," MacArthur was suspending the bombing as ordered, but it would have a "disastrous effect, both physical and psychological. . . . I trust that the matter be immediately brought to the attention of the President," he continued, "as I believe your instructions may well result in a calamity of major proportion for which I cannot accept the responsibility without his personal and direct understanding of the situation. Time is so essential that I request immediate reconsideration of your decision." (MacArthur to JCS, cable no. 8618, November 6, 1950, ibid.; reproduced from Truman's memoirs in *FRUS, 1950*, 7: 1058.)

Bradley called Truman in Missouri and read MacArthur's message to him, whereupon the president approved the bombing. That evening at approximately 9:00 p.m. Marshall met with the JCS, Acheson, and Lovett, after which MacArthur was given permission to bomb Sinuiju and other targets at the "Korean end of Yalu bridges" if neither Chinese nor Soviet air space was violated, but not "any dams or power plants on the Yalu River," which they incorrectly believed to be critical factors in Chinese decision making. (JCS to MacArthur, cable no. 95949, November 6, 1950, NA/RG 218, Geographic File, CCS 383.21 [Korea, Sec. 38]; Schnabel and Watson, *History of JCS*, 3, pt. 1: 125–30.) The JCS also repeated their previous request for an estimate of the situation, which MacArthur provided on November 7. He warned that Chinese ground units had "seized the initiative in the west sector and . . . materially slowed the offensive in the east sector." If reinforced they could threaten any further UN advance and even force a retreat. The bombing campaign was therefore "essential." In another telegram that day he noted the increasing number of hostile aircraft emanating from Manchuria, complained that "present restrictions imposed on my area of operation provide a complete sanctuary for hostile air immediately upon their crossing the Manchuria–North Korean border," and requested "instructions for dealing with this new and threatening development." (MacArthur to JCS, cables no. 8731 and 8674, November 7, 1950, NA/RG 218, Geographic File, CCS 383.21 [Korea, Sec. 38]. See also Schnabel and Watson, *History of JCS*, 3, pt. 1: 126–30.)

All of this led Marshall to send MacArthur a special message on November 7. ★

148

To General of the Army Douglas MacArthur — November 7, 1950
Radio No. DEF-95961. *Top Secret* — Washington, DC

Personal for MacArthur from Marshall

This is a very personal and informal message to you from me. I have just talked to the President in Independence Missouri. Though absent from Washington he has been kept almost hourly aware of the latest developments as reported by you. The discussions and decisions here are heavily weighted with the extremely delicate situation we have before the Security Council of the UN at the present time whose meeting tomorrow may have fateful consequences.[1]

We all realize your difficulty in fighting a desperate battle in a mountainous region under winter conditions and with a multi-national force in all degrees of military preparedness. I also understand, I think, the difficulty involved in conducting such a battle under necessarily limiting conditions and the necessity of keeping far distant headquarters closely informed of developments and decisions. However this appears to be unavoidable but I want you to know that I understand your problem. Everyone here Defense State and the President is intensely desirous of supporting you in the most effective manner within our means. At the same time we are faced with an extremely grave international problem which could so easily lead to a world disaster.

Incidentally for my personal information do you feel that the hydroelectric and reservoir situation is probably the dominant consideration in this apparently last minute move by the Chinese Communists incited by the Soviets to protect their interests in Vladivostok Dairen and Port Arthur?[2] No distribution.

GCMRL/G. C. Marshall Papers (Secretary of Defense, Selected)

1. See the next editorial note.

2. "Appreciate deeply your cordial and understanding msg and am in complete agreement with the basic concept of localizing, if possible, the Korean struggle," MacArthur responded. "I do not believe that the hydro-electric system is the dominant consideration animating the Communist intervention in Korea. . . . I believe that the motivating influences are far more fundamental." These focused on "changes in Chinese character and culture over the past fifty years," which MacArthur described in terms of the growth of

a militarized Chinese nationalism. "I have from the beginning believed that the Chinese Communist support of the North Koreans was the dominant one. Their interests are at present parallel to those of the Soviet, but I believe that the aggressiveness now displayed not only in Korea but in Indo-China and Tibet and pointing potentially toward the south reflects predominantly the same lust for the expansion of power which has animated every would-be conqueror since the beginning of time." (MacArthur to Marshall, cable no. 9061, November 8, 1950, GCMRL/G. C. Marshall Papers [Secretary of Defense, Selected].) "Thanks for your comprehensive analysis of the causes and effect of the present situation," Marshall responded. "I think you misunderstood my query re hydroelectric installations. I was referring only to the sudden developments of the past week. Don't bother to acknowledge this." (Marshall to MacArthur, November 8, 1950, ibid.)

IN ADDITION to sending his November 7 message to MacArthur, Marshall also met with Truman when the president returned to Washington that afternoon. On November 6, Deputy Undersecretary of State H. Freeman Matthews had forwarded to Major General James H. Burns (USMA, 1908), special assistant to the secretary of defense for foreign military affairs and assistance, the draft of a resolution regarding Chinese intervention that the State Department intended to submit to the UN Security Council, along with a request for comments "as well as the views of the Department of Defense of the military significance of the Chinese intervention." (*FRUS, 1950*, 7: 1058–59.) On November 9, Marshall informed Acheson that the Defense Department had no objection "from the military point of view" to the draft resolution. (Ibid., 1116–17.) On the following day, he forwarded to Acheson a lengthy November 9 JCS memorandum on the subject which he had requested on November 6 and which had been presented to the National Security Council. In his cover letter Marshall quoted the three JCS conclusions, with which he concurred:

"a. Every effort should be expended as a matter of urgency to settle the problem of Chinese Communist intervention in Korea by political means, preferably through the United Nations, to include reassurances to the Chinese Communists with respect to our intent, direct negotiations through our Allies and the Interim Committee with the Chinese Communist Government, and by any other available means.

"b. Pending further clarification as to the military objectives of the Chinese Communists and the extent of their intended commitments, the missions assigned to the Commander in Chief, United Nations Command should be kept under review, but should not be changed.

"c. The United States should develop its plans and make its preparations on the basis that the risk of global war is increased." (Marshall to Acheson, November 10, 1950, NA/RG 330, CD 092 [Korea]. The JCS memo is reproduced in *FRUS, 1950*, 7: 1117–21.) ★

149

To Brigadier General Charles G. Dawes[1] November 9, 1950
Washington, DC

Dear Dawes: I have intended writing you for the past week to tell you that I have finished reading your Journal of the McKinley Days, and I found it intensely interesting.[2] It revived a period when I was a very young fellow. As a matter of fact, my examination for a commission in the Army was delayed one month by Mr. McKinley's assassination, as General [John R.] Brooke, then in command of the Department of the East, had gone to Buffalo for the funeral and he was the President of my Board of Examiners.[3] The fact that I have visited your home in Marietta and had the great pleasure of meeting your Mother and other members of your family, in addition to intimate contact with Beeman and his wife and to a lesser degree Henry, and then later on with your brother Rufus and his wife, and too, my knowledge of the Lincoln days made it all intensely interesting to me.[4] I would have understood you much better in those early days of my acquaintance with you had I known of the build up of your association with people like Knowlton Ames and the part your uncle Mr. Mills played in the drama of your life.[5] Altogether, the Journal made intensely interesting reading to me and I was only sorry that you had not carried it on a few years later.

Affectionate regards to Mrs. Dawes and you.[6] Faithfully yours,

GCMRL/G. C. Marshall Papers (Secretary of Defense, Number Indexed, M214-1-24)

1. Charles G. Dawes was a banker, politician, and old friend of Marshall who during World War I had served with the AEF as chief of supply procurement and risen to the rank of brigadier general. In 1921, he was appointed the first director of the Bureau of the Budget and from 1925 to 1929 was vice president of the United States. He was also co-recipient of the 1925 Nobel Peace Prize for the Dawes Plan to stabilize the German economy and reparations payments and from 1929 to 1932 served as US ambassador to Great Britain.

2. Dawes had sent Marshall an inscribed copy of this book in late October. (Charles G. Dawes, *A Journal of the McKinley Years*, ed. Bascom N. Timmons [Chicago: Lakeside Press, R. R. Donnelley & Sons Company, 1950].) Marshall assured Dawes that he would "certainly seek an early opportunity to read your account of the contributions to this country of that great man." (Marshall to Dawes, October 24, 1950, GCMRL/G. C. Marshall Papers [Secretary of Defense, Number Indexed, M214-1-24].)

3. Marshall's examination had been scheduled for early September 1901, but was delayed until September 23 because of President William McKinley's assassination on September 6. See *Papers of GCM*, 1: 16.

4. Beeman, Henry, and Rufus Dawes were brothers of Charles Dawes. Their mother, Mary Gates Dawes, died on October 28, 1921. Charles Dawes had practiced law from 1887 to 1894 in Lincoln, Nebraska, where he befriended then Lieutenant John J. Pershing, a military instructor at the University of Nebraska who would become commander of the AEF, in which Dawes and Marshall served during World War I. ("Gen. Dawes at Dying Mother's Bedside When His War Colleagues Celebrate Here," *New York Times*, October 29, 1921, p. 1; Bascom N. Timmons, foreword to Dawes, *Journal of the McKinley Years*, vii–viii.)

5. Knowlton "Snake" Ames, a second cousin of Dawes, was a record-setting fullback on Princeton University's football team from 1886 to 1889. William Webster Mills had been president of the First National Bank of Marietta, Ohio, and led several railway and utility companies in Ohio and Illinois. In September 1920, Marshall had traveled with

General Pershing, Dawes, Mills, and Ames to tour the Pure Oil Company in Dawes, West Virginia, of which Mills was director. ("Col. K. L. Ames a Suicide in His Car in Chicago," *New York Times*, December 24, 1931, p. 1; "Pershing Visits Pure Oil Co.'s Properties," *Oil and Gas News* 8, no. 5 [September 16, 1920]: 12; Pogue, *Education*, 223–24.)

6. Dawes responded to Marshall on November 15, "What you say in your letter about my book also reaches my heart. . . . As Stimson once said 'You are the most selfless man I have ever known.' I remember General Pershing's great anxiety that you remain Chief of Staff during the First [*Second*] World War and not go as a Commander in Chief of the American Army in Europe. Your declination of that crowning honor was also characteristic." (Dawes to Marshall, November 15, 1950, Northwestern University Special Collections/Charles G. Dawes Papers.)

150

SPEECH TO THE CONSULTANTS OF THE RESEARCH AND DEVELOPMENT BOARD[1]

November 9, 1950
Washington, DC

Dr. Compton and Gentlemen: I appreciate your response to our call. We need the benefit of your knowledge and experience to help us solve the twin problems of money and manpower in connection with our program of research and development.

The fiscal problem appears to be the less difficult. The Department of Defense has maintained a substantial research and development budget, and Congress shows every evidence of continuing to recognize our needs in this effort. Already we have increased our 1950 budget of some 500 million for research and development by 120 million, or more than 20 per cent.

How to divide the money we get between research and immediate production is the first of our basic problems. The present military situation is grave. We need equipment immediately, and in some cases cannot wait for research to bring added improvements. At the same time there are some items on which the planned research and development will not bring results until 1955. We may need those weapons before that date. Furthermore, there are some long range ideas which have particular promise and which should be pushed at the highest possible rate.

Our next fiscal question is to determine whether we are asking for enough money. Demands for new and improved weapons add to a huge total for research, and suggestions have been made that present effort should be doubled or even tripled. So much for the fiscal problem.

The manpower problem presents an even greater challenge. The limitation on research appears to be the number of scientific and engineering personnel available for the military program, either within the government laboratories or in the laboratories of our contractors. We have no reliable figures on the scientific manpower of the country or even how much the country at large can profitably spend on research and development.

An increased military research effort of the magnitude under consideration cannot be accomplished without seriously affecting the civilian economy. How severe a strain might this increase in military research place on industrial growth and expansion? Will it be tolerable? Is the rapid rate of growth we are considering feasible? Or should we plan to reach the same level of effort in a longer time? To answer these questions we need your expert help and advice.

Dr. Compton has pointed out that the problem of manpower cannot be attacked through statistics alone. We have asked you here today in order to learn your thoughts and ideas on the most effective scale of effort possible for military research in the immediate future.[2]

Thank you again, Dr. Compton, for responding to our call for help and persuading so many able citizens to come here to consider this problem with us.[3]

GCMRL/G. C. Marshall Papers (Secretary of Defense, Speeches and Statements)

1. Drafts of this document contain typed notes stating that it had been prepared and edited by OSD staff members and that it constituted "drafted remarks from which SecDef made off-the-cuff address of welcome." (Address of Welcome to the Compton Group, draft, and attached memorandum, November 9, 1950, HSTL/A. Robert Ginsburgh Papers [Speech File]; memorandum attached to draft of address, GCMRL/G. C. Marshall Papers [Secretary of Defense, Speeches and Statements].)

The seven-member Research and Development Board advised the secretary of defense on developments in scientific research relating to national security. It had gained some authority to make decisions rather than purely advise through 1949 amendments to the National Security Act, but Secretary Johnson had restricted this power. (Condit, *Test of War*, 22.) The current chairman of the RDB, William Webster, had asked his predecessor, Karl Compton, president of the Massachusetts Institute of Technology Corporation, to organize a committee to review the board's budget and determine additional appropriations required for upcoming fiscal years. Twenty-seven people joined Compton at the committee's meeting on November 9. ("Dr. Karl T. Compton Dies Here; Led in Atom Bomb Development," *New York Times*, June 23, 1954, p. 1; memorandum for the file, "Research and Development Board—Dr. Compton's Group Conference on Potential Budget Expansion," November 9, 1950, American Association for the Advancement of Science Archives/Memoranda of William T. Golden.)

2. Compton had also been the chairman of the President's Advisory Commission on Universal Training, which met for the first time on December 20, 1946. Marshall testified before this committee on May 23, 1947. In its report submitted to the president on May 29, 1947, the commission labeled UMT "an essential element in an integrated program of national security." (President's Advisory Commission on Universal Training, *A Program for National Security* [Washington: GPO, 1947], 89.)

3. William T. Golden, a special consultant on science and technology to President Truman and the Bureau of the Budget, commented that the "session was undoubtedly helpful to all concerned, although no answer to the question was arrived at; as the group represented scientists, university professors and presidents, engineers, industrial presidents, and others, varied viewpoints were present. As a minimum, the conference was valuable in helping to inform and bring up to date the individuals present on the magnitude of scientific research in the military organization." (Memorandum for the file, "Research and Development Board—Dr. Compton's Group Conference on Potential Budget Expansion," November 9, 1950, American Association for the Advancement of Science Archives/Memoranda of William T. Golden.)

151

Remarks about Anna Rosenberg's Visit to the Pentagon

November 10, 1950
Washington, DC

I am delighted that I was successful in persuading Mrs. Rosenberg to undertake the office of Assistant Secretary of Defense. During my few weeks as Secretary, I found tremendous pressures regarding manpower coming to me from no less than five different offices in the Defense Department and it was evident that the pressures would increase both from within and without the Department relating to manpower in industry, manpower in the military forces and manpower in the administrative system and with relation to specialists in the scientific, engineering and allied fields. Preparing for this problem, I found the consensus of opinion was that one of the outstanding experts in the United States was Mrs. Anna Rosenberg.[1]

There was still another factor involved in this recommendation of mine. The Defense Department is confronted with the formalization of the proposals to the Congress regarding our system for raising and maintaining our armed forces. This involves the question of Universal Military Training and the Selective Service Act procedures. I knew of no one who had had more experience regarding these issues than Mrs. Rosenberg because of her previous contacts both within and without the Army and her six months service on the Compton Commission.[2]

Therefore, I feel that I personally and the Defense Department have been very fortunate in securing her reluctant agreement to serve as Assistant Secretary of Defense with special relation to manpower and personnel.

GCMRL/G. C. Marshall Papers (Secretary of Defense, Speeches and Statements)

1. See pp. 206–7. Rosenberg met with Marshall on November 1 and agreed either before or after this meeting. Marshall later wrote that he discussed her nomination with Truman on November 7. It was announced to the press on November 9, and on the following day Marshall submitted his recommendation to Truman and gave these remarks at a press conference. (Marshall to Truman, November 10, 1950, NA/RG 330, SD 040 [Manpower and Personnel, 1950].) For Rosenberg's Senate confirmation hearings, see pp. 262–63 and 296–97.

2. Rosenberg had been one of the nine individuals to serve on the President's Advisory Commission on Universal Training. For more on the Compton Commission, see the previous document, n2.

152

To Mrs. Claire E. Hutchin — November 10, 1950
Washington, DC

Dear Katharine: I am answering your postal both for Mrs. Marshall who has difficulty in writing because of her shingles, and for myself. We were much concerned to learn of Hutch's wounds but very deeply impressed by his courageous conduct. I hope his recovery has been rapid and not complicated by his refusal to drop out of the action on September 16.[1]

The Korean War presents very sudden changes to the individual—from a peaceful setting in this country to a dreadful one with great hazards over there.

Please let us hear from you when you know definitely about Hutch's recovery.[2] With congratulations on his fine performance, Affectionately,

GCMRL/G. C. Marshall Papers (Secretary of Defense, Number Indexed, M200-5-36)

1. Katharine Hutchin's husband, Lieutenant Colonel Claire E. Hutchin Jr. (USMA, 1938), was Marshall's assistant executive officer during his mediation mission to China from May to November 1946. He had been wounded in Korea while commanding the Twenty-third Infantry Regiment, First Battalion. Katharine Hutchin had written to Katherine Marshall on November 5 that her husband "had received the Purple Heart for wounds in hip & knee." Colonel Hutchin received the Distinguished Service Cross on December 14, 1950, for his effective command of his battalion in the face of a heavy North Korean ambush near Changyong on August 31, 1950. For more on the Chinese Communists' entry into the war, see 226–28. (Katharine Hutchin to Katherine Marshall, November 5, 1950, GCMRL/G. C. Marshall Papers [Secretary of Defense, Number Indexed, M200-5-36].)

2. Mrs. Hutchin replied to Katherine Marshall on December 2, "Your letter was appreciated so very much.—it amazes me how you both do so much for so many. Hutch has assured me the hip and knee wounded in Sept. are completely healed—I am thankful it wasn't more serious." (Katharine Hutchin to Katherine Marshall, December 2, 1950, ibid.)

153

To W. Averell Harriman

November 10, 1950
Washington, DC

Dear Harriman: Pace has just told me of Walters' promotion to the temporary grade of Lieutenant Colonel on November 3rd.[1]

The old army custom is to drop the new insignia in a glass of hard liquor, drink the liquor, and then fasten the insignia on the tunic. As Walters is a teetotaler, it looks like you will have to use milk or water!

I am glad to be able to pass this word on to you. Faithfully yours,

I am sending along the necessary insignia, I doubt if these leaves can stand hard liquor.[2]

NA/RG 330, SD 210.2

1. On October 24, Marshall had forwarded to Army Secretary Pace a copy and an endorsement of Harriman's October 2 request that his military assistant, Major Vernon A. Walters, be promoted to his reserve grade of lieutenant colonel. "I hope very much that this request of Ambassador Harriman can be granted," Marshall wrote. "I have known Major Walters since he was a Lieutenant. He rendered important service to me in Brazil during the meeting at Petropolis, at Bogota in Columbia [*Colombia*], and finally in Paris at the United Nations meeting in 1948. These services went far beyond the mere business of interpreting." Marshall also commented on Walters's service during World War II as aide-de-camp to Lieutenant General Mark W. Clark (USMA, 1917), who had commanded the Fifth Army during the Italian campaign, and noted that "In our first landing in Africa November 9, 1942," Walters had "acted with great courage in the confused situation involved in the first landing in the dark from a destroyer at Safi." (Harriman to Marshall, memorandum, October 23, 1950, and Marshall to Pace, memorandum, October 24, 1950, with Marshall's handwritten draft, NA/RG 330, SD 210.2.) Walters was an accomplished linguist who had served Marshall during the latter's 1947–1949 tenure as secretary of state. (See *Papers of GCM*, 6: 589–90 and photo #31.) Walters had also accompanied Harriman to the recent meeting between Truman and MacArthur on Wake Island. (See pp. 186–87.) For more on Walters's service in North Africa and Italy during World War II, and with Harriman as well as Marshall, see his memoir, *Silent Missions* (New York: Doubleday, 1978), 28–45, 86–89, 168–69, and 188–89.

2. Walters reproduced the original of this letter in *Silent Missions*, with the last sentence handwritten by Marshall. (Ibid., 208 and photo insert between 322 and 323.)

154

Remarks at the Graveside of General John J. Pershing[1]

November 11, 1950
Arlington, Virginia

This ceremony this morning is of deep personal significance to me because I was closely associated with General Pershing when he commanded the First Army during the San Mihiel and Meuse-Argonne Battles. Later, after the cessation of hostilities, I became his aide and served him for four years.[2]

When I returned to Washington in the summer of 1938 to become Deputy Chief of Staff of the Army and later Chief of Staff, I saw the General frequently; as a rule, regularly about once a week, and talked over the critical world situation or the progress of hostilities in which for a time we were not engaged.

General Pershing left a lasting impression on our Army and also on our people. He was a great soldier, without evasions, cool and determined in every crisis and capable of tremendous powers of command and control.

On his death I succeeded him as Chairman of the Battle Monuments Commission. He devoted the last twenty years of his life almost exclusively to the direction of the work of that organization in establishing our National Military Cemeteries abroad.[3]

As Chairman of the Battle Monuments Commission, I am concerned with the final resting places of our deceased veterans in sacred plots of ground all over the world. There are twenty-two such cemeteries overseas, and in each we have erected, or are in process of erecting a beautiful chapel containing a permanent graphic record in stone, bronze and mosaics of the achievements of the American forces that fought in these regions. Memorial references are included for those tens of thousands of missing or unidentified dead to whom the tragedies of war denied a known and honored burial. Their names will be inscribed on the walls for all to read.

These memorials will serve to remind the peoples of Europe, Africa and the Far East that American men fought, bled, and died side by side with their own sons to make life more abundant for all of us.

These chapel tributes to the heroism and sacrifices of our men and women are national in character and therefore far more enduring then any individual could provide. They are the product of the finest work of the most noted architects, sculptors, artists and landscape authorities in this country. As a nation we are entrusted with the honor of perpetuating these shrines and keeping them always beautiful.

Each year official representatives of our Government and of the governments of the friendly countries in whose lands our men served and died, visit these cemeteries. Thousands of visitors from home and abroad also visit the cemeteries, especially during the summer months. These visits will be in increasing numbers when all the splendid structures and plantings are completed.[4]

Armistice Day this year has for us unusual significance. Earlier occasions were marked by special homage to those who gave their lives in the First World War, and later to the fallen in the recent world conflict. November eleventh this year we are also doing honor to four thousand or more of our men who recently gave their lives in Korea, and today at this very moment other names are surely being added to this list of sacrifices in our behalf.

Each of these casualties represents precious life, precious to the individual and precious to his family and friends. We can do nothing to restore life to those men, but we can keep faith with them, remembering and honoring their sacrifices and doing our very best to support the ideals they courageously represented. They will not be forgotten. Their Government will see that their last resting place is kept beautiful and peaceful, and a reminder to all peoples that we believe in the dignity of the individual and stand ready to make any sacrifice in defense of his inalienable rights.

GCMRL/G. C. Marshall Papers (Secretary of Defense, Speeches and Statements)

1. Marshall delivered this Armistice Day address in Arlington National Cemetery at 9:45 a.m. He then visited in his office with commander of the American Legion Erle Cocke Jr. and his wife at 10:23 a.m. (see p. 253n1) and returned to Arlington Cemetery at 10:50 a.m. to attend a wreath-laying ceremony at the Tomb of the Unknown Soldier. He arrived back at the Pentagon at 12:07 p.m. before departing immediately for Princeton, New Jersey, for the Princeton-Harvard football game. (See the next document.)

"It was a very cold and damp day," Marshall later confided to Charles Dawes, "and I consider myself fortunate in escaping a cold. The services at General Pershing's grave were dignified, though simple and brief." (Marshall to Dawes, November 22, 1950, GCMRL/G. C. Marshall Papers [Secretary of Defense, Number Indexed, M200-5-18].)

2. For more on Marshall's relationship with Pershing during and after World War I, see *Papers of GCM*, 1: 104–260, and George C. Marshall, *Memoirs of My Services in the World War 1917–1918* (Boston: Houghton Mifflin Company, 1976).

3. Pershing died in the early morning on July 15, 1948. See *Papers of GCM*, 6: 503. Marshall accepted the chairmanship of the American Battle Monuments Commission (ABMC) on January 27, 1949.

4. For more on the construction and dedication ceremonies of the various World War II military cemeteries, see pp. 289–90, 618–19, 706–7, 724–29, 740–41, and 969–70.

155

To Mrs. Harold W. Dodds — November 13, 1950, Washington, DC

Dear Mrs. Dodds: First I want to thank you and Dr. Dodds again for your kindness in arranging for me to barge in on the game Saturday. We thoroughly enjoyed it. It was a restful trip both ways and we were back in our apartment at 6:00 P.M.[1]

Now as to your Pinehurst visit. I want to go into details for your information because we are very serious in our desire to have you take advantage of our invitation.[2]

The cottage has two double bedrooms and one single, two bathrooms, a large living room, a dining room, a little breakfast room and an efficient kitchen set up;

also a servant's room and bath. It is within walking distance of the Golf Club.

We have to open it very shortly for our own convenience, so you need not feel that whatever trouble we go to in opening it up for your occupancy is in any degree an imposition. If you will accept, I think you and your Washington friends will find it a very nice set up.[3] I would send down an orderly sergeant of mine several days in advance to get the place opened up, to engage a cook, if you want one, preferably our old cook ($50.00 a week), see that the furnace is going, and to orient you. He would leave a station wagon at your disposal.

If you did not wish to do more than have breakfast in the cottage, there are convenient places nearby to have meals and particularly luncheon at the Golf Club, which Mrs. Marshall and I did very frequently.

I do hope we may be able to make your visit pleasanter in this way.[4] With warm regards, Faithfully yours,

GCMRL/G. C. Marshall Papers (Secretary of Defense, Selected)

1. On November 2, Marshall had asked if Dodds would allow him and Mrs. Marshall to fly to Princeton after the Armistice Day ceremonies in order to attend the Princeton-Harvard football game on November 11. (See the previous document.) Dodds responded by telegram on November 6 that he was "overjoyed" the Marshalls were coming to the game. (Marshall to Dodds, November 2, 1950, and Dodds to Marshall, telegram, November 6, 1950, GCMRL/G. C. Marshall Papers [Secretary of Defense, Number Indexed, M214-3-39].)

2. Apparently Katherine Marshall had offered the Dodds the use of their Pinehurst home after Thanksgiving. After initially declining the invitation, Dodds saw Marshall at the Pentagon on November 20 and accepted the offer at that time, if not earlier. (Dodds to Marshall, November 13, 1950, and Carlson to Yeager, memorandum, November 20, 1950, GCMRL/G. C. Marshall Papers [Secretary of Defense, Selected].)

3. Neville Miller, president of the Federal Communications Bar Association, and his wife stayed in Pinehurst with the Doddses. (Miller to Marshall, December 7, 1950, GCMRL/G. C. Marshall Papers [Secretary of Defense, Number Indexed, M200-6-1].)

4. Margaret Dodds sent Katherine Marshall a telegram from Pinehurst on November 24, informing her, "Everything perfectly lovely and very welcoming. Extremely grateful." Marshall responded to the Doddses' telegram on November 29 that they were "glad to know that you found everything at the lodge satisfying and comfortable. We hope that you will enjoy a pleasant and restful vacation." (Margaret Dodds to Katherine Marshall, November 24, 1950, and Marshall to Dodds, November 29, 1950, ibid., M200-5-9].)

Dodds reported to Marshall on December 4 that they had returned "from Liscombe Lodge greatly refreshed and with most pleasant memories of a delightful time. Your house was comfortable all the time, even on the coldest days, although I fear we consumed an inordinate amount of fuel oil. The comfort of the house with all its conveniences was far superior to any hotel, and we are profoundly grateful to Mrs. Marshall and you for trusting it to us." (Dodds to Marshall, December 4, 1950, ibid.) For the Marshalls' summer 1951 vacation at a cottage owned by Dr. and Mrs. Dodds on Cape Cod, see pp. 603–4.

In his November 29 letter cited above, Marshall also informed Dodds that he had been elected on November 19 to the Red Cross Board of Governors as a member-at-large and thanked him for his willingness to accept the position. For more on Marshall's resignation from the Red Cross and his address to this board of governors meeting, see pp 220–22, 247–51, and 283–84.

156

Memorandum for the Record — November 13, 1950
Secret — Washington, DC

Subject: Interview between Secretary of Defense Marshall and Ambassador Muccio[1]

Ambassador Muccio thanked Secretary Marshall for the excellent cooperation received by him in Korea from all military personnel with whom he had dealings. Conversation then turned to the question of UN rehabilitation plans for Korea and Mr. Muccio noted the tendency to progress too fast and to attempt to raise the Koreans too quickly from a primitive and agrarian economy.

Mr. Muccio described the effective work of KAMAG.[2] Through previous training efforts there now exist in the Korean army a large number of officers whose primary loyalty is to the Government and not to any individuals. This is the result of discarding the older Japanese-trained officers.

Secretary Marshall expressed satisfaction at learning of this and discussed briefly the problem of a country the size of Korea supporting a ten-division army as proposed in current studies on the subject. While an establishment of that size would be necessary for the immediate future after the cessation of hostilities, he considered it essential not to overburden the country with too large an army which would either collapse or become a threat to civil authority and to financial stability of the country. The problem therefore to be solved is to adjust downward from ten divisions to some plan which can endure for a long time involving perhaps a truly strong quickly-mobilized unit on a national reserve basis. Our own National Guard does not become available quickly enough and should not be a pattern.

A. C. Murdaugh

NA/RG 330, CD Memorandum of Conversation

1. In addition to Marshall and US Ambassador to South Korea John J. Muccio, U. Alexis Johnson, director of the State Department's Office of Northeast Asian Affairs, and Navy Captain Albert C. Murdaugh of the Defense Department's Far East Bureau, who wrote this memorandum, attended this meeting.

2. KAMAG (more commonly spelled KMAG) was the United States Military Advisory Group to the Republic of Korea and was under the operational control of Ambassador Muccio. It was created when the United States recognized the ROK in early 1949, and it replaced the army advisory mission in Korea that had reported directly to the commanding general of US Army forces in Korea.

157

To Elmer G. Davis — November 13, 1950
Personal — Washington, DC

Dear Davis: I received your letter of November 8 with its invitation to Mrs. Marshall and myself to become sponsors for the Third Annual Roosevelt Day

Dinner on January 26.[1]

I am somewhat embarrassed on finding myself between two impulses. One is the desire to honor Roosevelt and the other, to my mind, is the very important necessity for me, at this particular time, to keep as clear of any matters of plain political significance as possible. In everything I do these days I appear to be accused of participating in a political maneuver—that I have no intention of serving as Secretary of Defense beyond the election and that I merely accepted the post in order to facilitate the political rearrangement, and now in recommending Anna Rosenberg I am again accused of conniving at the behest of the political group in the administration. Nothing could have been further from the truth in both of these cases, but nevertheless, these attacks make it all the more difficult for me in prospect in my dealings with the Congress.[2]

I think you will understand my reason for regretting your invitation.[3] Faithfully yours,

GCMRL/G. C. Marshall Papers (Secretary of Defense, Number Indexed, M214-4-17)

1. Davis, director of the Office of War Information under Roosevelt and chairman of the Washington Committee for Roosevelt Day, had invited the Marshalls "on behalf of the Washington Chapter, Americans for Democratic Action [ADA], to become sponsors for the Third Annual Roosevelt Day Dinner, which will be held this year on January 26, 1951." The purpose of this dinner was "to foster and promote the program and principles enunciated by Franklin D. Roosevelt," particularly the United Nations. (Davis to the Marshalls, November 8, 1950, GCMRL/G. C. Marshall Papers [Secretary of Defense, Number Indexed, M214-4-17].)

2. For more on the Rosenberg nomination, see pp. 206–7, 232–33, 262–63, and 296–97.

3. Marshall Carter directed that Secretary Marshall's letter be "*hand-carried direct* to Mr. Davis." (Carter to Commander Barry, memorandum [November 13, 1950], ibid.) "I thoroughly understand your reasons for declining the ADA invitation," Davis replied on the same day. "Indeed if I had seen the list of people to whom my letter was to be sent I should have asked them to strike you off, as I know your feelings." (Davis to Marshall, November 13, 1950, ibid.) Katherine Marshall similarly turned down a January 1951 invitation to join the Woman's National Democratic Club "for evident reasons. General Marshall has felt it necessary to follow a similar course and I must do so on my side of the house." (Katherine Marshall to Mrs. William E. Warne, January 12, 1951, ibid., M217-2-17].)

158

To Mrs. James J. Winn — November 15, 1950
Washington, DC

Dear Molly: Your Mother has talked to you over the telephone, but I'd better confirm the set up for you.

Sergeant Heffner will meet you at the boat at 7:45 Saturday morning. It will not be necessary for you to start out to Walter Reed until about 8:20.[1] The morning traffic slows movement considerably. You can arrange with Heffner as to when he picks you up and brings you back to our apartment. I am telling your Mother to give him a key to the apartment for you so that you can certainly get in if Anna happens to be out at the time.

The jeep will be parked in the rear of the apartment unless a previous invitation of ours to the President of Princeton and his wife to utilize the cottage at Pinehurst for two weeks, is accepted. In that case, Heffner will be obligated to motor down in the jeep and open the cottage and have it ready for them. However, the Oldsmobile will be at your disposal. I do not know exactly when the Dodds plan to go to Pinehurst, but I fear it is the end of this week. I will hear from them presumably tomorrow and then I can rearrange plans accordingly.[2]

I understand that Aline is coming into the apartment Saturday to spend one night.[3] Sunday she gets a room at the Sulgrave Club.

There is an excellent restaurant in the apartment house across the street and a quarter of a block up the hill for dinners. Down the hill a block and a half on the far side of the street is a blue front restaurant that is excellent and moderate. Of course Anna will do the breakfast.

From our apartment the way to Walter Reed is out Connecticut a short distance to Military Road and then a cut through the park, debouching on Sixteenth Street right near the entrance to Walter Reed.

We will return to Washington probably about 7:00 o'clock Sunday night, so your Mother will be there at the time of Jimmy's operation on Tuesday.[4]

I don't think I have omitted any necessary details.[5] Hastily and Affectionately,

GCMRL/G. C. Marshall Papers (Secretary of Defense, Selected)

1. Marshall's stepdaughter was scheduled to take her ten-year-old son, James, to Walter Reed Hospital for minor surgery.

2. Marshall called Dodds on November 15 as well. For more information on these arrangements, see pp. 236–37.

3. This may be a reference to Katherine Marshall's sister, Allene Lacy. Marshall often misspelled the names of Allene Lacy and her husband, Sterling.

4. The Marshalls were in Chicago for the American Red Cross convention. They departed from Washington on Thursday, November 16, and returned in the evening of November 19. See pp. 247–51.

5. Marshall had written to Colonel James C. Kimbrough of the Army Medical Center to verify that "Mrs. Winn will arrive with her son Jimmie—the patient—around 8:30 Saturday morning" and that Sergeant Heffner would "bring them right up to your office." (Marshall to Kimbrough, November 15, 1950, GCMRL/G. C. Marshall Papers [Secretary of Defense, Number Indexed, M200-4-17].)

159

MEMORANDUM FOR COLONEL MARSHALL S. CARTER — November 15, 1950
Washington, DC

I have in mind a luncheon for some of the old boys in Washington, my friends, here at the Pentagon, and including the three secretaries and the Chiefs of Staff, and, of course, Lovett. I have made a tentative list which follows. Maybe you will think of some other names, but particularly I'd like to get your reaction to the procedure.[1]

1 General John L. Hines
Brig. General John McA. Palmer
Lt. Gen. C. D. Herron
Maj. General James Ulio
5 Colonel Julius Conrad
Lt. Gen. Stanley Embick
Maj. Gen. William Bryden
Brig. Gen. Royden E. Beebe
Maj. Gen. Frank McCoy
10 Maj. Gen. Fox Conner
Maj. Gen. W. D. Connor
Maj. Gen. Walter Reed
Gen. Conger Pratt[2]
Gasser Lorenzo
15 Dewitt John L
Arnold Arch
Tyner
Thompson C
Wilson Arthur
20 Ely Hanson
Stark
King
Collins James L
Halstead Larry
25 Grant, Walter
Milling, Thos D
Land, Emory[3]

GCMRL/G. C. Marshall Papers (Secretary of Defense, Number Indexed, M206-1-23)

1. Carter replied by warning Marshall that "the whole project could get out of hand without much trouble," but he attached nonetheless "a list of the Army, Navy, and Air Force retired General and Flag officers living in the Washington area" for Marshall to verify against his own typed and handwritten list reproduced above. (Carter to Marshall, memorandum, November 21, 1950, GCMRL/G. C. Marshall Papers [Secretary of Defense, Categorical, Memoranda, Marshall S. Carter, 1950–1951].)

2. General John L. Hines (USMA, 1891) was a former army chief of staff. Lieutenant General Charles D. Herron (USMA, 1899) was an old friend of Marshall and former commanding general of the Army Hawaiian Division. Major General James A. Ulio had been army adjutant general during World War II. Colonel Julius T. Conrad (USMA, 1892) was a former adjutant general of the Philippine Department as well as the Second and Third Corps Areas. Lieutenant General Stanley D. Embick (USMA, 1899) had been chief of staff of the American division of the Allied Supreme War Council during World War I, army deputy chief of staff before World War II, and a senior military adviser to Marshall and the rest of the JCS as a member of the Joint Strategic Survey Committee during World War II. Major General William Bryden (USMA, 1904) had been deputy army chief of staff prior to US entry into World War II and commander of the Fourth Service Command. Brigadier General Royden E. Beebe Sr. was an old friend from Marshall's days as a student at Fort Leavenworth Infantry and Cavalry School in 1906 and a former commanding general of

Fort Jackson. Major General Frank R. McCoy (USMA, 1897) was another old friend and a soldier-diplomat who had held a series of high-level politico-military assignments, including membership on the Roberts Commission investigating the Pearl Harbor attack during World War II and chairman of the postwar Far Eastern Commission (see pp. 869–71, 935–36. and 942–43). Major General Fox Conner (USMA, 1898) had been chief of operations for the AEF during World War I, army deputy chief of staff, and a mentor of Marshall and Eisenhower. Major General William D. Connor (USMA, 1897) served in the Operations Section of the AEF during World War I and as commandant of the Army War College and superintendent of West Point. Major General Walter L. Reed was former inspector general of the army. Major General Henry Conger Pratt (USMA, 1905) had been a member of the office of the army chief of staff under Marshall.

These first thirteen names were typed; those that follow were handwritten by Marshall after Pratt's name. The numbers were also handwritten.

3. Major General Lorenzo D. Gasser was a former assistant army chief of staff for personnel, acting deputy chief of staff after Marshall became chief of staff in 1939, and a member of the War Department Manpower Board during World War II. General John L. DeWitt commanded the Western Defense Command after the Pearl Harbor attack. Major General Archibald V. Arnold (USMA, 1912) was a former commanding general of the Seventh Infantry Division and military governor of Korea. Brigadier General George P. Tyner was a former assistant chief of staff for supply (G-4). Major General Charles F. Thompson (USMA, 1904) had been commanding general of the Military District of Washington. Major General Arthur R. Wilson had served in the supply division of the War Department General Staff and as a supply officer in the Pacific, Mediterranean, and European theaters of operation during World War II. Major General Hanson E. Ely (USMA, 1891) had commanded the Twenty-eighth Infantry Regiment, First Division, at the battle of Cantigny during World War I and ended the war as commanding general of the Fifth Division. Admiral Harold R. Stark (USNA, 1903) was chief of naval operations (CNO) from 1939 to 1942. Fleet Admiral Ernest J. King (USNA, 1901) had been commander in chief of the US Fleet and chief of naval operations during World War II. Major General James Lawton Collins (USMA, 1907), brother of Army Chief of Staff J. Lawton Collins, had been aide-de-camp to General Pershing during World War I and commander of the Second Division at Fort Sam Houston prior to World War II. Brigadier General Laurence Halstead (USMA, 1899) had been chief of staff of the Eighty-fourth Division during World War I, chief of operations for the First Army after the war, and a member of the chief of infantry office from the outbreak of war in Europe in 1939 until his retirement in 1940. Major General Walter S. Grant (USMA, 1900) had worked with Marshall at AEF General Headquarters in planning the St. Mihiel and Meuse-Argonne offensives during World War I and was a former member of the secretary of war's personnel board. Brigadier General Thomas D. Milling (USMA, 1909) was an early pilot and associate of General Henry H. Arnold before the war who had served as commander of air service of the First Army during World War I. Vice Admiral Emory S. Land (USNA, 1902) had been chairman of the US Maritime Commission during World War II and former chief of the Navy Bureau of Construction and Repair.

By early April the list had expanded to fifty-eight retired officers, at which point Marshall deleted twenty-six names. Sixteen actually attended the luncheon on April 25, 1951: Bryden; Collins; Conner; Conrad; DeWitt; Ely; Embick; Gasser; Herron; Major General Guy V. Henry (USMA, 1898), chief of cavalry prior to World War II and member of several Allied defense boards during the war; Major General Albert W. Kenner, chief surgeon in the European theater of operations; McCoy; Lieutenant General Eugene Reybold, chief of the army corps of engineers during World War II; Brigadier General Charles D. Roberts (USMA, 1897), a Medal of Honor winner during the 1898 war with Spain and chief of staff of the Eighty-first Division during World War I; Tyner; Ulio; and Major General Charles M. Wesson (USMA, 1900), chief of army ordnance at the outbreak of World War II and a former assistant to then Lend-Lease administrator Edward R. Stettinius Jr. Generals Grant, Halstead, Hines, Milling, Pratt, and Reed declined the invitation due to illness. (George to Marshall, memorandum, April 5, 1951, GCMRL/G. C. Marshall Papers [Secretary of

Defense, Number Indexed, M206-1-23]; Ackerman to Marshall, memorandum, April 24, 1951, GCMRL/G. C. Marshall Papers [Secretary of Defense, Chronological, Secretaries, Ackerman].)

160

To Colonel William M. Spencer

November 15, 1950
Washington, DC

Dear Spencer: I have not had time up to this moment to answer your letter of July 12, regarding incidents leading up to my appointment as Chief of Staff in 1939.[1] I really have not the time now, but here goes:

a. The Devers you refer to should be General Hugh Drum. The same correction applies to any mention of Devers later on.[2]

b. I have no recollection of this reference to Eisenhower. What I do recall is that a few days after Pearl Harbor, I saw fit to order Eisenhower into Washington where I was assembling some of the most able officers I knew of in the Army.[3]

c. I have no recollection of this.[4]

d. The statement regarding General Pershing is correct, but there should be added to it the very heavy influence exerted by Harry Hopkins who I only met once, that being during the Christmas holidays of '38 for an interview of one hour, regarding WPA [Works Progress Administration] employment in connection with expansion of air power. I had outlined the entire situation, trying to put the various factors in proper perspective—I am referring to artillery, ammunition, tanks, planes, bombs, personnel to train, etc.[5]

e. Is correct, and I participated with Mr. Woodring, then Secretary of War and General Arnold in a rather intense debate with Morgenthau.[6]

f. I attended no Cabinet Meeting at that time or during my entire service as Chief of Staff. I did attend meetings in the Cabinet Room or in the President's office or in his sitting room upstairs, but they were not Cabinet Meetings. What is evidently being is referring to in f. is a meeting in the President's office in which, among others, as I recall, Morgenthau, Jackson, then an official for the Department of Justice, Oliphant, Woodring, Malin Craig, I think Louis Johnson, maybe Sumner Welles, though I doubt it, Pa Watson and myself. What happened as regards me was that the President, after delivering his comments on the building up of air power and questioning various members, turned to me and assumed my agreement. I disagreed with a flat no but was given no opportunity, as I recall, to state the case as I saw it. Later on, however, at a meeting with the President, in company with Woodring and Malin Craig, then Chief of Staff, I did find an opportunity to talk.[7]

Some ten days before a public announcement of my appointment was made or before even the Secretary of War Woodring was advised of it, the President sent for me on Sunday afternoon and greeted me with the statement that he intended to appoint me his Chief of Staff. We had about a half hour of conversation in which I got in a few of my conceptions but in very sketchy form.[8] Faithfully yours,

GCMRL/G. C. Marshall Papers (Secretary of Defense, Number Indexed, M200-4-46)

1. Spencer was a Chicago businessman and friend who had known Marshall since 1934, when Spencer was an intelligence officer in the Illinois National Guard and Marshall its senior instructor. On July 12, Spencer had written to Marshall to request verification of what Frank McCoy had recently told Spencer regarding how Marshall had become army chief of staff in 1939. On July 27, Spencer sent a second letter after a visit with Marshall in Leesburg, enclosing another copy of the letter outlining "exactly what General McCoy told me" and reiterating his comment at Leesburg that Marshall's appointment was "an historic episode in the life of this nation" for which there was no historical record. He asked Marshall to review the July 12 letter and then, "preferably in your own handwriting, point out discrepancies." (Spencer to Marshall, July 12 and 27, 1950, from the personal collection of Colonel William M. Spencer, used with permission of his grandson, Robert Faurot. Further use requires his permission.) On August 2, Major George informed Spencer that "the General did not have the opportunity to write himself as your letter arrived shortly before he and Mrs. Marshall departed for New York and Huron Mountain. He will drop you a line after his return about the first of September. While motoring to the airport," George added, "the General asked me to tell you in my acknowledgment, that some of the incidents you mentioned he couldn't recognize at all and that others have been transplanted from the consideration of quite different matters to that of his appointment." (George to Spencer, August 2, 1950, GCMRL/G. C. Marshall Papers [American Red Cross, General].)

Marshall's response was typed rather than handwritten, but in the margin of Spencer's July 12 letter, which he returned as requested, he hand-lettered each paragraph "a" through "f" to correspond with his responses. All statements and quotes in the subsequent footnotes except for factual identifications of individuals and references to previous volumes of the Marshall Papers come from Spencer's July 12 letter.

2. Spencer had written that according to speculation in army circles in 1938, "the most prominent candidates" to replace General Malin Craig (USMA, 1898) as chief of staff were General Jacob Devers (USMA, 1909), then chief of staff of the Panama Canal Department, General McCoy, and Marshall himself. Instead of Devers, as Spencer had stated in his letter, the third prominent candidate to replace Craig was General Hugh Drum, who at that time commanded the First Army in New York.

3. According to Spencer, Marshall, McCoy, and Craig informally discussed the matter of succession at the Chevy Chase Club in suburban Washington, DC, with McCoy and Craig feeling that Devers (Drum as per Marshall's correction above) was the most likely choice. Marshall supposedly then told them, "I want you to keep your eyes on a man down the line named Eisenhower. He has everything the job requires, and if it is in my power to do so, I am going to see that he is promoted over the heads of plenty of officers who now rank him."

4. Spencer reported that McCoy recalled that "while the discussion was going on" at the Chevy Chase Club, Marshall was "called to the telephone" and was "gone for some time. Upon your return you stated that you had been called to the 'W.H.' (White House) and so left immediately."

5. Spencer had written that the two "outstanding" factors in Roosevelt's decision to appoint Marshall were the recommendation of General Pershing and "an extraordinary event which occurred in the President's office a few weeks before his conversation with General Pershing in which you played the primary role," about which Spencer wrote in his paragraphs e and f. Marshall's Christmas meeting with Hopkins is recounted in Pogue, *Education*, 325–26.

6. According to Spencer's letter, Secretary Morgenthau had received President Roosevelt's approval, "without the War Department having much to say in the matter," to invite a French Air Force officer to the United States to consult with an American counterpart

on "new developments." The French officer and his American pilot crashed in California in late January 1939, which led to speculation that the United States was sharing secrets with the French. Spencer recounted that Roosevelt resolved that "something must be done to counteract" the intense criticism the administration was receiving. (For more on this incident, see Mark S. Watson, *Chief of Staff: Prewar Plans and Preparations*, in *United States Army in World War II* [1950; repr., Washington: Center of Military History, US Army, 1991], 131–34.) Harry H. Woodring was secretary of war from September 25, 1936, to June 20, 1940.

7. Spencer had mistakenly suggested that as a result of the January 1939 airplane crash discussed in n6, Roosevelt "called a meeting of his Cabinet," at which Acting Chief of Staff Marshall represented the War Department. Roosevelt, Spencer said, "delivered a monologue on the subject under discussion" and asked each man present "if he agreed." All did except for Marshall, who spoke "frankly" and told the president that he "entirely disagreed with it."

Marshall recalled in his response a different meeting, held on November 14, 1938. (See *Papers of GCM*, 1: 650–51; *Interviews*, 108–9; and Pogue, *Education*, 322–23.) Robert H. Jackson was at the time of this meeting assistant attorney general. Herman Oliphant was professor of law at Columbia University and chief counsel to the Treasury Department. Sumner Welles was the undersecretary of state, and General Edwin "Pa" Watson (USMA, 1908) was senior military aide to President Roosevelt.

8. See *Papers of GCM*, 1: 713.

161

To Owen J. Roberts

November 16, 1950
Washington, DC

My dear Justice Roberts: Thank you for sending me the views of your Committee on the problem of an integrated defense for the Atlantic community.[1]

Any program in general accord with the aims of the North Atlantic community, whether in or outside the treaty organization, which will strengthen our political unity, is naturally of great importance. The question in my mind is the risk, so far as the time element is concerned, in reaching out for the goal of a political federation when the plan under immediate consideration for securing a program of mutual defense has made progress and appears near to realization. Experience from 1775 to 1789 in forming a federal union out of thirteen states with a common language and a common tradition as a basis gives some idea of what may be expected in the way of legal and constitutional problems in trying to effect a political federation among the diverse nations in the North Atlantic community.

Time today is the dominant factor in our mutual defense program, and time is the one element that we cannot spare. We are trying in every way to find immediate and effective answers to the military needs.

We have just completed a discussion of this crucial question with the Defense Ministers of the North Atlantic Treaty countries.[2] I feel that important progress was made in spite of the disagreement, entirely French, on the point of a German contribution to eastern European defense.[3] The Defense Ministers have now defined, and recommended adoption by the countries concerned, of principles which should be followed to insure the effectiveness of military training and mobilization procedures; and to provide a continuous flow of trained manpower to the military forces. They have, furthermore, determined from the military point of view what forces each member country should contribute.

If the North Atlantic community is to be prepared in time, we must work with the national governments and the institutions empowered by them which alone can provide the men, the equipment, and, most important, the determination necessary to establish an effective military force in the immediate future. I am to call another meeting of the Defense Ministers, presumably in a few weeks, to confirm the work of the military men and the political deputies which is now being rushed to bring about an agreement on the German issue.[4] That done we will be well underway since the basic agreements on practically all other points have already been reached and drafted into final form as to integration, command and the necessary directives as to responsibilities.

Under these conditions, with the great pressure for speed, I would hesitate to introduce a new element into our deliberations at this time. Faithfully yours,

NA/RG 330, SD 092

1. Roberts was a former associate justice of the US Supreme Court who had headed the Roberts Commission investigating the Pearl Harbor attack in 1941 and 1942. At this time he was president of the Atlantic Union Committee, which he had organized in 1949 with the goal of persuading Congress to call for a federal convention, similar to the one that had written the Constitution in 1787, to explore the possibility of a union among all the democratic countries of Europe and North America.

On October 29, Roberts had written a public letter to Marshall enclosing a public statement, signed by twelve members of the committee, all of whom had previously held high positions in government and/or the armed forces, that called for a single, unified NATO defense and foreign affairs department. (Roberts to Marshall and attached statement, October 29, 1950, NA/RG 330, SD 092.) "As soon as possible get me some view of the State Dept.," Marshall wrote on the bottom of Carter's October 30 memorandum forwarding this material. (Carter to Marshall, memorandum, October 30, 1950, with Marshall handwritten comment, ibid.; H.) Although drafts of this response were written and edited by Douglas MacArthur II, deputy director of the State Department's Office of European Regional Affairs, and H. Freeman Matthews as well as Ginsburgh and Carter, Marshall very heavily edited the final version, in effect rewriting it and adding much of the last two paragraphs. Leva, General Bradley, and the State Department also reviewed it before it was sent. (Carter to Lovett, November 9, 1950, ibid.)

2. See pp. 204–6 and 218–20.

3. "General Marshall signed this letter to you just prior to his departure for Chicago," Marshall Carter informed Roberts in a cover letter. "As he was leaving he asked me to tell you that he had dealt very frankly with the problem, particularly as to the French, and hoped that the letter would not be made public. In any event, no general dissemination of the letter should be made with the French reference as contained in the 4th paragraph, and the words, 'entirely French,' should be deleted without indicating that a deletion has been made." (Carter to Roberts, November 16, 1950, GCMRL/G. C. Marshall Papers [Secretary of Defense, Chronological, Director, Executive Office (Marshall S. Carter), 1950–1952].)

4. In December, the Military Committee met in London and the Defense Committee and North Atlantic Council met in Paris. Pace represented Marshall, who remained in the United States.

162

Speech to the Board of Governors of the American Red Cross[1]
Confidential

November 19, 1950
Chicago, Illinois

When I took office as President of the Red Cross a year ago, my knowledge of the organization was limited to observations as Chief of Staff of the Army and to what Mrs. Marshall had told me of her Red Cross experiences.[2] Immediately I became aware of how very much more I had to learn. That in itself was somewhat disconcerting. But what was more disconcerting, however, was the fact that I found that many leaders and most active workers in the Red Cross suffered from a similar limitation in knowledge, having concentrated on activities that were within their own special interest.

I have endeavored during the past year to correct this serious weakness, to secure better-informed interpreters of what the Red Cross is and does and why. Progress has been made, but not nearly enough. There seems to be a general agreement with me as to this weakness, but little is really done to correct the matter. Distributing pamphlets is not enough, it is only a beginning. I told the Chairman of our approaching fund drive, General Sarnoff, that this was his most serious problem.[3]

I must report to you today that I still find too little appreciation and acceptance of what the Red Cross does today, too little recognition of the threats that would—if successful—seriously impair the efficiency of Red Cross.

Less than six months ago, we were proceeding in accordance with your instructions to reduce expenditures and to gear the program downwards in line with diminishing contributions. Real progress was made. Then came the Korean conflict and the action of the United Nations by which it is to be hoped, peace will be restored. As an auxiliary to the government of the United States and especially to the armed forces, the Red Cross had to gear it work as quickly as possible to the needs of changed conditions, expanding certain of its activities immediately. Demands for expansions have been carefully analyzed by a special group, and none has been undertaken except as it was strictly necessary to meet our obligations. The results of this careful screening and planning are evidenced by the small amount of additional budget that will be required to complete this fiscal year. It is further evidenced by the modest budget under present circumstances which is projected for the coming fiscal year. Yet the five major programs that are under way, following the outbreak of conflict in Korea, are very *heavy* responsibilities. If they are to be successful and justify the confidence placed in the organization, the full resources of the Red Cross must be effectively put to work.

Acting on requests from the Department of Defense and the National Security Resources Board, the Red Cross is giving top priority to:

1. Rapid expansion of Red Cross services to the armed forces to meet the needs of a 3,000,000-man fighting force called for by President Truman.[4]
2. Procuring blood for meeting whole blood needs on the Korean fighting

fronts and for processing into plasma and other derivatives for military and civil defense requirements.[5]

3. Taking a leading part in training 20,000,000 persons in first aid, including treatment of atom bomb attack injuries.
4. Training 250,000 nurse's aides and hundreds of thousands of housewives in home nursing to help meet the critical shortage of professional nurses which would probably occur in event of a national emergency.
5. Assisting civil defense authorities in plans for the provision of food, clothing, and shelter during any emergency period.

I think I am accurate in saying that the Red Cross is mobilized for Defense—for ourselves, our homes, and our country.

We must bring the people of this country to a realization of this, for if they but knew what the Red Cross is doing and is preparing to do, there would be no question about the adequacy of their response.

Obviously, the 1951 Red Cross Fund Campaign must be for an increased amount of money. Our expenditures must necessarily increase. Unfortunately our reserves have all but vanished. Yet we are still operating on deficit financing.

The report of the Finance Committee today should not be as alarming as might well have been expected. The fund goal recommended will be much less than we had expected. As a matter of fact, due to economies already perfected, it will represent but a small increase over the present budget of approved expenditures, but with no large reserves to reduce the amount of the total call on the public. Nevertheless, to reach that goal will not be an easy job. The campaign next March will not be successful unless it is carefully organized, aggressively directed, and reaches all people in every community. But as I am about to explain I am sure it will be so organized and directed.[6]

Nationally, the Chairman of the campaign will be General David Sarnoff, Chairman of the Board, Radio Corporation of America. Already he has been working with our National Headquarters staff for several weeks and spent these past several days with us, getting better acquainted with what the Red Cross does, why and how. He has demonstrated his lively interest in Red Cross many times. He has already made evident his devotion to the country of his adoption. Now, at my request, he generously comes forth to give us the best of his services. His ability as a leader, his well-known organizing ability, his capacity to interpret, his resourcefulness are outstanding among the great figures in American life. His acceptance of the responsibilities I have entrusted to him cause me to have the highest hopes or the success of our 1951 campaign.[7]

However, I think I probably should thank Mrs. Sarnoff for a large part of the energy and enthusiasm he is putting into this new task.[8]

Now he cannot do the job alone. He must have the real help, the active support of all of us who are closest to the needs and to the problems of the Red Cross. There are several ways by which you, as members of the Board of Governors, can assist.

Speakers will be needed for state and regional meetings. You can be of great value as such, and you should work out in advance your treatment of the subject. These meetings will bring together the top leadership of our chapters. It is essential that they receive clear and complete interpretations of the increased responsibilities of the organization and the resulting need for additional funds.

You can help in making special approaches to corporations aimed at securing larger contributions. Through your representation on corporation boards, many of you may be able to make important contributions in this particular field.

A letter from you to the chapters within your own individual states should provide a healthy stimulus to their campaign operations.

The area managers will contact you as specific developments indicate a need for your help. I want General Sarnoff to leave here feeling confident of your active support.

Significant steps were taken a few years ago by the Advisory Committee on Organization, of which E. Roland Harriman was chairman, which culminated in May 1947 when the President of the United States signed the legislation popularly described as that which democratized the Red Cross.[9] Of course, democracy does not come into being by fiat or legislation. It comes about only as the responsibilities it imposes are accepted and fulfilled by the people which democracy seeks to benefit. And so it is no small wonder that the American Red Cross is not yet completely democratized. Much progress to that end has been made. Let no one say otherwise. But in two major respects, at least, much more must be made. Labor—organized labor—has given strong support to Red Cross, not only by engaging in our activities but especially in financial support to the extent of about thirty percent of our total budget, and in blood donations. But labor has not had a sufficient part in responsibility for giving Red Cross leadership and in the determination of Red Cross policies and practices. Labor lacks interpreters from its own ranks and for its own personnel of what the Red Cross is and does. Adequate representation of all groups within organized labor is quite impractical. I would hope, however, that Red Cross—just as it has found solutions to so many other problems—will find the way to have representation of labor on the Board of Governors nationally and especially on chapter Boards of Directors.

We are all agreed that Red Cross must not only serve without regard to race, color, religion, or politics; it must also be served by those who are representative of every segment of our society. The day will be welcome and a great further contribution will have been made when Red Cross not only serves but *is* served by total cross-sections of our people.

No organization in the country has numerically more popular support than Red Cross. An examination of its present program will prove that Red Cross activities are practically universal. Support and participation, however, lag behind.

We need a more-extensive, better-planned program of participation, information, and interpretation. I strongly endorse steps recently taken and about to be implemented that should help to bring this about. If the people of this country but knew what Red Cross is doing and has undertaken to do—especially because of critical world conditions—there could only be one response—universal acceptance, participation, and support.

I must report in good conscience that I have failed to contribute to a more effective employment of the Junior Red Cross. I feel that we have barely tapped this great potential. I have talked about it a great deal and done about it very little. I hope you and my successor can really do something big in this field. Perhaps General Sarnoff may point the way.[10]

Red Cross has become very close to me. There was a time and not so long ago when I could think of nothing so satisfying as to close my years of active work in the field of the Red Cross. Events have decided otherwise. Even so, I had hoped that before leaving the organization I could make certain that what I had started—especially with respect to present service to the armed forces and for civil defense—would be totally implemented. There remains, however, much that needs to be done before these results are achieved. Since the appointment of my successor, I have had no qualms. The job will be done and well done. I have assured him—and I do so again here and officially—that he can count on me to assist him in every feasible way. I know that his task the next year will be far from an easy one. He will need all our help, and the strong support of every chapter.[11]

GCMRL/G. C. Marshall Papers (Secretary of Defense, Speeches and Statements)

1. Marshall was in Chicago for this and other Red Cross meetings from November 16 to 19. All meetings took place at the Palmer House, where Marshall stayed. During his time in Chicago, the Marshalls also visited Charles Dawes and "made a tour of our 'old stomping grounds'" where he had been a senior instructor with the Illinois National Guard from 1933 to 1936. Although he had "little time for myself" in Chicago due to "almost continuous meetings . . . , I did have the golden opportunity of going down to Champaign to see the Ohio State–Illinois game, thanks to the thoughtfulness of Adlai Stevenson," the Democratic governor of Illinois, who had invited Marshall to join him at the football game. (Marshall to Dawes, November 22, 1950, GCMRL/G. C. Marshall Papers [Secretary of Defense, Number Indexed, M200-5-18]; Stevenson to Marshall, September 25, 1950, and Marshall to Stevenson, December 15, 1950, ibid., [M214-1-34].)

2. Marshall had discussed the Red Cross on several occasions during his time as chief of staff. For an example of what Katherine Marshall told him and his ensuing action, see Katherine Marshall, *Together*, 60; and *Papers of GCM*, 3: 121.

3. Radio and television pioneer David Sarnoff had been president of the Radio Corporation of America (RCA) since 1930. He held the reserve rank of brigadier general for service in World War II. On November 8, Marshall had written that he was "particularly glad to hear" that Sarnoff would join him in Chicago for the meeting of the large city chapter chairmen on November 17 and that he hoped "it would be possible for you to stay over for the meeting of the Board of Governors on Sunday. I believe you know most of the members, but I would like to have you meet them all and tell them of your plans." (Marshall to Sarnoff, November 8, 1950, GCMRL/G. C. Marshall Papers [Secretary of Defense, Categorical, Organizations, American National Red Cross, 1950–1951].)

4. Truman announced during an evening radio broadcast on September 1, 1950, that US military plans would require an increase of troops "to close to 3 million, and further increases may be required." (Harry S. Truman, *Public Papers of the Presidents of the United States: Harry S. Truman, 1950* [Washington: GPO, 1965], 612.)

5. See, for example, pp. 113–22 and 136–42. On July 20, 1950, Secretary of Defense Johnson had named the Red Cross the "official coordinating agency for the procurement of blood and blood derivatives for the Armed Forces." (Speech at a Volunteer Services Meeting, September 27, 1950, GCMRL/G. C. Marshall Papers [American Red Cross, Speeches

and Statements].)

6. Edward Dana, chairman of the finance committee, reported to the board of governors that the total net fund goal for the March 1951 fund campaign was $85 million. (Minutes of the Red Cross Board of Governors Meeting, November 19, 1950, GCMRL/G. C. Marshall Collection [Minutes, Statements, American National Red Cross, G. C. Marshall Presidency, 1949–1950].)

7. Born in Russia in 1891, Sarnoff had come to the United States as a child in 1900. ("Sarnoff Retires as RCA's Chairman," *New York Times*, January 8, 1970, p. 54.) On December 11, Marshall thanked Sarnoff "very especially for the highly effective and vigorous manner in which you have undertaken this special job for the Red Cross—at my request. I am very sorry I cannot go along and work with you because it would be very satisfying, and I do want you to feel that I am deeply appreciative of how and what you are doing even though I am no longer in a responsible position with regard to the matter." (Marshall to Sarnoff, December 11, 1950, GCMRL/G. C. Marshall Papers [Secretary of Defense, Number Indexed, M200-6-8].)

8. Sarnoff had married Lizette Hermant in 1917.

9. The Advisory Committee on Organization, commissioned in March 1946 under the leadership of E. Roland Harriman, recommended measures to democratize the Red Cross, including elections of members of the board of governors. President Truman signed these changes into law on May 8, 1947. ("Advisory Unit to Meet," *New York Times*, March 10, 1946, p. 17; "Red Cross Bill Signed," *New York Times*, May 9, 1947, p. 3.)

10. The Junior Red Cross was founded in 1917 to coordinate aid and relief activities between the Red Cross and schools across the country during World War I. Membership had diminished since the end of World War II.

11. Marshall's resignation was effective December 1, 1950. "This work has become very close to me," he admitted on November 29. "In a few days I will turn over the reins to Roland Harriman. . . . He is a fine man." (Marshall to Dodds, November 29, 1950, GCMRL/G. C. Marshall Papers [Secretary of Defense, Number Indexed, M200-5-9].) See pp. 220–22 and 283–84.

163

Remarks at a Dinner in Honor of Erle Cocke Jr.[1] — November 24, 1950
Fort Benning, Georgia

It is both natural and a happy circumstance that we have come to Fort Benning today to express our affection for Erle Cocke and our faith in his leadership as National Commander of the American Legion.

It is very natural because Fort Benning is the home of the Infantry School and Erle Cocke one of its most distinguished graduates. It was the battle performance of company officers like him that gave this school its great reputation.

Not merely as Secretary of Defense, but as a doughboy of long standing and one time director of this Infantry School I have a personal pride in Erle Cocke and in the quality of leadership he displayed in combat.[2] I predict for him an unusually successful administration as National Commander of the American Legion.

This meeting is fortuitous because it gives me the opportunity to make some observations on our military history, which I hope the National Commander of the Legion and his people will take to heart.

The history of national defense in this country has been a succession of feasts and famines, that have followed each other in demoralizing sequence. For a nation that prides itself on its logic, business precocity and its practical common sense, we have given the world quite an opposite impression of these qualities when it came to the matter of national defense. Speaking frankly, I fear that we have given a demonstration somewhat of emotional instability.

Consider the history of national defense in your own lifetime, particularly in the lifetime of those of you who are veterans of the first World War. There was the unpreparedness of 1916, the magnificent Army and Navy of 1917–18, the demobilization of 1919, the attempt to set up an enduring system of national defense in 1920, followed quickly by its emasculation in the twenties and thirties, the sudden resurrection in 1939, the rise to world preeminence in the second World War, and an almost violent dip to a new low in the midst of a dangerous world. The drastic demobilization that followed the cessation of hostilities in 1945 is now succeeded by a long swing of the pendulum back to the demand for the immediate build up of great strength.

It is always when our national defense is weakest that we most feel its need. I recall in 1947, as Secretary of State when our country urgently needed military strength to support our international responsibilities I found that my position was supported by but one and one-third Infantry divisions in this country available for duty. Yet, as some of you may recall, I was being urged from many sides to pour it on the Soviets and give them hell.

Despite the failings I have just is referring to in our swings toward stronger national defense we have hung up amazing records, in making up for lost time. Our great resources, our varied and abundant skills, and our dynamic spirit once geared into action accomplished miracles. But always the cost was great, much of which could have been avoided with a little prudent foresight. And always the aftermath of the battle was followed by recriminations, investigations, and demands for accounting—an accounting for precious lives that might have been saved, for money and resources that might have been used to better advantage, for waste that might have been avoided. And always there has been a drive to find scapegoats to shoulder the blame. The basic error, however, has always been with the American people themselves. The fault has been their refusal to sanction an enduring posture of defense that would discourage aggression, and if war came, would reduce the casualties, the sacrifices, the excessive costs, and the needless waste.

This alternate cycle of strength and weakness in national defense must stop. No longer can we count upon years or even months in which to prepare after the war is on. In Korea for the first time we were called upon to fight the first day. That will certainly be the case hereafter. At best we are to face a period of tension of long duration. We must grow stronger to defend ourselves against the risk of aggression wherever it may develop.

We must work, and hope, and not merely pray that we can avoid another World War. Our people are ready to give our armed forces what they need. They will sacrifice. They will produce. They will give us the men and munitions we need. They will probably break many new speed records.

But what then? What will happen after this immediate crisis passes and we are involved in a long and less spectacular tension? Will we again lapse into weakness, an invitation to trouble or will we read the warning of history and set up a system of defense consistent with our democratic ideals, a system which will give us *enduring* security in peace and the immediately available potential strength we need for war, if war becomes necessary?

I know which of these alternatives Erle Cocke will favor. I am confident that the American Legion will line up solidly behind him. Let us, therefore, take the time now and make the effort during his administration to set up an *enduring* system of national defense, a system that will not collapse at every change of wind and temperature, a system that will keep us prepared for any emergency, yet will not sap the economic strength which is of maximum importance to the democratic people of the entire world.[3]

GCMRL/G. C. Marshall Papers (Secretary of Defense, Speeches and Statements)

1. Cocke, a farmer and railroad executive of Dawson, Georgia, had been elected to be the national commander of the American Legion at the organization's October 12 meeting in Los Angeles. Cocke was twenty-nine at the time of his election and had been a POW of the Nazis and escaped on three occasions during World War II. ("Legion Excoriates State Department," *New York Times*, October 13, 1950, p. 16.) Prior to this dinner, Marshall had introduced Cocke at his homecoming celebration in Dawson, Georgia, and had commented that in spite of his wartime imprisonment by the Nazis, Cocke recognized "not only the gravity of the present crisis but the compelling necessity it imposes of allowing Germany . . . to contribute to the defense of Western Europe." (Remarks at the Homecoming Celebration of Commander Erle Cocke Jr., November 24, 1950, GCMRL/G. C. Marshall Papers [Secretary of Defense, Number Indexed, M214-3-29].)

2. Marshall had been assistant commandant of the Infantry School at Fort Benning from 1927 to 1932. See *Papers of GCM*, 1: 319–78.

3. Marshall would repeat these sentiments on numerous occasions as secretary of defense in his efforts to obtain UMT. See, for example, pp. 269–75.

164

MEMORANDUM FOR THE DIRECTOR OF CENTRAL INTELLIGENCE[1]
Top Secret

November 27, 1950
Washington, DC

Subject: Present Status of United States Intelligence[2]

In the overall planning for our national security, an adequate and timely intelligence capability is felt to be a first priority consideration. In order to prevent strategic and tactical surprise we would wish to have:

(a) A 7- to 10-day warning of the imminence of hostilities during which period our defense systems could be alerted and forces deployed or positioned as required.

(b) ~~Provide~~ additional warnings at least 12 to 48 hours prior to the initiation of hostilities which will indicate the location of bases on which atomic attacks are mounted and which will report the approximate time of launching of these attacks.[3]

The foregoing provisions are obviously beyond our capabilities and possibly for a long time to come. However, they do provide a clear-cut target toward which your agency and the Department of Defense should point their intelligence efforts.

Satisfaction of these requirements necessitates detailed, comprehensive and continuing knowledge of the disposition, organization and state of readiness of the Soviet Armed Forces and the supporting economy. The current basis of estimates concerning the Soviet armed forces seems dangerously inadequate.

Because of the extraordinary security program of the Soviet Union virtually no intelligence contribution to these requirements is available through normal channels available to Service intelligence agencies.

In view of the basic requirement to prevent strategic and tactical surprise, our limited capability to meet this requirement and the potential for improvement of this capability through operations by the Central Intelligence Agency [CIA] within the USSR and the satellites, particularly in the covert and defector fields, the Department of Defense is prepared to place support of CIA operations in these fields in Priority One.

In view of the foregoing, a statement of your foreseeable quantitative and qualitative requirements in as much detail as possible is requested in order to enable the Department of Defense to arrange for this support.

With special reference to the matter of military equipment it is further requested that your requirements in this field be forwarded as soon as possible and separately from the more general requirements in support of the broader intelligence programs.[4]

NA/RG 330, CD 350.09

1. Lieutenant General Walter Bedell Smith had become director of the CIA on October 7, 1950.

2. The Joint Chiefs of Staff had sent Marshall a draft of this memorandum and proposed that he send it to Smith. On November 22, Marshall informed Bradley that he did "not understand the phraseology of the first paragraph. It seems obvious that the intelligence capability 'required' for the national security, as indicated by the JCS, is beyond anything we have at present and anything that we are remotely liable to get in the future. The implication, therefore, is at least from the JCS wording, that if we do not have such an intelligence capability, provisions for our national security could be ineffectual. I do not believe that the JCS had any intention of apparently writing for the record, but this statement is puzzling." Marshall admitted that he might be "unduly sensitive in my reaction, but I think I can realize Smith's unenviable position." He attached a new version of the first two paragraphs containing his revisions and requested Bradley's "very personal views on it." Bradley wrote that he concurred under Marshall's signature, though the final version of the memorandum sent to Smith contained further revisions and additions. (Marshall to Bradley, November 22, 1950, NA/RG 330, CD 350.09.)

3. "Provide" has a line through it in this version of the document, but the version printed in *FRUS* does not. (*FRUS, 1950–1955: The Intelligence Community, 1950–1955* [Washington: GPO, 2007], 85.)

4. "This Agency will make a maximum effort and will coordinate the collective efforts of all intelligence agencies toward attainment of the objectives set forth" in Marshall's memorandum, Smith replied on December 26. Smith cautioned that "Defense plans cannot be based, however, on the assumption that timely warning of Soviet attack can be assured" and thus requested the implementation of several policies to increase the assignment of

military personnel to the CIA and to ensure a seamless flow of information between the JCS and the CIA. (Smith to Marshall, memorandum, December 26, 1950, NA/RG 330, CD 350.09.) See pp. 484–85.

A Pretty Tough Business

November 28, 1950–March 26, 1951

It is not a peaceful world and when you are at the hub, it is a pretty tough business.

—Marshall to Marie Singer
March 5, 1951

ON NOVEMBER 7, Communist Chinese forces broke off their attacks on UN forces and withdrew. (See pp. 226–29.) Their intervention the preceding week had clearly worried America's UN allies as well as Washington, however, and the Joint Chiefs consequently asked MacArthur to comment on a possible reexamination of his directives and plans. MacArthur strongly opposed any such reconsideration, responding on November 9 by comparing Britain's desire to halt south of the Yalu and establish a buffer zone as appeasement similar to what London had practiced at Munich in 1938 and insisting that he could stop further Chinese reinforcement with his airpower and reach the Yalu with a mid-November offensive. "Any program short of this," he warned, "would completely destroy the morale of my forces and its psychological consequence would be inestimable." The JCS concurred but recommended to Marshall that Washington also try to resolve the situation politically through the UN, plan for the possibility of a global war, and keep MacArthur's mission under review. Marshall agreed, as did Acheson. (*FRUS, 1950*, 7: 1097–98, 1107; Doris M. Condit, *History of the Office of the Secretary of Defense*, vol. 2, *The Test of War, 1950–1953* [Washington: Historical Office, OSD, 1988], 78–80.)

On November 18, MacArthur informed the Joint Chiefs that he intended to begin his offensive on November 24. At a November 21 meeting of Marshall, Lovett, Harriman, Army Secretary Pace, the Joint Chiefs, Acheson, and other State Department officials, Marshall "expressed satisfaction that Mr. Acheson had stated his belief that General MacArthur should push forward with the planned offensive" and "expressed some doubt" regarding the British proposal to establish a demilitarized zone just south of the Yalu. (*FRUS, 1950*, 7: 1204–5.)

MacArthur's "home by Christmas" offensive began on November 24, but by the following evening it faced fierce counterattacks by a Communist Chinese force estimated at two hundred thousand. "We face an entirely new war," MacArthur informed the Joint Chiefs on November 28 as he went on the defensive. On that same day, Truman called an extraordinary 3:00 p.m. meeting of the National Security Council (see next document), to be followed by a meeting of the cabinet.

Prior to the NSC meeting, Marshall spent the morning in a series of meetings with Lovett, Bradley, Ginsburgh, Rosenberg, Averell Harriman, Rusk, and the Armed Forces Policy Council. He received an intelligence briefing at noon, met with Truman in the White House at 12:30, and then addressed the Women's National Press Club luncheon in the Hotel Statler at 1:00 p.m. Here he publicly labeled the Korean situation "very critical" but cautioned that "I know of no time when it is more important, though, that we are very calm and very careful and very wise in forming our conclusions. . . . The intense desire of all is to proceed in such a way that we can avoid a full world war," and that required both maintaining "a posture of sufficient strength" and making certain that "what we do must be very soberly thought out in the coldest, calmest, most calculating way we can handle and meet the matter." (GCMRL/G. C. Marshall Papers [Secretary of Defense, Speeches and Statements].) ★

165

NOTES ON NSC MEETING
November 28, 1950 Washington, DC

ACCORDING to the notes taken by Ambassador-at-Large Jessup, Acheson asked Marshall and Bradley to explain the military situation in Korea. Bradley said the JCS did not believe MacArthur presently needed a new directive, though he might in another two or three days. They also opposed military moves across the Yalu River border, with Bradley noting there were three hundred enemy aircraft in Manchuria that "could strike a severe blow" against vulnerable UN airfields and road convoys.

Marshall referred to a 10:00 a.m. meeting that morning he had held with Rusk and Harriman as well as the three service secretaries and the JCS (see previous document), during which he had asked the secretaries and Joint Chiefs to state and then to formulate their views. He then read the service secretaries' memorandum, which "proceeds on the following assumptions: We are engaged with other members of the UN in suppressing a Korean aggression. We are now faced by a new Chinese aggression. We should act through the UN and not individually. It is possible to hold a line. While the Chinese action is dictated in large measure by the Politburo we should not publicly hold the USSR responsible now. Our purposes are to fulfill our UN obligations but not to become individually or as a member of the UN involved in general war in China with Chinese Communists. To do this would be to fall into a carefully laid Russian trap. We should use all available political, economic and psychological action to limit the war. Strong military support is needed for the localized action. We should not go into Chinese Communist territory and we should not use Chinese Nationalist forces. To do either of these things would increase the danger of war with the Chinese Communists." Instead, he said, Washington needed "a more rapid build-up" in Western Europe and should increase the number of non-American UN troops in Korea "regardless of whether we have to pay for them." The administration should also press Congress immediately for the second supplemental 1951 appropriation, make clear more would be needed, revise the 1952 budget, and "accelerate production and production facilities as a matter of special emphasis." (This summary of assumptions is in Jessup's memorandum of the NSC meeting in *FRUS, 1950*, 7: 1243; the actual service secretaries' memorandum is in NA/RG 330, CD 092 [Korea].)

Marshall then commented on the paper by asserting that "There should be no cuts in the estimates of personnel and materiel needed. In the next two weeks we should work in the UN and maintain our position in Korea. We should not now try to change our budgetary figures. We should find a way to go along with the UN approach without involving injury to our troops. A very difficult question is the danger of Chinese aerial bombardment to which our troops are not accustomed. This would pose a most difficult question. The question on how to line up our allies in the UN is for the State Department. He stressed once more the view of the three secretaries that we should not get into war with the Chinese Communists.

He suggested that the general attitude in the UN would probably not complicate our decision in that respect." Bradley added that the JCS "feel just as strongly as the three secretaries that we should not be pulled into a war with the Chinese." Marshall then noted that while this was "a problem to be considered here in Washington . . . it would not be helpful to interfere in MacArthur's operations on the spot." (*FRUS, 1950*, 7: 1243–44.)

Discussion then shifted to MacArthur's "home by Christmas" statement, which Marshall labeled "an embarrassment which we must get around in some manner." He stated that the number of Chinese troops in Korea was "very much in excess of previous estimates." In response to Vice President Alben Barkley's fear of the Chinese sending even more men in, Marshall said that "we want to avoid getting sewed up in Korea" and did not know in that eventuality "how could we get out with honor." Acheson warned that "we were much closer to the danger of general war" and that the Soviets were behind the Chinese attack. Korea must be considered "not in isolation but in the world-wide problem of confronting the Soviet Union as an antagonist." He also "thought the memorandum of the three secretaries and the comments by General Marshall were very wise" and concurred with their conclusions. The United States needed to terminate the Korean conflict, not expand it, and must "find a line that we can hold, and hold it" as well as "liquidate the French objection to the development of a European Army." Truman mentioned what he labeled "the campaign of vilification and character assassination which has been going on in this country and that would constitute the best asset of the Soviet Union." He did not think it was presently desirable to send a special message to Congress "or have an individual approach to the problem pending UN action," but that he should "meet the campaign of vilification and lies in the United States." Later in the discussion Marshall defended MacArthur's decision to launch his offensive as "necessary in order to find out what the Communists were up to. Now we know." (Ibid., 1244–48.)

In line with the global strategy and emphasis on Western Europe expressed at this meeting, Marshall in a November 29 letter to Senate Foreign Relations Committee chair Tom Connally (D-TX) strongly supported Truman's request for funds to provide emergency food aid to Yugoslavia on the grounds that the existing food shortage would negatively affect the Yugoslav armed forces. "It appears desirable," Marshall noted, "that the largest armed force on the continent of Europe (over 30 divisions) outside of the USSR should remain militarily effective and friendly to the Western Powers." (Marshall to Connally, November 29, 1950, NA/RG 330, SD 091 [Yugoslavia].) ★

166

MEMORANDUM FOR
GENERAL OF THE ARMY OMAR N. BRADLEY
Confidential

November 29, 1950
Washington, DC

The President just telephoned me expressing the desire that all instructions to

General MacArthur from the Chiefs of Staff be processed through the Secretaryof Defense to the President personally. It is therefore directed that this procedure be followed. Please advise the Chiefs of Staff accordingly.[1]

NA/RG 330, CD 092 (Korea)

1. On November 29, MacArthur proposed to the JCS the use of Chinese Nationalist troops in Korea and asked that he be allowed to negotiate directly with the Nationalist government on this matter. On the same day, the press published a special communiqué he had issued that summarized his November 28 message to the JCS, including his statement that "we now face an entirely new war." (James F. Schnabel and Robert J. Watson, *The History of the Joint Chiefs of Staff: The Joint Chiefs of Staff and National Policy*, vol. 3, *The Korean War*, pt. 1 [Washington: Office of Joint History, Office of the Chairman of the Joint Chiefs of Staff, 1998], 152; Senate Committee on Armed Services and Committee on Foreign Relations, *Hearings to Conduct an Inquiry into the Military Situation in the Far East* [hereafter *MSFE*] . . . , 82d Cong., 1st sess., 3495.) It is unclear whether Truman's call to Marshall resulted from just the previous November 28 message and NSC meeting (see previous document), or these November 29 statements as well.

In consultation with the State and Defense Departments as well as the White House, the JCS informed MacArthur that his proposal was "being considered" but that it involved "world-wide consequences," including possible extension of the war to Formosa "and other areas" and rejection by the Allied powers that would leave the United States diplomatically isolated. The American "position of leadership in the Far East is being most seriously questioned" in the UN, and "utmost care will be necessary to avoid the disruption of the essential Allied line-up in that organization." (Schnabel and Watson, *History of JCS*, 3, pt. 1: 152–53; Harry S. Truman, *Memoirs*, vol. 2, *Years of Trial and Hope, 1946–1952* [Garden City, NY: Doubleday & Company, Inc., 1956], 384–85.)

167

To Millard E. Tydings — November 29, 1950
Radio. — Washington, DC

Lovett informs me your committee asked him the circumstances surrounding Mrs. Rosenberg's appointment as Assistant Secretary of Defense. I want you to know that I personally thought of her and selected her for the position without suggestion, or recommendation, or consultation from anyone. I advised no one, other than Lovett and Mrs. Rosenberg, of my selection until I talked to the President on Election Day.[1]

GCMRL/G. C. Marshall Papers (Secretary of Defense, Selected)

1. Marshall had probably informed Truman on November 7 of his intention to nominate Rosenberg during a 3:00 p.m. meeting at the White House. He then told the press on November 9 and 10. (See pp. 232–33.)

Rosenberg had been serving on a recess appointment since November 15. See photo #6. Congress received her nomination as well as that of Lovett, who had been serving on a recess appointment since October 4, when it reconvened on November 27. On November 29, the Senate confirmed Lovett after the Armed Services Committee had unanimously recommended that it do so. That afternoon at 3:45 p.m., the committee opened its hearings on Rosenberg, during which Tydings announced that he had received this telegram from Marshall earlier in the day and inserted it into the record, along with Marshall's November 10 statement to the press and the November 9 press release. (Senate Committee on Armed Services, *Nomination of Anna M. Rosenberg to be Assistant Secretary of Defense*, 81st

Cong., 2d sess., 8–9.) The committee recommended Rosenberg's confirmation, but then reconsidered in December as a result of allegations regarding supposed communist associations. (See pp. 296–97.)

168

STENOGRAPHIC TRANSCRIPT OF INFORMAL REMARKS AT THE DINNER IN HONOR OF CHAIM WEIZMANN

November 29, 1950
New York, New York

Mr. Chairman, Ladies and Gentlemen: I am very much impressed with this gathering, setting, music, general effect and purpose, this twin anniversary of the birthday of your great leader, Doctor Weizmann, and the anniversary of the decision of the United Nations three years ago.[1] I believe all the friendly people of the world were deeply touched by the drama of the return of the children of Israel to their Promised Land, a return which was made with great courage and determination, and a powerful purpose and will to succeed. It carried with it pioneers who entered into the problem of the development and settlement of very desolate lands in a most remarkable manner. I find that automatically I always turn in my own mind to events in the history of their country in order to measure an appreciation of somewhat similar events that are occurring today.

And in thinking of the three short years of the existence of the sovereign State of Israel, I look back to refresh my mind as to the first three years of our country under its present Constitution, which began in 1789. They were years beset with difficult, baffling problems of literally every kind, and at the end of the three year period—this being the end of the three year period of the life of the sovereign State of Israel—in this country in 1792 there were frontier difficulties of tremendous importance. Along the Great Lakes there were military posts that had not yet been evacuated by our recent opponent in the Revolutionary War. The treaty of peace was still two years distant, three years after we started in business, as it were.[2]

In the South, Spain was contesting for frontiers in Florida, and was also contesting with us the right to navigation on the Mississippi River. This was happening at the end of the first three years of our struggle into our present position in the world. And there were areas greatly disturbed by Indian uprisings, and there was every conceivable problem of currency, taxes, tariffs, pensions, a world of other difficulties.[3]

So it is against that background that I try to measure in my mind what has occurred in the State of Israel and conclude that truly remarkable progress has been made (Applause).

The people of Israel have had great problems, political, economic and sociological in nature, and many others that remain to be overcome before you approach the ideal of those who have built this great prospect. Dr. Weizmann, in whose honor this dinner is occurring tonight, I first came to know in Washington in the very depressing, dangerous years of 1942 and, as I recall, I was introduced to him by the gentleman who just introduced me tonight, the then Secretary of the Treasury.[4]

Dr. Weizmann had come to this country to add his voice to the urgent requests of the British Parliament and British leaders for assistance and materiel to meet the threat to the Middle East, to Cairo, to Oran in Africa. We had very little to offer there. We were in dire necessity of materiel for our army that we were attempting to build up. However, we managed to scrape together some important materiel and dispatch it with all possible speed to the Middle East. The fact that a great victory was won was ample, bountiful reward for whatever we were able to do at the time.[5]

I might interject here this comment, this additional comment, that I have made a number of times recently. This seems to be where I came in before. When I talk about materiel even now I feel the same pressure. The same necessities that were urgent then exist again, and I am at the recipient end of many requests. In many respects there has been very little change.

I think many have forgotten the very honorable and courageous part that was taken by units of the Jews of Palestine in the fighting that occurred at that time ("Applause"). And how much was done from Palestine by the Jews of that region to assist and contribute to the general effort to suppress the Nazis. And, further than that, the numerous acts of real gallantry of the Jews who were parachuted in the rear of the Nazi lines to carry out the most dangerous missions! All of that is part of history, too apt to be forgotten in the present struggles. But it all goes into the makeup and toward the future development of a nation which will build up in strength, I feel certain, to resist Communist aggression, to maintain the peace in its region, and to make a very genuine contribution in the world for peace and security generally.

I hope, in conquering the remaining preliminary difficulties of national life, that the State of Israel will early arrive at that degree of independence where it can sustain itself out of itself, and where its prosperity will enable it to raise the standard of living of its people to the point that they would desire. Along with that prosperity will come a benevolence in attitude which will enable them to forget the scars of the strife and tribulations leading up to the organization of the State which will lead to the contribution of their great developments to the other peoples nearby who are in so much need of the same general developments, to develop productive land, where now it is arid and desolate.

That brings me to the main purpose, I understand, of this dinner meeting, this gathering which is for the benefit of your three higher schools, and the one of which I have particular interest—the Weizmann Institute of Science. There I understand very special efforts are being made to develop a technique and an ability to convert arid districts into bountiful lands.[6]

I know you are all intensely, I might say desperately, interested in events in Korea. I am restrained from making very general comments because of the fact that the issues are now under immediate consideration here in your neighborhood at Lake Success, and it would be most inappropriate for me to be commenting at any length as to the details of the various points of view.[7]

The situation is critical. We must do everything we can to get it in hand, and I am sure everything will be done, but we look with the most intense interest to the consideration and decision, action, stand, of the United Nations.

Our forces in Korea consists of representatives of a great many countries. Our own United States troops, naturally, are the larger part, along with those recently organized Korean units. And they all suffered throughout the campaign very heavily in casualties, both battle casualties and other casualties incident to the particular characteristics of that campaign, both as to its movements and as to terrain.

All of this, and the tension that has been created in the world by the incidents that have developed there, by the fact of the invasion of South Korea, have produced a very critical issue for us here, and for all the world.

Our Congress has just come into session, and it will be necessary for its members to consider immediately certain measures to enable us, in this country, to carry out the actions that seem urgently required at this particular time. We are very much in need of an intelligent understanding on the part of the public as to just what the situation is as to ourselves, and as to our abilities—our capabilities I should say—at this time, and what is needed from the Congress of the United States and the administration. I am going to take a moment of your time to try, if I can, to make clear to you several points that I regard of great importance.

In the first place, we are in a situation which is different, I believe, from any in which we have ever been situated heretofore. And it imposes something for which we were not prepared. I am talking about what we call a partial mobilization. Now to the average person, it would seem a very simple proposition, that if you build on a basis of either peace on the one side, or total mobilization for war on the other, ~~a simple proposition~~ to scale that down the ladder to a temporary point of partial mobilization.[8] It is not at all so. It is an intensely complicated and difficult proceeding, and requires the action, in a great many particulars, of the Congress of the United States. Our laws and regulations growing out of those laws, pertaining to what is the largest part of any definitive force that we have must be adapted to fit the present situation. Our civilian components, for instance, are based on a peacetime setting or a full war mobilization. Those laws never anticipated that we would have a long period of tension in which we take our men away from their homes, their families, their business, and do not know for how long—in a period that is not war.

It is quite evident that at the very best we are faced by a long period of tension. All the agreements in the world that we seek to get, and that we are trying most earnestly to get, we could not accept them all in a moment, and abandon our defensive posture. We would have to wait until good faith is demonstrated.

So I say, at the very best, we have to face a long period of tension. That is something the American public has never been called upon to do. We had a tension, a tension in 1939 and 1940 and 1941. It was a tension during which there was a world war. All of Europe was swamped, as you know so tragically, as pertaining to the Jews in particular, and yet in the midst of that tension, in the midst of the measures we took which actually were a full mobilization, both as to men and materiel, we only saved those forces by a single vote in August of 1941.[9] Now we are facing a tension which we hope and pray will not involve any great destructive war such as was going on at that time. How will our public respond to that?

We are involved in the procedure of a partial mobilization in a setting which must see itself automatically and almost instantaneously to a full mobilization if that becomes necessary, but which, at the moment, I would think would be ill-advised.

How do we go about it? How do we set up such a procedure that the American public will continue to accept and to support? By adopting an enduring system of national defense.

I have used the word "enduring." We have got to have something that is "enduring," that the public will continue to support even when there is not the great excitement, the great tragedies that bring about an emotional rise for the moment. We must not create mountains and then drop down into valleys again.

We are unanimous—yes, I think there is complete unanimity, in the feeling that we must immediately build up our strength. But we must be very careful not to set up a mountain which will inevitably slough off into a valley of weakness. We must find an enduring method that pertains to the materiel proposition. Putting it briefly, we must have a setting that is rapidly expandable. That means assembly lines of a nature and the tools and the dies and jigs and everything of that sort that will enable us quickly to increase production as it is now needed, and not just set about building up great piles of things, you might say, in numbers and then having them grow obsolescent.

Great standing forces of this country, we have never had except in the state of full mobilization as in 1941, and then we almost lost them right in the middle of a great crisis. We have to have some system that will have the support of the American public always. We know what is required in such a system. It must be of such a nature that it provides the reserves that you need almost instantly, prepared to act, and yet is of such a nature that it does not beggar us financially. I can illustrate that a little bit by what happened in Korea, and I can talk rather frankly about that because I was not a part of it. I did not come into the Government until the effort of the Northern Koreans had nearly collapsed because of the landing near Seoul. In fact, I came in, ~~I think about ten days, two weeks or three~~ five days after that.[10]

So I was not a party to that campaign. What happened presented a dilemma that approached the catastrophic because we did not have available trained reserves. I am not talking about numerous divisions. I am talking about men, individuals. We only had four divisions, in Japan, and, of course, those were the first moved into Korea. It was quite a time before any other troops came to their assistance, other than the South Koreans themselves. Those four divisions were about half-strength, but if they had been of full strength they would have numbered about 72,000 men.

General MacArthur had to put into the ranks of those American units 30,000 quickly trained South Koreans. We took 17 weeks during the war to train replacements, individuals, and that was about a twelve hour day. In fact, I received many complaints from individuals, from parents, and from leaders in political life that this was too strenuous, and yet that was 17 weeks and it was thought to be too little. MacArthur had to put 30,000 Koreans into a 72,000-man organization with three weeks training. He had to create South Korean divisions in four weeks, yet it took some of our divisions in World War II two years before we thought they were in shape to send to Europe.

Our Selective Service Act which is in effect a compulsory service act, produces the authority but is afflicted by the number of deferments under the law and under the regulations which limit very decidedly the number of men that can be called. Certain changes, I think, will have to be made, and I don't anticipate much difficulty in their being made.[11]

I was rather interested to have brought to my attention in relation to this gathering tonight, that apparently, historically Moses was the architect of compulsory service. However, this amused me a little bit, and I'll explain later why. He had deferments that would not be at all acceptable today. In the first place he deferred—let out—all those weak in spirit, quite evidently feeling that there were not too many of them and they would not be worth much anyway. He deferred the builder of the house if he had not yet dedicated it. He deferred even the young man who was betrothed to the young lady, but had not yet taken her over.[12]

I was thinking when this was brought to my attention of the immediate problem of the new Assistant Secretary of Defense, your protegee, Anna Rosenberg. When I left her today, she was in the middle of a struggle of deferments and she would have disagreed completely with Moses. We are suffering from a plague of deferments.

I might say in regard to her that she has already done very fine work and is on the way to do very splendid work. I had known her, had been aware of her ability, personality, courage, her necessary toughness and the fact that quite evidently she was the leading individual in this country in relation to manpower. There was some surprise when her name was put forward. There is less surprise now around the Pentagon. I have been sorry to learn that there have been various rumors and allegations as to the influences that put Anna Rosenberg in office. The truth is I selected her because she, quite evidently to me, was the leading individual I know of to do what I found was a very pressing and magnificent job. I found on my back at least five different sections of the Pentagon coming at me in relation to manpower—manpower for the military forces, manpower for the Munitions Board, manpower to industry, manpower in relation to the various personnel we had outside of the fighting forces, manpower in relation to the scientists, to the engineers, to the doctors, all of those various groups, and their relation to the National Guard and to research. It was a phantasmagoria of various influences in connection with manpower. Anna Rosenberg seemed to be the person for the job. I did not consult anybody.[13]

So she came into office in the Defense Department in a very critical operation and in a very critical time through her own ability, pure and simple.

I have been very much touched by the generous references to me here tonight. I have enjoyed renewal of associations I have had in the past here among many of those at this table and I am very appreciative of the reception that you have given me.

Thank you.

GCMRL/G. C. Marshall Papers (Secretary of Defense, Speeches and Statements)

1. Weizmann had been the president of Israel since the nation declared independence on May 14, 1948. (See *Papers of GCM*, 6: 459–60.) The UN General Assembly had approved the partition of Palestine on November 29, 1947. This dinner in Weizmann's honor, held at the Waldorf-Astoria Hotel in New York on his seventy-sixth birthday and the third anniversary of the General Assembly vote, was organized by the American Committee for the Hebrew University, the Weizmann Institute of Science, and the Technion, Israel's three institutes of higher education. The three were known collectively as UIT (University-Institute-Technicon), which had been organized under its president, Albert Einstein, in January 1950 "to enlist support in this country for Israel's three institutions of higher learning." ("Marshall to Speak Here," *New York Times*, November 26, 1950, p. 31.)

2. Marshall is referring here to Jay's Treaty, signed in 1794 and ratified in 1795, in which the British agreed to evacuate these posts.

3. Spain at this time controlled both Florida and Louisiana. It claimed that the boundary between Florida and the United States was the 33rd parallel of latitude, not the 31st as the Americans claimed, and it denied American citizens the right to navigate the Mississippi River or deposit their goods at the port of New Orleans. Britain and Spain also supported Indian resistance to American westward expansion.

4. Henry Morgenthau Jr. had been the secretary of the treasury during World War II.

5. Weizmann had met with Marshall on July 4, 1942. See *Papers of GCM*, 3: 267–68. For the war materiel sent after German General Erwin Rommel's conquest of Tobruk, which took place during a June 1942 Anglo-American summit conference in Washington, see ibid., 245–50. Consisting of three hundred new tanks and one hundred self-propelled guns sent by fast convoy, this materiel helped the British halt Rommel's advance through Libya and Egypt and achieve a decisive victory at the October battle of El Alamein.

6. The Weizmann Institute of Science had begun discussions with associates at Harvard University to develop a method for purifying the wealth of brackish water beneath the Negev, a vast desert in southern Israel, to support the growing population of the country. ("Scientific Work in Israel Praised," *New York Times*, April 29, 1951, p. 26.)

7. See pp. 259–61.

8. These words—and those crossed out below and discussed in n10 below—were deleted in the source text by use of the "x" letter of the typewriter.

9. In August of 1941, the bill to extend the service of draftees, which was about to expire, passed the House of Representatives by a vote of 203–202.

10. The Inchon landing near Seoul took place on September 15; Marshall was sworn in as secretary of defense on September 21 (see pp. 167–68), which probably accounts for the crossed out words in this sentence.

11. President Truman had signed into law the Selective Service Act of 1948 on June 24, 1948, which required one year of peacetime military service from those men inducted into the armed forces between the ages of nineteen and twenty-five. For more, see pp. 325–29 and 338–47.

12. Also deferred were those under the age of twenty, those who had planted a vineyard but not yet harvested it, and those who had been married less than a year. See Numbers 1:1–4 and Deuteronomy 20:1–9 and 24:5.

13. See previous document.

169

Transcript of Remarks at the National Preparedness Orientation Conference[1]

November 30, 1950
Washington, DC

I might say in starting, gentlemen, that I do not think of anything at the moment that I will say that may not be repeated. If anything comes up of that nature while I am talking, I will refer to it at the time.

I also would like to explain that I am only going to skim over the surface because I do not want to be covering a subject in a very rough manner that is going to be covered in rather exact detail later on by General Gruenther and by Mr. Nitze of the State Department. I will not go into the economic problem myself.[2]

I think probably the best way for me to start is to explain that we are in a very difficult situation, militarily. There are world-wide hazards because we have had no basis of preparation for a partial mobilization.

Now, that seems to be a very innocent statement, but it is one representing tremendous difficulties, complications, irritations, and public reactions at the present time.

Heretofore, in our history we have been either on a peace basis—however weak that was—or on a full mobilization basis.

When we go to full mobilization, which is a terrific undertaking in so many respects, it is necessarily somewhat wasteful and very disturbing to the whole public. Yet, when we go into that, we all go together and, in one respect, it is a rather simple procedure because it is all-out everywhere. How long we can maintain that all-out state is something else in relation to the public reactions, which I'll refer to later. When we are on peacetime status, you of course are familiar with our difficulties in procuring the necessary funds, the struggles we have, the criticisms of military expenses in this field or in that field, and things of that nature.

Now, today, we are confronted by a situation—very, very critical and of an increasingly critical nature—We could meet it by all-out mobilization which would be a relatively simple adjustment for the Department of Defense but I think it would be too precipitate to take that line of action.

I feel that we should develop a workable system of partial mobilization from which we can move with great rapidity into a full mobilization. The degree of partial mobilization is something else. It becomes a matter of degree, once we can set the base and get the laws rearranged and take other steps that will permit us to do this.

The background of all of this is the fact that our whole military system or posture, is based on a citizen Army. We have a National Guard of 27 divisions and some 20 combat teams. A combat team consists of about 5,000 men, an infantry, regiment, artillery, engineers, to make a little independent machine in the next degree below a division. It is different from a brigade, as those of you know who have some military experience, in that a brigade is one unit all infantry, or all artillery, but a combat team is a composite unit of about 5,000 men of war strength of all ground troops. So there are 27 divisions and 20 combat teams and a great many special units of one kind or another excluding the air components, that is the large part of our great citizen soldiery. We have a considerable number of Reserves, of individuals, as officers, and then we have the necessity of bringing into the armed forces by means of the Selective Service Act, whatever its terms are at the time, the necessary men to fill these units up, to keep them filled after you once get them going, and to organize all new units. That is a long time-consuming process, but the basis of all our procedure has been a citizen Army.

At the present time in considering any degree of a partial mobilization, we find the laws are not adapted to that purpose. I am not criticizing Congress. I am not criticizing the public. I am not criticizing the Pentagon. Nobody had quite the vision to see that we were going to be faced with a period of long tension requiring partial mobilization. We hope—because the very best that we can hope for at the present time as I see it and as my associates see it—is a prolonged tension. That is the best we can hope for. And even if we got every agreement in the world in the next six months, we would be very foolish to drop our guard immediately until there was time to prove good faith. So our best hope is a "tension."

How long will the American public carry themselves through this tension, making the necessary contributions and sacrifices to maintain what we feel is a necessary military set-up, both as to individuals and as to materiel? Well, when it comes to that, I find differences of opinion.

I can best explain one of them by a conversation that took place shortly after I came into the building here and that has been very recent. I might say at this point that I was completely cut off—not exactly cut off, but I held myself apart from defense activities when I was out. I was going to stay out and not be halfway in and halfway out. Now, I am all the way in! In that conversation—a high official here in the building said, "Do you consider that I am naive to say that the American public has learned its lesson?" We were disagreeing as to what had to be done. I will come to that later when I am talking about an enduring system. And I said, "I don't think you are naive. I just think you are incredibly naive, because when you come to this tension and it becomes a monotonous tension without all of the excitement that keeps booming up such tensions, the bottom will drop out, unless we have completely changed."[3]

I have gone through, personally, some very destructive periods. Maybe I have been bumped too often and am not a good guide, but I saw the destruction of 1920, when General Pershing, with all his prestige, was utterly unable to do anything to save even the remnants of what we call a ground force. I was with him at the time. He could not do anything and at times could not even see the President, because during the greatest period of false prosperity—I do not want to get into political—economic difficulties here—which blew up in '29, we had the Army in some places living in tents with their wives and families and they had been in tents from 1919 to 1932 through that booming period of prosperity. We could not get anything. We just had, literally, no Army at all.[4]

Then, when we had a buildup of the air force due to the Baker Board, Congress did not provide the added personnel required.[5] We had to take them out of this vanishing ground force and reductions kept on. We lost the third battalion of the infantry regiment. We lost half the companies. We lost the headquarters companies, and finally lost the bands. In one case, we had no money to move a regiment which we wanted to get to Fort Snelling, Minnesota—And at Fort Sill, Oklahoma it lost one battalion. A little further it lost half the strength of the companies and, finally, after five or six days it lost 1,200 more men. It never even reached Fort Snelling! It simply went out of existence.

You forget all that but that happens often with the American public. If you doubt that statement, let me recite this. I took over a command after this complete debilitation when we could not even really train. It was like having a football team with a center and quarterback and no guards, tackles, or ends. You can not practice much of a game on that basis. That is about what we had. That was the command I had.

When I had been head of the big infantry school in Georgia we had 400 or 500 officers in training from brigadier general, down to second lieutenant. Now I went off to a big command. It was independent. That was good, but it had only 200 or 300 men in it. I had the command closed down as a unit and put all the men together. I took all the cooks, truck drivers, and men of all sorts and actually got a company of 140 men out for drill. I had no communications. I had none of the radio devices everybody is so insistent on now, none of the small guns, even the little Stokes mortars, weapons of that sort. We had no men for that. That was the kind of a force we had.[6]

Later in the fall of '38 I came in and inherited the responsibility for that mess as Deputy Chief of Staff. Then I became Chief of Staff in the summer of '39 so I know a good bit about American changing attitudes toward national defense. I have been with the "patient" through some very strenuous, difficult days in his illness.[7]

Then we came to another example in August 1941 when the insistent demand all over the country was for the return of the National Guardsmen to their homes, the return of the Selective Servicemen to their homes. Had we complied, we would have had nothing left. We protected the National Guard against having its men drawn away from it, gave it a full year to train, and filled its ranks with Selective Service men. The Regular Army was entirely ripped to pieces. It had to provide men to the Pacific Islands, to this place, and to that place, and only had from 20 to 75 men of the original stock in any regiment and almost no equipment. The average antiaircraft regiment only had part of one battery for training. We had to send men to the Hawaiian Islands, the Philippines—we had to send National Guard units because we had used up our regular forces on other equally important assignments. In August 1941, in the middle of a World War with all Europe under the Nazis and with this situation in the Army that I have described, we saved that Army from complete, utter, entire disintegration by one vote in Congress. So when I say that it was incredibly naive to believe that America has learned its lesson I create my own lesson, but I had a graduation exercise, too.[8]

When I came in as Deputy Chief of Staff and later as Chief of Staff, we had 15 flying fortresses without enough money to maintain them or enough gasoline to do the appropriate flying. In my last week as Chief of Staff here in the fall of 1945, I signed the agreement for the destruction of 2,700 of these fortresses. That is a considerable bracket—from 15 and not enough money for them, to the destruction of 2,700 of them for very evident, logical reasons.

And then the great demobilization was on with which you are all familiar. I am more familiar with the pressure to produce that demobilization than you are because I had to go before Congress twice to try to save this situation in some way. It was a tidal wave for demobilization.[9]

Now, we are confronted at the very best with a period of long tension, we hope—we hope.

Now, what do we do about it? First what is the situation? That will be described to you in detail here. What do we do about it? That is the next issue.

There are several factors to consider. I have said a little about partial mobilization, which is such a critical matter. It has gotten us in trouble with the National Guard and gotten us in trouble with the Reserves. They pour letters in to us every day, and our latest—I can't call a "recruit," because she's far above that—our latest recruit here though, Anna Rosenberg—she has that manpower problem all in her lap. . . .[10]

I have just given you the items of our own deficiencies of our own soldiers at the present time. You can not get soldiers in a minute. It is not a question of "springing to arms over night," as Mr. Bryan once said.[11] It is a long tedious process and you have to have a system. You have to have a method or you are sunk, especially if we get into any large affair. We got out of this one by a miracle, as far as we have gotten out.

General MacArthur was also creating divisions of Koreans. The tendency is to look at the title "division" and think of it as a great big, powerfully trained unit like these with which Patton swept through France in 1944.[12] We were, in some cases, almost two years getting our units over to France, almost two years getting them up to the point where they could give a satisfactory account of themselves. MacArthur was organizing a division every four weeks, and those are the Korean divisions you read about. And when you see they have given back here and given back there—remember that they have done pretty well to do what they have done. They are good fighters.[13]

It has been a desperate procedure from start to finish because, for the first time—*for the first time*, we had to fight the first week, and we know that, if there's a second time, it will be the first day. These developments give you some idea of what our situation is in a relatively "little" campaign, how critical it is, how great the losses are despite the fact that we are engaged, with complete naval control of the waters, with complete air on our side, and yet we have the troubles that you read about in the paper.

Now, what seems to me so important—and this gets into the whole procedure of material procurement which interests the industrialists and interests labor—is that we do not pick up an emotional wave, just build a mountain and then slide right off into a valley again. We have got to figure out how long the people will be able to carry the load. Of what nature must it be in order for the American public to carry it along? We must have an enduring system. We have got to build up. There is a complete unanimity about that. We have got to build up now as rapidly as we can. But we have got to have a system, in doing so. We just must not fall of our own weight with the boredom of the public to a prolonged tension into another catastrophic state of great weakness, which in the present state of the world would be terrible.

What is an enduring system that will endure through these various fluctuations and through this evident period of long tension that is in front of us? If we are thrown under the necessity of full mobilization in one respect, terrible as it is, we can meet it but we have to have an enduring system, one that can be taken and carried on without a collapse of public support.

As to materiel, we have got to procure great quantities of materiel and get them quickly, as rapidly as we can, for ourselves, Western Europe and ourselves, and others, but particularly for Western Europe and ourselves.

Now, there are ways of doing that. We can just pile it up, you might say, and get into the numbers racket, which is what we were pressed with, all the time in 1939 and 1940. What we do want is a basis of rapid increase of production. I will express it in simpler terms this way—It is far better for us to begin at once with existing assembly lines on a 40-hour week, an eight-hour day, and double or treble the shifts to get production going rather than wait for the construction of new lines which in their stride could increase the flow of munitions 600 per cent. We have got to get materiel quickly, right now, and build up a certain peak,—but in such a way that we do not get to the top and then fall to the bottom. Everybody wants some security in the continuity of the procedure. We are more interested in such continuity even than the industrialists and even labor. We have got to get—I keep repeating that word—an "enduring" system.

We have another aspect in addition to the partial mobilization and the enduring system of defense which requires great understanding on the part of all the leading citizens in this country that you will hear about in detail later. That is the United Nations. I just want to make one or two comments about it. You could almost say we are fighting in Korea under a committee of about fifty nations. It was tough enough when we were fighting in World War II under a committee of two nations with the Combined Chiefs of Staff.[14] We rode through all of our troubles. One of the most notable examples pertained to the Battle of the Bulge, which we had to work out together.

Now, we are in a situation where it is paramount, as I see it and my associates see it, that we have a common front among many nations, if there is any conceivable way to find it, because we must not be alone in the world. We must have allies with us, and they have a world of different ideas, a world of different confidences, and when you get into trouble—we are in difficulty now; anybody who reads the paper can find that—that makes unity all the more difficult. We have got to maintain a solid front.

I remember when I was Secretary of State I was being pressed constantly, particularly when in Moscow, by radio message after radio message to give the Russians hell. It looked like a regular message where they put "No. 2" and then send it. When I got back, I was getting the same appeal in relation to the Far East and China. At that time, my facilities for giving them hell—and I am a soldier and know something about the ability to give hell—was 1 1/3 divisions over the entire United States. That is quite a proposition when you deal with somebody with over 260 and you have 1 1/3. We had nothing in Alaska. We did not have enough to defend the air strip up at Fairbanks. We had to do something and got into arguments of every kind. We started rebuilding, being Americans, and got into all kinds of discussions, remember—the B-36 and the big carriers and all that stuff.[15]

Actually, the great problem was how you were going to manage the maintenance and the replacement of those great air fortresses. Battleships, fortunately, last a considerable period of years, and carriers presumably last a long time. A degree of obsolescence or complete obsolescence is always possible particularly if the other fellow develops something that is more effective. So your great problems was basically an economic problem, how you were going to meet the problem of replacements. You must proceed in some way that the country can support. The controversies of a year ago reflect the way we get off on all kinds of tangents. That is natural and likely to prove very difficult in the next few months while we are trying to find ourselves and get together because that is very important. Understanding is the most important aspect of the problem. I am trying to contribute a little bit along that line. What I have been saying is a rather heterogeneous approach to the general problem, but, if I had made two points clear to you—the question of the complications involved in partial mobilization and the necessity of an enduring procedure—why, then I have discharged my functions so far as this particular meeting is concerned.

I appreciate very much—and I know your Chairman here, Symington, does—your coming down here. I think it can have a tremendous beneficial, important effect generally in this country. Thank you.

GCMRL/G. C. Marshall Papers (Secretary of Defense, Speeches and Statements)

1. The conference would include off-the-record discussions with ninety members of industry, labor, and agriculture "to give information to the leaders of these three groups on the seriousness of the situation in order to have a better understanding of our military and international problems and their effect on civilian economy." It took place in the Pentagon and began at 10:00 a.m. with brief welcoming remarks by Symington, followed by Marshall. (Rosenberg to Marshall, November 22, 1950, NA/RG 330, SD 337 [National Preparedness Conference].) According to a *New York Times* account on the following day, 125 individuals attended this all-day closed meeting. ("Symington Notes Defense Speed-up," *New York Times*, December 1, 1950, p. 11.)

2. Paul H. Nitze and Lieutenant General Alfred M. Gruenther (USMA, 1918), deputy army chief of staff, spoke after Marshall on the international political and military situations, respectively. Also scheduled to speak were Lovett and Leon Keyserling, head of the Council of Economic Advisers. ("Symington Notes Defense Speed-up," *New York Times*, December 1, 1950, p. 11; memorandum for Marx Leva, November 27, 1950, NA/RG 330, SD 337 [National Preparedness Conference].)

3. This conversation took place with Frank Pace following his return from the October 15, 1950, Wake Island conference. (See pp. 186–87.) In an oral history interview with Marshall's biographer, Forrest C. Pogue, Pace recalled Marshall confessing that MacArthur's statement that the Korean War would "'be over by Thanksgiving and the boys home by Christmas . . . troubles me,'" because "'The American people have not learned the meaning of a cold war. They are not aware of the fact that we're going to be engaged in this kind of struggle in one way or another over a long period of time and that our old determinations of what war means have to be revised in the light of the world in which we live.' 'And,' he said, 'the American people need to learn the nature of permanent war and permanent strength in a society.'" When Pace asked if he was "'naive if I said the American people had learned their lesson'" regarding the rapid demobilization after World War II, Marshall "looked at me with those cold blue eyes and said, 'No, Pace, I wouldn't say you were naive, I would say that you're incredibly naive.'" (GCMRL/Oral History Collection, tape 42, interview with Pace, April 1, 1959, and March 23, 1975, p. 28.)

4. For Marshall's work under Pershing and the controversies regarding army reorganization legislation that culminated in the National Defense Act of 1920, see *Papers of GCM*, 1: 182–83, 193–94, 200; and Forrest C. Pogue, *George C. Marshall*, vol. 1, *Education of a General, 1880–1939* (New York: Viking, 1963), 203–15.

5. See p. 166n3.

6. See p. 253n2. After he left Fort Benning in June 1932, Marshall was appointed commander of a battalion of the Eighth Infantry at Fort Screven in Georgia.

7. Marshall had been appointed deputy army chief of staff on October 16, 1938, and chief of staff on September 1, 1939, though he had been acting chief of staff since July 1.

8. See the previous document n9.

9. For Marshall's testimonies on demobilization, see *Papers of GCM*, 5: 229–31 and 311–13.

10. Seven paragraphs regarding Anna Rosenberg, Moses, draft deferment, and MacArthur's use of Korean soldiers that repeated statements Marshall made in his remarks in the previous document have been omitted here. See pp. 266–67.

11. The claim that "a million men would spring to arms overnight" if the United States was endangered has been attributed to William Jennings Bryan of Nebraska, three-time Democratic presidential candidate and secretary of state under Woodrow Wilson.

12. General George S. Patton (USMA, 1909) commanded the Third Army in 1944 and 1945.

13. For more on the Korean divisions, see pp. 341–42.

14. The Anglo-American Combined Chiefs of Staff directed the war effort of all US and British ground, naval, and air forces during World War II.

15. Marshall is referring here to the conflict between the air force and navy culminating in the so-called "revolt of the admirals" that took place in 1949 under former Defense Secretary Johnson.

"EVERYTHING leads to the conclusion the Chinese forces have as their objective the complete destruction of United Nations forces and the securing of all of Korea," MacArthur warned the JCS in the early morning hours of November 30. (*FRUS, 1950*, 7: 1260.) In a press conference later that morning, Truman responded to a question regarding the possible use of the atomic bomb by stating that "There has always been active consideration of its use," though "I don't want to see it used." (Ibid., 1260–61; Harry S. Truman, *Public Papers of the Presidents: Harry S. Truman, 1950* [Washington: GPO, 1965], 727.) That led British Prime Minister Clement Attlee to propose an immediate visit to Washington to confer with Truman. (See pp. 284–87; *FRUS, 1950*, 7: 1269.) Simultaneously

Acheson met with Lovett and requested a meeting with Marshall, the JCS, and CIA Director Smith. (Ibid., 1270–71.)

That meeting took place at 8:30 a.m. the following morning, December 1, in the Pentagon. Also in attendance were Harriman and numerous State Department officials. Acheson warned of a "state of panic which seemed to exist among our friends" at the UN that needed to be addressed and asked "if a line could be established from a military point of view." Bradley responded that it was too soon to tell and that much depended upon whether the X Corps in eastern North Korea at Wonsan could successfully regroup. Collins concurred and said "someone" should be sent to Japan immediately to assess the situation. Marshall agreed that Collins should go and that it would be "hard to establish a line" and "not a practicable proposition." After additional discussion of that along with the possibility of obtaining and accepting a cease-fire—which Marshall thought "would represent a great weakness on our part," Smith asserted that the Russians' primary aim was to "defeat European rearmament. They probably do not plan on war now but are willing to have it if they can bog us down in Asia. They will never accept a Korea in hostile hands. We should get out of Korea even though we do not solve the problem by getting out." (Ibid., 1279.) Lovett then summarized "a consensus on two points: first, that Korea is not a decisive area for us; and second that while the loss of Korea might jeopardize Japan and bring about its eventual loss, Western Europe was our prime concern and we would rather see that result than lose in Western Europe." It was "best to hold in Korea for political moves" if possible, but Western Europe came first. (Ibid., 1276–81.) In line with this conclusion, conversation then shifted to the defense of Western Europe, a discussion "capped," according to Acheson, by Marshall's "abrupt, authoritative statement that it was no use talking about divisions, integrated forces, or commanders until we faced and solved the problem whether we wished to moderate our present determined ('one package') stand." (Dean Acheson, *Present at the Creation: My Years in the State Department* [New York: W. W. Norton, 1969], 473.) See also pp. 167–68 and 184.

Marshall then attended a cabinet meeting at the White House, followed by an executive session meeting regarding Korea that the president held with House and Senate leaders. He then returned to his office for a series of afternoon meetings and at 1:35 p.m. departed for the Capitol. ★

170

House Testimony on the Second Supplemental Appropriation Bill for 1951
December 1, 1950 Washington, DC

ON DECEMBER 1, Marshall, Lovett, the JCS, and Brigadier General Robert S. Moore, USA, special assistant to the Defense Department comptroller, testified before the Special Subcommittee on National Defense Appropriations of the House Committee on Appropriations, which was then considering Truman's request for an additional and speedy appropriation of $17.98 billion. (House Committee on Appropriations, *Hearings . . . on Second Supplemental Appropriation Bill for 1951*, 81st Cong., 2d sess., 1–15.) These funds were to be used not only for increased expenditures in Korea due to the Chinese intervention, but also for the major and global military buildup proposed in April in NSC 68 and approved by the National Security Council and Truman at the end of September. (Condit, *Test of War*, 227–40.)

Marshall informed the subcommittee that he had no prepared statement and agreed with chair George H. Mahon (D-TX) that Bradley should speak first to provide "an outline of the situation"—to include not only Korea, but also Europe, Indochina, and the Middle East as well. Bradley did so off the record, after which Marshall, Lovett, and the members of the JCS answered a series of questions from Mahon and other committee members. Marshall made clear that there would probably be additional requests for funds during the remainder of the fiscal year, with Lovett noting that this was "not a war or a full mobilization budget. It is an initial step in a planned 4-year effort to restore our military posture" so as to provide both a deterrent and a base for a rapid buildup "in case of all-out war." It had been prepared in mid-November—before the most recent Chinese attacks in Korea—and would not be sufficient "if we suffer reverses in Korea or elsewhere." (*Hearings*, 16–20, quotes on 20.)

When Mahon asked if the government was "doing everything in its power to avoid an all-out shooting war with Red China," Marshall said yes and added that this had involved "considerable sacrifice." Did Marshall agree, Mahon then asked, that such an all-out war was something the United States "cannot permit to happen." Marshall responded that "We are trying to avoid, in every way that is conceivably within reason, being projected into an all-out war; and at the same time we realize that an all-out war can be initiated by a single word from the other side." Was there hope that such an all-out war could be averted? Marshall replied affirmatively with the saying "While there's life there's hope." He also emphasized the psychological as well as financial costs of a lengthy full-scale mobilization without full-scale war and made clear that he "would feel very much concerned if we plunge into an all-out wartime mobilization until we clearly have to do it," but "even more concerned if we did not establish a well-laid foundation and base for a very rapid mobilization if that becomes necessary."(Ibid., 24–25.)

Other questions concerned specific appropriations for such matters as the research and development program, with Marshall noting that it had led to the bringing of about fifty leading scientists to Washington to advise on whether the proposed sums could be "usefully expended" as well as how to handle "the question of perfection—of scientists wishing to achieve perfection. We do not have time for perfection on some of these things." (Ibid., 22–23. See also pp. 231–32 [Document 150].) He and the others in attendance also answered congressional questions concerning such matters as the army's extensive logistical tail, the buildup after the start of the Korean War, the calling up of reserves and National Guard units, the length of the work week, and even the size and depth of the Yalu

River. Many of the answers and discussion, however, were off the record. For Marshall's later testimony on this bill before the Senate Committee on Appropriations, see pp. 291–93. ★

171

To J. Churchill Newcomb — December 1, 1950, Washington, DC

Dear Newcomb: I received your letter of the 25th and was interested in the extract regarding horses.[1] Confidentially, I feel that the Army went too far in the elimination of the horse. It had been my feeling as I finished my term as Chief of Staff that we should maintain one two-squadron Cavalry Regiment with an attached battalion of horse and pack artillery. I had in mind that a third of the officers would be detailed for four years and the remaining two-thirds would come in in increments for six months service only, in order to keep alive in the Army the knowledge of the horse, care, riding, draft, etc.; also that at certain places in the Army, notably Fort Benning, Ga. and West Point, a few horses should be kept for officers to ride so we would always have men who had that facility. This, in a manner, was pointed up two days ago when we found the Chinese Communists were reported to be bringing in 2,000 mounted men, mounted infantry in effect, I presume. My original idea was somewhat influenced by the fact that we had to utilize horses in the mountains of Italy.[2] The trouble, I think, regarding the Army action, not only was the economical factor but the fact that the horse proponents were so intense and the inevitable horse show build-up so aggressive, that a clean sweep was made of everything.

I was interested in what you had to say about Charlotte Coles and Donna Lloyd. I saw them both last summer.[3]

Now that I am here in Washington I do not find it possible this season of the year to attend any of the meetings of the Catoctin Club. In the spring, when I hope to be based more at Leesburg, I will resume my attendance because I always enjoy these meetings.[4] Faithfully yours,

GCMRL/G. C. Marshall Papers (Secretary of Defense, Selected)

1. Newcomb, a well-known landowner near Leesburg, Virginia, had forwarded to Marshall on November 25 "a clipping regarding the place of the horse in defense," as some farmers were "beginning to express their fear also that, if we should suffer an all-out attack which disrupted the free flow of fuel oil and gas, our farmers, left without horses, would be unable either to plant or harvest their crops." (Newcomb to Marshall, November 25, 1950, GCMRL/G. C. Marshall Papers [Secretary of Defense, Number Indexed, M200-5-35].) The newspaper clipping, "Draft Horses—Will They Come Back Strong?," lamented that "In 1920, there were more than twenty million horses. In 1940, just before the war, there were fourteen million, despite great strides on the part of tractors and mechanical farm equipment. But in 1948, the records show that only seven and a half million horses were left on the farms, or less than one team for each farm in the country." ("Draft Horses—Will They Come Back Strong?," unknown publication, n.d., ibid.)

2. For the use of horses during the World War II Italian campaign, see Mary Lee Stubbs and Stanley Russell Connor, *Armor-Cavalry*, pt. 1, *Regular Army and Army Reserve*, in

Army Lineage Series (Washington: Office of the Chief of Military History, US Army, 1969), 72–73.

3. Newcomb had "very much enjoyed seeing Mrs. Lloyd and Miss Charlotte together at a party down in the Green Mountain section. Miss Charlotte is actually getting out these days and enjoying it very much. They both had many questions to ask, which I could not answer, and both sent their affectionate regards." (Newcomb to Marshall, November 25, 1950, GCMRL/G. C. Marshall Papers [Secretary of Defense, Number Indexed, M200-5-35].) Charlotte Coles was the aunt of Marshall's first wife, Lily. She and her husband lived in New York City and the Green Mountain area of Albemarle County, Virginia, where her family had a cluster of estates. Donna Lloyd was the widow of Arthur H. Lloyd, the former vice president of Old Dominion Soapstone Company, based in Esmont, Virginia. After addressing the VMI graduates in Lexington on June 13, 1950 (see pp. 108–10), Marshall had driven to a hotel in Charlottesville and had dinner with Coles and Lloyd.

4. Newcomb had "been out of the County at the late fairs and purebred livestock sales" and "failed to have the pleasure of seeing you at recent meetings of the Catoctin [Farmers' Club]," a group established in 1868 to develop solutions to agricultural problems plaguing northern Virginia. (Newcomb to Marshall, November 25, 1950, ibid.)

172

STATEMENT FOR THE ARMY-NAVY GAME PROGRAM[1] December 2, 1950
[Philadelphia, Pennsylvania]

In watching a cricket match about 125 years ago, Lord Wellington was reported to have remarked, "The battle of Waterloo was won on the playing field of Eton."[2]

This famous statement by Lord Wellington has special significance at this Army-Navy football game here in Philadelphia today. Those who are wearing the Army grey and the Navy blue on the gridiron today, and those who stand behind them in support, are all part of the greater All-American team which we count upon for victory in battle.

Among those who played on this field a year ago and those who sat in these stands and supported their teams were many young men who today are taking part in the tough game of war thousands of miles from here. You will find them in the snow covered mountains of Korea, in the mine infested waters nearby, and in the dangerous skies overhead. A glance at last year's program compared with the overseas rosters of our Armed Forces taken a short time before publication of this program shows that seven players of the Classes of 1949 [*1950*] at West Point and Annapolis are now serving in the Far East: Galiffa, Henn, Kellum, Maladowitz, McDaniel, Purvis, and Trent.[3]

Even in the midst of these great festivities, let us keep in mind these men and all of our American young men of today and other years who learned on our athletic fields the lessons of strength, loyalty, courage and leadership.[4]

GCMRL/G. C. Marshall Papers (Secretary of Defense, Speeches and Statements)

1. Marshall had approved this statement—to be printed in the program for the December 2 game in Philadelphia—in Washington on November 9.

2. Arthur Wellesley, later the Duke of Wellington and commander of the forces that defeated Napoleon Bonaparte in June 1815 at Waterloo, was an alumnus of Eton, the prestigious all-male British preparatory school.

3. The members of the USMA class of 1950 were Arnold Galiffa, William Henn, William Kellum, Ray Maladowitz, Paul McDaniel, and John Trent. Elvis Purvis was a member of the US Naval Academy's class of 1950.

4. Marshall left Union Station in Washington, DC, for Philadelphia at 8:00 a.m. with his party, but returned to Washington by Military Air Transport Service (MATS) that afternoon, arriving at 2:37 p.m., and met with Lovett and Carter at 2:50 p.m. For more on Marshall's plans for the Army-Navy game, see pp. 204 and 225–26.

173

Meetings on the Chinese Intervention in Korea

December 2–4, 1950 Washington, DC

DURING the late afternoon or early evening of December 2, Acheson went to Marshall's apartment to coordinate recommendations to Truman. (Acheson, *Present at the Creation*, 473.) At 8:00 p.m., they and Bradley met with the president, who had by then returned from the Army-Navy game in Philadelphia (see previous document). After talk of new recommendations to the UN General Assembly in light of the Chinese military intervention in Korea, discussion shifted to the likely Chinese "price" for a settlement. According to Acheson's recollections immediately after the meeting, Marshall then said "that we were in a great dilemma of determining how we could save our troops and protect our national honor at the same time. He thought it would be difficult for us to abandon in good conscience the South Koreans. All agreed that we must think a long time before we come to any such conclusion." (*FRUS, 1950*, 7: 1310–11.) According to Jessup, who also attended the meeting, "Marshall said the situation looked very bad indeed. General Bradley also took an extremely pessimistic view of the military situation and thought that not more than 48 to 72 hours would elapse before it reached a crash state." (Ibid., 1312.)

Discussion then turned to possible evacuation of the X Corps, with Marshall warning "that even a Dunkirk type of evacuation might be prejudiced if the Chinese brought in their air." Truman "raised the question of General MacArthur's view about the need of operations across the frontier." Acheson then repeated what he had previously told Marshall: "that decisions should be based solely on whether it would help or hurt our troops. We need a very good military judgment as to whether knocking out the Chinese airfields would bring in the Russians. This decision should not be made by MacArthur but by General Marshall on the advice of General Collins, who should stay in Tokyo. We should not take this action for the purpose of holding Korea or merely for the purposes of retaliating against the Chinese but only for the purpose of permitting the evacuation of our troops if necessary." He also "stressed the importance of having at least the appearance of consultation with Attlee before definitive action was taken," but Marshall warned "that we might have only 48 hours in which to reach a decision and we could not wait" for Truman's first scheduled meeting with the British prime minister on December 5. He also said that "it would be better to have Mr. Attlee suggest a settlement rather than having us bear the burden of making the suggestion." (Ibid.,

1313. See also pp. 284–87.)

Acheson further proposed that Truman declare a state of national emergency to make the public aware of how serious the situation was and consider using his powers to freeze prices and wages as well as establish production controls. Truman agreed. The three then discussed "the urgency of getting our armed forces built up as quickly as possible" and concurred that additional appropriations beyond the amount requested the previous day would probably not be needed in the near future (see pp. 276–78). (Ibid., 1311–12.) They also agreed that Acheson and others from the State Department should meet with the JCS the following morning, to be followed by another meeting among Truman, Marshall, Acheson, and Bradley.

The first morning meeting at 9:30 a.m. on December 3 took place at the Pentagon and included Harriman as well as Acheson, Marshall, the Joint Chiefs, and numerous additional officers and State Department officials. It had been preceded by receipt of a very pessimistic report from MacArthur and began with a somber briefing by Ridgway, who warned that the ability of the X Corps to withdraw was "questionable" as was the ability of the Eighth Army to get to Seoul before the pursuing Chinese did. US/UN forces would be able, however, to hold beachheads at Inchon in the west, Hamhung in the east, and Pusan in the south "for some time," Ridgway added, and until a decision was made on their evacuation—if those troops could get into the beachheads. Acheson then asked whether Ridgway's information provided "the answer to the questions asked at the meeting last night with the President; namely, has the military situation reached a point at which it is necessary for us to get a cease-fire?" Bradley said a cease-fire "would be fine" if possible, but wondered what the Chinese "price" would be, perhaps including total withdrawal from Korea, withdrawal of the Seventh Fleet from the straits of Taiwan, and agreement to grant Mao's government a seat in the UN and a role in negotiation of a Japanese peace treaty. Citing Marshall's previous points about both "the security of our troops" and the effect of a request for a cease-fire "on the position of the United States in the Far East and the whole world," Acheson warned of the "danger of our becoming the greatest appeasers of all time if we abandon the Koreans and they are slaughtered" and bluntly stated that "we are presented with a bitter choice." He favored a cease-fire if it could be limited to withdrawal to the 38th parallel but doubted the Chinese would agree. He also warned, twice, that "if we get into a general war with China and there are grave chances of general war with the Soviet Union soon then we would fight without allies on our side." Bradley countered that "we must weigh that against Korea and against the loss of prestige in Asia and Europe. We would lose Indochina and Formosa. The Germans are already saying we have proved that we are weak. Appeasement is gaining in Europe." The "great trouble," Acheson said, "is that we are fighting the wrong nation. We are fighting the second team, whereas the real enemy is the Soviet Union." In that regard, devoting US resources to a full-scale war against China would preclude building up strength against the Soviets in Europe. It would also lead European allies to "quit us and deal with the Soviet

Union." (Ibid., 1323–26; Schnabel and Watson, *History of JCS*, 3, pt. 1: 159–62; Acheson, *Present at the Creation*, 475.)

At this point Marshall "raised the question of Indochina and the dilemma of the French there and the resulting French attitude." Acheson responded that "the French are so weak and shell-shocked they are anxious for a deal which would give them the illusion of safety" and asked Rusk for his opinion. Rusk concurred that France "would try to get a deal" with Ho Chi Minh, the Communist leader of Vietnam, "and then withdraw." He also amplified on Acheson's "bitter choice" by noting that "we cannot sustain here the theory of an absolute priority for Europe if we surrender the Far East." Bradley questioned in this regard whether the Europeans would believe that we would go to war with the Soviets should even a platoon of US soldiers be attacked if the United States did not "react to the Chinese attack." (*FRUS, 1950*, 7: 1327.)

Marshall asked if a cease-fire could be confined to "a line at the 38th parallel." He considered the "attitude" in the UN "illogical, amounting to almost bad faith, but that one had to recognize that such situations do arise in international relations." In this regard he compared the present situation to British press reactions during the 1944–45 Battle of the Bulge. "We must accept the UN procedure and try to improve it but not expect perfection." He supported an effort to obtain a cease-fire at the 38th parallel before the present retreat reached the South Korean capital, but emphasized that "the line-up with the British Commonwealth is most important." Bradley asked whether it was time to begin the evacuation of civilian dependents from West Berlin "and other exposed places," while Marshall "kept pressing the questions of whether we need more money to do more than we are doing." Acheson "asked whether anyone doubted the desirability of a cease-fire at the 38th parallel if some other country suggested it." No one did. He also called again for a presidential declaration of national emergency, but then noted that the military situation "looked better" than it had the previous evening. Marshall concurred that "it did look slightly better," asked why MacArthur had not been ordered to get his troops into the three beachheads, but noted that Truman "should talk with Attlee before final decisions were made." He also expressed concern for the fate of the South Koreans. (Ibid., 1327–34.)

Acheson summarized most of these points during the ensuing meeting with Truman. He also repeated his call for a presidential declaration of national emergency, and asserted that "it was essential to get some kind of censorship in the Far Eastern Command immediately" in order to halt MacArthur's public statements attacking the limitations imposed upon him—limitations he labeled "without precedent in military history." Truman agreed that he "might" have to order censorship, but Marshall responded that "this would be a rather difficult thing to do." Acheson reported later that day his feeling that Truman would want to hear what Attlee had to say and "see what the general temper is of our allies," as well as his certainty that "the President was not prepared, at this point at least, to negotiate with anyone, or to ask for a cease fire." Truman was prepared, however, to approve a new JCS directive to MacArthur asserting that "preservation of your forces is now the primary consideration" and that "Consolidation of forces into beachheads is concurred in." On the following morning, December 4, during a meeting with Kennan, Rusk, and Matthews, Marshall compared the present situation to the one the United States had faced in the Philippines after Pearl Harbor and, according to Kennan, "cited this as an example of the virtue of hanging on doggedly for reasons of prestige and morale." Acheson also informed the three upon their return to the State Department that "the President had no patience with the suggestions that we resolve to abandon Korea and had felt that we should stay and fight as long as possible." (Ibid., 1336–39; Acheson, *Present at the Creation*, 471–73, 475–76; Schnabel and Watson, *History of JCS*, 3, pt. 1: 162–63; Frank Costigliola, ed., *The Kennan Diaries* [New York: W. W. Norton & Co., 2014], 275.)

In line with Acheson's December 3 recommendation regarding the need to stop MacArthur's public attacks on administration policies in Korea, Truman on December 5 directed that all public statements by government officials relating to foreign or military policies were henceforth to be cleared in advance with the State or Defense Department, and that advance copies submitted for clearance should also be submitted to the White House. He further directed Acheson and Marshall to order overseas officials, "including military commanders and diplomatic representatives, . . . to exercise extreme caution in public statements, to clear all but routine statements with their departments, and to refrain from direct communication on military or foreign policy with newspapers, magazines, or other publicity media in the United States." These two directives can be found in NA/RG 330, CD 350.001; they are also quoted and discussed, along with the behavior by MacArthur that led to their issuance, in Truman, *Memoirs*, 2: 383–84; and James F. Schnabel, *United States Army in the Korean War*, vol. 3, *Policy and Direction: The First Year* (Washington: Office of the Chief of Military History, US Army, 1972), 284–85. ★

174

Remarks to the Staff of the American Red Cross — December 4, 1950, Washington, DC

A leave-taking is a difficult occasion at best. It is doubly so when one must break-off a pleasant and memorable association in such ominous times as these.[1]

I cannot confine myself to the conventional good wishes for your continued success and happiness although you have them in full measure. This moment in history is too grim for conventional felicitations.

We have lived with danger for some years. Now that danger has become acute. The events of the next few weeks—or even days—may determine the course of our civilization for long years to come.

As I have watched the forces of despotism and aggression grow more reckless with human happiness each passing month, my association with the Red Cross has been a tonic to my spirit. I have learned that there are great reserves of simple goodness and altruism in human beings that, when catalyzed by an agent like the Red Cross, create good will, friendliness and helpfulness. Knowing that these qualities exist, even when dormant, is about the only proof we have that some day man will learn to live in peace.

Meanwhile real peace is only a hope for the future. We face an indefinite period of acute tension, hard work and great sacrifice.

From you of the Red Cross, particularly, much will be expected. I know that as I leave you, you face one of the most critical tasks in Red Cross history—the training of the American people in the skills and attitudes that will make them self-confident and calm no matter what trials they may have to endure.

The time is past when only the military forces of a nation must bear the brunt of enemy aggression. In this age there are few communities that are not potential targets. Every man and woman should be prepared to help if the blow falls. The Red Cross has the experience and the organization in being to give the American people the training that may be essential to survival.

I know you will not fail because it is not in the Red Cross tradition to fail.

I have an added measure of confidence in your success because of the superior qualifications of the distinguished man who, today, takes over the leadership of the American Red Cross. Unlike myself, for I was a raw recruit when I took office last year, Mr. Harriman is a Red Cross veteran. He knows the Red Cross, he has lived with it and loved it for many years as a member of the Board of Governors, as Manager of the former North Atlantic Area, and as a National Fund Chairman. His Red Cross experience has been so extensive that one wonders how he has found time to be one of the country's outstanding bankers and Chairman of the Board of the Union Pacific Railroad.

It gives me great pleasure to introduce your next President of the American Red Cross, Mr. E. Roland Harriman.

GCMRL/G. C. Marshall Papers (Secretary of Defense, Speeches and Statements)

1. For more on Marshall's decision to resign from the Red Cross, see pp. 220–22 and 247–51.

175

Meetings with President Truman and Prime Minister Attlee
December 4–8, 1950 Washington, DC

AFTER President Truman's November 30 remarks concerning the possible use of atomic weapons against the Chinese in Korea, British Prime Minister Attlee quickly arranged a trip to Washington (see p. 275). This resulted in a series of high-level Anglo-American conversations from December 4 to 8, many of which included Marshall as well as Truman, Attlee, Acheson, and other US and British officials. The primary topic was how to respond to China's military intervention in Korea, both militarily and diplomatically in the UN, but that in turn led to discussion of broader defense issues focusing on NATO as well as Anglo-American policy differences in Asia regarding Formosa and recognition of the Communist Chinese regime, whose request for UN membership the British favored but the Americans did not.

Acheson did most of the talking on the American side, with Marshall only occasionally commenting—usually in response to a request that he do so by Acheson or Truman. During the first meeting on December 4, he admitted that X Corps would probably have to be evacuated in the northeast but overall he was "much more hopeful than he had been four days ago." (*FRUS, 1950*, 3: 1713.)

Marshall as well as all the others who spoke at these meetings agreed that Korea should continue to be defended if militarily feasible, but that the war should not be expanded and that defense of Western Europe remained the primary consideration. As Attlee summarized this consensus, "we must not get so involved in the East as to lay ourselves open to attack in the West," to which Acheson responded, "we had to bear in mind that the central enemy is not the Chinese but the Soviet Union." But whereas Acheson insisted that "all the inspiration for the present action comes from there" and that the Chinese were "subservient to Moscow," Attlee saw the Chinese acting on the basis of their own perceived interests and favored attempting to obtain a cease-fire with them. Acheson disagreed, noting that this was "the worst" moment for negotiation with the communists since 1917 and that if they were successful in Korea it could lead to French withdrawal from Indochina and the possible loss of the entire Western position in Asia and the western Pacific. Referring back to his 1945–46 mediation mission and meetings with both Mao Tse-tung and Chou En-lai, Marshall emphasized the Chinese leaders' insistence that they were Marxist Communists, not agrarian reformers, and that they had "made not the slightest attempt to conceal their Moscow affiliations. They regarded the Russians as co-religionists." (Ibid., 1711–15.) The following day, in response to a question as to whether the strategic importance of Formosa could be separated "from the question of the recognition of Chiang Kai-shek" as well as a request from Acheson that he speak as an "expert" on Chiang, Marshall emphasized the importance of the island, stated that it would be "very dangerous" strategically to give it up, warned it would be difficult to find a replacement for Chiang given his stature and the corruption of his followers, and asked what would happen to Formosa if no replacement was found. (Ibid., 1736–37.)

On December 6, Truman turned the discussions to the primacy of Europe while maintaining the US position in the Pacific, asserting in this regard that "we are almost in the same condition in which we found ourselves in the middle of World War II." Discussion then turned to the still-linked issues of German rearmament and appointment of a supreme commander, as well as US and French troops for NATO. The Chinese intervention had postponed plans to move two US divisions to Europe that summer and fall, Truman and Marshall noted. Marshall was also worried that French plans for "ten divisions with five more divisions later" would be seriously disrupted by the loss of regular officers in Indochina. He had been informed that the French "were losing more officers than they normally had graduating from St. Cyr," their military academy, raising the question of "what they would have left to train the new divisions in Europe." (Ibid., 1748.) He was also concerned over congressional belief that present plans were impractical and could not stop the Soviets. He compared the situation to the one that had existed in 1940 and emphasized the need to move forward. When the British suggested for morale-boosting purposes the sending of untrained US divisions that could be trained later in Germany, however, Marshall related his World War I experiences with untrained troops who had to have their guns taken away on board the ship "because they couldn't handle their guns and their feelings at the same time." When they arrived in France and a French officer approached one of these soldiers and inquired about his weapon, the soldier "immediately handed him his rifle and went off and sat down on a log. . . . [I]t took us one and a half years to correct the impression this had made on the French." (Ibid., 1750–52. For more on Marshall's World War I story, see *Papers of GCM,* 1: 646–47; Marshall, *Memoirs of My Services*, 13; and Pogue, *Education*, 147.)

By this time Marshall had succeeded in modifying the US military's insistence that all these issues must be resolved in a "single package" so as to allow for the appointment of an American in supreme command of an integrated NATO force on the condition that German rearmament and participation were accepted in principle and begun. The American "Spofford Plan" called in this regard for a French commitment to this package with German troops at the level of a regimental combat team of approximately six thousand men—smaller than the division size that French Defense Minister Moch had previously rejected, but clearly larger and more independent than the one the French had proposed in the Pleven Plan. (See pp. 218–20.) The long-term goal was to be an integrated European army, which Acheson labeled "a refinement and improvement of the Pleven Plan." (Acheson, *Present at the Creation,* 485–86; Robert L. Beisner, *Dean Acheson: A Life in the Cold War* [New York: Oxford University Press, 2006], 372.) While there was general agreement to proceed with the appointment of a supreme commander on this basis, Marshall warned of the problems that the commander would have with a multinational force.

Simultaneously Marshall directed the Joint Chiefs to review a proposed course of action for the NATO Defense Committee and Council on the issues of German rearmament, reorganization of the NATO military structure to include creation of an integrated European defense force and establishment of a headquarters for a supreme commander (Supreme Headquarters Allied Powers Europe, or SHAPE), and the appointment of such a commander. The United States would then inform the Defense Committee, he continued, "if expedient, its intention to assign to SHAPE those United States combat forces in Continental Europe and, at the earliest feasible date, to increase United States forces in Europe to about four infantry divisions and the equivalent of one and one-half armored divisions, eight tactical air groups and appropriate naval forces. In addition to the above, the United States should dispatch to Europe, on the outbreak of hostilities, further forces." (Marshall to JCS, memorandum, December 5, 1950, NA/RG 330, CD 091.7 [Germany].)

During an after-dinner meeting on December 6 that lasted from 9:30 p.m. to midnight, Attlee "raised the question of General MacArthur's direction of the effort in Korea," noting the European feeling that MacArthur "was running the show" and the other nations "had little to say in what was done." Marshall and Bradley responded that MacArthur "was doing what he was required to do by the United Nations." Marshall explained the joint control of MacArthur by the State and Defense Departments and asserted that "the British could not say they were not consulted." Bradley bluntly rejected a British proposal for the establishment of a committee to direct the war with the comment that "a war could not be run by a committee." (*FRUS, 1950*, 3: 1759–60.)

Throughout the meetings Marshall had deferred to Acheson and refrained from commenting on political as opposed to military issues, stating at one point during a rather heated December 7 discussion and continued Anglo-American disagreement over policies toward Communist China that "the problem of world reaction and attitudes in the United Nations were not in his field and it was not for him to discuss them." After Acheson quipped that Marshall "had been in that field a lot longer than he had," Marshall said that "if there were any reasonable means by which we could avoid war with Communist China, we would want to take them because we were faced with the threat of a global war." But "it was almost impossible to negotiate" with the Chinese, and it would be "intolerable" to have Formosa "in enemy hands." He shared the fear of general war breaking out and presently opposed expanding the conflict by bombing Manchuria, but he was still thinking through all the options. (Ibid., 1767–70.)

By this time, Collins had returned from his trip to Japan and Korea (see pp. 276 and 280) and reported that MacArthur was pessimistic about holding any part of the peninsula without reinforcements. Collins himself was more optimistic about the situation, and this had a major impact on both Marshall and Truman. (Schnabel and Watson, *History of JCS*, 3, pt. 1: 179; Condit, *Test of War*, 89.)

In the midst of these sessions, Marshall confided to Thomas Watson Sr. that he had "very few moments any more to call my own. I have been sitting in meetings almost continuously, and if it keeps up I will have to take out of storage the rubber cushion" Stimson had given to Marshall following his December 1948 kidney operation. (Marshall to Watson, December 5, 1950, GCMRL/G. C. Marshall Papers [Secretary of Defense, Number Indexed, M200-3-18]; *Papers of GCM*, 6: 682–83.) ★

176

MEMORANDUM OF CONVERSATION — December 7, 1950
Secret — Washington, DC

SUBJECT: Korean Views on Present Situation

Ambassador Chang called on Secretary Marshall at 1030 this morning on instructions from President Rhee, to present the views of the Korean Government in the present situation.[1] The Ambassador informed the Secretary that he had had the great pleasure of meeting with the President yesterday to present these views and that the President had suggested to him that he see Secretary Marshall.[2] According to the Ambassador, President Rhee wishes President Truman and Secretary Marshall to know that he is determined to carry on the struggle as long as necessary, and that he has no intention of giving up. Secondly, President Rhee believes that Chinese Communist conquest of Korea will result in the massacre of all anti-Communists in Korea, and indefinitely delay the recovery and reconstruction of Korea. Accordingly, President Rhee requests the U.S. Government to consider arming the approximately 1,000,000 able-bodied, young men in Korea who now have no arms and the desire to resist the Communists. Ambassador Chang explained that the Korean "Youth Corps" has been in existence for several years. Its members receive a modified form of military training but they have no arms. He believed that if they could be supplied with light arms, they could help turn the tide in this hour of need.[3] The Ambassador gave the Secretary a copy of the aide-memoire containing President Rhee's views.[4] After reading this aide-memoire, Secretary Marshall stated that he was gratified to learn of President Rhee's determination to resist, and that he fully agreed with President Rhee's estimate of the probable consequences of Chinese Communist conquest of Korea. The Secretary stated that the U.S. was fully together with Korea in this critical moment, and was determined to make every effort to meet the situation.

Turning to the Korean request for light arms, the Secretary summarized the present supply of military equipment to the Koreans. He said that everything possible was being done urgently to supply our forces, as well as the Koreans, in Korea, even including certain drastic actions. Secretary Marshall noted that the U.S. has provided equipment for the 10 [*9*] divisions that are now operating in Korea, for some 20 to 30,000 Koreans attached to American divisions, and for training cadres. He pointed out that equipment for the Koreans has the same priority as equipment for American forces in Korea and that that priority is the very highest for the supply of American materiel anywhere in the world. He reassured the Ambassador that the Koreans were receiving exactly the same consideration. Secretary Marshall explained that the distribution of this equipment was the responsibility of the Theatre Commander and asked if President Rhee had communicated his request to General MacArthur. Ambassador Chang replied that he presumed President Rhee had informed General MacArthur.

Secretary Marshall referred to the present military difficulties in Korea, and described the regrouping of the Korean and American divisions in the northeastern area.[5] He pointed out that retention of their heavy equipment would be one of the important supply problems that would have to be considered in the whole question of providing the U.N. forces with sufficient materiel.

The Secretary stated that the situation was extremely difficult since the Communists seemed bent on the conquest of Asia. Secretary Marshall concluded by saying that the U.S. Government was doing everything it possibly could to safeguard and maintain South Korea, leaving aside for the moment the question of

North Korea.

He cautioned the Ambassador on the necessity for preventing any disclosure of the situation in the northeast, and on several other matters discussed in the conversation.

Ambassador Chang thanked the Secretary for the opportunity of presenting the Korean Government's views, which he again summarized on departing.[6]

K. T. Young

NA/RG 330, CD Memorandum of Conversation

1. Chang had been confirmed as the new ROK premier on November 24 but on Rhee's instructions stayed in the United States as ambassador until late January. Also attending this meeting were ROK Colonel Young Kang and Kenneth T. Young, who was assistant to the director of the Defense Department's Office of Foreign Military Affairs, and who took these notes.

2. For Chang's meeting with Truman, see *FRUS, 1950*, 7: 1425–26.

3. Chang had made the same request to Dean Rusk on December 4, 5, and 6, and to Truman during their December 6 meeting, and he was seeing Marshall to discuss it further on Truman's suggestion. (Ibid., 1350, 1387, 1424–25; Burns to Marshall, memorandum, December 7, 1950, NA/RG 330, Briefings, CD 092 [Korea].)

4. The aide-memoire warned that should the United States and UN withdraw forces from Korea, "the nations in Asia which have looked to the United States and the United Nations for leadership in a time of constant threats from communist hordes, will lose their confidence in the United States and the United Nations." Such failure "to demonstrate continued determination to repel the new armed aggression in Korea" could lead to "a loss of prestige of unspeakable magnitude" and an "immediate massacre of our democratically inclined people and leaders." This document went on to assert that South Koreans "would rather die than be subjugated to the evil forces of these inhuman communists." In light of these views, the South Korean government would "put an additional one million Koreans of fighting age into immediate military service," but they would require the United States to provide them with "arms and ammunition to defend their mother soil" and to provide "reassurance to calm their fears." (Aide-memoire, n.d., NA/RG 59, Decimal File, 1950–1954, 795.00/12–650.)

This may have been the same aide-memoire Chang gave to Truman on December 6. See *FRUS, 1950*, 7: 1426.

5. Marshall is referring here to the withdrawal of the US X Corps and the South Korean I Corps to ports in the east, from which their evacuation would begin on December 10.

6. On December 12, Marshall had the army request the views of MacArthur on Chang's request, and on December 14, he asked the JCS for their "views and recommendations, as a matter of priority." (JCS 1776.175, "Proposed Arming of the Korean Youth Corps," NA/RG 218, Geographical File, CCS 383.21 [Korea].) For their negative assessments as forwarded by Marshall to Acheson on January 19, 1951, see *FRUS, 1951*, 7: 105–7.

177

Memorandum for Frederick J. Lawton

December 7, 1950
Washington, DC

I have your memorandum of November 14 regarding the Battle Monuments Commission appropriations.[1] Your directions in regard to the procedure will be carefully observed.

I would like to make this comment. First I am disturbed by the effect on mothers, wives and families going to Europe on finding that some cemeteries have been completed, and the development of others where their sons or husbands are buried is not being carried forward. This produces inevitably very serious reactions.

Now as to the curtailments imposed. It seems to me that your letter of November 14 and its enclosure are inconsistent. The letter contemplates that the construction of *all* memorial features scheduled for fiscal year 1951 *but not now* in progress shall be deferred until after 1952. The enclosure contemplates that the starting of at least three memorials shall be deferred until after 1952, and that all others shall be deferred indefinitely.[2]

I am asking General North, the Secretary of the American Battle Monuments Commission, to go over the matter with your representative.[3]

GCMRL/G. C. Marshall Papers (Secretary of Defense, Categorical, ABMC)

1. Lawton, director of the Bureau of the Budget in the White House, had reported to Marshall on November 14 that Truman had approved only $775,000 for salaries and expenses and $4,000,000 for the construction of memorials and cemeteries for the ABMC's fiscal year 1952 budget. He noted that "the change in the situation with respect to national defense and the domestic economy" since the original budget proposals made in June 1950 had necessitated a reexamination that resulted in "budget allowances on a more restrictive basis." (Lawton to Marshall, November 14, 1950, GCMRL/G. C. Marshall Papers [Secretary of Defense, Categorical, ABMC].)

2. In his November 14 letter, Lawton had stated that "construction of memorial features at five locations scheduled to be started in 1952 will be deferred and that construction of memorial features at all other locations in Europe where construction was scheduled for 1951 but is not now in progress will be deferred until after 1952." (Lawton to Marshall, November 14, 1950, ibid.)

General Thomas North, secretary of the ABMC, had pointed out this inconsistency to Marshall on November 27. The ABMC had protested the curtailment of its program to no avail. North listed the nine cemeteries scheduled to begin construction in 1951, and he recommended that Marshall "suggest to the President verbally that the Budget directive be amended to omit, at least, the details of how many memorials to start, and when." (North to Marshall, memorandum, November 27, 1950, ibid.) For more on North's long association with the ABMC, see p. 735n2.

3. North reported to Marshall on December 13 that a representative from the Bureau of the Budget had met with him on the previous day and believed "that the most logical method in our case is to defer work on memorials on which architects' plans are not far advanced" but "conceded" that ABMC would be allowed to proceed "with all work, except memorials, at *all* cemeteries" as well as memorials at nine while construction of memorials at six others would be deferred until after fiscal year 1952. (North to Marshall, December 13, 1950, ibid.)

He added that "we may have to explain to relatives why we are not now preparing to record the names of certain of the Missing (i.e. on those memorials to be deferred)" and noted that ending contracts with the architects would be "difficult." (Ibid.)

For more on the ABMC budget and construction of cemeteries, see pp. 618–19.

178

Remarks and Senate Testimony on the Second Supplemental Appropriations Bill for 1951
December 8–11, 1950 New York, NY, and Washington, DC

DURING "a very rushed trip" to New York City, Marshall addressed the annual dinner of the Mobilization Congress of American Industry of the National Association of Manufacturers at the Waldorf-Astoria Hotel. (Marshall to Connie Berry, December 11, 1950, GCMRL/G. C. Marshall Papers [Secretary of Defense, Selected].) He cautioned the nearly three thousand attendees that in order to endure the present "period of the greatest tension" without it "deteriorating into something dreadful to contemplate—another world war," the United States "must quickly reach a high plateau in the mountain range of preparedness from which we can look in all directions, firm in a position of readiness to act in whatever way may be necessary, rapidly, but deliberately and effectively." Manpower had to be built up "from the low state of last June" at the outbreak of the Korean War. In the field of munitions, Marshall was "particularly anxious not only that production be gotten underway as quickly as possible and pushed as rapidly as possible but even more concerned to see that we do this in such a manner . . . so that we can quickly and greatly accelerate production as it becomes necessary." These goals were part and parcel of "the development of a system new to American practice that will be enduring, not a system that will collapse at any surface relaxation in the tension I refer to or because our people far distant from Western Europe and the Continent of Asia grow indifferent to the consequences of a relaxation in our measures of preparedness." (Speech at the Annual Dinner of the Congress of American Industry, December 8, 1950, GCMRL/G. C. Marshall Papers [Secretary of Defense, Speeches and Statements].)

Marshall expanded on this argument and the need for the second supplemental appropriation of nearly $18 billion as the first witness in executive session hearings before the Senate Appropriations Committee the following day. As he had stated to the House Appropriations Committee (see pp. 276–78), this supplemental appropriation was first prepared to create the defense structure envisioned in NSC 68, but the Chinese intervention in Korea required revision of budget estimates that "involves virtually as many men in the Army in fiscal year 1951 as was originally contemplated for the build-up through 1954." The funding requested, Marshall asserted, "establishes a base of departure, a base from which we develop increasing momentum—from which if necessary we can pull out the stop and then go ahead very, very rapidly," particularly in regards to manpower and materiel, and to do so "much more economically than otherwise." (Senate Committee on Appropriations, *Hearings . . . An Act Making Supplemental Appropriations for the Fiscal Year Ending June 30, 1951, and for Other Purposes*, 81st Cong., 2d sess., 2.)

Marshall informed the committee that the initial Defense Department budget for fiscal year 1951 projected an army of 630,000 men. The second supplemental appropriation request now planned for a 1,263,000-man army by July 1, 1951. The other services would see similar increases in manpower goals: the navy from 375,000 to 684,000; the marines from 72,000 to 166,000; and the air force from 416,000 to 651,000. The total authorization "for major items of war materiel" among the initial and supplemental budgets for the Defense Department would reach almost $19 billion. (Ibid., 2–3.) Despite these large increases from initial plans during the period of partial mobilization, Marshall had "heard objections" that the Defense Department budget "does not show evidence of the seriousness of the situation; that we should do this more quickly." Marshall felt "very strongly that that is a delusion. The thing to do is to get this under way, to get the momentum established, which is the difficult part of it, and then have it set in such a manner that we can if necessary just pull the lever, and spread out and go very rapidly." He concluded by cautioning against forcing "a too rapid expansion," which leads to "skim milk and a great many other weaknesses. So I think it is much better not to try to rush things beyond the immediate capability of expansion." (Ibid., 3–4.)

Senate committee members then asked Marshall a series of questions regarding specific aspects of the request for supplemental funds. Marshall answered some of these questions directly, but relied for most of the detailed responses upon officials who had accompanied him to the hearings: Lovett; Wilfred J. McNeil, assistant secretary of defense and comptroller; and Generals Bradley, Haislip, Vandenberg, Robert Moore, and William Reeder (USMA, 1917), army assistant chief of staff for logistics (G-4). Marshall himself did explain why more than 50 percent of the requested funds were allocated to the army, emphasizing that ground forces "were in a woeful state of deficiency" in terms of both equipment and numbers. (Ibid., 6–7.) He also reiterated that he was not recommending appropriations for full mobilization, but rather sufficient funds to put the armed forces into position to move quickly to full mobilization if and when required. More than one senator felt full mobilization should take place immediately. "How can we delude ourselves that we are not in world war III?," Senator Joseph C. O'Mahoney (D-WY) asked; "the time is here for full mobilization," and Truman should issue a declaration of emergency. Other senators concurred. (Ibid., 14–16.)

The hearings continued on Monday, December 11, at 2:00 p.m. Marshall made no statement and let others respond to most of the senators' remaining questions. He left before the hearings ended in order to attend a 3:30 p.m. NSC meeting.

Marshall wrote to a childhood friend on the second day of these hearings that he was "having a pretty tough time of it as to a mountain of work of the most critical nature, but more particularly as to oppositions, prohibitions and accusations. We have not yet stepped into full mobilization in the military way but we certainly are going strong in a democratic way." (Marshall to Armstrong, December 11, 1950, GCMRL/G. C. Marshall Collection [Armstrong].) He later divulged in a letter to General Sir Hastings Ismay: "Confidentially, I am having a perfectly delightful heluva time!" (Marshall to Ismay, December 15, 1950, GCMRL/G. C. Marshall Papers [Secretary of Defense, Number Indexed, M200-5-29].)

Congress authorized $16.795 billion in the second supplemental appropriation, which Truman signed on January 6, 1951. (Condit, *Test of War*, 239–40.) ★

179

MEMORANDUM FOR FRANK PACE

December 12, 1950
Washington, DC

A telephone message just came to me from Congressman Spence, Chairman of the Banking and Currency Committee, regarding the construction of quarters for families. He stated that he was under considerable pressure in the matter, particularly from Senator Benton regarding Camp Pickett where Connecticut National Guard Division is stationed.[1]

I told him I would telephone him what the policy was, that I did not have a clear understanding of it but thought that we had decided that in this emergency, funds, materiel and labor should not be directed to such developments.

There is attached hereto a hastily prepared memo giving me the supposed situation.[2] However, I assume that the Army Department has this matter under full consideration and I therefore wish that Congressman Spence be telephoned today (if he is not in his office, information to be dictated to his secretary) regarding the exact status in this matter.[3]

NA/RG 330, CD 628

1. Representative Brent Spence (D-KY) had written to Marshall about Camp Pickett, located in Blackstone, Virginia, which had been reactivated in August 1950.

2. According to a December 12 memorandum from Major George, "there has been no construction of family quarters by the Army since the 1949 budget," the "last time funds were available for this purpose." The only exception was in Alaska. George told Marshall that the army planned to request funds for housing in the 1952 budget and explained the Wherry Act, "a military version of the National Housing Act which provides for temporary housing on or off military installations" funded privately. No such projects were "in effect at Camp Pickett." (George to Marshall, memorandum, December 12, 1950, NA/RG 330, CD 628.)

3. Pace replied later on December 12 that one of his general officers had called Spence that afternoon and dictated a memorandum for him in his absence indicating that "no construction of family housing in the Zone of the Interior has been authorized for the Army since 1949." The Wherry Act required that housing projects "can be authorized only at permanent installations and must be so certified by the Secretary of the Army," and therefore Camp Pickett, "not an installation for the permanent establishment," did not qualify. Given the present situation, "the Army is not justified in seeking funds for family housing at other than permanent Army installations." (Pace to Marshall, memorandum, December 12, 1950, ibid.) For more, see pp. 561–62.

180

TO RALPH A. BARD

December 14, 1950
Washington, DC

Dear Bard: I read your letter of December 6 with great care and later talked over your suggestions and comments with Lovett. As to your Paragraph 1, I cannot go into this in an open letter at this time, but all the factors you mention are being considered.[1]

Your 2 we are already doing, and very urgently, and the matter comes to a head in most points at the meetings occurring in Brussels commencing next Monday.[2]

As to 3, we are engaged, especially with regard to Korea, in a severe test of the United Nations' stability at this time. We are doing everything in our power to strengthen the organization. At the same time we are naturally having our difficulties in critical matters regarding a large assemblage of representatives of different peoples.[3]

As to your 4, there are already three civilian advisory committees, one to each Department of the Defense Establishment and in addition there are certain specialties which have expert civilian coordination,—the guided missiles for example with Keller. I think this phase of the matter is very effectively covered and in addition I am in constant consultation with groups of civilians regarding many of our affairs.[4]

Thank you for writing as you did. It is very helpful. Faithfully yours,

GCMRL/G. C. Marshall Papers (Secretary of Defense, Number Indexed, M200-2-23)

1. Bard, assistant secretary of the navy from 1941 to 1944 and undersecretary of the navy from 1944 to 1945, had written to Marshall with "a suggested definite program of procedure to help solve the critical situation in which our country finds itself at this time." First, if Chinese Communist forces were "in Korea to stay" and if "unlimited numbers of reenforcements are available in Manchuria, . . . we should at once make plans to evacuate our forces to Japan," sign a treaty with that country "to create for us a strong ally in the Asiatic Theatre," and both finance and rearm the Japanese "so that they will be an effective barrier against Communistic aggression in this area." Such action would require the USSR to build up forces "in the Manchuria area, and thereby weaken the Russians in any program which they may attempt to carry on in Europe." (Bard to Marshall, December 6, 1950, GCMRL/G. C. Marshall Papers [Secretary of Defense, Number Indexed, M200-2-23].)

Marshall had asked Lovett to "read Bard's pars. 1 and 4 and let me have, later on, your oral reaction." (Marshall to Lovett, memorandum, n.d., ibid.)

2. Second, Bard proposed that the US assess whether the other NATO members were "prepared and ready to assume their full obligations under this pact" immediately. If not, "we should not become further involved, as it is perfectly apparent that we cannot carry this load ourselves." (Bard to Marshall, December 6, 1950, ibid.) The NATO member nations were scheduled to meet in Brussels beginning on December 17, 1950.

3. Third, Bard proposed clarifying to the American people "whether the United Nations can be made into a strong operating unit as a result of the complete cooperation by the great majority of the members of the United Nations who stand for its program as approved during the past few years by this majority," including "the creation of an armed force to carry out its decisions and edicts" as provided in the charter. (Ibid.)

4. Fourth, Bard recommended the establishment of "a strong civilian advisory committee to the Secretary of Defense . . . composed of industrialists, scientists, labor-leaders, and representatives from the Senate and the House," that would develop "a program which will determine the relative importance of the several units of the Armed Forces of the United States," given prevailing "economic considerations, and also the limitations based on common sense and the realization that we cannot compete on a manpower basis with our enemies all over the world." (Ibid.)

On October 24, 1950, Marshall had appointed K. T. Keller director of guided missiles and "a consultant and advisor" to the chairmen of the RDB and the Munitions Board.

(Marshall to the service secretaries, et al., memorandum, October 24, 1950, NA/RG 330 [OSD Index, 201–Marshall, George C.].)

181

To Edith Nourse Rogers

December 14, 1950
Washington, DC

Dear Mrs. Rogers: This is in reply to your communication of 20 November 1950 concerning the recommendation of the American Gold Star Mothers that the remaining sons and daughters of Gold Star Mothers who have lost one or more sons or daughters in the service of their country shall be exempt from foreign combat duty and be retained in the United States.[1]

I can assure you that the Department of Defense fully appreciates the importance of recognizing the sacrifice and contributions made by families whose sons or daughters have been lost in the service. Accordingly, on 20 September the Department of Defense announced the following policy covering those cases where one or more sons or daughters of a family have as a result of hazards incident to their service in the Armed Forces since 16 September 1940, been killed, died as a result of wounds, accidents, or diseases, or are in a captured or missing in action status:

"The sole surviving sons of such family who is serving in the Armed Forces of the United States, upon his own request or upon the request of one of his parents, will not be assigned to duties normally involving actual combat with the enemy. The individual concerned may waive his rights to this policy if he wishes.

"Sole surviving sons now serving in duties involving actual combat with the enemy will be reassigned provided they meet the requirements of this policy.

"This policy shall not be interpreted to mean that sole surviving sons will not be assigned to overseas commands, but rather that they will be assigned to appropriate areas as designated by the Major Commanders concerned."[2]

The recommendation of Chapter 31 of the American Gold Star Mothers goes far beyond the policy of the Department of Defense which is directed toward giving reasonable assurance that all of the sons or daughters of a family will not be lost by reason of combat or other unusual hazard incident to military service. I believe that the Department of Defense policy provides sufficiently for the safety of those classes of survivors which are, or will be, given special consideration with respect to their military service. Faithfully yours,

NA/RG 330, SD 200.3

1. The American Gold Star Mothers was founded on June 4, 1928, as a service and support organization for mothers who had at least one child die as a member of the armed forces. Chapter 31 of this organization (the Department of Massachusetts) had passed a resolution at its September 1950 convention proposing that the "remaining sons and daughters" of Gold Star Mothers "when inducted into service shall be exempt from foreign combat duty and be retained in the United States, for service assigned to them." Representative Edith Nourse Rogers (R-MA) forwarded this resolution to Marshall on November 20 and requested "that the request made therein be complied with, if possible." (Rogers to

Marshall, November 20, 1950, and attachment, NA/RG 330, SD 200.3.)

2. Ralph N. Stohl, director of administration, had announced this policy in a memorandum for all personnel in the Office of the Secretary of Defense dated September 29, 1950, but signed on September 20. (Stohl to OSD personnel, memorandum, September 29, 1950, ibid.)

182

To A. Willis Robertson — December 15, 1950, Washington, DC

Dear Robertson: There has just been handed to me the Congressional Record–Senate of November 28th. I appreciate very much your remarks regarding my fifty-yard dash on the gridiron a half century ago. I have received quite a number of clippings from the people in the Lexington area who noticed it in the Rockbridge County News and were thoughtful enough to cut it out and send it to me. The ball I am carrying today is a little heavier than the ordinary football, but the goal is the same.[1] Faithfully yours,

GCMRL/G. C. Marshall Papers (Secretary of Defense, Number Indexed, M200-5-46)

1. Senator A. Willis Robertson (D-VA) of Lexington had inserted into the *Congressional Record* on November 28, 1950, a column from the *Rockbridge* [Virginia] *County News* that reproduced its report of fifty years earlier on VMI's November 17, 1900, football game with neighboring Washington and Lee University. "The final score was 41 to 0 in favor of the Cadets," the newspaper had reported, and "George Marshall's run of 50 yards for a touchdown for the Cadets was the feature of the game." Robertson added that "if we reach the goal of peace George Marshall may have to make another 50-yard run. I am glad that he is carrying the ball for our team." (*Congressional Record* 96, pt. 12, 81st Cong., 2d sess., 15918.) "It is hard to believe now," Marshall wrote to one of those who had previously sent him the clipping, "that I ever ran fifty yards with eleven intent young men trying to stop me!" (Marshall to Faulkner, December 5, 1950, GCMRL/G. C. Marshall Papers [Secretary of Defense, Number Indexed, M200-5-46]; *The Bomb* [Lexington, VA: VMI, 1901], 97–98.)

183

To Harry S. Truman — December 18, 1950, Washington, DC

My dear Mr. President: I believe the full Senate consideration of the nomination of Mrs. Anna Rosenberg is to take place today, however, we feel here in the Defense Department a great sense of satisfaction in the unanimous report of the committee recommending her confirmation.[1]

The major factor in bringing about this unanimous report was the highly effective work of the F.B.I. [Federal Bureau of Investigation] Through the services of Mr. Hoover's organization we were able to locate the source of all the false accusations and to bring the facts to the immediate attention of the Senate Committee.[2]

I must express my appreciation of your direct action in making it possible for me to work effectively towards the favorable consideration of the nomination by the Senate Committee. And I also want to express my keen appreciation of the energetic and full out assistance which the Defense Department received from the Department of Justice.[3]

With great respect, Faithfully yours,

GCMRL/G. C. Marshall Papers (Secretary of Defense, Selected)

1. Although the Senate Armed Services Committee had in late November recommended that Rosenberg be confirmed as assistant secretary of defense for manpower and personnel, it decided in early December to reconsider in light of charges that she had in the 1930s belonged to the John Reed Club, an American Communist association (see pp. 262–63). "I was almost his [Marshall's] Dreyfus case," Rosenberg later stated in reference to the notorious case of French anti-Semitism during the 1890s. She said that she went to Marshall and told him she was "willing to resign. It was the only time I saw him get mad. He said I told you this would happen. They are not after you, they are after me. We will stick this out. It is aimed at me." Rosenberg added that "this was not completely accurate. Part was the fact that I was a New Dealer." (GCMRL/Oral History Collection, Notes 71N, copy 2, interview with Rosenberg, December 30, 1957.)

Now under the chairmanship of Richard B. Russell (D-GA), the committee began to investigate the charges on December 5. On December 14, the committee members voted unanimously to recommend Rosenberg's confirmation to the full Senate after several witnesses recanted their testimony, others denied the claims of an ex-Communist that they had accused her, and the FBI reported that another woman bearing the same name had belonged to the John Reed Club. ("Committee Clears Anna M. Rosenberg," *New York Times*, December 15, 1950, p. 24. For more information on this episode and Marshall's efforts to defend Rosenberg, see Forrest C. Pogue, *George C. Marshall*, vol. 4, *Statesman, 1945–1959* [New York: Viking, 1987], 431–36.) Rosenberg later recalled that on the day of the vote Marshall "was impatiently waiting for word" and told her, before beginning a meeting with the JCS, to "just come right on in" if she heard anything. When she received word of the committee vote, she rushed in and found Marshall and the chiefs, with their coats on, about to depart for a White House meeting. "I was choked up," she recalled, and when she told him the result, he said "That's good. Go home and get a facial. You look like Hell." According to Rosenberg, "the Joint Chiefs looked shocked that General Marshall would know anything about a facial." (Pogue, *Statesman*, 435–36; GCMRL/Oral History Collection, Notes 71N, copy 2, interview with Rosenberg, December 30, 1957.) A one-page summary by Pogue of his oral interview with Rosenberg provides the following and somewhat different version of what took place: "I flew into office, where all Joint Chiefs assembled. Told him. Kissed, said Anna, that's fine. He realized suddenly he was too sentimental . . . 'Now get out of here and get a facial . . . you look like HELL.' I didn't know he knew about facials." ("Tape of Mrs. Anna Rosenberg for Marshall Biography. Page Transcript," GCMRL/Xerox 3289 [Dr. Pogue].) According to the official history of the OSD, Rosenberg was "the only Pentagon official Marshall addressed by first name." (Condit, *Test of War*, 489.)

2. Marshall sent a copy of this letter to J. Edgar Hoover, director of the FBI. Hoover replied on December 19 that he was "glad that we could be of service," but "regarded our efforts in this case as a part of the routine operation of the FBI," since such accusations were "similar to those which our Agents are dealing with every day of the week." (Marshall to Hoover, December 18, 1950, and Hoover to Marshall, December 19, 1950, NA/RG 330, SD 040.1.)

3. Truman replied on December 19, "I am certainly most happy that it worked out as it should have in the first place. The attack on Mrs. Rosenberg has not been one that would reflect honor on those who brought the attack." (Truman to Marshall, December 19, 1950, GCMRL/G. C. Marshall Collection [Harry S. Truman].)

The full Senate confirmed Anna Rosenberg's nomination on December 21. ("Mrs. Rosenberg Wins Confirmation," *Washington Post*, December 22, 1950, p. 1.)

184

Memorandum for Record — December 20, 1950[1]
Restricted — Washington, DC

Subject: Visit of Mr. Moshe Sharett, Israeli Foreign Minister on 18 December 1950[2]

After being greeted by General Marshall Mr. Sharett stated that he had come again to talk about the changed world situation since their last meeting. General Marshall stated that he had seen Mr. Sharett in New York recently and he did not understand that there had been any major change in the world situation since he last saw him.[3]

General Marshall stated that he would like to tell a story to Mr. Sharett on the position the U.S. took in regard to the defense of Korea. Mr. Acheson proposed to poll countries fighting in Korea to determine whether Russian-type planes would be pursued across the Manchurian border. Foreign Minister Attlee concurred in the proposal. He firmly pointed out that these planes were in combat with U.S. planes and were menacing U.S. nationals fighting in Korea, but that the U.S. accepted the decision by vote not to pursue such planes across the Manchurian border. The Secretary stated that he brought this to the attention of Mr. Sharett to show the personal sacrifices that were made by the Americans after being voted down by other 10 forces then participating in Korea.[4]

Mr. Sharett then outlined the material needs of Israel and told of the part Israel could play in manufacturing of war materials in the time of emergency. He stated that his factories have a great capacity and what they need most is technical advice and guidance from the U.S. in bettering production. He further stated that in view of the imminence of another world struggle, it would seem advantageous to the U.S. to stockpile food and other materials in Israel that may not be readily taken there in time of war. Such materials he stated could be withdrawn from time to time by the Israelis, with the permission of the U.S., and be paid for by the Israeli Government.

Mr. Sharett then went on to tell of the strategic location of Israel in the Middle East. He spoke of the necessity of enlarging Haifa harbor as a war supply port for the Middle East. He spoke of the communication lines to Israel from the Indian Ocean through the Gulf of Aqaba which would be a necessity in view of the probability of damage to the Suez Canal. He felt that some expert from the U.S. should come over and quietly talk to them about how they should develop such a line of communication. He felt that if the U.S. did not do all of these things she would be found wanting one day and it would not be the fault of Israel.

Mr. Sharett next stated that Israel was not receiving all of the arms necessary for the proper security of Israel. The U.S. had turned down many things that were essential and others were slow in coming. The Secretary then referred to the list which was appended as item B of the briefing notes and stated that a 300-ton patrol craft was about to be released, also mosquito aircraft and 200 Browning machine guns. This Mr. Sharett appeared not to know about but was very pleased to hear. The Secretary then said—you know we cannot release 75mm recoilless rifles, jet planes, tank guns and Sherman tanks as they are needed for our commitments in North Atlantic Treaty Organization.[5] Mr. Sharett then requested to know what had happened about the 100,000 rifles they had requested. The Secretary referred the question to Captain Patrick who stated that he had no knowledge of such a request. Ambassador Eban said that he was not sure the request had been forwarded to the Department of State yet although he did have such a request which was associated with standardization of arms in Israel. Mr. Sharett further stated that by standardizing arms with the U.S., Israel would be in the position to help the U.S. by manufacturing these items in time of war. He further stated that some new machinery would be required by Israel to conform to U.S. standards.

Mr. Sharett told General Marshall it was very important that he know at this time what the plans of the U.S. and U.K. are for the Middle East in the event of war with Russia.[6] General Marshall regretted that he could not readily answer that questions, would have to refer it to the Joint Chiefs of Staff, and hence would not attempt to answer at this time. The Secretary further stated that such information would have to be obtained through the Department of State.

Mr. Sharett spoke of his appreciation for the increase in allotment of Israel nationals to U.S. service schools, but they still desired to have several allocations to our staff colleges. He further stated that the British had already offered them such a schooling, but now they need an insight into the U.S. military in order to better their position. The General stated that he would keep this in mind.

Just prior to departure, Mr. Sharett stated that he had one very important request to make of General Marshall. He stated the military attache from Israel had been permitted to sit in on certain restricted briefings concerning the progress of the war in Korea. He did not wish to ask for highly classified material, but felt that there was much restricted information that the U.S. services could perhaps release to their school personnel which they are not obtaining at this time.[7]

G. Serpell Patrick
Captain, USN
Office of Foreign Military Affairs

NA/RG 330, CD 092 (Israel)

1. The report for this December 18 conversation was submitted on December 20.
2. Ambassador Eban accompanied Sharett to this meeting. Also in attendance were an army and a navy officer, who wrote this memorandum.
3. Marshall may have been referring to his November 29 appearance and speech at the UIT dinner in New York honoring Israeli President Chaim Weizmann's birthday and the third anniversary of the UN General Assembly vote to partition Palestine into separate Jewish and Arab states. See pp. 263–68.
4. For more on this issue, see pp. 499–501 and 505–16.
5. See Murdaugh to Marshall, memorandum, "Visit of Israel Foreign Minister, Moshe Sharett," December 18, 1950, NA/RG 330, CD Briefings.
6. Sharett had asked this question during his October 19 meeting with Marshall. See pp. 205–6.
7. On December 23, Sharett sent Marshall a detailed memorandum covering all the points he had raised during this meeting. See pp. 329–30.

THE CHINESE military intervention in Korea in November and the ensuing discussions with visiting British Prime Minister Attlee in early December precipitated a major reassessment of American defense policies (see pp. 259 and 284–87). On December 14, the NSC reported to Truman that the four-year military buildup envisioned in NSC 68 would have to be accelerated on the grounds that "the period of greatest danger is directly before us," not in 1954 as originally projected. Truman consequently directed Acheson and Marshall "to undertake immediately a joint review of the politico-military strategy of this Government" and to submit their recommendations through the NSC "as soon as possible." (*FRUS, 1950*, 1: 467–69.) On December 21, Marshall informed the service secretaries, the JCS, and the chairman of the Munitions Board that a joint working group would be established for this purpose; that the Defense Department would be represented by General Burns and Robert LeBaron, chair of the Military Liaison Committee to the Atomic Energy Commission (AEC); and that the Joint Chiefs were to participate in the working group's deliberations. (Marshall to service secretaries, JCS, and Small, memorandum, December 21, 1950, NA/RG 330, CD 381 [Gen.].)

Truman also announced and issued a proclamation on December 15–16 declaring the existence of a state of national emergency. As part of this declaration, he established the Office of Defense Mobilization (ODM) within the Executive Office of the President and appointed Charles Wilson, president of General Electric, to serve as its director. ("Wilson Resigns as G.E. President; Cordiner Is Named His Successor," *New York Times*, December 17, 1950, p. F1.) On December 18, Marshall informed the service secretaries that Truman's proclamation allowed them to authorize the negotiation of purchases and contracts. Previously he had instructed the secretaries "to accelerate procurement actions in connection with 2nd Supplemental 1951 Funds." Now he issued guidelines for broadening the industrial base of the procurement program. (Marshall to service secretaries, memorandum, December 18, 1950, GCMRL/G. C. Marshall Papers [Secretary of Defense, Number Indexed, M200-3-26].) Marshall considered creation of this broadened base vitally important and had so informed the House Appropriations Subcommittee and the Senate Appropriations Committee during his December 1 and 9 testimonies (see pp. 276–78 and 291–93). He reiterated these points to the public in a recorded segment for an end-of-year program broadcast on December 31, 1950, on the Columbia Broadcasting System (CBS). (Ibid., [M200-3-28].) As he later wrote to Senator Margaret Chase Smith (R-ME), "To my mind it could spell the difference between survival and disaster. My experiences during World War I and World War II led me to the conclusion that the creation of an adequate expansible industrial base in advance of actual requirements was more important than the hurried accumulation of vast quantities of military materiel." (Marshall to Smith, April 29, 1953, GCMRL/G. C. Marshall Papers [Retirement, General].) For more from this letter, see pp. 757–59.

Also in process at this time was a change in policy regarding Formosa. As early as December 4, Acheson in a letter to Marshall had agreed that the NSC should review US policy regarding the island, noted that recent JCS comments regarding its military importance appeared to be a "substantial modification" of their previous position, and consequently recommended a JCS review of the issue so that the NSC could have their current views. (*FRUS, 1950*, 6: 587–88.) Citing this letter along with numerous other relevant documents, Marshall informed the Joint Chiefs on December 20 that "the question of the strategic importance of Formosa has come up in several different policy decisions now in the planning stage" and requested their "views and recommendations . . . on the short-term and long-term U.S. strategic interests in Formosa, from the military point of view." (Marshall to JCS, memorandum, December 20, 1950, NA/RG 330, CD 092 [China].) On that same day, he met with Brigadier General Peter T. K. Pee, the Nationalist Chinese military attaché, and sent him a letter the following day. ★

185

TO BRIGADIER GENERAL PETER T. K. PEE — December 21, 1950
Confidential — Washington, DC

Dear Pee: I have not yet had time to go into the matter of military materiel for Formosa, but I find a program of such assistance has been developed but has not yet been finally passed on. Final action has not yet been taken by the Joint Chiefs of Staff, which is an absolutely essential preliminary.[1]

I tell you this most *confidentially* (which means specifically for the Generalissimo only and not for any of your officials in Washington.) Faithfully yours,

GCMRL/G. C. Marshall Papers (Secretary of Defense, Selected)

1. After his December 20 meeting with Pee (see previous editorial note), Marshall contacted Major General Charles L. Bolté, assistant army chief of staff for operations (G-3), to obtain information on military assistance to Chiang's forces on Formosa. Bolté responded both verbally and in writing on the same day that the JCS, after requesting and receiving a survey by MacArthur on the military assistance required to prevent Communist capture of the island, had prepared a program of military assistance totaling $71.2 million but that this program still awaited final JCS action. (Bolté to Marshall, memorandum, December 20, 1950, GCMRL/G. C. Marshall Papers [Secretary of Defense, Selected].)

Marshall had also recently received a letter from General Sun Li-jen (VMI, 1927), a commanding general of the Chinese forces who had fought under US General Joseph Stilwell in the China-Burma-India Theater during World War II and was at this time the head of Chiang Kai-shek's ground forces on Formosa. Sun wrote on November 8 of the urgent "necessity of forging a modern army for the Chinese people." He reported that he had trained thirty thousand "intelligent and well-disciplined men," but they were "very much under-nourished and almost unpaid and unclothed." Marshall Carter forwarded Sun's letter to the State Department for suggestions on a response. Dean Rusk advised replying to Sun "in as friendly and encouraging terms as is possible without either putting General Sun on the spot or committing ourselves too deeply" and enclosed a draft response. Using Rusk's draft as a guide, Marshall replied on December 19 that he was "interested" in Sun's report and progress, which "is a pretty large undertaking and I can appreciate some of the difficulties with which you undoubtedly had to contend." (Sun to Marshall, November 8, 1950; Rusk to Carter, December 18, 1950; and Marshall to Sun, December 19, 1950, GCMRL/G. C. Marshall Papers [Secretary of Defense, Number Indexed, M200-8-44].) See pp. 438–39.

186

To Madame Chiang Kai-shek

December 21, 1950
Washington, DC

Dear Madame: I received your note of November 28 transmitting the summary of intelligence which the Generalissimo asked you transmit to me. I immediately had it considered by the agencies dealing with the subject and while a considerable portion of the information had already come in, there were valuable additional facts included in the summary. All of this, of course, goes to the better appreciation of the situation.[1]

Will you please be good enough to express to the Generalissimo my personal appreciation of his sending me this information.

Though the foregoing is decidedly of a business nature, I cannot refrain from making some reference to personal things. Katherine has written you, she tells me, and she very recently heard from you.[2] Actually she is in better shape now than for sometime, but still has a shingles reaction if she allows herself to get tired or develops a cold. She finds the small apartment—and it is very small, a great relief from housekeeping cares. We take a good many of our meals out as quietly as can be managed and we have succeeded so far in keeping our location quiet and our telephone number is not in the book, which is a great protection to her.

We had hoped to spend a few days at Pinehurst for Christmas, but do not know today whether or not it will be possible to leave the day after tomorrow. In any event, I will have to be back here at 10:00 o'clock the morning after Christmas and will probably return Christmas eve.

A gentleman recently returned from Formosa came in to see me the other day and told me he had seen you personally and the Generalissimo and that you both are looking very well, as a matter of fact he was most complimentary and I can only hope that you are in as good shape as he indicated.[3] So far, I am getting along, but there are about a million pressures each day and I have to spend a great deal of my time with the Congress.

General Pee came in yesterday to talk to me about Formosa equipment and I have just sent him a confidential note on the subject.[4]

With Christmas greetings to you and the Generalissimo and our very heartfelt wishes for you both in the critical New Year.[5] Faithfully yours,

GCMRL/G. C. Marshall Papers (Secretary of Defense, Selected)

1. Madame Chiang had sent Marshall an intelligence summary from the numerous intelligence reports that her husband had received regarding the Chinese Communist intervention in Korea. This attachment, titled "Instructions on the participation of the Korean War Given by the Chinese Communist Central Political Bureau to its branch Bureaus on November 1, 1950," listed the Communists' supposed purposes and plans. (Madame Chiang to Marshall, November 28, 1950, NA/RG 330, CD 092 [China, Communist].)

2. The most recent letter from Madame Chiang to the Marshalls was dated November 28. (GCMRL/© Marshall-Winn Collection [Katherine Tupper Marshall Collection, Correspondence].)

3. The editors have been unable to identify this person.

4. See the previous document.

5. Madame Chiang replied on February 6, 1951, "The Generalissimo and I both deeply appreciate your efforts in helping China and us. . . . I am helping on the project which the gentleman who visited Taipeh and returned to America mentioned to you upon arrival in America. I hope that all will go well." (Madame Chiang to Marshall, February 6, 1951, GCMRL/G. C. Marshall Papers [Secretary of Defense, Selected].) See also pp. 426–27 and 438–39.

187

To General of the Army Dwight D. Eisenhower — December 21, 1950, Washington, DC

Dear Eisenhower: I will not attempt the detailed answer to your letter of December 12, which I had prepared to give until I saw you personally. Most of the matters you discussed with me were included in your letter and most of them have reached a degree of understanding or solution acceptable to you.[1]

The best I can tell you right now at this moment is that I am at your disposal in anyway I can find to be helpful. I believe you are taking over my old office and I am only sorry that I cannot really give you a great many of the things you so urgently require immediately.

I repeat again what I told you the other day that I think your attitude in the matter and the sacrifice you are making is a very great offering to your country, and I am certain you will acquit yourself with the highest honor, which is so greatly to the national interest and the interest of the world generally.

There are a great many men of wisdom and of courage, men of reputation in the world, but your combination of these qualities together with a rare ability to work harmoniously with other people and control their efforts, capped by an outstanding quality in the high degree of integrity which has characterized your every action, makes you rather unique in the world.[2] Faithfully yours,

GCMRL/G. C. Marshall Papers (Secretary of Defense, Selected)

1. Eisenhower had written to Marshall on December 12 to express some of his thoughts and concerns about the prospects of his becoming Supreme Allied Commander, Europe of NATO. He reiterated his previous agreement to Truman and Marshall that he would "undertake the responsibility of Supreme Command in Europe if I am requested unanimously by the Governments concerned, and designated by the President," but noted that Truman had "indicated that he would not ask me" to do so "unless the advance political and military arrangements were such as to give justifiable promise of success." From Eisenhower's perspective they were not. He had met with the JCS on December 9 and had found "a readiness to rush the United States into a responsibility, namely that of taking over Command in Europe, without a careful evaluation of the situation and without clear comprehension of all that this assumption of responsibility might mean." Of particular concern to him were: the assumption that the Germans would accept any Anglo-French-US agreement on their rearmament; the fact that no NATO nation was pledged "to do its maximum in order to make sure that the project succeeds"; the evidence to the contrary he found in the limitations many of the NATO papers sought to place on a unified command, such as separation of the Mediterranean from his command; the "uncertainty" that the United States could send more than three or four divisions to Europe; and the negative impact this would have on other member nations. (Eisenhower to Marshall, December 12, 1950, GCMRL/G. C. Marshall Papers [Secretary of Defense, Selected].) For more, see *Papers of DDE*, 11: 1467–71.

Eisenhower had seen Marshall at a luncheon hosted by David Sarnoff at the Bankers Club in New York on December 8, and they had a discussion with Lovett on the evening of December 14 in Washington. Marshall Carter had on that day handed to Marshall a four-page draft response to Eisenhower "based on very rough notes of your conversation" and Eisenhower's reiteration to Carter of his "deep concern" about two of the problems mentioned in his December 12 letter: the lack of commitments from other NATO member nations and the burden that places on the United States, and the "complete lack of sense in having a separate Mediterranean Command." If the Mediterranean was not part of his command, "and a very vital part, then he did not understand the setup and they had better get somebody else who did." Carter's draft response had urged Eisenhower to "take on face value the promises that other nations have already made to us" and had expressed confidence "that by designating an American Commander at this time we would have somebody on the spot to push these matters along and see them through." It also clarified that "the present thought of our Chiefs of Staff is that the Mediterranean is so large, and part of the mission of the Mediterranean Fleet will be so far removed from Western Europe, that it may be better to keep the Mediterranean as a separate command" while recognizing "that the Mediterranean's principle mission will be to support the defense of Western Europe." (Carter to Marshall, December 14, 1950, ibid.)

Whether Marshall used any of these points in his evening conversation with Eisenhower and Lovett, which lasted approximately thirty minutes, cannot be determined. On December 15, however, Lovett telephoned Acheson and said that Eisenhower "had been reassured" and "was willing to accept the appointment." (*FRUS, 1950*, 3: 578–80.) On December 18–19, the NATO Council and Defense Committee meeting in Brussels approved a compromise arrangement on German rearmament and requested the United States name Eisenhower as SACEUR. Truman did so on December 19. (Ibid., 604–5; Condit, *Test of War*, 331–34.)

For more on the development of the SACEUR position and Eisenhower's appointment, see pp. 167–68, 199–203, 204–6, 218–20, 245–46, and 284–87.

2. Eisenhower replied on December 29 that he was "most grateful for the sentiments you express" and that he was "certainly determined to do the very best I can in the extraordinary task assigned me." He anticipated discussing that task with Marshall in early January before departing for an exploratory trip to Europe. (Eisenhower to Marshall, December 29, 1950, GCMRL/G. C. Marshall Papers [Secretary of Defense, Selected].) See photo #7.

188

To Queen Frederica of the Hellenes — December 21, 1950
Washington, DC

Your Majesty: I have never acknowledged your letter of July 20 suggesting certain action relative to the crisis developed by the outbreak of the fighting in Korea. At the time I sent it to our senior military official, General Bradley, in order that he might have the benefit of your ideas regarding Western Europe and Greece in particular. As you suggested in your letter, it was not permissible then for me to make any formal comments. Since then, however, my status has changed, as you know, and all these matters come to my official attention.[1]

I had a lengthy talk with General Van Fleet and had him submit to me later his written views on the situation. You can well imagine just what they were. Since then I have been very much in the thick of the struggle of building up our military power as rapidly as possible, and have spent a considerable part of my time before the appropriations committees of Congress and in meetings concerned with rearmament of Western Europe. As a matter of fact, I stepped into the latter problem at a formal meeting in New York with Bevin, Schumann, Shinwell and Moch just a few hours after I took over this present office of mine.[2]

Naturally I have been heavily involved in matters pertaining to fighting in Korea and the very threatening situation that is developing there.

I had a rather lengthy talk with your ambassador the other day just prior to his return to Athens. I knew him and was entertained by him in Moscow in 1947 during one of those periods of futile negotiations.[3]

In this extremely dangerous world situation and with emotions aflame, it is very difficult to manage a calm and deliberate approach to the necessities of the day. I have been through similar periods. They present many trying difficulties.

I was happy to see the other day that a beginning had been made, however minute, in the returning of your children to Greece. I can only hope this will expand into large numbers with the consequent tremendous effect on the morale of your people.[4]

Mrs. Marshall appreciated very much your inquiry regarding her and her eye trouble. She still has to be careful or she suffers a temporary return, but she appears to be in very good health, though this present turn in our affairs has ruined our home life and all our plans. We have closed up our place at Leesburg, Virginia, and have not been able to open our little place at Pinehurst, North Carolina, merely living in a very small and at present hidden apartment here in Washington.

She was particularly pleased with the reference to your children and the little pencils she gave them, and with the affectionate greeting you sent us.[5]

With our prayers for you and His Majesty and your people in the New Year, believe me, always, Faithfully yours,

GCMRL/G. C. Marshall Papers (Secretary of Defense, Number Indexed, M200-6-41)

1. For Queen Frederica's July 20 letter, see pp. 134n5 and 149n3.

2. Marshall had met with Van Fleet on October 4, 1950. Van Fleet, now the commanding general of the Second Army at Fort Meade, Maryland, wrote to Marshall on November 9 that he concurred with the opinions expressed in Frederica's July 20 letter. (Van Fleet to Marshall, November 9, 1950, GCMRL/James A. Van Fleet Papers [Greece, Correspondence, General]; H.) For more on Van Fleet, see pp. 133–34. For more on Marshall's meeting with the European foreign and defense ministers, see pp. 167–68.

3. On November 29, 1950, Marshall had met with Panagiotis Kanellopoulos, chief of the Greek delegation to the United Nations, and Greek Ambassador to the US Athanase Politis. Kanellopoulos delivered a message of appreciation to Marshall from King Paul and Queen Frederica for his visit to Greece in 1948 and "for the great help the U.S. is giving to Greece in the form of military aid and assistance." As secretary of state, Marshall had visited Greece from October 16 to 18, 1948. (See *Papers of GCM*, 6: 591–94.) Marshall thanked Queen Frederica through Kanellopoulos for Greece's support of the West and asked him to inform the queen that she would soon be receiving his response to her July 20 letter. (Memorandum of conversation with Kanellopoulos and Politis, November 29, 1950, NA/RG 330, CD Memorandum of Conversation.)

4. The Yugoslav government had returned sixty-three children to Greece on November 22, 1950, after the two countries resumed diplomatic ties the day before. The Greek government estimated that the Yugoslav government had kidnapped around twenty-eight thousand children since the outbreak of the Greek civil war. ("Greek Youth to Return,"

New York Times, November 23, 1950, p. 10.) For the background on this situation, see pp. 132–34.

5. Frederica hoped "this letter will find you and your wife in good health. I hope her eye trouble has passed and she is well and happy again. My children still treasure the small pencils she gave to them." (Frederica to Marshall, July 20, 1950, GCMRL/G. C. Marshall Papers [Secretary of Defense, Number Indexed, M200-6-41].)

189

MEMORANDUM OF CONVERSATION — December 21, 1950
Secret — Washington, DC

General Romulo and Ambassador Elizalde came to see Secretary Marshall at 2:15 today, by appointment.[1] General Romulo informed Secretary Marshall that he had asked for this appointment in order, first, to pay his respects to Secretary Marshall, whom he had not seen for some time, and to discuss the greatest concern of his Government, Philippine security.

General Romulo asked two questions: first, Did the United States intend to shorten its lines in the Far East and pull back? Secretary Marshall replied that, if the Philippine Government meant by that question the possibility that the United States would pull out of Asia, the Philippine Government need have no concern whatsoever in this regard. Secondly, General Romulo raised the question of what support the United States intended to provide the Philippines in the present situation? He informed the Secretary that the Philippine Congress had just appropriated 29 million pesos (about $15 million) for equipping ten additional BCT's [battalion combat teams]. General Romulo stated that these funds were not nearly enough to take care of the needs, and, therefore, the Philippines would need assistance from the United States.[2]

Secretary Marshall asked whether the Philippine Government had any specific requests to make. Ambassador Elizalde then read, from his rough notes, a telegram from Manila which he had just received by telephone from the Embassy. While it was not easy to follow the Ambassador's notes, they did mention equipment for a jet fighter squadron, mobilization of ground divisions, and certain naval combat vessels.

Secretary Marshall suggested to Ambassador Elizalde that this information be put in its proper form and presented to the Department of Defense so that it might give it the consideration it deserved. General Romulo and Ambassador Elizalde agreed that they would have this done immediately. Secretary Marshall then told the Philippine representatives that the United States Government was very much concerned with security of the Philippines, in which the United States has a close and continuing interest. The United States is providing aid to the Philippines within the limits of its capacity to meet needs all over the world. The Secretary stated that the current United States military assistance program had been well over half-delivered, and that more assistance was being developed, although he was not in a position to give them exact figures.

Secretary Marshall then stated that he wished to have a very frank and confidential discussion with General Romulo and Ambassador Elizalde on the question of military leadership in the Philippines. Secretary Marshall explained that the Chinese Communist leaders were all very tough and able men and that Philippine leadership would have to be of a high quality. He asked General Romulo whether there was a real military leader in the Philippines who was not politically influenced and who could develop the fighting strength of the Philippine people. General Romulo replied that he recognized that Philippine military leadership was poor and the problem needed a good deal of attention. He and Ambassador Elizalde mentioned that the aggressive, non-political military officers were not in a position of command for the very reason that they remained out of politics. Secretary Marshall inquired about the Philippine Scouts.[3] Romulo replied that they had been disbanded and completed many years service, in any event. Romulo and Elizalde both referred to the loss, during the Japanese occupation, of some top Philippine military leaders who had been trained at West Point.

Secretary Marshall then returned to the question of leadership in the Philippines. He stated that this was one of the most important questions facing the Philippine Government today. Therefore, he requested General Romulo to convey a personal message to President [Elpidio] Quirino along the following lines:

Secretary Marshall personally would do everything he could to help the Philippine Government in the present situation. However, this help would be nullified without strong military leadership. There must be good leadership in the Philippine Armed Forces or United States equipment would not be effective.[4]

General Marshall stressed to General Romulo the necessity for such leadership. General Romulo assured him that he would convey this message to President Quirino.[5]

K. T. Young

NA/RG 330, CD Memorandum of Conversation

1. Carlos Romulo, the Philippine secretary of foreign affairs and delegate to the UN, was president of the General Assembly during its 1949–50 fourth session. Joaquim Elizalde was the Philippine ambassador to the United States.

2. The Philippine government was contributing troops in Korea while simultaneously battling the Communist-led Hukbalahap guerrillas (Huks).

3. Originally formed to help the US Army during the Philippine-American War of 1899–1902, the Philippine Scouts were authorized by Congress in 1901 as official military units in the US Army. These units were composed of Filipino volunteers led primarily by US Army commissioned officers. They were disbanded after the Philippines became independent in 1946.

4. "This is but a tactful interpretation of what I said," Marshall wrote in the left margin. According to the minutes of a January 22, 1951, conference between US Ambassador to the Philippines Myron M. Cowen and Philippine Secretary of National Defense Ramon Magsaysay, Cowen had read the minutes of this December 21 meeting among Marshall, Elizalde, and Romulo. Based on his reading, Cowen reiterated to Magsaysay that Marshall "did not wish to have the same experience that he had had in China in supplying arms to an Army which was guided by political interests." (*FRUS, 1951*, 6: 1504.)

5. For more see pp. 429–31.

190

To Lieutenant General Richard J. Marshall — December 22, 1950
[Washington, DC]

Dear Marshall: I have been making inquiries in various directions and have arrived at the firm conclusion that the situation on the Board of Visitors is not at all satisfactory. What has happened seems to be very much what I predicted and arises out of the fact that there is no firm leadership because of my absences and inability to get intimately into the business week by week with you. As a matter of fact, the situation, in my opinion, has developed more seriously than even I anticipated.[1]

My reaction to this is that I must resign as President at the meeting on January 15, and I am giving you notice so that you can take whatever steps seem advisable to lead up to a desirable successor, and incidentally and *most confidentially*, it is possible that I may be in Tokyo at the time of this meeting. I don't think it is probable, but it is possible.

This is a very short note because I am deeply engaged, but I wanted to send you this word as quickly as possible.[2] Faithfully yours,

GCMRL/G. C. Marshall Papers (Pentagon Office, Selected)

1. George Marshall had been appointed to the VMI Board of Visitors effective July 1, 1946. He had been elected president of the board on September 23, 1950, to fill the vacancy left by James S. Easley, and was supposed "to serve until next January, when a regular election is to be held." ("Gen. Marshall Invited to Join VMI Board," *Washington Post*, May 15, 1946, p. 7; "V.M.I. Names Marshall," *New York Times*, September 24, 1950, p. 26. See also pp. 172–73.)

2. Superintendent Richard Marshall responded on December 24 that he was "very sorry" that Secretary Marshall felt he had to resign but thanked him for the advance notice. (R. J. Marshall to Marshall, December 24, 1950, GCMRL/G. C. Marshall Papers [Pentagon Office, Selected].) At Superintendent Marshall's urging, Secretary Marshall did attend the January 15 board meeting in Richmond, Virginia, where he resigned as president of the board. George Marshall later wrote to Leonard K. Nicholson (VMI, 1901), Marshall's four-year roommate at VMI and president of the New Orleans–based Times-Picayune Publishing Company, that he "found it necessary to resign the presidency of the Board not so much because of myself personally, . . . but because the situation was giving, in my opinion, rise to dissatisfaction that possibly the interests of the Institute were suffering" due to Marshall's "failure to give active leadership to the business of the day." Marshall reported that he had declined the board's requests to "reconsider" and to serve as "Chairman of the Board—a new office," or "Honorary President." The board elected Earnest A. Sale (VMI, 1919), president of the Sale Knitting Company in Martinsville, Virginia, and former president pro tempore of the VMI Board of Visitors, to succeed Marshall. (Marshall to Nicholson, January 31, 1951, GCMRL/G. C. Marshall Papers [Secretary of Defense, Number Indexed, M200-4-36].)

191

To Lieutenant General Walton H. Walker — December 22, 1950
[Washington, DC]

Dear Walker: You are facing a very hard Christmas. I am sorry I cannot contribute something material to assist you and provide a little cheer. I have been on the verge of writing you a number of times since I became Secretary of Defense and each time just as I was about to write the situation changed materially and somewhat violently. Now, I want you to at least have my holiday greetings and all of my most sincere wishes for the New Year along with which I want to tell you that I feel that you have done a magnificent job. I don't think anyone has had a tougher campaign, a longer strain and a greater series of difficulties than you have encountered since last June. And as the year draws to a close, you are faced with a mounting strain.

I do hope that physically and mentally you have been able to rise above the natural fatigues which must ordinarily be yours. You have our very real prayers for yourself and your men.[1]

With my affectionate regards, Faithfully yours,

GCMRL/G. C. Marshall Papers (Secretary of Defense, Number Indexed, M200-7-1)

1. Walker was killed on December 23 in an automobile collision north of Seoul on the way to present a distinguished unit citation to the Twenty-fourth Division, in which his son, Captain Samuel Simms Walker, commanded an infantry company. General Walker was the highest-ranking officer to die in the Korean War. Lieutenant General Matthew B. Ridgway, then deputy army chief of staff, succeeded Walker as commander of the Eighth Army. ("Gen. Walker Killed Driving to See Son," *Washington Post*, December 24, 1950, p. M3.)

Marshall released excerpts from this letter to the press when news of Walker's death broke and sent a telegram to Mrs. Walker to express Mrs. Marshall's and his condolences. They attended the funeral at Arlington Cemetery on January 2. (Press release, December 23, 1950, and Marshall to Mrs. Walker, December 23, 1950, GCMRL/G. C. Marshall Papers [Secretary of Defense, Number Indexed, M200-7-1].)

192

To Mrs. George C. Marshall — December 26, 1950
Washington, DC

Dearest: I had them telephone you on my arrival here and I am adding this note to outline the prospects.

I have to meet the President at 5:30 on the field and then have dinner at Blair House at 7:30 this evening—informal. Just what will come out of all this I, of course, don't know.

Tomorrow I have a very important hearing, over which I preside, here in the Pentagon at 2:00 P. M. which Lovett is organizing. That means there is small chance that I can fly down to Pinehurst tomorrow evening. Apparently the best I can do is Thursday noon if I find it is not necessary for me to attend the Cabinet meeting Friday morning.[1]

I just talked to Sterling. He said Allene is in bed with a cold. I think long underwear is the cure for her and not nylons! Sterling was well.

I have not yet gotten in touch with ~~Catherine~~ Clifton or Anna [Wong].

Enclosed is a copy of the release I made on poor Walker.[2]

GCMRL/G. C. Marshall Papers (Secretary of Defense, Selected)

1. The Marshalls had left Washington on Friday, December 22, to spend Christmas at Pinehurst. Marshall arrived back in Washington on the morning of Tuesday, December 26, while Katherine Marshall remained in Pinehurst. At 2:00 p.m. on Wednesday, December 27, he met with Rosenberg, Pace, Finletter, Secretary of the Navy Francis P. Matthews, Leva, Assistant Secretary of the Army Earl D. Johnson, General J. Lawton Collins, Air Force Deputy Chief of Staff for Personnel Lieutenant General Richard E. Nugent, US Air Force Vice Chief of Staff General Nathan F. Twining (USMA, 1918), and Defense Department Personnel Policy Board Chairman J. Thomas Schneider, to discuss combat duty pay. Marshall did attend the cabinet meeting at 10:00 a.m. on Friday, December 29, and departed for Pinehurst again that afternoon.

2. See previous document n1.

193

To Brigadier General Robert E. Wood — December 26, 1950
Washington, DC

Dear General Wood: I read your letter of November 18 very carefully. You have a pretty accurate analysis of the conditions against which we struggle financially. Unfortunately, so far as I am concerned, I always arrive on the scene when we are in deep trouble which makes it an extremely difficult time to bring about sound changes in policy procedure.[1]

With regard to Universal Military Service, I find that the situation now is so demanding as to speed and quantity that a backlog of reserve which would have been brought about by Universal Military Training at small expense cannot be managed in this particular emergency, but I am determined that we will weld this principle to whatever measures we find it necessary to take immediately—I am referring to amendments to the Selective Service Act.[2]

As to the Germans, the question of their contribution has been before the North Atlantic Treaty Organization and the full agreement reached is now a matter of public knowledge. The difficult part, of course, is the implementation, and our three high commissioners, John McCloy for us, are now at work with the head of the West German government, endeavoring to find a basis acceptable for the speed up of defenses preparations. This is exceedingly difficult business because of the unfortunate publicity that has taken place during the past four months;—unfortunate in its effect on the German people who are human like the rest of us in their reactions.[3]

As to Japan, we are involved there at present by the decision of the Far Eastern Commission which adopted a policy for the tentative disarmament of Japan which will have to be repealed. The directive implementing this policy decision was sent to MacArthur in 1948, so there are these factors to be overcome.

Our government proposals regarding a treaty of peace with Japan have been handled openly in the press. These proposals contain nothing which would restrict any efforts the Japanese may make after the treaty is signed to provide for their own defense. Just what we can do to proceed rapidly in this matter in the present emergency remains to be seen.[4]

All matters pertaining to defense that I touch these days cost extraordinarily large sums and inflationary effects reduce the buying power of the monies appropriated. Since the declaration of a national emergency, it may be that some of this may be gotten under control, but it all makes for numerous difficulties.

I was much interested in your letter and thank you for writing. Faithfully yours,

GCMRL/G. C. Marshall Papers (Secretary of Defense, Chronological, Secretaries, Ackerman)

1. Wood (USMA, 1900) had been chairman of the board of Sears, Roebuck & Co. since 1939. He had attended the November 5 Business Advisory Council meeting at Sea Island, Georgia, during which Marshall had outlined a defense production program of at least four years in duration that would require increased defense spending. ("Marshall Reveals a Defense Program of 4 Years or More," *New York Times*, November 6, 1950, p. 1.)

Wood thought that Marshall had placed his "finger on the root of our greatest present difficulty," namely that the nation could not afford an armed force of three million given the high living standard Congress had mandated for US forces. Wood was willing to support UMT to reduce costs, but he also suggested rearming Germany and Japan to achieve that same goal. (Wood to Marshall, November 18, 1950, NA/RG 330, SD 381.)

2. For more on Marshall's changed approach to UMT, see pp. 207–9, 325–29, and 338–47.

3. In the aftermath of the December 18–19 agreement by the NATO foreign ministers to establish a unified defense force that included West German forces under a US commander, the three Western high commissioners for Germany had met with West German Chancellor Konrad Adenauer on December 21 to begin discussions regarding the transfer of more sovereignty to West Germany from the Allied occupation and the scale of West Germany's contribution to the new European defense force. ("Allies and Bonn Set Stage for Treaty and Arms Talks," *New York Times*, December 22, 1950, p. 1.)

4. For more on US concerns about an independent Japan and the directive sent to MacArthur, see *Papers of GCM*, 6: 366–67. For more on the Japanese peace treaty, see pp. 324–25.

194

To John McSweeney

December 27, 1950
Washington, DC

Dear McSweeney: Since your visit on December 4, I have informed Secretary Pace of your desire to serve and asked him to let me know if there was an appropriate assignment in which your services could be utilized.[1]

He informs me that, with regard to recall to active duty as a Reserve officer, the present policy of the Department of the Army, in accordance with pertinent law, precludes recall of reservists who have reached their sixtieth birthday. However, present age-in-grade policies pertaining to military government work are being reviewed with a view to increasing utilization of older officers during full mobilization.

Mr. Pace further stated that at the present time there are no available vacancies in a civilian capacity for a man of your wide experience and background, but he will certainly keep you in mind if a suitable position should open up in the near future.[2]

I regret that I cannot give you a more favorable reply at this time, but I do appreciate your willingness to serve and shall certainly let you know if an appropriate assignment becomes available in the future. Faithfully yours,

NA/RG 330, SD 326.02

1. Informing Marshall earlier in December of his service in both world wars and the fact that "recent physical examinations show me to be in good health," Representative John McSweeney (D-OH) had asked "that some opportunity be given to me for service at home or abroad." (McSweeney to Marshall, December 4, 1950, NA/RG 330, SD 326.02.)

2. C. J. George had informed Marshall on December 6 that McSweeney held an inactive reserve rank of lieutenant colonel, and that his request on August 30, 1949, to receive an appointment to the active reserve had been turned down based on the fact that at fifty-eight he was beyond the age limit of fifty-five. Marshall handwrote at the top of this memo: "Is there any duty appropriate to his experience and age he might be given?" (George to Marshall, memorandum, December 6, 1950, and Marshall to George, n.d., ibid.) On the following day, he asked Pace to look into the matter. Marshall summarized Pace's December 23 response in this letter to McSweeney. (Pace to Marshall, memorandum, December 23, 1950, ibid.)

195

To Mrs. John B. Wilson — December 27, 1950
Washington, DC

Dear Rose: Your Xmas note re Page's contribution to my happiness and the cute card with your photographs I found at the apartment last night when I returned from three days at Pinehurst. You were sweet to send us the card and to write me about Page. I am sending him a note of thanks direct.[1]

Katherine and I flew down to Pinehurst for the Xmas week end and I left her there and flew back yesterday morning. I hope to go back for the New Year's week end but it looks doubtful. With the lame duck Congress holding its final, and vitally important session New Years day and General Walker's funeral probably on Saturday I don't see my way out of the Pentagon.[2]

I think I owe you a reply to your fine long letter of some weeks back. Evidently you are delightfully situated now and your family delightfully amusing, or exciting judging from what you told me of the youngest gentleman. I hope to get to see you and them this winter or spring.[3]

With my love, Affectionately,

G.C.M.

GCMRL/J. Page Wilson Collection; H

1. The editors have been unable to locate Rose's Christmas card to Marshall.

Marshall wrote to Rose's elder son, Page, on December 29 to thank him for his "Christmas card and also the little souvenir of paper doll cutouts. I appreciate your including me on your list this year. That was a very attractive Christmas card your mother sent with the pictures of you and your brother and your mother and dad. I hope you all had a very merry Christmas and that Santa Claus was especially good to you and your brother." (Marshall to Page Wilson, December 29, 1950, GCMRL/J. Page Wilson Collection.)

2. For more on Marshall's visit to Pinehurst around Christmas, General Walker's death,

and Marshall's interest in the new session of Congress, see pp. 309–10, 325–29, and 338–47.

3. Rose had written a lengthy letter to Marshall on December 7 "to remind you that I think of you." She understood Truman's need for Marshall, but asked "how many more big, tough jobs are you going to accept? You really have broken all records for the patriot so now I know that you will never, never retire and raise tomatoes." She also expressed her opinions on Korea and MacArthur and provided details on other members of her family. Her son Page had "reached an age when he will listen to reason" and was "completely absorbed in playing football," and she described her younger son, Tom, as "a terror, he is full of beans, he is incorrigible, and he is very, very funny." Her husband, John, had consequently "set aside a budget to cover damages done by Tom." She also informed Marshall that John had received a raise and "now makes $25,000—we were married on $2500." (Wilson to Marshall, December 7, 1950, GCMRL/G. C. Marshall Papers [Secretary of Defense, Number Indexed, M200-6-31].)

Marshall wrote to Rose again on January 5 that he "was thinking about you this morning as I drove down to the office through the park, which is my usual route. I go by so many of the places that Celeste and you explored with me on Saturday or Sunday afternoons when we were all living at 2400 Sixteenth Street. That was all a great many years ago and you and Celeste have scattered quite a bit to other points of the compass. I, however, am back on the old terrain. I hope your family were all well over the holidays and that the youngest has not yet burned down the house." (Marshall to Wilson, January 5, 1951, ibid.) See pp. 146–47 and 422–23.

196

To Errett P. Scrivner

December 28, 1950
Washington, DC

My dear Mr. Scrivner: I have read your letter of December 26 with reference to the reasons for public reactions regarding national defense, particularly the impressions made by the attitude of the members of the Defense Department in Washington.

Referring to your first paragraph "A statement attributed to you by the Press indicates your concern over the general apathy of the public to defense needs", my concern specifically related to the apathy of the public during periods when no crisis appeared imminent. It did not refer to times like these when actually there is a general pressure to do more or at least to do things faster than at present seems wise from the viewpoint of efficient accomplishment.[1]

My statement related to the public apathy at other times when there is no emotional charge such as exists today. I was referring to the 1920's and early 30's, to the period after the close of hostilities in 1945 for several years and not to the reactions of today.

As to the personnel in the Pentagon, I think you would find that the principal actors and they constitute a very large number, are overworked decidedly to such a degree that it has awakened my concern. There are many hundreds of others who have appointed tasks that fall within specific hours unless something most unusual occurs. Then, of course, they must keep to their posts. But for most of this latter group, merely to hold them to their desks over longer hours without adequate tasks would not promote efficiency. In my long experience in the War

Department, which included both the air and ground forces, and my more recent experience in connection with the Navy, I have never found any vestige of unwillingness to work through long hours and over weekends. When there is work to do, they do it. And when there is not work to do, I would not be one to insist that they hang around. Quite the contrary. That has never appealed to me as an effective procedure towards efficient accomplishment.[2] Faithfully yours,

GCMRL/G. C. Marshall Papers (Secretary of Defense, Selected)

1. Representative Scrivner (R-KS) believed that "some of the apathy" of the public to national defense policies was a result of the behavior of the military, particularly due to reports in the press of parties and receptions for officers during normal working hours. (Scrivner to Marshall, December 26, 1950, NA/RG 330, SD 330.14.)

2. Scrivner also blamed the apathy on the fact that the public "sees the Pentagon and other military buildings at a stand-still" outside of normal working hours for a civilian office. (Ibid.)

197

MEMORANDUM FOR ROBERT A. LOVETT

December 28, 1950
Washington, DC

Herewith is a diagram outlining the organization of the Office of Defense Mobilization under Wilson. It provides for a Defense Production Administration under an administrator who will be nominated by the President and confirmed by the Senate.[1]

The change that is made in pencil in the outline of the Defense Production Administration duties was made at my request.[2]

There is also attached a proposed Executive Order establishing the Defense Production Administration.

It was agreed that any objections to this order should be turned in to Mr. Wilson before 5:00 P.M. tomorrow, Friday. Otherwise, it will be assumed that the form and content of the order are acceptable.[3]

It was also agreed that the first meeting of the Board would be held at 11:00 A.M., January 10. At first there will be weekly meetings, to be reduced later to two meetings a month.

NA/RG 330, SD 040 (Defense Mobilization, Office of)

1. Marshall had previously met with Wilson and did so again at 10:25 a.m. on the day he wrote this memorandum. After the first meeting, Marshall wrote to Edmund Coles, who was an old friend of Wilson, that he "had Charles Wilson in for lunch the other day and afterwards he and I got together for a talk. As a matter of fact, we talked so long that of the two appointments I had following, one had to be canceled and the other was delayed almost an hour. He has a very important job to do, but he has all the necessary qualifications with it." (Marshall to Coles, December 22, 1950, GCMRL/G. C. Marshall Papers [Secretary of Defense, Number Indexed, M200-2-11].)

2. The attached diagram had listed the duties of the Defense Production Administration: to establish production priorities; estimate labor supply needs to meet these production goals; represent the United States on combined boards; and determine production plans, methods, and procedures for all agencies. Marshall had crossed out the final item and

replaced it with: "secures production plans from all agencies and develops methods and procedures for their execution." (Marshall to Lovett, attachment, December 28, 1950, NA/RG 330, SD 040 [Defense Mobilization, Office of].)

3. The attached six-page draft of the executive order, dated December 27, 1950, expanded on the duties of the administrator of the Defense Production Administration as listed above. (Ibid.)

198

To Arthur H. Vandenberg

December 28, 1950
Washington, DC

Dear Arthur: Katherine and I have had you much in our minds, particularly during this Christmas period. I do hope that you are feeling much better.[1]

There is no one I can think of today in whose breadth of vision and quality of integrity I have more respect. I can imagine the interest with which you follow the national and international picture at this time. Certainly it is all very difficult,—in one sense confusing but in another crystal clear.

Lovett and I have been hard at it since our return to duty. If he was an important factor in the State Department, he is an absolutely invaluable force here in the Defense Department. I was amazed at the rapidity with which he got into action. Within an hour after his taking office, he was under full steam and instantly converted an office which was primarily one of mere public relations into the executive coordinating and directing force for the entire department. Everyone received him with open arms, and my only fear is that he works too hard, but he claims he enjoys it.

I managed to get the Christmas weekend at Pinehurst, but I flew back early Tuesday morning, leaving Katherine there. Whether I can spend the New Year's weekend there or not, I am not able to tell now, but I very much hope so.

I know if Katherine were here she would join me in all our best wishes and prayers for you in the New Year. Please feel that my admiration and affection for you have increased with the months.[2] Faithfully yours,

GCMRL/G. C. Marshall Papers (Secretary of Defense, Number Indexed, M200-7-15)

1. Vandenberg had been undergoing treatment for cancer at Butterworth Hospital in Grand Rapids, Michigan, since late November. ("Vandenberg Better, Hopes to Work Soon," *New York Times*, December 25, 1950, p. 22.)

2. Vandenberg replied on January 2, 1951, that he was "still in the hospital," but the doctors were "definitely optimistic." He was glad "you have Bob Lovett whose courage and capacity and integrity can be your everlasting reliance." (Vandenberg to Marshall, January 2, 1951, GCMRL/G. C. Marshall Papers [Secretary of Defense, Number Indexed, M200-7-15].)

Vandenberg died on April 18, 1951. See pp. 490–91.

THROUGHOUT December the US/UN position in Korea had continued to deteriorate in the face of the Communist Chinese offensive. While the State and Defense Departments discussed the merits and terms of a possible cease-fire, attention also continued to be focused on the primacy and defense of Europe. On December 11, Marshall noted in an NSC meeting "that we were just on the verge of launching the NATO armed forces and that our entire international position depended on strengthening western Europe. We could not rush into measures for Korea and the Pacific that would cause such Russian reactions that our European allies would be scared away." (Truman, *Memoirs*, 2: 419.)

Marshall was also concerned with the defense of Japan in light of the paucity of US forces remaining in that country after the Eighth Army deployed to Korea. During a December 19 meeting of his Armed Forces Policy Council along with Rusk, whom he had invited to attend, Marshall stated that he had "been concerned for a week or ten days about the extreme vulnerability of Japan in the event of a sudden Russian onslaught." While the American people were familiar with the problems the United States would face in defending Western Europe against a Soviet invasion, an attack on Japan "would disclose a degree of vulnerability which would surprise the American people and the resulting shock would produce a very serious situation." In the middle of this meeting Marshall was brought a telegram from MacArthur to the JCS requesting four National Guard divisions for the defense of Japan. Marshall then asked the group "whether there was any way in which we could 'withdraw from Korea with honor.'" (*FRUS, 1950*, 7: 1571–73.)

On December 22, the Joint Chiefs told MacArthur that they would postpone their decision on the four National Guard divisions he had requested on December 18 pending high-level discussions in Washington. Those discussions, centering on whether or not to withdraw entirely from Korea, took place during the last week of December. By December 24, the evacuation of the X Corps from Hungnam had been completed, and the Chinese had both rejected a UN-sponsored cease-fire proposal and made clear that they would not stop at the 38th parallel. On the evening of December 26, Truman met with Marshall, Acheson, and Bradley to discuss the situation. At that meeting, Acheson opposed withdrawal. Marshall and Bradley felt that MacArthur could hold at the Kum River, but only by using all of his available forces and thereby leaving none to defend Japan. All agreed that for this reason MacArthur could not risk the destruction of his forces. On December 27, the Joint Chiefs informed Marshall of their belief that MacArthur should be ordered to evacuate if the Kum River line could not be held. Acheson and Rusk objected during a meeting with Marshall and Lovett on the following day and called for revision of the proposed JCS message to MacArthur so as to emphasize the political importance of remaining in Korea as long as possible. Marshall then edited their proposed draft, with the final version approved by Truman as well as the State and Defense Departments. (Schnabel and Watson, *History of JCS*, 3, pt. 1: 179–81. Marshall's editing of the State Department draft is in NA/RG 218, Geographic Files, CCS 381 [Far East].) Sent to MacArthur by the Joint Chiefs on December 29, that message rejected his calls for an expanded war, bluntly stating that "Korea is not the place to fight a major war" and that "we should not commit our remaining available ground forces to action against Chinese Communist forces in Korea in face of the increased threat of a general war." Nevertheless, continued resistance in Korea "would be of great importance to our national interests, if this could be accomplished without incurring serious losses." Consequently the JCS modified MacArthur's basic directive, ordering him to defend successive positions but stating their belief that he should evacuate the peninsula if unable to hold the Kum River line. They then requested his views "as to the above-outlined conditions which should determine a decision to initiate evacuation, particularly in light of your continuing primary mission of defense of Japan for which only troops of the Eighth Army are available." (*FRUS, 1950*, 7: 1025–26.)

In his December 30 response MacArthur bluntly disagreed with the administration's Europe-first strategy and argued strongly for expansion of the war in Korea via blockade of the China coast, air and naval bombardment to destroy China's war-making capacity, use of Chinese Nationalist troops in Korea, and "diversionary action (possibly leading to counter-invasion)" by Chiang against the Chinese mainland. (Ibid., 1630–33.) See pp. 323–24 for subsequent events. ★

199

To Winston S. Churchill

January 3, 1951
Washington, DC

My dear Mr. Churchill: I have waited until I had finished reading your last volume, which you were good enough to send me, before thanking you, which I do now. (That's a pretty long sentence and not after your pure English style, but expresses the idea), and now Mrs. Marshall and I also have to thank Mrs. Churchill and you for that very handsome Christmas card.[1]

I would like an opportunity to see you these days and talk over things with the frankness of the past, but reactions, criticisms and pressures seem very much a repetition of those war years. I can only pray that we will have a repetition of the success of those same days.

I was called back into service at a rather difficult time and fortunately was able to obtain the services of my old first assistant in the State Department and former Pentagon companion, Bob Lovett. We have very complete coordination these days in contrast with some of our struggles in other years and, of course, in one sense we are far better prepared. However, in another, particularly as to the time element and the over-all development of the communist threat with its hordes of people, its knowledge of the organization and leadership of great armies and its industrial set-up, the situation is, I fear, far more serious.

This was to be a pleasant New Year's note, or to pun a little bit, it was to carry a pleasant note, but I can't escape the urge to make a few comments to you.

With warm regards to both Mrs. Churchill and yourself, and with great respect and affection. Faithfully yours,

GCMRL/G. C. Marshall Papers (Secretary of Defense, Number Indexed, M200-5-29)

1. Churchill was currently the leader of the Conservative opposition in the British House of Commons. He had released the fourth volume of his *Second World War* series in

October 1950. See Winston Churchill, *The Second World War*, vol. 4, *The Hinge of Fate* (Boston: Houghton Mifflin Company, 1950). Neither Churchill's correspondence transmitted with the book nor the Christmas card is in the Marshall Papers.

200

TO BERNARD M. BARUCH

January 3, 1951
Washington, DC

Dear Baruch: I have you to thank for a note and several messages, particularly the birthday greetings which reached me in Pinehurst just as I was returning to Washington.[1]

Katherine and I were really very very sorry not to pass the end of the year with you and Navarro, and, of course, I missed the shooting tremendously.[2] However, things were on such an edge I felt I had to be within a few minutes of the telephone and sitting virtually against an airfield.

Katherine got a very nice rest because she stayed through two weekends and the intervening week. I simply flew in and out.

My week here in Washington was particularly strenuous and very critical in many respects. Incidentally, Lovett and I went over your sage suggestions very carefully.

With my thanks and affectionate regards, Faithfully yours,

I'll urge your suggestion on the President and Wilson.[3]

GCMRL/G. C. Marshall Papers (Secretary of Defense, Selected)

1. Baruch had written to Marshall on December 24 and again on December 25, 1950. The first letter was in response to a December 22 letter from Marshall thanking him for a package of Christmas gifts but warning that "it looks very doubtful as to whether I can make my shooting engagement with you" at Hobcaw Barony, Baruch's South Carolina estate, due to his need to be near airfields and in telephone communication with Washington in the midst of the present crisis. Despite Baruch's assurances that there would be airfields and telephones nearby, the Marshalls declined his invitation. (Marshall to Baruch, December 22, 1950, Baruch to Marshall, December 24 and 30, 1950, GCMRL/G. C. Marshall Papers [Secretary of Defense, Selected].) See p. 743.

In his December 25 letter, Baruch had suggested sending the "best possible industrialist" to assist Eisenhower in persuading "European countries to give up [their] march to better economic conditions for immediate preparedness through use of much of their man power and resources." (Baruch to Marshall, December 25, 1950, ibid.)

2. Elizabeth Navarro was Baruch's nurse and companion for the last twenty years of his life.

3. On January 8, Marshall Carter asked John Small to "advise me as to what action the Munitions Board has taken, and what action, if any, General Marshall should take to follow up" on Baruch's suggestion to send an industrialist to assist Eisenhower in Europe, as discussed in n1 above. (Carter to Small, memorandum, January 8, 1951, GCMRL/G. C. Marshall Papers [Secretary of Defense, Number Indexed, M200-4-3].) The editors have been unable to locate any related correspondence among Marshall, Truman, and Charles E. Wilson.

201

To Jesse H. Jones

January 3, 1951
Washington, DC

Dear Jones: I really greatly appreciated your birthday note. Also I am in need of encouragement and support these days because, as you can well imagine from your long experience, things are pretty difficult at times like these.[1]

I was interested in your "if", that is if I had certain people with me. As a matter of fact, I have them all and what is more interesting the five of us—Wilson, Lovett, Clay, Weinberg and I sat down together last week and went over the preliminaries of modus operandi. I had previously had Wilson over here for lunch with the leading newspaper men of the country—some fifteen of them.[2]

It will not be difficult for you to conjure up the general procedure here in Washington—wheels within wheels—the pressures of enthusiasm and of criticism, and with a personal protective purpose. It is all the same atmosphere that we experienced together in '40 and '41.

It was good of you to think of me and write this note. And I send you my thanks and appreciation, and also my very affectionate regards to Mrs. Jones and you for the New Year. Faithfully yours,

GCMRL/G. C. Marshall Papers (Secretary of Defense, Number Indexed, M200-6-39)

1. Jones had been head of the Reconstruction Finance Corporation under Roosevelt and secretary of commerce from 1940 to 1945. His letter is not in the Marshall Papers.

2. Marshall and Wilson had met on December 28 to discuss the Office of Defense Mobilization (see pp. 314–15). Sidney J. Weinberg, a senior partner at Goldman, Sachs, and Company, and wartime vice chairman of the War Production Board, and General Lucius D. Clay (USMA, 1918), former military governor of the American sector in Germany and chairman of the New York State Civil Defense Commission, were Wilson's special assistants. Marshall had hosted twelve newspaper editors and radio broadcasters along with Wilson for lunch in his Pentagon dining room on December 18, 1950.

During the December 28 meeting, Marshall and Wilson may also have discussed who should head the newly established North Atlantic Defense Production Board that the NATO defense ministers had, during their December 18–19 meeting in Brussels, agreed to establish in order to maximize military equipment production. On the same date that Marshall sent this letter to Jones, he sent Truman a memorandum stating that he had consulted with Wilson, Clay, and Weinberg, as well as Harriman, Foster, Small, Assistant Secretary of State for European Affairs George Perkins, and Assistant Secretary of the Army Karl R. Bendetsen representing Army Secretary Pace on the matter. They had agreed on three nominees, but Marshall informed Truman that they strongly preferred William Rogers Herod, president of the International General Electric Company. (Marshall to Truman, memorandum, January 3, 1951, and Dawson to Carter, January 8, 1951, NA/RG 330, CD 092.3 [Defense Production Board].) Truman expressed no objection to Herod's appointment, whereupon Marshall offered the position to Herod, who accepted a few days later on a short-term basis and with other conditions to which Marshall agreed. (Herod to Marshall, telegram and letter, January 10, 1951; and Marshall to Herod, telegram, January 12, 1951, NA/RG 330, CD 092 [NATO, William Herod].)

202

To Frank McCarthy

January 3, 1951
Washington, DC

Dear Frank: We appreciated very much your thinking of us Christmas with those fine records for "your" machine, and also for your Christmas radio.[1]

I wonder what sort of a Christmas you had in your present surroundings. Of course, you had many associates of more or less distinction and I presume some beauty. I picture you as living in the midst of female hazards. Possibly it would be best for your future if you would appoint me referee in the matter in any possible engagement. I certainly would consider your best interests whatever furies might arise.

Katherine and I spent the Christmas and New Year's weekend at Pinehurst. She remained during the intervening week. I had to return to Washington and then fly back. We returned to town early yesterday morning and are in our little apartment, very comfortably established but resentful of losing the right to laze about in Pinehurst or other pleasanter places.

With our love to you and every good wish and hope for you in the New Year, Affectionately,

GCMRL/Frank McCarthy Collection (Additions)

1. At McCarthy's request, C. J. George had purchased recordings of five musicals for the Marshalls. (George to William McCarthy, December 23, 1950, GCMRL/G. C. Marshall Papers [Secretary of Defense, Number Indexed, M212-3-20].) McCarthy's Christmas telegram to the Marshalls is not in the Marshall Papers.

Also on January 3, Marshall thanked Margaret Emerson for her gifts of a diary and pen. He also commented that he and Mrs. Marshall were "enjoying the television set," which Emerson had given to them, "very much, rather to our surprise because we paid almost no attention to the machine we had at Leesburg except during a football game or a prize fight. This one works beautifully and as we are in close to the principal sending station, I suppose it adds to the clearness of the picture." (Marshall to Emerson, January 3, 1951, ibid., [M212-3-18].)

203

Memorandum of Conversation[1]
Top Secret

January 5, 1951
Washington, DC

Monsieur Bonnet opened the interview by stating that he had been instructed to deliver personally to General Marshall a message from Monsieur Pleven, which he handed to the Secretary. This message thanked General Marshall for the delivery of B-26 aircraft to Indochina.[2]

The Secretary acknowledged the thanks and informed Monsieur Bonnet that 7 of the B-26's were now in Saigon, 18 were at Hawaii, and 5 were still under modification in the United States.[3] He noted recent dispatches concerning the fighting in Indochina and asked Monsieur Bonnet what he thought had been the effect of the arrival of General de Lattre de Tassigny.[4] He further queried Monsieur Bonnet as to whether, in his opinion, pressure on Bao Dai to form and leave a government of national union which could take effective action would influence the situation.[5]

In reply, Monsieur Bonnet extolled General de Lattre de Tassigny's qualities as a soldier and leader and affirmed that he had been an undoubted inspiration to all concerned in Indochina. With regard to pressure on Bao Dai he expressed the opinion that nothing that Bao Dai could do would have appreciable effect in increasing confidence in him by the people of the Associated States. Nevertheless, he was confident that the French and Vietnamese would hold Indochina unless there was intervention by "volunteer" divisions of Chinese Communists.

General Marshall noted the change in meaning which the Communists had now given the word "volunteer", particularly with reference to Chinese Communist "volunteers" in Korea. He compared it with their distortion of the meaning of the word "democracy" and expressed the hope that some of our able writers would play this up in the public press. He agreed as to de Lattre's fine qualities as a soldier and recalled his resistance work in France. This brought to mind another leading French military figure and he asked Monsieur Bonnet about the present status of General Juin.[6]

Monsieur Bonnet informed the Secretary that Juin's status was not yet finalized but that it was hoped that General Juin would become President of the French Chiefs of Staff, in which position he would be the counter-part of General Bradley. General Marshall expressed the view that the position of Chief of Staff of the French Army was not one of real authority and influence and hoped that the appointment in mind for General Juin was such. Monsieur Bonnet assured the Secretary that this was so and took occasion to express the determination of the French Government to build up a military force on the Continent which would be a real deterrent to aggression.

General Marshall expressed the view that we had been too long governed, both in the Far East and elsewhere, by fear of what Soviet reaction might be; whereas, the Soviet forces went ahead and did what seemed best to them without regard to our possible reaction. He thought that the time had now come for us to do likewise. During the last war, in supporting the bombing of Germany and Japan, he had felt that the all-important reason for doing so was that the lesson must be impressed upon the world that the democracies, when once aroused, were tougher than anyone else to deal with. He had confirmation that this lesson had been impressed upon the Japanese Ambassador in Berlin and believed that the rest of the world likewise realized it.[7] For his part, he would see that swift and powerful retaliation was visited upon Russia, both in Europe and the Far East, if they started anything.

General Marshall concluded the interview by saying that he would reply directly to Monsieur Pleven's message and would take action to expedite the delivery of the remaining B-26's.

A. C. Murdaugh

NA/RG 330, CD Memorandum of Conversation

1. This conversation between Marshall and French Ambassador Henri Bonnet took place at 2:45 p.m. Also in attendance was the author of this memorandum, Captain Murdaugh.

2. See pp. 194–99. Bonnet wrote on January 2 to convey the thanks of the French government and Pleven's "personal feelings of gratitude" for a message from Marshall on December 26, 1950, which had informed the French that nine of the B-26 aircraft had left the West Coast on the previous day and were en route to Indochina by air, that fifteen others were being unloaded in Hawaii and would depart by air on January 2, and that six were still in US depots "undergoing final overhauling." Pleven's government recognized Marshall's personal role in this decision and "deeply" appreciated "this new gesture of solidarity" by the American government with the French concerns in the Far East. Marshall thanked Pleven by telegram soon after this meeting. (Bonnet to Marshall, January 2, 1951, and Marshall to Pleven, cable no. DEF-36867, January 6, 1951, GCMRL/G. C. Marshall Papers [Secretary of Defense, Number Indexed, M200-7-43]; Carter to Marshall, memorandum, December 26, 1950, NA/RG 330, CD 091.3 [MDAP, Indochina].)

Marshall had been informed that the primary purpose of this visit was to thank him in person for delivery of the aircraft. (Murdaugh for Burns to Marshall, memorandum, January 5, 1951, NA/RG 330, CD Briefings.) He had pressed for their delivery "Over JCS opposition and even at the 'expense of the Korean pipeline,'" the official history of the OSD noted. (Condit, *Test of War*, 209. See also *History of the Joint Chiefs of Staff: The Joint Chiefs of Staff and the First Indochina War, 1947–1954* [Washington: Office of Joint History, Office of the Chairman of the Joint Chiefs of Staff, 2004], 57.)

3. This information came from the memorandum cited in the previous note, Murdaugh for Burns to Marshall, January 5, 1951, NA/RG 330, CD Briefings.

4. Commander of the Free French First Army during World War II and West European land forces from 1948 to 1950, General Jean de Lattre de Tassigny had in December been appointed high commissioner and commander of French forces in Indochina.

The January 5 memorandum cited above in notes 2 and 3 had informed Marshall of this appointment and its positive effect on French and Vietnamese morale, but had warned that the immediate military situation was "discouraging" and that there were "many indications of impending intervention in Indochina by the Chinese Communists" who had 185,000 troops nearby. It also summarized a December 29 CIA estimate that warned the Viet Minh could force the French out of North Vietnam in six to nine months if Chinese Communist aid continued and French strength and material were not increased; that there was "only a slight chance" the French could hold their position long enough to build up Vietnamese forces and contain the Viet Minh; and that Chinese intervention could occur "at any time" and would make the French position "untenable." (Ibid.)

5. Bao Dai had been emperor of Vietnam from 1926 until he was ousted by the Communist-led Viet Minh after World War II. He returned under French urging in 1949 to head the new State of Vietnam that they established in January 1950.

6. For his resistance work, General de Lattre de Tassigny had been imprisoned by the Vichy French government but had escaped in September 1943 and joined the Free French. For Marshall's relationship with Juin, see p. 188n2.

7. The Japanese ambassador in Berlin during World War II was Baron Hiroshi Oshima.

204

MEMORANDUM FOR THE PRESIDENT

January 5, 1951
Washington, DC

SUBJECT: Inscription for the Tomb of the Unknown,
Arlington National Cemetery

1. While the selection and interment of World War II Unknown has been postponed until such time as the international situation stabilizes, the inscription

for the Tomb of the Unknown should be decided upon.

2. As the Department of the Army is the executive agency for national cemeteries, Secretary Pace has recommended that the present inscription which reads

   "Here Rests in Honored Glory an American Soldier Known But to God."

   be amended to read

   "Here Rest in Honored Glory American Heroes Known But to God."[1]

   This recommendation has been concurred in by the Secretaries of the Treasury, Navy, and Air Force, the Fine Arts Commission, and the Arlington Memorial Amphitheater Commission.[2]

3. The suggested change appeals to me greatly and I submit it for your consideration and approval.[3]

NA/RG 330, SD 293.8

1. Pace had previously suggested this change, and on November 21, Marshall informed him that the change "appeals to me greatly." He had also asked Pace to "take the necessary action to process your recommendation through all the appropriate agencies and, if general agreement is obtained, prepare the necessary draft memorandum for me to get Presidential approval." (Marshall to Pace, November 21, 1950, NA/RG 330, SD 293.8.)

2. Pace reported that the military services, the Commission of Fine Arts, and the Arlington Memorial Amphitheater Commission had approved the language. (Marshall to Pace, November 21, 1950, and Pace to Marshall, memoranda, December 15 and 28, 1950, ibid.)

3. While unknowns from World War II, Korea, and Vietnam were eventually added to the tomb, the inscription was never changed and still reads "Here Rests in Honored Glory an American Soldier Known But to God."

ON DECEMBER 31, the Chinese resumed their offensive in Korea, forcing Ridgway to abandon Seoul on January 4. On January 9, the Joint Chiefs informed MacArthur that his December 30 proposals (see pp. 315–17) would be "given careful consideration" but in effect warned that there was little possibility his recommendations for an expanded war against China would be accepted. They also directed him to defend successive positions in South Korea but to withdraw to Japan if he deemed it "essential to avoid severe losses in men and material." On January 10, MacArthur again objected and asked for clarification regarding exactly what was desired in Korea. He warned that he could not with present forces simultaneously hold Korea and defend Japan. He also concluded that "under the extraordinary limitations and conditions imposed upon the command in Korea its military position is untenable, but it can hold for any length of time up to its complete destruction if overriding political considerations so dictate." (Schnabel and Watson, *History of JCS*, 3, pt. 1: 185–87.) MacArthur further warned that the morale of his troops "will become a serious threat to their battle efficiency unless the political basis upon which they are asked to trade life for time is clearly delineated, fully understood, and so impelling that the hazards of battle are cheerfully accepted," leading Marshall, according to Acheson's later recollections, to tell Rusk "that when a general complains of the morale of his troops, the time has come to look into his own." (Ibid., 187; Acheson, *Present at the Creation*, 515.) "We were at our lowest point" at this time, Marshall would later state. (*MSFE*, 329.)

The desperate situation in Korea and the possibility of evacuation and/or expansion of the war to China deeply upset the British, with Attlee writing to Truman on January 8 that he was "greatly disturbed." (*FRUS, 1951*, 7: 37–39.) Truman's response on January 9, drafted by the State Department and amended by Marshall and the JCS, sought to reassure the British prime minister that there had been no change in the policy to which they had agreed during Attlee's December 4–8 visit (see pp. 284–87), and that there was no US intention to expand the war, MacArthur's recommendations to that effect notwithstanding. (Carter to Davis and Carter to Rusk, memoranda, January 9, 1951, GCMRL/G. C. Marshall Papers [Pentagon Office, Selected]; *FRUS, 1951*, 7: 39–40.)

Throughout this time of crisis, attention had also centered on the defense of Japan, which the Joint Chiefs continued to define as MacArthur's primary mission. By mid-December, the administration was preparing to send John Foster Dulles to Japan to negotiate a peace treaty, and on January 3, the Joint Chiefs requested MacArthur's views. He responded that "the desirability of a Japanese peace treaty from both a military and political stand point is of such urgency that all practical measures should be taken without delay to negotiate such an agreement." (*FRUS, 1951*, 6: 780–81.) On January 8, Acheson and Marshall discussed the matter at the Pentagon with Bradley, Harriman, and Lovett, and agreed that Dulles's mission should not be delayed by the crisis in Korea. On January 9, they jointly signed and sent to Truman the next document, which Acheson had drafted. ★

205

Memorandum for the President — January 9, 1951
Top Secret — Washington, DC

You will recall that on September 8, 1950, you approved a Joint Memorandum from the Secretaries of State and Defense concerning the general basis upon which progress should be made looking toward a peace treaty with Japan. The Secretaries of State and Defense have now agreed that the time has come to implement paragraph 5 of that memorandum, which provided that after the initial discussions with the friendly powers "a United States political representative will go to Japan to discuss confidentially with General MacArthur the proposed treaty and by arrangements through and in cooperation with General MacArthur will discuss the proposed treaty with the Japanese Government and also seek a procedure for Japanese participation in the treaty-making process which will assure genuine acceptance by the representatives of all important, non-Communist political groups in Japan."[1]

It is recommended that Mr. John Foster Dulles, who has been conducting the preliminary negotiations concerning the Japanese peace treaty, be appointed by you as Special Representative of the President with the personal rank of Ambassador to carry on these negotiations and to head a Presidential Mission to Japan for the purposes outlined above.

There is enclosed a draft letter to Mr. Dulles informing him of his designation and setting forth the terms of reference of his Mission.[2] It is recommended that this draft letter be approved and transmitted to Mr. Dulles through the Secretary of State who, in cooperation with the Secretary of Defense, will take the necessary steps to implement this recommendation. Signed: Dean Acheson, Secretary of State, and G. C. Marshall, Secretary of Defense

HSTL/Harry S. Truman Papers (President's Secretary's Files, Subject File, Foreign Affairs–Japanese Peace Treaty)

1. See *FRUS, 1951*, 6: 1293–96. The quote is on 1295.
2. The draft letter is reproduced in ibid., 788–89. Truman approved it on January 10 with only one minor change which is explained in ibid., 788n3. The letter included a statement that Dulles should keep in mind during his negotiations that the United States intended to commit troops to assist in the defense of Japan, that it desired that Japan should eventually be able to defend itself, and that the US would enter into mutual assistance agreements with Australia, New Zealand, the Philippines, Japan, and perhaps Indonesia to "resist aggression from without" and from within should Japan "again become aggressive." (Acheson and Marshall to Truman, memorandum and enclosure, January 9, 1951, NA/RG 330, CD 387 [Japan].) See pp. 427–29.

MARSHALL had long been a strong proponent of universal military training and, since becoming secretary of defense, had spoken and written on numerous occasions about the need for such a system (see, for example, pp. 164–66, 174–75, 177–78, 180–82, 207–14, 233, 251–53, and 263–75). As army chief of staff he had attempted in 1945 to obtain it but had been unable to do so. Truman had been equally unsuccessful in his efforts to obtain congressional passage of a universal military training bill, and in August 1950 he asked the committees involved to halt their hearings on the grounds that UMT could not be implemented in the midst of the Korean War. Instead the administration relied upon Selective Service, which Congress had reinstituted in June 1948 and extended for one year at the beginning of the Korean War.

Given these facts, and with Anna Rosenberg finally confirmed in December as assistant secretary of defense for manpower and personnel (see pp. 296–97), Marshall moved forward on his long-desired UMT bill, now combined with a continuation of Selective Service in light of the immediate need for additional forces in Korea. On December 27 and 28, he described to the service secretaries and the Joint Chiefs "the urgency and importance of the subject of universal military service and training and the need for a long-range definite plan" that would both meet immediate manpower needs and create "an enduring system which will remain in effect over the years. . . . [W]e cannot continue with our present policy. We cannot continue to make short-term plans for emergencies which are followed by periods of radical demobilization and the termination of authority to train men for military service. We must take constructive action now." He and Rosenberg then outlined their proposal, which called for twenty-seven months of service and training, followed by three to five years in the reserves or National Guard, for all able-bodied males (and national service for those unfit for military service), with presidential authority to raise, lower, or eliminate the period of service required after training depending on needs at the time. He also requested their comments on the proposal "as soon as possible" and the immediate designation of personal representatives to form an ad hoc committee "to meet at the call" of Rosenberg. On December 29, he described his proposal to Truman and the cabinet and sent the president a copy. (Marshall to service secretaries and JCS, memorandum, December 28, 1950, NA/RG 330, CD 353 [UMT]; Marshall to Rosenberg and Marshall to Truman, memoranda, December 29, 1950, GCMRL/G. C. Marshall Papers [Secretary of Defense, Chronological, Secretaries, Ackerman]; Marshall to service secretaries and JCS, memorandum, January 4, 1951, GCMRL/G. C. Marshall Papers [Secretary of Defense, Number Indexed, M200-3-26].) At the same time, Lovett sent an approved final draft of a national manpower mobilization policy to the NSRB for submission to the NSC. (Lovett to Symington, December 29, 1950, NA/RG 330, SD 370.01.) On January 10, Marshall appeared before the Preparedness Subcommittee of the Senate Armed Services Committee to explain his proposal. ★

206

STATEMENT BEFORE THE PREPAREDNESS SUBCOMMITTEE OF THE SENATE ARMED SERVICES COMMITTEE[1]

January 10, 1951
Washington, DC

Universal Military Service and Training represents what I believe is the best way to meet our immediate need for enlarged combat forces and at the same time, to provide an enduring base for our military strength. It is a vital element in a long-range program of national security. I know of no other that will give us so much protection at a cost in men and money that is within the capacity of our economy to bear.

The tensions that unsettle the world may persist through the lifetime of many of us. We must husband our military and industrial manpower with utmost care; we must foster our scientific and technical resources; we must avoid waste of the productive energies that have helped make our nation powerful.

Maintenance over the years of a military establishment so large that it makes impossible the continuance of a fruitful civilian economy will defeat itself. Unless we now proceed to put into effect a program realistically geared to our immediate needs and our capacities and our future requirements, I fear that we will once again throw aside all our military power whenever our sense of urgency subsides. Personally I have gone through some very destructive periods in the history of our unpreparedness. We must not continue to make short-term plans for immediate emergencies to be followed by abrupt demobilization and the withdrawal of authority to train the men necessary to a reasonable posture of defense.

The objective of our present program must be adequate forces in being, backed up by a vitalized National Guard and Reserve. An assured flow of trained men into the Guard and Reserve on a basis established by law is the key to transforming these Reserve components into an integral part of our first-line defenses. That is the distinctive virtue of Universal Military Service and Training.

It makes it possible to get the trained manpower and to build a balanced military structure at minimum cost. It is at once the most effective, the most economical and the most democratic way to safeguard our nation. I do not present it as a cheap solution, for there is no cheap or easy solution to our security problems. But I do recommend it as the one that will give us the necessary security at a cost that we can sustain.

The program proposes that young men reaching the age of 18 fulfill their obligation for the nation's defense by entering the armed forces for twenty-seven months of service and training. Immediately thereafter they would enroll for a specified term in a Reserve component.

When our urgent need for a large military force in being abates somewhat, the President would have the right to reduce or to cut the requirement for military service and to retain the training features. There would remain at all times a requirement that these young men reaching 18 devote from four to six months to training so that they could take their place in the Reserve and be ready to fit into units. This would give us a durable layer of military protection that would survive the alternate moods of public alarm or complacency.

The calling of men of 18 to prepare for their own defense and the defense of their country is not new in our history. It happened in both World Wars and the young men summoned to duty acquitted themselves with the same distinction as their comrades in arms. In my biennial report as Chief of Staff at the end of the second World War, I said: ". . . Men of 18, 19, and 20 make our finest soldiers. The excellent Marine divisions are made up largely of men of these age groups. They have stamina and recuperative power far beyond that of older men and this physical superiority often determines the issue in heavy and prolonged fighting."[2] I believe the record of the millions of veterans of all ages who have returned to civilian life during the last five years offers to the parents of America heartwarming evidence of the success of the Army, Navy, Air Force and Marine Corps in preserving the moral and mental, as well as the physical, strength of their sons even under the most severe conditions of combat or the more trying periods of less exciting service.

I feel certain that the young men of 18 who would come into the services under the proposed conditions would learn much to make them sturdier and better citizens. At the same time they would make the major contribution to our national security and greatly improve their own chances of survival.

I hope that your committee will promptly approve a program that will meet our needs, one that can be borne financially as part of the reasonable price a resolute people will be willing to pay for their liberties. The sooner it is put into effect, the greater will be our security and our ability to assert effective leadership toward a lasting peace.

The concept of Universal Military Service and Training reaches back more than 150 years. The Father of Our Country recognized the need for a citizen's army based on reserve of trained manpower. He asked Congress to approve a plan for universal training.[3] In every National emergency since that time our military efforts have been hampered, our very National existence has been imperilled by the lack of trained Reserves. We cannot afford to delay any longer in correcting this deficiency. In view of our preeminent position in the world, corrective action, it seems to me, is mandatory.[4]

GCMRL/G. C. Marshall Papers (Secretary of Defense, Speeches and Statements)

1. Marshall began his testimony before the subcommittee, chaired by Senator Lyndon Johnson, at 10:30 a.m. Given the "considerable indication that the three Services are not yet completely in agreement on the Universal Military Service and Training Bill" and out of fear that "someone will either intentionally or inadvertently mess up the works by indicating a split opinion" at the Pentagon, Marshall Carter had forwarded to Marshall on January 9 Anna Rosenberg's recommendation that he "state in clear and unequivocal terms at the Armed Forces Policy Council Meeting this morning that the completed program as presently worked out is the policy of the Department of Defense." Carter had also noted that President Truman concurred with Rosenberg's recommendation, saying that "'the program to be advanced by Gen. Marshall will be an Administration plan and that Gen. Marshall will speak for all agencies of the government.'" (Carter to Marshall, memorandum, January 9, 1951, GCMRL/G. C. Marshall Papers [Secretary of Defense, Memoranda, Marshall S. Carter, 1950–1951].)

2. See *General Marshall's Report*, 106.

3. See *General Marshall's Report*, 122–23.

4. See the next editorial summary.

207

Senate Testimony on the Universal Military Service and Training Bill of 1951

January 10, 1951 Washington, DC

FOLLOWING his testimony Marshall was asked a series of questions dealing with such matters as when the proposed bill would be available, whether the military establishment was in agreement on it, whether the training and use of youth from other nations such as Germany was under consideration, and what the proposed numerical breakdown of forces between the different services would be. During his responses he emphasized that the bill "combines the present emergency" via universal military service "with the future enduring program" of universal military training. (Senate Committee on Armed Services, *Hearings . . . on S. 1: A Bill to Provide for the Common Defense and Security of the United States and to Permit the More Effective Utilization of Manpower Resources of the United States by Authorizing Universal Military Service and Training, and for Other Purposes*, 82d Cong., 1st sess., 28.) When he responded positively to the question of whether other departments were in accord on the bill, Senator Lyndon Johnson remarked that if true, "it would be like a breath of fresh air." Such accord, Marshall admitted, "would be a miracle, of course, but I think you will find a reasonable agreement." He also responded affirmatively when asked whether he thought the early existence of UMT could have avoided US participation in the two world wars and the present war in Korea, which he labeled "these tragedies." (Ibid., 32.) His most extensive reply came in response to a question from Senator Styles Bridges regarding the very large number of support troops needed by American divisions. Two primary causes of this large "division slice," Marshall responded, were the "vast distances" American troops had to be transported and the services they needed once they arrived. In addition, the numbers needed had been underestimated during World War II: "our greatest drain is in these long hauls we are involved in, and the fact that all of our policy is built on fighting outside of this country, so long as it is possible to conduct ourselves in that fashion, and the Soviets have nothing like that at all." The same was true of the Communist Chinese, whose soldiers in Korea were provided with only twelve pounds of rice and ammunition and were on their own after these were exhausted. "Well, we cannot do things that way at all," he noted. (Ibid., 35. See also pp. 391–93.) When asked whether his proposals would lead to sending eighteen-year-old Americans overseas—which present legislation prohibited—Marshall replied that the training period would keep them in the United States until they had reached the age of nineteen. He then responded affirmatively when asked if Assistant Secretary Rosenberg would speak for the Defense Department while noting that others would testify as well. Rosenberg then followed with her prepared statement.

As he had estimated during this testimony (ibid., 27), Marshall forwarded the draft UMT bill to Senator Johnson one week following the Senate hearings. In a five-page letter which accompanied the draft bill, Marshall informed Johnson that the UMT bill was "the principal proposal in the Department of Defense Legislative program for 1951" and had received the approval of President Truman, "the Bureau of the Budget, the Director of Selective Service and all the civilian agencies concerned with manpower problems." Marshall, the JCS, and the service secretaries thus urged "prompt enactment by the Congress." (Marshall to Johnson, January 17, 1951, NA/RG 330 [OSD Index–201, Marshall, George C.].) See also pp. 338–47, 369–71, 409–13, and 423–26. ★

208

TO MOSHE SHARETT

January 11, 1951
Washington, DC

Dear Sharett: Thank you for your letter of 23 December 1950, summarizing the views you presented to me during your recent visit.[1] In that connection I am sure the appropriate officials in the Department of Defense will be glad to see Ambassador Eban and Colonel Herzog to discuss the matters further.[2] If any complications develop in such arrangements, or if Eban wishes to see me personally, I shall be glad to have my office make the necessary arrangements.

I have sent copies of your memorandum to General Bradley, the Chairman of the Munitions Board, and the three Service Secretaries for preliminary study and appropriate action where possible by their staff agencies. As you know some of the proposals contained in your memorandum are of considerably broader interest than to the Department of Defense alone. I think it would be helpful to both our governments if you would have your people forward the proposals, broken down into individual papers on separate subjects through the appropriate State Department diplomatic channels. This will insure that all interested agencies of the Government are fully apprised of, and can take appropriate action on your suggestions. I have, of course, already initiated within the Department of Defense the necessary studies based on our conversation, and your memorandum will be most helpful in this regard. The suggestion I have made above will provide the necessary follow up and U.S. governmental coordination to insure the fullest consideration of your proposals.

I want you to know in a rather personal way that I am acutely aware of the problems facing the State of Israel and that I am sympathetic to many of the proposals you make. I also know that you in turn are fully aware of the many problems facing this country at the present time, particularly in the military and production fields, which have a direct bearing on your proposals.

Thank you again for your letter and memorandum, and more personally for your good wishes. I send you mine for the New Year. Faithfully yours,

NA/RG 330, CD 092 (Israel)

1. Sharett had met with Marshall on December 18 (see pp. 298–99). His December 23 letter thanked Marshall for his "courteous and sympathetic attention" and enclosed a two-part memorandum summarizing the matters they had discussed, including Israel's need and desire to have the United States stockpile food and raw materials in the country and "the service Israel could render, if its military potential were developed and organized in good time." Sharett consequently requested "urgent consideration" of eight measures he had previously discussed with Marshall, including the ability to obtain US arms and expertise so as to expand and improve Israel's military capabilities. (*FRUS, 1950*, 5: 1077–82.)

2. Chaim Herzog was Israeli defense attaché in Washington and former head of Israeli military intelligence. Sharett had requested such discussions in his December 23 letter to Marshall.

Eban met with Lovett on February 19 to discuss further some of the issues that Sharett had raised during his December 18 discussion with Marshall and in his December 23 letter. (Memorandum for record, February 19, 1951, NA/RG 330, CD Memorandum of Conversation.)

MACARTHUR'S January 10 message caused consternation and dismay in Washington (see pp. 323–24). A series of conversations and meetings among Marshall, Acheson, and Truman as well as the JCS and the NSC ensued and resulted in a new JCS directive to MacArthur on January 12, followed on the next day by a message to the Far East commander from Truman himself. The JCS admitted that it was "infeasible under existing conditions" to maintain a position in Korea for an extended period of time but nevertheless reiterated their previous instructions that MacArthur hold out if possible, inflict maximum damage on the

Chinese, but withdraw to Japan if absolutely necessary to prevent the destruction of his forces. Truman's message asserted that even if forced to withdraw from Korea, the United States "would not accept the result politically or militarily until the aggression has been rectified"—a statement MacArthur interpreted as a rejection of evacuation unless absolutely necessary. (*FRUS, 1951*, 7: 57–79; Condit, *Test of War*, 94–95; Schnabel and Watson, *History of JCS*, 3, pt. 1: 188–91.)

While Marshall appears not to have favored the presidential letter, he did favor—and indeed had proposed—the dispatch of General Collins, this time accompanied by General Hoyt S. Vandenberg (USMA, 1923), US Air Force chief of staff, on another mission to Japan and Korea to evaluate troop morale in light of MacArthur's January 10 comments. After meeting with him in Tokyo and reading him a recently approved JCS paper on US objectives in the Far East and possible actions, they flew to Korea just as General Ridgway was launching a limited and successful counterattack with one corps of the revived Eighth Army. Contradicting MacArthur's January 10 warnings, they reported both good morale in the army and Ridgway's conviction that he could hold for at least two or three months. (*FRUS, 1951*, 7: 71–72; Schnabel and Watson, *History of JCS*, 3, pt. 1: 189–90, 193–94; and Condit, *Test of War*, 94–95.) The JCS paper that Collins and Vandenberg had taken to Tokyo would become a major point of contention between MacArthur and Marshall during the hearings that followed MacArthur's relief. (See pp. 478–81, 499–501, and 505–16.)

In addition to concerns about the defense of Japan and Formosa as well as the crisis in Korea caused by the Chinese intervention, administration officials in Washington also had to deal at this time with a deteriorating military situation for the French in Indochina and ensuing French requests for increased aid and tripartite military staff talks. ★

209

To Dean G. Acheson — January 16, 1951
Secret — Washington, DC

Dear Mr. Secretary: With reference to your letter of 16 November 1950 regarding proposed United States-United Kingdom-French military talks concerning the defense of Indochina, I am transmitting herewith, for your information, a memorandum of 10 January 1951 from the Joint Chiefs of Staff on this subject. In this memorandum the Joint Chiefs of Staff refer to a previous memorandum to me, dated 8 December 1950, in which they then stated that "additional military staff talks should not be undertaken at this time." I am also enclosing that memorandum for your information.[1]

In view of the opinion which the Joint Chiefs of Staff have reaffirmed in their memorandum of 10 January 1951 that, from the strictly military point of view, no additional military staff talks are desirable at this time, I believe that the holding of such talks now depends on whether or not the Department of State believes that there are overriding political considerations. I realize that the opinion of the Joint Chiefs of Staff would have the effect of indefinitely postponing your agreement reached with Mr. Schuman and Mr. Bevin on 14 September 1950. Yet, I believe that, in the light of the views of the Joint Chiefs of Staff, the Department of Defense can only recommend that, unless there are overriding political considerations, the French and British Governments be informed of the present U.S. military position regarding these talks.[2] Faithfully yours,

NA/RG 330, CD 092 (Indochina)

1. During a September 14 meeting with Bevin and Schuman, Acheson had agreed to tripartite "operational military talks" regarding Indochina. On November 15 (according to *FRUS, 1950*, 6: 346n1) or 16 (according to Marshall in this letter), Acheson had suggested to Marshall that preparations be completed so that these talks could take place as soon as possible, but the JCS, citing the dramatically changed military situation resulting from the Communist Chinese military intervention in Korea, had on December 8 recommended that these talks not take place. On the recommendation of two of his advisers, Marshall had on December 21 informed the JCS that he was "reluctant at this time to proceed with your recommendation without further advice, since it would have the effect of reversing the position of the United States Government, and delaying indefinitely a decision of the three Foreign Ministers." He therefore requested "as a matter of urgency, your additional advice." (Murdaugh and Burns to Marshall, memoranda, "JCS Decision Against Military Talks with French and U.K. on Defense of Indochina and Southeast Asia," December 20, 1951; and Marshall to JCS, memorandum, "Proposed Military Talks Regarding Defense of Indochina," December 21, 1950, NA/RG 330, CD 092 [Indochina].) On January 10, the JCS reaffirmed their opposition to the talks as well as any commitment of US military forces to Indochina "from the strictly military point of view," while recognizing that the "political considerations" Marshall had noted on December 21 "may be regarded as overriding." (Davis to Marshall, memorandum, "Proposed Military Talks Regarding Defense of Indochina," January 10, 1951, ibid. See also *FRUS, 1951*, 6: 346–48.)

2. On January 26, Acheson responded that his prior commitment to hold these talks "constitutes, as a practical matter, an overriding political consideration" and therefore requested that the Defense Department initiate these talks "as soon as possible" in light of Pleven's forthcoming visit. (*FRUS, 1951*, 7: 365.)

On February 9, Marshall directed the JCS to do so. The JCS official history notes that they "complied but resolved to limit the scope of the discussions and not permit them to deal with 'matters of strategy affecting United States global policies and plans.'" The conference took place in Singapore on May 15. (*The Joint Chiefs of Staff and the First Indochina War*, 76–77.)

210

To Benjamin M. McKelway — January 17, 1951, Washington, DC

Dear McKelway: Thanks for your note of the 12th. I will be very glad to meet with your group some convenient date in February, which I do not think we will have any difficulty in arranging as I seldom go out at night.[1]

With warm regards and looking forward to seeing you.[2] Faithfully yours,

GCMRL/G. C. Marshall Papers (Secretary of Defense, Number Indexed, M214-6-50)

1. McKelway, editor of the Washington *Evening Star* and *Sunday Star*, had asked Mar-

shall to meet with around eighteen old wartime newspapers friends over dinner, which "would, of course, be completely private." He also requested Lovett's presence. (McKelway to Marshall, January 12, 1951, GCMRL/G. C. Marshall Papers [Secretary of Defense, Number Indexed, M214-6-50].)

According to his authorized biographer, Marshall as wartime chief of staff "had learned that the best way to keep a secret out of the newspapers was to reveal it to responsible newsmen and then explain why it could not be printed." (Forrest C. Pogue, *George C. Marshall*, vol. 2, *Ordeal and Hope, 1939–1942* [New York: Viking, 1965], 201–2. See also *Papers of GCM*, 2: 676–79. For one journalist's wartime reports on these meetings with Marshall as well as Admiral Ernest J. King and others, see Glen C. H. Perry, *"Dear Bart": Washington Views of World War II* [Westport, CT: Greenwood Press, 1982].)

2. McKelway later suggested a list of nineteen guests, including himself, to have dinner with Marshall and Lovett at the Hotel Statler on February 5. (Ackerman to Marshall, memorandum, January 18, 1951, GCMRL/G. C. Marshall Papers [Secretary of Defense, Number Indexed, M214-6-50].)

Marshall Carter informed Marshall that the "consensus was that . . . this served to deny all of the rumors and allegations that have previously appeared about your health and stated senility. . . . They had the feeling that you thought you were telling them a lot of deep secrets—things which they said they already knew. In other words, the evening was enjoyable, but relatively uninforming and not particularly productive." (Carter to Marshall, memorandum, February 6, 1951, GCMRL/G. C. Marshall Papers [Secretary of Defense, Categorical, Memoranda, Marshall S. Carter, 1950–1951].) See pp. 367–68.

IN LATE 1950, Republicans opposed to the administration's European focus in foreign and military affairs initiated what became known as the "Great Debate" in Congress. On December 20, former President Herbert Hoover publicly called for an alternative "Western Hemisphere Gibraltar" policy based on unilateral defense with air and sea power of the Western Hemisphere, the Atlantic Ocean (including Great Britain), and the Pacific along the line of Japan, Formosa, and the Philippines. In Congress, Republicans led by Senator Robert Taft of Ohio attacked not only the administration's "Europe first" policy and decision to commit US forces to NATO, but also the president's constitutional authority to commit those troops without congressional consent. (Condit, *Test of War*, 339; see also Acheson, *Present at the Creation*, 488–93.)

Although these attacks focused on Truman and Acheson, Marshall and the JCS were not spared criticism. Indeed, according to the *New York Times*, Taft asserted on December 29 in Cincinnati that "he had no great confidence in the judgment of many of the top military leaders of the nation" and assessed the sentiment in Washington as "'a kind of wavering between panic and reassurance that goes right up to the Pentagon.'" He criticized the performance of military leaders in light of the "'setback'" in Korea and the administration's focus on protecting Europe ("Taft Says He Lacks Trust in Pentagon," *New York Times*, December 30, 1950, p. 3.)

Prior to a private dinner at which both Marshall and Taft would be present, Marshall Carter on January 4 reminded Marshall of Taft's statement that he "had lost faith in the high military leaders of this country, or words generally to that effect," and then informed Marshall that Taft "has never met Admiral Sherman, has not talked to General Vandenberg for five years, and has not talked to General

Bradley or General Collins for at least the last two years." Marshall responded, "Do you mean to suggest that I tell him this -!!" (Carter to Marshall, memorandum, with Marshall and Carter handwritten responses, January 4, 1951, GCMRL/G. C. Marshall Papers [Secretary of Defense, Categorical, Memoranda, Marshall S. Carter, 1950–1951].) Carter replied with similar humor, but others did not. To the contrary, they were deeply concerned and wanted Marshall to respond. ★

211

To Mrs. Franklin D. Roosevelt — January 18, 1951
Radio No. DEF-40390. — Washington, DC

Reference your telegraphic invitation to discuss the international military situation on your NBC [National Broadcasting Company] radio program the weekend of January twenty sixth, I am sorry that I cannot accept.[1] My public statements are now intimately involved with both timing and frequency, and more particularly now, with my appearances on the Hill. I am already committed for several public statements during the next few weeks and in fact am making a major address to the Womens Patriotic Conference on National Defense on Thursday evening, January twenty fifth.[2] I am confident you will understand my situation in this connection. With warm personal regards,[3]

GCMRL/G. C. Marshall Papers (Secretary of Defense, Number Indexed, M214-7-10)

1. "At this time of a widening isolationist trend and a spreading of fear," Eleanor Roosevelt had informed Marshall, "I feel that the peoples of the United States need a greater reassurance from our government and military leaders, a reassurance on a more personal basis than public pronouncements." She consequently invited Marshall "to record with me a discussion" for her radio program, *The Eleanor Roosevelt Show*, while she would be in Washington on January 26 or 27. (Roosevelt to Marshall, telegram, January 17, 1951, GCMRL/G. C. Marshall Papers [Secretary of Defense, Number Indexed, M214-7-10].)

2. See pp. 350–54.

3. On January 19, Marshall replied similarly but with more detail to James B. Carey, secretary-treasurer of the Congress of Industrial Organizations (CIO), who on January 10 had written warning Marshall that "liberalism and internationalism" were being threatened by "reactionary elements," which were endangering the UN and forcing the "abandonment of our allies throughout the world." He asked for Marshall's comment on a January 6 speech in which Carey charged that "Isolationism is Communism's fifth column." Marshall declined Carey's request, stating that he was avoiding "getting in the midst of the political fight" as it would limit his ability to work with Congress. (Carey to Marshall, January 10, 1951, and Marshall to Carey, January 19, 1951, GCMRL/G. C. Marshall Papers [Secretary of Defense, Number Indexed, M215-1-3].) Marshall Carter had summarized Carey's speech as "a sort of rabble rouser" and gave Marshall a reply drafted by Ginsburgh and to be signed by Marshall's acting executive secretary "to get you off the hook from" replying directly. (Carter to Marshall, memorandum, January 19, 1951, ibid.) Marshall instead sent his January 19 letter.

212

To Charles P. Nelson

January 19, 1951
Washington, DC

Dear Mr. Nelson: Thank you for your thoughtful letter of 20 December in which you suggest that a selective program be set up so that disabled former military personnel who volunteer to serve may be used in the Armed Services.[1] This is a subject of much interest to me both as Secretary of Defense and as an associate member of the President's Committee on National Employ the Physically Handicapped Week. In endorsing the program for the selective placement of physically handicapped persons in industry and government I pointed out that in the Armed Services we already have thousands of disabled persons, especially veterans, on civilian jobs and in certain categories of military assignments. Still greater use of this type of personnel is planned as the needs for their services develop.[2]

Because of the pertinency of your letter, however, I have referred it to the Chairman of the Personnel Policy Board. That Board is continually considering questions involving policies with respect to the determination of standards for the procurement, induction and utilization of military and civilian personnel. Recently as a result of a review of the physical induction standards by a committee of representatives of the Armed Services studies have been initiated regarding certain other aspects of the physical standards problem. One study pertained to the greater utilization of individuals who become psychiatric casualties or incur static defects while in the Service. Although your letter confined itself to the use of disabled personnel who had been discharged or retired, the points made therein would be helpful in connection with that study.[3] Faithfully yours,

NA/RG 330, SD 201.601

1. Representative Nelson (R-ME) had written to Marshall to suggest the creation of a program to make use of "disabled personnel of the Armed Forces who wish to volunteer," as he believed that such a program would save money and would serve as a "tremendous boost to the morale of the Nation and to the men involved when the Armed Services recognize the need for their assistance in this emergency." (Nelson to Marshall, December 20, 1950, NA/RG 330, SD 201.601.)

2. Employ the Physically Handicapped Week was celebrated during the first full week of every October as per an August 11, 1945, resolution by the Seventy-ninth Congress. Truman had established the President's Committee on National Employ the Physically Handicapped Week in 1947 to coordinate events and generate publicity for the week and handicapped issues in general. Marshall had written a statement for the December 1950 issue of the committee's publication, *Performance: Story of the Handicapped*, in which he expressed support for employing the physically handicapped in industry and government to support national defense needs. (Article for *Performance*, October 26, 1950, GCMRL/G. C. Marshall Papers [Secretary of Defense, Speeches and Statements].)

3. J. Thomas Schneider, director of the Office of Personnel Policy, had informed Marshall on January 11 that the board was exploring the "possibility of greater utilization of individuals who become psychiatric casualties or incur static physical defects while in the military service," stated that Representative Nelson's recommendations would "be helpful in connection with that study," and recommended that Marshall sign the attached letter. (Schneider to Marshall, memorandum, January 11, 1951, NA/RG 330, SD 201.601.)

213

Remarks at a Tribute to Henry L. Stimson[1]

January 21, 1951
Washington, DC

Henry L. Stimson was a great American. We have come here, to the church he attended when he made Washington his home, to pay homage to his memory and perpetuate in our small way the record of his outstanding achievements.

Mr. Stimson carried into his public life the basic ideals of Christianity which made him a devoted husband, a courageous soldier, a great lawyer, a profound statesman, and an inspiring leader. He had great faith in the spiritual quality of our people and fostered this quality throughout his life.

He kept himself physically fit and mentally alert. The creation of a healthy environment for our soldiers was one of his major objectives as Secretary of War. He thoroughly understood the values of discipline. He recognized the importance of training. He set for himself high standards of devotion to duty, and greatly influenced others by his shining example. With a deep sense of moral values, he held before himself, his friends and associates and the American people, the principle that the right will and must triumph, but only if all those devoted to its cause give themselves courageously to its service. He had great faith in the ultimate values of life, in the reign of law, in the victory of good over evil, and he patterned his actions to the maintenance of these ideals.

It was my honor and great good fortune to serve under Mr. Stimson's leadership during the war years. I watched him in those difficult days of 1940 and '41 when, in a divided America, he fought for an adequate national defense. I observed him in the very dark days of 1942 when we were suffering a succession of defeats. His faith was unbounded, his determination fixed, and his confidence in final victory unshaken. I recall his inspiring reactions during the exhilarating moments of the great victories in the final triumph over our enemies. Then Mr. Stimson turned immediately to thoughts of defense in enduring terms and urged that we must continue strong and therefore adopt some method by which we could maintain ourselves before the world as a strong people determined to enforce the peace.

Mr. Stimson brought to the office of Secretary of War a brilliant record of public service. President Theodore Roosevelt used him as a United States attorney at a time and in a place of great importance. President Taft called on his services as Secretary of War. President Coolidge appointed him Governor-General of the Philippine Islands and made him the President's personal emissary to settle the civil war in Nicaragua. President Hoover appointed him Secretary of State. Later in his seventies he was again to serve as Secretary of War under President Roosevelt and President Truman before his final retirement in his seventy-eighth year.[2]

Wherever he served, Mr. Stimson's administration was always clearly in the public interest. His was always the voice of courage. As Secretary of State he strongly urged the use of moral sanctions to halt the first steps of the aggressors in Manchuria and Ethiopia, which, allowed to go unchecked, led us to a world-wide disaster.[3] Later as Secretary of War he courageously assumed responsibility for the security of this nation when only skeleton forces existed, and those largely unequipped, to meet the tide of highly organized aggression. It took moral courage to lead in the demand for the Selective Service law. His was always the honest approach. He had a way of dipping into a stream of facts and ideas, and coming up with a simple and direct course of action, a course easy to understand and practical to carry out.

In the present crisis Mr. Stimson would have been a rock of support for all of us. The logic of his views on war and peace, on international morality and national security, on universal service and common sacrifice, on hemisphere solidarity and world government, all should be re-stated in the face of the present crisis. Those views are as sound and appropriate today as they were at the time they were first uttered. They should be re-affirmed now as a living memorial to him. They should inspire us to continue his good fight for the right and the just to help preserve our country and the ideals for which he so completely devoted himself.[4]

GCMRL/G. C. Marshall Papers (Secretary of Defense, Speeches and Statements)

1. The eighty-three-year-old Henry Stimson had died on October 20, 1950. In a public statement the following day, Marshall called him "a great American, a model citizen. I found him a tower of strength throughout the war. He showed the highest integrity in his every purpose. I feel that I have lost a very dear friend." (GCMRL/G. C. Marshall Papers [Secretary of Defense, Speeches and Statements].) Marshall attended the funeral at Stimson's Long Island estate, Highhold, the afternoon of October 23.

Major George advised Marshall that Frank McCoy, who headed the committee planning a memorial service for Stimson, had suggested that the ceremony be held on January 7 at the National Cathedral and that Marshall, first vice president of the National Cathedral, was "the natural choice to make a talk." Marshall noted that shifting the date to "later in the month would help." The date of January 21 was set on November 23, and the location shifted around December 15 from the National Cathedral to the National Presbyterian Church in Washington. Mrs. Stimson planned to be present; she had requested a very short service, and "asked that there be two tributes paid to the late Colonel; the first by the old pastor of the church, and second a short talk by you. She also wants you to unveil the bronze plaque which has been installed in the church." (George to Marshall, memoranda, November 14 and December 15, 1950, and George to Carter, memorandum, November 24, 1950, GCMRL/G. C. Marshall Papers [Secretary of Defense, Number Indexed, M214-6-10]; George to Marshall, memorandum, December 15, 1950, GCMRL/G. C. Marshall Papers [Chronological, Secretaries, Carlson].) Marshall wrote to Mrs. Stimson on December 16 that he was "not only glad, but highly complimented" to speak at the service. (Marshall to Stimson, December 16, 1950, GCMRL/G. C. Marshall Papers [Secretary of Defense, Number Indexed, M200-1-1].)

Edward L. R. Elson, pastor at the National Presbyterian Church, had extended a formal invitation on December 19 for Marshall to speak at the service along with Albert J. McCartney, minister emeritus of the church and Stimson's longtime pastor. Marshall accepted on January 2 but asked for guidance on what he should address in his remarks. Elson replied that McCartney would be speaking about Stimson "as a churchman," and he suggested that Marshall speak about Stimson's "life, character, public service . . . on behalf of the Government." (Elson to Marshall, December 19, 1950, and January 10, 1951, and Marshall to Elson, January 2, 1951, ibid., [M214-6-10].)

Other attendees at the service included Mrs. Stimson, President and Mrs. Truman, W. Averell Harriman, Lovett, and several ambassadors including Sir Oliver Franks. ("Plaque Dedicated to Honor Stimson," *New York Times*, January 22, 1951, p. 36.)

2. Stimson was US attorney for the southern district of New York, 1906–9; secretary of war, 1911–13; presidential emissary to Nicaragua, 1927; governor-general of the Philippines, 1927–29; secretary of state, 1929–33; and secretary of war, 1940–45.

3. For the Manchurian and Ethiopian crises, see pp. 32–33n5 and n6. As secretary of state during the Manchurian crisis of 1931–32, Stimson had initiated, in what became known as the Stimson Doctrine, the US policy of nonrecognition of changes in the status quo accomplished by force and in violation of international agreements.

4. Elson later wrote to thank Marshall for his tribute and to share Mrs. Stimson's expression of "special gratitude for that which you did." (Elson to Marshall, January 26, 1951, GCMRL/G. C. Marshall Papers [Secretary of Defense, Number Indexed, M214-6-10].)

214

Statement Before the House Armed Services Committee[1] January 23, 1951
Washington, DC

Today no voice is listened to in our troubled world unless it has adequate steel to support it.

The most effective contribution we can make to our own security and the preservation of peace is to provide clear-cut unequivocal proof that we can, first attain, and second, maintain, the military strength we need as long as world peace remains insecure.

The practical solution to both our immediate and our long-range problems lies in the adoption of a system of universal military service and training. The bill we have submitted to your committee would give us the authority to create the strength that is needed today. It would give us the authority to provide, for the first time, the assurance that our long-term requirements could be met on an adequate basis.

The first part of our job, that of building up our forces to the level made necessary by the existing crisis, must be carried forward rapidly. The Joint Chiefs of Staff have set 3,462,000 men as the goal we must reach by June 30. This is roughly 1,000,000 beyond our present strength, but we will have to increase our forces beyond this strength if the situation worsens.

The second part of our job, that of providing now for the maintenance of a strong military posture on an enduring basis, is equally imperative.

In the past it has been our habit after victory to emasculate our military power and leave ourselves impotent before the world, impotent to defend the peaceful principles that have always been in our American tradition.

If we give the other nations of the world any basis for believing that we may again weary of the need for keeping our strength at a high level, the inevitable result will be to encourage those who plot against us and discourage all of those who have made common cause with us.

It is the terrible and continuing threat of aggression that makes universal service and training the imperative response of our democratic Nation today.

Without such a program we would risk again having our defenses reduced in periods of complacency to a level far below our needs and then be obliged to race uphill again in turbulent, wasteful rearmament in the emotional resurgence after danger again becomes glaringly apparent. There have been too many such occasions in the past. That mistake we must now correct, and at the same time set our guard against its repetition. There must be no repetition of past invitations to disaster.

The speed and destructiveness of present methods of warfare makes it imperative that we place our security on a firm base. We should proceed with the development of our military strength in personnel on the same basis that we are arranging for matériel, to make possible a tremendously rapid expansion of our military forces in an effective manner whenever that becomes necessary.

The program we have developed is within our capacity to support through the years of tension that we may have to endure. It will permit us to meet our urgent immediate military necessities and also will set us on a course for the first time in our history that will give us a reasonable prospect of an enduring posture of military strength, and without bankrupting us in the process.

Under its provisions no man physically able to share in the common military defense will be free to stand aside and ignore his obligation as a citizen. The period for entering upon service and training would be the year between a man's eighteenth and nineteenth birthdays. This age is recommended because it represents the judgment of educators, industrialists and others who are expert in their field, that this is the period in a man's life when there would be least dislocation if he is called up for service and training. Few men of 18 are married or have children; fewer probably have entered college or started on their life work. From the standpoint of the men and from the standpoint of the community—industry, agriculture, education, science and family responsibilities—this appears to be the logical year in which the national obligation for military service should be fulfilled.

From my own experience I can state that men of 18 are among our best soldiers. They are brave; they are strong; they perform their duties with patriotic dedication and understanding. Thousands of them volunteer each year because of their eagerness to participate in the great mission of national defense. Then also, when these young men come out of the Armed Forces, they are much better equipped, I am sure, to enter upon useful lives as good citizens in every field of civilian endeavor. I do not present this as a reason for calling them into service; it is cited as an objective fact well supported by the records of the millions of young veterans who are now making a tremendous contribution to our national life.

It is our desire, it is our intention that none of the men between the ages of 18 and 19 who are inducted at the start of the Universal Military Service and Training program would be sent into combat areas until they have passed their nineteenth birthday. I shall not go into the details of these plans. They will be outlined fully by Secretary Rosenberg and the military authorities. When you hear them, I think you will be satisfied that it is unlikely, barring a dire emergency, that anyone will be sent into combat before he is 19.[2]

But I must say in this connection, that I very much hope you will not impose a legal limitation barring the assignment of such men to combat duty. No one can foretell the character and degree of hostile action that might be launched against us, except that certainly it would be in a manner to gain the tremendous advantage of surprise, and certainly it would be utterly ruthless in conception and execution. In such a dire emergency we should be free to act instantly and as effectively as possible, that is without strings attached. We must not be handicapped by limitations of virtually any kind at such a moment when our national existence is at stake.

There is one other phase of our proposal which I should like to bring especially to your attention. It is the recommendation to extend the period of service for men inducted through Selective Service from 21 months to 27. From a purely military point of view, it would have been desirable to request an even longer period of service than 27 months. Our forces need many specialists and technicians today and it takes a long time to make them expert in their work. To return most of these men to civil life just as they reach the period of greatest value to the Government is a definite and really severe handicap to the efficiency of the military effort.

We realize that we cannot well insist on holding men simply because it is desirable from a military viewpoint, or because it would result in a considerable saving of tax funds by obtaining this increased return on the training investment. The important consideration is that the 27-month period represents the minimum term we consider consistent with the urgent needs of an efficient military organization in the present period of world tension. We feel that the 27-month period should apply until the continued operation of universal military service and training has enabled us to reduce our forces on active duty and to transfer a larger share of responsibility to the Reserve.

The bill allows for this flexibility. It authorizes the President to reduce the period of service whenever the national security permits. He could eventually withdraw the service requirement entirely, but the obligation for training would remain, so that young men would always be coming forward to build up a vigorous, strong Reserve. Such a system would give us, I feel, the kind of basic protection we need to keep us strong with minimum drain on our productive energies.

Universal military service and training is in the best democratic tradition. It is within our capacity to support through the years. It will permit us to build up our strength quickly in the present emergency. It will provide a system for procuring and maintaining a reserve of trained manpower. It will give us the enduring system of national defense that our country has always needed, a posture of strength to discourage aggression, a reserve of power to marshal in an emergency.[3]

I think, Mr. Chairman, it might save in later questioning if I describe now a little of the situation which has developed during the past 6 months and where we are at the present time, because it is related to everything I have just said. Possibly if I sketched an outline of the situation now, a better understanding of these proposals would be in the hands of the committee.

The CHAIRMAN. Before you start, general, the photographers will have to stop making pictures while the general is testifying. It is annoying to everyone. Go ahead.

Secretary MARSHALL. To go back to the beginning of this crisis last June, I assume most of you know the dilemma in which the Army found itself, and General MacArthur's command in particular. The troops out in Japan, some four divisions, were at about half strength in size of units and matters of that kind. So they went into Korea in this partial strength condition. You cannot appreciate the meaning of that merely on a basis of arithmetic, that they had 50 percent and not 60 or 40 and not 50, because the moment you go into campaign aside from the bullet, shell, and bomb casualties you have casualties of sickness particularly under the conditions in Korea, those that get lost and those that completely give out, particularly in a terrific retreat situation as developed at the beginning of fighting.

So the fighting power of the unit would always be below the strength of the unit in numbers of men as they grow more fatigued and more fatigued and there is nothing to stimulate them such as the arrival of replacements to fill all the vacant places that are occurring daily.

In that dilemma, General MacArthur made a very courageous decision and moved into the ranks of those four divisions some 30,000 Koreans. So, in order to save ourselves in that critical situation of combat, we had to depend on men that had only had 3 weeks of training, men of another country and put them into American units to a tune of some 36 percent. And as late as November I found those units were still 20 percent short in American manpower. In addition to that, there were created 10 divisions of South Koreans. General MacArthur undertook to create one every 4 weeks. Well, when one remembers that it took us almost 2 years to get our divisions ready for heavy fighting in Europe and in the Southwest Pacific, you must realize what it was to turn out a division of South Koreans with their difficulty of understanding our weapons and our conceptions of discipline and tactics in only 4 weeks' time. Nevertheless, that was done and the fight was made on that basis.

The interesting fact I would like to point up to you now is that we still have not made good the deficiencies. And I am informed, when I have checked through all the records, it will be next April before we make good on the men required to bring General MacArthur's existing force up to its strength.

Now in order to understand that—and it has a tremendous bearing on what we are proposing here—I want to sketch for you the procedure the Army has gone through these past 6 months. We had, I find, in the summer, four training centers for giving men the basic training, disciplinary training, the weapon training in the various weapons that they would be called upon to use, including tanks and artillery and the various special techniques involved particularly in the way of radio communications and equipment of that sort. The Selective Service Act, I believe, was reenactivated in July. But the first men did not begin to go into the camps until September.[4] The camps could not then be used for basic training. Those four camps as a beginning had to be used for processing the men, that is getting them into uniform, giving them their injections and getting them organized so they could be moved around in some sort of order, classifying them in groups and matters of that sort. They had to be immediately sent into units in this country to take the place of the men in the ranks of those units in this country who had been stripped out and sent to Korea. Virtually every unit we had in this country was just wiped of privates, probably 50 percent of the noncommissioned officer and officer strength, to meet the immediate requirements in Korea—first to build up the strength of the units over there and also to try to make good on the casualties of campaign—casualties of bullets, shells and bombs—and casualties of sickness and happenings of that character.

I find in going back through the developments of last summer and fall that throughout the months of September, October, and November, practically all the selective service men were being put into the ranks of units in this country to meet the continued draft on those ranks for men to be sent to Korea. So it was not until in October that the first small beginning was made of assigning men to normal basic training camps, to provide the manpower that we needed. It could only be a small beginning. The number of camps was increased from 4 to 19. Nine of those I think were the basic camps where the first 6 weeks of training was given and the others were the camps where the men took the final 8 weeks for whatever their arm assignment was to be—the Artillery, the Engineers, the Signal Corps, the tanks, and so on—to complete that 14 weeks' training. They held to the policy throughout that no men should be sent out from the selective service draft who had not had 14 weeks' training. That meant, of course, we had to put these men in units in this country, take the men out of the units in this country and ship them to General MacArthur. His needs in various categories have averaged from month to month about 15,000 a month—not new units but replacements. As I say, under the present situation, it appears to be about the 1st of April before they will have fully filled the ranks with American soldiers in the American units in Korea.

As an example, in one division, the Seventh Division, there were 7,800 Koreans put in its ranks before it left Japan for Korea. That is a very large percentage of the whole and it represents quite a predicament in which the United States Government should find itself regarding the support of its Armed Forces.[5]

Those things I think are lost sight of in the debate of why we did this and why we did that. What I am talking about exclusively are the military factors of why we were in this predicament in connection with our military forces and how we can avoid the repetition of these happenings in the future, along with the authorization that will permit us to build up strength as rapidly as possible as the present time.

By the 1st of December they began assigning recruits to these training camps for basic training in larger numbers. I think the December quota that was sent directly into these training camps was some forty-odd thousand. But the interesting point to me is that the first normal graduates of that fundamental basic training will not graduate until the last week in January. In the present situation—I am rather hesitant talking about this publicly, but I think it is better to do so because the manpower bill is so important to us that we should have as complete an understanding as possible in your minds—under the present situation the product of normal basic training, which is the foundation of any unit, will be about 5,000 at the end of January, 6,000 or so in February, increasing gradually to about 35,000 in June and, we hope, reaching the average level of 50,000 late in the summer. At the same time we will be taking in during January, February, and March—that is as far as we have gone in announcements—80,000 men a month through the medium of selective service. There is a difference here which represents men that have gone into officer training camps and men who are to be given certain special courses, but our necessities will continue to require that we take men out of units in this country for General MacArthur and, of course, they will have to be replaced by men from the selective service draft who therefore cannot be sent directly into basic training camps.

The first return from the selective service was in September. We went up as high as, I think, 70,000 in November. Then the take was lowered to 40,000 in December, But commencing in January we started up again, with 80,000 in each of the next 3 months. I am not in a position to state accurately what will be the call in remaining months of this fiscal year.

One of the difficulties in this matter, I think, has been the difficulty of understanding how long it takes to get a man started in this business if it is going to develop into a durable, dependable machine. The National Guard units were called in, for example—four of them—last summer. They began assembling in September. They had from 45 to 50 percent of their strength. Some of the Organized Reserve units were as low as 10 percent of their strength. They began a preliminary training of those men in the basic disciplinary weapon requirements which cannot be effectively managed in ordinary National Guard training at home.

The ranks of these units were not filled up until sometime in November. Then they started on the complete course of basic military training. That will be completed about the 1st of March.

Now how much further training and time is going to be required to develop effective battalions, regiments, and brigades, and the division is something else again. Meanwhile here in the United States we are in a position in the world, with factors of this sort facing the responsible authorities in meeting the critical situation of today. The background of it all has been and is the lack of a military system that has some prospect of enduring through the days when people are least interested in military matters except as to costs, which of course are always very great.

Our tendency today is to think in terms of divisions as a measure of strength. That is not an accurate unit of measurement. Divisions differ. Our division, for instance, is twice the size of a Soviet division. It is about the same—twice the size—of a Chinese Communist division. The Korean divisions are a little smaller than the Chinese Communist divisions. Divisions are not all alike. Then you must consider what is behind them, what degree of corps troops and army troops. Corps troops as a rule consist of additional artillery, additional tanks, engineers, all other special troops which it would be wasteful to put into the division until actually needed. With the pool in the corps they can be assigned in large numbers to the division that urgently needs them for a particular operation. All of those factors are involved in using the division as a unit of measurement of strength.

I should imagine, without knowing anything definite about it, that the Chinese Communist troops have very few corps and army troops at their disposal. They have been able to realize on utilizing tremendous numbers of infantrymen with a complete disregard of human life. That cannot be kept up indefinitely and go over a wide range of territory.

Again, we have considerations involved in this matter which are of interest to many here in the Capitol; that is, what we call the divisional slice. It has been stated that it takes about 65,000 men to produce one division of 18,000 men. That seems a rather extravagant set-up, but when you stop to consider 19 training camps alone which we have to use to get these men ready and each one necessary has an overhead almost equivalent to the numbers they are training, when you consider that our logistical requirements involve the maintenance of lines of communications, of supply lines, from, we will say, 8,000 miles on the one side, taking in half the continental width, and about 3,000 on the other side across the Atlantic—all of these requirements and many others in the way of staging areas, and so forth, the size of the division slice becomes more understandable.[6] Incidentally, it wasn't until the spring of 1943 that we caught up with our replacement necessities for divisions. And the effective result became evident with the resumption of a general offensive in Italy on May 11. In the fighting that followed each division every morning was at 100 percent strength and they were able to go, some of them, as much as 150 kilometers or more without relief. Whereas theretofore they had been so worn down with losses because their ranks were continually thinning, that morale was adversely affected. We could not get sufficient men for the ranks for a wide variety of reasons and one of them was the 18-year-old problem.

So the real measure of our military strength, our military potential at the present time is to be measured in trained men. For example, two National Guard divisions are now concentrating. They started, I think, the 15th of January. In their ranks are 45 to 50 percent of men who have not had the necessary basic military training because they could not obtain it under the conditions of service in time of peace within the ranks of the National Guard at home. Everyone understands that. So those men have to be trained. But in addition to that, it is necessary to put into their ranks an additional 50 or 55 percent of men from selective service at the present time.

Now I think you can readily understand the tremendous difference that would be brought about if we could put 50 or 55 percent of basically trained men in those same ranks. It would shorten the time of their development for service by at least 3 or 4 months. That is General Collins' estimate. That would be my guess. I cannot talk with the assurance in regard to the National Guard that I once could because it is under different conditions now in that, fortunately, the officer personnel are mostly veterans and there are a great many veterans among the noncommissioned officers. This makes a training prospect a much more favorable condition than was the case in 1940 and 1941.

The millennium, aside from peace, that I would like to see is one surplus trained man. It would be the first time in our history that we ever had one. I would like to see him. That would represent the greatest measurement of our development for security, for power, that is so necessary in the world today. I am sorry to have talked at such length, Mr. Chairman.[7]

House Committee on Armed Services, *Hearings . . . on H.R. 1752: A Bill to Provide for the Common Defense and Security of the United States and to Permit the More Effective Utilization of Manpower Resources of the United States by Authorizing Universal Military Service and Training, and for Other Purposes*, 82d Cong., 1st sess., 8–14.

1. Marshall was the first witness to testify before the committee, chaired by Representative Carl Vinson (D-GA), which was considering the now-completed universal military service and training bill. For Marshall's previous testimony before the Senate subcommittee considering such a bill, see pp. 326–29.
2. Rosenberg testified before the committee the following day.
3. Marshall's reading copy and press version of his testimony ended at this point. (Both are in GCMRL/G. C. Marshall Papers [Secretary of Defense, Speeches and Statements].) What follows is only in the printed congressional hearings and apparently was delivered extemporaneously.
4. See pp. 325–26.
5. According to *The Encyclopedia of the Korean War*, there were 8,625 Korean soldiers attached to the Seventh Infantry Division before the unit left Japan in August 1950. (Spencer C. Tucker, *The Encyclopedia of the Korean War: A Political, Social, and Military History*, 2d ed., vol. 1, *A–L* [Santa Barbara, CA: ABC-CLIO, 2010], 486.) See also Allan R. Millett, *The War for Korea*, vol. 2, *They Came from the North, 1950–1951* (Lawrence: University Press of Kansas, 2010), 158–59; and pp. 180–81 and 181–82n2, 193–94, and 287.
6. For more on the division slice, see pp. 391–93.
7. See the next editorial summary and pp. 409–13.

215

House Testimony on the Universal Military Service and Training Act of 1951

January 23, 1951 Washington, DC

IN THE lengthy session that followed his testimony before the House Armed Services Committee (see previous document), Marshall was questioned on numerous points. For many of these he suggested the committee members ask Assistant Secretary Rosenberg, who was with him at this hearing and who was to testify the following morning.

Marshall emphasized once again his belief that UMT "was the only method I could see, both as a military man and as a taxpayer and as a citizen, that we could financially manage a real effective posture of strength. I couldn't think of any other method procedure that would do it. Therefore I was considering the financial phases of it." He also made clear that while the Joint Chiefs dealt only with "purely military" factors, he as secretary of defense had to consider political factors that affected the armed forces as well. (House Committee on Armed Services, *Hearings . . . on H.R. 1752*, 16.) In response to a series of questions, he asserted the importance of and reasons for training and drafting eighteen-year-olds instead of older men—an issue that concerned many of the committee members. He referred back to the problems he had had on this issue during World War II, bluntly stating that older men "could not do the things required. They lacked the resiliency of youth and also they required increased hospital service." (Ibid., 19.)

Marshall then explained "the build-up of this bill. There have been a series of day and night conferences among the services, among educational groups, among the labor groups, among other groups, that has really run about 18 hours a day." He had not attended all the meetings, but had insisted on "certain fundamental things." Beyond that, he informed the committee members, "I have had to turn to somebody else, and he or she can give you an accurate and complete answer." (Ibid., 19–20.) He did explain the reasons the proposed bill gave the president the power to reduce the pay of those being trained to thirty dollars per month. He also explained, as he previously had to the Senate subcommittee (see pp. 325–29), the reasons for the large number of support troops needed for an American army division (the "division slice") as compared to the numbers needed by the Chinese and Soviet divisions, noting in particular the length of American supply lines overseas and their relationship to the US policy "to keep the war as far away from our shore as it is possible to manage." (Ibid., 21–24, quote on 24.) See pp. 391–93.

Numerous representatives then questioned Marshall as to whether military service and training should be combined in the same bill, since one dealt with present needs and the other with the future, with Representative Paul J. Kilday (D-TX) suggesting that the bill be divided into two titles: one for the present emergency and one for future training. Marshall made clear that he was primarily responsible for the combination and strongly voiced his opposition to any division. "I lower my voice so as not to sound overemphatic," he told the committee, "that if you ever divorce this phase [UMT] from the bill we are sunk again. I do not want to be involved in that disaster." When asked about the number of divisions the administration intended to send to Europe, Marshall stated that he was "not in a position here to answer that because that goes above me." (Ibid., 25 and 28.)

After a question about whether illiterate trainees would be educated, the committee members returned to previous questions regarding the proposed size of the armed forces and the training and drafting of eighteen-year-olds as well as their registration at seventeen. Some committee members were concerned about the impact on the morals of these young men when they were exposed in camp, as Representative Clyde Doyle (D-CA) put it, to "the use of liquor, . . . prostitution and other problems that arise out of mass military effort." (Ibid., 30–37, quote on 37.) When asked what the impact of earlier passage of a UMT bill would have had on the present situation on Korea, Marshall forthrightly said it "would have completely metamorphosed the situation" and that on the global scene, "we would not be threatened with war today." (Ibid., 33.) He also dismissed fears that UMT would militarize society by noting the speed and totality of demobilization after previous wars—including World War II when "the Army was dissolving literally in my lap. I couldn't find the Army one day to the next. I don't think you can change the American boy. He doesn't change very readily into a military automaton. . . . [E]very indication that we have is that you can't enforce a military feeling on our people unless there is an immediate objective before them that all can recognize is of vast importance to the country." (Ibid., 37–38.)

When Dewey Short (R-MO), the ranking minority member of the committee, labeled the tying of UMT to the draft a "shotgun wedding," Marshall bluntly stated, "I did it." Short responded that he was glad Marshall had "the courage to admit it." Marshall retorted, "I am not admitting it. I am telling you. I did it." Short stated, "There are no apologies to be offered," to which Marshall repeated, "I am not admitting it. I did it." Short then reminded him that committee members nevertheless "were entitled to our views and the right to interrogate," to which Marshall responded, "I know that from past experience. . . . You almost made me feel 10 years younger this morning. It is kind of like old times." (Ibid., 41.) See also pp. 369–71 and 409–13. ★

216

GRADUATION REMARKS AT THE ARMED FORCES STAFF COLLEGE
January 24, 1951 Norfolk, Virginia

MARSHALL FLEW TO Norfolk, Virginia, on January 24 to address the graduates of the Armed Forces Staff College, which had been established in 1946. He began by admitting that "the popular conception" of military education is "that it ends at Annapolis or West Point. I won't characterize just what is there; but there is a great deal that comes after, and a very intense effort, because a man's whole career is at stake every step of the way in the various institutions." Despite this lack of public knowledge, Marshall found the additional education provided by these schools to be "of tremendous value" throughout his career, particularly during World War II, when mobilization was so nascent and critical. While Marshall did not "want to go through the hackneyed reiteration regarding unity" in this speech, he intended to "make several references to it here" at the school which had played "a great part" in fostering such unity. (Graduation Remarks at the Armed Forces Staff College, January 24, 1951, GCMRL/G. C. Marshall Papers [Secretary of Defense, Speeches and Statements].)

Marshall recalled congressional efforts in the early 1920s "to try to bring about some greater cohesion" between the services, which resulted in the creation of a board consisting of Marshall and Theodore Roosevelt Jr., the eldest son of President Theodore Roosevelt and then assistant secretary of the navy. (Roosevelt Jr. had fought alongside Marshall during World War I. With the rank of brigadier general during World War II as assistant commander of the Fourth Infantry Division, he accompanied the Eighth Infantry Regiment onto Utah Beach during the D-Day invasion, though he died of a heart attack on July 12, 1944. See *Papers of GCM*, 4: 522.) While serving on this board, Marshall proposed that the army employ a naval officer in "every section of the General Staff" and that the navy reciprocate with army officers. Marshall recalled that this plan "only developed opposition" from both services, and he "learned a good bit . . . as I went through that procedure." Considering that "status of things" in the 1920s, "today the developments have been prodigious, and very satisfying." (Ibid.)

Following Marshall's appointment as chief of staff, he and Admiral Stark were able to organize a large joint army-navy exercise in the Pacific Ocean in 1940. (See *Papers of GCM*, 2: 93–94, 101, 133, 137–38, 141, 150, 154–55, 157, and 257.) Witnessing the confusion in the command structure that became apparent during this operation, Marshall was determined to "'change the whole damn organization'" of the army staff "'right quickly.' And that's what we did. We reorganized the entire War Department" and did so "in a great hurry" in early 1942. "We did it and it worked. We were able to deal with some 8 1/2 million men all over the world." Marshall expressed praise for the members of his General Staff, including Omar Bradley; J. Lawton Collins; Walter Bedell Smith, who had been on Marshall's general staff since September 1939 and left to become Eisenhower's chief of staff in September 1942; and Frank McCarthy who, as secretary of the General Staff at the end of the war, operated "one of the most successfully run affairs I have ever seen. As we approached demobilization we had to bring in regular officers so they could see how the system had developed and we wouldn't lose it." (Ibid.)

In response to "probing" from Congress regarding Korea and the efficiency among the services there, Marshall concluded by responding that he thought "we are doing it beautifully together. Everybody is in accord, . . . and it is a most satisfying thing, and this school represents a crux of that very business." (Ibid.) ★

217

To Dean G. Acheson — January 25, 1951
Restricted — Washington, DC

Dear Acheson: The attached letter with its inclosure was prepared for me by the Personnel Policy Board of the Department of Defense which includes representatives of the three services.[1]

I particularly want to expand on point 4 of the inclosure which I consider the most forceful argument against curtailing our present authority to make awards to foreign personnel.[2]

The battlefield morale value of on-the-spot decorations for gallantry in action is tremendous. It is particularly impressive from both a morale and foreign relations viewpoint, when performed by the United States commander. I have in mind the recent bayonet charge gallantry of the French Battalion and the continued high fighting qualities of the Turkish Unit.[3] The point is that these units and numerous others from our allies are because of their size attached to larger United States units. Under these circumstances, the foreign commander cannot very well recommend himself to his own Government for a decoration, and the chances are that the foreign commander does not have his Government's authority to award *on-the-spot decorations* to his own nationals.

I would deplore any curtailment of this authority under the conditions now existing in Korea. At the same time, of course, I have no desire that United States decorations be issued to foreign nationals as a standard component of the field rations, and I am reasonably certain that this is not being done.

As for the British Brigade, in particular, since it is a self-contained unit not attached to a larger U. S. combat unit, I have no objection if the British wish to take unilateral action in the case of United States awards to their nationals. Faithfully yours,

NA/RG 330, SD 200.63

1. On October 18, Acheson had requested the Defense Department's reaction to a British proposal that each nation with forces in Korea confine the awarding of decorations to its own personnel. In the formal reply attached to the letter reproduced above, Marshall reported that the military departments did not agree and that he concurred in their conclusions. (Marshall to Acheson, January 25, 1951, NA/RG 330, SD 200.63.)

2. Point four of the enclosure noted that MacArthur was a US as well as a UN commander, that troops of participating nations were attached as units to US organizations and served under US commanders, and that it was therefore "natural" for US commanders to provide these forces with "prompt recognition of heroism or meritorious service." (Ibid.)

3. Both the French battalion and the Turkish brigade in Korea were known for their bayonet charges. The French battalion had arrived at the end of November and made such a charge on January 10; it did so again on more than one occasion in the following months and won three US presidential citations for bravery. Some of the officers and men of the Turkish brigade, which had arrived in October, received the US Silver and Bronze Stars. Noting the fact that these charges raised the morale of UN forces, Ridgway "decided to have all infantry units fix bayonets to their rifles." (Tucker, *Encyclopedia of the Korean War*, 1: 277, and 2: 867–68; Stanley Sandler, ed., *The Korean War: An Encyclopedia* [New York: Garland Publishing, 1995], 114–16, 338–40; Millett, *The War for Korea*, 2: 260–61.)

218

To Mrs. James J. Winn

January 25, 1951
Washington, DC

Dear Molly: I was sorry I could not find it possible to arrange to see you on my brief trip to Norfolk yesterday. When, the evening before, your mother found where I was going, she made a rather sly approach to the proposition of flying down with me. But I was going to proceed on a very rush basis as I had to be back here for an important meeting that afternoon at the White House and I did not think it wise to take her. She can't walk as fast as I do nor break away from gatherings with the rapidity that I do and I have to make every minute count.[1]

I am delighted that you are pleased with the house and that you found it possible to arrange for an immediate rental. This will give you a firm base for the future and I think one that will be self-sustaining. Don't concern yourself now about the money involvement. I will explain the status of that so far as I am concerned when I see you.[2]

With my love to all of you. Affectionately,

GCMRL/G. C. Marshall Papers (Secretary of Defense, Number Indexed, M200-4-17)

1. James Winn, Molly's husband, had been promoted to colonel earlier in January. He

was stationed in the Office of the Chief of Army Field Forces at Fort Monroe in Hampton, Virginia. Marshall had traveled to Norfolk to speak at the Armed Forces Staff College. See pp. 347–48. He attended the National Security Council meeting that day at 3:30 p.m.

2. The Winns signed a mortgage and agreed to pay Marshall a $10,000 principal sum plus interest between January 15, 1951, and January 15, 1956, for a house in Pinehurst, North Carolina. (Mortgage arrangements, January 15, 1951, GCMRL/G. C. Marshall Papers [Secretary of Defense, Categorical, Winn Mortgage, 1951].) Marshall later wrote to Rose Page Wilson that the Winns bought the house "against the possibility of Colonel Winn's having to go over seas at any moment. She got a rare bargain, five bedrooms, three baths, long living room, and equally long sun porch, all completely furnished china, glassware, frigidaire, toasters, washing machine, new oil furnace, etc. and one acre." (Marshall to Wilson, February 10, 1951, GCMRL/J. Page Wilson Collection; H.)

219

Remarks to the Women's Patriotic Conference on National Defense[1]

January 25, 1951
Washington, DC

The title of your organization is very appropriate to the present situation, for these are days when the patriotic impulse should dominate our lives.

We are in a period of critical tension, a tension which, unhappily, is perhaps the best we can hope for in the years ahead, and America urgently requires the support of its women to deal with this situation effectively. I have always felt, and on occasion have expressed, the conviction that "if I could get the understanding support of the women of America I would be at least half way along the road toward winning the support of the men generally and the political branches of the government particularly."

During the agonies of the last war I corresponded with thousands of women who had suffered casualties in their own families. They proved understanding and tolerant to a remarkable degree. This surprised me because I thought, and quite naturally, that the reactions of a wife or mother who had suffered a loss would be unforgiving toward officials in my position. Instead, I found more of courage, more of generous understanding among those women who had suffered, than in any other group in this country, male or female.

We need the understanding support of American women today on every matter vital to the national defense.

Let me outline a few fundamentals of American military policy.

America wants to avoid war. All of us, and particularly you women, mothers of sons or wives of men who may have to suffer the hazards of battle, all want to avoid war. War is abhorrent to me and I pray that we may avoid it, for I have lived with daily casualty lists and that is a truly awful experience. I have gone through hospital after hospital and viewed the human wreckage of war. Always I left with the feeling that we had failed miserably in our efforts to avert the cause for such sacrifices.

All agree that we must make every endeavor to maintain the peace. The question is, the problem is, how do we proceed in order to avoid wars. Clearly it must be evident to all these days that we must first develop, and then maintain strength, material as well as moral.

Another fundamental objective of our military policy today is to build up strength as rapidly as possible so that in the event that a war is thrust upon us we will be able in concert with our allies to defeat the enemy conclusively. Keeping these two objectives in mind—to prevent war if possible and to win it if it is thrust upon us—let us consider the character of our present mobilization, its degree and its rapidity both as to men and materiel, and then take a look at some aspects of the campaign in Korea.

Congress has recently taken two important steps in building up our military strength. The first additional appropriation, that is—the first beyond the routine yearly budget appropriation—voted by the Congress was approved by the President on September 27. The Department of Defense immediately got underway with the expansion of the military forces and the build-up of materiel permitted by that appropriation. Altogether some twenty-five billions were made available.

On New Year's Day, the second additional military appropriation became available. It involved nearly 17 billions. The two taken together provide the funds for large increases in men and about nineteen billions of dollars for heavy materiel, such as guns, tanks, ships, and planes, which gives us a broad base of departure.[2]

Our first great task as to materiel was to make the necessary contracts and get production started. That we are doing as expeditiously as conditions permit and by April we will need to secure additional funds for the continued accelerated expansion. I think that we are spending wisely as well as rapidly and making every effort to see that each dollar counts.

The same rapid rate of acceleration applies to men. We have increased the demands on the Selective Service System to 80,000 men a month, and we are steadily ordering to active duty men and units of the reserve components. There are now on active military duty some 6 divisions and over 70 other separate combat units of the National Guard; more than 200,000 Naval and Marine reservists; and personnel from 47 Air Guard and Reserve wings and organized air units. These measures will permit us to build rapidly to a total strength of approximately 3 1/2 million men on active duty by July of this year.[3]

We are building very much faster than had been planned originally. Last spring in accordance with the plans of the North Atlantic Treaty Organization it was intended that we would not have that many men in our Armed Forces even by the summer of 1954. In other words, we have increased the total and advanced the date of our build-up by three years.

What is far more important than these general observations regarding personnel is the Universal Military Service and Training bill now before Congress, which involves the much discussed recommendation of the Defense Department for the inclusion of men between the ages of 18 and 19. This bill carries what to me is of vital importance to the future of this country in the kind of world in which we are now living. It provides for a system of maintaining our military strength through the years, particularly the next ten, without bankrupting us financially. In the employment of our manpower the eighteen to nineteen year old group is the largest factor in this plan for an enduring system, although it is necessary today unless we turn to the alternative of drafting veterans and married men.

Many protests are received expressing disapproval of the plans for the eighteen to nineteen year old group. Considering the mothers of the land, the number heard from percentagewise is small but these are very emphatic in their objections. My own feeling is that our failure to provide for Universal Military Training in 1920 and the tragic repetition of that error in 1945 and 46 are largely responsible for the call we must make on our young men today. I am convinced that it would not now be necessary to interrupt the normal course of their lives if we had taken the conservative, wise action, an effort that was defeated largely by emotional, rather than logical, reactions.

It is very difficult for me to understand the tremendous influence on the public of those emotional waves and vocal minorities which have invariably defeated us in efforts to make war highly improbable. War would have been and would still be improbable, I think, if the American military posture commanded the respect of nations who threaten us today. Our job at this moment is to hasten the build-up to such a posture.

I want you to understand the objectives of our mobilization program. I want your understanding, too, of the conduct of our campaign in Korea. I want especially to make you aware of the near tragedy that developed in that campaign, how it was met and what a lesson it should teach us, particularly in the light of the present consideration by Congress of our manpower proposals.

When the trouble developed in Korea we had four divisions in Japan. They were sent with little or no delay to meet the crisis that threatened the life of the Republic of South Korea. These divisions were greatly under strength and it was necessary immediately to reinforce their ranks, not only to fill the vacancies that already existed, but more importantly to fill those that were bound to develop quickly through campaign casualties from battle and sickness.

Our divisions are supposed to have a strength of about 18,000 men. Behind them are expected to be corps troops, that is, special groups of tanks, artillery and engineers, and behind them, army troops of many kinds. But the four divisions in Japan were faced with the necessity of going into action with less than 60% of the required strength, and with little by way of Corps and Army support. It was foreseeable that wastage of campaign might cut even this 60% strength down to 50, 40 or even 30% of their fighting effectiveness. There were absolutely no trained replacements immediately available anywhere to fill up their ranks or those vacancies that would soon occur, except by emasculating the few units of the regular army on duty in this country, stripping them of virtually all of their privates and many of their non-commissioned and commissioned officers. That was done. One team was ruined to save another but even that drastic procedure failed to provide the divisions in Korea with the strength they urgently needed.

In this critical dilemma, General MacArthur made the courageous decision to assign South Koreans in large numbers to the ranks of American units. In those early days last summer 36% of the strength of American units was made up of

South Koreans to a total of some 30,000. In the Seventh Division alone, some 7,800 Koreans were absorbed. But even now these divisions are still short of their American quota.[4]

In addition, General MacArthur was creating South Korean divisions at the rate of one every four weeks. When you pause to consider that it took us almost two years to properly prepare our American divisions to fight in Europe and in the Pacific, and it was 2 1/2 years—from December 7, 1941 to June 6, 1944—before we were able to mount an invasion of Europe, you can understand how much could fairly be expected from a division which had but four weeks of preparation. It is to the credit of the leadership of our officers, the training techniques that had been developed in the army over the years and to the unfailing good sense and judgment of our non-commissioned officers that these divisions were organized, equipped and prepared to take their position beside us in combat in such record breaking time. They have given a very creditable performance under the circumstances but that fact does not relieve us of blame for having placed General MacArthur in such a dilemma. You and I are responsible, I feel, because we had not seen to the adoption of a system that would have made available a reserve of trained men that could be called upon instantly to report to the colors when an emergency arose.

The trouble started in Korea last June. It is now the end of January and we have not yet been able to fill the ranks of our few divisions to full strength. As to that basic training which is the very foundation of any battle worthy unit it will be the last of this month before we graduate the first few trainees who have been given a normal course of training.

We have twenty training camps now underway in the Army, only a few in full operation, and about one-half have just sufficient staff to carry out the immediate task of training the few available trainees assigned to them. The product of these camps available for the Army under present conditions will be about 5,000 in January, 8,000 in February, and will increase to about 35,000 in May and we hope will reach 50,000 in the summer.

Our objective under the present 21 month term of service for selectees is to reach a monthly production figure of about 50,000. Meanwhile, we must take our chances in the world.

We are paying a price, no one yet knows how great a price, for our failure to use foresight and good judgment in this vital matter. We failed to provide a system for steadily maintaining a reserve of trained men to permit the rapid build-up of units, especially the National Guard, or for the creation of new units, and to meet the casualties of any campaign in which we might suddenly become involved. For that failure all of us are responsible.

I have referred to a reserve of trained men. For the moment, at least, there can be no reserve. Availability is the urgent requirement today and will be until we reach a point in mobilization of manpower where we can quietly and effectively allocate men to reserves and hold them in a ready state of availability in that status. When we reach that point and only then will we have created a sufficiently strong military posture to deter aggression by making plain to the world our ability to carry out a very rapid and efficient expansion of our military forces.

When our reserve strength in readily available trained men matches our tremendous reserve strength in the ability quickly to produce war materiel,—then this country will be so powerful that its views on peace will be compelling.[5]

GCMRL/G. C. Marshall Papers (Secretary of Defense, Speeches and Statements)

1. The twenty-fifth meeting of the Women's Patriotic Conference on National Defense, an organization that brought together representatives of thirty-six women's groups, occurred from January 25 to 27 at the Hotel Statler in Washington. ("Gen. Marshall Will Address Women's Patriotic Conference," *Washington Post*, January 1, 1951, p. B2.)

Florence H. Becker, national president of the Patriotic Women of America and chair of the conference, had invited Marshall and his wife to their opening evening banquet and "to bring a word of greeting." Mildred Carlson, a secretary in Marshall's office; Margaret S. Banister, a member of the National Organizations Branch of the Office of Public Information at the Defense Department; and General Ginsburgh agreed that Marshall should attend. On December 7, Marshall accepted the invitation "with pleasure." (Becker to Marshall, November 24, 1950; Carlson to George, memorandum, n.d.; Banister to LeBailly, memorandum, December 1, 1950; and Marshall to Becker, December 7, 1950, GCMRL/G. C. Marshall Papers [Secretary of Defense, Number Indexed, M214-5-31].)

2. See pp. 276–78 and 291–93.

3. See pp. 440–41.

4. See p. 345n5.

5. Becker wrote on February 10 to thank Marshall for his "splendid address," assure him of the support of all women represented at the conference, and inform him that the "Conferences passed a resolution in favor of Universal Military Training." (Becker to Marshall, February 10, 1951, ibid.) See also pp. 361–63 and 376–77.

220

TO MAJOR GENERAL ORLANDO WARD — January 27, 1951, Washington, DC

Dear Ward: Thanks for your letter of January 18th with Robinett's reaction to General Palmer's papers. I too am sorry that the infirmities of age caught up with him before he could finish his work.[1]

I have been looking for an opportunity to visit Palmer at Walter Reed—he has been there for several days now. I understand that there is nothing seriously wrong with him, just fatigued.[2]

With my thanks to you and Robinett for looking into this matter for me, and with warm regards, Faithfully yours,

GCMRL/G. C. Marshall Collection (Miscellaneous)

1. John McAuley Palmer had written to Marshall on December 17, 1950, that his failing health prevented him from completing his "book on national military policy," and he was transferring the "unfinished manuscript and other papers" to the Library of Congress. Palmer offered "the use of all my papers" to the Defense Department, since a younger officer "might find something pertinent to the present crisis or to a better and more economical military system after the crisis." Marshall had replied on December 22 that he would assign an officer to review the manuscripts, and he forwarded a copy of Palmer's letter that day to General Ward to ask him to designate a qualified officer. Ward informed Marshall that

his office had been studying demobilization and that he would assign Brigadier General Paul M. Robinett, a former member of Marshall's army staff and at this time chief of the Special Studies Division of the Office of the Chief of Military History, to review the papers. (Palmer to Marshall, December 17, 1950; Marshall to Palmer, December 22, 1950; Marshall to Ward, December 22, 1950; Ward to Marshall, December 26, 1950, GCMRL/G. C. Marshall Papers [Secretary of Defense, Number Indexed, M200-6-43].)

Ward later informed Marshall that the material Palmer deposited in the Library of Congress manuscript divison consisted of unfinished memoirs and supporting papers that Palmer had hoped to use to present once again his views on military policy. While these views were well known, Ward nevertheless considered it "a pity" that Palmer could not complete his manuscript. Although it included nothing new, the combination of Palmer's "vast store of knowledge" and "sound observations . . . would be of benefit to the officers of the United States Army and to the people of the United States." The draft memoir ended, however, before Palmer "finished work on any of the more important periods of his career." (Ward to Marshall, January 18, 1951, GCMRL/G. C. Marshall Collection [Miscellaneous].) See p. 176.

2. Marshall wrote on January 27 that the duties of his office had consistently prevented his visiting Palmer at Walter Reed. He added that Palmer's papers "will be used in future studies of military policy and allied subjects" and that he was "very, very sorry that you were unable to finish your memoirs for they would have been of great interest and help to many." (Marshall to Palmer, January 27, 1951, GCMRL/G. C. Marshall Papers [Secretary of Defense, Number Indexed, M200-6-43].)

Palmer's wife, Maud, told Carter on February 3 that she was "anxious" to speak to Marshall "so that she could tell John she had heard from you." While "there was a 'No Visitors' sign on his door," she assured Carter that Marshall could visit Palmer at any time. His memory had deteriorated, so "there would not be much point in discussing anything unless John himself brought it up," but Mrs. Palmer said that "he hangs his friendship" with Marshall "as the bright spot in his life." (Carter to Marshall, memorandum, February 3, 1951, ibid.) Marshall later wrote to Palmer that he was still unable to visit Walter Reed among his "fairly full days. You are lucky to be able to take it easy, and I do hope you are getting along well." He assured Palmer that he would visit at the "first opportunity I get." (Marshall to Palmer, February 15, 1951, ibid.)

221

MEMORANDUM FOR ASSISTANT SECRETARY ROSENBERG | January 29, 1951
Washington, DC

Apropos of my suggestion this morning that we prepare a brief digest of the line of questions being asked us regarding the manpower bill as to ages and length of service in Western Europe, General Eisenhower just gave me over the phone this example. The French Government has so cracked down on its people that even a widow with five sons, four of whom have been killed, gets no exemption for the fifth son.[1]

Please treat this as confidential because he gave it to me merely in an illustration of the firmness of the present French Government and he must be the one to quote it if it is to be quoted. But it does impressively support my replies to the Committee regarding ages of induction, when I said I must know their policy of deferments before I could answer the questions.[2]

I told General Eisenhower we were preparing a digest for him which I would send up to West Point. He told me he was now preparing his radio broadcast, so the earlier we get the digest to him the better it will be.[3]

NA/RG 330, CD 381

1. Marshall met with Rosenberg twice on the day he sent this memorandum. Eisenhower was at this time visiting the US Military Academy at West Point. He would later praise the French for "one of the strictest, most inclusive conscription laws that would be possible to devise." (*Papers of DDE*, 12: 29.)

2. See pp. 325–29, 338–47, and House, *Hearings . . . H. R. 1752*, 31, 39–40.

3. The editors have been unable to locate any such digest. A handwritten comment by Marshall Carter in the margin of this paragraph says "by telephone done." Eisenhower made his broadcast on February 2.

222

Memorandum for the Executive Secretary of the National Security Council[1]
Top Secret

January 29, 1951
Washington, DC

Subject: United States Policy toward Spain

I am forwarding herewith for the information of the Members of the National Security Council the views of the Joint Chiefs of Staff with respect to NSC 72/2, subject as above.[2]

The Joint Chiefs of Staff are convinced that, in the face of the well-known objectives of the Kremlin and the ever increasing military capabilities of the USSR, lack of military collaboration between the signatory nations of NATO and Spain is adversely affecting not only the security position of Europe but also that of the United States.

The Joint Chiefs of Staff, from the security point of view which they believe should be overriding, recommend that the United States policy toward Spain be as follows:

a. That the United States now propose the acceptance of Spain as a member of NATO; and

b. Regardless of whether or not Spain soon becomes a member of NATO, the United States propose to NATO that authority be given for the military agencies of NATO to establish military association with Spain, and the necessary political arrangements be made at the earliest possible moment for United States military planners to enter into conversations with Spanish military planners.

In NSC 72/2 the Department of State takes the position that United States sponsorship at this time of Spanish membership in NATO would endanger our fundamental policy objectives in Western Europe. The fact is, however, our security interests require, as a minimum, early military association between NATO and Spain, immediate military association in the planning field between the United States and Spain, and provision of military assistance by the United States to Spain. Timing is a very important consideration today and for this reason I think our Government's attitude toward Spain should reflect more of a sense of urgency in securing our objectives with respect to that country.

With the foregoing considerations in mind, there are proposed in the enclosure certain amendments to NSC 72/2.[3]

NA/RG 59 (Records Relating to the National Security Council, NSC 72/3 [United States Policy Toward Spain])

1. Burns had forwarded to Marshall a draft version of this memorandum to James S. Lay Jr., executive secretary of the NSC, with the recommendation that Marshall sign it. (Burns to Marshall, memorandum, n.d., NA/RG 330, CD 092 [Spain].) He did so, but only after editing it by hand. For this memorandum and its two enclosures reproduced in full, see *FRUS, 1951*, 4: 782–86.

2. The JCS and State Department had previously expressed divergent views on appropriate policy toward Spain, with the JCS favoring that nation's membership in NATO and the State Department opposed because of the likely Western European reaction. (*FRUS, 1950*, 3: 1570–72.) In NSC 72/2, the State Department continued to oppose Spain's immediate entry into NATO but agreed that its eventual participation should be "our ultimate objective" and thus listed a series of measures to be taken to facilitate that eventual entry. (Ibid., 773–76.)

3. Unlike the JCS, the service secretaries thought that NSC 72/2 represented "a significant advance in thinking by the State Department" and proposed a series of amendments to the document. Burns informed Marshall that "the effect of these corrections is to defer to State's position that we should not sponsor Spanish membership in NATO now, but to state early Spanish membership in NATO as an objective and to incorporate other action desired by JCS, such as U.S.-Spanish planning, and military assistance for Spain." (Burns to Marshall, memorandum, n.d., NA/RG 330, CD 092 [Spain]. The amendments are in *FRUS, 1951*, 4: 785–86.) One State Department official informed Acheson on January 30 that they were "apparently prepared after consultation" with Marshall. (Ibid., 788.) They, together with this memorandum by Marshall and the enclosed JCS memorandum, became NSC 72/3. On February 1, the NSC approved these amendments and forwarded the revised State Department paper, now numbered NSC 72/4, to Truman, who approved it the following day. (Ibid., 789–90.) See pp. 493–94.

223

Meetings with Truman, Acheson, and French Prime Minister Pleven
January 29–30, 1951 Washington, DC

ON JANUARY 29 and 30, Marshall as well as Acheson and others participated in three conferences with Truman and visiting French Prime Minister Pleven. By this time Ridgway had succeeded in halting the third Chinese offensive in Korea and had launched successful, limited counteroffensives of his own. Combined with a positive report on the military situation and troop morale by Generals Collins and Vandenberg after a visit to Korea and Japan (see pp. 330–31), this ended talk of a possible immediate withdrawal from the peninsula. The better news from Korea sharpened the American decision to support Chiang Kai-shek and defend Formosa, to continue to oppose the People's Republic of China (PRC) diplomatically as well as militarily, and in Marshall's words "to penalize the Chinese Communists for their aggression" in ways that would "lead to the subversion and depletion of their military strength." (Marshall to Acheson, January 27, 1951, NA/RG 218, Geographical File, CCS 381 [Far East].) Telegrams from Truman as well as the JCS also appeared to calm MacArthur and provide him with at least part of the directive he had desired. (See Condit, *Test of War*, 94–95; Schnabel and Watson, *History of JCS*, 3, pt. 1: 188–91, 193–99; and James, *Years of MacArthur*, 3: 554–59.)

Discussion during the first meeting with Pleven on the afternoon of January 29 centered on Indochina as well as China and Korea, with the French premier requesting additional US material and financial aid as well as naval air support for the Vietnamese battalions France was creating and warning of the possibility of Communist Chinese military intervention there as well as in Korea. At Truman's invitation, first Bradley and then Marshall described Ridgway's present military action, with Marshall emphasizing that it constituted "an inconvenience to us insofar as it affected other things which we felt should be done"—such as building up strength in Japan, whose present military weakness "would be very dangerous if the USSR started a general war." (*FRUS, 1951*, 4: 304–10; quote on 309.) Marshall apologized for the delay in sending promised transport planes to Indochina (see pp. 194–99 and 320–22) but indicated that there was "no prospect" of sending additional planes at this time, though "we were still looking at the whole problem of strengthening the entire position in Indochina." In response to Pleven's renewed request for the loan of an aircraft carrier to provide the desired air support in Indochina, he emphasized that the US Navy was "very reluctant" to release one "since it needed everything we have to carry out its task in Korea." Such a loan would also require congressional consent that would be problematic. Nevertheless his officers were examining the request again "with the view to trying to work out something." Truman in turn said that Marshall would see what could be done about the French request for additional arms for Indochina, while Marshall said that additional help in the event of a Chinese attack and forced evacuation from Indochina "was under discussion with the French." (Ibid., 311 and 313.)

The second meeting on January 30 focused on Europe. Pleven first reassured Truman that France still supported German integration—economically via the Schuman Plan and militarily via its previous agreement to accept German forces within NATO and its proposal for a European army (see pp. 201, 203n4, 218–20, 284–87, and 303–4). He then asked bluntly about the American ability to defend Europe with atomic weapons should the Russians attack before completion of the NATO military buildup—specifically "whether the United States' predominant position in the atomic field is being maintained." (*FRUS, 1951*, 4: 315–18; quote on 318.) Truman assured him "that our advance in the atomic field was phenomenal" and invited first Acheson and then Marshall to comment. Acheson emphasized the importance of all present at these meetings being "able to say that there had been no discussion of the atomic bomb" and therefore responded indirectly, emphasizing the importance of building up NATO military forces as well as "the terrific and immediate retaliatory power which is now in being in the United States" and its "immense" military potential. (Ibid., 318.) Marshall asserted that the rapid buildup of military forces in Europe was the only alternative to submission to the Russians, once again expressed concern about the "drain on training personnel needed in France which is occurring in Indochina" (see pp. 280–83 and 284–87), and explained (as he recently had to Congress) the US policy of creating now the "productive capacity to turn out war material so that in case of need a tremendous reserve power could be brought quickly to bear." (See pp. 276–78 and 291–93.) "He concluded that for the moment time is on our side but that this may not be the case in one and one-half to two years from now. During this period we must go forward with all possible speed to build up our defenses." When Pleven asked whether this was a reply to his question about continued American atomic superiority, Marshall replied affirmatively. Pleven and General Alphonse Juin, now inspector general of the French armed forces, then concurred with Marshall on the drain being caused by the war in Indochina—a situation Truman compared to the drain on US forces being caused by Korea. (Ibid., 319–20.)

Marshall then questioned Pleven on the political reaction in France to the extension of military service from twelve to eighteen months, with Truman mentioning that Marshall "is up against the same problem in the current session of Congress" and Marshall asking the French prime minister to avoid discussion during his meeting with the National Press Club later that day of the differences between the French length of service and the longer length of twenty-seven months that he was proposing to Congress. The prime minister predicted that the length of service in France would in all likelihood be increased to twenty-one or twenty-four months and said that his government was committed by existing plans to have by 1953 an army of nine hundred thousand—a statement Marshall considered "the greatest reassurance Mr. Pleven could give him." (Ibid., 321–22.) But Pleven wanted to know what reinforcements the United States could send during the first ninety days of a war with the Soviets. Marshall responded that the air power buildup would be very rapid but that the number of troops would be limited by the shipping available, which "depended to a large extent on our premonition of approaching war." Bradley added that once military equipment was "plentiful," the United States would ask for permission to ship to and store in France large quantities of such equipment so that in the event of war all available shipping could be used to transport soldiers. Juin then asked about the advance stationing of US divisions in Europe as called for in NATO plans, with Truman acknowledging congressional questioning of his power to do so but asserting that he did have such power. (Ibid., 322–24.) Discussion then shifted first to French fears of NATO being run by Britain and the United States and then to the Soviet proposal for a four-power conference, discussions in which Marshall apparently did not participate.

During the third and final meeting on the afternoon of January 30, Marshall informed the other participants that Bradley had told Juin "that we are studying the problem of emergency evacuation of French forces in Indochina and that we will do whatever we can in the event this action becomes necessary." Marshall also stated that the Defense Department had "looked again" into providing the French with another aircraft carrier, "but that he had nothing new to add to what he had said yesterday. He repeated that the two difficulties were that (1) the only carrier available would have to be one taken out of moth balls which was a long process and (2) Congress would have to approve any transfer." He added that "we might be willing" upon French request to "ease" some of the present restrictions on French use of the USS *Langley,* an escort carrier that was in the process of being transferred to France for service in the Mediterranean, and reported that while he had asked the air force to "look again for any transport planes that might be turned over to the French for use in Indochina," he was "very doubtful" they would find any. (Ibid., 333–34. On the *Langley,* see Condit, *Test of War*, 211, and *FRUS, 1951*, 6: 366.)

Shifting back to Europe, Marshall then asked Juin "to do anything he could" to facilitate negotiation of an agreement for American use of a Moroccan air base, emphasizing that the "fastest build-up" of US forces in the event of war would be via air "and that it was very important for us to be all set to do this." In regard to four-power negotiations with the Soviets, he questioned "whether you could believe the Soviets and rely on their agreements even if they accepted agreements. He said that in his experience on this question he favored making no change in our policies until a year or two after the Soviets had accepted agreements, during which time we could see if we could believe that they had honestly changed their intentions. He argued that the Soviets must prove their good faith by deeds and that we would be foolish to alter our programs until we were convinced by their action that we were safe in believing them." (*FRUS, 1951*, 4: 334, 337–38.)

In line with his comment to Pleven on the importance of available shipping in determining the number of US troops that could be sent to Europe during the first ninety days of hostilities, Marshall on January 29 informed Office of Defense Mobilization Director Wilson that the Defense Department was "vitally interested" in the functions and responsibilities of a proposed Emergency Shipping Agency and its relationship to the Defense Department's existing Military Sea Transportation Service. (Marshall to Wilson, January 29, 1951, NA/RG 330, CD 334 [Defense Mobilization Board].) On the next day, and again in line with the continuing emphasis during the discussions with Pleven on building up NATO ground forces as rapidly as possible, Marshall informed Acheson in response to a previous query that the Joint Chiefs favored efforts to obtain additional ground forces for Korea from other UN states but not from Great Britain or other NATO members. Lovett had labeled such efforts a "futile exercise" but agreed that the JCS views should be "passed along." His comment led to the deletion from this letter of Marshall's concurrence with this JCS recommendation. (Marshall to Acheson, January 30, 1951; Lovett handwritten note on Murdaugh to Burns, memorandum, January 26, 1951; and Carter to Marshall on Murdaugh to Carter, memorandum, January 29, 1951, NA/RG 330, CD 092 [Korea].) ★

224

To James A. Lyle

January 30, 1951
Washington, DC

Dear Lyle: I have your undated letter in which you request my assistance in your desire to pursue a career in the Army. I remember your father very well from my days at the Virginia Military Institute and I am glad to do what I can in the matter and that is to pass your letter to Secretary Pace of the Army for his consideration of your request and also to write you directly of your possibilities of being commissioned.[1]

I wish you would express to your father my very best wishes as it has been many years since I have seen him.

I appreciate very much your interest in desiring to be of service, and with best wishes,[2] Faithfully yours,

GCMRL/G. C. Marshall Collection (James A. Lyle)

1. Lyle was a twenty-five-year-old African-American resident of 113 Diamond Street, Lexington, Virginia. The editors have been unable to locate his letter to Marshall.

Lyle's father, Austin H. Lyle, had worked as a mess hall attendant at VMI from 1929 to 1944 and again from 1947 to 1954 and "had occasion to encounter General Marshall during the latter's return visits to the Institute after his graduation in 1901." ("Letter Given by Lyle Adds to Marshall Items," *Rockbridge Weekly*, November 1964.)

2. Lyle later decided to pursue a career in teaching rather than in the army and taught social studies at Lexington's Lylburn Downing High School. (Ibid.)

225

To Mrs. Oveta Culp Hobby

January 31, 1951
Washington, DC

Dear Mrs. Hobby: The other day when we were talking at lunch here in the Pentagon, you suggested the gathering of a certain representation of women such as we had in the last war. I have forgotten just who they were and how it was managed and I would appreciate your advice.[1]

I have just had a long conversation with Mrs. [Hiram C.] Houghton, President of the General Federation of Women's Clubs. She came in to talk to me about the attendance of four service women leaders at the meeting of the Federation in Texas, I think next month. But the conversation ran on to the question of the organization of a committee of women to help us in the general relationship with American women. She had been much shocked by the resolutions which were passed by the Women's Patriotic Conference on National Defense. I must confess I have not yet read them but I understand they were very extreme in their condemnations and in their evident tendency towards isolationism. They did endorse the Defense Department's stand towards building up our military strength. I was shocked to find that I had been injected into a meeting with Sokolsky as the principle speaker, to be followed the next evening by Senator McCarthy as the principle speaker and to

~~then~~ be preceded by another individual who is of the extreme variety but whose name I have forgotten. The Chairman, Mrs. Becker, appeared to be very pleasant, but the unanimous adoption of the resolutions is to me a very shocking piece of business.[2]

Mrs. Houghton has a group of fifty women from all over the country here who have been briefed by the State Department in an all-day session regarding foreign policy. She tells me they were very enthusiastic and most of them had completely changed their point of view. They are up on the Hill today talking to their senators. I am taking over a similar group at a later date here at the Pentagon for a general briefing on the military posture, legislation and developments.[3]

I know you will give me your attention in this matter and I apologize for imposing this burden on you. I appreciated your note regarding the meeting at Eugene Meyer's.[4] Affectionately,

GCMRL/G. C. Marshall Papers (Secretary of Defense, Number Indexed, M200-8-50)

1. Hobby had met with Marshall and Rosenberg and had eaten lunch with Marshall, Lovett, and Rosenberg on January 9.

One such conference of women's representatives on UMT was held at the Pentagon on April 26, 1945. For Marshall's remarks to this gathering, see *Papers of GCM*, 5: 153–58.

2. Marshall had met with Mrs. Houghton at 10:55 a.m. on January 31.

The Women's Patriotic Conference on National Defense had adopted thirty-eight resolutions at its January 25–27 session. One resolution supported UMT, but others opposed the designation of any American troops to NATO defense forces without explicit congressional approval; rejected "any form of World Government, or partial World Government such as Atlantic Union, which would in any way impair the sovereignty of the United States"; called for investigation of the State Department and the removal of Dean Acheson as secretary of state; and praised Joseph McCarthy "for his courageous delineation of the events and personages responsible for the country's present plight, with assurance that we dedicate ourselves to the imperative task of house-cleaning the State Department." ("Resolutions Adopted by the Twenty-Fifth Women's Patriotic Conference on National Defense," pamphlet, January 25, 1951, Columbia University Rare Book and Manuscript Library/Herbert H. Lehman Papers [Special Correspondence Files].)

Marshall had addressed the Women's Patriotic Conference on National Defense at its January 25 opening dinner (see pp. 350–54). George Sokolsky, a staunch anti-Communist, wrote a nationally syndicated newspaper column entitled "These Days." Other speakers at the conference included Senator McCarthy; Rabbi Benjamin Schultz, executive director of the American Jewish League Against Communism; and former US Army Air Forces Major George Racey Jordan, who had accused President Franklin Roosevelt's adviser Harry Hopkins of allowing uranium and secret papers to pass to the Soviet Union during World War II. (Program, Twenty-fifth Women's Patriotic Conference on National Defense, GCMRL/G. C. Marshall Papers [Secretary of Defense, Selected]; "Defense Meet Will Attract 1500 Women," *Washington Post*, January 21, 1951, p. S4.) See pp. 376–77.

3. The participants in this briefing session had heard from high-ranking State Department officials on Monday and Tuesday, January 29 and 30; and their local congressmen, members of the Senate Foreign Relations Committee, and Marshall on Wednesday, January 31. Marshall's briefing took place at 4:05 p.m. at the Pentagon. They were scheduled to spend February 1 and 2 in New York to visit the UN headquarters. ("Clubwomen Briefed on Foreign Policy," *Washington Post*, January 30, 1951, p. B5; "Federation 'Clarifies Its Thinking.'" *Washington Post*, February 1, 1951, p. B5.)

Marshall's remarks to this group are not in the Marshall Papers. Houghton wrote on February 2 to thank Marshall for both his remarks to the group and their morning meeting. She offered "the services of our organization in every way that we can be helpful" and wondered "if you came to any decision about a Woman's Advisory Board to the women in the Armed Services." Marshall informed her on March 6 that Rosenberg was "exploring the possible establishment" of such a board and she would "keep in touch with you on this matter." (Houghton to Marshall, February 2, 1951; and Marshall to Houghton, March 6, 1951, GCMRL/G. C. Marshall Papers [Secretary of Defense, Number Indexed, M200-8-50].)

4. Marshall, Lovett, and the JCS had cocktails on the evening of January 8 at the home of Eugene Meyer, a former governor of the Federal Reserve and publisher of the *Washington Post* and current chairman of the Washington Post Company, to "meet newspaper people." Meyer later forwarded to Marshall a copy of a letter Hobby had sent to Meyer, thanking him "for the evening spent in your house. You have performed a real service for the country and your publishing colleagues." (Meyer to Marshall, January 27, 1951, with attached Hobby to Meyer, January 24, 1951, ibid., [M200-8-14].)

Hobby replied on February 5 that she was "preparing the information that you requested" and would mail it from Houston later that week. She sent Marshall a "list of National Women's organizations" on February 9, and Marshall responded he was "hopeful that we will soon be able to organize an advisory council and schedule an early meeting of this group" under Anna Rosenberg. (Hobby to Marshall, February 5, 1951, and Marshall to Hobby, February 15, 1951, ibid., [M200-8-50].) See pp. 639–47.

226

To Frank L. Weil

February 6, 1951
Washington, DC

Dear Mr. Weil: I read with great interest your letter of January 9th, reporting the favorable progress of negotiations between United Service Organizations [USO] and Associated Services for the Armed Forces [ASAF] for the purpose of developing a united voluntary national agency.[1]

I feel that the successful attainment of this highly desired objective was due to the foresight, energy, and good judgment of the President's Committee on Religion and Welfare in the Armed Forces, and you have my congratulations and gratitude.

While I shall regret the suspension of operations by the President's Committee, I am glad that the Committee has added another accomplishment to those which have already placed all members of the armed forces under obligation to it.[2] Faithfully yours,

GCMRL/G. C. Marshall Papers (Secretary of Defense, Chronological, Secretaries, Carlson)

1. A New York lawyer involved in numerous social, religious, and cultural activities, Weil headed the President's Committee on Religion and Welfare in the Armed Forces that had been established in the fall of 1948. On September 19, 1950, this committee submitted a report, "The Welfare of Armed Forces Personnel in 1950," which emphasized the dramatic changes in needs brought about by the Korean War and recommended a series of private and governmental actions to address them. Marshall and Weil discussed this report on October 10, and Weil wrote Marshall the following day to offer to continue their conversation at his earliest convenience. Marshall replied on October 17 that he looked forward to doing so following the NATO defense ministers' meeting in late October 1950 (see pp. 218–20). Marshall had also signed letters to Weil and President Truman in which he expressed his agreement with the committee's finding regarding the need for a united national voluntary organization, in addition to the Red Cross, "covering the entire field of

recreation and hospitality services to the members of the armed forces." ("The Welfare of Armed Forces Personnel in 1950," HSTL/RG 220, Records of the President's Committee on Religion and Welfare in the Armed Forces; Weil to Marshall, October 11, 1950, GCMRL/G. C. Marshall Papers [Secretary of Defense, Number Indexed, M200-3-47]; Marshall to Weil and Marshall to Truman, October 13, 1950, NA/RG 330, SD 334 [President's Committee on Religion and Welfare in the Armed Forces].)

Weil's January 9 letter is not in the Marshall Papers, but in response to Marshall's request for his reaction to it, Secretary Matthews wrote that the USO-ASAF merger was finalized on January 31. (Marshall to Matthews, memorandum, January 31, 1951, and Matthews to Marshall, February 2, 1951, GCMRL/G. C. Marshall Papers [Secretary of Defense, Chronological Files, Secretaries, Carlson].) The ASAF had been established in mid-April 1950 as a "voluntary, interdenominational agency, to provide services to armed forces personnel in communities near their stations." By December 1950, the Associated Services had called for the reopening of all the facilities previously administered by the USO, which had been deactivated by that time. ("New Agency Set Up to Aid Service Men," *New York Times*, May 1, 1950, p. 3; "Marshall Urges Troops Fund Aid," *New York Times*, December 31, 1950, p. 19.)

Marshall had long supported this merger, asserting on December 19 that it was "essential that a united voluntary agency (in addition to the American Red Cross) be developed to cover the entire field of recreation and hospitality services to the members of our armed forces." (Marshall to Firestone, December 19, 1950, GCMRL/G. C. Marshall Papers [American Red Cross, General].) He reiterated his support for a unified agency on December 30 in a recorded statement supporting the United Defense Fund (UDF), which had been established on November 28, 1950, with the support of Weil's committee to coordinate national fundraising for all charitable organizations, except for the Red Cross, that supported the armed services. (Statement for the United Defense Fund, December 30, 1950, GCMRL/G. C. Marshall Papers [Secretary of Defense, Number Indexed, M214-6-2].) See also pp. 535–36.

Following the reactivation of the USO, Marshall appeared on Eddie Cantor's NBC television show, the *Colgate Comedy Hour*, on March 25 to solicit fundraising support for the USO, which Marshall said provided for the "proper religious, social, recreational, and cultural facilities for our young men and women in the armed forces when they are off duty." ("United Services Organization," March 25, 1951, GCMRL/G. C. Marshall Papers [Secretary of Defense, Speeches and Statements].) Two days following this appearance, Marshall signed a memorandum of understanding with the president of the USO, Lindsey F. Kimball, in which the Defense Department recognized the USO as "its official contact" with all USO-affiliated organizations. The USO would be the "principal but not exclusive channel" for public participation "in a total war or emergency program for the Armed Forces," as the Defense Department would maintain its existing relationships with the Red Cross and similar agencies. ("Memorandum of Understanding between the Department of Defense and the United Services Organizations, Inc.," March 27, 1951, NA/RG 330, SD 080 [United Services Organization].)

2. Due to a lack of funding by Congress, a longstanding problem for the President's Committee on Religion and Welfare in the Armed Forces, the committee was disbanded on February 28, 1951. (Harry S. Truman, *Public Papers of the Presidents of the United States: Harry S. Truman, 1951* [Washington: GPO, 1965], 115.)

227

TO DARRYL F. ZANUCK

February 6, 1951
Washington, DC

Dear Zanuck: Thanks for your letter of January 25th enclosing Lichtman's letter to you of the 23rd. I was interested in what you both had to say about the film “Why Korea?”, and of your circulation plans for the future.[1]

As you probably know, Tony Muto of your New York office showed the film here in the Pentagon to a fairly large gathering of ranking people of the three services. I personally enjoyed it very much and think it will answer many questions which now occupy the minds of millions of people at home and abroad. There is enclosed a copy of the message General Ridgway circulated to his command on the subject of why we are in Korea. To my mind, it is an excellent statement and I think it will interest you.[2]

I received in this morning's mail a letter from Frank McCarthy, in which he tells me of his plans for the next several months. He especially wrote of the work to be done in connection with the filming of “The Desert Fox”, and the satisfaction he received from contributing to “Decision Before Dawn”.[3]

With my thanks again for telling me about “Why Korea?”, and with warm regards, Faithfully yours,

Please make my compliments to Mrs. Zanuck[4]

GCMRL/G. C. Marshall Papers (Secretary of Defense, Number Indexed, M200-8-23)

1. Zanuck, vice president of production at Twentieth Century–Fox Film Corporation in Beverly Hills, California, had informed President Truman in August 1950 of his plans to exhibit in movie theaters within three weeks this brief film made of documentary newsreels. (“Documentary on Korea,” *New York Times*, August 15, 1950, p. 25.)

Zanuck had shared with Marshall a note from Al Lichtman, vice president and director of distribution at Twentieth Century–Fox in New York, that bookings for the film were “moving along very well.” Zanuck added that at least ten thousand theaters would show the film and that it was “being translated into 40 foreign languages.” (Lichtman to Zanuck, January 23, 1951, and Zanuck to Marshall, January 25, 1951, NA/RG 330, SD 062.2.)

Release of the film had caused controversy, with some theater owners believing that the White House was pressuring them to show the film after Truman's presidential assistant John R. Steelman urged theaters to screen it. (“White House Backs Korea Movie Action,” *New York Times*, January 27, 1951, p. 10.)

2. Anthony Muto, the Washington, DC, representative of Twentieth Century–Fox, had shown the film at the Pentagon for Marshall and other Defense Department officials on December 20, 1950. On January 21, Ridgway had sent a memorandum to his commanders entitled “Why We Are Here” for dissemination by each of them “to every single member of his command at the earliest possible moment.” (Ridgway to Eighth Army commanders, memorandum, January 21, 1951, USAMHI/Matthew B. Ridgway Papers [Series 3, Official Papers, Eighth US Army, Dec. 1950–Apr. 1951].)

3. Zanuck had written previously on January 16 to thank Marshall for the cooperation from all of the services in Germany during the filming of *Decision Before Dawn*. Zanuck also praised McCarthy, who “has done such a splendid job on this picture that I am holding him in Germany to do the preliminary work on THE DESERT FOX which, as you know, has to do with General Rommel.” Marshall replied that he appreciated Zanuck's comments and was “especially interested in what you had to say about Frank McCarthy, and your evaluation of the job he did on this picture.” Twentieth Century–Fox released *The Desert Fox: The Story of Rommel*, starring James Mason, and *Decision Before Dawn*, a World War II drama that McCarthy produced, in late 1951. (Zanuck to Marshall, January 16, 1951, and Marshall to Zanuck, January 22, 1951, GCMRL/G. C. Marshall Papers [Secretary of Defense, Number Indexed, M200-8-23].) McCarthy's letter is not in the Marshall Papers. See also pp. 170–71n4, 183–84, and 562–63.

4. This postscript was handwritten by Marshall.

228

MEMORANDUM OF CONVERSATION[1] February 6, 1951
Confidential Washington, DC

Since the Colombian Embassy had indicated this to be primarily a social visit on the part of the Colombian Minister of War, Dr. Urdaneta, the majority of the interview was devoted to reminiscences and informal discussion. Secretary Marshall recounted recent achievements in the Korean war on the part of the United Nations Command, and Dr. Urdaneta informed him of the latest progress at the United Nations, where he is Colombia's principal delegate.

At the close of the interview, however, Dr. Urdaneta raised with Secretary Marshall the question of appropriate U.S. assistance in training and equipment for the Colombian battalion accepted for service in Korea, and also for such units as might be designated in connection with the "Uniting the Peace" resolution adopted by the United Nation General Assembly on 3 November 1950. It appeared that a request concerning the battalion for Korea had already been made to the United States by Colombia, but that the Colombian Embassy had not yet formulated a specific proposal in connection with "Uniting the Peace". General Marshall indicated that he would be very much interested in seeing this latter item; Dr. Urdaneta and General Bayona assured him that it would be submitted to the United States in the near future.[2]

Philip E. Barringer
Office of Foreign Military Affairs

NA/RG 330, CD Memorandum of Conversation

1. Colombian Minister of War and chairman of the Colombian delegation to the UN Roberto Urdaneta, Colombian Ambassador to the US Eduardo Zuleta-Angel, and Colombian Military Attaché General Ricardo Bayona met with Marshall, Marshall Carter, Captain Ramon E. Benedetti of the office of the assistant army chief of staff for intelligence (G-2), and Philip E. Barringer of the Office of Foreign Military Affairs, who took these minutes, at 3:13 p.m. on February 5.

2. In the briefing notes for this meeting, General Burns "suggested that you may wish to comment favorably upon Colombian military action in support of the United Nations action in Korea." Colombia, the only Latin American to join the UN effort, offered the battleship *Almirante Padilla*, formerly the USS *Groton*, and one battalion from the Colombian Army, which did not reach Korea until June 1951. (Burns to Marshall, memorandum, n.d., NA/RG 330, CD Briefings; Tucker, *Encyclopedia of the Korean War*, 1: 169.)

The Uniting for Peace resolution, passed on November 3, 1950, in response to the inability of the UN Security Council to take stronger action against the North Korean invasion due to Soviet vetoes, authorized the General Assembly to take action on any issues on which the Security Council could not reach a unanimous decision. (For more on developments in light of the Uniting for Peace resolution, see *FRUS, 1951*, 1: 616–20, 628, 636–45, 658–65, 668–78, and 682–84; *FRUS, 1951*, 2: 18; Schnabel and Watson, *History of JCS*, 3, pt. 1: 102, 192, 200, 226–28; and Tucker, *Encyclopedia of the Korean War*, 2: 886, 893–94.)

229

TO ALEXANDER "CASEY" JONES — February 7, 1951
Washington, DC

Dear Casey: I was glad to get your letter and find that my comment regarding you sent you to bed happy. I took the liberty of showing your letter to General Brooks and he was much gratified and pleased by your approval of his talk. He is a fine fellow. He was one of my first associates when I started out in the War Department in 1939.[1]

The night before last I talked to about twenty-five of the old crowd at a private dinner at the Statler. It was the first time I had seen some of them for a considerable period. Incidentally, I discovered later that an appreciable number had fallen victims to the rumor that senility had overtaken me. I wouldn't attempt to run a hundred yards with any of them though I might be a temporary victor with some, but I think my average day's activity would produce considerable exhaustion. Along this line, Lovett amuses me by taking over all the irritations that might otherwise be mine. Every now and then he comes in red-faced and states his outraged feelings at another attack on me along the line, as he phrases it, of "synthetic solicitude."[2]

The game here has not changed. I suppose it will always be the same. I am in the usual struggle with Congress—on the one side meeting the reaction that the dangers of the situation are not fully realized by the Defense Department and on the other a multitude of objections to the proposals I make for prompt action. I don't need to expand on this. You are well aware of the democratic processes.

Mrs. Marshall and I are both feeling fine and comfortably established in a small apartment about fourteen minutes drive through the park to the Pentagon, though during the recent storm it took me two and a half hours to get home one night.

With warm regards. Faithfully yours,

P.S. I answered your letter yesterday, and enjoyed it so much that I sent for it again today and now wish to expand on the points I have already mentioned to you.[3]

GCMRL/G. C. Marshall Papers (Secretary of Defense, Number Indexed, M200-9-23)

1. Jones, executive editor of the Syracuse *Herald-Journal* and former managing editor at the *Washington Post*, had written to Marshall on February 2 to express his appreciation for "your very kind reference to me" in his remarks at the dedication of the new *Washington Post* building on January 28. According to an article on Marshall's speech in the *Washington Post*, he began with an unprepared "preface," during which he "spoke fondly" of Jones, who had "'repeatedly comforted me during the war years.'" In his prepared remarks, Marshall praised the free press as "one of the most delicate instruments in America's arsenal for freedom" and commented that despite the "opposite points of view" of a journalist and a military censor, he felt "that the traditional gap between the censor and the correspondent has greatly narrowed. . . . The result is more accurate and more interesting reporting for the benefit of all of us." (Jones to Marshall, February 2, 1951, GCMRL/G. C. Marshall Papers [Secretary of Defense, Number Indexed, M200-9-23]; Remarks at the Dedication of the *Washington Post* Building, January 28, 1951, GCMRL/G. C. Marshall Papers [Sec-

retary of Defense, Speeches and Statements]; "Marshall Dedicates Post's New Building," *Washington Post*, January 29, 1951, p. 2.)

Jones reported that Lieutenant General Edward H. Brooks, assistant army chief of staff for personnel (G-1), had spoken before the "almost solidly Republican" New York State Publishers Association and "made a terrific impression." Jones remarked that he "could almost see the isolationism melt away" and that "the change in their viewpoint" of their reporting since the speech "has been marked." (Jones to Marshall, February 2, 1951, GCMRL/G. C. Marshall Papers [Secretary of Defense, Number Indexed, M200-9-23].)

2. See pp. 332–33. "The General has made it a practice," C. J. George had recently informed a correspondent, "not to comment on recommendations or statements allegedly made by him, or on writings of correspondents or columnists in which he is mentioned, regardless of the lack of substantiation therein or the source wherefrom they came." (George to Muehlberg, January 30, 1951, ibid., [M204-1-46].)

3. In his February 6 letter, Marshall had praised Jones's work at the *Washington Post*, confessed that "our work here would be a lot easier if more people understood the problems with which we are faced," as Brooks had made clear in his speech, and stated that he was pleased by the positive reaction to Rosenberg's appointment, which Jones had said was "excellent." (Jones to Marshall, February 2, 1951, GCMRL/G. C. Marshall Papers [Secretary of Defense, Number Indexed, M200-9-23]; Marshall to Jones, February 6, 1951, GCMRL/G. C. Marshall Papers [Secretary of Defense, Chronological, Secretaries, Hawkins].)

230

To Jimmy Winn

February 7, 1951
Washington, DC

Dear Jimmy: I was glad to get your letter and the evidence of your good grades in school. Your November 3rd spelling test showed a strong sign of heredity, but I was happy to see that by January 19th you had developed into a grade 90 speller. This beats Nana's record all to pieces! Your arithmetic marks are really something to be proud of—keep up the good work![1]

Nana is feeling fine, and so am I. We spent last week-end at Pinehurst and it was almost as cold there as the Washington weather we left behind us. You should have been with us on that airplane ride—it was an adventure which would put "Sky King" to shame.[2]

Did you have enough snow there last week for sledding?

I have not seen Tupper for some time, but your Grandmother saw him just last week. He is getting along swell, and so is his little brother.[3] With love to all from both of us,

GCMRL/G. C. Marshall Papers (Secretary of Defense, Number Indexed, M200-4-17)

1. Marshall's stepgrandson had reported on January 27 that he had received "a good report this month" and had attached "two arithmatic, one reading, one Language and two Spelling Test." He had received scores of 94 and 100 on the arithmetic tests, an "S" on a recent English test, a "C-" on the language test, a 70 on a November 1950 spelling test, and a 90 on a January 1951 spelling test. (Winn to Marshall, January 27, 1951, and attachments, GCMRL/G. C. Marshall Papers [Secretary of Defense, Number Indexed, M200-4-17].)

2. Winn had wondered, "Is nano all right? I hope you are all right." (Ibid.)

Sky King was a thirty-minute, twice-weekly radio show about an adventurous airplane pilot who chased evil-doers in a Cessna plane called "Songbird."

3. Winn had asked in his January 27 letter if Marshall had "seen Tupper," another of Marshall's stepgrandsons, recently, and had left a blank space within the handwritten letter on which Marshall could write his reply to that question. (Ibid.)

Marshall had recently received a letter from Tupper Brown thanking him for a book on woodworking. He knew Marshall was "busy and it was too bad that I didn't see you when I was visiting Grandmother. . . . I have got a lot more homework this year and have not much time for letters." Marshall replied on February 16 that he appreciated Tupper Brown's letter "and also the fact that you have gotten along so well in your schooling as the letter indicates." While Marshall did not expect Brown "to become a carpenter," he would "have some use for the knowledge that is in that little book" for years to come. "I am seventy years old and I still have to saw and hammer at times," Marshall concluded." (Brown to Marshall, n.d., and Marshall to Brown, February 16, 1951, ibid., [M200-10-2].)

231

Senate Testimony on the Universal Military Service and Training Act of 1951
February 8, 1951   Washington, DC

MARSHALL had previously testified before the Preparedness Subcommittee of the Senate Armed Services Committee regarding the Universal Military Service and Training Bill (see pp. 326–29). At the personal request of Subcommittee Chairman Lyndon Johnson, he now made a second appearance, accompanied by Assistant Secretary Rosenberg, to discuss in executive session some of the features of and proposed changes to the bill on the afternoon of February 8. (George to Marshall, February 7, 1951, GCMRL/G. C. Marshall Papers [Secretary of Defense, Number Indexed, M214-7-41].) Also in attendance were representatives of the National Guard Association, the Reserve Officers Association, and the American Legion.

The session, which lasted nearly three hours, focused on draft ages, length of service, relationship of the National Guard to the draft, and deferments. As had previously occurred when Marshall was questioned by the House committee considering the bill (see pp. 345–47), a great deal of time was devoted to the issue of drafting eighteen-year-olds, with Marshall objecting strongly to a proposed limitation that would require the drafting of all men aged nineteen to twenty-six before any eighteen-year-olds. He emphasized in this regard the importance of training eighteen-year-olds in order to create a young trained reserve force for the future. "Our great hope is to have one surplus trained man some day," he told the committee. "That is what I hope to see before I die." (Senate Committee on Armed Services, *Hearing held before Preparedness Subcommittee of the Committee on Armed Services, S. 1 National Security Training Act of 1951, Executive Session, Thursday, February 8, 1951* [Washington: Ward & Paul, 1951], 89.) He also emphasized how disruptive the calling up of older men would be to their lives and to morale in the armed forces. He considered it a "terrible thing" that in World War II "we uprooted" men over thirty "because I could not get 18-year-olds." Furthermore, these older soldiers "were not valuable to me as fighting men." (Ibid., 93.) "I think I understand your political situation as a practical proposition," he admitted in regard to the public opposition to the drafting of eighteen-year-olds; "I just do not like it." (Ibid., 95.) He also asked for repeal of draft law provisions that allowed eighteen-year-olds to avoid induction via enlistment in the National Guard or the Organized Reserves, pressed for a lengthy term of service for draftees, and strongly opposed the creation of a civilian commission that would control military training as opposed to being an advisory body. Such training, he and Rosenberg insisted, had to remain the responsibility of the military.

Near the end of his remarks Marshall returned to the central theme he as well as John McAuley Palmer had emphasized on numerous occasions over the last thirty years: that the lack of preparedness via universal military training had lengthened America's wars and increased the number of deaths suffered. "Yes, we did it," he said in regard to victory in World War II, "but the hand of God was in part of the procedure, and the length of the war bore a very direct relation to our failure to do these things at the time we should have, and we suffered and suffered all the way through." To argue, as members of a House committee had done a few days previously, that this victory illustrated that a universal military training bill was not necessary Marshall considered "no argument at all. It was merely, you might say, advocating a repetition of the errors we made in the past, which would cost us, goodness knows, how many billions and how many casualties." (Ibid., 145.)

Marshall also asked the committee members "to be very solicitous as to the possible effect of any limitations that are imposed in the active debate on the bill, when you are on the floor. . . . [D]o not tie the hands of the commanders" into whose hands "you put the life and the lives of all these men. . . . All these limitations are dangerous," he concluded, especially in this time of "great emergency . . . [E]ither fire us and get somebody you have more faith in or take over operations yourselves, because it is a terrible thing to work against these complications." (Ibid., 145–46.)

On the day after Marshall's testimony, the press reported that neither he and Rosenberg nor the subcommittee had been "able fully to convert the other" to their point of view. "We were closer together when they left than when they came," Johnson told the press, "but we are not together." ("Limits on Service of Men 18 Likely," *New York Times*, February 9, 1951, p. 6.)

In early February, Marshall also addressed the related issue of full national manpower mobilization, non-military as well as military, by forwarding to appropriate individuals throughout the Defense Department the broad policy on this matter that Truman had approved on January 17, and by designating Rosenberg as "my representative to act for me in coordinating, assisting, and advising addressees on the implementation of this directive." (Memorandum, "Implementation of National Manpower Mobilization Policy," February 1, 1951, GCMRL/G. C. Marshall Papers [Secretary of Defense, Number Indexed, M200-3-26].)

In a lengthy February 19 letter to Senator Henry Cabot Lodge Jr., Marshall amplified many of the points he had made in this session in regard to the drafting of eighteen-year-olds. (Marshall to Lodge, February 19, 1951, NA/RG 330, Office of the Assistant Secretary of Defense for Manpower and Personnel [Chronological File].) See also pp. 409–13. ★

AS ARMY chief of staff and as secretary of state, Marshall had reorganized both the War Department and the State Department. As secretary of defense he set out to reorganize the Defense Department as well and in a somewhat similar manner. According to the official history of his office, Marshall "did not seek drastic organizational change." (Condit, *Test of War*, 483.) Nevertheless, his efforts to improve efficiency led to some significant changes.

Lovett later noted that there had been in the State Department "some 19 different offices reporting directly to the Secretary," with coordination between them "haphazard, and in some cases studiously avoided." Marshall found a similar situation in the Defense Department and quickly moved to rectify it in the same way he had at State: via the creation of a "permanent executive office." Consequently he brought Marshall Carter back to Washington from Japan (see pp. 175–76) to serve as his executive officer and to organize and direct a new Executive Office of the Secretary (EXOS). Lovett labeled EXOS "an essential extension of the Secretary's own personality," with its duties stemming "from the dual concept of a 'Secretariat' operation and a 'Chief of Staff' operation." In the latter role it provided "the final audit to insure completeness, accuracy, coordination, quality, and all other related factors, to insure that the Secretary takes appropriate action when, as, and if required—and equally important, to provide that final review designed to protect the Secretary from ill-considered or unilateral actions." As such it would "protect" the secretary "against low standards, unsuspected departures from policy, inaction, disjoined action, delayed action, and precipitous action." (Lovett to Wilson, December 23, 1952, GCMRL/G. C. Marshall Papers [Retirement, General]; see also Condit, *Test of War*, 483–84.) To make all of this clear to the entire Defense Department staff, Carter in late November 1950 suggested the preparation of a directive informing Department of Defense chairmen and directors that "all matters of policy" were to be brought to the attention of EXOS and that "any correspondence or action" taken "in the name of the Secretary or Deputy Secretary" was to be sent to him before distribution. (Carter to Stohl, memorandum, November 28, 1950, GCMRL/G. C. Marshall Papers [Secretary of Defense, Chronological, Director, Executive Office (Marshall S. Carter), 1950–1952].)

Also of critical importance in the running of the Defense Department was Deputy Secretary Lovett, who "carries out the policies I have announced," Marshall asserted. "He is in complete charge of operations." The official history of the OSD labeled Lovett "Marshall's alter ego," but the press noted that Marshall also delegated substantial duties and authority to the deputy secretary, as well as to the service secretaries, that they had not possessed under Louis Johnson. (Condit, *Test of War*, 36; "Huge Defense Machine Functioning Smoothly," *New York Times*, December 3, 1950, p. E10.)

For assistant secretaries Marshall retained comptroller Wilfred J. McNeil, and

Marx Leva for legal and legislative affairs. He replaced the retiring Paul Griffith with Anna Rosenberg but changed the position she would hold from assistant secretary for administrative and public affairs to assistant secretary for manpower and personnel. (See pp. 206–7, 232–33, 262–63, and 296–97.) According to the official history, this constituted Marshall's "only major change in OSD organization and personnel." (Condit, *Test of War*, 35.) Marshall also supported McNeil's efforts to gain greater control over management of defense funds, directing on September 27 that the service secretaries appoint assistant secretaries or undersecretaries for fiscal management and departmental comptrollers and deputy comptrollers and giving McNeil control over comptroller activities within each service. Marshall also used the staff council to coordinate staff work, with Lovett meeting with those at the rank of assistant secretary or lower. (Ibid., 485–87.) See also p. 169n3.

In early 1951, Marshall took additional actions to improve the efficiency of the DOD. These included a reorganization of the Munitions Board and replacement of the Office of the Director of Medical Services and the Armed Forces Medical Advisory Committee by an Armed Forces Medical Policy Council, to be chaired by a civilian physician and composed of both service surgeons general and civilian physicians. ("Munitions Board Reorg.," *Army Navy Air Force Journal*, January 13, 1951, p. 542; Condit, *Test of War*, 495.) On January 12, he also established the OSD Domestic Security Coordinating Council to organize the activities of staff groups that dealt with civil defense as well as "internal security." (Marshall to service secretaries, JCS, assistant secretaries, chairmen of OSD boards, councils, and committees, and directors of OSD offices, memorandum, January 12, 1951, GCMRL/G. C. Marshall Papers [Secretary of Defense, Number Indexed, M200-3-26].) On February 1, he issued a directive redefining the duties of the RDB and allowing it to issue directives in his name in order to implement its policies and decisions. (Marshall to service secretaries, JCS, assistant secretaries, chairmen of OSD boards, councils, and commitees, and directors of OSD offices, memorandum, February 1, 1951, ibid.; Condit, *Test of War*, 507.) Then on February 9, Marshall informed one of his assistants of additional actions to improve efficiency that he had taken and planned to take in the near future. ★

232

To Miss Katharine Foley

February 9, 1951
Washington, DC

Dear Miss Foley: I hope that you have gotten well rested up and that you and your Mother are gradually getting back on an even keel after your Father's death. I must admit that this is somewhat of a selfish hope too because I have a very critical job to be done—for which I know you are eminently qualified.[1]

At the moment we are slowly but surely consolidating a number of the separate agencies which reported directly to the Secretary before you started your leave. We have already issued new charters and instructions for the Armed Forces Medical Policy Council and the Management Committee, designed to place them more in the policy and less in the operating field.[2] Confidentially I contemplate in the very near future splitting up some of the functions of the Director of Administration so that they will be channeled through Mrs. Rosenberg and Mr. McNeil. I am also in the process of strengthening and expanding the functions of the Executive Secretariat along the lines of the one I set up in the State Department, with which I know you are familiar.

As you know we do not have at the present time any formal body of material which expresses the various policies, plans, programs and procedures issued by the Office of the Secretary of Defense. Nor do we have a formal system for disseminating such plans, policies, etc. to appropriate agencies. In addition we do not have a screening process by which proposed papers of this type are fully coordinated and checked against past policies prior to their issuance. In order to overcome this fault I intend to issue in the very near future a directive which will pull all of this problem into proper line in accordance with the following purpose:

"It is the purpose of this directive to establish a system to assure that all interested officials are informed of all *proposed* directives which may affect their responsibilities, and to assure that proper distribution is made to all interested officials of all *confirmed* directives. The system also provides for a central review of such documents prior to issuance to avoid duplications, inconsistencies and conflicts in the subject matter."[3]

You can see from the foregoing that a high degree of continuity of thought is required, in addition to an intimate knowledge of what has gone on in the Department in prior years.

I have now gotten to the purpose of this letter. I want very much for you to head up the office assigned responsibility to implement this policy issuance directive. The office would probably initially be a free-wheeling organization working directly under me and Mr. Lovett, but utilizing the available material presently in the office of the Director of Administration and the Executive Secretariat. Eventually I would expect the functions of the office to become a major portion of the expanded control organization we contemplate the Executive Secretariat will develop into. In any event I hope I have made the initial task clear and an indication of what the future might hold in this immediate office.[4]

I know you can do the job that I want done and it is my very real hope that you will let me know when you can start it. With warm regards to you and your Mother.[5] Faithfully yours,

GCMRL/G. C. Marshall Papers (Secretary of Defense, Selected)

1. Katharine Starr Foley had been personal secretary to James Forrestal for ninc years, including his tenure as the first secretary of defense, and a secretary to Secretaries of Defense Johnson and Marshall. In mid-November 1950, Marshall had approved a leave of absence for Foley, whose father had fallen ill, and on December 4, he assured her that she could "take as much leave as you need." Foley's father died on December 6, 1950, in St. Petersburg, Florida. (Carter to Stohl, memorandum, November 17, 1950, GCMRL/G. C. Marshall Papers [Secretary of Defense, Selected]; Marshall to Foley, December 4, 1950, GCMRL/G. C. Marshall Papers [Secretary of Defense, Number Indexed, M200-2-37];

"Obituary, Edward H. Foley Sr.," *New York Times*, December 7, 1950, p. 33.)

2. See the previous editorial note.

3. The editors have been unable to locate a directive using this or similar language. On February 15, however, Marshall did establish within EXOS a central registry "for all official correspondence" to and from the JCS. (Marshall to assistant secretaries, chairmen of OSD boards, committees, and councils, and directors of OSD offices, memorandum, February 15, 1951, NA/RG 330 [OSD Index, 201–Marshall, George C.].)

4. Marshall on March 15 officially established EXOS and appointed Carter its director and Colonel Kenneth R. Kreps (USAF) its deputy director, with Carter to determine the office's functions, duties, and internal organization. Via a separate memorandum that same date, Marshall also authorized only EXOS to use the "For the Secretary of Defense" signature line as authenticated by the director or deputy director, with its use indicating that the action had his approval. In a third March 15 memorandum, he attached the director of administration, Ralph N. Stohl, to EXOS and broadly defined his responsibilities. (Marshall to the service secretaries, JCS, assistant secretaries of defense, chairmen of OSD boards, committees, and councils, and directors of OSD offices, memoranda, March 15, 1951, GCMRL/G. C. Marshall Papers [Secretary of Defense, Categorical, Memoranda].)

5. Foley informed Marshall on February 28 that she would be unable to commit until her father's estate was settled, which she hoped would be completed by May. (Foley to Marshall, February 28, 1951, GCMRL/G. C. Marshall Papers [Secretary of Defense, Selected].) Foley was officially still employed by the Defense Department on May 31, 1951, as Marshall's secretary, according to the *Official Register of the United States, 1951*, and she met with Marshall on June 19, 1951.

233

MEMORANDUM OF CONVERSATION[1] February 13, 1951

Secret Washington, DC

The Prime Minister of New Zealand called on General Marshall, by appointment, at 1130, 9 February 1951.

At the end of Major Turk's briefing of the immediate Korean military situation, General Marshall gave the Prime Minister a full and detailed exposition of the major factors concerning the Korean situation and the problems facing the United States.[2] General Marshall highlighted the following points:

General Ridgway had rightly decided to move north from Line D in order to probe Chinese Communist intentions and to keep UN forces in activity—an essential factor from the morale point of view.[3]

Chinese forces were undoubtedly facing difficult conditions, since their losses from military action had been very large, according to actual counts, and typhus definitely had taken a large toll. General Marshall said that he and General Bradley felt that the Chinese Communists would have to take the offensive sooner or later in order to regain face. This offensive might resume in Korea, or it might break out elsewhere. He suggested Formosa. When Ambassador Berendsen suggested Indochina, General Marshall replied that the losses in Korea and the supply situation was already making it difficult for the Chinese in Indochina, and the situation in Indochina had improved.

The morale of the US troops in Korea was very high. South Korean forces fought well against Koreans but were afraid of the Chinese. The disintegration of certain Korean units had contributed to the UN retreats. This situation had been improved by interspersing Korean units along the line with US or non-Korean units to back them up.

The US faces a very difficult problem in replacements. Divisions in the process of formation in the US had to be ripped up to provide replacements for the units in Korea. The basic training schedule was just getting started and would not reach the monthly output of 35,000 men until early summer. The US hoped eventually to be able to replace units in Korea with those formed in the US.

The air situation had definitely improved. The air forces now are able to strike hard and constantly against Chinese troop concentrations and lines of supply. In this connection, General Marshall pointed out that if the Chinese Communists mounted massive—he emphasized the word massive as against strong—air attacks, the UN forces would be compelled to strike at the bases from which air attacks were mounted.[4]

The UN forces were using air fields in Korea but the problem there was congestion of air fields in Japan. General Marshall then told the Prime Minister that the situation in Japan gave him great concern because there was no garrison at all at this time in Japan. The island of Hokkaido is wide open to attack, as is the rest of Japan, from an airborne or amphibious invasion. There was a certain amount of information that the Russians were collecting forces along their Siberian coast and in Sakhalin. If the US Air Force in Japan could hold together for six hours after a Russian attack, they could cause a great deal of damage to Vladivostok, Port Arthur, etc. It would be difficult to move troops fighting the Chinese Communists to Japan. Such a Soviet attack would create an entirely new situation in the Pacific. The Prime Minister agreed.

In general, the situation in Korea was greatly encouraging and had definitely improved during the past month from many points of view. The Prime Minister was very interested in this statement and General Marshall repeated it for emphasis.

General Marshall then briefly discussed the possible outcome of the present situation. He thought the first thing to do was inflict the greatest loss possible on the Chinese Communists without injury to our forces. In the meantime, Korean strength should be increased in every way to put them along the line, and leave a few US units behind the Koreans for reinforcement. General Marshall emphasized that this was his personal point of view and, since so many other countries were concerned, it was difficult to see how the situation would turn out. He felt greatly concerned over the way this problem had been handled, with so much emphasis on so-called US aggression and practically nothing said about all the terrible things that the Chinese Communists were doing—breaking every law, committing all sorts of inhuman acts. The Prime Minister and the Ambassador vigorously agreed.

General Marshall noted that we all had to remember the consequences for the Koreans if they were abandoned. They would suffer a horrible fate, which the prestige of the Western world could not afford to suffer. The Prime Minister and the Ambassador appeared to agree emphatically with this statement.

General Marshall briefly touched on the bearing which the American domestic political situation had on our foreign policy in general, and particularly on the Korean problem.

Prime Minister Holland told General Marshall that he was happy about the political situation in New Zealand where international affairs did not enter into party politics and where there is close cooperation between the two parties and their leaders on foreign policy matters. The Prime Minister said that he wished to convey General Marshall's remarks to Mr. Nash, the leader of the opposition, and that he would do so with due discretion to the nature of some of General Marshall's remarks. He said that he was sorry New Zealand was such a small country and could not contribute more in Korea. General Marshall expressed appreciation for what New Zealand had done and particularly for the staunch and dependable support of New Zealand. In departing, the Prime Minister and the Ambassador expressed great appreciation for the valuable and comprehensive account which General Marshall had given them.[5]

Kenneth T. Young

NA/RG 330, CD Memorandum of Conversation

1. New Zealand Prime Minister Sidney Holland, New Zealand Ambassador to the US Sir Carl Berendsen, and Air Commodore J. L. Findlay, chairman of the New Zealand joint staff mission to the US, met with Marshall and Kenneth T. Young. Although the meeting took place on February 9, Young submitted this memorandum on February 13.

General Burns reported that Holland, who was on his way back to New Zealand from the prime ministers' conference in London, had no urgent issues but wished to speak with US officials on "matters of mutual interest." (Burns to Marshall, memorandum, February 7, 1951, NA/RG 330, CD Briefings.)

2. Major L. A. Turk was part of the Joint Staff's Joint Intelligence Group.

3. In early January Ridgway's Eighth Army had retreated to Line D, which ran from a position forty-five miles south of Seoul on the Yellow Sea northwest through Wonju to Wonpo-ri on the coast of the Sea of Japan. On January 25, however, he had launched a major offensive (Operation THUNDERBOLT) that forced the Chinese to withdraw north of the Han River in western Korea, and by February 9 north of Seoul. (Billy C. Mossman, *United States Army in the Korean War*, vol. 5, *Ebb and Flow: November 1950–July 1951* [Washington: Center of Military History, US Army, 1990], 152, 160–61; Millett, *The War for Korea*, 2: 386–92.)

4. For details on this matter, see pp. 505–16.

5. In the briefing notes for this conversation, General Burns informed Marshall that Holland's "National (conservative) Party" government had surpassed its predecessor in maintaining "the closest relations with the U.S. and has supported our position in the United Nations with respect to Communist aggression, even to the extent of opposing Commonwealth leadership." Sir Walter Nash was the leader of the opposition Labour Party. (Burns to Marshall, memorandum, February 7, 1951, NA/RG 330, CD Briefings.)

234

To Mrs. William A. Becker — February 12, 1951
Personal — Washington, DC

Dear Mrs. Becker: I was very much surprised and I am frankly shocked at some of the resolutions passed by the Women's Patriotic Conference on National

Defense.[1]

While your group endorsed the Department of Defense program for Universal Military Service and Training, an action which I hope will be helpful to us, I feel that the conference has taken very harmful action in other ways.

To be very frank with you, I was much surprised to find that I had been inserted into a program which included some of the leading extremists in the United States, extremists whose irresponsibility, I think, is a matter of common public knowledge. This arrangement was not disclosed to me. As some positive evidence of the irresponsibility I mentioned, there are attached some resolutions from the dominant Jewish organizations in the United States.[2]

I am writing you this note quite personally and quite frankly, because I was so impressed with you that I would be interested in your reactions. I intend to keep your views entirely between the two of us.[3] Faithfully yours,

GCMRL/G. C. Marshall Papers (Secretary of Defense, Selected)

1. See pp. 350–54 and 361–63.
2. See p. 362n2 for identification of the individuals to whom Marshall is referring.

On February 6, Bernard Weitzer, national legislative director of the Jewish War Veterans of the United States of America, had met with Marshall and handed him a statement approved and signed by leaders of seven national Jewish organizations. They condemned the attacks by Rabbi Benjamin Schultz "on the patriotism and moral character" of Marshall, whom Schultz referred to "as a 'fall guy' in a plot to shield pro-Red activities," and Admiral Nimitz, whom Schultz said was "a foil 'in a deliberate attempt to whitewash an evil, pro-Communist situation.'" The statement concluded that the organizations "repudiate and condemn his repeated resort to vilification and slander of reputable Americans on the pretext of combating Communism." (Resolutions, January 30, 1951, and Lovett to Carter, memorandum, February 9, 1951, GCMRL/G. C. Marshall Papers [Secretary of Defense, Selected].)

3. Becker regretted the incident and reported that while she was "distressed" by the remarks, the speakers had been selected by committee of which she was not a member. She had not read any of the resolutions until they were announced to the gathering, and she felt that Marshall's speech counteracted any "detrimental" statements. She asked Marshall to accept her "most humble apology." (Becker to Marshall, February 24, 1951, ibid.)

235

REMARKS TO THE COMMITTEE OF THE GOVERNORS' CONFERENCE

February 12, 1951
Washington, DC

I am particularly glad that you gentlemen have come here today because the strengthening of our National Guard is an indispensable element in our plans for a military program that will provide genuine security for our country.[1]

You, the Governors, are the directing heads of the National Guard. Your inspiration and leadership has been invaluable in increasing the readiness of Guard units to fulfill their key function in our first line of defense. You have had to struggle against one almost insurmountable handicap—the impossibility of getting a dependable flow into the Guard of well-trained young men, who could keep their military skills fresh and their unit effectiveness high with necessarily limited periods of Guard training.

It is urgent that that handicap to a fully-effective National Guard be eliminated. You should be assured that the Guard will have at all times an ample number of men who start with sufficient military knowledge to be of real value to your organizations. That is a primary goal of the Universal Military Service and Training [UMST] program, which the Department of Defense is sponsoring in Congress.

It represents, in our judgment, the soundest way to accomplish the immediate expansion in our armed forces that is needed and, at the same time, to provide an enduring base for our future security. Its basic premise is that our regular military establishment—Army, Navy, and Air Force—should and must be held to the smallest number consistent with our needs, and that the balance of our strength should be represented by a trustworthy National Guard and civilian Reserve.

This is the democratic way to plan our national defense. It shuts out the danger that a protracted state of emergency would lead to militarization of our country. It distributes the obligation for protecting our country fairly among all young men.

This is the economical way to plan our defense. It avoids the ruinous cost in men and money that would be involved in putting all our trust in a huge force in being. By transferring responsibility to the Reserve, it reduces the cost to a level that is within the capacity of our economy to bear for as many years as may be necessary.

This is the effective way to plan our defense. It guarantees that we will have a striking force adequate to cope with any sudden enemy thrust. At the same time it provides a sound machinery for calling up the Guard and other Reserve components speedily, with assurance that they will be prepared to render effective service when they are called.

Because of the essential role of the National Guard, the proposed legislation makes specific provision that the Secretary of Defense is to have the right to release inductees under the U.M.S.T. program before they have completed their full 27 months of training and service, provided they volunteer and are accepted in the Guard. This clause gives men an extra incentive to go into the Guard and thus fulfill the plans you have had so long for attaining the peak effectiveness in your Guard units.

We are most eager to have the benefit of your ideas on how the job can be done most successfully. I hope when this meeting is completed and you have heard in somewhat greater detail what our plans are, you will designate a subcommittee to work with us on building a better and stronger National Guard—one of which you and we can be eternally proud.[2]

GCMRL/G. C. Marshall Papers (Secretary of Defense, Speeches and Statements)

1. Adlai Stevenson had informed Marshall by telegram on January 31 that he would be receiving a request from Frank Bane, secretary-treasurer of the Governors Conference, to set up a meeting "about February 12" with the executive committee of the conference "to discuss National Guard and reserve policy." Bane telephoned Marshall Carter on February 1 and followed up with a letter on February 2 to finalize plans for this February 12 meeting at the Pentagon between Marshall and several members of the committee: Frank J. Lausche (D-OH); Gordon Browning (D-TN); Frederick Payne (R-ME); Elbert Carvel (D-DE); and Sherman Adams (R-NH). Bane and Stevenson would attend, as well. Others in attendance

included Lovett; Rosenberg; General Bradley; General Vandenberg; Major General Maxwell D. Taylor (USMA, 1922), assistant army chief of staff for operations (G-3); and Major General Raymond H. Fleming, acting chief of the National Guard Bureau in the office of the army chief of staff. (Stevenson to Marshall, telegram, January 31, 1951; Carter to Marshall, memorandum, February 1, 1951; Bane to Carter and Carter to Bane, telegrams, February 7, 1951; Bane to Carter, n.d.; and memorandum for Marshall, February 12, 1951, GCMRL/G. C. Marshall Papers [Secretary of Defense, Number Indexed, M206-1-18].)

2. Bane wrote to Marshall on February 16 to thank him for participating. (Bane to Marshall, February 16, 1951, ibid.)

236

MEMORANDUM FOR THE SECRETARIES OF THE MILITARY DEPARTMENTS, THE ASSISTANT SECRETARIES OF DEFENSE, THE JOINT CHIEFS OF STAFF, THE CHAIRMEN OF THE BOARDS, COUNCILS AND COMMITTEES, OSD, THE DIRECTORS OF OFFICES, OSD

February 13, 1951
Washington, DC

At Armed Forces Policy Council recently, I discussed the subject of Saturday work and overtime work generally. As was pointed out in the course of the discussion of this subject, many officials of the Department of Defense have been working, over a period of many months, hours far in excess of the normal work week. The purpose of this memorandum, therefore, is to restate, in writing, the considerations that should govern hours of work, as outlined orally at Armed Forces Policy Council on 6 February.[1]

In order to conserve manpower to the maximum extent, it shall be the policy of the Department of Defense to extend the work week from 40 to 44 or 48 hours, as may be required by the increasing workload resulting from the present emergency. Authority to determine when workload justifies the extension of the work week may be delegated to appropriate commanders of field installations or heads of the activities concerned.

To provide continuity at the top level of the affairs of the Department of Defense, I am asking my principal assistants and such supporting staff as may be necessary, for the time being, to increase their official work week from five to five and one-half days. This shall apply to all personnel in the Office of the Secretary of Defense and associated agencies, except those who the heads of the principal offices and agencies concerned determine are not required for Saturday duty to carry out the purposes of this directive.

It is requested that the Secretaries of each military department similarly direct the extension of the work week for all top officials and supporting staffs in Washington departmental or headquarters activities whose opinions or decisions are required on matters of major policy in connection with the war effort.

Nothing contained herein shall be construed to change or limit present policies with respect to the authorization of intermittent or occasional overtime work as required. The extension of the work week at this time shall not affect those personnel on whom Saturday work imposes an undue hardship, such as married women with families who are required to make special arrangements for their children on Saturday.

GCMRL/G. C. Marshall Papers (Secretary of Defense, Numbered Indexed, M200-3-26)

1. "It has been obvious to me for some time that important decisions in connection with the present emergency cannot wait from Friday until Monday," Lovett had written to Marshall on February 5. Consequently he had recommended an extension of the work week to Saturday, with four additional hours for "top officials and their staffs" at this time and possible extension to a full day at a later time. He also recommended a similar policy for agencies working with Defense Department, such as the State Department, CIA, and Office of Defense Mobilization, and suggested that Marshall discuss the matter at the next cabinet meeting. On the same date, Rosenberg sent Marshall similar recommendations, along with a draft of the above memorandum. Marshall wrote on the bottom of Lovett's memorandum that he had discussed the matter with the cabinet on February 5 and with the Armed Forces Policy Council on February 6, and that "informal decision" had been reached in the cabinet "that the departments concerned maintain Saturday hours." He also edited Rosenberg's draft of this memorandum. (Lovett to Marshall and Rosenberg to Marshall, memoranda, February 5, 1951, and Randall to Stohl, memorandum, February 6, 1951, NA/RG 330, SD 230.44.)

237

To Lyndon B. Johnson — February 15, 1951, Washington, DC

Dear Johnson: I just want you to know in this rather personal and informal way that I think you did a magnificent job in conducting the Committee hearings on the manpower legislation.[1]

I am most appreciative of your outstanding efforts. Faithfully yours,

GCMRL/G. C. Marshall Papers (Secretary of Defense, Chronological, Director, Executive Office [Marshall S. Carter], 1950–1952)

1. The Senate Armed Services Committee had approved the UMT bill on February 14 and was referring it to the full Senate for debate. See pp. 325–29 and 369–71. ("The Proceedings in Washington," *New York Times,* February 15, 1951, p. 23.) On that same day, Marshall was scheduled to attend a luncheon at the Capitol. George suggested that when called upon to say a few words at the luncheon he express "strong appreciation to Senator Johnson for his constructive efforts on behalf of UMST. You might also give them your thoughts on the Wherry resolution, on which you will testify tomorrow." (C. J. George to Marshall, memorandum, February 14, 1951, GCMRL/G. C. Marshall Papers [Secretary of Defense, Chronological, Secretaries, Carlson].) See the next document and editorial summary.

238

Statement before the Senate Foreign Relations and Armed Services Committees[1] — February 15, 1951, Washington, DC

In regard to the question under consideration this morning, it seems to me that fundamentally the real issue is what should we do, the United States, in our own self-interest as a nation.

Whatever we do in the way of giving military assistance to Western Europe naturally requires the wholehearted support of the nation. The trouble seems to be somewhat a state of confusion in the public mind, and for evident reasons, as to just what the situation is and, more specifically, what are the military necessities.

In one sense, this is not a new issue for you gentlemen to be discussing in this room because many of you considered much the same issue when the Senate Foreign Relations Committee was considering the Vandenberg Resolution S. R. 239 of the 80th Congress.[2]

Much the same issue also was before you a few months earlier when I was called to testify here in support of the European Recovery Program.[3]

The action of the Senate in 1949 when it voted 82 to 13 in favor of the North Atlantic Treaty, and then 55 to 24 in favor of the Military Aid Program was, I took it to be, a confirmation of the view that the independence of the North Atlantic Community of Nations was of vital importance not only to the further development of free and democratic governments but also to the security of this country. To be more specific, in enacting the Military Aid Program, your Committee added to the basic legislation a requirement that the bulk of the funds to carry out the program would not be available until there had been prepared and then approved by the President integrated plans for the defense of the North Atlantic area.[4]

Since then there have been five meetings of the Defense Ministers of the North Atlantic Treaty Nations, at the fourth of which I presided.[5] In addition, there have been numerous meetings of the Military Committee in which General Bradley represented the United States and a number of meetings of the North Atlantic Council at which the Secretary of State represented the United States. Further, the Standing Group consisting of one representative from the United Kingdom, one from France, and one from the United States—General Bradley representing this country—has been in almost daily session.

Out of all of these meetings has emerged, as Congress expressly stipulated, a plan for the integrated defense of the North Atlantic Area—a plan that will succeed or will fail, depending upon two fundamental factors: first, the support which it receives from this country and the other nations associated with us; and second, the ability with which it is carried out by General Eisenhower and the staff he is now assembling. Regarding the second point, I am sure I am right in the belief that none of you have any misgivings. It is the first point to which your deliberations here appear to be addressed.

Please permit me to state the issue as I see it, in a rather different form. I assume that no one will differ from my belief that the United States will be safer—that is, more secure—if governments friendly to the United States are in power throughout the North Atlantic Community. If this is correct, the question then resolves itself into the problem of how the nations of the North Atlantic Community can best protect their independence. This is the problem to which the North Atlantic Treaty was addressed and it is the problem to which all of our discussions under that Treaty have been addressed.

In my opinion, the course outlined by our planning is the logical one. We are building up in the United States and in each of the nations of the North Atlantic Community stronger armed forces. We are not building up these stronger forces for any aggressive purpose, but in order to enable us to defend ourselves if we should be attacked. Also our aim is primarily to deter aggression if that be possible and to defeat aggression if, in spite of all our efforts, the actions of the Soviet Union or its satellites should precipitate another world war.

Fundamental to all of our efforts in this regard is the immediate start towards the creation in Western Europe of strong and integrated forces—land, sea, and air—in such proportions to one another as appears reasonable and practicable.

As General Eisenhower pointed out in his recent testimony here, the United States forces will constitute only a minor portion of these proposed integrated forces—the major portion being furnished by Western European nations.[6] This is particularly true in the matter of ground forces. Because of the great amount of discussion which has been centered on the subject of ground forces, I have obtained the express permission of the President to discuss with you the specific strength of the ground forces which the United States has planned to maintain in Europe in the present emergency.

I take this step reluctantly because of the security considerations involved—but I have reached the conclusion that there is a greater peril to our security through weakening the morale of our allies by a debate based upon uncertainties, than there can possibly be through the public disclosure of our planned strength figures.

To be specific, the Joint Chiefs of Staff have recommended to me, and I have so recommended to the President—and the President has approved—a policy with respect to our forces in Europe which looks to the maintenance by us, in Europe, of approximately six divisions of ground forces.[7]

We already have there, on occupation duty, about two divisions of ground forces. Our plans, based on the recommendation of the Joint Chiefs of Staff, therefore contemplate sending four additional divisions to Europe. While this number does not appear to represent in pure fighting power a large contribution to the immediate defensive strength of Western Europe, it does represent a small Army unit of high efficiency and we believe a tremendous morale contribution to the effectiveness and build up of the projected ground forces the North Atlantic Treaty nations are undertaking to develop under General Eisenhower's direction and command.

As President Truman pointed out in his announcement on September 9, 1950, "The basic element in the implementation of this decision is the degree to which our friends match our actions in this regard. Firm programs for the development of their forces will be expected to keep full step with dispatch of additional United States forces to Europe."[8]

General Eisenhower outlined to you the responsibility which he possesses, and which he intends to exercise, to assure that all members of the North Atlantic Treaty contribute the maximum amount of strength which their geographic, economic, and manpower situations permit. In the key position to which he has been named at the request of the nations which make up the North Atlantic Treaty Organization, General Eisenhower will be in a position to insist that all members of the North Atlantic Treaty play their full parts in this vital undertaking.

Proportionately, the American contribution will be greater in air and in naval forces than in ground forces, for the greater strength of the United States is in the air and on the sea. Proportionately also, our contribution will be greater in the production of munitions, than in the provision of manpower—for the industrial capacity of the United States is the greatest of any of the member nations of the North Atlantic Treaty.

In all that we are doing, as just outlined, we are specifically carrying out the instructions of the Congress with respect to the preparation, and the approval by the President, of integrated plans for the defense of the North Atlantic area. As a result of the various steps I outlined earlier, these plans are now well advanced and General Eisenhower as you know has assumed Supreme Command.

In order for him to succeed in this most difficult and critical of assignments, it is essential that he not be deprived of that freedom of action which is so necessary to a military commander. I realize, of course, that whenever this issue of flexibility is raised, some people will say, "If the fighting starts in Europe, the military commanders will be given complete freedom of action."

But what we want above everything else is something infinitely more important,—namely, a certain freedom of action to establish a deterrent against the development of a general war.

Moving in an international setting in a military way is at best frought with many and often great difficulties. We had them throughout the last World War but we successfully overcame the problems and proceeded to a victorious conclusion of the war. In this situation, though, we have a far more delicate and more dangerous situation to deal with. The most important, the greatest factor in the creation of military strength for Western Europe in my opinion is the build up of morale,—of the will to defend,—the determination to fight if that be necessary. And because of the events of the past few years and the increasing threat presented by the Soviet Union, we have an exceedingly difficult situation with which to deal, in the way of preparations which we hope will enable us to avoid war and will help us to take the necessary action, if war is thrust upon us. Under these conditions, having in mind the various measures which have been taken by the Senate in regard to the North Atlantic Community, the fewer limitations you impose upon the Military Establishment the better off we will be. And incidentally, I would say, Gentlemen, that it is not a question today of having large bodies of troops ready to march down to the docks and embark for Europe. Our problem is the creation of troops. The limiting factor today, by far the most critical factor, is the long time yet required to do this.

Those of you who are members of the Armed Services Committee have been addressing yourselves to this problem for many weeks and I will therefore not repeat here the things we are doing to achieve this build-up as rapidly as possible.[9]

GCMRL/G. C. Marshall Papers (Secretary of Defense, Speeches and Statements)

1. As part of the "Great Debate" in Congress on US foreign policy (see pp. 333–34), Senator Kenneth S. Wherry (R-NE) had on January 8 introduced Senate Resolution (SR) 8

directing the Senate Armed Services and Foreign Relations Committees, under the chairmanship of Senators Richard Russell and Tom Connally, respectively, to issue a report that would determine if "'it is the sense of the Senate that no ground forces of the United States should be assigned to duty in the European area for the purpose of the North Atlantic Treaty pending the formulation of a policy with respect thereto by Congress.'" The joint committee began this process on January 23. (Condit, *Test of War*, 339; Carter to Marshall, memorandum, February 13, 1951, GCMRL/G. C. Marshall Papers [Secretary of Defense, Categorical, Memoranda (Marshall S. Carter), 1950–1952].)

2. By a vote of 64–4, the Senate had passed SR 239, submitted by Arthur Vandenberg, on June 11, 1948, to express the Senate's affirmation of collective self-defense under Article 51 of the UN Charter, as had been expressed in the March 1948 Brussels Pact among the UK, France, Belgium, the Netherlands, and Luxembourg, and called for US adherence to such collective security arrangements. This led to the formation of NATO with US membership on April 4, 1949. ("International Peace and Security through the United Nations," SR 239, *Congressional Record* 94, pt. 6, 80th Cong., 2d sess., 7791, 7846.)

3. See *Papers of GCM*, 6: 309–28.

4. The Senate had ratified the North Atlantic Treaty on July 21, 1949, and approved the Mutual Security Assistance Act of 1949 on September 22, 1949.

5. See pp. 218–20.

6. On February 1, Eisenhower had addressed a joint session of Congress and a meeting of the joint Senate Foreign Relations and Armed Services Committees following a tour of NATO countries in Europe. (Senate Committees on Foreign Relations and Armed Services, *Hearings on S. Con. Res. 8, A Concurrent Resolution Relative to the Assignment of Ground Forces of the United States to Duty in the European Area*, 82d Cong., 1st sess., 1–35.)

7. See Condit, *Test of War*, 340.

8. Truman issued this statement upon approving an increase in US forces in Western Europe on September 9, 1950. ("Statement by the President Upon Approving an Increase in U.S. Forces in Western Europe," Truman, *Public Papers, 1950*, 626.)

9. Marshall had testified before the Preparedness Subcommittee of the Senate Armed Services Committee regarding the universal military training bill. See pp. 326–29 and 369–71.

239

Senate Testimony on the Wherry Resolution
February 15, 1951 Washington, DC

MARSHALL'S REVELATION in his statement to the Senate committees that only four additional divisions would be sent to Europe "took a great deal of the wind out of the sails of the opposition," according to the official history of his office. (Condit, *Test of War*, 340.) Indeed, many of the ensuing questions and comments were phrased in a manner designed to support him and required only a yes or no answer. Senator Connally, for example, asked whether passage of the Wherry Resolution and ensuing congressional control of the disposition of US troops would result in the enemy knowing US plans in advance, whether "that would not be to our advantage," and whether George Washington during the War for Independence had been "hampered a great deal" by the interference of congressional committees. Did he understand correctly, Connally continued, that Marshall believed US national security would be "immensely increased and strengthened" by the sending of US troops as part of the rearming of Western Europe? Marshall responded affirmatively to each question and emphasized that the impact of these troops on European morale would be considerable, that "morale right now is the greatest factor," that "the time element is a deadly important factor," and that "our position of security will be proportionately increased by what we do to build up the morale and the military strength of Western Europe and the speed with which we do it." (Senate Committees on Foreign Relations and Armed Services, *Hearings . . . on S. Con. Res. 8*, 42.) After commending Marshall for his "forthright statement" and asserting that it was "a very significant thing . . . when the Secretary of Defense of a great Nation such as ours will come out and tell the entire world just exactly what our plans are," Russell asked Marshall whether the sending of these US divisions would improve European morale and "will to fight." Not sending them, Marshall replied, "would have a very disastrous effect on morale." Nor was the defense of Western Europe against the huge Red Army a hopeless task. The situation in 1940, Marshall asserted, "in many respects looked far, far more hopeless than this situation today." (Ibid., 44–46.)

After refusing to comment on diplomatic matters and asserting that "When I walked out of the door of the State Department I ceased to be Secretary of State" (ibid., 47), Marshall reassured the committee members that US divisions would remain separate within NATO defense forces and that there were no plans to send additional divisions or to create a large army. Instead the Universal Military Service and Training bill then under consideration was designed to provide a large trained reserve to be used as and when needed. (Ibid., 47–49 and 54. For Marshall's testimony on the UMT bill, see pp. 326–29, 338–47, 369–71 and 409–13.) Presently the manpower situation was so serious that "we had a great deal of difficulty in working out" how to send just four divisions to Europe. "Of course, I suppose I react a little bit," Marshall admitted, "to a period while I was Secretary of State when we had one and a third divisions in the whole United States." (Ibid., 55.)

Other questions enabled Marshall and his Senate supporters to point out that the total number of troops in these six divisions would constitute a very small percentage of the US armed forces, which presently stood at approximately 2.5 million and were projected to rise to nearly 3.5 million, and that not supporting the Europeans by refusing to send the four additional divisions would require an even larger force to defend the nation. In the process of answering questions on these matters Marshall revealed as an aside that as secretary of state he had in 1948 delayed the sending of B-29 aircraft to England in hopes of reaching a settlement with the Soviets during the Berlin blockade crisis. (Ibid., 56–59.) Other Senate questions enabled him to point out that air and naval forces alone were insufficient to protect Western Europe and that such protection was, in the words of Senator Wayne Morse's question, "of vital importance in protecting the security of the United States." That was "very decidedly so," Marshall responded, "and affecting the whole civilization of the world for years to come." (Ibid., 64.)

Given his opposition to the Wherry Resolution, more than one senator asked Marshall what he thought the extent and limit of congressional powers were in the realm of military affairs. Congress certainly had an important role in a democratic society, he responded, as his very appearance and testimony on this resolution and previously on the Universal Military Service and Training Bill and during World War II illustrated. Indeed, he and the senators were presently having "a very frank discussion of plans, so frank that it is rather remarkable in the way of disclosing every strategic conception that we have in advance, while we learn nothing whatever of what the other fellow may do or plans to do. All of that produces, it seems to me, a rather normal basis of going ahead in this matter." (Ibid., 65; see also ibid., 52–53.) Senator Knowland asked how restricted military testimony might be in light of Truman's December order that all public statements by officials in the executive branch concerning foreign or military affairs had to be cleared by the White House as well as the State and/or Defense Departments (see pp. 282–83). "Of course that is an age-old problem we always have," Marshall responded, "where you want to get the personal opinion of the individual, and there has been a policy decided upon. A great deal depends upon the individual, and a great deal depends on the political significance of the policy." In general he did not believe Truman's directive would deprive Congress of individual opinions, especially from higher-level officials and officers, but the senators needed to remember that in this democratic society, "when you get on to debatable questions you can get just about as many debatable opinions as people." (Ibid., 70–71.)

At one point in his testimony Marshall linked the sending of four divisions to join the two already in Europe to the highly successful European Recovery Program that he had proposed as secretary of state. "We first moved to restore their morale related to their table, related to their everyday life," he pointed out in this regard, "and that has been pretty well done. Now we have to meet the situation where they are under duress, are under a continuous threat and a very terrible threat." (Ibid., 67.)

Wherry himself had been unable to attend the session but had asked Knowland to submit to Marshall a series of questions, twenty-seven of them, Knowland noted, filling three pages. Rather than take up more time in the hearing, Knowland proposed to submit them for the record and to Marshall for his later response. "I will be very glad to do so," Marshall said. (Ibid., 71–72.)

Connally concluded the session by referring once again to past US history, this time citing congressional interference during the Civil War and asking whether that interference had "greatly hampered, greatly embarrassed, and greatly interfered with" Abraham Lincoln's conduct of the war. "Yes, sir," Marshall replied. (Ibid., 75.) ★

240

Memorandum of Conversation[1] — February 15, 1951
Restricted — Washington, DC

The visitors were introduced to the Secretary at approximately 1440.

The Secretary observed that it must have been quite educational and beneficial for the German visitors to have been present while he testified that morning before the Senate Committees which were conducting hearings concerning the deployment of additional troops to Europe.[2] He commented that hearings of that type had probably never been held in Germany, at which comment the Germans laughed in agreement. The Secretary explained that throughout the period of the war he appeared before congressional committees three or four times a week and that in so appearing his objective always was the same, namely to try to insure that the required action was taken in time. The Secretary pointed out that General Bradley and the Chiefs of Staff of the three Services would soon appear before the Senate Committee and that upon the completion of the Senate hearings it would be necessary for the witnesses all to appear again to testify for the House Committees. This procedure, the Secretary commented, meant that everything we wanted to do became public knowledge and for this reason there could be no conniving.

The Secretary then discussed at some length the manpower problem in the U.S. and outlined the steps which should be taken in order that a pool of basically trained manpower would be readily available in the event of an emergency. The Secretary then indicated he would be glad to answer any questions.

Mr. Euler stated that he could inform the Secretary on behalf of his colleagues that Germany was definitely on the side of the West. He then pointed out that the Occupation Statute prevented Western Germany from making an appropriate contribution to the security of Western Europe and stated that if these restrictions were lifted it would prove a great help to Western German confidence and morale. The Secretary asked if this matter had been raised with Secretary Acheson, to which Mr. Euler replied in the affirmative.[3]

Each of the other five German visitors then successively expressed a few views concerning the necessity of the Western Allies establishing a protective umbrella on the Elbe to guarantee Western Germany's security while it rearmed.[4] One visitor expressed appreciation to the Secretary concerning the deploying of four additional divisions to Europe. Another mentioned that his constituents had inquired of him where Germany was to procure the necessary arms and equipment to enable Western Germany to form armed units.

The Secretary did not respond directly to the subject of a protective umbrella on the Elbe, but directed his comments toward the query concerning the availability of equipment. He outlined in some detail our plans for industrial expansion and in this respect mentioned the assistance Mr. Lovett was giving him in this field. The Secretary stated that our current efforts were directed toward meeting our immediate requirements while, at the same time, creating a broad base on a high level which would permit very rapid expansion of industry in the event of an emergency. As an example, he mentioned that we would make 5,000 planes of a certain type this year, 20,000 the next year, and if the situation required we would be able to make 50,000 the following year. During this discussion the Secretary emphasized the importance of subcontractors and mentioned specifically that 10,000 subcontracts had been let in support of the Oak Ridge project during the last war.[5] He also mentioned our efforts to plan our industrial expansion in an orderly efficient manner in order not to over-produce in certain fields. As an example, the Secretary referred to the necessity of making a large cut back in the production of airplanes in the middle of 1944.[6] The Secretary stated that our production effort was geared to provide as soon as possible the equipment necessary to meet MAP [Military Assistance Program] requirements. He referred to the fact the $5,000,000,000 was to be spent for foreign military aid before the end of June and that part of the projected $70,000,000,000 FY 52 budget would be allocated for the same purpose.

The Secretary then asked if the German visitors had been briefed on the Korea situation. When they replied in the negative the Secretary conducted a map briefing on this subject.

The visitors departed at approximately 1520.

E. S. Hartshorn, Jr.
Colonel, USA
Office of Foreign Military Affairs

NA/RG 330, CD Memorandum of Conversation

1. Marshall met with six members of the West German Bundestag, the lower house of the German parliament, who were visiting the US for two weeks as guests of the State Department: Heinrich von Brentano, leader of the Christian Democratic Union–Christian Social Union (CDU-CSU) party caucus; August Martin Euler, chairman of the Free Democratic Party (FDP) caucus; Dr. Gerhard Leutkens, national secretary of the Social Democratic Party (SPD); Dr. Hans Muehlenfeld, leader of the German Party caucus; Hermann Punder, a member of the CDU; and Erich Ollenhauer, deputy chairman of the SPD and an aide to SPD chairman Kurt Schumacher. Also in attendance were the following US officials: Geoffrey W. Lewis, State Department deputy director for German affairs; Anton F. Pabsch, a State Department interpreter for John McCloy; Frank Nash, deputy US representative to the UN Commission for Conventional Armaments; Colonel E. S. Hartshorn Jr. of the Defense Department Office of Foreign Military Affairs, who took these minutes; and Major J. G. Miller, representing G-3 in the Department of the Army.

2. See the previous two documents.

3. The international Occupation Statute of West Germany, passed on April 11, 1949, authorized the Allies to administer the disarmament and demilitarization of Germany. In a summary of his February 12 meeting with the German representatives and other meetings they had had while in Washington, Acheson informed McCloy that "all members expressed solidarity" of the overwhelming majority of the German people with the West and that they were prepared to contribute to NATO on two conditions: repeal of the Occupation Statute so as to give the Germans "substantial polit[ical] equality including complete 'autonomy' in internal affairs," and an increase in Allied military forces in Germany. (*FRUS, 1951*, 3: 1321.)

After receiving assurances from Konrad Adenauer that his government would accept responsibility for prewar and postwar debts, the Allied Powers agreed to amend the Occupation Statute effective March 6, 1951, which they had been discussing since the foreign ministers meeting in September 1950. The revisions authorized the establishment of a German foreign ministry to handle direct diplomatic relations and the relinquishment of some of the powers of the Allied High Commission in the fields of review of state laws and distribution and oversight of funds, food, and foreign trade. The entire Occupation Statute was not repealed until May 26, 1952. ("Germans Receive Wide New Powers, *New York Times*, March 7, 1951, p. 1; "Occupation to End," *New York Times*, May 27, 1951, p. 1.)

4. In his summary to McCloy, Acheson mentioned as a condition for German contribution to European defense an "increase in Allied Military strength in Ger (SPD mentioned

10–15 Divisions) to provide protective screen or umbrella permitting safe development Ger defense plans." Acheson "did not respond directly" to the Germans' request when asked. General Burns had forwarded to Marshall the minutes of Acheson's February 12 meeting with the Germans and had recommended that if they raised this subject with Marshall, he should reply that "a considerable period of time will be required for NATO to create sufficient forces to permit the establishment of a defensive line any place in Western Europe." The aim, however, was to provide "sufficient forces to permit the adoption of a 'forward defensive strategy,'" and to ensure that other nations "concerned with security against a Soviet attack" would progress in their rearmament programs. (*FRUS, 1951*, 3: 1321; Burns to Marshall, memorandum, n.d., NA/RG 330, CD Briefings.)

5. Oak Ridge, Tennessee, was the center of uranium enrichment for the Manhattan Project to develop an atomic bomb during World War II.

6. Marshall may have been referring to the navy's abrupt cancellation on May 20, 1944, of a contract with the Brewster Aircraft Company for fighter planes. (Byron Fairchild and Jonathan Grossman, *The Army and Industrial Manpower*, in *United States Army in World War II* [Washington: Office of the Chief of Military History, Department of the Army, 1959], 126.)

241

MEMORANDUM FOR THE PRESIDENT — February 16, 1951
Personal and Confidential — Washington, DC

SUBJECT: Recommendations with Respect to Appointments to the Court of Military Appeals

During the nine months since the Uniform Code of Military Justice was enacted, the Department of Defense has been compiling information on all of the names that have been called to our attention, for possible appointment to the Court of Military Appeals. As you know, this Court comes into existence at the end of the current month, and at any time thereafter you may name three judges to the newly created positions on this judicial body.[1]

Names have been submitted to the Department of Defense, for our consideration, by the Department of Justice, members of the White House Staff, members of the Senate and the House of Representatives, and private citizens. We have carefully reviewed each name that has been called to our attention, and based on this review, the following recommendations are submitted for your consideration:[2]

The first name that I want to call to your attention in this connection is that of Edmund M. Morgan, Jr. He was the able and energetic chairman of the committee which drafted the Uniform Code of Military Justice, and was one of the most effective witnesses in support of the Code, before the Armed Services Committees of the House and Senate. Of all of the names that have come to our attention in connection with the Court, his represents the first choice, and the first recommendation, of the Department of Defense.[3]

In view of Morgan's age, it is our recommendation that you consider him as a possible appointee for the five year term—the initial three appointments, as you know, running for five, ten, and fifteen years. A biographical sheet giving Morgan's background is attached. You will note that he served in the Army in World

War I, and was Acting Dean of Harvard Law School during World War II, and is generally regarded as the country's outstanding authority in the field of evidence.

The second name that I wish to call to your attention is that of Benjamin A. Matthews. He has been highly recommended by, among others, Judge Learned Hand, Judge Bolitha J. Laws, and former Secretary of War Robert Patterson. His record includes extensive private practice, plus six years of service in the United States Attorney's Office for the Southern District of New York. He is sixty years old, and I recommend him to your consideration, in connection with the ten year term.[4]

It is my belief that you should consider a younger man for the fifteen year term. A number of outstanding younger men have been called to our attention. In addition to the biographical sheets on Morgan and Matthews, which are attached, there is attached biographical material on seven others—some of them falling into the younger category, and some of them falling into a somewhat older bracket. In submitting these additional names, no effort has been made to arrange them in order of preference. Morgan and Matthews are the top men in our opinion for first and second choices, but all of the other names are submitted in alphabetical order.

In addition to the nine names referred to above, on each of which there is attached a biographical sheet, I am attaching a list of all of the names that have been called to our attention. This list consists of more than fifty names, together with the address of each of the individuals. The complete files on any or all of the individuals whose names are contained in this list are available.[5]

It appears of the utmost importance that men of clearly outstanding ability be named to this newly created Court. Your initial appointees to this Court will set the tone for the Court for many years to come. The Court will be the ultimate authority over the three and a half million men and women we expect to have in the Armed Forces in the near future, and of the vastly increased force that would be organized in the event of full mobilization.[6]

GCMRL/G. C. Marshall Papers (Secretary of Defense, Correspondence, Selected)

1. The Uniform Code of Military Justice, passed on May 5, 1950, and signed by President Truman on February 9, 1951, would go into effect on May 31, 1951. Article 67 created a Court of Military Appeals, administered under the Department of Defense, that would consist of three judges, no more than two of whom were of the same political party, to be appointed by the president. The first set of judges would serve terms of staggering expiration at five-year intervals, and their successors would each serve fifteen-year terms. (Uniform Code of Military Justice, Public Law 506, 81st Cong., 2d sess., May 5, 1950.)

2. Lovett informed Marshall that while the American Bar Association was not willing to submit names, it was willing to screen the candidates. Truman declined the offer, and Marshall so informed Leva, although "a leading member of the Bar Association" had offered some informal advice. Marshall asked Leva to arrange the Defense Department's recommendations "into final form of a proposal by me to the President. I think that it would be best to submit six names in alphabetical order with a brief resume of the qualities of each individual." Marshall requested that he include "a list of all the men who have been recommended" as well as "a brief digest of the legal aspects as to term of appointment" and the department views on "initial appointees, having in mind particularly Professor Morgan." (Marshall to Leva, memorandum, February 13, 1951, NA/RG 330, SD 250 [Court of Military Appeals].) The order in which Leva ranked the names for Marshall differs from the

order forwarded by Robert Haydock Jr., counsel for the Office of Foreign Military Affairs in the Legal Services Division under Marx Leva.

3. The only Republican under serious consideration, the seventy-two-year-old Morgan was a law professor at Vanderbilt University. (Haydock to Leva, memorandum, January 24, 1951, ibid.; Marshall to Truman, February 16, 1951, and attachments, GCMRL/G. C. Marshall Papers [Secretary of Defense, Selected].)

4. The sixty-year-old private practice lawyer and former assistant US attorney for the southern district of New York had received a number of endorsements, including Patterson, Judge Learned Hand of the US Court of Appeals, Second Circuit, and Judge Bolitha J. Laws of the US District Court for the District of Columbia. (Haydock to Leva, memorandum, January 24, 1951, NA/RG 330, SD 250 [Court of Military Appeals].) Marshall thanked Hand on January 26 for his recommendation of Matthews, adding that the new Court of Military Appeals was "a most important feature of the new Uniform Code of Military Justice." (Marshall to Hand, January 26, 1951, GCMRL/G. C. Marshall Papers [Secretary of Defense, Number Indexed, M200-8-38].)

5. This list, which totaled sixty names, included the nine candidates whose biographical information Marshall had transmitted to Truman.

6. Marshall wrote to Truman on March 7 to request that Representative Overton Brooks (D-LA), whose name had appeared on the general list mentioned in n5, "be moved up from the list of candidates, to the list of seven others I previously recommended for the fifteen-year judgeship," mentioned in the sixth paragraph of this document. (Marshall to Truman, March 7, 1951, ibid.)

Truman announced on May 22 that he would nominate Paul Brosman, dean of the Tulane Law School who had been on Marshall's list of seven names mentioned in the sixth paragraph of this document, to the five-year term; George W. Latimer, a Republican justice on the Utah Supreme Court who had been on the list of sixty names mentioned in n5, to the ten-year term; and Robert E. Quinn, a Rhode Island Superior Court justice and former governor of that state who was not on Marshall's original list of sixty names, to the fifteen-year term. The Senate Armed Services Committee approved of them unanimously on June 16. ("Named to Court of Military Appeals," *New York Times*, May 23, 1951, p. 30; "3 Backed for Court of Military Appeals," *New York Times*, June 17, 1951, p. 17.)

242

To Charles E. Potter

February 19, 1951
Washington, DC

Dear Mr. Potter: This is in further reply to your letter of 24 January, requesting comparative data on the ratio of non-combatant to combat personnel and the ratio between civilian and military personnel within the military departments for the United States and a number of other countries. There is attached a brief statement on the proportion of U. S. combat personnel to total personnel.[1]

I agree that it is essential that we make the best possible use of our resources. The Department is taking vigorous action to insure a full utilization of manpower. It is important to recognize that increased combat effectiveness does not come about merely through increasing the proportion of combat troops.

To consider one extreme, an army, navy or air force consisting entirely of combat troops could not maintain a fight for more than a few days. It would lack the men to tend the sick and wounded, service operational equipment, repair damaged equipment, provide food, clothing and ammunition to the fighting troops, train replacements, transport fresh troops, supplies and equipment to the combat area, return the wounded to hospitals outside the combat areas, etc. Combat troops are at their maximum effectiveness only when supported by adequate numbers of well-trained service and other supporting troops.

Comparisons of the ratio of combat troops to total numbers in other countries is very apt to be misleading and confusing. The Chinese Communist Army, for example, apparently has a very high ratio of combat troops to total. They send an infantryman into action with his weapon, ammunition, and twelve pounds of rice. Little or no attempt is made to care for the sick or wounded and to replenish supplies of food and ammunition on the battlefield. Complete disregard of human life by Chinese Communists has led to staggering casualty rates among their troops and has represented a really extravagant use of their manpower resources.

One of the factors that limits the proportion of combat troops in our armed forces is the service support necessary to maintain the long lines of communications between the United States and possible overseas combat areas. The USSR is not faced with this situation and can place a larger proportion of its troops in combat divisions. Were we to fight a war within the boundaries of the United States we could dispense with part of our service troops and achieve a higher proportion of combat troops in relation to our total forces. It is our purpose, however, to see that we confine the fighting, so far as possible, to lands beyond our bordering oceans, and we must, therefore, be prepared to build up and maintain long lines of communication involving a considerable number of men for that purpose.

For your information, attached is a copy of a recent monograph on "The Division Slice" which outlines additional factors involved in comparative utilization of combat troops. Also attached is a statement on the "Relationship of Military and Civilian Personnel" for the Department of Defense. Comparable data on civilian personnel are not available, however, for the countries you mentioned.[2] Faithfully yours,

NA/RG 330, SD 050

1. Representative Charles Potter (R-MI) had written to Marshall on January 24 to express his concerns over the "extravagant" use of manpower and to ask for "the ratio of non-combatant to combat personnel" as well as "civilian and military personnel" in Russia, France, England, and China as compared to the United States. (Potter to Marshall, January 24, 1951, NA/RG 330, SD 050.)

Marshall attached a statement to this February 19 response that indicated a combat potential for the army of "64 percent combat troops and 36 percent service support troops." By summer the navy would have "54% of its personnel in its operating forces"; the marines, 65 percent; and the air force between 45 and 50 percent. (Marshall to Potter, February 19, 1951, and attachments, ibid.)

2. The summary page to the attached monograph defined the division slice as a measure used to quantify "the strength of a specific force divided by the number of combat divisions contained in the force." This attachment also cautioned against a comparison of US and Soviet division slices, since the smaller Red Army slice was at least partially the result of less training and medical care, increased periods of service, and shorter lines of communication, among other factors. Marshall also included a chart detailing the ratio of military personnel per civilian employee in the US between June 30, 1939, and December 31, 1950, which was 2.4 at the end of 1950, compared to 5.1 at its peak on June 30, 1944. The attachment warned, however, that this was "a very crude measure of civilian personnel

utilization" that did not "take account of variations in civilian employment unrelated to the size of the armed forces." (Marshall to Potter, February 19, 1951, and attachments, ibid.)

243

Statement to the American Association of School Administrators[1]

February 19, 1951
Atlantic City, New Jersey

A philosopher, I am told, was asked what he thought boys should be taught. He replied simply, "Those things which they will use when men." Certainly the fundamental duties or obligations of citizenship are involved in this alleged reply.[2]

Our American schools have carried out their responsibilities, and the Defense Department now proposes a system of military training to prepare young men to discharge their obligations as citizens in times of great emergency. It is a part of the proposal for military service and training which is now before the Congress.

In my youth and for the following decade such training was generally neglected. Most of my generation and especially the younger generations came up to the crisis of 1917 completely unprepared for the critical and dangerous duties they were suddenly called upon to perform. And, incidentally, please have in mind that a year and a half elapsed after that call-up before our first American army could be put in the field. And also remember that during that year and a half of delay France and England were fighting desperately for our mutual cause and had been doing so for three long years before our entry into the war.

The same error, or failure, was repeated and the same crisis developed before our entry into the last war. Only one in my position who is directly held heavily responsible for failures, defeats, disasters, and casualties can fully realize the agony of struggling against the heavy odds built up out of our national past neglects.

Six months ago, our present generation was caught in the same dilemma. But on this occasion we were involved in the necessity of fighting during the first week, not two or three years later. Our young men paid a heavy price ~~of~~ for this latest example of national neglect or, to put it more bluntly, lack of wisdom and foresight.

Our future as we foresee it these days will be beset with such dangers. The crises will be sudden and the perils great. In all likelihood, there will be little or no time for preliminary training. It is, therefore, imperative in my opinion that we turn back to one of the fundamentals of early American life and adopt the proposal of General Washington for some form of universal military training as a definite obligation of citizenship in our democracy.

I say "return to fundamentals" because the obligations of universal military training and service have always gone with the rights of citizenship under the English common law which our ancestors brought with them to the new world. In the early Colonial days, for example, all able bodied men were compelled to train and serve and those who absented themselves were fined.[3]

On the frontier in those days, the danger of attack was always present. An enemy lurked in the nearby forests ready to take instant advantage of any relaxation of the Colonial defenses. Somewhat the same situation has developed today, but the possibilities are far more alarming.

It is generally conceded that the fear of our present great atomic power is the principal deterrent to Communistic Soviet aggressions. It is generally admitted, I think, that our well-known military weakness encouraged Communist aggression in Korea. If we had had immediately available a trained reserve that could have quickly been brought into action, that Korean attack would never have been made. But if made, it would have been suppressed, I think, long before this time. And, incidentally, the temptation to hunt for scapegoats supposedly responsible for our predicament in the dilemma of such crises tends to divert us from a sober consideration of the proper measures to be taken to avert a repetition of these war tragedies.

The present emergency is critical. We need armed forces on active duty of three and one-half million men by next summer. We may need forces of that size for years to come. We need trained men for assignment to our reserve forces, especially the National Guard.

In the spirit of our democratic institutions, it would seem that every man should carry a fair share of this burden of responsibility.

The danger of Communist attack is not transitory. There is reason to believe that it will continue for years, until the popular strength of democratic institutions is again firmly established in the world. It therefore behooves us to set up a system that we can sustain during the next decade without bankrupting ourselves. Common prudence should dictate such a decision.

In Colonial days it was sufficient to train a man to use a musket, take cover and respond to simple command. As a matter of fact, most men were good shots to start with, always on the alert to defend their homes and frequently engaged in procuring game for the table. Today, weapons are complicated. The rifle is merely one, and the simplest one of many, and the average boy today knows little about its use. Then too, the ability to take care of one's self involves more than hiding behind a tree or a rock. Modern discipline calls for the development of great powers of endurance and the coordination of a wide variety of skills. Preliminary or, as we term it, basic military training, therefore, must be thorough, and four months, we believe, is the absolute minimum period for the teaching of these fundamental principles.

I take it that all school administrators appreciate the character of the times we live in and the dangers we face. I take it, also, that all of you feel that our young men should be prepared to face the vicissitudes of life in this critical period. The time when the military training should best take place is the subject of some differences of opinion and, in a country like ours, such differences must be fully considered. That is why I wish to explain to you the reasons for our recommendation to the Congress on this subject.

I am not going into the details of the universal military service and training bill which Congress is now considering. I assume that its principal features are now well known to most of you. But I do want to assure you that in the Department of Defense we have given a great deal of study to the determination of what age bracket would best serve the defense of our country and at the same time meet the requirements of our young men. We have discussed the question with a large number of groups from the fields of education, labor, industry, veterans' and women's organizations, as well as with the various service organizations concerned. We have tried to avoid interference, so far as possible to do so, with the well-established pattern of American education. The problems that confront school administrators are, I think, thoroughly appreciated. We know what you are doing to provide a solid standard of education for our young people. We, perhaps more than others, realize the part that education has played in the moulding of the character of our young men which makes them such superb soldiers once they are trained. For our purpose we prefer men who are high school graduates and we want to make it reasonably possible for every young man to have his high school diploma before he might be called up for military training.

The majority opinion of a wide variety of well-informed citizens, especially college and university officials seems to be—and almost unanimously, that the period between high school and college or high school and a job would be the least disturbing to our national life and to the careers of the individuals concerned. That is why we recommend calling up 18-year olds for training. There is nothing magic about the year 18. Some boys are just as mature at 17. Others are still not mature at 19. But after a careful analysis of all the factors involved and with special consideration for the needs of education, it appears that the 18th year comes nearest to meeting the situation for the average young man and for the schools that are responsible for his education.

The system proposed is American in character and consistent with our principles of education. I think it is fair. I am certain that it is democratic. It would be universal in application. There would be no privileged groups because of birth or wealth.

Instead of simply an interruption or an interlude in education, this course in military training and the service to follow may turn out to be an actual boon toward further learning. The experience with GI's after the last war gives convincing evidence of the stimulation among veterans of a determination to continue their studies upon completion of military service. Expanded horizons resulting from their military experience evidently stimulated their ambition to learn. The returned GI's almost invariably proved themselves serious, eager, hard working students, much more so as a matter of fact than the young men who entered college at the same time but with no military background.

While in service, all young men would be encouraged to study. The Armed Forces Institute recently reported 95,000 young men of the Army, Navy, Marines and Air Force, taking correspondence courses on their own time. The University of Maryland in Germany and the University of California in Japan have several thousand GI's in resident study.[4]

Under the system recommended to the Congress 75,000 young men among those called up for training would be selected on merit, selected by civilian direction to continue in college. Thousands of others would be sent to schools and colleges for training in some specialties needed in our Armed Forces and many more of them, high school graduates, would be selected to take courses conducted in their services to prepare them for specific military assignments. In these cases the training would definitely be an extension of their education, in many cases the opening for a career in civil life for talented young men.

The requirement for trained men in the Armed Forces is not only urgent today but is continuous and the qualities of leadership, which are most frequently found among educated men, are in great demand. Time and again during World War II we met the urgent demands of our leaders in the field for men who could command—men who had the ability to lead. The demand came not only for officers but for sergeants and corporals and even for 1st class privates who demonstrated the character and the courage to accept responsibility and to inspire confidence. It is that type of young men that the high schools have been producing for years and it is upon them that we would place heavy responsibility in our defensive structure.

In devoting myself in this talk so largely to the needs for trained manpower I must not appear to slight the vital importance of munitions, war materiel. I know what American industry can do. I saw its performance during the last war. Our goal today is to get immediately the most modern munitions for the 3 1/2 million men we are now forming up and for our reserves and allies and to set up the munitions industry in a position of stand-by readiness to meet whatever additional demands of an all-out mobilization might be. But I feel it necessary again to emphasize the present critical need for trained manpower in our armed forces. We need a trained reserve now as we never have needed it before, though in fact we have needed it pretty desperately time after time in our brief history as a nation.

That need has been emphasized time and again since our earliest days as a Federal Government. No one advocated universal military training more clearly and specifically than did George Washington. To quote his words: "It may be laid down, as a primary position, and the basis of our system that every Citizen who enjoys the protections of a free Government, owes not only a proportion of his property but even of his personal services to the defense of it, and consequently that the Citizens of America (with a few legal and official exceptions) from 18 to 50 years of age should be borne on the Militia Rolls, provided with uniform arms, and so far accustomed to the use of them, that the total strength of the Country might be called forth at a short notice on any very interesting emergency." He also stated: "There is a rank due to the United States among nations which will be withheld—if not absolutely lost—by the reputation of weakness . . . If we desire to avoid insult, we must be ready to repel it; if we desire to secure peace—one of the most powerful instruments of our rising prosperity—it must be known that we are at all times ready for war."[5]

Three days from now we shall celebrate Washington's birthday as a national holiday. I hope, in that connection, we will finally, at long last endorse his wisdom and sound common sense.[6]

GCMRL/G. C. Marshall Papers (Secretary of Defense, Speeches and Statements)

1. Dr. Worth McClure, executive secretary of the American Association of School Administrators, had met with Marshall on October 25, 1950, and invited him to address the February 19, 1951, evening session of its annual gathering of around fourteen thousand school superintendents, principals, and some university presidents and executive officers. McClure and Warren T. White, president of the Dallas-based association, asked for the assistance of Senators Tom Connally and Lyndon Johnson as well as Speaker of the House Sam Rayburn (D-TX) in urging Marshall to accept the invitation. It would be a venue for Marshall to address the attendees' "genuine misgivings about universal military training," White informed Connally. Marshall tentatively accepted the invitation on October 28 and confirmed this decision on January 9. (McClure to Marshall, October 25, 1950; McClure to Johnson, October 19, 1950; White to Connally, October 19, 1950; Marshall to McClure, October 28, 1950; and McClure to Marshall, January 10, 1951, GCMRL/G. C. Marshall Papers [Secretary of Defense, Number Indexed, M214-3-28].)

While preparing this speech, Marshall sent identical letters on February 3 to James Conant and Harold Dodds to ask for advice on what to say regarding "the manpower problem" during the speech. Conant urged Marshall to appeal to the concept of UMT as "a democratic, fair system; there are no privileged groups (this audience is very fearful of privileged groups). . . . I believe they can all be made to see that UMST at 18–20 is far superior to the alternative—Selective Service with its erratic and unfair deferment policy as administered by local boards in times of peace or partial mobilization." Dodds thought "it would be most advantageous to concentrate on the emergency and the democratic and moral values of universal service as against selective service," since many secondary "[e]ducators have an allergy towards military service." Marshall thanked each of them in identical letters on February 20 and attached a copy of his speech. (Marshall to Conant and Dodds, February 3 and 20, 1951; Conant to Marshall, February 7, 1951; and Dodds to Marshall, February 6, 1951, ibid.) See also pp. 409–13.

2. A variation of this quote is attributed to Aristippus of Cyrene, a student of Socrates. According to Diogenes Laertius, "Again, when Aristippus was asked what are the subjects which handsome boys ought to learn, his reply was, 'Those which will be useful to them when they are grown up.'" (Diogenes Laertius, trans. R. D. Hicks, *Lives of Eminent Philosophers*, vol. 1, rev. ed. [1925; repr., Cambridge: Loeb Classical Library, Harvard University Press, 1972], 209.)

3. Marshall is referring here to the colonial militia system.

4. Based in Madison, Wisconsin, the US Armed Forces Institute, formerly the Army Institute, produced educational materials and coordinated courses for officers preparing to go overseas. The University of Maryland–European Command College of Special and Continuation Studies, established in October 1949, offered on-base courses for military personnel as well as civilian employees of the armed services and the State Department from centers in West Germany and West Berlin. ("Seven Maryland U. Professors To Start GI Courses Overseas," *Washington Post*, October 3, 1949, p. 2.) The University of California Extension's Far East Command Program, launched in 1950, offered similar services in Japan, Guam, and the Philippines.

5. See George Washington to Alexander Hamilton, enclosure, "Sentiments on a Peace Establishment," May 2, 1783, in John C. Fitzpatrick, ed., *The Writings of George Washington from the Original Manuscript Sources, 1745–1799*, vol. 26, *January 1, 1783–June 10, 1783* (Washington: GPO, 1938): 389; and George Washington, "Fifth Annual Message to Congress," in Theodore J. Crackel, ed., *The Papers of George Washington, Presidential Series*, vol. 14, *1 September–31 December 1793* (Charlottesville: University Press of Virginia, 2008): 464.

6. White wrote to Marshall on February 21 that he was "delighted with your frank, informal approach to your subject," which "was universally applauded by all of the administrators." (White to Marshall, February 21, 1951, GCMRL/G. C. Marshall Papers [Secretary of Defense, Number Indexed, M214-3-28].)

244

MEMORANDUM FOR GENERAL MARSHALL FROM COLONEL MARSHALL CARTER

February 20, 1951
Washington, DC

The Democratic National Committee called to determine the circumstances under which you were awarded a Soviet medal. Apparently, one of their speech-makers got into a public debate with a Republican in this matter, which involved you and General Eisenhower. They wanted the information so that they could brief their people as to how to rebut the Republican's accusations, since they felt it might develop into something further.[1]

I told them that I felt sure it would be highly inappropriate for the Democratic National Committee to take up the cudgel in your regard, or for you to be involved in this thing at all. He said he understood perfectly but wanted me to look into it. I said I would look into it but doubted very much if I even mentioned it to you.

We can pass the buck and still keep them happy by referring them to the Decorations Branch, AGO [Adjutant General's Office].

MSC

[*Handwritten by GCM*]: As a matter of fact I *opposed* the business and Harriman in Moscow urged it on Mr. Roosevelt. I received the medal the evening our troops landed in Normandy, ~~tho the Soviets~~

GCMRL/G. C. Marshall Papers (Secretary of Defense, Categorical, Memoranda, Marshall S. Carter, 1950–1951)

1. The Soviet Union had expressed a desire during World War II to award Marshall its highest military honor, the Order of Suvarov, First Degree. Marshall had refused to accept any foreign decorations during the war, but since Harriman, then ambassador to the USSR, had failed to discourage the Soviets from bestowing this award, Roosevelt thought Marshall should accept it so as not "to offend the Russian Government." Marshall received the medal from Soviet Ambassador Andrei A. Gromyko, at the Soviet embassy in Washington, DC, on June 5, 1944. Eisenhower had been the only other non-Russian recipient of the award. See *Papers of GCM*, 4: 339–40 and 469–70.

245

STATEMENT TO THE HOUSE PUBLIC WORKS COMMITTEE

February 21, 1951
Washington, DC

Mr. Chairman, Gentlemen: The Department of Defense, including the Joint Chiefs of Staff, supports the House Joint Resolution now before your Committee which would permit implementation of the St. Lawrence Seaway and power project and recommends its adoption by the Congress.[1]

Our support is based on the advantages to national defense that this project offers.

First, the Seaway, when completed, will increase the flow of high grade iron ore for the production of steel for munitions and other purposes from the Labrador-Quebec area which is now being developed. Unless the Seaway is built, obtaining ore from this new source will present serious problems of transportation including the hazards of wartime sea transportation. On the other hand, the accessibility of the Labrador-Quebec area made possible by the Seaway would supplement our present supply and would furnish a substantial additional source if our present primary source should be seriously reduced. Freedom from submarine attack does not, of course, mean full security. The risk of interruption of the new Seaway by enemy sabotage must be faced. The danger of sabotage, however, is already of critical importance at the locks at Sault Ste. Marie, through which our Lake Superior ores are brought in such vast quantity. Until the Seaway is built, almost the whole of our iron ore supply is subject to interruptions by a single act of sabotage there.[2]

Second, the power project in connection with the Seaway will provide additional sources of cheap and independent power so necessary, especially in the case of an all-out mobilization.

Third, the Seaway will facilitate the transportation of munitions to overseas bases. Moreover, in case of atomic attack, transportation could be diverted from one city to another. It is realized that the Seaway will be closed for months every year because of ice conditions but that is equally true of the present Great Lakes transportation route from the Mesabi Range to which all interested parties have successfully adjusted their operations.[3]

Fourth, the Seaway will afford access to additional shipbuilding and repairing facilities always very necessary in time of war to the maintenance of our supremacy on the high-seas.

Finally, it should increase the capabilities of mutual defense between Canada and the United States.[4]

I have brought with me Mr. Small, Chairman of the Munitions Board, who can explain in some detail the industrial mobilization aspects of the project.

For the record, I want to add that the project has had the approval of the Department of Defense in the past and that I supported it before a Committee of Congress as Secretary of State.[5]

We are still in the fortunate position of being able to buy time insofar as this project is concerned. We have not yet run short of iron ore in Continental United States. Our annual supply from the Lake Superior region is declining, however, in a period when our requirements are mounting rapidly. We must have other sources readily available. It is urgent that this project be begun promptly, so that by the time we must depend heavily on foreign sources of ore supply it will be ready.

GCMRL/G. C. Marshall Papers (Secretary of Defense, Speeches and Statements)

1. Marshall had been scheduled to deliver this statement at a hearing on a series of House resolutions recommending congressional approval of a joint venture between the United States and Canada to construct a seaway along the St. Lawrence River. He fell ill, however, so John Small, chairman of the Munitions Board, read this statement on Marshall's behalf. See pp. 404–5 and 426–27.

2. For more on the Labrador iron ore deposits, see pp. 203–4.

3. At the time of the discovery of a twenty-four-thousand-square-mile iron ore deposit in Labrador and Quebec in 1947, the Mesabi Range in northern Minnesota contained eight hundred square miles of ore. By the time of this testimony, there were concerns that the

Mesabi Range would be depleted within a decade. ("New Iron Range Rivals Mesabi," *Washington Post*, March 2, 1947, p. B6; "Truman Demands Action on Seaway," *New York Times*, January 27, 1951, p. 9.)

4. For more on the Permanent Joint Board on Defense, Canada–United States, see pp. 434–35.

5. See *Papers of GCM*, 6: 138–39.

246

To Harry S. Truman — February 22, 1951
Secret — Washington, DC

Dear Mr. President: Reference is made to your instructions at the Wake Island conference that the Department of the Army, in collaboration with the Department of State, investigate the advisability of initiating a pay-as-you-go system in Japan and submit appropriate recommendations to you.[1]

As the result of a study of the above proposal made by the Department of the Army, with assistance from the Departments of State, Navy, and Air Force, the Secretary of State and the Secretary of Defense concur in the recommendation that a partial pay-as-you-go policy be adopted by all United States occupation forces in Japan, effective 1 July 1951.

It is considered psychologically and politically appropriate that this policy provide for the payment of approximately fifty percent of the yen costs of maintenance of all United States occupation troops in Japan, the remaining yen costs to be met by the Japanese Government, and this policy will apply during United States fiscal year 1952.

Future policies in respect to the principle of partial pay-as-you-go, as it is applied to Japan, and the specific percentage distribution of maintenance costs will be covered in a bilateral agreement to be effective simultaneously with the Japanese peace treaty after further study of and consultation with regard to the related factors.

The foregoing arrangement will not be applied to other areas in which troop costs are involved without careful study and consultation among interested government departments.

Funds required to support the pay-as-you-go in the forthcoming fiscal year may total $180 million, assuming that the number of United States troops stationed in Japan reaches the currently planned maximum strength by 1 July 1951. It is probable, however, that the actual funds required to support a partial pay-as-you-go program for the United States Armed Forces would not exceed $140 million in fiscal year 1952 because of probable delays in reaching peak troop strength and the competing demands of other strategic areas. For fiscal year 1952, therefore, it is not anticipated that there would be any additional expense to the United States, since adoption of the above program would make possible elimination of the Japanese economic aid request for $140 million, as submitted to the Bureau of the Budget by the Department of the Army. Only in the event of substantial augmentation of troop strength in Japan would a request for additional funds for their support be required.

The Japanese Government has already budgeted the equivalent of $280 million for the support of the occupational forces for approximately the same period as that covered by the United States fiscal year 1952. The adoption of the proposed partial pay-as-you-go policy would permit the Japanese to release a substantial portion of yen savings for the strengthening of their own security forces.

It is suggested that you approve the recommendation in paragraphs two and three above.

The Treasury Department concurs in the above recommendation.[2]

Respectfully yours,

NA/RG 330, CD 092 (Japan)

1. General MacArthur had advocated the transition to a "pay-as-you-go" system for the Japanese occupation on several occasions. On June 23, two days prior to the North Korean invasion, MacArthur affirmed his belief that the Japanese "would welcome the contribution to their national economy reflected from a 'pay as you go' basis," which would have totaled around $300 million at that time. (*FRUS, 1950*, 6: 1228.) In discussing the possibility of a peace treaty with Japan during the Wake Island conference on October 15, 1950 (see pp. 186–87), General MacArthur asserted again that once a treaty was negotiated, the Japanese should no longer be responsible for paying for the American occupation; instead, adopting a "pay-as-you-go" system rather than using "GARIOA [government and relief in occupied areas] funds . . . might be a satisfactory arrangement if it can be worked out." Secretary Pace agreed that such a plan could be beneficial. Truman then requested that the Department of the Army and State Department work on a proposal to implement this plan. (*FRUS, 1950*, 7: 955–56.)

On December 29, 1950, U. Alexis Johnson recommended to Livingston T. Merchant, deputy assistant secretary of state for Far Eastern affairs, that a partial "pay-as-you-go" system be initiated for fiscal year 1952 whereby the US government would reimburse "the Japanese Government for 50% of the expenses incurred by it out of the Termination of War account," from which the Japanese had been funding the entire occupation. After the first year, the US would provide funds directly rather than reimbursing the Japanese government. (*FRUS, 1950*, 6: 1395–96.) Acheson approved this proposal in a letter to Marshall on January 30, and he included a draft letter to the president on these developments. (*FRUS, 1951*, 6: 809; Acheson to Marshall, January 30, 1951, NA/RG 330, CD 092 [Japan].)

In a conversation with John Foster Dulles on January 27, MacArthur "was emphatic in his opposition" to this plan should a peace treaty be negotiated in the interim. Once a treaty had been signed, MacArthur stressed, it would be "essential that arrangements for the support of our forces be the same as with other sovereign countries where our troops are stationed." (*FRUS, 1951*, 6: 821.) For more on the Japanese Peace Treaty, see pp. 323–25 and 427–29.

Marshall had written to Acheson on the pay-as-you-go system on January 22, but the editors have been unable to locate this document.

2. Truman replied on February 24 "approving paragraphs two and three as suggested in your letter." (Truman to Marshall, February 24, 1951, GCMRL/G. C. Marshall Collection [Harry S. Truman].)

ON FEBRUARY 23, Marshall informed Lovett—by telephone from his Washington apartment, where Marshall was recuperating from flu—that Truman had approved the sending of the Fortieth and Forty-fifth National Guard divisions to Japan. Marshall also acknowledged that he "was most anxious to have action taken on this matter immediately, particularly as regards the preparation and approval of an appropriate press announcement," which he wanted released before his scheduled appearance before Congress on Monday, February 26. The army made the announcement on February 24. (Lovett to Bradley, memorandum, February 23, 1951, GCMRL/G. C. Marshall Papers [Secretary of Defense, Chronological, Director, Executive Office (Marshall S. Carter), 1950–1952].)

MacArthur had requested additional divisions to defend Japan in December, and Collins in late January had recommended to the JCS that these two divisions be sent. Marshall informed Bradley on February 7 that he and Acheson had discussed the matter with Truman on February 6 and that "agreement had been reached with the President and Secretary Acheson that two additional divisions should be sent to Japan" and one to Europe, that the division to Europe should be announced before the two to Japan, but "that nothing should be allowed to leak out concerning these movements until the resolution on troops to Europe had been settled in the Congress, and, if possible, the Manpower Bill passed, too." (Bradley to Davis, February 8, 1951, NA/RG 218, Geographic File, CCS 381 [Far East].) Marshall may have received Truman's approval to make the announcement during a February 20 meeting with the president or via a possible telephone conversation with Truman from his apartment on February 23.

Marshall's February 23 telephone call to Lovett may have resulted from a memorandum Carter wrote to him on that same day reporting that despite Truman's reluctance, the Joint Chiefs and House Armed Services Committee chair Vinson desired immediate action on the matter and that "a number of differing opinions on this exist in Government." (Carter to Marshall, memorandum, February 23. 1951, GCMRL/G. C. Marshall Papers [Secretary of Defense, Categorical, Memoranda, Marshall S. Carter, 1950–1951].) Because of his illness, Marshall did not testify before Congress on February 26. ★

247

To Margaret Chase Smith — February 23, 1951
[Washington, DC]

Dear Senator Smith: In further reference to your letter of 11 December 1950, the current plans and programs of the Department of Defense, including the military departments, for the utilization of women in the various stages of a national emergency, have been reviewed.[1]

Briefly, the current position of the Department is as follows: The women members of the Army, Navy, Marine Corps, and Air Force are now being recruited under the present limitations of Public Law 36 (Army-Navy Nurses Act of 1947) and Public Law 625 (The Women's Armed Services Integration Act of 1948) and are being used in many suitable assignments for which qualified personnel are available.[2] As a result of the emergency created by the conflict in Korea, the Army has more than doubled the quotas for enlistment of WACs. The basic training of

WAC personnel has been accelerated and a program for the call to active duty of WAC officer and enlisted personnel for female medical officers of the organized reserve has been initiated. The current WAC strength is approximately 9,000 and a recruiting campaign has been launched to reach an objective of 30,000 as soon as possible. The present strength of female medical officers on active duty is approximately 4,200. This number is to be increased to 9,000. Women in the Navy are being utilized in 28 of the 68 military ratings covering 7 major occupational fields. They are still being utilized on a nucleus basis which the law established for peacetime planning. Under the present emergency, it is contemplated that the number of women in the Air Force shall not exceed the 2 per cent established by law. All recruitment for the women in all branches of the military service is on a voluntary basis.

The Department of Defense has recommended the revision of the limitations imposed on women's services in order to permit a greater number of women to be brought into active military service. It has been determined that women will be used to the maximum extent possible in case of mobilization.[3] Under full mobilization conditions, the Navy can probably utilize women to supply up to 15 per cent of the officer, and up to 12 per cent of the enlisted strength of the Navy. The Marine Corps estimates an appropriate maximum utilization of 7 per cent of the strength of the Marine Corps. The Air Force in full mobilization would like to increase the use of women up to 10 per cent of total military strength. The precise degree and nature of the utilization of women will depend on many factors: such as the urgency of the national manpower situation, the numbers of women who respond to the voluntary recruitment program and the needs of the services.

Civilian women are being utilized extensively by the Department of Defense, its boards and agencies, and the military departments. About one-quarter of the total civilian force or approximately 200,000 women are being used in a wide variety of assignments.

The Department of the Army has in process a plan for surveying the needs of the various installations and individual missions to determine the way in which women may be more extensively utilized. Facts will also be gathered as to the problems which will arise in hiring women and the adjustments and adaptations which may have to be made to bring them into full and effective performance. In the Department of the Navy similar studies have also been initiated by the Office of Industrial Relations. In the Department of the Air Force, as of 30 November 1950, women made up 25.47 per cent of the total civilian personnel complement.

During the period of peak civilian employment in World War II women made up 47.52 per cent of the total civilian complement. A phased building up of its civilian female work force at least to World War II level is anticipated as well as increased job dilution and extension of training programs for women for positions which call for skill and responsibility. Under present conditions, Headquarters USAF has been encouraging its commands and installations through conferences and training materials to make increasing use of women employees.

Although the operation of the Veterans' Preference Act has in the past served to reduce the ratio of female to male employees, the stringencies of the over-all manpower situation may compel the widest possible preference for the employment of women.[4]

Planning for the utilization of women is being given increased attention by military and civilian personnel officers.[5] Of particular concern to them at this time is a reappraisal of occupational specialty requirements for the various military and civilian assignments in order to establish the maximum extent to which women may be used. The studies of the military occupational classification project apply to all of the divisions of the Department of Defense.

These comments are necessarily general. Should you desire more details with respect to any particular aspect of the problem, the information will be furnished so far as possible. Faithfully yours,

NA/RG 330, SD 370.01

1. Senator Smith had asked Marshall to advise her of any specific plans that were "being made for the utilization of women in the war effort—not only in the event of all-out war but in the event of a limited emergency, a full emergency, or the period which you refer to as months of tension." Marshall acknowledged receipt of this letter on December 18 and informed Smith that he would send a detailed reply "as soon as that information is compiled." (Smith to Marshall, December 11, 1950, and Marshall to Smith, December 18, 1950, NA/RG 330, SD 370.01.) He rewrote an earlier draft of this letter on February 21, before the onset of his flu.

2. The Army-Navy Nurses Act of 1947 created permanent women's nurse corps in the army and navy and provided commissioned officer status for their members. The Women's Armed Services Integration Act of 1948 gave permanent status to women in the regular and reserve branches of all of the services but restricted total female active duty strength to 2 percent. (Bettie J. Morden, *The Women's Army Corps, 1945–1978* [Washington: Center of Military History, US Army, 1990], 50.)

3. For more on Marshall's attempts to overturn the ceiling on women serving on active duty, see pp. 412–13.

4. The Veterans' Preference Act of 1944 required the government, when hiring new employees, to favor returning veterans.

5. See pp. 361–63 and 639–47.

248

To General Matthew B. Ridgway — February 27, 1951, Washington, DC

Dear Ridgway: This is not a case of "out of sight, out of mind", but rather that events have been moving with such rapidity that I have not been able to do what has been in the back of my mind for some time and that is to tell you that I think you are doing a magnificent job amidst many hardships.[1]

I have been checking directly and indirectly on your family, and I understand that Penny and little Matt are getting along in splendid fashion. Please don't concern yourself about them too much as they are in excellent shape and being looked out for. My only regret is that you are not with them.[2]

Mrs. Marshall was struck down by an attack of flu last Saturday and the bug got around to me Tuesday last. I have been laid up since then but am hopeful of returning to the office, at least for a short period, tomorrow.[3] The weather is really spring-like and should I have a breather on one of these nice week-ends I hope to get down to Leesburg and sow some seeds!

As you probably realize, the game is pretty much the same here at the Pentagon. At times, Potomac fever seems to run rampant but so far I think I have been able to escape it. However, after reading some of the mail that has been coming into my office, I may have absorbed a larger dose than many of the others around here!

I am hopeful of early action on UMST legislation, but we are still having our trials and tribulations with the House Committee. They have temporarily amended some of our recommendations but I think that before the bill is moved to the floor we will get pretty much what we have been after from the start.[4]

I thought the picture of you in LIFE Magazine was quite good—at least it indicated that while there are many things running through your mind you still are able to relax.[5]

With my appreciation for a job that is being well done, and with affectionate regards,[6] Faithfully yours,

GCMRL/G. C. Marshall Papers (Secretary of Defense, Selected)

1. For Ridgway's military successes in Korea during February, see pp. 407–8.
2. Penny was Matthew Ridgway's wife, and Matthew Jr. their son.
3. Marshall dictated this letter on Monday, February 26, while he was still in his Washington apartment with flu, and signed it the next day.
4. See pp. 338–47 and 409–13.
5. The February 19, 1951, issue of *Life* included a photograph of Ridgway, "as artillery shells burst against the hills behind him," sitting "perilously close to the front, completely alone as he contemplates the next move of his advancing Eighth Army." ("GIs Become Soldiers—And It Pays Off," *Life*, February 19, 1951, p. 29.)
6. Ridgway replied on March 12 to thank Marshall for his letter and to express his "profound respect, admiration and deep affection" for Marshall. He looked forward to "the pleasure of being able to talk to you, when in a few minutes I can crowd in far more than is possible when writing." (Ridgway to Marshall, March 12, 1951, USAMHI/Matthew B. Ridgway Papers.)

249

Remarks at the American Red Cross 1951 Fund Campaign Kick-Off[1] — February 27, 1951, New York, New York

Thank you, General Sarnoff.[2]

Ladies and Gentlemen: I am here tonight to fulfill a promise I made to General Sarnoff last fall. Shortly after my acceptance of the job of Secretary of Defense, General Sarnoff wrote me a very friendly letter in which he indicated that his services were at my call just as they were throughout World War II. Knowing his remarkable qualities of energy, initiative, cooperation and leadership, I thought immediately that he would be the ideal choice to head the National Red Cross Fund Appeal for 1951, which, incidentally, is no easy task.

This was very much on my mind at that time. As you may recall I was still

President of the American Red Cross. The day that General Sarnoff visited me in my office at the Pentagon I asked him to take on this job. He said he never backed down on a promise and would undertake the assignment with the stipulation that I agree to take part in this Mobilization Rally with him tonight. Well—here we are.[3]

I had the opportunity to talk briefly with General Sarnoff after his recent return from an extended and really arduous trip around the country as National Fund Chairman. Just a year ago I had taken a similar trip of some 35,000 miles. He found the same devotion to the purposes of the Red Cross as I did. He reported that appreciation and understanding of the Red Cross is becoming much clearer today in view of the world situation.[4]

We Americans have always been a peace-loving people. Even today, with our sons in combat our thinking and our efforts are directed toward peace.

The achievement of this peace, we know, lies in strength—all the strength we can mobilize. And we are building that strength now with all the power and might at our disposal.

The government has assigned an important part of this gigantic task to the American Red Cross. For many years the organization has been looked to as the source of aid to the distressed in great disasters of peace and war. But seldom, if ever, in its long history has it faced a larger test of responsibility than it does today. Having played a part in accepting these responsibilities for the Red Cross, I speak with some authority and deep feeling on this point.

Let me outline for you briefly the scope of some of these new obligations:

First, the Red Cross must provide blood and blood products for all of the Armed Forces. It must provide these same life-giving products for civil defense stockpiling in case of attack upon this country. At the same time it must continue to provide whole blood and blood derivatives to the civilian sick and injured in communities served by the Red Cross Regional Blood Centers. All this is a tremendous operation in which the Red Cross must coordinate the activities of other blood banks and agencies, as well as establishing new blood centers in key communities where none now exist.[5]

In the second phase of the defense mobilization the Red Cross, through its disaster and health and safety services, is obligated to train millions of volunteers in skills that are essential to the preservation of life and the relief of suffering in a time of great emergency.

A third responsibility concerns the Armed Forces. The Red Cross must expand its services rapidly to increase the numbers of service personnel, both at home and overseas.

I know officially and through long experience of the importance of the Red Cross to the well-being of the servicemen and women of our democracy. The countless services performed by the Red Cross are an important factor in their morale. The serviceman has in the Red Cross an understanding counselor and an ever-present friend, working with the military, but not an organic part of it.

One helpful arm of this great civilian agency extends into the serviceman's setting, the other reaches into his home. One arm is made up of Red Cross Field

Directors and their staff at military stations and hospitals in the United States and overseas. The other consists of the wide network of Red Cross chapters throughout the country.

These essential services must be expanded to keep pace with our rapidly growing military strength.

The added tasks of the Red Cross which I have enumerated are public responsibilities. Their execution requires active participation and generous support from the American people.

America will be a better America, a stronger America—if it rallies to the support of the Red Cross in this critical hour.

GCMRL/G. C. Marshall Papers (Secretary of Defense, Number Indexed, M214-3-28)

1. Marshall delivered this address at a rally at Madison Square Garden that began at 8:45 p.m. The event, which included a statement by President Truman delivered in Washington and appearances by celebrities such as comedians Milton Berle and Bob Hope, singers Perry Como and Kate Smith, boxing champion Sugar Ray Robinson, and the Radio City Rockettes in New York, was broadcast on all radio and television networks from 10:30 to 11:00 p.m. Collections for the 1951 Red Cross fund campaign, the goal of which was $85 million, would begin on March 1. (Press release, February 28, 1951, GCMRL/G. C. Marshall Papers [Secretary of Defense, Number Indexed, M214-8-45].)

Marshall had recently expressed his support of the Red Cross fund campaign in a program featuring appeals from himself and Generals MacArthur, Eisenhower, and Bradley, and in a statement released to the press on February 15. (Press release, February 15, 1951, GCMRL/G. C. Marshall Papers [Speeches Binder #12]; "Appeal by Four Generals," *New York Times*, February 20, 1951, p. 4.) See photo #8.

2. Sarnoff (see p. 250n3), national chairman of the 1951 fund campaign, had introduced Marshall as "the man who knows most about the nation's needs and the ability of the Red Cross to meet them." (Remarks by General Sarnoff, February 27, 1951, GCMRL/G. C. Marshall Papers [Secretary of Defense, Number Indexed, M214-8-45].)

3. Prior to his resignation as president of the Red Cross (see pp. 247–51 and 283–84), Marshall had made "a verbal agreement" to Sarnoff that he would speak at this event, and he formally accepted the invitation on February 9. (George to Marshall, memorandum, February 12, 1951, ibid. [M214-8-2]; Marshall to Boothby, February 9, 1951, ibid. [M214-7-50].)

4. Sarnoff had told Marshall that he had toured eleven cities for the Red Cross campaign. Marshall commented that "the wealth of information gained and the acquaintances made on my 35,000 mile trip last year was a very interesting experience for me and I am sure you will think so, too, when you look back at it." Sarnoff does not appear in Marshall's appointment calendars between the time of this exchange and the 1951 fund campaign rally. (Sarnoff to Marshall, January 13, 1951, and Marshall to Sarnoff, January 19, 1951, ibid. [M200-6-8].) See pp. 19–21 and 47–48 for more on Marshall's Red Cross–related travels.

5. The Red Cross board of governors had voted at its November 19, 1950, meeting in Chicago to start twelve new regional blood programs across the country during 1951 and 1952. (Minutes of the Board of Governors, American National Red Cross, November 19, 1950, GCMRL/G. C. Marshall Collection [Minutes, Statements. American National Red Cross, George C. Marshall Presidency, 1949–1950].)

ON FEBRUARY 11, the Chinese launched their fourth offensive against UN forces in Korea. Their failure in major battles at Chipyong-ni and Wonju marked a turning point in the war, with the strategic initiative now shifting to

Ridgway. On February 21, his forces counterattacked (Operation KILLER) and were able to force the Chinese to retreat north of the Han River in central Korea. (Tucker, *Encyclopedia of the Korean War*, 1: 161–62, 166–68, and 407–8.)

Ridgway's successes raised the question of whether to attempt to cross the 38th parallel again. On February 23, Acheson asked Marshall for his views on a draft memorandum to Truman that asserted it was "undesirable for United Nations forces to attempt a general advance north of the general vicinity of the 38th parallel" and recommended the JCS and MacArthur be so informed. (*FRUS, 1951*, 7: 189–94, quote on 193.) The service secretaries mostly agreed but the Joint Chiefs did not, labeling the memorandum "from the military point of view, an unsound approach to the problem of determining future *military* courses of action." Marshall sided with the chiefs in this disagreement, informing Acheson on March 1 of his concurrence with the JCS "that there is a risk of disclosure to the enemy of a United States military decision, that freedom of action and freedom of maneuver must be maintained for U.N. ground forces, and that it is now premature, from a military point of view, to determine the action to be taken by U.N. forces with respect to the 38th parallel." He did agree with Acheson that the United States should "abide" by UN decisions regarding Korea, but concluded, as had the JCS, "that it is urgently necessary to formulate U.S. political objectives in Korea and China." Once this was done, the Defense Department would "recommend proper military courses of action. Therefore it appears to me that the political and the military factors should be worked out" by the NSC with conclusions forwarded to Truman. In the meantime the president should be informed that the matter was being studied by the State and Defense Departments, that the NSC was "urgently preparing recommendations for his approval on an integrated political and military position with respect to Korea and China," and that making any decision now respecting the 38th parallel was from a military point of view "premature." (Ibid., 202–6, quotes on 202–3; see also Condit, *Test of War*, 100, and Schnabel, *Policy and Direction*, 351–54.)

Marshall also agreed with the JCS in mid-February that MacArthur should be granted permission to bomb Rashin, a port city near the Soviet border on Korea's east coast, but he altered his opinion after discovering that Acheson opposed the attack. After Marshall discussed the matter with Bradley, the JCS rejected MacArthur's request for such permission. On March 1, they also turned down his February 26 proposal to destroy the entire North Korean power complex, including plants on the Yalu River. (Condit, *Test of War*, 99.) See pp. 505–16.

Ridgway's successes in Korea also affected congressional opinion of the proposed UMT bill, albeit in a negative manner from Marshall's perspective. He made this clear in his congressional testimony on March 1—the same day he sent the above-mentioned memorandum to Acheson regarding the 38th parallel. ★

250

Statement for the House Armed Services Committee[1]

March 1, 1951
Washington, DC

A month ago I appeared before you gentlemen and gave you a frank report of our military situation. Because I felt the matter was one of great urgency, I took it upon myself to tell you things about the status of our forces in Korea that up to then had been classified "top secret." I told you how short we were of trained military manpower and how costly that had been. That situation has not changed. We still have not made good the deficiencies with which we started in the Far East, nor have we been able to fill the holes we were forced to tear in our units elsewhere in the world because of our acute need for Korean reinforcements and replacements.[2]

It has been my hope that this committee, which is so familiar with the great price this country has paid for its past unpreparedness, would be quick to understand the importance of putting our defenses on a sound and enduring basis in this critical period.

I recall that in my first appearances before committees of the House and Senate in the weeks after my appointment as Secretary there was a considerable feeling that we were not building our Armed Forces up fast enough, that we had set our sights too low on what was needed.[3]

Most of the questioning indicated a belief that we should ask for more men, more money, more facilities. Our troops were in retreat in Korea and the demand was insistent that we do something, anything, provided we did it fast and on a gigantic scale. Today the atmosphere is quite different. Now the questioning is not how much more do we need, but why are we asking so much.

I am not unfamiliar with these abrupt changes in sentiment. I have lived through them before. I saw the Army disintegrate in General Pershing's lap after World War I. I saw the Selective Service Act come within a single vote of repeal only a few months before Pearl Harbor. I saw us cast aside our strength again after VJ-day. These things are familiar to me, but I must confess that I was not prepared for the speed with which the present shift in sentiment has developed.[4]

Only 2 months ago I was being criticized for not requesting a force in being of 5 or 6 million. There were even suggestions that the force should be equal to our wartime peak of 12,000,000. We resisted these suggestions because we felt it would be dangerous for the United States to overload its productive economy with a force that was beyond our immediate needs. We felt it was far wiser to draw our security plans on a foundation that would involve minimum disruption of the civilian economy, while at the same time insuring our ability to invoke the needed military strength quickly in a crisis that might develop this year or 20 years from now.

We have submitted to your committee a universal military training and service bill that represents a realistic answer to that need in my opinion. It enables us to expand our immediate combat strength to the number deemed necessary by the

Joint Chiefs of Staff. It assures a dependable flow of trained manpower into the National Guard and our other civilian Reserve components so that we can maintain maximum available strength with the smallest necessary expenditures of men or dollars.

This is the sensible, the practical way of meeting our military requirements now and in the future, in my opinion. It is effective, it is economical, it is democratic.

I do not pretend that the bill we submitted was perfect in all its details. Many improvements have already been suggested by the members of your committee. We welcome these changes. But we cannot view with favor proposals that would strike at fundamental principles of this legislation or that would seriously restrict the ability of the Armed Forces to fulfill their mission.

I am particularly concerned with your suggestion that no man be made eligible for induction until he is 18 ½, rather than 18, as we have recommended. Let me give you my reasons.

I believe we can agree that there is no real mental or physical difference between 18-year-olds and 18 ½-year-olds. Some 18-year-olds are mature beyond their years. Some 18 ½-year-olds are often young for their age. So far as capabilities are concerned, there is little, if any, choice between 18-year-olds, 18 ½'s, or 19's. So far as needs for the man and service to the country are concerned, there is a big difference.

We believe that 18 is the most desirable age for the individual. Consultation with representatives of management, labor, education, and extended in our own Armed Forces in an effort to determine an age most convenient to the greatest number of American young men for training and service, resulted in our conclusion that 18 was the ideal age.

Eighteen and one-half is not as good an age because eighteen is the normal age for graduation from high school. To postpone training for 6 months until the young man becomes 18 ½ would offer no substantial benefit to him.

On the contrary, he would be reluctant to take a job knowing that he would be in uniform 6 months later. Nor would his employer be very eager to start him off. And the prospect of starting college only to have it interrupted at the end of 1 year would not be appealing either.

All the testimony that has been offered from men prominent in education, science, industry, mental health, and community life has supported the idea that 18 is the best time to induct a young man. This is based on what is best for the man and what is best for the country.

Now, let us examine the arithmetic in the problem. We estimate we need 3 ½ million men in our Armed Forces today. As a reasonable precaution, we must leave ourselves a margin for expansion in case world conditions worsen. We want to be in such a position that we may be able to expand to 4 million, if necessity requires. That would seem like reasonable defense planning and the kind of planning that I hope your committee will support.

We cannot meet that 4 million figure out of the present 19 to 26 pool even after we reduce our physical and mental standards to the greatest practicable extent. We fall short 245,000 men below the minimum reserve pool required in the selective service operations under General Hershey. If we include 18-year-olds, we get a margin of safety of 76,000.

I submit to you that that is a reasonable margin of safety for an organization that must consider the possibilities of a 4 million man force. We hope it will never be necessary to go above the 3 ½ million figure, but we must prepare for the probability.

The drafting of 18-year-olds has another strong argument in its favor, it seems to me. It will give us enough men to enable us to equalize the sacrifices incident to military service. It would permit us to give our reservists on active duty fairer consideration. When the present emergency broke out we called to active duty many reservists who already had served faithfully in war, many of them under arduous field conditions.

Moreover, a large number of the recalled are past the age limit we have set for men coming in now through the selective service. These reservists should be allowed to return to civil life at the earliest practicable date. We cannot let them go home now because we cannot spare them. If we do not get a sufficient expansion of our pool of available manpower, we will have to continue them in uniform. I hope we will not be forced to do that. With 18-year-olds available we will not have to do that. We will be glad to return reservists to civil life after they have performed a reasonable period of service.

We are strongly opposed to the committee's plan to remove from the bill the proposal that up to 75,000 young men a year may be deferred in the first 3 years of the program in order that they may pursue college courses. We are opposed because we realize that our own strength lies not only in the number of men we have in uniform. We appreciate the importance of science and technology in national defense. It is in full recognition of that fact that we have provided for the deferment of such 75,000 men.[5]

The men to be selected, it should be emphasized, are deferred and in no way exempted from their military obligations. They will have to perform their services after their college courses are completed. Nor is 75,000 a mere arbitrary figure. It, too, represents the consensus of constructive consideration by leaders in the fields of science, industry, and education. They helped us arrive at this figure.

Nor is 75,000 a fixed figure for an indefinite period. It operates for but 3 years. It is intended to bridge a gap that might have developed if we withdrew all of our men from college during the early period of the operation of this act.

Of all of the provisions for universal military training and service, this provision for the education of the 75,000 has received the fullest support of the American people and especially of our educators and scientists. The fact that the selection of the 75,000 and of the courses that they will pursue in the colleges will be made under civilian direction assures us that our established democratic principles of liberal education will not suffer. No one need fear that under our system either the colleges or the students will become militarized nor will the operation of the act necessitate the wholesale closing of colleges and universities because of a lack of students.

There are two other provisions I should like to mention briefly. One is the committee's unwillingness to lift the 2-percent ceiling that now exists on the voluntary recruitment of women into the permanent military services. At a time when we want the broadest assumption or responsibility for meeting our national needs, I am at a loss to understand why we should keep out of the services any woman who wants to come in and who can be usefully employed in the Military Establishment and offer them the chance of a permanent career in the services. The more women we have within our needs, the more we will be able to release for field duty. That is as true now as it would be under conditions of total mobilization. I hope the ceiling will be removed.[6]

I am also concerned over the proposal for a mandatory legal requirement that we reduce our minimum standards of physical acceptability to those that we applied in January 1945. It is important to remember that we were scraping the bottom of the manpower barrel by January of that year.[7]

We were obliged to take men of marginal military utility because there were just no other men we could take without doing irreparable damage to other phases of our total effort. What is more, we were able to distribute these men among a force of nearly 12 million, as against the 3 ½ million force we now anticipate.

With a force of that size, it is much easier to accommodate a considerable number of men who could not ordinarily be used even for the most limited duty that it is under present conditions. It should also be borne in mind that the efficiency of those men was very low, and the medical and pension costs their employment ultimately involved was very high. These considerations make it highly inadvisable to force us to go too far by statute at this time.

We have already assured your committee of our determination to do everything that can be done, consistent with military efficiency, to utilize men in limited-service work and to bring down our physical and mental requirements. We ask you not to tie our hands by removing any flexibility in our operations.

It is equally our determination to reduce the costs of our Armed Forces once we get them properly equipped. We believe that once the equipment job is completed we will be able to maintain an armed strength of 3 ½ million men at the cost of 35 billion dollars annually, provided, of course, present price levels prevail, and the international situation does not deteriorate.

As a result of the operation of universal military training and service over a number of years, we believe we would build up our reserves in such strength as to enable us to reduce our Armed Forces below the 3 ½ million figure. When such a reduction takes place, the annual cost of our Armed Forces will be reduced in general in approximate proportion to the principle of the 35 billion dollars cost for 3 ½ million men.

You have charged us with a great responsibility. We believe we have put forward a constructive program for carrying out that responsibility on a basis that is within the capacity of our economy to support and that will be adequate to cope with any emergency. Our survival depends on the carrying forward of that program decisively and effectively.[8]

House Committee on Armed Services, *Hearings . . . on H.R. 1752*, 436–439.

1. Marshall began his testimony with off-the-record and unpublished comments in executive session that the editors have been unable to locate.

2. See pp. 338–47.

3. See pp. 276–78 and 291–93. See also Marshall's testimony before the joint Senate Armed Services and Foreign Relations Committees, pp. 380–86.

4. See p. 268n9.

5. Section 1, subsection r of the proposed legislation authorized the president "until June 30, 1954, to provide for the temporary removal from active training and service upon completion of their initial periods of basic training in the Armed Forces" of up to seventy-five thousand people to allow them pursue university studies in any field determined "to be in the national interest." A new version of the bill, H. R. 2811, submitted after an analysis of the Senate version of the bill, eliminated this provision. (House Committee on Armed Services, *Hearings . . . on H.R. 1752*, 3, 295–301.) See pp. 393–97.

6. See p. 404n2.

7. A Senate amendment to the bill required the Defense Department to reclassify one hundred thousand men who had been designated as "4-F," ineligible to serve due to failing to meet the established physical and mental standards. ("390,000 Draft Pool Seen in Bid to Call 4-F's and Childless," *New York Times*, January 30, 1951, p. 1.)

8. Following Marshall's statement, Carl Vinson recognized that Marshall "and a great many members of the committee have been sick with the flu, so we are not going to tax your strength unduly." Vinson wanted to clarify to Marshall, however, that "the way the committee bill is written there is only 3 months' difference between 18 year olds and what the committee proposes"; that "the President has [a] right to put in 75,000 or 150,000, whatever number he wants to, for education purposes" and deferment; and that "in regard to removing the percentage of women in the service, this, as we visualize it, is a draft law and we want to confine it only to drafting," although he was "satisfied the committee will entertain favorably just as soon as a bill is sent here to deal with that in a separate bill." (House Committee on Armed Services, *Hearings . . . on H.R. 1752*, 440.)

251

To Erle Cocke Jr.

March 2, 1951
Washington, DC

Dear Cocke: Thank you for serving on our Citizen's Advisory Committee on Armed Services Training Installations which is to report to me on the adequacy of the physical plants, living standards and the health and welfare of personnel in the various Armed Services Training Installations.[1]

As you know, the Committee was formed for the purpose of making certain that the Armed Forces have the benefit of the fullest citizens guidance and advice in developing their facilities and personnel programs. In establishing the Committee, I assured the members that they would have full and free access to every part of the training program and that they would have every opportunity to talk to individual men and women in training and receive first hand their reactions and suggestions.

Now that you are about to leave on an extended trip abroad, I hope that you will utilize as much time as possible during your journey to examine those aspects of the Committee's area of interest which you encounter at overseas installations.[2] Faithfully yours,

GCMRL/G. C. Marshall Papers (Secretary of Defense, Number Indexed, M200-10-20)

1. On February 26, Marshall had announced the creation of the Citizens Advisory Committee on Armed Services Training Installations, an organization of "seven outstanding citizens" asked to "inspect Armed Services' training installations and, on the basis of their study, advise him as to their adequacy and to suggest possible improvements." The committee would investigate housing, living standards, and personnel related to their nearby communities during the recruits' time in training. Lovett, Bradley, and other officials met with the seven-member committee on February 26. (Press release, "Committee of Prominent Citizens to Study Adequacy of the Armed Services' Training Installations," February 26, 1951, GCMRL/G. C. Marshall Papers [Secretary of Defense, Speeches and Statements].)

Marshall informed Senator Lyndon Johnson on March 20 that the committee had been formed shortly after Rosenberg joined the Defense Department. (Marshall to Johnson, March 20, 1951, NA/RG 330, Office of the Assistant Secretary of Defense for Manpower and Personnel, Chronological File [November 1950–December 1951].)

2. Cocke's tour took him to Japan, the Philippines, Formosa, and Korea, as well as stops in Europe that included audiences with Pope Pius XII in Rome and Generalissimo Francisco Franco in Madrid. ("Legion Chief to Inspect Bases," *New York Times*, March 3, 1951, p. 11; "Legion Chief Goes to Orient," *New York Times*, p. 10.)

In late March and early April, the other six members of the committee toured installations around San Diego, California, and the Great Lakes Training Station near Chicago, Illinois. (Rosenberg to Marshall, memorandum, March 28, 1951, NA/RG 330, Office of the Assistant Secretary of Defense for Manpower and Personnel, Chronological File [November 1950–December 1951].)

252

To Dean G. Acheson — March 5, 1951
Top Secret — Washington, DC

Dear Mr. Secretary: In view of the world situation, the Joint Chiefs of Staff consider it of military importance to use the occasion of the forthcoming Meeting of Consultation of Ministers of Foreign Affairs of the American Republics, scheduled to open in Washington on 26 March 1951, to press for the achievement of certain military objectives in Latin America. In this connection, the Joint Chiefs of Staff reaffirm the validity of the military measures and objectives outlined in both the Analysis and the Conclusions of NSC 56/2, "United States Policy Toward Inter-American Military Collaboration," dated 18 May 1950. They consider, therefore, that those points should be pressed in general and in detail.[1]

From the military point of view, action to achieve the following purposes appears to be particularly important at this time:

(a) The acknowledgment by the American Republics of the necessity for self-help and mutual aid in preparation for meeting and defeating aggression. The principle that each nation has a moral obligation to prepare itself to contribute its full share to defense of the hemisphere should be emphasized. Likewise, the necessity for assisting neighbor republics through mutual aid should be stressed.

Some of the forms of mutual aid contemplated are the use of military bases, the provision of strategic raw materials, assistance in the procurement of military equipment and the provision of military training facilities;

(b) Approval by the several Latin American nations of the "Common Defense Scheme for the American Continent." This scheme, adopted by the Inter-American Defense Board (IADB), has as yet been approved only by the governments of the United States and Cuba;[2]

(c) Willingness on the part of the Latin American Republics to proceed urgently with ADDITIONAL military plans to assure effective collective hemisphere defense. Such plans would include statements of the strategic military objectives of the American States, of the roles and missions of the several states in meeting such objectives, and of the strategic military requirements of the several states as derived therefrom. The development of military assistance programs for Latin America, if they are to be both effective and economical, must be based upon a foundation of such objective military planning;

(d) Acknowledgment of the necessity as a primary matter for using contingents of the armed forces of the several American Republics within the boundaries of the Western Hemisphere in order to maintain the security of the hemisphere. Its defense with Latin American forces operating in Latin America should be regarded as the initial task for the Latin American nations. The machinery of the hemispheric regional organization should not be used to provide armed forces for service outside the region. Further, the Joint Chiefs of Staff would find serious military objection to the establishment, for the Western Hemisphere, of a military organization parallel or similar to that of the North Atlantic Treaty Organization, because such an organization would not be in consonance with the Joint Chiefs of Staff concept of operations in the Western Hemisphere and in fact would otherwise seriously interfere with the effective conduct of a global war;

(e) Agreement that the several Latin American Governments will support actively the work of the IADB and will consider promptly the plans and recommendations of that body. In this connection, however, the Joint Chiefs of Staff would not acquiesce in any arrangement for the command participation of the IADB in Western Hemisphere strategy or operations; and

(f) Establishment of the principle of the maintenance of national armed forces tailored to meet the requirements of hemisphere defense. Such a principle is in direct contrast to the existing nationalism in Latin America which dictates a policy of military power balance in all arms vis-à-vis neighbors. Each nation should be encouraged to strengthen those military forces best adapted to the execution of the tasks which it accepts in the defense of the hemisphere.

The Joint Chiefs of Staff assume that the processes used in the subject conference relating to the approval, from the military point of view, of position papers or draft resolutions will follow the procedures already established in connection with other Meetings of Heads of State or with the Councils of Foreign Ministers.

I am in full accord with the preceding recommendations of the Joint Chiefs of Staff, and urge that this Government take every advantage of the opportunity offered by the forthcoming Inter-American Meeting to secure their adoption by the other participating nations, as primary military objectives of the United States.

On the other hand, these present recommendations of the Joint Chiefs of Staff do not, in my opinion, preclude a determined effort by this Government to awaken the Latin American nations to their responsibility to provide ground forces for service in Korea in the near future, as recommended by the Joint Chiefs of Staff and set forth in my letter to you of 30 January 1951, to which your reply of 23 February 1951 refers.[3] Such action in support of the United Nations will be consonant with the Program of United Nations Action to Stop Aggression, approved by the President as U.S. Governmental policy on September 16, 1950, following consideration in the National Security Council. Subparagraph (d) above postulates that the machinery of the Organization of American States, including the Inter-American Defense Board, should not be used to provide armed forces for service outside the Western Hemisphere. Any steps in this connection should therefore be pursued by the United States in its capacity as executive agent for the United Nations in accordance with the Security Council resolutions of June 25, June 27 and July 7, 1950, rather than within the framework of the Inter-American System.[4] Faithfully yours,

NA/RG 330, CD 381 (Inter-American Collaboration)

1. In light of the Chinese intervention in Korea, Acheson on December 16 had called for a consultative meeting of the foreign affairs ministers of the member states of the Organization of American States (OAS), pursuant to the charter agreed to at the Bogota conference in April 1948, to discuss economic and manpower policies to ensure the defense of the western hemisphere. On December 20, the OAS Council agreed to hold such a meeting in Washington. (*FRUS, 1951*, 2: 928–29; "U.S. and Latin American Nations Set Parley to Bolster Hemisphere Defense," *New York Times*, December 21, 1950, p. 16.) For more on the Bogota conference, see *Papers of GCM*, 6: 426–38.

To ensure hemispheric security in the event of a global war and the ensuing planned "transoceanic projection of major U.S. offensive power," NSC 56/2 concluded that "the United States should make every effort" to use "indigenous armed forces in Latin America" and to encourage "inter-American military collaboration" and "development of agreed collective defense plans." It consequently recommended that the Inter-American Defense Board create a Western Hemisphere Defense Scheme, and that the United States, in order to maximize efficiency in collective defense, should "assist Latin American nations to obtain from U.S. sources the armaments required" to maintain "only those armed forces necessary to meet their obligations for collective defense." (*FRUS, 1950*, 1: 628–37, quotes on 635–36.)

2. Marshall had forwarded a copy of this common defense scheme to Acheson on December 16, 1950, and on January 15, 1951, the State Department approved use of the plan as the basis for the development of a collective defense agreement at the upcoming foreign ministers meeting. For Marshall's letter, see *FRUS, 1950*, 1: 679–80.

3. For these letters, see *FRUS, 1951*, 7: 147, 194–95.

4. These resolutions called on UN member states to provide any assistance possible to the ROK and authorized the US to command the international UN forces in Korea. General Burns, Director of the State Department's Office of Regional American Affairs Ivan B. White, and Edward A. Jamison, officer in charge of special political problems under White, added this final paragraph since they believed the JCS views listed above "would be a serious bar to achieving the common State-Defense aim of securing additional ground force units from Latin America for service in Korea." (Burns to Marshall, memorandum, March 2, 1951, NA/RG 330, CD 381 [Inter-American Collaboration].)

Acheson replied on March 20 that he believed it was possible "to stimulate political support and more active backing" by Latin American countries for UN collective security measures and the Uniting for Peace resolution (see p. 366n2), in addition to addressing the JCS military objectives, without using OAS pathways and thus not contradict JCS recommendations. He attached a position paper in preparation for the upcoming conference which called on the US to foster the approval of a resolution that would affirm the responsibility of Latin American countries as UN member countries "to support UN action against aggression in other parts of the world." (Acheson to Marshall and attachments, March 20, 1951, ibid.)

Acheson replied further to Marshall on April 26 that "the views of the Joint Chiefs of Staff and the Department of Defense on proposals and position papers" of the recently concluded OAS meeting were "accurately reflected in the resolution finally approved on the pertinent subjects." (Acheson to Marshall, April 26, 1951, ibid.)

One country the United States unsuccessfully attempted to convince to send troops to Korea was Brazil. Despite efforts by Marshall, Truman, and the State Department, Brazil never sent troops. (*FRUS, 1951*, 7: 383; "Brazil Would Vote Curbs on Red China," *New York Times*, May 2, 1951, p. 4; "Brazil May Send Troops," *New York Times*, June 27, 1951, p. 4.)

253

To Major General Forrest Harding — March 5, 1951
Washington, DC

Dear Harding: I sent you and Eleanor a telegram from Katherine and myself the other evening expressing our sympathy, and this morning on my return from Pinehurst, I found your letter written I believe the same day little Eleanor [*Anne*] died.[1]

I was relieved to learn that her final days were peaceful and I suppose the end was really a blessing under the circumstances. However, I know what a terrific shock and sorrow this is to Eleanor and you. It's pretty hard to understand such things. I remember Anne Hayne's case. It seemed so wholly unnecessary and cruel and yet she had had some opportunity at an interesting life.[2]

I hope Eleanor can bear up in this distress. Give her my love.

Katherine and I were down at Pinehurst for a weekend two weeks ago and flew back to Washington just in time to go to bed with the flu,—the first attack I have had for six or eight years, but unfortunately not her first attack. It kept us down for about ten days and she has quite a ways to go before she fully recovers. I was under the necessity of getting out of bed and going before committees of Congress and returning to bed which is not a very happy way of convalescence. I also had to go up to New York and speak before some twenty thousand people at Madison Square Garden. The railroad gave me a car so I stayed in bed all the way up and went to my hostess' home and went to bed there and just got up in time to go to the Garden and immediately on making my talk I headed for the train and went to bed again. Unfortunately the next morning I had to go before a committee of Congress and that is an ordeal.[3]

I left Katherine at Pinehurst. Thank goodness! And she already showed considerable improvement because it is beautiful down there.

With all of our sympathy and affection.[4] Faithfully yours,

GCMRL/G. C. Marshall Papers (Secretary of Defense, Number Indexed, M200-1-43)

1. Major General Edwin Forrest Harding (USMA, 1909) had been a friend of Marshall since their service together with the Fifteenth Infantry in Tientsin, China, from 1924 to 1927 and had been the editor of *Infantry Journal* from 1934 to 1938. (For more on Marshall's relationship with Harding, see *Papers of GCM*, 3: 477–78, 553.) Harding's younger daughter, fifteen-year-old Anne, had been diagnosed with osteogenic sarcoma, a form of bone cancer, in 1950. Harding's other daughter, Elinore, whom Marshall had known since his time with Harding in China, had returned home to be Anne's companion and nurse. Marshall wrote on December 26 to offer his prayers and to ask Harding to keep him informed of his daughter's condition. Marshall, who regularly referred to people by incorrect names, confused the names of Harding's two daughters and wrote "little Eleanor" instead of the child's correct name, Anne, in both his December 26, 1950, and March 5, 1951, letters. (Leslie Anders, *Gentle Knight: The Life and Times of Major General Edwin Forrest Harding* [Kent, OH: Kent State University Press, 1985], 306–7; Marshall to Harding, December 26, 1950, and Harding to Marshall, February 28, 1951, GCMRL/G. C. Marshall Papers [Secretary of Defense, Number Indexed, M200-1-43].)

General Harding wrote on February 28 to inform Marshall that Anne Harding died that day. Marshall cabled the Hardings the following day to express his and Mrs. Marshall's sympathy. (Harding to Marshall, February 28, 1951, ibid.; Marshall to Hardings, telegram, March 1, 1951, GCMRL/G. C. Marshall Papers [Secretary of Defense, Chronological, Secretaries, Carlson].)

2. Anne Dulany Hayne was the wife of Colonel Frank B. Hayne, who had served in the Fifteenth Infantry with Harding and Marshall in Tientsin, China. (See *Papers of GCM*, 1: 386–87 and 540–41.) She had died in 1933 at age thirty-three. Marshall had also known her parents, who lived in Upperville, Virginia, and had served as a pallbearer at the funeral of Anne's father in 1940.

3. The Marshalls had spent February 16–18 at Pinehurst. He addressed a Red Cross rally on February 27 at 8:45 p.m. in New York City, returned to Washington at 7:15 a.m. on February 28, and testified before the House Armed Services Committee on March 1 on the UMT bill. See pp. 405–7 and 409–13.

4. General Harding's wife, Eleanor, replied on June 9 to thank Marshall for his sympathy. "It was hard for me to write coherently for a long time afterward." (Harding to Marshall, June 9, 1951, GCMRL/G. C. Marshall Papers [Secretary of Defense, Number Indexed, M200-1-43].)

254

TO MRS. JOHN SINGER

March 5, 1951
Washington, DC

Dear Marie, Katherine and I have been battling with the flu for the past two weeks. But I had to get out of bed to go to New York to make a talk in Madison Square Garden and then get out of bed to go before a committee of Congress and back to bed.[1]

We flew down to Pinehurst Friday and it was perfectly beautiful there,—shrubs and some of the trees are in bloom. I left her there and flew up here this morning. Have to go to New York this afternoon to talk at Columbia University.[2] She will stay at Pinehurst I hope for two weeks, and I hope I can go back there this week-end again. But it will depend on our struggles here with Congress, strikes, etc. It is not a peaceful world and when you are at the hub, it is a pretty tough business.[3]

My love. Affectionately,

GCMRL/G. C. Marshall Papers (Secretary of Defense, Number Indexed, M200-4-6)

1. Marie Marshall Singer was Marshall's sister. For this speech and testimony, see pp. 405–7 and 409–13.

2. For Marshall's speech at Columbia University, see the next document.

3. Singer replied that reports of pending snow around her home in Greensburg, Pennsylvania, were "nothing in comparison to the bad war news and also the stupendous job you are doing—I only hope it will not wear you down. I am very much concerned about you all the time." (Singer to Marshall, n.d., GCMRL/G. C. Marshall Papers [Secretary of Defense, Number Indexed, M200-4-6].)

255

REMARKS AT COLUMBIA UNIVERSITY

March 5, 1951
New York, New York

The subject assigned for my talk tonight, as you already know, is "The Citizen Looks at his Country."[1]

In the very early days of our history as a nation, a distinguished American citizen and a student of the original Kings College, took a similar look at our country of that day and age. He described it in a letter for the benefit of the American Minister to Great Britain, who then was living in London. That letter from Alexander Hamilton to Rufus King in October 1798 explored the state of the American public mind, discussed the temper of Congress and commented upon the efficiency of the Executive Departments. It contained one paragraph that seems of special significance for us.

"I anticipate with you," wrote Hamilton, "that this country will ere long assume an attitude correspondent with its great destinies—majestic, efficient and operative of great things. A noble career lies before it."[2]

Today, 153 years later, it may well be said that we have assumed such an attitude. We are leading the free world in a united effort to realize man's cherished hopes of peace and security. If we and those who are aligned with us succeed, and succeed we must, a noble career will lie ahead of us for this country and all of mankind.

The free world is waging a struggle for peace and vigorously working for security on many fronts. Under the banner of the United Nations it is striving to establish an international order for the peaceful discussion and solution of world problems. It is now engaged in fighting the forces of aggression in Korea. In the Western Hemisphere it is promoting unity of action through the organization of the American states. In the North Atlantic and Western European area it is mobilizing men and munitions to discourage aggression and to defeat it if that becomes necessary. In all of these efforts the United States is playing a leading and courageous role.

It is the last of these closely inter-related projects that has an especial interest for you Columbia men today. The success of the plans for the defense of Western Europe will depend to a great extent upon the leadership of your President, General Eisenhower, who has again donned his uniform in the service of the country.

We all realize that his assignment is one of exceeding difficulty. We know that it is hard to get the members of the armed forces of the same country to work together as a team. It was harder to get allies in time of war faced with a common and great danger to forget their differences and submit themselves to over-all plans of operation. Now to whip into shape a team of twelve sovereign states, in a period short of all-out war, and secure their acceptance of certain roles and their wholehearted support in carrying out their assigned missions is a responsibility for the leader without historic precedent. We believe General Eisenhower can do that job; and what is far more important, everyone of the other North Atlantic Treaty states shares that belief. They have pledged him their support. They are willing to place their troops under his command and let them become part of the integrated force necessary for the defense of Western Europe.

It will be up to every one of the members of this team of soverign states to contribute its full part to this common undertaking.

The development of an effective system of mutual defense for Western Europe calls for the full support of the American people. We are assigning Army, Navy, and Air Forces to the program—much more support on sea, and in the air, than on the ground. But we are not neglecting the latter for experience of battle from earliest times down to the current campaign in Korea points to the continued and decisive role of ground forces, and there is no new development on the horizon that would relegate the foot soldier to limbo in the near future.

We are going to send to Europe four Infantry divisions and their supporting troops not only because of the psychological effect on the ground troops of the other nations who are contributing so many more men, but because we believe such a force would help make free Europe hard to conquer. The combined and integrated ground forces of the North Atlantic Treaty states properly deployed and heavily supported from the air and aided from the sea should give an imprudent aggressor something to think about before he dare set out on a hostile venture.[3]

There are people who fear that the very augmentation of our troops, and particularly ground troops, will give the aggressor the excuse that he is looking for to justify an attack. That threat exists, of course. It existed when we set out to help restore the economy of Western Europe. It existed when we gave military aid to Greece and to Turkey.[4] There is always a risk in positive action but the risk becomes far greater if we hesitate to act with courage, intimidated to the point that we become paralyzed and do nothing. Our antagonist needs no excuse, that government will strike whenever it chooses. It has no tempering public opinion to consider. It has few standards of integrity or honor to observe.

In the early days of our country France, under Napoleon, which then threatened the peace of the world, tried such tactics and Rufus King, our American Minister to Great Britain to whom I referred earlier, cautioned his friend, Alexander Hamilton, against its influence. He wrote: "France. . . . .has believed that our government like that of every country that she succeeded to overturn and enslave, would act with such timidity and in so qualified a manner, that the affections and support of the people would be easily withdrawn from and even turned against it. If the Government continues to speak and act with decision, the people will become more and more united, and still better inclined to execute its purposes."[5]

That was the proper reaction to intimidation 150 years ago. That is good sense today. We and all the nations who have made common cause with us are a formidable array of potential might and genius. We are not yet as strong as we would like to be but we are making rapid progress toward that end. Already we may be giving our enemies some occasion to pause. There is no excuse however for even a suspicion of complacency. On the other hand, there is certainly no reason to lose faith in our ability to meet any challenge ultimately. But before we can achieve ultimate success there may be a period of many sacrifices, but they will be unavoidable. We seem to have planned it that way, or I should say, by failing to act when we had the time for action we have made it inevitable.

Throughout our history we had the chance to develop a system of Universal Military Training to give us reserves available for emergency. We have deliberately rejected these opportunities. In a much more limited fashion that opportunity still exists. I hope we can take advantage of it this time. I hope we can set up an enduring system of national defense to support us through the years especially when the tide flows in our favor and the temptation to relax develops.

The citizen who looks at his country today should find great encouragement in the sincerity and intensity of our readiness to face reality and to prepare and train accordingly. Of course he notes signs of dissension, jockeying for position, some carping criticism, and some real and fancied bewilderment. These faults seem to go with democracy but the democratic process continues sound. We must not lose patience. In a democracy we prefer to thrash out the matter of the 18 year olds, for instance, and give hearings to every point of view. We lose time and valuable time, but we must give heed in a democracy to those who disagree. It is only countries like Russia that know exactly what to do with 18 year olds and any other young men and when to do it. I doubt if they or their parents or even their nominal representatives have much of anything to say in the matter, or can dare to look at the proceedings with a critical gaze. In America the citizen may look at his country at any time and criticize it freely.

The most important word in the title of my address is the citizen himself. If the citizen exercises his rights, performs his duties and accepts his responsibilities as a citizen, he will always have a great country—a wonderful democracy to be proud of. The code for his conduct was laid down by our first President and is still worth repeating.

George Washington asked that "All of us act the part of good citizens; contributing our best endeavors to maintain the Constitution, support the laws, and guard our Independence against all assaults from whatsoever quarter they may come. Clouds," he said, "may and doubtless often will in the vicissitudes of events, hover over our political concerns, but a steady adherence to these principles will not only dispel them but render our prospects the brighter by such temporary obscurities."[6]

The obscurities that followed World War II, I hope have proved temporary. "A noble career still lies before" us.[7]

GCMRL/G. C. Marshall Papers (Secretary of Defense, Speeches and Statements)

1. On July 10, 1950, Eisenhower, then president of Columbia University, had invited Marshall to deliver in early 1951 one of a series of six public lectures "designed to stimulate and to inform, to arouse our people from their political apathy and blind prejudices, to focus public interest on the grave issues now confronting us as a nation." Eisenhower understood that because of the state of world affairs, Marshall might have to make a tentative acceptance. "I will give you now a tentative acceptance," Marshall responded on July 17. "I emphasize to 'you' for I am giving it to you and not to Columbia and I am purposely handling it on that basis when I have to explain myself regarding a number of regrets I have made to similar invitations." On February 22, Marshall confirmed the date of March 5 and requested that his $150 honorarium check "be made out in favor of the American National Red Cross and credited to the Leesburg Loudon County Fund Campaign." Approximately fifteen hundred people attended the 8:30 p.m. speech. (Eisenhower to Marshall and attached press release, July 10, 1950; Marshall to Eisenhower, July 17, 1950; Marshall to Potter, February 22, 1951; George to Marshall, memorandum, February 28, 1951; and Potter to American National Red Cross, March 6, 1951, GCMRL/G. C. Marshall Papers [Secretary of Defense, Number Indexed, M214-8-43].)

2. For the full letter from Hamilton, the first secretary of the treasury and at the time a practicing lawyer in New York, to Rufus King, the American minister to Great Britain, dated October 2, 1798, see Harold C. Syrett, ed., *The Papers of Alexander Hamilton*, vol. 22, *July 1798–March 1799* (New York: Columbia University Press, 1975): 192.

3. The Senate was currently deliberating a plan to send four divisions to Europe. For Marshall's testimony on this debate, see pp. 380–86.

4. For more on the European Recovery Program and US military aid to Greece and Turkey, consult the index of volume 6 of *Papers of GCM.*

5. For the full letter, dated July 31, 1798, see *Papers of Alexander Hamilton*, 22: 44.

6. This statement comes from Washington's letter to the citizens of Alexandria, Virginia, on March 23, 1797. See John C. Fitzpatrick, ed., *The Writings of George Washington from the Original Manuscript Sources, 1745–1799*, vol. 35, *March 30, 1796–July 31, 1797* (Washington: GPO, 1940), 423.

7. Russell Potter, director of Columbia University's Institute of Arts and Sciences, which hosted the lecture, thanked Marshall on March 6 for his "most memorable" address. (Potter to Marshall, March 6, 1951, GCMRL/G. C. Marshall Papers [Secretary of Defense, Number Indexed, M214-8-43].)

256

To Mrs. John B. Wilson — March 6, 1951
Washington, DC

Dear Rose: I received your letter of February 27 this morning enclosing that old letter of mine of twenty-six years ago. The letter is being returned to you under this cover.[1]

Last night I talked to Columbia University. One of the professors—I think he is a dean—told me that your Mother had planned to attend this talk but had not been feeling well enough. He said he was from Durham and had been a great friend of your Father and I believe of your Mother's Father.[2]

I hope you and your family are all well.

Give my regards to John. Believe me, always with love, Affectionately,

P.S. I think your Red Cross talk was excellent. I am returning that manuscript to you also.[3]

GCMRL/G. C. Marshall Papers (Secretary of Defense, Number Indexed, M200-6-31)

1. See pp. 312–13. Wilson had written to thank Marshall for several letters he had written over the winter, "one about driving to your office through our old 'playground' and the other from Pinehurst. It's nice to receive letters like those, it reminds me that you are the same Col. Marshall you were those years and years ago when I was little (not little, I guess!, young) and you were just a brilliant young Army officer and not the famous General and Statesman you are today." (Wilson to Marshall, February 27, 1951, GCMRL/G. C. Marshall Papers [Secretary of Defense, Number Indexed, M200-6-31].) Rose Page Wilson referred to Marshall as "Colonel Marshall," his rank when she first knew him as a child, as a term of endearment long after he was promoted.

Wilson had enclosed with her letter Marshall's twenty-six-year-old letter with a request that it be returned, along with a Red Cross speech she had recently written. The "twenty-six-year-old letter" may be the January 10, 1924, note from Marshall to young Rose Page in GCMRL/J. Page Wilson Collection.

2. See the previous document. The editors have been unable to identify this professor.

3. Wilson had told Marshall that she "was asked to write a speech for . . . our Fund Chairman here," who had asked for something to counteract the "unfavorable publicity" that the Red Cross had received in North Carolina over its separate fundraising drive, its home service program, and disaster assistance. (Ibid.) For more on Wilson's involvement with the American Red Cross, see pp. 146–47.

257

To the Members of the United States Senate

March 6, 1951
Washington, DC

My dear Senator I am informed that the Senate will be asked to vote on a proposal that all sections relating to Universal Military Training be eliminated from the Universal Military Training and Service bill, now under discussion.[1]

In my opinion this is not just another amendment, to be given hasty consideration. Scrapping the Universal Military Training provisions would cut the heart out of the bill. The distinctive contribution the bill makes to our national security would be removed. This single action would be sufficient to cancel the assurance that our defenses would have, for the first time, an enduring base that would guarantee us adequate military strength at a cost we could bear for the years of critical world tension that we now face.

I have been fearful that the long debate over many details of this legislation would dim the fundamental conception which is the basis of the bill. I believe it is important to restate that purpose now so that every Senator may realize exactly what will be the result of voting to remove the Universal Military Training features from this measure.

This bill is intended to enable us to maintain the strength we need to curb aggression and safeguard peace. We must expand our forces in being with all possible speed. At the same time we must assure a dependable flow of trained young manpower into our civilian reserve components so that we can transfer a larger part of the future responsibility for our security to these citizen groups and thus cut down the size of our professional military establishment, of the troops on active duty.

No man is wise enough to know how long the present emergency will last. One thing we do know. Unless we give unequivocal proof now of our determination to organize our defenses on a sound, long-range basis, our potential enemies will be encouraged to believe that we will, sooner or later, relax our vigilance and provide them with an opportunity to achieve their goal of world domination.

Our past history is a fever chart of panicky mobilization in periods of crisis, followed by too hasty disarmament when the sense of urgency subsided. So long as our enemies have any ground for believing that we will again weary of the cost of preparedness or that we will wreck our economy by attempting to support a standing military organization of large proportions, we can have little hope that they will abandon their aggressive policies and seek an honest peace at the conference table. By the same token, our allies will find it hard to place any confidence in the durability of our support and their will to stand fast against totalitarian pressure will be correspondingly reduced.

Universal Military Training is not a step toward militarizing our country. Its effect in my opinion is precisely the opposite. By building up the civilian reserve and cutting down the regular military establishment or troops on active duty it offers maximum assurance that we can reduce the number of men who must leave their families, their jobs and curtail their education to serve in the Army, Navy and Air Force. It would require fewer men under arms, while giving us a vastly greater number of trained men quickly available for duty in a sudden emergency.

It would distribute the obligation for national defense equitably and democratically among all our young men at the time when fulfillment of this obligation would involve minimum hardship for them, for their communities and for our productive economy. It would permit the maintenance of a strong educational system and prevent any interference with the scientific and technical leadership that is so vital to our total security. It is the common-sense answer to our defense problems in a world situation that may remain tense for a long period of years.

Because this legislation is designed to meet needs that are so unpredictable, the establishment of a fixed expiration date would wipe out much of its value. Any date that was set would represent a marker for those who conspire against us to anchor their hopes that we would revert once again to our old state of vulnerable unpreparedness. Instead of peace, their strategy would be directed toward creating a synthetic atmosphere of calm so that we would strip ourselves of available trained reserves without putting anything in their place.

I am not suggesting that the Congress should adopt this program on a permanent basis and then abandon all concern with its effectiveness or administration. On the contrary, I believe it should be the obligation of the Department of Defense and also of the independent control commission, to be appointed by the President with the advice and approval of the Senate, to render regular reports to the Congress on all aspects of the program.

It is my conviction that any program of such fundamental importance to the

American people should have a full review by the Congress at regular intervals to make certain that it is accomplishing the purpose for which it was set up and that it is being administered in a democratic, economical and effective manner. Such a review should go beyond the comprehensive appraisal that every Governmental program receives each year in the course of its Congressional budget hearings.

My experience in a lifetime of association with the military departments has convinced me that Universal Military Training is an essential element in any genuine program of national security for this country. It is not a new idea. It has been advocated by many thoughtful, peace-loving Americans in all of the years since George Washington first proposed a program of this type 150 years ago.

There are always people who feel that this is not the right time to consider Universal Military Training. In periods of emergency, it is argued that we must concentrate all our attention on building up our immediate strength, not waste energy on long-term plans. In periods of apparent peace, it is argued that we must scale down our strength almost to the last degree.

We have a great national decision to make, a really historic decision. We need Universal Military Training as a fundamental and inseparable part of the bill you are now considering. We cannot draw a line between the problems we must face today and those we may have to face tomorrow. I hope the Senate will not follow the line of evasion or delay. I hope you will vote to approve the basic provisions of this legislation, as reported out by the Senate Armed Service Committee.[2] Faithfully yours,

NA/RG 330, Office of the Assistant Secretary of Defense for Manpower and Personnel, Chronological File (November 1950–December 1951)

1. The Senate considered two amendments on March 9 that would have eliminated provisions for UMT from the bill. The first was proposed jointly by Edwin C. Johnson (R-CO) and John W. Bricker (R-OH), and the second by William Jenner. Each would have essentially extended provisions for Selective Service inductions, which were due to expire in July 1951. (*Congressional Record* 97, pt. 2, 82d Cong., 1st sess., 2174–86, 2202–5.) Marshall sent this letter opposing the amendments to each member of the Senate (ibid., 2184–85).

2. The Johnson-Bricker amendment failed by a vote of 20–68–7, and the Jenner amendment failed by a vote of 18–64–13. (Ibid., 1186, 2205.)

Marshall had been concerned for some time about the large number of amendments that were being proposed during debate on the Senate UMT bill, several of which were offered by Wayne Morse. In response to General Bradley's testimony before the House Armed Services Committee that any man between the ages of eighteen and nineteen would make a "grand" soldier, Morse proposed one amendment that would set the induction age at eighteen and six months. Marshall and Bradley both wrote letters to Senator Lyndon Johnson on February 27, which Johnson inserted into the *Congressional Record*, to express their opposition to this amendment, reiterate their opinion that eighteen was the best age for induction, and clarify Bradley's testimony. The Senate debated Morse's amendment for several days and finally rejected it by a vote of 31–55–10 on March 5. (*Congressional Record* 97, pt. 2, 82d Cong., 1st sess., 1590–98, 1600–1602, 1710, 1897–1910; Marshall to Johnson, February 27, 1951, NA/RG 330, Office of the Assistant Secretary of Defense for Manpower and Personnel, Chronological File [November 1950–December 1951].) See also pp. 325–29, 338–47, 369–71, 393–97, and 409–13.

On March 7, Marshall sent a second letter to Lyndon Johnson opposing another amendment proposed by Morse that would have restricted the total strength of the active duty armed forces to 3.5 million men. "A statutory ceiling on the size of the armed services at this time would be, in effect, a direct gamble with national security in the present chaotic world situation," Marshall warned. The JCS and the president should be free to determine "the country's minimum defense need," and they "cannot fulfill their responsibility if an arbitrary limit is set on the size of our forces. . . . The armed forces have never been throttled with a mandatory ceiling in the midst of a period of great emergency. To do so now would be serious, I believe, far beyond the conception of many who might favor such a procedure in the heat of debate." (Marshall to Johnson, March 7, 1951, NA/RG 330, CD 320.2 [Strength, Military].)

During the floor debate on the Morse amendment, Senator Johnson read this letter and excerpts of similar letters from the JCS opposing the establishment of a ceiling on the strength of the armed forces. He also had the letters in their entirety inserted into the *Congressional Record* and reminded his colleagues that the members of his subcommittee had unanimously declined to include a ceiling in its version of the bill. (*Congressional Record* 97, pt. 2, 82d Cong., 1st sess., 2042–43, 2052–53 [Johnson quote on 2052].)

Morse's amendment was further amended to establish a four million–man ceiling. This version passed by a vote of 49–41–6. With this ceiling, the entire bill passed the Senate on March 9 by a vote of 79–5–11. (Ibid., 2054–57, 2207–10; "Senate Votes to Draft at 18, Sets Service at 24 Months; Fight to Delete U.M.T. Fails," *New York Times*, March 10, 1951, p. 1.)

258

To Madame Chiang Kai-shek

March 6, 1951
Washington, DC

Dear Madame: I am going to dictate this letter because it is both easier for you to read and easier for me to prepare. I received your note of February 6 together with the present of the lovely handkerchiefs that you generously sent me by the hand of General Pee. You are always so generous and thoughtful that I am under great obligations.[1]

As to Katherine, she and I simultaneously developed flu about two weeks ago immediately upon our return from a weekend at Pinehurst. It was of course harder for her to deal with than for me. But it took me all of ten days to work up to the point where I could leave the apartment. As it was I had to get out of bed and go before committees of Congress and from the hearings straight back to bed.[2] Last weekend we returned to Pinehurst and I came back yesterday morning. Katherine remained there and I hope will stay for several weeks in order to regain her strength in that delightful climate and in those lovely surroundings. Things are generally in bloom there now though it is very wintery up here in Washington. A heavy cold spell is sweeping east from the middle west.

General Pee gave me the memorandum from the Generalissimo with his views on certain matters which I am having considered by appropriate officials here in the Defense Department. Please give him my thanks.[3]

Katherine and I are always worried about you,—just how you are getting along. We hope you are not troubled with your nervous reactions that develop so uncomfortably and that climatic conditions are agreeable.

I send you my affectionate regards, with my respects to the Generalissimo.[4]
Faithfully yours,

GCMRL/G. C. Marshall Papers (Secretary of Defense, Selected)

1. For Madame Chiang's February 6 letter, see p. 303n5. In early December, she had sent Marshall for his birthday some handkerchiefs, but they were "still being delayed by the American customs" as of her writing him on February 6. (Madame Chiang to Marshall, February 6, 1951, GCMRL/G. C. Marshall Papers [Secretary of Defense, Selected].)

2. See pp. 409–13.

3. Pee had met with Marshall on February 15 and delivered an oral message from Chiang. At Marshall's request, Pee dictated a report on the strength of Chiang's forces on Taiwan, and on February 21, Pee handed Carter a copy of a two-page list of Chiang's military requirements that had already been submitted to the State Department. (Handwritten memorandum, n.d.; Pee to Marshall, memorandum, February 15, 1951, with Marshall's handwritten comments; Carter to Matthews, memorandum, February 22, 1951, and attachment, NA/RG 330, CD 092 [China].) See pp. 300–301.

Marshall also received a report on Taiwan from Colonel David D. Barrett, army attaché at the American embassy in Taipei, Taiwan, who had known Marshall since serving in China together in the 1920s and again as acting military attaché during Marshall's postwar mission to China. Barrett wrote that "Definite progress on the road toward Democracy had been made in the recent elections in Taiwan," but it had also "become a complete police state, in which the safeguards of personal liberty as we understand them are almost non-existent. The Generalissimo is aging fast, and his contacts are almost altogether with aged reactionaries" who were "rotten to the core." Since the United States was "unwilling to do anything to force a change for the better in this government," though, Bennett felt that "we have no other course than to give" Chiang's government "full military support." Marshall thanked Barrett for his letter "reporting on occurrences at Taiwan" without significant comment. (Barrett to Marshall, January 29, 1951, and Marshall to Barrett, February 21, 1951, NA/RG 330, CD 300-1-3.)

4. Madame Chiang replied on March 29 that she hoped the Marshalls had "fully recovered" from their illnesses and reported that her brother was sending a dehumidifier to counteract the coming humid weather which last year "played havoc with my skin." She added that US Ambassador to Formosa Karl Rankin had informed her "that the fifty million dollars' worth of military equipment for the army is being sent out." There remained a desperate need for shipments of "gasoline both for trucks and planes," which she requested Marshall assist in expediting. (Madame Chiang to Marshall, March 29, 1951, GCMRL/G. C. Marshall Papers [Secretary of Defense, Selected].)

Marshall responded that the US and Formosa governments were cooperating "in formulating import requirements" for gasoline, and the Defense Department was "assisting and procuring from commercial sources gasoline and oil for normal military operating requirements." 1.3 million gallons "of aviation gasoline" had departed the West Coast two weeks prior, and an additional two million "gallons are expected to be concluded within the next three days." (Marshall to Madame Chiang, April 25, 1951, ibid.)

259

Memorandum for General of the Army Omar N. Bradley — March 7, 1951
Secret — Washington, DC

Subject: Negotiations Regarding Pacific Pact
(Re: Japan Peace Treaty)

Mr. Dulles has just gone over the various aspects of his trip to the Far East. He tells me that so far as he knows there has been a general agreement in connection with the bilateral arrangements with Japan as to military provisions of one kind and another. Mr. Earl Johnson, General Magruder and Colonel Babcock were involved in these with General MacArthur and his staff.[1]

What is troubling Mr. Dulles is the fact that the future negotiations regarding the Pacific Pact cannot be carried out in a normal manner due to the complications which would instantly be provoked regarding Communist China or Nationalist Formosa China positions in the matter. Therefore the buttoning up procedure (he tells me that in general things are about 90% agreed to with the British, Australians, New Zealanders) must be carried out in a step by step manner, day by day almost, as a matter of fact. He would like to have someone from the Defense Department alongside him throughout every phase of this feature in order that he can be certain that he is not getting involved in commitments that would be objected to by the Defense Department.

So Dulles wants very much Colonel Babcock to be designated as this man since Babcock enjoys the confidence of General MacArthur and has been with Dulles every step of the way from the Security Council through the Far East. He visualizes Babcock keeping track of what he, Dulles, is doing and in turn keeping this Department, presumably the Chiefs of Staff, constantly informed of the steps being taken or about to be taken, so that we will have the opportunity to advise Dulles at any time this appears necessary.

I am attaching a copy of a letter of February 25 from Dulles to me which I had not seen before, and incidentally, Dulles wishes to have it returned to him because he thinks it is his only copy. This explains the matter somewhat.[2]

It seems to me the arrangement with Babcock is a logical one, though I imagine some other name may be suggested, proposing an officer of more rank and prestige. However, I think in this matter Babcock would better serve the general purpose than another.

Please discuss this with the Chiefs of Staff and let me have your reaction.[3]

NA/RG 330, CD 387 (Japan)

1. See pp. 324–25. On December 12, Dulles had informed Marshall that he would be resuming negotiations on the Japanese peace treaty and wished to have a representative from the Defense Department to accompany him. Dulles requested that Marshall approve the assignment of Colonel C. Stanton Babcock of the army's office for occupied areas, who had been working with Dulles "for the past three months" and had been a participant in the talks with representatives from the Far Eastern Commission member countries. Marshall had replied on December 14 that he would discuss his request with the JCS and service secretaries and noted his support of Babcock. On January 10, Marshall had informed Acheson that he had appointed Assistant Secretary of the Army Earl Johnson to represent the Defense Department with the assistance of both Colonel Babcock and Major General Carter B. Magruder (USMA, 1923), deputy for programs for the assistant army chief of staff for logistics and former chief of the office for occupied areas under the assistant secretary of the army. (Dulles to Marshall, December 12, 1950; Marshall to Dulles, December 14, 1950; and Marshall to Acheson, January 10, 1951, NA/RG 330, SD 092.2 [Peace Treaty].)

Marshall met with Dulles at 10:30 a.m. on March 7.

2. In this February 25 letter, Dulles had explained that due to the progress being made on the negotiations of the Japanese peace treaty and "a possible Pacific Island Pact," full-time Defense Department representation at the talks was crucial. As Magruder and Johnson would not have sufficient time to work on both treaties, Dulles urged Marshall to assign Babcock to his permanent staff, as he had lengthy experience serving on General MacAr-

thur's staff and was the only Defense Department official who had been involved with the Japanese peace treaty negotiations since they began. (Dulles to Marshall, February 25, 1951, ibid.)

3. Marshall's response to Dulles on March 21 affirmed that Babcock was available to Dulles as needed and had been "instructed to keep the Department of Defense informed regarding the work of your Mission." However, if Babcock became "a permanent member of your staff he would become only a working member of your Mission and not a representative of the Department of Defense, and he could no longer serve as an official liaison officer." Marshall believed that from Dulles's perspective, "it might be better to leave Colonel Babcock with his present instructions, which include direct liaison with the various agencies of the Department of Defense in your behalf." Dulles replied later on the same day that Marshall's proposal was "satisfactory" and that he appreciated the cooperation of the entire Defense Department in this matter. (Marshall to Dulles and Dulles to Marshall, March 21, 1951, ibid.)

260

MEMORANDUM OF CONVERSATION — March 7, 1951
Secret — Washington, DC

General Romulo met with Secretary Marshall by appointment at 2:30 this afternoon.[1] First of all, Romulo informed Secretary Marshall that the reorganization of the Philippine Armed Forces had been completed along the lines that Secretary Marshall had previously supported. Romulo then stated that, inasmuch as he had seen President Truman to tell him of the critical situation in the Philippines, he now wished to tell Secretary Marshall that it is so very critical that the Philippines immediately needs more military equipment, and, especially, $50 million of assistance.[2]

Secretary Marshall asked what the $50 million was for. Romulo was not specific and replied somewhat tentatively that the money was needed to pay the troops and would not be used to purchase military equipment. He believed that the $50 million would be over and above the MDA programs planned by the U.S. Government.

Secretary Marshall said that a good portion of the military assistance programs was delivered, and that the U.S. Government would do all it could to continue these deliveries. However, the request for $50 million had many aspects which were quite different from the MDA programs and lay beyond his scope. Therefore, he could not give General Romulo any answer to the request today. Secretary Marshall made it very plain that he could give Romulo no answer at this time.

Secretary Marshall emphasized that he was fully aware, from General Hobbs' reports, of the critical situation in the Philippines, as was the entire U.S. Government. He wanted to do everything he could to help the Philippines and was looking for ways to reinforce their defense against the Huks. He mentioned specifically the problem of defending Clark Field.[3] He pointed out to Romulo that the United States was under great pressure in Korea, where he had hoped for a respite but where he was now anticipating a real crisis coming up soon.

Secretary Marshall asked Romulo to tell President Quirino that he was gratified over the turn of events in the Philippines and hoped that President Quirino would keep working to maintain these improvements. Secretary Marshall stated that he had received encouraging reports on the effective activities of Secretary of National Defense Magsaysay and the Acting Chief of Staff.[4]

The Secretary asked Romulo to tell him frankly of the loyalty of subordinate officers under General Duque. Romulo replied that he returned to Manila a few days after seeing Secretary Marshall in December, at which time he had reported to President Quirino on the need for honest and competent leadership. He had attended a conference with Quirino, Secretary Magsaysay and the Acting Chief of Staff, at which time Quirino had ordered Duque to proceed with the complete reorganization of the Philippine Armed Forces. Romulo assured Secretary Marshall that, as a result, subordinate staff officers were now competent and completely loyal officers with West Point or U.S. Service training. In answer to Secretary Marshall's question, Romulo stated that these officers were not undergoing any political harassment and that they were conducting their work with efficiency and vigor. Romulo also stated that General Hobbs was extremely pleased with these developments.

The Secretary asked General Romulo what he thought about Indonesia. Romulo replied that he was very disappointed with Indonesia which seemed to be following India's general line in the United Nations. Secretary Marshall pointed out that there seemed to be quite a difference between Nehru's attitude in the U.N. and the situation facing India in the north. Romulo agreed with Secretary Marshall's statement that never in political history had there been such a performance as the treatment of Chinese aggression in Korea—calling black white.[5]

At the conclusion of the meeting Romulo handed Secretary Marshall an aide-memoire. The Secretary read this aide-memoire but did not comment on it.[6]

Kenneth T. Young

NA/RG 330, CD Memorandum of Conversation

1. Besides Marshall and Romulo, no other Philippine or Defense Department officials attended this meeting except Kenneth T. Young, who took these minutes.

2. Following their December 21, 1950, meeting (see pp. 306–7), Romulo on December 26 had informed Marshall that President Quirino had signed an executive order to reorganize the Philippine military and announced "major changes in the high-ranking personnel." Romulo believed these actions made it clear that Quirino "is desirous of carrying out your suggestion and has acted most expeditiously." With this in mind, Romulo reasserted the urgency of his request of "United States assistance amounting to fifty million dollars" to create and equip additional battalion combat teams "as well as immediate shipment of the 1951 MDAP" funds. Marshall replied on December 29 and repeated his "suggestion to you at our meeting on 21 December that your Government submit its specific requests through the usual MDAP channels." (Romulo to Marshall, December 26, 1950; and Marshall to Romulo, December 29, 1950, NA/RG 330, SD 091 [Philippines].)

Marshall also had sent Acheson on December 29 a copy of Romulo's December 26 letter. Acheson replied a few weeks later that the changes Romulo reported "are in effect little more than a reshuffling of the present incompetent and corrupt leadership. . . . For political reasons of his own, President Quirino still appears unable to decide on that kind of sweeping change which alone can prove effective." (Acheson to Marshall, January 18, 1951, NA/RG 330, CD 091.3 [MDAP, Philippines]. See also *FRUS, 1951*, 6: 1491–92.)

In the briefing notes for this meeting, General Burns had informed Marshall that "Romulo will probably press for your favorable consideration" of the Philippine request for additional military aid, as Quirino was "extremely critical" of Romulo's "alleged failure to obtain sufficient aid from the United States, and has been on the point of recalling Romulo to Manila." Burns also noted improvements in Philippine military leadership showed a "slow but sure trend toward greater efficiency." (Burns to Marshall, memorandum, March 7, 1951, NA/RG 330, CD Briefings.) Romulo had previously met with Truman on February 28, 1951.

3. Major General Leland S. Hobbs (USMA, 1915) was chief of the Joint US Military Assistance Group (JUSMAG) to the Philippines. Clark Air Force Base, formerly Clark Field, was located near Manila.

4. In early January 1951, Quirino had relieved his chief of staff, Major General Mariano Castañeda, and replaced him with Brigadier General Calixto Duque.

5. Under the leadership of Prime Minister Jawaharlal Nehru and Permanent Representative to the UN Benegal Rau, India had supported the June 1950 resolutions condemning the North Korean invasion but had not offered substantial support to the UN effort since then. India attempted on several occasions to begin cease-fire negotiations that would include admission of Communist China to the UN. Simultaneously, India and Pakistan were disputing their border and claims to power in the provinces of Jammu and Kashmir. During negotiations in early 1951 on a UN resolution condemning the Chinese intervention in Korea, the US representative to the UN, Warren Austin, reported to Acheson that he believed India and Indonesia would be the only two nations of the Arab-Asian group that would not support such a resolution. (William Stueck, *The Korean War: An International History* [Princeton, NJ: Princeton University Press, 1995], 152, 196–97; Tucker, *Encyclopedia of the Korean War*, 1: 357–59, and 2: 723–24; *FRUS, 1951*, 7: 9–13.)

6. Romulo's aide-mémoire summarized the points he had made during this meeting with Marshall and emphasized "the extreme urgency of our request for military assistance." (Romulo aide-mémoire for Marshall, March 7, 1951, NA/RG 330, CD 091.3 [Near East to South Africa].) Retired Major General Harry J. Malony (USMA, 1912), a consultant on southeast Asian affairs in the Defense Department and a representative on the Southeast Asia Aid Policy Committee, reported to Marshall on March 19 that in response to Romulo's aide-mémoire, a State-Defense-Treasury committee "favored giving at least a portion of the amount requested, possibly "10 million dollars applicable to the general project . . . while an additional 11.8 million might be used for purposes not including pay and maintenance of Philippine troops." Marshall in turn requested on March 20 JCS views on this proposal "as a matter of priority" and informed Romulo on the same day that his request for $50 million was under consideration. He also praised the steps taken to reorganize the armed forces and "secure competent, non-political military leaders." (Malony to Marshall, memorandum, March 19, 1951; Marshall to JCS, memorandum, March 20, 1951; and Marshall to Romulo, March 20, 1951, NA/RG 330, CD 091.3, MDAP [Philippines].) See pp. 486–87.

261

To General of the Army Dwight D. Eisenhower — March 8, 1951
Secret Personal — Washington, DC

Dear Eisenhower: We have all been concerned here over the necessity for delay in announcing the movement of troops to Europe. We are ready to come out with a statement that a division is going in April, another in June and two others in the Fall, as soon as the developments regarding the Wherry Resolution will permit. The feeling at the present time is, particularly in the State Department, that an announcement today would have a very unfortunate affect with regard to the action of the Senate.[1]

I am sending you this note merely to advise you that we are very anxious here not only to come out with a statement as indicated above, but to alert the divisions and get things well underway.

We made the announcement regarding the divisions to Japan because we dared not delay any longer because of the wide open situation in Hokkaido. The Chiefs of Staff wanted to include the European announcement the same time but it was felt that would be ruinous to our interests in the Senate. Strange to say, the announcement regarding the two divisions to Japan gave rise to very few comments—none adverse.[2]

I deplore the fact that we cannot hasten our steps in supporting you in your mission.[3] Faithfully yours,

GCMRL/G. C. Marshall Papers (Secretary of Defense, Chronological, Secretaries, Ackerman)

1. For the "Great Debate" and Wherry Resolution, see pp. 333–34 and 380–86. On March 2, Marshall had informed Bradley that he had discussed the announcement with Harriman and Acting Secretary of State James Webb, who was also concerned with the possible impact of the announcement on a forthcoming deputies meeting in Paris to prepare the agenda for a meeting of the Council of Foreign Ministers. All three agreed that the announcement should be made early in order to limit complications with the deputies meeting and that it would be best to announce the complete timetable rather than just the one division in April. Marshall told Bradley regarding the Wherry Resolution "that we will have to wait a few days" to see how the debate is resolved, but once it was "out of the way," he thought "the full announcement should be made." (Marshall to Bradley, memorandum, March 2, 1951, NA/RG 330, CD 371 [Europe].)

On March 6, Carter informed Marshall that the State Department no longer had "any concern" in regard to the impact of an announcement on the deputies meeting, although it believed the announcement would be "catastrophic" to a successful conclusion of the Wherry Resolution debate and the UMT bill. (Carter to Marshall, memoranda, March 6, 1951, ibid.)

2. US officials feared, particularly after the inception of the Dulles presidential mission to negotiate a Japanese peace treaty and with it the possible rearmament of Japan (see pp. 324–25 and 427–29), that the Soviet Union might invade Hokkaido, the northernmost of Japan's four main islands and one containing no American troops. Consequently they reversed a previous decision not to announce the sending of two additional divisions to Japan until after announcement that additional divisions were being sent to Europe. (*FRUS, 1951*, 6: 778–81, 805–9; Bradley to Davis, memorandum, February 8, 1951, NA/RG 218, CCS 381 [Far East].)

3. "I just received your note of the 8th," Eisenhower wrote at the end of a lengthy March 12 letter to Marshall. "I fully understand your reasons—and I concur." (*Papers of DDE*, 12: 121.) For more on the shipment of troops to Europe and Eisenhower's March 12 letter to Marshall, see pp. 455–56 and 472–74.

262

TO HARRY S. TRUMAN — March 8, 1951
Top Secret — Washington, DC

Dear Mr. President: Reference is made to your memorandum of 2 February 1951 concerning the safety, in the event of hostilities, of the American civilian population in Germany and Japan, and expressing your desire that the possibility of their evacuation in case of serious danger should be examined.[1]

At the present time there are approximately 380,000 nonmilitary citizens of the United States in foreign countries. It is estimated that this figure will be increased by about 115,000 during the coming summer tourist season. In this connection it is noted that there are approximately 70,000 nonmilitary United States citizens in Germany and 55,000 in Japan.

The responsible military and civil authorities in Germany and Japan, as in other areas throughout the world, have prepared plans for the emergency evacuation of all United States citizens therein, should the circumstances require.

Factually, it must be stated that transportation and other necessary facilities are inadequate for simultaneous evacuation from those areas which might be reasonably expected to be subject to Soviet action in the event of general hostilities. Additionally, a mass exodus of indigenous refugees, as well as direct enemy action, could be expected to reduce appreciably our capability of evacuation. Accordingly, it must be realized that in the event of general hostilities only a relatively small portion of these people could be evacuated safely.

From the military point of view the Joint Chiefs of Staff consider that the presence of large numbers of United States nonmilitary citizens overseas in potential combat areas constitute a grave military liability in the event of sudden hostilities, and that it would be highly desirable to have a minimum number of nonmilitary personnel in any combat area upon the outbreak of hostilities. It would be militarily desirable that a minimum of military potential be diverted from combat duties in order to execute evacuation plans.

The Joint Chiefs of Staff believe that a number of factors must be considered before reaching a decision relative to an evacuation of nonmilitary personnel from overseas areas prior to an outbreak of hostilities. Among them are:

(a) The political implications regarding our relations with the USSR, with our allies, and with the governments of occupied areas;

(b) The economic effects of tourist travel; and

(c) The effects on United States business interests abroad.

A fourth consideration which is of special importance to the Armed Forces is the adverse effect on morale and the consequent marked reduction in military efficiency resulting from protracted separation of military personnel from their families.

In view of the above, the Joint Chiefs of Staff recommend, and I concur, that at this time action be limited by departments and agencies of the Government to:

(a) A study of the possibility of reducing the number of U.S. civilian employees in sensitive areas, replacing them to the extent practicable by indigenous personnel.

(b) A study of the possibility of reducing business and tourist travel to sensitive areas.

(c) Continuing review by the Joint Chiefs of Staff of recommendations by overseas commanders on policies regarding dependents of military personnel in each of the areas concerned, with recommendations as appropriate by the Joint Chiefs of Staff to the Secretary of Defense.

I concur with these recommendations of the Joint Chiefs of Staff, and have directed that subparagraphs (a) and (c) be explored from the standpoint of the Department of Defense. Subparagraphs (a) and (b), however, also raise a broad question of national policy affecting other government agencies, particularly the Department of State and the Economic Cooperation Administration. I therefore suggest that you may wish to have this question considered by the National Security Council.

The Secretary of State is in accord with this suggestion. If you approve, we will jointly be prepared to consider and discuss the matter at an appropriate future meeting of the Security Council.[2]

With great respect,[3] Faithfully yours,

NA/RG 330, CD 370.05

1. Truman had informed Marshall on February 2 that he had been thinking about American civilians in Germany and Japan should hostilities erupt and asked Marshall to examine "the possibility of their evacuation in case of real danger." Marshall replied on February 5 that he had asked the JCS to look into the matter. (Truman to Marshall, February 2, 1951, and Marshall to Truman, February 5, 1951, NA/RG 330, CD 300-1-2.)

2. Burns reported to Marshall on March 1 that "nonmilitary citizens in potential combat areas overseas constitutes a grave military liability." The JCS recommended further study by the NSC, as these measures should extend to all US nationals living abroad. The JCS recommendations in the letter above had been "fully coordinated with the Washington Liaison Group, the interdepartmental planning agency concerned with protection and evacuation of U.S. nationals overseas." (Burns to Marshall, memorandum, March 1, 1951, NA/RG 330, CD 370.05.)

Lovett asked on a memorandum transmitting a draft of the above letter if the US should "use the introduction of 4 new Divs. to Germany as the excuse to bring out the Army civilians and families." Colonel Carey A. Randall, Lovett's executive officer, had responded on March 6 that the JCS had rejected this idea, as they thought that the six divisions would "share the space now being utilized by two divisions and that no over all increase of dependents is involved." With this response, Lovett approved of the above letter. (Lovett to Burns, memorandum, [February 28, 1951], and Randall to Carter, March 6, 1951, ibid.)

3. Truman approved Marshall's suggestion that the NSC consider this matter and so advised the council secretary. That approval as well as Marshall's original letter are in NSC 106 dated March 12, 1951. The NSC report, dated August 31, 1951, received presidential approval on September 13, 1951. See NSC 106/1 and 106/2. (NSC 106, "The Safety of the American Civilian Population in Germany and Japan in the Event of Hostilities," March 12, 1951; NSC 106/1 and NSC 106/2, "The Possibilities of Reducing the United States Civilian Population in Sensitive Areas Abroad," August 31 and September 13, 1951, in Paul Kesaris, ed., *Documents of the National Security Council: First Supplement* [Frederick, MD: University Publications of America Inc., 1981], text-fiche, reel 1, frames 403–56.)

263

To Dean G. Acheson — March 8, 1951
Top Secret — Washington, DC

My dear Mr. Secretary: At the request of the U. S. Joint Chiefs of Staff and the Canadian Chiefs of Staff Committee, the Permanent Joint Board on Defense, Canada–United States at its meeting on February 1, 1951, considered the subject of combined Canada–United States air defense exercises and operations.[1] To provide for the coordinated defense of contiguous areas in Canada and the United States, it is necessary that the air defense forces of both countries be trained in combined exercises in order to be prepared to reinforce each other on short notice.

In these circumstances the Board recognized the desirability of providing the two air defense forces with general authority to arrange for combined air defense exercises without the necessity of obtaining approval through diplomatic channels in each case. These arrangements would apply only to fighter forces. The Board therefore recommended:

That the air defense forces of Canada and the United States be given authority to carry out on local notification combined air defense training exercises.

I am in agreement with the foregoing recommendation, and request the Department of State, in coordination with United States members of the Board, to prepare an implementing agreement for negotiation with Canada, in order that the conduct of combined air defense training exercises between the United States and Canada may be expedited. Faithfully yours,

NA/RG 330, CD 334 (Permanent Joint Board on Defense Canada)

1. The Permanent Joint Board on Defense, Canada–United States (PJBD), had been established by President Roosevelt and Prime Minister William Lyon Mackenzie King in August 1940 to study and address issues relating to the military defense of North America. During the months preceding Marshall's March 8 letter to Acheson, the board as well as the JCS and representatives of the two air forces had been exploring expanded air defenses. On February 23, Marshall informed Acheson that the PJBD, at the request of the JCS, had considered a plan for a radar net in Canada and reported that it was "acceptable and feasible of implementation." The JCS agreed, and Marshall therefore requested Acheson's approval and submission to Truman of the board's recommendations, which he enclosed, as well as negotiation of an agreement with the Canadian government once presidential approval had been obtained that would allow for "prompt implementation of the plan for the extension of the presently authorized air defense system." (Marshall to Acheson, February 23, 1951, NA/RG 330, CD 334 [Permanent Joint Board on Defense Canada].) On March 2, Acting Secretary of State Webb requested Truman's approval of the plan, which "had been developed by the Air Forces of the two countries" and approved by the Defense Department. He attached Marshall's February 23 letter as well as a letter to Truman from the acting chairman of the US section of the board, retired Major General Guy V. Henry (USMA, 1898). Webb informed Truman of his belief that the plan provided "an equitable and feasible basis for cooperation in this joint defense project" and stated that following the president's approval, the State Department would "initiate action to put the Board's Recommendation into effect through an exchange of notes with the Canadian Government." Truman approved of this plan on April 14, "'subject to the availability of required funds.'" (*FRUS, 1951*, 2: 875–76.)

264

To General of the Army Omar N. Bradley — March 13, 1951, Washington, DC

Dear Bradley: In addition to my other duties, I still seem to be Chairman of the American Battle Monuments Commission.[1]

I note from the attached memorandum for members of the Commission that the JCS has determined that the overseas officer personnel for the ABMC should be cut in half.[2]

My personal concern has mainly to do with the possible adverse reaction in the event this reduction in officer personnel creates conditions of poor maintenance in the existing cemeteries and poor supervision of construction work on our new cemeteries. The number of parents visiting our overseas cemeteries has been considerable during the past few years and I anticipate no great reduction in those visiting this summer.

I would appreciate your informal comments on the attached memorandum and my views above.[3]

GCMRL/G. C. Marshall Papers (Secretary of Defense, Number Indexed, M208-1-27)

1. See p. 54.

2. General Thomas North had written to Pace on February 14 to protest a 50 percent reduction (from ten to five) in army officers assigned to its overseas stations, stating that it would "cripple" the commission's activities. On March 7, Pace responded that the reduction had resulted from a JCS study initiated before the Korean War and that "in consideration of our many other priority missions, I do not feel that it is advisable to recommend" to the JCS a restoration of the five officer spaces. On March 13, North had informed the committee members of the reductions. (North to Pace, February 14, 1951; Pace to North, March 7, 1951; and North to members of the ABMC, memorandum, March 13, 1951, GCMRL/G. C. Marshall Papers [American Battle Monuments Commission, General].)

3. One of Bradley's subordinates informed him that the reduction "is a direct result of a memorandum" by General Joseph R. McNarney (USMA, 1915), chairman of the management committee in the OSD. All Marshall needed to do in order to reverse these cuts is to direct McNarney "to authorize ten officers for overseas duty" with the ABMC. "In fact," the memorandum's author continued, from the information I have it is suggested you may want to make it 15" officers. (Memorandum for Bradley, March 15, 1951, ibid.)

On March 16, Marshall wrote to McNarney (who during World War II had been first Marshall's deputy chief of staff and then deputy Supreme Allied Commander in the Mediterranean Theater as well as postwar commander of US occupation forces in Germany) that he was "deeply concerned" about morale if the cemeteries were not maintained and suggested an increase in the personnel assigned to the ABMC. (Marshall to McNarney, March 16, 1951, ibid.) McNarney sent a memorandum to the service secretaries on March 20 authorizing the assignment of sixteen army officers, two navy officers, and four air force officers to the ABMC. (McNarney to service secretaries, memorandum, March 20, 1951, GCMRL/G. C. Marshall Papers [Secretary of Defense, Number Indexed, M208-1-27].)

265

TO EDWARD H. REES

March 13, 1951
Washington, DC

Dear Mr. Rees: I was glad to receive your letter of March 6, expressing your interest in the relief of personnel now serving in the Armed Services in Korea.[1]

I can well understand the feelings of the families of men who have been in the Korean area for an extended tour of duty. The Department of the Air Force and the Marine Corps have announced a policy for the rotation of Marine Corps and Air Force personnel in that area. Copies of the pertinent press releases are enclosed.[2]

The Army and the Navy have not, as yet, announced a similar policy, but it is being considered on a most urgent basis. The trouble is at present to find the noncommissioned and first class private grades to enable a rotation procedure to be gotten underway.[3]

It is expected however that we will be able to rotate personnel in the combat areas in the very near future. In the meantime, I want you to know that we here feel what these men are doing in Korea must be recognized by relief at the earliest possible date. Faithfully yours,

NA/RG 330, SD 370

1. Representative Rees (R-KS) had relayed the deep concern of many of his constituents who had been in service since July 1950 and were asking why they have not been replaced. Rees requested information on Marshall's "policy with respect to this extremely important problem." (Rees to Marshall, March 6, 1951, NA/RG 330, SD 370.)

2. The Marine Corps had announced a "small scale" rotation program on February 24 but warned against "over-optimism" since the continuation of personnel rotation would depend on consistent favorable operations in Korea. The Air Force began rotations in May 1951. ("2 Guard Divisions Alerted for Japan," *New York Times*, February 25, 1951, pp. 1, 43; Historical Studies Branch, USAF Historical Division, "Combat Crew Rotation, World War II and Korean War," [Maxwell AFB, Alabama: Air University, Aerospace Studies Institute, 1968], 23.)

3. On the same day Marshall wrote this letter, he and Lieutenant General John E. Hull, deputy army chief of staff for administration, had discussed policies on press releases regarding the army's rotation plans at that morning's Armed Forces Policy Council meeting. Hull noted that prior to that meeting, the Department of the Army stated in a press release that it would "exchange 50 company grade officers and 100 non-commissioned officers now on the Korean battlefront with a similar number of officers and NCOs serving as instructors and trainers in the United States" around April 1. Hull pointed out that the release "carefully avoided using the word 'rotation.' However, the stories as carried by the press immediately tabbed it with the word 'rotation.'" (Hull to Marshall, memorandum, and press release 336-51, March 13, 1951, NA/RG 330, SD 370; "Troop Rotation Planned," *New York Times*, March 14, 1951, p. 6.) For more on the army's rotation plan, see pp. 463 and 488–89.

266

TO GENERAL JULIUS OCHS ADLER[1] March 15, 1951
Washington, DC

Dear Adler: Many thanks for your assurance that Raskin may stay with us until April 1. His work on the Universal Military Training and Service bill has been invaluable and it would have handicapped us severely to have had him leave now. The hardest part of our fight for a good bill is still ahead, and we cannot afford to break up our first team at the time we need all our experts most.[2]

If it were not for the knowledge that Raskin's future lies with The Times and that you are reluctant to have him stay away longer, I would have urged that he remain here beyond April 1, or until the UMST bill is made law.

Raskin has also started to create a basic framework for the Industrial Relations Division, which we need very badly. He is ideally fitted to carry forward this important work, and my only reason for not asking you to make him available for it full-time was Mrs. Rosenberg's insistence that we had made a commitment to you not to ask for him beyond April 1, except on a one-day-a-week consultant basis. I know Raskin can provide substantial guidance to his successor by coming down one day a week after he returns to the newspaper, and I certainly hope you will allow him to do so.

He has managed to make himself indispensable here in a very brief period. I can understand your eagerness to have him back, and must I say I envy your prior lien on his services.

With my thanks again, and warm regards[3] Faithfully yours,

GCMRL/G. C. Marshall Papers (Secretary of Defense, Chronological, Secretaries, Ackerman)

1. Adler was the general manager of the *New York Times.*

2. Abraham H. Raskin, a well-respected *New York Times* reporter on economics and labor relations, had been a consultant to President Truman on UMT and had been helping to develop the Defense Department's Division of Industrial Relations. Carter had informed Marshall on March 12 that Raskin was under pressure to return to the *New York Times*. Rosenberg was paying the difference between his *New York Times* salary and his Defense Department pay "out of her own pocket" as he was "the most essential element in Mrs. Rosenberg's operations on the UMT business." Carter urged Marshall to "call Adler (a telegram will accomplish little if anything) and request that you be allowed to keep Raskin *until* UMT is passed by Congress. If you get a complete negative reply, then you could settle for 1 April." ("A. H. Raskin, 82, Times Reporter and Editor, Dies," *New York Times*, December 23, 1993, p. B6; Carter to Marshall, memorandum, March 12, 1951, GCMRL/G. C. Marshall Papers [Secretary of Defense, Categorical, Memoranda, Marshall S. Carter, 1950–1951].)

3. Adler's March 19 reply is not in the Marshall Papers, but on March 27 Marshall wrote to express his appreciation that Adler could continue until April on a part-time basis with the understanding that his other duties might limit his time at the Defense Department. (Marshall to Adler, March 27, 1951, GCMRL/G. C. Marshall Papers [Secretary of Defense, Number Indexed, M200-11-42].)

267

TO GENERAL SUN LI-JEN

March 19, 1951
Washington, DC

Dear Sun: Thanks for your letter of February 19th. As to your thoughts on who should head the military mission, several of the names you mention will in all probability not be considered because of their present very important positions.[1] For instance:

General Lucius Clay is now a special assistant to Mr. Charles E. Wilson, Office of Defense Mobilization. This is probably the most important organ of the Executive Department at this particular time for it has responsibility for the mobilization of labor, industry, and manpower.

General Mark Clark, as you know, is Commanding General of the Army Field Forces and his duties are as manifold as those of the Chief of Staff, with induction, training, equipping, housing, etc.

General Ridgway and General Almond are in command of the Eighth Army and Tenth Corps respectively, and their hands are full with the Korean situation.

However, I have passed your letter down to General Bradley and the Joint Chiefs of Staff for their consideration of your suggestions. The entire military problem is receiving a great deal of study and I am sure you will be kept abreast of all developments.[2]

I hope everything is going well with you, and with warm regards, Faithfully yours,

NA/RG 218, Geographic File, CCS 381 (Far East)

1. In his February 19 reply to Marshall's December 19 letter (see p. 301n1), Sun had expressed gratitude for the US decision to send a military mission to Formosa along with increased military aid, and had suggested that the head of the mission be one of the "great generals" like Clay, Clark, Ridgway, Almond, or retired Lieutenant General Gerow (VMI, 1911), who had been commanding general of the V Corps and the Fifteenth Army during World War II and commanding general of the Second Army from 1948 until his retirement in 1950. (Sun to Marshall, February 19, 1951, NA/RG 218, Geographic File, CCS 381 [Far East].)

2. On March 23, Major General William C. Chase was appointed head of the Military Assistance Advisory Group for Formosa, "pending his ultimate assignment as Chief of the Joint U.S. Military Advisory Group in Formosa." (Lalor to chief of staff, US Army, memorandum, March 23, 1951, ibid.) For more on US military aid to Formosa, see pp. 300–301 and 426–27.

268

Memorandum to the Joint Chiefs of Staff — March 19, 1951
Secret — Washington, DC

The Secretary of State is concerned over the strong reaction of the French to the reports of another British-American meeting in Malta. He feels that it will be necessary to take this matter up with Minister Schumann [*Schuman*] during the visit of the President of France, and therefore that we have a very clear understanding of just what has happened in connection with the two meetings in Malta and exactly what should be the procedure in the future.[1]

Mr. Acheson also feels that we must take up in some manner with Mr. Schumann [*Schuman*] the question of security of communications.

Mr. Acheson feels that we must get together with the French and that probably there should be a proposal for a meeting here or in Europe with the British, French and ourselves for a discussion along military lines, presumably I suppose with very specific regard to the Mediterranean.[2]

GCMRL/G. C. Marshall Papers (Secretary of Defense, Chronological, Secretaries, Ackerman)

1. Admiral Robert Carney (USNA, 1916), commander in chief of the US naval forces in the eastern Atlantic and Mediterranean, had met with General Sir Brian Robertson, commander in chief of the British Middle East forces, on January 23 and 24 to discuss Middle

East defenses as part of larger deliberations on the establishment of a NATO command structure. (See pp. 455–56.) On January 30, French Premier Pleven expressed to Truman his frustration that a French representative had not been invited to participate, asserting that "the French did not want NATO to be an Anglo-Saxon show." Truman and Bradley tried to reassure Pleven that this was not the case, with the president noting that "there were no conversations going on with the British about Middle East problems" and that neither Acheson nor Marshall intended to cut "the French out of any conversations." (*FRUS, 1951*, 4: 324–25, 358.)

Carney announced publicly on March 8 that he would meet again with Robertson on March 13, and on March 10, Ambassador Bonnet requested that the French be allowed to participate. This request was denied, and the US Navy declared on March 12 that the meeting would discuss only defense strategies for the Middle East and other non-NATO areas, not the question of the Mediterranean command. Foreign Minister Schuman sent notes to the US and UK on March 16 expressing the outrage of the French cabinet at the situation and requesting that the US clarify France's role in defense plans for the Middle East. French President Vincent Jules Auriol, accompanied by Schuman, would be visiting the US in late March and would be meeting with both Truman and Acheson. In its background memorandum for this visit, the State Department recommended that the US express "regret" for the publicity surrounding these recent meetings but also remind the French that the US "believes that there are many questions that can be best handled on a bilateral basis," including several matters which had been resolved recently in US-French bilateral talks. (*FRUS, 1951*, 4: 358–62; *Papers of DDE*, 12: 130; "Malta Talks Limited to Mid-East," *New York Times*, March 13, 1951, p. 8.) For Eisenhower's and Truman's reactions to this controversy, see *Papers of DDE*, 12: 128–29.

2. Vice Admiral Arthur C. Davis (USNA, 1915), director of the Joint Staff, informed Marshall on March 21 that the JCS had reached an agreement on the Mediterranean NATO command at their meeting that morning and recommended that their views be sent to Eisenhower for comment after consultation with the State Department. Following this, the JCS would coordinate with the British chiefs of staff through the British Joint Services Mission in Washington and propose to the British and French a tripartite meeting in Washington where, "subject to a three-cornered agreement on the Mediterranean setup, the French Chiefs of Staff would be informed fully as to what transpired at the Malta conference." (Davis to Marshall, memorandum, March 21, 1951, NA/RG 330, CD 337 [Malta].)

At his March 30 meeting with Acheson, Schuman insisted that France must participate in any talks about the defense of the Middle East. While maintaining the belief "that there was room for both multilateral and bilateral approaches" to address these issues, Acheson suggested a tripartite meeting in Washington in accord with the JCS recommendations mentioned in the previous paragraph. Schuman expressed his "full satisfaction" with this plan. (*FRUS, 1951*, 4: 370–72; Burns to Marshall, memorandum, April 9, 1951, NA/RG 330, CD 337 [Malta].)

269

To Harry S. Truman — March 20, 1951
Radio No. DEF-26824. *Personal* — Washington, DC

Personal for the President from Secretary of Defense Marshall

As of tomorrow, 21 March 1951, the strength of our Armed Forces will be exactly double what it was on 25 June 1950. This doubling of our strength has been accomplished less than nine months after the Communist aggression against the Republic of Korea. For your information the strength we have already attained—a total strength in excess of 2,900,000—was not attained in World War Two until more than twenty one months after our build up started in June 1940 following the fall of France and more than three months after Pearl Harbor.[1]

NA/RG 330, CD 320.2 (Strength, Military)

1. Truman, who was on vacation at the Little White House in Key West, Florida, replied the same day congratulating Marshall and his staff for making "such growth possible. . . . I am confident that, under your wise leadership, the Department of Defense will continue to build the strength we need, fully supported by the Congress and by the American people." (Truman to Marshall, March 20, 1951, *Public Papers, 1951*, 194.)

Marshall sent identical letters to Senators Kenneth McKellar (D-TN), chairman of the Appropriations Committee, and Joseph O'Mahoney; and Representatives Carl Vinson, Clarence Cannon, and George Mahon. (NA/RG 330, CD 320.2 [Strength, Military].)

The Marshall-Truman telegrams were released to the press on March 21. The *Washington Post* reported that "the telegram exchange was obviously intended to produce a dual psychological effect abroad—warn Russia and assure America's friends. It also appeared to have a message for critics of the Administration's rearmament program at home." ("U. S. Has Doubled Armed Force Since Korea," *Washington Post*, March 22, 1951, p. 3.)

270

INTERVIEW FOR THE APRIL 13, 1951, ISSUE OF *U.S. NEWS & WORLD REPORT*[1] — March 26, 1951, Washington, DC

Q *Mr. Secretary, what has caused the "letdown" in the public attitude toward the defense program?*

A I should say that is one of the few cases where you can put your finger on the fellow who is responsible, and that's General Ridgway, our field commander in Korea. His successes have dulled the public interest and urge as to the defense program.

Q *Do you think the public, Mr. Secretary, has attached too much importance to our military successes in Korea?*

A I wouldn't say they had attached too much importance—they have just relaxed in their interest.

Q *Is there much danger now in such a "letdown?"*

A The world situation is just as serious if not more serious than it was last November. Every indication we have from abroad is of increasing build-up. It has been noticeable particularly in the satellite countries. The situation not only hasn't changed in the matter of being less tense, it is really more tense than before.

Q *The world situation, as you see it, requires us to build up to whatever tensions exist, yet most people don't know what these tensions are because we don't get any expression from the Government as to the degree of tension that does exist—*

A I would differ with you on that because I think that in the statements that were made in the President's national-emergency declaration practically all of that came out, but the trouble is, we must say it once a week—I think that's the problem.[2]

Q *When you are essentially taking a long-range view of our defense requirements and are not being affected by the changes from day to day in Korea?*

A That's it, exactly.

Q *Do you consider then that what people have got to do is to bear in mind the over-all picture constantly instead of some little lessening of tension in Korea or perhaps some other part of the world?*

A Put it this way—the best we can hope for, as I see it, is a prolonged tension rather than an all-out war. What we hope and pray for at the present time is that, as between the two, it might be a prolonged tension, rather than war, during which we can build up our strength and our resources, get organized in Western Europe, which General Eisenhower, Supreme Commander in Europe, is trying to do—get straightened out, we hope, in the Far East—but that's the best hope at present. If we should get a complete agreement with the Soviets, we would be perfect fools to relax our military strength until we had evidence of good faith. Unfortunately, the tendency already is to relax. That's what we have to fight against.

Q *How long will it be before we have a big enough club behind the door so that we don't have to worry too much about these tensions?*

A At the rate we are going now, by the time we get to the summer of 1952 we will be very strong. The problem then is how do we continue without imposing too great a financial burden on our economy and our people? How do we maintain our forces? That is why I argue that we must find a way that is within our financial capabilities. That's the reason I think the fundamental concept of our man-power bill is of such great importance.[3]

Q *Universal training is vitally important?*

A It's vitally important. But the way we've gotten into this situation makes what we could have done very simply a couple of years ago not practical under conditions of today. Unless we get some basis, some system that has an enduring quality, we will be guilty, I think, of a tragic and possibly fatal error.

As to matériel, what Deputy Secretary Lovett and I have been striving for—and I think we've been fairly successful—is facilities. Of course we must have certain matériel immediately and we're getting that. But what we want to avoid is accumulating a tremendous number of planes, for instance, and having them deteriorate in open storage. We do want the capacity to produce planes at a very high rate of speed. The same way with other items—such as tanks. Tanks change all the time. We don't want thousands of tanks in excess of immediate and reserve requirements, but we do want the capacity to turn them out very rapidly.

Q *Can you illustrate that concretely?*

A To give a rough example, with a particular type of plane, this year we will get 5,000, and next year we can get somewhere between 15,000 and 20,000—if we want them. And the next or third year we could get 50,000. What we are after is resources, both in additional assembly lines and additional plants, but particularly additional assembly lines, and orders so placed that we don't demand great quantities now, right off. We want to leave a requirement sufficient to keep the plants in operation through a considerable period of time without submerging us in equipment and matériel. But yet we want facilities available so that we can turn on a full blast in 24 hours. The problem, then, would be in raw materials.

Orders are being placed at the rate of 4 or 5 billions a month, and that is a very rapid negotiation of contracts. We are trying to shorten the period between the time the contract is placed and the time the actual procurement under that contract is gotten under way. There are many requirements under law and many procedures. We are trying to boil those down somewhat.

The Basic Need: Trained Men

The personnel part is an effort to put ourselves in the same position of rapid availability in personnel as we are in the matter of the production of matériel. Once we do that, we will be outstandingly the most powerful country in the world. But unless we can approximate our personnel situation—I don't mean in great standing forces, but in rapid availability in case of necessity—with respect to matériel, we will be weak without realizing the reason. What we need then is wisdom and vision in getting a program that will not break our backs financially and yet will maintain the proper military posture.

Q *How do we do that?*

A That is the fundamental conception of this manpower bill which is under fire at the present time.

Q *Mr. Secretary, you made a point about tensions. I was wondering whether this might not be a fair question to ask you: In this period of prolonged tension to which you have referred, could we as a nation accept some paper agreement that might be made and then relax our efforts? Do you think we should wait and see that the agreement is kept in good faith?*

A I think that is essential. We would be quite foolish if, in accepting a paper agreement, our efforts are immediately completely relaxed. The tendency to relax will be great without even a negotiatory basis of justification.

Q *In other words, this is an era of deeds and acts of good faith?*

A We must have confirmation of good faith. Once we have a basis of good faith, we have solved most of the world's problems.

Q *So that the solution doesn't lie in writing something on a piece of paper?*

A That's correct. When you get something on paper, you've made a beginning. Then you've got to see confirmation in actions which indicate good faith.

Q *We've learned that from experience, haven't we?*

A I think we have.

Inconvenience Now or War Later

Q *What the people have got to face then, as you see it, is a choice between a period of prolonged tension with a great deal, perhaps, of inconvenience, and a war in which there will be real losses of life? Isn't that the alternative?*

A Those are the alternatives that I see at the present time.

Q *This period of tension may be costly to us, or may be inconvenient to us, but it is necessary to prevent the war itself?*

A I would address my thinking to the immediate build-up to a position of readiness based on an enduring system. I hope we can maintain ourselves in a position of strength, and at a decreasing cost as we reduce the size of the active forces as rapidly as we get trained men into the ranks of the Reserve units.

Q *When might universal training be applied?*

A Well, the training phase could not get under way, purely as such, much before the fall of 1952, but the procedure should be gotten under way immediately.

Q *A lot of people say why have military training when you've already got a draft—you're going to have a draft for three or four years—why then have military training?*

A We are going to have the training going on and as men from the 18–19 age group become available, they will go into that training. But what we want is to work steadily into the real universal-military-training phase. Once we have that well developed, we can begin the reduction of the service phase to the point where we can depend on volunteers for the active forces and not need to depend on a Selective Service. At that point, we would be building up a reserve of trained men and putting them in the ranks of the National Guard and Reserve units not on active duty.

Q *And that might be in 1952?*

A That would be the earliest time I would estimate—the fall of 1952. We can't reduce the size of the active forces until we have gotten at least a few units of the National Guard that are not on active duty, in a state of real readiness so that they could quickly be made available for active-campaign service.

Changes for Reserve Program

Q *Mr. Secretary, what is the outlook for Reservists and National Guardsmen who are still at home—are they going to be called in large numbers?*

A We are trying to avoid calling large numbers and we are trying very hard to get a basis for relieving the Reservists who have already been called and who really are suffering hardship—men with families, men who are losing their businesses, and men that never visualized a partial mobilization—and we are developing a bill in relation to the entire Reserve program. We already have the proposals of the Civilian Components Policy Board, and the staff is working hard on the matter. The first congressional hearing will be after the passage of the man-power bill. It is a very difficult matter, and we have to be careful that no such radical action is taken as to completely emasculate the Reserve system in our national defense. One of the provisos of the House proposal in the man-power bill is that, at the end of twelve months' service, veteran Reservists will be released.[4]

We do want to release veteran Reservists called involuntarily, just as fast as we can, but if the proviso of one year's service went into effect we would be faced with a large-scale and sudden exodus beginning in June and most of them leaving the service by the first of September. There is not much point in sending National Guard divisions to Japan and have them dissolve over there two, three or four months after arrival.

Q *In getting up to this state of readiness, is it going to be necessary to go* *beyond the 3.4 million figure?*

A I don't know. We hope not. That will depend on the world situation this summer, as we estimate it then. We hope to avoid that necessity. We wish to avoid calling in additional reserve troops—National Guard units.

Q *Is there any evidence that Russia is less determined?*

A Not that I know of.

Q *You've been Secretary of Defense for about six months now, and have had a chance to get an over-all view of the Department—how do you think it is functioning?*

A Both Lovett and I were very greatly surprised when we took over to find the degree of co-ordination and co-operation that existed. After the trials and vicissitudes of the early days, we found the procedure entirely different from what we anticipated. I knew, of course, the progress that had been made, but I didn't realize the degree of progress. It appeared to me that you might say the ship had found itself—the growing pains were about over.

Q *That's the integration being done inside the Department?*

A The operations of the Defense Department as a whole.

Q *Do you visualize your chief function as co-ordinating the three departments or setting up a special function?*

A I can't answer that quite as you put the question. I am charged, under the law, with direction, control and authority over the entire Department of Defense, which, as you know, includes the military departments of the Army, the Navy and the Air Force. There are some specific limitations of the exercise of this direction, authority and control. For instance, there is a provision in the law against merging the departments. There is a provision that the combatant functions assigned to the military department should not be transferred from one department to another, or abolished, or consolidated. There is a stipulation, by law, that in matters of supply, other than combat affairs, alterations in the way of proposed transfers, or re-assignments of functions, must be reported to the armed services committees of Congress. I think there are one or two other minor limitations, but those are the principal ones.

New Status of Defense Department

Q *So you've got what you might call an integrated department now?*

A Yes, I suppose you would call it that. Each one of the three services is a military department, and is to be administered as such by its Secretary. They formerly were executive departments, and now they are military departments. Under the original terms of the act of Congress, the present Defense Department was not an executive agency. It was an organization for general co-ordination. Now it is the executive agency, and the Army and Navy and Air are military departments, and not executive agencies—that's a great change that has been made.

Q *You have had experience with the Joint Chiefs of Staff, and now you have experience as civilian Secretary—how are you satisfied with the setup? Would you recommend any changes to Congress?*

A No, as a matter of fact, on the whole I would say that I see no changes in the organization of the Defense Department indicated now of sufficient importance to get involved in legislative debate—and I think it is too soon, anyway. We ought to go along and find ourselves, as it were. So far as the Chiefs of Staff are concerned, the organization I think is quite satisfactory. The position of the Chiefs of Staff, however, is not, I think, clearly enough established in the public or the legislative mind. I fear it is bad practice to have them called before Congress as Chiefs of Staff. It's all right for each one to go up there as representative of his service, but not as a representative of the Joint Chiefs—the strategy-planning body.

How Joint Chiefs Operate

Q *Isn't the conception of the Joint Chiefs of Staff, as far as the public is concerned, rather inadequate anyhow? Isn't there a lack of definition in the public mind as to just what part the Joint Chiefs play in this whole thing?*

A That is so to a degree, but I think it has come out of all of the legislative battles in getting the organization built in the manner that it is now constructed. I think people will come along into a common acceptance of the Chiefs of Staff as being a very sound source of military advice.

In my own personal experience with the Chiefs of Staff we never made a public appearance of any kind that I recall. Of course, it was during wartime when we got out of the old joint-board status and into the Chiefs-of-Staff status organization. We not only never appeared publicly, but we never had a directive, which is a rather interesting fact. All of our subordinates always wanted directives. I think they drafted about a half a dozen which we debated. Each time we thought it was the part of wisdom to leave well enough alone. So that's the way we went through the war period, you might say with an "unwritten constitution." Various practices grew up and were confirmed by repeated action and formed the accepted procedure.[5]

Q *But the Joint Chiefs had a great deal of authority in that period? Their decisions usually were unanimous?*

A We didn't vote on decisions. We avoided voting.

Advice for the President

Q *Might it not be said that the Joint Chiefs, as you visualize it, is a body which gives military advice to the President primarily, and doesn't act as an institution separate from the Defense Department in its relations with Congress?*

A That's it. It makes recommendations to the President, to the National Security Council and to the Secretary of Defense.

Q *And that's its primary function?*

A That's its primary function. As to the Chiefs of Staff organization today compared to what it was during the war years, in the first place, it is operating under quite different conditions. During those years there was a war on and that changed the complexion of practically everything. Now we are in a very difficult period when there is no war—there is a fear of war, but even that fear, at least in the public mind, has relaxed in the last six weeks to an extent that has made it very difficult to get the action by Congress that we feel is now essential.

Q *Isn't that always true?*

A I never expected it to develop with this rapidity.

Q *Is it more rapid than after the last war, when people just dropped everything?*

A Yes, but we are in the middle of a fight today. If you asked any of those fellows in Korea—if you said, "The war's over," they'd differ with you.

Q *So, even though the war is going on, there is an apathy here?*

A What we are thinking about is possibly a 10-year tension—but the tension has relaxed here in six weeks. I was certain it would relax by 1952. And in my recommendations to Congress, I built the whole conception on the basis of having to meet exactly that sort of public and legislative reaction. That is, for example, the fundamental concept of this man-power bill that is now before the Congress. I wanted something enduring, something that would hold through the years, and that would be within our financial capabilities and also within the radius of our tolerance—let's put it in that manner.

That view was the subject of a great deal of criticism because I wasn't thought to be viewing the picture in large-enough terms, as to personnel in particular, and also as to matériel requirements. The amounts we asked for were believed to be insufficient, the numbers of men were believed to be insufficient. We were told the whole National Guard should be called in.[6] What I was trying to avoid was calling out a mass of men that actually would interfere with the efficiency of our immediate build-up. Certain things we have to do very fast now. It's almost a speed proposition. We must get these divisions together and train them as rapidly as possible to meet the immediate requirements of the situation.

Demands for Faster Build-up

Q *They were saying then, last November, that, in effect, you were not preparing fast enough?*

A They said we didn't see the whole picture. I was specifically criticized on the ground that this was a very serious situation and that I should meet it head on and recognize its larger picture. Now, of course, we've received our vindication, but a little too soon for me. The best we can hope for in this present world of ours is a long period of tension.

Q *Rather than a war, you mean?*

A Yes. The only other alternative would be a full-fledged war. If impatience develops that quickly, what will it be in 1952 and 1953 and 1954 and 1955? If we should put large numbers of men in uniform, as was frequently proposed, what's going to be the reaction? The man himself presents quite a problem, because you know how restless Americans would be standing around under conditions of that kind. To meet such problems is the fundamental conception of the man-power act now under debate. We must develop some system that will permit us to reduce the standing force without weakening our military posture.

Q *And that's universal military training, you think?*

A It's a combination of that and other things. We plan to put into the ranks of the National Guard basically trained men—that is, those who have had at least four months' military training. And the replacements for the veteran officer personnel that they have now should come out of a Reserve Officers Training Corps which has its foundation based on drawing its material from this same group of basically trained men.

To illustrate: The National Guard divisions which were called last September came in at about 45 per cent strength. Selective Service then had to provide 55 per cent. Under the necessity of receiving the reinforcements in small lots, it was November before they got their full strength. And it was the middle of March before they completed their basic training, and it will be June before they get their complete training. The world situation does not permit of such a lengthy procedure as that.

High Cost of Standing Army

Q *How do you meet that requirement?*

A One way is to have a large force on active duty. How long will that be tolerable—because it would cost a tremendous amount of money? I think when we figure everything in, by and large, it's almost $10,000 a soldier. No country in the world can stand such an expense.

But if we can build up a posture of military strength without having a large number of men on active duty, then there is some possibility of weathering this long period of crisis we anticipate in a sufficiently strong position to be the determining factor militarily in the world.

Q *And we can pay for that?*

A It must be in terms that we can pay for. So the fundamental conception of our plan isn't just universal military training. Primarily it is to vitalize our reserve system.

The National Guard as part of that reserve system have the equivalent of 34 divisions of ground troops. Now if those units can be gotten in a state of availability, with their 50 per cent strength, all having had basic fundamental training, and a system that would always have available to carry them to war or full strength with the remaining 50 per cent already trained, you can see what a tremendous difference in time of preparation that would make. And after we got out the first group—say six divisions—the others would have had time to catch up with the necessities of the situation in trained troops. So we would have a large ground force available, but one which had not been on the daily pay roll and yet would be quickly available. That is the fundamental purpose of this present proposed legislation.

Q *Wouldn't you have to sell the country the idea that you need ground troops? Aren't there a great many people who feel that with the new gadgets you don't need ground troops?*

A Any thought that you can conduct a war with any special gadget and exclusive of ground armies is in my mind utterly indefensible. We have had all sorts of proposals. If you go back to 1940 and 1941 you will find me being criticized then for supposedly raising a mass army. The claim was all troops should be mechanized.[7] And then, when we landed in Normandy, there was a clamor for infantry divisions. And the misfortune of the German defense in Normandy was that they got caught with their *Panzer* divisions in the first line, and the infantry divisions far back. It was a very costly mishap for them. War may, and probably will, start in the air, or maybe on the sea, but it's going very soon to be in the mud. You can't get and hold air bases without ground action. Whatever you may win by air or naval action you must hold with ground troops. Take the present situation in Korea, where we are up against unlimited man power. There we have another great difficulty demanding ground troops—you can't evade this.

I was very much struck with the public reactions to the atomic bomb on its first appearance. I had been thinking about its effect on warfare for about two years and a half, and yet the decision on its effect seemed to be settled in the press in about 24 hours. What we had to do in ground warfare in order to be in the position to use the bomb was completely overlooked. There was a reaction in favor of a sort of push-button warfare. People overlooked the tremendous number of men that would be involved before we could get the necessary fields from which to use the bomb. Take Saipan, for example—or Guam—those were gained in big, costly battles. And they were preceded by Tarawas and Kwajaleins—all necessary to acquire the fields from which we launched the bombs. There were many people involved in those operations.[8]

Q *So, broadly speaking, you need ground troops to support all the services, really?*

A Yes. And then they have to carry out operations these other services can't possibly manage by air or sea.

Q *Because in the end you have to defeat the enemy on the ground, you have to bring him to his knees?*

A Yes.

Factors in 'Balanced Forces'

Q *Going back to the basic concept of the Department of Defense, the phrase has been used, "balanced forces." Is there any other phrase that you can think of that expresses the need for three military services today as essential to any operations in which we may become engaged?*

A "Balanced forces" is a precise phrase, but has become somewhat of an irritant to Congress and others as it has been used. One must consider many factors. The greater rapidity with which a force can be organized is one factor. Costs are a factor, in relation to a peacetime setup, or to a position of readiness, if we may term it that way. The rate of build-up is a very critical consideration when we come to peacetime appropriations.

Q *Isn't perhaps the key word "joint"—that is, "joint operations"?*

A "Balanced forces" is really the correct term. But it involves a great many considerations in relation to the rapidity of the build-up, the costs, etc.

In that connection, I might explain further my own view. The test of the Defense Department in its present organization is not that of today. However, the rapid progress that has been made since last June would not have been possible without the unification that had been achieved in the Department. I think all of us are in agreement in the Defense Department as to that. Since I have become Secretary of Defense, in the latter part of September, the development of unity budgetwise has been very pronounced. For the first time, I think, the budgets have been developed on the basis of national necessity, rather than on imposed limitations. After we first got the estimates prepared on that basis, we proceeded to see how sound they were.

It was quite a time, of course, before the representatives of the three services could reach a satisfactory agreement as to what actually were the requirements in the light of the world situation. And rather than impose on them a monetary limitation, we decided to go ahead and work this out initially on the basis of what we thought were the national requirements.

Q *You mean they didn't start with a lump sum?*

A No lump sum was indicated.

Q *Wasn't that a change from the previous approach?*

A This was the first time, I think, that had been done.

Unification Aids Budget

Q *And when you removed the lump sum and let each service decide what it had to do to meet the national necessity, then you took a lump sum later, didn't you?*

A It was converted into a lump sum afterwards. There had to be a general estimate. We then examined into the basis of these various estimates, and decided just how far we thought that we could go along with the general over-all proposal for our defensive build-up. I don't think it would have been possible to manage these matters as I have indicated and to do as we are doing right now in getting up the 1952 budget, except on the basis of present unification. And also I know it would have been very difficult to manage if I hadn't had somebody as able and understanding, as astute in harmonizing procedure as Lovett, who thoroughly understands this business from a long experience both in and out of the Government and keeps not only good will but a businesslike efficiency in the direction of matters.

But the real test of the Defense Department and its organization, in my opinion, is not under present conditions. Confronted by a very dangerous situation, you always find solutions. We found it in the last war without even a written directive for the Chiefs of Staff. There were overlappings, and situations that we didn't like. But we were able, on a wartime basis, to get things done. The real test of the matter is what the Defense Department is able to do to maintain a reasonable military posture for this country in times of profound peace, which is what we are all searching and praying for. Each time we've had a period of profound peace, the whole military force has been emasculated, and we sank into such a position of weakness and impotence that we got into the very trouble we wished to avoid.

The greater our position in the world—we seem to have gotten into a situation where we can't evade the responsibility that comes to us in an economic and military sense—the greater will be our responsibility for the maintenance of peace.

Q *Recently after the Korean war began, there was an announcement in the papers that a committee or board had been created of the three civilian secretaries. Is that board still functioning?*

A Yes, that meets each Thursday morning with Mr. Lovett—the three civilian secretaries and the Deputy Secretary of Defense, who is chairman.[9]

There is the Armed Forces Policy Council, which consists of the Secretary of Defense, who has the power of decision, the Deputy Secretary, and each of the secretaries of the three services, with General Bradley, Chairman of the Joint Chiefs of Staff, and the three Chiefs of Staff. They meet once a week and go over all general considerations. We met this morning, for example.[10]

Q *How is that related to the National Security Council?*

A There is no formal relationship, but we may discuss issues that are to come up in the National Security Council.

Q *Do you make recommendations to the National Security Council?*

A Not necessarily recommendations—as a rule, those come from the Chiefs of Staff, but they may come both ways.

Civilian Role in Defense

Q *There has been a lot of talk as to whether we are being dominated by military or by civilians—I wonder whether you could give us the answer to that?*

A The Defense Department (exclusive of the three military departments) is quite large—it includes upwards of 2,700 people. And the large majority are civilians. The Deputy Secretary, the under secretaries, assistant secretaries, chairmen of the various boards—the Research and Development Board, the Munitions Board, the Personnel Policy Board, and the Civilian Components Policy Board—are civilians. The last named board is headed not only by a civilian, but by a man who has had no military experience—he's a railroad man. He is leaving shortly, and his successor is a man very carefully chosen who has also had no military experience.[11] The board includes Reserve officers, National Guard officers—it has seemed best that it be presided over by a civilian who has no alignment with any one of the various services.

Q *I think the point sometimes relates more particularly as to whether the Defense Department or foreign policy defines the obligations which the military must carry out.*

A Foreign-policy proposals come from the State Department. The reaction of the Defense Department comes mainly from the Joint Chiefs of Staff, but also, of course, from the Secretary of Defense, and the three service secretaries.

Carrying Out Foreign Policy

Q *You don't actually initiate foreign policy anywhere in the Defense Department?*

A No. We execute it so far as it involves matters of a military nature, and we bring our influence to bear when the foreign policy proposed has military implications.

Q *And your influence is as to whether you can execute the policy satisfactorily?*

A Whether it is a practical proposition. For example, yesterday afternoon, the Secretary of State and one under secretary met with Lovett and myself and the Chiefs of Staff in the latter's board room from 3 o'clock until almost 6. Here was the State Department with its proposal, with an outline of the situation and the United Nations considerations, asking what was the military reaction.[12]

Q *Could you deliver such a reaction?*

A Not only could we deliver—but did it put us in a dangerous situation—were we overreaching—or did the proposal weaken our position—all of those questions would enter the discussion. When finally we come to an agreed proposal, that usually goes to the National Security Council for final decision.

Q *And that is the President and yourself and other Cabinet members?*

A That is the President, the Vice President, the Secretary of State, the Secretary of Defense, and the chairman of the National Security Resources Board.

Q *Of course you two would dominate that, wouldn't you—if the Secretary of State and the Secretary of Defense have already agreed—*

A In a sense that might be the case, but as a rule it is carried out in this fashion: An issue comes up—say, they want an agreed estimate on a certain situation or with regard to a certain area. The State Department would ordinarily prepare the draft, and then it is sent over and the Chiefs of Staff take a look at it, the three service secretaries take a shot at it, and it is also being looked over by NSRB and the Secretary of the Treasury. Out of that come the various reactions—reactions of the three service secretaries, the reactions of the Chiefs of Staff, and my forwarding a reaction to their proposals. That goes over to the State Department and they may agree to most of proposed changes, so that by the time it gets to the formal Security Council meeting there has been a general agreement on the modifications of the original paper. But before that is done—I omitted one procedure—we have a senior staff of the National Security Council. They sit down together—including a representative of the Defense Department and a representative of the State Department—they sit down together and work through the suggestions to develop what unanimity there seems to be. Finally here is the original proposal, here are the proposed amendments of the Chiefs of Staff, the amendments of the secretaries, and here are the revisions by the senior-staff group—and the issue gets whipped into shape. The Security Council then formally decides what the decision shall be in these various matters.

Q *And the President makes the final decision?*

A Yes.

Q *I'd like to develop that point a little bit further. All that the Defense Department does on these matters of policy is evaluate the military consequences of the policy. It doesn't create the policy, does it?*

A No, it does not.

Q *It doesn't initiate any action from the standpoint of foreign policy or relations with other nations?*

A It does not initiate action unless the particular situation has gotten into a serious state where we feel something has to be done.

Q *I was speaking of policy action—*

A I'm speaking of that, too. In other words, we may become impatient because there hasn't been a change of policy and the situation has tended to grow more dangerous or difficult in a military way.

Q *That is a military consideration, primarily?*

A Yes, it is, exactly that.

Military Readiness: Improving

Q *Could you give us an evaluation of the Army, Navy and the Air Force as you see them in their state of readiness, or the progress each of these three services has made?*

A Let me first say this: We started in June from a state of bankruptcy as to available trained reserves. Whatever reserve organizations we had were only 40 or 50 per cent of strength, and that strength only partially trained. We had no resources, no established system for the creation of trained man power. I might say that I told the staff that when they had produced the first surplus trained man I'm going to hold a ceremony here in Washington to celebrate that event. They would be seeing something that had never been seen before in time of peace in the history of our Government.

With that beginning from zero, with 30,000 South Koreans in the ranks of four American divisions out there—that means about 36 per cent of the enlisted strength was South Koreans—we were in a serious dilemma. And we haven't worked out of it yet. This month, I think, is the first time we will begin to see a little light.

Better Off in May

Q *How would you describe the present situation?*

A We are getting to the point now where for the first time we have a little leeway in trained men. In May we will be much better off. As we work out of our troubles or deficiencies, we are steadily getting into a stronger position. We now have just exactly doubled the strength of the military forces since June, about 2.9 million.[13] To get a basis of comparison, that is more men than we obtained from the time we started mobilization in August, 1940, up to three months after Pearl Harbor, or March, 1942.

Q *That's for the three services?*

A That's for the three services—2.9 million. By the 30th of June we ought to be up to the figure we were after, about 3.4 million. The fact that we were able to double our numbers in this short time, and I think in an orderly manner, is encouraging.

What we are now trying to do is overcome this complete deficiency of trained men that we've had. And it hasn't been a problem of getting additional divisional units so much as getting trained men to put into units. We are now getting on a basis of what might be called a position in readiness, both in personnel and in matériel from which we can go forward very rapidly to whatever degree is required by the sudden development of the situation.

We are getting on a very solid basis as to the future, and without overextending ourselves. What we've got to watch, very carefully, I think, is that we don't do as some propose—build up a tremendous organization and then have it fall flat when public interest slacks, and congressional support, as a consequence, might fail us.

Q *What would you say of the state of readiness of the Air Force?*

A It has made very rapid progress and it has gone ahead just as rapidly as it can possibly absorb the men. It has constantly increased. And the navy has been taking ships out of moth balls and manning them in a very effective manner.

Q *Are they getting the personnel, both those forces?*

A Yes, they are getting the personnel.

Q *Then we are a much stronger country now than we were six months ago?*

A Yes.

GCMRL/G. C. Marshall Papers (Secretary of Defense, Speeches and Statements); used under license

1. Marshall, accompanied by Clayton Fritchey, director of the Defense Department's Office of Public Information (OPI), participated in an almost two-hour interview with David Lawrence, editor of *U.S. News and World Report*, on March 20 at 2:30 p.m. The Defense Department reserved the right to edit the transcript of this interview, which it did substantially before publication in the magazine's April 13, 1951, issue. The document above is a March 26 transcription of the interview as it was published and is reproduced under license by *U.S. News and World Report*.

2. See pp. 300–301.

3. See pp. 325–29, 338–47, 369–71, 409–13, and 423–26.

4. The Civilian Components Policy Board (CCPB) was charged with developing and coordinating policies for the Department of Defense with regard to the National Guard and other reserve forces. See pp. 185–86.

5. The Joint Chiefs of Staff came into existence in early 1942 to replace the old Joint Army-Navy Board and match the organization of the British Chiefs of Staff Committee on the new Anglo-American Combined Chiefs of Staff. They reported directly to President Roosevelt and existed at his discretion, functioning without any charter or formal directive throughout World War II and until the passage of the National Security Act in 1947.

6. See, for example, pp. 409–13.

7. See *Papers of GCM*, 2: 163–64, 248, 309–10.

8. For similar comments by Marshall after the detonation of the atomic bomb, see *Papers of GCM*, 5: 259–60, 313.

9. The *New York Times* reported on July 18, 1950, that Pace, Francis Matthews, and Finletter had formed the "Joint Secretaries," an "'executive committee' . . . to deal with the political-military aspects of the Korean fighting and cold war" that would serve "as a counterpart at the civilian level to the Joint Chiefs of Staff." ("Service Secretaries Form Organization," *New York Times*, July 18, 1950, p. 2.)

10. For more on Marshall's reorganization of the Department of Defense, see pp. 371–72 and the chart on p. 1006.

11. Edwin H. Burgess, a former vice president and general counsel of the Baltimore & Ohio Railroad, had become chairman of the CCPB on May 1, 1950. At Marshall's behest, the CCPB became the Reserve Forces Policy Board under Rosenberg on June 13, 1951, and Charles H. Buford, a former president of the Chicago, Milwaukee, St. Paul, and Pacific Railroad companies as well as federal manager of railroads when Truman nationalized the industry in May 1946 in an attempt to avoid a strike, replaced Burgess. (Condit, Test of War, 498; "New Head Named for Defense Post," *New York Times*, April 13, 1950, p. 22;

"Charles Buford, Railway Official," *New York Times,* August 19, 1960, p. 23; Marshall to Lovett, memorandum, January 18, 1951, NA/RG 330 [OSD Index, 201–Marshall, George C.]; Marshall to Burgess and Marshall to Buford, February 8, 1951, GCMRL/G. C. Marshall Papers [Secretary of Defense, Number Indexed, M200-7-3].)

12. For a record of this March 19 meeting by Paul Nitze, see *FRUS, 1951*, 7: 246–47.

13. See the previous document.

271

To General of the Army Dwight D. Eisenhower — March 21, 1951
Top Secret — Washington, DC

Dear Eisenhower: Many thanks for your highly informative letter of 12 March. I showed it to Bradley, who in turn read it to the Joint Chiefs at their meeting on the 16th. The Joint Chiefs in turn instructed their representative on the Standing Group to fully back your plan when the Standing Group meets on it. I have also let General Lindsey, Chairman of the JCS Committee working on this problem, read your letter and make pertinent notes so that there will be no misunderstanding as to what you want.[1]

We seem to be heading for trouble in the house on our Universal Military Training and Service Bill, but have hopes that if we do not make out too badly there, we will be able to get the important things ironed out in conference.[2]

I cannot guarantee that "no American official, military or other, may upset these delicate negotiations through lack of understanding, etc.," but I will do my best. Many complications in our business here are frequently traced to just such lack of understanding and it seems that we spend about half of our time chasing them down and correcting them.[3]

With warm regards, Faithfully yours,

NA/RG 330, CD 370.21 (SHAPE)

1. In his five-page letter to Marshall, Eisenhower had outlined some of his general concerns about the structure and command hierarchy of NATO, including the subpar public relations department, the need to appoint officials of multiple nationalities in high-ranking positions to appease political considerations, and the controversy surrounding the establishment of a Mediterranean–Middle East command and its relationship with the European command (see pp. 439–40). He labeled NATO "more an idea or concept than it is a real organization" and told Marshall that "The situation is more complicated than it was in World War II because of the increased number of nations, and is further confused because the economic and political factors enter into *everything* we do." Eisenhower asked Marshall to share this letter with Bradley, who informed Marshall on March 16 that the JCS had instructed its "representative on the Standing Group to fully back General Eisenhower's plan" for the organization and command of NATO. (Eisenhower to Marshall, March 12, 1951, and Bradley to Marshall, memorandum, March 16, 1951, NA/RG 330, CD 370.21 [SHAPE].) For more, see pp. 431–32.

"I had a letter from Eisenhower just the other day," Marshall informed Lord Tedder on March 19, "and he and his top-level staff are experiencing pretty much the same problems of several years ago. However, I fear the military and political problems will be much more complex." (Marshall to Tedder, March 19, 1951, GCMRL/G. C. Marshall Papers [Secretary of Defense, Chronological, Secretaries, Carlson].)

Major General Richard C. Lindsay, USAF, was the deputy director for strategic plans of the Joint Staff.

2. See pp. 409–13, 423–26, 462–63, and 481–84.

3. For more on NATO appointments and the development of command structure, see pp. 472–74.

Determined to Be Strong

March 27–September 11, 1951

There should be no doubt in the world's mind that we are determined to be strong enough to stand up in this present crisis in the world's history.

—Testimony on the Mutual Security Act of 1951
July 2, 1951

BY MID-MARCH 1951, Ridgway's latest offensive (Operation RIPPER) had resulted in the recapture of Seoul and was on the verge of forcing the Chinese to withdraw north of the 38th parallel, thereby providing the administration with an opportunity to propose armistice negotiations. On March 20, the Joint Chiefs informed MacArthur that the State Department was planning a presidential announcement (which Acheson had discussed with Marshall and the JCS on March 19) stating "that, with clearing of bulk of South Korea of aggression, United Nations now prepared to discuss conditions of settlement in Korea" and that there was "strong UN feeling . . . that further diplomatic effort should be made before any advance with major forces north of 38th Parallel." (*FRUS, 1951*, 7: 246–54; quote on 251.)

MacArthur, however, rejected such limits and continued to press for expansion of the war into China. On February 13 and again on March 7, he had violated Truman's December 5 directive to clear all public statements in advance (see pp. 282–83) and had denounced the limits placed upon him, in particular his inability to attack the Chinese "sanctuary" in Manchuria. He did so again on March 15 by publicly criticizing the halting of Ridgway's advance at the 38th parallel or short of "accomplishment of our mission in the unification of Korea." (James F. Schnabel, *United States Army in the Korean War*, vol. 3, *Policy and Direction: The First Year* [Washington: Office of the Chief of Military History, US Army, 1972], 373; Dean Acheson, *Present at the Creation: My Years in the State Department* [New York: W. W. Norton, 1969], 518.) Now on March 24 (March 23 in Washington), he once again violated Truman's directive—and subverted the administration's plan to propose armistice negotiations—by issuing a press release that called upon the Chinese to accept a cease-fire agreement or risk expansion of the war across the Yalu River to China's "coastal areas and interior bases," an expansion that he warned would "doom Red China to the risk of imminent military collapse." (Senate Committee on Armed Services and Committee on Foreign Relations, *Hearings to Conduct an Inquiry Into the Military Situation in the Far East* [hereafter *MSFE*] . . . , 82d Cong., 1st sess., 3541–42.) Marshall later stated that at the time MacArthur issued this statement, "the clearance of the proposed Presidential statement with the other thirteen nations having forces in Korea had very nearly been completed. In view of the serious impact of General MacArthur's statement on the negotiation with these nations, it became necessary to abandon the effort, thus losing whatever chance there may have been at the time to negotiate a settlement of the Korean conflict." (*MSFE*, 344.) See pp. 505–16.

At 11:00 p.m. on March 23, Washington time, Lovett, Rusk, and two of his State Department associates brought the text of this press release to Acheson at his home. According to Acheson's later recollections, Lovett "was angrier than I had ever seen him" and said that MacArthur "must be removed and removed at once. After reading the statement I shared his sense of outrage." They discussed the matter until 1:00 a.m., with Acheson sending it to numerous US embassies and making clear that it "was not authorized, expected or representative of the views of this Govt." (Acheson, *Present at the Creation*, 518–19; *FRUS, 1951*, 7:

264–65.) The following morning Acheson, Rusk, and Lovett (acting for Marshall, who was in Pinehurst for the Easter weekend) met with Truman, who, according to Acheson, "although perfectly calm, appeared to be in a state of mind that combined disbelief with controlled fury." Truman later labeled MacArthur's statement an "ultimatum" as well as "open defiance" of his orders that "left me no choice—I could no longer tolerate his insubordination." Consequently he had Bradley remind MacArthur of the December directive. (Acheson, *Present at the Creation*, 519; Harry S. Truman, *Memoirs*, vol. 2, *Years of Trial and Hope* [Garden City, NY: Doubleday & Company, Inc., 1956], 441–43.)

On the afternoon of Monday, March 26, Marshall returned from his weekend in Pinehurst and had three separate meetings with Lovett, followed by additional meetings with him on the morning of March 27 as well as the service secretaries and the army, navy, and air force chiefs. At 12:30 p.m. he met with the president, and at 3:00 p.m. he held what appears to have been his first full press conference since becoming secretary of defense the previous September. ★

272

Remarks at a Press Conference
March 27, 1951 Washington, DC

"NOW, for your convenience, if not your pleasure," Marshall began, "I'll tell you right at the start that I assume that you'd all wish to question me on relation to this recent statement by General MacArthur, and, judging from the papers, some of you know more about it than I do, but, in any event, I'm going to make no comment so there is no use in asking me the question." (Transcript of remarks at a press conference, March 27, 1951, GCMRL/G. C. Marshall Papers [Secretary of Defense, Speeches and Statements].) Carter had informed Marshall prior to the press conference that Truman and Acheson urged that Marshall offer "'no comment' on the MacArthur business," but Carter added that "there is unquestionably a lot of talking behind the scene," as James Reston, a reporter with the *New York Times* who had published two articles on MacArthur's statement prior to Marshall's press conference, "has the whole story." Carter thus recommended a statement similar to how Marshall began his press conference. (*FRUS, 1951*, 7: 265–68; Carter to Marshall, memorandum, March 27, 1951, GCMRL/G. C. Marshall Papers [Secretary of Defense, Number Indexed, M204-2-9]; James Reston, "Washington and MacArthur Clash Anew on Truce Offer," *New York Times*, March 25, 1951, pp. 1, 3; James Reston, "Joint Chiefs Tell MacArthur To Clear Future Statements," *New York Times*, March 27, 1951, pp. 1, 6.) See the previous editorial note.

Marshall presumed "also that some of you at least would wish to question me now about the problem of the 38th Parallel and the Korean campaign. As to that, the question of any full advance north of the 38th Parallel is a political question, as has already been stated, particularly by General MacArthur. The compelling factor there, the dominant instruction there is that he will proceed in accordance with the necessities to safeguard the security of his command. That dominates his actions." (Transcript of remarks at a press conference, March 27, 1951, GCMRL/G. C. Marshall Papers [Secretary of Defense, Speeches and Statements].) According to Reston's March 27 article cited in the previous paragraph, Truman's advisers agreed that MacArthur should be allowed to cross the 38th parallel "whenever necessary to keep the enemy off balance and to protect the security of his international army."

Marshall also explained "that the military issue, which is the governing one, involves a very difficult and delicate situation in the event that the enemy breaks off contact. General MacArthur or General Ridgway, rather, is then confronted with the problem of whether or not he attempts to resume contact. Normally, in any military campaign contact is of first importance. In Korea, he has the problem of how far he might proceed with patrols, to what distance, without the danger of their being cut off. The only remedy for that is to move forward the divisions. He is then confronted with the problem of how far he chooses to move his divisions forward, so it makes a rather difficult situation for a military decision. But the guiding principle, as I have already stated, would be the security of his command." (Ibid.)

In the Far East, Marshall supposed "you already know that the two National Guard Divisions that are to go out to Japan are scheduled to sail the latter part of this week, possibly Thursday: the 45th from New Orleans and the 40th I think from San Francisco, anyway from the West Coast. I was cautioned by some of my staff that this probably was top secret but it's no longer such and I imagine that everybody in that vicinity knows pretty well what's going on." Emphasizing that these comments were "Very much off the record," Marshall added that these "divisions have not completed their full training. They could not well be sent to Japan until they had completed at least their basic training. They are a very good example of our present problem under the existing scheme of national defense whereby our largest ground forces are bound to come from the National Guard." It had taken these divisions seven months, from their call to "service in September . . . until the middle of March" to "complete their basic training," and they had not yet completed their training "in the regimental, brigade and the divisional basis." Marshall remarked: "Naturally, in a world situation like that today such a procedure does not fit the circumstances." (Ibid.; George to Marshall, memorandum, March 27, 1951, GCMRL/G. C. Marshall Papers [Secretary of Defense, Number Indexed, M204-2-9].) See pp. 431–32.

Marshall then asked for any questions, stipulating that his responses were "for background, and I will specifically mention if it is otherwise." When asked if MacArthur could "go all the way to the Yalu River under his present directives" if he thought "it's necessary to safeguard the security of his command," Marshall replied negatively, as such action would "be a little extreme" and "would be the peril of the command" rather than its security. He declined to comment on a question as to whether a "mutual zone set up" would be established "in Korea or north of the Yalu River" should a truce be accomplished. Shifting to Western Europe, Marshall maintained that there were no plans to provide more than six army divisions to support Eisenhower's NATO command, and he agreed to provide information on naval and air contributions, which had "never been very debatable." (Transcript of remarks at a press conference, March 27, 1951, GCMRL/G. C. Marshall Papers [Secretary of Defense, Speeches and Statements].)

Using briefs of sample questions and answers on the Defense Department budget and UMT provided by Marshall Carter, Marshall began a lengthy explanation about the budget requests by the Defense Department currently under consideration by Congress, both a third supplemental request to the fiscal year 1951 budget of approximately $10 billion to address the Korean War, and a nearly $60 billion request for fiscal year 1952. The supplemental request was necessary for "very easily understandable items such as pay and rations" but also to ensure the "uninterrupted" manufacture of certain materiel critical to national defense. During his December 1950 testimony on supplemental appropriations (see pp. 276–78 and 291–93), Marshall recalled, there was an informal agreement by members of Congress "that there'd be no objection if we over-spent in that fiscal year." The congressmen believed the Defense Department was "not asking for enough," but Marshall and other Defense Department officials "thought we were going ahead on the right basis to spend the money efficiently, expeditiously, and that we could over-spend as the occasion demanded." (Ibid. See Carter to Marshall, memorandum and attachments, March 27, 1951, GCMRL/G. C. Marshall Papers [Secretary of Defense, Number Indexed, M200-4-9]; and Doris M. Condit, *History of the Office of the Secretary of Defense*, vol. 2, *The Test of War, 1950–1953* [Washington: Historical Office, Office of the Secretary of Defense, 1988], 240 and 252.)

Another consideration at this time was the UMT bill which would come "into a general debate in the House in a few days." (See pp. 481–84.) Marshall hoped that "crippling amendments" to the bill would be stopped and believed that the debate on the bill and the appropriations requests were exposing the radical shift in public opinion and that of Congress over the previous several months. In late 1950, "There was a general feeling of the majority of the people with whom we came in contact publicly and on the Hill, that we were not seeing the problem in its enormity and danger and, therefore, not asking for enough." Now, however, "There's been a relaxation," so it was "of monumental importance" to redouble efforts to build "an enduring program" of national defense "to protect us against these mountains they want built up and these valleys that we slide into through relaxation." Marshall noted that "in this particular instance you can put your finger on the man that is responsible for the whole business": General Ridgway, whose "efficiency" and "leadership" brought successes in Korea and were causing "trouble back here" for Defense Department proposals. "Of course, I think he'd be very much startled to learn that, but he's been through a little of this with me at other times and I wouldn't want to deter him from any further successes!" (Transcript of remarks at a press conference, March 27, 1951, GCMRL/G. C. Marshall Papers [Secretary of Defense, Speeches and Statements]; Carter to Marshall, memorandum and attachments, March 27, 1951, GCMRL/G. C. Marshall Papers [Secretary of Defense, Number Indexed, M200-4-9].)

Marshall believed that passage of the UMT bill was critical "because, if we're going to live through this period of the next—whatever it is—five or ten years and grow negligent and careless in the first six weeks, what is there to expect?—unless we have some basis that is within our possibilities financially that permits us to retire the number of men on active duty and still maintain an effective defense posture." A key purpose of the bill was "to enable us to build up the availability and efficiency and vitalize the National Guard." This was critical to allow the United States to send divisions wherever they were needed "without scalping units," as had been required at the outbreak of the Korean War until March 1951, when there were finally "enough graduates of basic military training to meet our immediate requirements." This would allow the initiation of "a rotation procedure for the Army" which would be announced shortly. (See pp. 436–37 and 516–17.) He added that the urgent need at the time was "not new divisions but trained men to meet our commitments of those that we now have under way." That need had been reduced by more "voluntary enlistments" than expected, although Marshall asked the reporters to consider that the Defense Department had not "just gone along and tried to hog a lot of men. We've taken what we think we needed at the time," and the department reduced the draft call in light of the higher level of enlistments. That "was a rather difficult thing to do because it didn't have a happy effect on the legislation," but the Defense Department "went along very honestly and exactingly, and we got more men than we anticipated, so we cut." (Ibid.)

Marshall later reiterated his frustration with the "emotional reaction" by the public and Congress in late 1950. He cautioned that Korea was "a very small peninsula" while "the Soviet Union's activities cover pretty much the whole world." Despite the improvements in Korea, "the situation now, as I see it, is more serious than it was" in the fall of 1950. This point was not resonating with the public, however, because of "some of the things you gentlemen write and the commentators, the political speeches, the general—television now. I can't compete with all of those and try to get a simple statement of the problem." When asked if he wanted "an emotional reaction," Marshall retorted: "I don't want an emotional reaction. That's the last thing in the world I want. I want cold-blooded calculation and wisdom and foresight. That's pretty hard to get." (Transcript of remarks at a press conference, March 27, 1951, GCMRL/G. C. Marshall Papers [Secretary of Defense, Speeches and Statements].)

After a lengthy exchange about whether Marshall's comments were on or off the record, Marshall and Clayton Fritchey agreed that two quotes could be attributed to Marshall: first, "The situation, as I see it, is more serious now than in November"; and second, "Any general advantages [*advance*]" north of the 38th parallel in Korea "is a matter for political decision." (Ibid.)

On March 28, Rear Admiral Richard E. Byrd (USNA, 1912), officer in charge of US Antarctic Programs, told Marshall that he agreed with Marshall's statements in the press conference. Marshall replied on April 2 that "In most cases the editorial reaction was good, but several took a crack at me for hollering wolf without further explaining my reasons for thinking the situation now is more serious than it was in November of last year." He also noted that "the Battle of the Potomac continues, and I find myself pretty much a part of it." (Byrd to Marshall, March 28, 1951, and Marshall to Byrd, April 2, 1951, GCMRL/G. C. Marshall Papers [Secretary of Defense, Number Indexed, M200-12-5].)

During an April 9 speech, while discussing this press conference, press demands for government transparency, and the difficulty in obtaining information about the Soviet military buildup, Marshall lamented that he sometimes felt like "a G-2 [intelligence officer] for Stalin. I am perfectly willing to be that if they make him a G-2 for me. We don't know anything about that side and have to tell everything on this side." (Speech to the Joint Civilian Orientation Conference, April 9, 1951, NA/RG 330, SD 353 [Joint Orientation Conference #8].) ★

273

To John D. Small | March 27, 1951
Confidential | Washington, DC

Dear Small: As part of our overall defense effort, both as to immediate operations and in our long-range planning, it seems to me that economic warfare, particularly vis-à-vis the Soviet Union, must be an important factor.

I realize that this matter ties in very closely with East-West trade which I understand is being handled by an interdepartmental committee, and with export controls under the Department of Commerce. However, I am not sure in my own mind as to just what organization and procedures, if any, are being used to develop plans and methods for economic warfare.

Will you please have one of your people prepare me a memorandum of information indicating who in the Executive agency of the government has primary responsibility, what the procedures for coordination are, and what the present status of our operations and plans is for economic warfare.[1] Faithfully yours,

NA/RG 330, CD 385 (Economic Warfare)

1. Small replied on April 3 that the NSC "is responsible for the initiation of economic warfare" and that the NSRB "is responsible for the development of over-all policies, plans, and programs for economic warfare, but is not responsible for the actual conduct of economic warfare measures." By that time, the NSRB and Department of Commerce had issued a total of nine reports on economic warfare policies. Small continued that the NSC's Special Committee on East-West Trade was currently considering "a comprehensive report" that recommended in part the creation of an "Economic Defense Strategy Board" under State Department chairmanship. Small did not know whether the Defense Department would be given "an opportunity to present its views on this part of the report" and added that the Munitions Board had prepared its own plan on economic warfare which proposed the establishment of a body within the NSC with the appropriate authority "to ensure the coordination of plans and operations." Elmer Staats, assistant director of the Bureau of the Budget, informed the Defense Department on June 21 that many different plans "were under consideration" and assured the department that it "would have further chance to be heard before a final decision is reached." (Small to Marshall,

April 3, 1951; memorandum to Lovett and attachment, June 22, 1951, NA/RG 330, CD 385 [Economic Warfare].)

274

TO MARGARET EMERSON

March 28, 1951
Washington, DC

Dear Margaret, Thanks for your very nice letter of March 16 [*15*]th and while I thought about sending my reply to Honolulu, I thought the time element would interfere as you would probably be enroute home, so this is just an addition to the batch which will probably be awaiting your return to the Park Lane.[1]

I am sorry that the weather was not good which no doubt caused you to spend many hours indoors while you probably would have preferred to be in the sun. I do hope that your trip home was pleasant and that you were not troubled with the usual inconveniences that go with making a long journey.

You have probably already learned that the Red Cross campaign here is not going so well either; as a matter of fact I think it is three or four percent below that of last year. However, to offset this they have extended the drive until the 15th of April.[2]

Katherine has been at Pinehurst now for several weeks and fortunately for me I have been able to join her every weekend so far. Leaving there on Mondays has been very difficult for me as for the most part the weather has been excellent and I have witnessed several fine golf matches. I get a great kick out of chasing the little white pill and at the same time get plenty of exercise. I have always thought that my work here at the Pentagon was difficult but it doesn't compare with what Katherine is experiencing at the moment. She is being cook, chambermaid, and housekeeper for her three grandchildren, together with their mother and father. In addition to this Sgt. Heffner has been down with the flu which required waiting on, as was her sister Mrs. Lacy. Fortunately her Florence Nightingale duties are over as the two sick ones are now back on their feet.[3]

Katherine and I are looking forward to your going with us to Lexington on May 14th. The plan is that you and Katherine will make your headquarters at the hotel and I will stay with the other members of the Board of Visitors at the barracks. I think many of our mutual friends will be there for the occasion, especially Mr. Bernard Baruch whom the Superintendent of the Institute is trying to sign up as speaker of the day.[4]

I am glad that you enjoyed the book, "American Guerrilla" and I hope you found the film version as interesting.[5]

With love from us both, Affectionately,

GCMRL/G. C. Marshall Papers (Secretary of Defense, Number Indexed, M200-7-47)

1. On March 6, Marshall had written to Emerson, who was vacationing in Honolulu, Hawaii, in response to her February 28 letter to Mrs. Marshall. Emerson replied on March 15 that she was sailing from Hawaii on March 31 and hoped to arrive at the Park Lane Hotel on April 8. She had "had the most *dreadful* weather, rain rain, then more rain—10¾ inches in

2½ days!" (Marshall to Emerson, March 6, 1951, and Emerson to Marshall, March 15, 1951, GCMRL/G. C. Marshall Papers [Secretary of Defense, Number Indexed, M200-7-47].)

2. Emerson reported in her March 15 letter that she was working with the Red Cross on "'odd' things. The 'drive' is *not* going well—but maybe it will pick up in a few days—Gosh, I hope it will. They have only *$38*,000 of their *200* odd thousand to raise!" (Ibid.)

The Greater Washington area drive had extended its fundraising deadline from March 31 to April 13. By April 3, the campaign had raised over one million dollars but was "still $300,000 short of the goal." ("Red Cross Fund Tops Million, Shy $300,000," *Washington Post*, April 4, 1951, p. B1.)

3. On March 23, Marshall had informed a neighbor in Leesburg of Heffner's illness as well as that of Katherine Marshall's sister, Allene Lacy, and had added that "Anna, the maid, is still on vacation." He also noted that Mrs. Marshall's eldest child, Clifton, who was going to join him in the trip to Pinehurst that day, had been ill as well but "seems to be allright now." (Marshall to Hayden Harris, March 23, 1951, GCMRL/G. C. Marshall Papers [Secretary of Defense, Number Indexed, M200-6-5].)

4. See pp. 518–23.

5. Marshall had sent a copy of Ira Wolfert's *American Guerrilla in the Philippines* (New York: Simon and Schuster, 1945), to Emerson in Hawaii on February 28. In her March 15 letter, she thanked Marshall "*so much* for the little book." The book had been developed into a screenplay in 1950, which Emerson had seen twice before receiving the book from Marshall. (Emerson to Marshall, March 15, 1951, ibid., [M200-7-47].)

275

To Jacob K. Javits — March 30, 1951
Washington, DC

Dear Mr. Javits: I appreciate your letter of March 10 commending the Army for the progress it has made at Fort Dix in providing equality of opportunity and treatment for all troops, regardless of race or color. I am certain that visits to other training installations would convince you that a similarly conscientious effort is being made in all Army training divisions to carry out the principles of non-discrimination.[1]

The combat experience of integrated units in the Korean fighting is currently being reviewed by a special board of Army officers to see what further action might be desirable to promote efficiency and morale among troops in this country and overseas. A great deal has already been accomplished along this line, as your own trip to Fort Dix has shown. I have asked the Army to prepare an analysis of some of the improvements that have been made in the period since V-J day. I shall send it to you in a few days so that you may have a fuller understanding of how much has been achieved.[2]

I share your concern over reports of discrimination and physical violence off the post against military personnel in uniform. As early as 1943 Secretary of War Stimson asked the Congress to pass a bill extending to members of the armed services the same protection that is accorded other classes of Federal officers against such abuses. I favor the passage of such a bill now as a matter of elementary fairness to our troops. However, I would urge that any legislative proposal to this end be considered apart from the University Military Training and Service bill in order that each of these important measures could be evaluated on its own merits.[3]

All of the other matters to which you refer in your letter are subjects of continuous study within the Army. The recommendations of the President's Committee on Equality of Treatment and Opportunity in the Armed Services have been a valuable guide in the progress that has already been made. I do not believe we need a new committee or a new blueprint at this time, but rather a continuation of the sincere effort that has been made in the ten months since the Fahy report to insure that every soldier will have a maximum opportunity to make his contribution to the effectiveness of our Army, without regard for his race or color.[4] Faithfully yours,

NA/RG 330, SD 291.2

1. Representative Javits (R-NY) had written to Marshall on several occasions since October 1950 regarding continued segregation in the armed services, particularly at Fort Dix, New Jersey, despite Truman's July 26, 1948, Executive Order 9981 calling for "equality of treatment and opportunity for all persons in the armed forces." ("Establishing the President's Committee on Equality of Treatment and Opportunity in the Armed Services," *Federal Register* 13, no. 146 [July 28, 1948]: 4313.) Marshall had initially advised Javits that he was giving his attention to further implementing Truman's directive. Citing this response, Javits informed Marshall on January 9, 1951, that he was considering submitting a resolution to "'authorize an investigation into segregation and discrimination in the armed services'" as he had done in the previous Congress. He thus requested a report on the status of desegregation efforts at Fort Dix and a review of such efforts among the services. Marshall replied on January 25 that "significant progress" was being made in each service and that he trusted that they had "the matter well in hand, within their zone of responsibility. There is, of course, a related community responsibility over which the services have no control." (Javits to Marshall, January 9, 1951, and Marshall to Javits, January 25, 1951, NA/RG 330, SD 291.2.)

In his March 10 letter to Marshall, Javits reported that he had recently visited Fort Dix with Representative Charles R. Howell (D-NJ). Integration at Fort Dix, begun by an order issued by Marshall "about six weeks" prior, was "working without difficulty and with colored troops in the training companies in percentages averaging 10% to 22%. There is also generally integration in barracks and messes." Javits indicated that "the morale of negro troops has been raised 100% by the integration order" and that facilities were now being used more efficiently. Despite this progress, he complained "that the Army still lags behind the Navy and the Air Force in the completeness of its integration." (Javits to Marshall, March 10, 1951, ibid.)

2. See pp. 474–75.

3. In June 1943 Stimson had submitted to Congress an amendment to a pending bill "providing punishment for killing or assaulting of Federal officers." (*Congressional Record* 89, pt. 4, 78th Cong., 1st sess., 5837.)

In response to Javits's March 10 letter, Leva had recommended to Assistant Secretary Rosenberg that "instead of a letter from Gen. Marshall," she call Javits personally "and tell him quite frankly that you would prefer to delay any reply until floor action on UMTS—for any letter we might send would be capable of being used against us on the floor." (Leva to Rosenberg, March 23, 1951, NA/RG 330, SD 291.2.) See pp. 481–84.

4. In his March 10 letter, Javits had urged "the reconstitution of a civilian committee equivalent to the President's Committee on Equality of Treatment and Opportunity in the Armed Services (which last reported May 22, 1950), to report on the actual status of equality of opportunity today." Named for its chairman Charles H. Fahy, solicitor general from 1941 to 1945 and former legal adviser to the State Department, this committee had been commissioned by Truman in Executive Order 9981. (Javits to Marshall, March 10, 1951, ibid.) See pp. 469–70.

276

To Brien McMahon April 2, 1951
Top Secret Washington, DC

Dear Senator McMahon: I refer to your memorandum, 12 February 1951, in which request is made for certain information concerning our atomic weapons, our ability to deliver them, the selection of targets, our atomic missile development, and other details.[1]

Most careful consideration has been given to a series of possible answers to the questions presented by you and, after consultation by the President with me and the Joint Chiefs of Staff, it has been decided that there is no practicable way in which this type of information can be made available without serious risk to our national security.

No question as to the integrity of anyone concerned in this matter has arisen. The risk to our national security arises from the fact that answers to the questions propounded cannot be complete in themselves; that is they can serve only to develop further fields for examination. Thus the ultimate result could only be a complete briefing of our most secret war plans including all the information upon which they are based.

Those mentioned above are unanimously of the opinion that this type of information must be held secret by the President, in his capacity as Commander in Chief, and his immediate subordinates. I believe that when you consider this matter from this point of view you will understand our reticence and agree with the conclusions reached.[2] Faithfully yours,

NA/RG 330, CD 600.96

1. The editors have been unable to locate the letter from McMahon (D-CT), chairman of the Joint Congressional Committee on Atomic Energy (JCAE), but according to a record of correspondence between Marshall and McMahon produced by Robert LeBaron, McMahon submitted a "list of questions" concerning the United States' "degree of military readiness in field of atomic energy," asked for a "written response," and implied "that written reply to these questions may give the JCAE sufficient data to satisfy their needs on this matter." (Robert LeBaron, "Log of Significant Events re JCS Proposed Response to Senator McMahon's Letter of 2 May 1951," June 19, 1951, NA/RG 330, CD 471.6.)

2. Much of the language of Marshall's reply comes from a March 27 memorandum from General Vandenberg, with input from LeBaron. (Vandenberg to Marshall, memorandum, March 27, 1951, NA/RG 330, CD 600.96.) General Bradley reported that Truman had "glanced through the list of questions" in McMahon's letter "and indicated that he fully concurred" with the response reproduced above. (Robert LeBaron, "Log of Significant Events re JCS Proposed Response to Senator McMahon's Letter of 2 May 1951," June 19, 1951, NA/RG 330, CD 471.6.)

CIA Director Walter Bedell Smith had also received a letter from McMahon which requested "a comprehensive estimate on Soviet capabilities 'to impair, prevent, or frustrate the delivery of atomic weapons to targets inside the USSR.'" Smith wrote to Marshall on February 5 to request "authorization for the Weapons Systems Evaluation Group," a body run jointly in the Defense Department by the JCS and RDB, to collaborate with the CIA in its preparation of a response to McMahon. Bradley informed Marshall on February 9 that the JCS did not approve of Smith's request. Marshall spoke with Smith about this matter on March 22, at which time Smith reported that several agencies, including the air force and the AEC, had "just about completed the preparation of a paper which answers most of the questions" in McMahon's letter. Marshall informed Carter that Smith felt "that certain portions of this certainly should" be eliminated before a response was sent to Congress, and he asked Carter "to see if it is not possible to draft a reply more or less on a technical level, which would not involve any statement of our war plans." Carter responded that he had referred the matter to the JCS, who were also "attempting to reply to a similar request from Senator McMahon to you." Marshall on April 17 forwarded to Smith a copy of the above April 2 response to McMahon and asserted security concerns forced him to prevent "Department of Defense participation in the project requested by Senator McMahon." (Smith to Marshall, memorandum, February 5, 1951; Bradley to Marshall, memorandum, February 9, 1951; Marshall to Carter, memorandum, March 22, 1951; Carter to Marshall, memorandum, April 2, 1951; and Marshall to Smith, April 17, 1951, NA/RG 330, CD 350.09.) For additional information on Marshall's involvement in nuclear issues during his year as secretary of defense, see pp. 559–60 and 616–17; Condit, *Test of War*, 456–77; and Richard G. Hewlett and Francis Duncan, *A History of the United States Atomic Energy Commission*, vol. 2, *Forging the Atomic Shield, 1947–1952* (University Park: Pennsylvania State University Press, 1969), 532–70.

277

MEMORANDUM FOR THE SERVICE SECRETARIES AND THE JOINT CHIEFS OF STAFF

April 2, 1951
Washington, DC

SUBJECT: Qualitative Distribution of Military Manpower[1]

1. The following policies are hereby promulgated to provide for the qualitative division of military manpower accessions among the Services on an equitable basis. These policies are applicable to the procurement of personnel through induction or by voluntary recruitment. They will be implemented 1 May 1951 by the Army, Navy, Marine Corps and Air Force.

2. *Policies of a general nature*

a. Each service may continue voluntary enlistment programs, subject to necessary limitations imposed by this and any other pertinent directives.

b. The same minimum physical standards for acceptance will obtain for each service. These acceptance standards will be identical for enlistment and induction of males except for officer candidates and aviation cadets.

c. Qualitative distribution of personnel enlisted and inducted under common physical standards will be accomplished by quota control of accessions to each of the services in each of the four major mental groupings.

3. Male acquisitions (with the exceptions cited below), whether obtained by induction or enlistment, will be charged against the qualitative and quantitative allocations of the respective services.

Exceptions

a. Officer candidates and aviation cadets.

b. Individuals *exempt* (as distinguished from *deferred*) from induction as set forth in Section 6 of the Selective Service Act of 1948 as amended or other applicable legislation.[2]

4. a. These policies will be administered under procedures prescribed by the

Office of the Assistant Secretary of Defense, Manpower and Personnel.

b. When special requirements support such action, a service may request of the Secretary of Defense specific exceptions to proportionate qualitative distribution.

5. Detailed policies are outlined in inclosure 1.[3]

GCMarshall

GCMRL/G. C. Marshall Papers (Secretary of Defense, Speeches and Statements)

1. This memorandum may have resulted, at least in part, from a congressional threat, during the debate over the UMT bill, of further investigation if the Defense Department failed to distribute equally among the military branches Selective Service draftees regardless of their mental aptitude. (James M. Gerhardt, *The Draft and Public Policy: Issues in Military Manpower Procurement, 1945–1970* [Columbus: Ohio State University Press, 1971], 169.) It was also relevant to the ongoing efforts to implement fully Truman's 1948 executive order regarding integration of the armed forces. See n3 below and p. 467n1.

2. The Selective Service Act of 1948 authorized the exemption from induction of several groups of men: those who served honorably for over twelve months from the initiation of the peacetime draft prior to World War II through the enactment of the 1948 law; those who served for over ninety days between the Pearl Harbor attack and V-J day; those who served on active duty for three or more years after the enactment of the 1948 law; ministers or those actively studying to become ministers; conscientious objectors; and sole surviving sons. (*Selective Service under the 1948 Act: June 24, 1948–July 9, 1950* [Washington: GPO, 1951], 28–31.)

3. The enclosure detailed how an inductee's performance on the Armed Forces Qualification Test (AFQT) would determine his mental group classification and the percentage quota from each classification that each service would be required to accept. (Marshall to service secretaries, memorandum and attachment, April 2, 1951, GCMRL/G. C. Marshall Papers [Secretary of Defense, Speeches and Statements].)

On April 10, Marshall appeared with Rosenberg and Ralph Sollott, a consultant to Rosenberg, at a press conference during which he announced this policy and distributed a coordinating press release that called this policy "'a further step in the progress of the unification of the armed forces.'" At the press conference, Marshall informed the reporters "that this was the first paper, the first task I gave Mrs. Rosenberg when she reported as Assistant Secretary, so it has been in the process of discussion, negotiation, you might call it, pretty much ever since." This policy was also "in accord very specifically with the opinion of the Armed Forces Committees of both the House and the Senate." (Transcript of press conference, April 10, 1951, GCMRL/G. C. Marshall Papers [Speeches Binder #13]; press release, April 10, 1951, GCMRL/G. C. Marshall Papers [Secretary of Defense, Speeches and Statements].)

This policy also had implications for the racial integration of the armed forces. According to the official history of the OSD, the order rejected both "the Navy's discriminatory selection standard and the Army's argument that its high proportion of poorly qualified men made segregated units necessary." (Condit, *Test of War*, 493–94.) In his study on the integration of the armed forces, Morris MacGregor called it "the single most significant contribution of the Secretary of Defense" to integration, because it "undercut the Army's most persuasive argument for restoring a racial quota and maintaining segregated units." (Morris J. MacGregor Jr., *Integration of the Armed Forces, 1940–1965*, in *Defense Studies Series* [Washington: Center of Military History, US Army, 1981], 618–19.) See pp. 474–75.

278

TO GENERAL J. LAWTON COLLINS — April 3, 1951
Personal — Washington, DC

Dear Collins: I note in this morning's press that Bradley is presenting four posthumous Congressional Medals of Honor [CMH], and further that the nine CMH's awarded so far by the Army during the Korean campaign have all been posthumous.[1]

It seems to me that in the normal course of events someone should perform a feat worthy of the Congressional Medal of Honor and live to tell about it. It may be that the awarding authorities have tended to consider death as one of the requirements.

It would be my first thought that as soon as a soldier had performed an act of heroism clearly indicating an award of the Congressional Medal of Honor we should withdraw him from combat and as soon as the award was approved, return him to the States for appropriate high level ceremonies.

Please look into this and give me your reactions.[2] Faithfully yours,

GCMRL/G. C. Marshall Papers (Secretary of Defense, Number Indexed, M200-12-7)

1. On April 3, Bradley awarded four posthumous Medals of Honor, the official name of the award. The editors have identified four other US Army recipients of the Medal of Honor during the Korean War up to this point. On January 9, 1951, President Truman awarded a Medal of Honor to Major General William F. Dean Sr., commanding general of the Twenty-fourth Infantry Division who had been captured early in the Korean War. Still listed as missing in action, he was being held as a POW. See pp. 792–93 ("Congressional Medals Given Parents of 4 GIs Slain in Korea," *Washington Post*, April 4, 1951, p. 1; Senate Committee on Veterans' Affairs, *Medal of Honor Recipients: 1863–1978*, 96th Cong., 1st sess. [Washington: GPO, 1979].)

2. Carter reminded Marshall of this issue on May 16 and informed him that the army would be awarding Medals of Honor to three living recipients on May 19. Marshall attended the ceremony. (Carter to Marshall, memorandum, May 16, 1951, GCMRL/G. C. Marshall Papers [Secretary of Defense, Number Indexed, M200-12-7]; Senate Committee on Veterans' Affairs, *Medal of Honor Recipients: 1863–1978*; "The President with Three Heroes of Korean Fighting," *New York Times*, May 20, 1951, p. 3.) There is no additional communication with Collins on this subject in the Marshall Papers.

279

TO JOSEPH SHORT[1] — April 5, 1951
Washington, DC

Dear Short: At the President's press conference the question will probably be brought up about the item in Newsweek regarding instructions from the Chief of Staff to MacArthur about bombing beyond the Yalu or the announcement in the paper this morning on the same subject.[2]

There is attached a slip with a suggestion for the President's reply.[3]

Incidentally, I think it would be dangerous for the President to expand on this.[4] Faithfully yours,

GCMRL/G. C. Marshall Papers (Secretary of Defense, Number Indexed, M200-2-29)

1. Short (VMI, 1925) was Truman's press secretary.

2. In its April 9, 1951, issue, *Newsweek* had stated that "the Joint Chiefs of Staff have given General MacArthur authority to unleash the U.S. Air Force and Navy against the Communists' Manchurian 'sanctuary' immediately if the enemy should send its air force—now estimated at 3,000 planes—all-out against U.N. troops in Korea. The Chiefs' feeling was that MacArthur should be in a position to act without delay to protect his command." ("He Can Hit Manchuria," *Newsweek*, April 9, 1951, p. 13; *MSFE*, 3546.) The actual number of planes in the Communist Chinese Air Force was closer to 1,050 by June 1951. (Robert F. Futrell, *The United States Air Force in Korea, 1950–1953*, rev. ed. [1961; repr., Washington: Office of Air Force History, USAF, 1983], 245.)

The editors have not located a newspaper article on this topic dated April 5. On April 6, however, the *New York Times* reported that on April 5, Lieutenant General George E. Stratemeyer (USMA, 1915), commanding general of the Far East Air Forces (FEAF), had commented on rumors that MacArthur had received new orders authorizing him "to launch an air attack on the enemy's 'protected sanctuary' in Manchuria if and when the Communists employed major air strength against the United Nations forces in Korea." Stratemeyer stated that FEAF was "'prepared to carry the air war to the enemy wherever he may be.'" ("Allies Go Deeper into North Korea," *New York Times*, April 6, 1951, p. 3.)

The JCS did approve a draft order to MacArthur on April 5 to be sent "if and when the enemy launches from outside Korea a major air attack against our forces in the Korean area" that authorized him to "'attack enemy air bases and aircraft in Manchuria and the Shantung peninsula in the immediate vicinity of Weihaiwei.'" Bradley later wrote that he "was now so wary of MacArthur that I deliberately withheld the message and all knowledge of its existence from him, fearing that he might, as I wrote at the time, 'make a premature decision in carrying it out.'" This message was approved by Truman, Marshall, and Acheson between April 6 and 7, but it was not transmitted to MacArthur prior to his relief from command (see pp. 478–81). (*FRUS, 1951*, 7: 309; James F. Schnabel and Robert J. Watson, *History of the Joint Chiefs of Staff: The Joint Chiefs of Staff and National Policy*, vol. 3, *The Korean War, 1950–1951* [Washington: Office of Joint History, Office of the Chairman of the Joint Chiefs of Staff, 1998], pt. 1: 220–21; Omar Bradley and Clay Blair, *A General's Life* [New York: Simon and Schuster, 1983], 630–31.)

3. The attached slip read: "For evident reasons there can be no comment on matters concerned with operational orders."

4. Truman was asked during his press conference whether MacArthur had "been authorized to bomb bases in Manchuria," to which Truman replied, "That is a question that cannot be answered because it is a military strategy question, and it is not a question that I can answer." (Harry S. Truman, *Public Papers of the Presidents of the United States: Harry S. Truman, 1951* [Washington: GPO, 1965], 217.)

280

MEMORANDUM FOR THE UNITED STATES REPRESENTATIVE, STANDING GROUP, NORTH ATLANTIC MILITARY COMMITTEE
Top Secret

April 6, 1951
Washington, DC

Subject: Allocation of National Forces to SHAPE

In my memorandum to you of the same subject, dated 30 March 1951, you were authorized to inform the Standing Group, North Atlantic Military Committee, of certain forces from the United States which are immediately available and are assigned to the operational command of the Supreme Allied Commander, Europe, to the extent necessary for the accomplishment of his mission.[1]

I desire that you inform the Standing Group that the United States plans to deploy the following additional forces to Europe during 1951 and, when such deployment is made, to allocate these forces to Supreme Headquarters Allied Powers Europe (SHAPE):

a. Scheduled for deployment in April 1951:

Army	1 Infantry Division[2]

b. Planned for deployment later in 1951:

Army	2 Infantry Divisions
	1 Armored Division
**Air Force*	3 Fighter Bomber Wings
	1 Tactical Recon Wing
	1 Lt. Bomber Wing
	1 Troop Carrier (Med) Wing

*These forces to be deployed only as facilities in Europe become available.

c. With respect to naval forces, it is planned to maintain the previously reported level of forces in the Eastern Atlantic–Mediterranean Area.

s/ G. C. Marshall[3]

NA/RG 330, Assistant Secretary of Defense for International Security Affairs, Office of "NAT" Affairs (Subject File, 1949–53, Organization NATO to US Special Representative in Europe)

1. General Bradley was the official US representative to the Standing Group; his deputy was Vice Admiral Jerauld Wright (USNA, 1917). The editors have been unable to locate this March 30 memorandum.

2. On March 27, General Burns had informed Larkin and Lovett that Eisenhower had asked for information about the proposed forces to be made available to him when he assumed formal command on April 1. (Eisenhower would officially open SHAPE on April 2.) With the JCS planning to decide on this matter within the next two days, Burns asked if Marshall could inform Eisenhower that the US will provide "additional forces . . . beyond those now stationed in Europe." Larkin responded that although the president, or the secretary of defense at his designation, maintained the legal right to inform Eisenhower of these orders, despite the ongoing debate in Congress, he cautioned against "exercising such authority" until the "troops to Europe" resolutions had passed. On April 4, the Senate passed a resolution approving the sending of additional US troops to Europe, and the following day, Burns recommended Marshall's signature on this memorandum, which had been "derived from the views of the Joint Chiefs of Staff." (Burns to Larkin, memorandum, March 27, 1951; Larkin to Lovett, memorandum, March 28, 1951; Burns to Marshall, April 5, 1951, NA/RG 330, Assistant Secretary of Defense for International Security Affairs, Office of "NAT" Affairs [Subject File, 1949–53, Organization NATO to US Special Representative in Europe]; "Text of the Senate's Troops-for-Europe Resolution," *New York Times*, April 5, 1951, p. 13.) See pp. 333–34, 380–86, 419–22, 431–32, and 462.

3. Carter had suggested to Marshall that during his April 6 meeting with Speaker of the House Sam Rayburn, he discuss the possibility of "issuing discreet movement orders" to send the Fourth Infantry Division to Europe, while keeping in mind that "public knowledge of this movement" would have an effect on amendments to the UMST bill under consideration in the House. (See pp. 338–47, 369–71, and 409–13.) Marshall and Secretary Rosenberg met at 9:20 a.m. in Carl Vinson's office, presumably with Rayburn in attendance. Marshall wrote that "Mr. Rayburn says OK" to this plan, and Carter further noted that all press releases on this issue were "to be cleared by GCM personally." (Carter to Marshall, memorandum, April 6, 1951, GCMRL/G. C. Marshall Papers [Secretary of Defense, Mem-

oranda, Marshall S. Carter, 1950–1951].) The press reported on April 12 that the Fourth Infantry Division had been ordered to Europe on April 11. ("4th Infantry Division Ordered To Europe to Join Pact Army," *Washington Post*, April 12, 1951, p. 12; "U. S. 4th Division Ordered to Europe," *New York Times*, April 12, 1951, p. 16.)

281

TO FREDERICK D. PATTERSON — April 6, 1951
Personal — Washington, DC

Dear Dr. Patterson: Thank you for your note of the 27th with the attached notes of your trip abroad and reactions.[1]

Since seeing you, something has come to my attention outside of the military with regard to the matter of segregation in Korea. I will recite what has been told me by a civilian who had been there for five months, on the assumption that this will be kept entirely confidential between the two of us.

He said that he had investigated this issue in a large number of organizations, usually companies, where white soldiers and Negroes were both in the ranks and had made an especial effort to see as many of these organizations as were commanded by southerners, particularly Texans. He found in every case expressions of satisfaction in the arrangement and complimentary references to the fighting of the Negro soldiers in the unit. He said this was particularly marked in several units commanded by Texans, and he concluded by expressing the thought that this should be written up. He—the writer, wanted to do this but had been discouraged at General MacArthur's headquarters in Tokyo, and one of the staff had told him confidentially that this was in accordance with instructions from the Pentagon. I have not located any such instructions so far.

~~Now~~ The other phase of the matter which is not pleasant to recite was that the regiment which was entirely composed of Negro soldiers had proved almost completely undependable in any heavy action, and therefore was given a very limited use.[2]

Now, I will not go into any analysis of these two contrasting reactions, but I would be much interested in hearing most confidentially your comments.[3] Faithfully yours,

GCMRL/G. C. Marshall Papers (Secretary of Defense, Selected)

1. On March 22, Marshall and James C. Evans, his special assistant on racial matters, had met with Patterson to discuss the latter's findings from a recent trip to Europe and Africa. Patterson attached to his March 27 letter to Marshall a report summarizing the points he had made in their meeting, which focused on the need to desegregate US military units in Germany. Patterson reiterated in his March 27 letter what he had told Marshall during their meeting and added that he did not expect any "definite statement or action" as a result of his report. (Patterson to Marshall and attachment, March 27, 1951, GCMRL/G. C. Marshall Papers [Secretary of Defense, Selected].)

2. On September 9, 1950, Major General William B. Kean (USMA, 1918), commanding general of the Twenty-fifth Infantry Division, had recommended to General Walker that the African-American Twenty-fourth Infantry Regiment, deemed by Kean to be "untrustworthy and incapable," be removed from combat due to poor performance in the Sangju

area and Battle Mountain and a successful breakthrough by the North Koreans into the regiment's sector between September 1 and 5. The Eighth Army inspector general agreed with Kean's assessment but recommended integration of all Eighth Army units up to 15 percent strength rather than the regiment's inactivation. Walker and the other leaders of the Eighth Army decided that due to the administrative burdens of integrating during war, it was better for the time being to focus on retraining the failing regiment and assigning additional officers. By 1951, the Eighth Army had begun to integrate units. (Roy E. Appleman, *United States Army in the Korean War*, vol. 2, *South to the Naktong, North to the Yalu (June–November 1950)* [Washington: Office of the Chief of Military History, Department of the Army, 1961], 485–86; William T. Bowers, William M. Hammond, and George L. MacGarrigle, *Black Soldier, White Army: The 24th Infantry Regiment in Korea* [Washington: Center of Military History, US Army, 1996], 175, 188–89; MacGregor, *Integration of the Armed Forces*, 436–38.)

3. On April 10, Patterson commented "on the adverse report" that he thought soldiers should be "measured on the basis of individual performance only. This could transpire only under those conditions where race would not be a factor in their assignment. . . . My point of view is that individual Negro soldiers should not have to bear this burden." (Patterson to Marshall, April 10, 1951, GCMRL/G. C. Marshall Papers [Secretary of Defense, Selected].)

C. J. George informed Marshall on April 18 that Evans had received a copy of Patterson's April 10 reply and requested to see Marshall's April 6 letter. Marshall declined the request because the letter was "very personal." (George to Marshall, memorandum, April 18, 1951, ibid.)

AS ARMY CHIEF OF STAFF during World War II, Marshall had issued three biennial reports to the secretary of war. (See p. 879n4 and *Papers of GCM*, 3: 71–73; 4: 105–7; and 5: 343, 350, and 357.) On March 6, Marx Leva recommended to Marshall the preparation of a similar report on the Korean War. (Leva to Marshall, memorandum, March 6, 1951, NA/RG 330, SD 091 [Korea].)

Marshall Carter informed E. T. Dickinson, assistant to the joint secretaries, on April 4 that Marshall approved of this proposal and desired that it "be completed in time for inclusion in the Department's semiannual report," planned for release on August 15, although the Korean War section of the report might be released as an earlier separate publication. (Carter to Dickinson, memorandum, April 4, 1951, GCMRL/G. C. Marshall Papers [Secretary of Defense, Chronological, Director, Executive Office (Marshall S. Carter), 1950–1952].) Marshall directed the service secretaries and the JCS on April 9 to begin "immediately" the preparation of this report and to each designate an officer for this task by the following day. (Marshall to service secretaries and JCS, memorandum, April 9, 1951, NA/RG 330, SD 091 [Korea].)

A draft of the report, which Carter referred to as "General Marshall's project," was completed by August 23, but it had not been revised or published when Marshall left office in September. The editors have been unable to locate this draft report. (Ginsburgh to Lovett, memorandum, August 23, 1951, and Carter to Winnacker, memorandum, September 14, 1951, ibid.)

On the same day Marshall instructed the service secretaries and JCS to begin preparation of this report, he also forwarded to Truman the recommendations of the JCS to address the military situation in Korea. ★

282

To Harry S. Truman — April 9, 1951
Top Secret — Washington, DC

Dear Mr. President: There is attached for your information a memorandum of 5 April 1951 from the Joint Chiefs of Staff giving their recommendations on the United States military position with respect to Korea.[1]

I believe that you might be interested in these recommendations which deal with basic military factors in the Korean situation. This memorandum is also being sent to the National Security Council for consideration.[2]

With great respect, Faithfully yours,

G C Marshall

GCMRL/G. C. Marshall Collection (Harry S. Truman)

1. Dated April 5, 1951, the JCS memorandum contained a series of recommendations regarding military action in Korea in light of Ridgway's approaching the 38th parallel. If the Soviets either precipitated a general war or committed ground combat units to Korea of sufficient size to threaten UN forces, those forces should be withdrawn from the peninsula, the memorandum stated. Even if Moscow did not precipitate a general war, the JCS warned, "The Korean problem cannot be resolved in a manner satisfactory to the United States by military action alone" or "by politico-military action which is confined to Korea." Indeed, "it is not to be expected unless and until there is a general relaxation of tensions." Given these facts, the JCS recommended continuation of the "current military course of action" in Korea "until a political objective for that country appears attainable without jeopardizing United States positions with respect to the USSR, to Formosa, and seating Chinese Communists in the United Nations." They also recommended creating "dependable" ROK units to replace UN forces, preparing for naval and air action against the Chinese mainland, and ascertaining "as a matter of urgency" the position of US allies regarding Korea, the Far East in general, and operations against China. (*FRUS, 1951*, 7: 295–96.)

2. At Marshall's request the memorandum was circulated to the NSC on April 10 and referred to the NSC staff for consideration in the revision of NSC 48/2 regarding US policy in Asia. (Ibid., 296n1.) NSC 48/2 underwent several revisions in light of ongoing deliberations within the NSC and this April 5 memorandum from the JCS. Marshall received the recommendations of the JCS on these revisions, and after further changes within the NSC, Truman approved a final version on May 17 as NSC 48/5. According to the official JCS history, this document, "a statement of understanding that had been reached by the Joint Chiefs of Staff and the Department of State," clarified that: "There was to be no attempt at forcible unification of Korea; military and political objectives were to be distinguished; the right of the theater commander to operate across the parallel was recognized, within limits. The prospective wider war urged by General MacArthur—the operations against mainland China—was ruled out." (Schnabel and Watson, *History of JCS*, 3, pt. 1: 212, 216–18; *FRUS, 1951*, 7: 387–88, 431–32, 439–42. For the full text of NSC 48/5, see *FRUS, 1951*, 6: 33–63.)

283

Meeting with Belgian Prime Minister Joseph Pholien
April 9, 1951 Washington, DC

PRIME MINISTER Pholien arrived at the Pentagon at 3:00 p.m., accompanied by Belgian Ambassador to the US Baron Robert Silvercruys. US Ambassador to Belgium Robert Murphy and Colonel E. S. Hartshorn Jr. of the Office of Foreign Military Affairs also attended this meeting. Pholien began by expressing his interest in the American "defense effort," as Belgium "was likewise improving its defense capabilities" and "had become the first Continental member of NATO to lengthen its term of military service to 24 months." Marshall praised this development, as this information "would be helpful to him in his appearances before Congressional committees." In attempting to defend a twenty-seven-month term of service before the House and Senate committees, Marshall stated that "Congressmen quoted statistics with respect to the shorter length of service in European nations." (Memorandum of conversation with Prime Minister Pholien, April 9, 1951, NA/RG 330, CD Memorandum of Conversation.) See pp. 325–29, 338–47, 369–71, and 409–13.

Pholien then questioned "the adequacy of the U.S. action in sending only four divisions to Europe." Marshall explained the recent congressional debate on this issue and added "that he had somewhat reluctantly disclosed publicly the exact number of divisions we intend to send to Europe" in order to dispel "some confusion in Congress." Marshall had said four divisions "simply because these divisions were all which we would have available to send to Europe in 1951," and it was unfortunate that "the public both in Europe and in the U.S." had become caught up in the number of divisions rather than the "main issue" of "the power of the President." When Pholien asked if "the four divisions were just a starter," to be supplemented by "whatever number of divisions was required," Marshall replied that such action "would be determined later." Ambassador Silvercruys stated his belief that the American people would support any level of assistance "toward the defense of Western Europe, provided they were convinced that the nations of Western Europe were making an all-out effort on their part." (Ibid.) See pp. 333–34, 380–86, and 472–74.

Marshall then provided background information on manpower and personnel problems facing the US since the outbreak of the Korean War in order to explain the importance of the UMST bill currently under consideration by Congress. Most of the problems Marshall mentioned "could be attributed to a shortage of basically trained individuals," the elimination of which was a "major purpose" of the UMST bill. This "continuous flow" of trained men would be assigned to the existing National Guard divisions, which would reduce expenses compared to assigning them to the Regular Army. Due to time constraints, Pholien declined Marshall's offer for a briefing "on the military situation in Korea," so Marshall concluded by suggesting that Belgium "maintain an overstrength of officers and non-commissioned officers in their battalion in Korea and that personnel in these grades be rotated so that as many as possible could obtain combat experience." (Ibid.)

In a subsequent meeting that afternoon with Secretary Acheson, Pholien expressed relief at Marshall's comment "that Europeans should not be worried about the Congressional resolution" limiting American troops in Europe. Acheson agreed but discouraged Pholien from sharing Marshall's comment with the European press, as "it might well create difficulties for General Marshall." (*FRUS, 1951*, 4: 269–73, quote on 269.) ★

ON APRIL 5, House Minority Leader Joseph W. Martin (R-MA) released and publicly read in Congress a letter that General MacArthur had sent to him on March 20. In that letter, MacArthur agreed with Martin that Chiang's forces should be allowed to attack the Chinese mainland and asserted that "here we fight Europe's war with arms while the diplomats there still fight it with words; that if we lose the war to Communism in Asia the fall of Europe is inevitable"; and that "There is no substitute for victory." (*Congressional Record* 97, pt. 3, 82d Cong., 1st sess., 3380.)

As with his March 23/24 statement (see pp. 459–60), MacArthur had sent this letter without prior clearance and thus violated Truman's December 5 directive to obtain such clearance in advance (see pp. 282–83). He did so with some of his other remarks, also published at this time, in which he once again attacked the limitations imposed upon him. On April 5, for example, the *New York Times* reported that British Lieutenant General H. G. Martin, a military correspondent for the London *Daily Telegraph*, had interviewed MacArthur, who "had told him in an interview in Tokyo that the United Nations could defeat the Chinese Communists easily if politicians would face up to realities." According to General Martin, MacArthur "'said it was not the soldier who had encroached on the realm of the politician but the politician [who] had encroached on that of the soldier.'" ("Briton Says MacArthur Deplored Political Curb," *New York Times*, April 5, 1951, p. 2; Acheson, *Present at the Creation*, 520; D. Clayton James, *The Years of MacArthur*, vol. 3, *Triumph and Disaster, 1945–1964* [Boston: Houghton Mifflin, 1985], 590–91.)

On the morning of April 6, Truman met with Marshall, Acheson, Averell Harriman, and Bradley to discuss the situation. No decision on how to proceed was reached at this meeting, though Truman later wrote that he suggested Marshall review all correspondence with MacArthur, and that he had already decided to relieve MacArthur but wanted further consultation with his advisers before officially doing so. (Truman, *Memoirs*, 2: 447–48.)

Recollections of the participants on what else was said at this meeting and ensuing ones differ (see James, *Years of MacArthur*, 3: 591–95, for these differing recollections). According to Bradley, Acheson and Harriman favored MacArthur's immediate relief at this meeting, while he and Marshall "recommended against such action." (Lalor memorandum for the record, April 24, 1951, enclosing Bradley memorandum, n.d., "Events in connection with change of command in Far East," NA/RG 218, CCS 013.36 [4-20-51], Sec. 2.) Acheson and Harriman later denied this version of their position, but "Everyone present later recalled that Marshall urged caution" at this meeting, Marshall's authorized biographer wrote, "pointing to problems that might arise concerning military appropriations in Congress." (Forrest C. Pogue, *George C. Marshall*, vol. 4, *Statesman, 1945–1959* [New York: Viking, 1987], 481–82.)

That afternoon Marshall met in his office with Acheson, Harriman, and Bradley from 4:35 p.m. until 6:30 p.m. Bradley wrote that each held to the position he had expressed in the morning meeting with Truman. Either at that meeting or the one with Truman the next morning, Acheson later recalled, Marshall "asked our opinion on the merits of calling General MacArthur home for consultation and reaching final decision after that. We were all strongly opposed." According to Bradley, they agreed that afternoon to recommend to Truman when they met with him again the next morning "that he not make his decision until we had all thought about it over the week end." (Bradley to Marshall, memorandum, April 18, 1951, GCMRL/G. C. Marshall Papers [Secretary of Defense, Selected, MacArthur]; Acheson, *Present at the Creation*, 521–22. Acheson incorrectly states that the afternoon meeting on April 6 took place in his office.)

On the following day, Saturday, April 7, Truman met with the same group from 8:50 a.m. until approximately 10:00 a.m., received this recommendation, and "indicated that he was going to confer with other leaders over the week end, including Chief Justice Vinson," Speaker Rayburn, and Vice President Barkley. He also directed Marshall to obtain the opinion of the JCS "from a purely military point of view." (Bradley to Marshall, memorandum, April 18, 1951, GCMRL/G. C. Marshall Papers [Secretary of Defense, Selected, MacArthur]; *MSFE*, 345.) In his memoir, Truman asserted that after reading the correspondence with MacArthur, Marshall now concurred with the judgment expressed by Harriman on April 6 that MacArthur should have been relieved two years earlier; but others disagree and maintain that Marshall remained "reluctant to agree to the relief of MacArthur throughout the weekend and did not give his assent" before the Monday morning meeting with the president discussed below. (Truman, *Memoirs*, 2: 447–48; Pogue, *Statesman*, 581n16.) Privately Marshall apparently agreed with Bradley's suggestion that he send "a personal and confidential letter to General MacArthur, pointing out the difficult position in which he was placing the government. We went so far as to draft a copy of such a letter," Bradley maintained. "I furnished part of the draft and General Marshall filled in the rest of it," but it was never sent. (Bradley memorandum, n.d., NA/RG 218, CCS 013.36 [4-20-51], Sec. 2; Condit, *Test of War*, 247.)

Since two of the chiefs were away, no JCS meeting took place until Sunday, April 8, when Bradley met with all the chiefs from 2:00 p.m. to 4:00 p.m. They all then met with Marshall in his office for an hour, during which the secretary asked each chief his opinion but did not express his own (Condit, *Test of War*, 105). "No written recommendation or report was made," Bradley later noted, though "all of them said in substance that from a military point of view only, they thought General MacArthur should be relieved." They realized, however, that "military considerations were only a small part of the question involved and, therefore they would refrain from making a specific recommendation to the President for the relief of General MacArthur, but merely express their views." (Bradley to Marshall, memorandum, April 18, 1951, GCMRL/G. C. Marshall Papers [Secretary of Defense, Selected, MacArthur]; Bradley memorandum, n.d., NA/RG 218, CCS 013.36 [4-20-51], Sec. 2.)

The following morning, April 9, immediately after a cabinet meeting at the White House, Truman again met with Acheson, Marshall, Bradley, and Harriman. (According to Truman's appointment log, Barkley also attended this meeting.) Bradley reported to Truman the view of the JCS, in which he concurred, that "from a purely military point of view" MacArthur should be relieved. Marshall "apparently concurred, stating that it was not a recommendation, but merely the views of the Joint Chiefs of Staff," while Acheson and Harriman again recommended that MacArthur be relieved. Truman then decided, "with the unanimous concurrence of those present," Marshall later stated, to relieve MacArthur of all his commands and replace him, on Marshall's and Bradley's recommendation, with General Ridgway. Similarly on their recommendation he agreed to replace Ridgway with General Van Fleet as Eighth Army commander. (Bradley memorandum, n.d., NA/RG 218, CCS 013.36 [4-20-51], Sec. 2; Billy C. Mossman, *United States Army in the Korean War*, vol. 5, *Ebb and Flow, November 1950–July 1951* [Washington: Center of Military History, US Army, 1990], 362; *MSFE*, 345.)

During the afternoon of April 10, Acheson, Harriman, Marshall, and Bradley met again with Truman, who signed the orders to be sent to MacArthur and Ridgway and directed that Short prepare, with Bradley's assistance, the statements that would accompany their public release. It was further agreed that Pace, who was then in Korea, would deliver the message to MacArthur in Tokyo on April 11 at 8:00 p.m. Washington time. (For Marshall's proposed message to Pace, see NA/RG 218, Geographic File, 383.21 [Korea].) After Bradley returned to the White House at 5:30 p.m. to help in the preparation of those statements, word arrived that rumors of MacArthur's relief had already leaked to the press and that the *Chicago Tribune* would publish them on April 11. Bradley then telephoned Marshall at dinner and contacted Truman at 10:00 p.m., who decided to have the messages delivered immediately and his decision announced at a special press conference, to be held at 1:00 a.m. Pace, however, was not reachable in Korea and did not receive his instructions, while Bradley's direct notification to MacArthur did not reach him until after one of MacArthur's aides had heard the news on the radio and telephoned Mrs. MacArthur, who informed him. (Bradley memorandum, n.d., NA/RG 218, CCS 013.36 [4-20-51], Sec. 2; *MSFE*, 345; Pogue, *Statesman*, 482–83; Truman, *Memoirs*, 2: 448; Condit, *Test of War*, 247–51; and Allan R. Millett, *The War for Korea*, vol. 2, *They Came from the North, 1950–1951* [Lawrence: University Press of Kansas, 2010], 422–23.) See also pp. 499–516.

Upon receipt of the news of MacArthur's relief and his own promotion,

Ridgway telegraphed Marshall his earnest "hope that great responsibilities entrusted to me may be discharged in manner to meet your approbation." (Ridgway to Marshall, cable no. SVC-2042 JC, April 11, 1951, GCMRL/G. C. Marshall Papers [Secretary of Defense, Selected].) Marshall handwrote his response on that message. ★

284

To General Matthew B. Ridgway — April 11, 1951
Radio. *Confidential* — Washington, DC

Reference your SVC 2042 JC, I have complete confidence in your ability and loyalty.[1]

G. C. M.

GCMRL/G. C. Marshall Papers (Secretary of Defense, Selected); H.

1. See the previous editorial note for Ridgway's initial message. "Grateful beyond words for your personal message," Ridgway responded on April 13. "You know you will have my utmost." (Ridgway to Marshall, cable no. SVC-575 J, April 13, 1951, GCMRL/G. C. Marshall Papers [Secretary of Defense, Selected].)

Also on April 11 the White House released the text of Marshall's order informing Ridgway of his new command. "It is realized that your presence in Korea in the immediate future is highly important," Marshall added, "but we are sure you can make the proper distribution of your time until you can turn over active command of the Eighth Army to its new commander. For this purpose, Lt. Gen. James A. Van Fleet is enroute to report to you for such duties as you may direct." (Press release of Marshall to Ridgway, April 10, 1951, ibid.)

285

To UMTS Conferees[1] — April 13, 1951
Washington, DC

This Congress has given long consideration to the various problems involved in providing adequate manpower for the armed forces. Both houses have endorsed the principles of Universal Military Training and Service, but fundamental points of difference have arisen on how this program is to be put into effect. These differences, in my opinion, go directly to the heart of the bill. The way in which they are resolved will decide whether or not we have a law that actually provides real security for our country.

I am particularly concerned about two provisions. One is the requirement in the House bill that a wholly new Act of Congress would have to be passed before Universal Military Training could be put into effect; the second is the power the House bill would vest in the National Security Training Commission to draw up a detailed program of basic military training without reference to the Joint Chiefs of Staff or the military departments.

The requirement that Congress would have to pass at some later date on the specific content of the Universal Military Training Program would make it impossible to proceed on the theory that we really had Universal Military Training. All the benefits Universal Military Training is designed to accomplish would have to be kept in a legislative deep freeze until both houses of Congress had acted on the program virtually all over again. From a practical point of view, the upshot of these months of discussion and debate that have gone into this legislation would be substantially the same as a mere extension of Selective Service.

Until we could be certain that the training plan had a full endorsement from Congress, we could never with any safety begin the cutting down of the size of our forces on active duty. It would be a betrayal of our security to shorten the period of service for our troops or reduce their number without solid assurance that we would have the kind of trustworthy National Guard and Organized Reserve that can only be built up through the functioning of a Universal Military Training procedure.

The absence of any real assurance on this point would make it essential that we continue to put our reliance on the men actually in uniform, with all the tremendous costs that entails in money and also in the productive time of our young men. Frankly, this is the course of improvident folly. It imposes a heavy burden on our economy; it disrupts industry, science and education and it creates unnecessary pressures on both our living standards and our democratic institutions. In a crisis that may last many years, it is important that we move with all possible speed toward a procedure that will transfer a steadily increasing share of the responsibility for defense to our citizen-soldier units. Universal Military Training is a vital necessity for such a defense system.

This is not a visionary program for the long-range future. It is my conviction that we would begin almost at once to reap tangible benefits from the introduction of Universal Military Training. The first benefits would come in speeding the rotation of men long in combat in the Far East and in returning to civilian life the veteran reservists who had to be called back in the early months of the Korean fighting. When these debts have been honored, we can begin cutting down the service periods and number of men called in through Selective Service. If there is no worsening in the tensions that now beset us, it should be safely possible within eighteen months to drop appreciably below our present strength requirement of 3,500,000 men on active duty. We could rely less and less on Selective Service until we reached the point where we could depend solely on volunteers to fill our regular forces, and I think personally, most of those volunteers would come from the ranks of the Universal Military Training group. All that would be required of other young men would be four to six months of basic training, followed by civilian duty in the National Guard or Reserve.

This is clearly the sensible, the economical and effective way to organize our defenses. It appears best for the country and best for the young men themselves. But we should not undertake it if Congress ties strings to the program in such a manner that it cannot gradually be put into effect and as rapidly as possible without all the delays and uncertainties involved in new legislation.

Apart from this element of paralyzing uncertainty, the requirement that Congress pass on what is to be taught in the Universal Military Training program, it seems to me, is basically unrealistic. The idea that any group, whether it be the National Security Training Commission or the Joint Chiefs of Staff or the individual military departments, can draw up a detailed program of military training that will operate effectively over a considerable period is contrary to all that we have learned as to the imperative necessity for keeping training methods flexible.

With weapons and theories of warfare changing constantly, the formal adoption by Congress of a training program would involve a Maginot-line approach to national security of a type that might lead to disaster.[2] No training plan is realistic unless the men charged with military responsibility are free to change it as rapidly and drastically as altered conditions require. A plan that had been voted upon by Congress, and that, therefore, could not be modified without new Congressional action, would serve as an iron collar around the necks of our military commanders. It could, I fear, convert the whole program into a bogus shield for the nation.

Even if the requirement for specific Congressional approval of the Universal Military Training program were deleted, there would be serious objections to vesting in the National Security Training Commission full power to "direct and control" Universal Military Training. The effect of this provision in the House bill would be to create a new agency that would be entirely independent of the Department of Defense, but that would have the power to "direct and control" a military program to be carried on by the military departments in military installations. The setting up of such a double-headed military organization would introduce such confusion and obscurity of authority in the military establishment that both Universal Military Training and the efficiency of our regular military forces would undoubtedly suffer.

There must be full integration between the training a man receives and the type of service he will be called on to give in a national emergency. Having a civilian Joint Chiefs of Staff for the training and a military Joint Chiefs of Staff for the service could create a fatal gulf. I am a firm believer in the principle of civilian authority over all phases of our military establishment. A lifetime of association with the armed forces has confirmed me in that belief. But that belief in no way contravenes my conviction that the specific content of a program of basic military training is not a matter on which civilians should be expected to render expert judgment.

Our own programs of basic training in two World Wars were drawn up by men who had made a career of studying military science and tactics and who were familiar with the capacities and requirements of troops in training for combat. In this manner our present program of basic training was drawn. It is the way we have always drawn our training programs. This has been true of armies in all countries in all periods of the world's history. This is the field in which military leaders are supposed to be experts. If they are not, they should not hold their jobs.

The reactions of the millions of veterans who have returned to their home communities since V-J Day is convincing evidence that military direction of military training does not have the effect of brutalizing or militarizing our men. The overwhelming majority have come back better able to make their way in civil life and to render useful service as citizens.

To guarantee that there will be no departure from this tradition, general supervision over the procedures, standards and surroundings and other phases of the Universal Military Training program should be vested in a civilian commission with direct access to the President. A commission of this type, with a civilian chairman and a civilian majority, should have primary responsibility over those aspects of the program that are not fundamentally military.

The Senate version of the bill does not contain the dangers I envisage in the House requirement. I hope that the conference committees representing the two houses will be able to reach agreement on a final draft that will permit realization of the historic gains that a well-conceived and functioning system of Universal Military Training and Service can bring to our safety and to the cause of world peace. The need is great and time is short.[3] Faithfully yours,

NA/RG 330, Office of the Assistant Secretary of Defense for Manpower and Personnel, 353 (UMT)

1. Each chamber of Congress had passed its own version of the UMT bill, the Senate on March 8 and the House on April 13, thereby necessitating the establishment of a conference committee to reconcile the two. The most significant difference was that while the Senate bill allowed the president to establish a UMT program pending a report by a civilian committee, the House bill endorsed only the principle of UMT and required another future vote following receipt of such a report in order to actually establish the program. Although Rosenberg listed twelve provisions of the House bill "disfavored" by the Defense Department, Marshall in this letter to the conference committee focused only on this point and the powers to be granted the National Security Training Commission. The *Washington Post* offered a concise comparison of the two bills prior to the conference committee's deliberations. (Rosenberg to Lovett, memorandum and attachment, April 19, 1951, NA/RG 330, SD 040 [Manpower and Personnel]; "Defense Dept. Hopes To Salvage UMT," *Washington Post*, April 15, 1951, p. M3.) The conference committee consisted of Senators Harry Flood Byrd (D-VA), Russell, Johnson, Bridges, and Leverett Saltonstall (R-RI), and Representatives Carl Durham (D-NC), Leslie Arends (R-IL), W. Sterling Cole (R-NY), Vinson, Brooks, Kilday, and Short. It convened on April 24.

2. The Maginot Line was a series of French fortifications along the French-German border built in the 1930s to deter or prevent a German invasion. It failed to do so in 1940, as Nazi Germany took advantage of the unprotected French-Belgian border to flank the Maginot Line and defeat the French in six weeks.

3. See pp. 551–53 and 558–59.

286

To General Walter Bedell Smith — April 13, 1951
Top Secret — Washington, DC
Personal and Informal...

Dear Smith: I have signed the attached letter to you which I understand is actually a communication between our respective staffs.[1]

I just want you to know personally and informally that you can count on us to give you every reasonable and possible assistance in carrying forward your heavy responsibilities. I am hopeful that our staffs, and the Joint Chiefs of Staff, can work out agreed arrangements to our mutual satisfaction, and know that if any difficulties arise which cannot be agreed by them, you will have no hesitancy in talking it over directly with me.

With warm regards, Faithfully yours,

NA/RG 330, CD 350.09

1. The attached letter was a response to CIA Director Smith's December 26, 1950, request for specific support from the Defense Department (see pp. 254–55n4). Marshall had forwarded Smith's letter to the JCS on January 22, 1951, and General Vandenberg replied on March 23 with a proposed letter to Smith, which Marshall's April 13 letter generally reflected. Among other points, it agreed to Smith's request for officers to aid the CIA in preparing national intelligence estimates but requested a "more detailed breakdown" of the numbers and types of enlisted and officer personnel requested "for use in clandestine intelligence and covert operations." It also stated that the JCS would "welcome" discussion regarding CIA use of certain army, navy, and air force installations as well as "any reasonable demands which will further national security." Use of "military cover" for covert operations and intelligence activities would be "authorized where practicable" and when consistent with paragraph 5 of NSC 10/2 "which enables the United States to disclaim plausibly any responsibility for them." The letter also addressed Smith's request for assignment of CIA representatives in military theaters of operations, arrangements to keep the CIA informed of JCS operational decisions and plans, and establishment of a permanent liaison between the CIA and the JCS. Marshall deferred replies to Smith's other proposals pending revision of NSC 10/2 and NSC Intelligence Directive 5, which dealt with CIA representation on and coordination with military theater general staffs and the JCS. (Vandenberg to Marshall, memorandum and attachments, March 23, 1951, and Marshall to Smith, April 13, 1951, NA/RG 330, CD 350.09.) See pp. 554–55.

WITH THE SENATE approving the US troop commitment to NATO on April 4 (see pp. 472–74), attention shifted to developing alliances with and ensuring the defense of key nations in the western Pacific and the Mediterranean in the event of all-out war with the Soviet Union. Acheson had asked Marshall on April 5 to review the draft of a proposed joint memorandum to Truman, who had previously supported "a mutual assistance pact among the Pacific Island nations (Australia, New Zealand, the Philippines, Japan, the United States and perhaps Indonesia)." The draft reported the belief of Dulles, who had returned from his peace treaty mission to Japan and visits to Australia, New Zealand, and the Philippines (see pp. 324–25 and 427–29), that "the desired results can be better achieved by a *series* of arrangements rather than a *single* arrangement." The joint memorandum consequently requested that Dulles's instructions be amended to allow for this. Acheson requested Marshall's urgent consideration of this memorandum due to the "political situation, particularly in Australia" where the peace treaty with Japan had become an issue in elections to be held in late April. Then on the following day, April 6, he informed Marshall of British opposition to a multilateral treaty as opposed to bilateral treaties and requested his comments on a draft statement on these developments to be given by the president. (Acheson to Marshall, April 5 and 6, 1951, NA/RG 330, CD 387 [Japan]; *FRUS, 1951*, 6, pt. 1: 183–85, 187–89.)

Marshall responded to both letters on April 13 by reporting and concurring with JCS recommendations for changes in the joint memorandum to Truman. The chiefs did not object to negotiating a series of agreements with the Pacific Island nations, but they "should be as few as possible." Furthermore, there should be no new arrangement with the Philippines to replace the present arrangement, which they considered "adequate and satisfactory," and any bilateral arrangement with Japan should "come into effect concurrently with the Japanese Peace Treaty." The JCS also opposed any formal pact with Australia and New Zealand, preferring instead a "simple understanding or public declaration," but if "political considerations" dictated the necessity of a formal pact, it should make no mention of "military plans, planning, or organizations." Marshall also informed Acheson that the service secretaries opposed a presidential statement in favor of a "less authoritative source." Dulles was able to redraft the proposed presidential statement in a manner acceptable to Marshall, and it was released on April 18. (Marshall to Acheson, April 13, 1951, NA/RG 330, CD 387 [Japan]; *FRUS, 1951*, 6, pt. 1: 202–4; Condit, *Test of War*, 192.) See pp. 567–69.

On April 14, Marshall responded to a lengthy March 24 letter from Acheson requesting Defense Department views on security arrangements with Greece and Turkey "as soon as possible." In that letter, Acheson reminded Marshall that at its September meeting in New York the NATO Council had concluded that the two nations should not be invited to become members of the alliance, but instead "should be invited to associate themselves with such appropriate phases of the military planning work" of NATO as were "concerned with defense of the Mediterranean." The JCS and Defense Department had at that time opposed full NATO membership for the two nations but recommended reconsidering the issue once defense of the present members was "reasonably assured." For numerous reasons, including Turkish dissatisfaction with this arrangement and the recommendation of the Middle East chiefs of mission, the State Department now believed that some form of security guarantee should be given to Greece and Turkey, be it through membership in NATO, bilateral agreements with each nation, a multilateral agreement with both and Great Britain, or "some other plan" that would "accomplish the purpose" of bilateral agreements. In his response, Marshall forwarded a summary of the JCS recommendation, with which he concurred, that the United States "propose and support early membership" for Greece and Turkey in NATO but that it first enter into negotiations with the British and French "to obtain their concurrence and co-leadership under whatever formula may be most palatable to nations reluctant to admit Greece and Turkey in full NATO membership." (Acheson to Marshall, March 24, 1951; Burns to Marshall, memorandum, n.d.; "Summary of Views and Bases for Joint Chiefs of Staff Position on Security Arrangements for Greece and Turkey," n.d.; and Marshall to Acheson, April 14, 1951, NA/RG 330, CD 092.3 [NATO, Gen.].)

On April 16, attention shifted back to the West Pacific when Marshall made clear his disagreement with the JCS over aid to the Philippines. General Romulo met with Marshall and General Malony for five minutes at 3:00 p.m. that day, when they discussed the "discouraging" position taken by the JCS. (See pp. 306–7 and 429–31, and *FRUS, 1951*, 6: 1526–28.) Marshall assured Romulo that "he was exploring every possible means whereby some aid could be obtained," and he hoped to designate "nine or ten million dollars which could be put at the disposal of General Hobbs for use in an emergency." Marshall agreed with Romulo that "the situation in the Philippines was very bad," so he was thus asking the JCS "to reconsider their position" prior to Romulo's departure for the Philippines later that week. (Memorandum of conversation, April 16, 1951, NA/RG 330, CD Memorandum of Conversation.) Bradley informed Marshall on April 19 that the JCS had reconsidered their earlier views and now recommended that "10 million dollars may be made available" to the Philippine Armed Forces through MDAP funds, even though they considered the use of such funds "outside their purview." Marshall "directed General Malony to prepare the necessary papers for his signature at once so he could present them to the President" to authorize the funds. (Bradley to Davis, memorandum, April 19, 1951, NA/RG 218 [Miscellaneous Papers from the Chairman of the JCS, General of the Army Omar N. Bradley, 1949–1953, Folder 091 Philippines].) Marshall also wrote to Thomas D. Cabot, chairman of the International Security Affairs Committee (ISAC) at the State Department, on April 19 to request his and Acheson's approval of the use of these MDAP funds, to be put under the control of General Hobbs. Marshall Carter later wrote Malony on April 25 that when Marshall noticed "tail dragging" on this topic, "he indicated that he was thinking about" discussing the matter "personally" with Acheson, Truman, and Treasury Secretary Snyder. Carter warned that "unless something definitive is done within the next 48 hours, all hell is going to break loose around this place," although Marshall recognized and supported Malony's "superhuman efforts to expedite matters." Following a discussion with Marshall on April 27, Truman and Acheson authorized these funds, and Marshall wrote to General Malony on May 2 "to insure that appropriate implementing action is taken without delay." (Marshall to Cabot, April 19, 1951, and Marshall to Malony, May 2, 1951, NA/RG 330, CD 091.3 [MDAP, Philippines]; Carter to Malony, memoranda, April 25, 1951, GCMRL/G. C. Marshall Papers [Secretary of Defense, Chronological, Director, Executive Office (Marshall S. Carter), 1950–1952].) ★

287

To General of the Army Douglas MacArthur — April 16, 1951
Radio No. DEF-35248. — Washington, DC
Personal for G/A Douglas MacArthur

The House of Representatives by unanimous consent invites you to appear before a joint meeting of the House and Senate. It is expected that the Senate will take similar action shortly.[1] The floor leader of the House, Mr McCormick [*McCormack*] has requested me to ascertain from you at what hour it would be convenient for you to accept the invitation to appear before the Congress on Thursday sometime after twelve noon. They would greatly appreciate this information so that appropriate announcement can be made by them.[2] Marshall Secretary of Defense

GCMRL/G. C. Marshall Papers (Secretary of Defense, Number Indexed, M200-2-29)

1. Truman's April 11 relief of MacArthur (see pp. 478–81) aroused a firestorm of public anger and partisan political attacks on Truman and his advisers, Marshall included. (See, for example, John Spanier, *The Truman-MacArthur Controversy* [New York: Norton, 1965], 211–13.) It also led to calls for a congressional investigation and MacArthur's appearance before a joint session of Congress.

On April 16, House Majority Leader John McCormack requested by telephone that Marshall arrange with MacArthur a time for the general to appear before that planned joint session on Thursday, April 19. (Marshall to McCormack, April 17, 1951, GCMRL/G. C. Marshall Papers [Secretary of Defense, Number Indexed, M200-2-29].)

The Senate unanimously agreed to the House invitation on April 17. (*Congressional Record* 97, pt. 3, 82d Cong., 1st sess., 3938.)

2. "Please inform Floor Leader McCormack of my deep appreciation for the action of the House of Representatives," MacArthur responded, "and suggest that the hour of my appearance be as soon after 12 oclock as may suit the convenience of the Congress." Marshall so informed McCormack on April 17 and attached this exchange of telegrams. (MacArthur to Marshall, n.d., cable no. 170052-Z, and Marshall to McCormack, April 17, 1951, GCMRL/G. C. Marshall Papers [Secretary of Defense, Number Indexed, M200-2-29].) MacArthur and his family arrived in Washington on April 19 at 12:15 a.m. and were met by Marshall, the JCS, and Truman's military aide, General Harry H. Vaughan, as well as approximately twelve thousand onlookers. (James, *Years of MacArthur*, 3: 612. See photo #9 and p. 501.

288

Memorandum for the President — April 17, 1951
Secret — Washington, DC

SUBJECT: Army Strength for Fiscal Year 1952

1. It has become increasingly apparent that the Department of the Army can no longer, and indeed for good reason should not remain within the average and end strengths previously approved by you for Fiscal Year 1952. An increase in authorized strength is required in order that the Army can carry out its program for the release of enlisted reservists, the rotation of men engaged in action in Korea, and have the essential mobilization base for the call up of additional National Guard divisions which the Chief of Staff of the Army feels will be necessary in FY 1952.[1] The separation of Army enlisted reservists called involuntarily to active duty, which is scheduled for completion in this calendar year, cannot begin until combat rotation and replacement has been effected in Korea. Thus reduction in strength through separations is not immediately advisable.

2. The Joint Chiefs have considered this matter and yesterday interposed no objection to an Army strength of 1,531,000 man-years and an end strength of 1,552,000* for Fiscal Year 1952. From the viewpoint of a sound National Defense

structure and in order to insure just military personnel policies, I recommend your approval of these strengths in lieu of your previously assigned ceilings.[2]

GCMarshall

* Present authorized strength—1,416,000 Army. G.C.M.[3]

NA/RG 330, CD 320.2 (Strength, Military)

1. Secretary Pace announced during testimony before the Senate Armed Services Committee on April 5 that the army would begin rotating about twenty thousand men from service on the Korean front back to the United States in the early summer. Pace emphasized that the number of men rotated out of active duty would depend on an adequate flow of replacements and continued high levels of combat effectiveness and training. ("Army to 'Rotate' G.I.'s from Korea," *New York Times*, April 6, 1951, p. 3.)

2. Acting Secretary of the Army Archibald S. Alexander had sent a memorandum to Marshall earlier on April 17 that asked for an increase in the maximum army strength compared to the 1.416 million figure approved in January 1951. He reported that the JCS "considered this matter on 16 April 1951 and interposed no objection to these increased strengths" and included a draft of this memorandum to Truman for Marshall's signature. Assistant Secretary Rosenberg marked her approval at the top of Alexander's memorandum to Marshall. (Alexander to Marshall, memorandum and attachment, April 17, 1951, NA/RG 330, CD 320.2 [Strength, Military].)

3. Marshall handwrote and initialed this addition.

Truman marked his approval on this document later the same day.

289

Conversation with Lord Tedder

April 18, 1951 Washington, DC

LORD TEDDER, accompanied by Air Chief Marshal Sir William Elliot, his successor as both chairman of the British Joint Services Mission and the British representative to the NATO Standing Group, met with Marshall and Colonel Beebe, now director of the Office of North Atlantic Treaty Affairs who took minutes of the meeting, on April 18. Following "a general conversation," Marshall compared the "difficulties in obtaining sufficient materiel" in World War II "and the present situation." He noted that it was a difficult process to understand "for those not acquainted" with production schedules; that criticism and calls for expanded production and deliveries grew quickly "When equipment lagged behind requirements," even if production was occurring more rapidly than expected; that "Governmental opinions as to the adequacy of programs, particularly on finances, would inevitably swing back and forth between too much and too little"; and that it was a struggle for citizens of the US "to understand conditions in Europe during this rearmament period." To reiterate this final point, Marshall "intended to present his point at the proper time to the United States public by asking them to imagine a reversal of the situation, where European forces were permanently stationed in the United States under a European commander, and ask them to appreciate the sacrifices that they would be called upon to make under such circumstances." (Memorandum of conversation, April 18, 1951, NA/RG 330, CD Memorandum of Conversation.)

Lord Tedder then mentioned "the difficulty the British Government was experiencing" in Parliament regarding the recommended appointment of Admiral William Fechteler as NATO's Supreme Allied Commander, Atlantic (SACLANT). The NATO Defense Committee had nominated Fechteler on February 19, which Prime Minister Attlee accepted. On February 22, however, Winston Churchill, leader of the Conservative opposition in the House of Commons, publicly objected. Attlee withdrew his support for the nomination, and Eisenhower, fearing a reversal of British support for the entire NATO structure, suggested that a British admiral be appointed as Supreme Allied Commander, Mediterranean (SACMED) prior to any further discussion of the SACLANT issue. Marshall responded to Tedder's concerns "along the lines of informal advice given him by the Joint Chiefs of Staff." Marshall "was non-committal and explained that he did not have full information on the problem." Following this meeting, Tedder "raised the same issue" with Beebe, indicated "that the situation was most embarrassing to the British Cabinet," and requested "further information" on the US position. (Ibid.; Walter S. Poole, *History of the Joint Chiefs of Staff: The Joint Chiefs of Staff and National Policy*, vol. 4, *1950–1952* [Washington: Office of Joint History, Office of the Chairman of the Joint Chiefs of Staff, 1998], 120–23.)

The JCS recommended to Marshall on April 24 that the entire debate on the appointment of supreme allied commanders be sent to the NATO Military Committee for resolution, but Acheson and Lovett, as acting secretary of defense, agreed to arrange for private discussions between British and American representatives to discuss the issue further, particularly the SACMED post. The issue stood unresolved through the remainder of 1951, due in part to the initiation of discussions to bring Greece and Turkey into NATO. On July 13, the JCS suggested that the NATO Council of Deputies reconsider Fechteler's nomination as SACLANT, but Fechteler was appointed as chief of naval operations, effective August 16, following Admiral Sherman's death. (Poole, *History of JCS*, 4: 123–25.) See pp. 595–96 and 619–20 and 621n4. ★

290

To Arthur Vandenberg Jr. — April 19, 1951
Radio No. DEF-36668. — Washington, DC
From Secretary of Defense General George C Marshall

Mrs Marshall and I were distressed to learn of your father's death.[1] You and your sisters have our deepest sympathy. This country and other nations of the world have suffered a truly great loss. Senator Vandenberg's contribution to the world has been historic and gives him a high position in history. His character and vision, his selfless efforts for the general good of mankind, and his final disregard of his own welfare in the interests of the public welfare place him on a high pedestal.

I feel I have lost a rare friendship and I know the people of this country have lost a giant who labored in the democratic field in their behalf.[2]

GCMRL/G. C. Marshall Papers (Pentagon Office, General)

1. Arthur Vandenberg Jr. was the son of Senator Vandenberg, who had died on April 18. The senator had undergone the removal of two tumors since October 1949 and suffered several relapses between then and his death. ("Vandenberg Dead; Bipartisan Leader on Foreign Policy," *New York Times*, April 19, 1951, p. 1.) See pp. 16n1 and 315.

2. Anna Rosenberg expressed her own condolences to the younger Vandenberg on April 30 and added that Marshall had spoken "at length and in the very highest terms" about Senator Vandenberg during his off-the-record remarks on April 20 to the American Society of Newspaper Editors. According to Rosenberg, he concluded by describing "the last letter he received from your Father expressing his desire to come back to Washington. Rarely have I had such a stirring emotional experience and I think it fair to report that everyone present shared this feeling." (Rosenberg to Vandenberg Jr., April 30, 1951, NA/RG 330, SD 032.3 [Vandenberg, Arthur H.]; Vandenberg to Marshall, March 7, 1951, GCMRL/G. C. Marshall Papers [Pentagon Office, General]; "TV Held No Brake on Sales of Papers," *New York Times*, April 21, 1951, p. 21.)

On June 6, Vandenberg Jr. thanked Marshall for his April 19 "gratifying" telegram, which was "a source of the greatest inspiration and comfort" to him and his sisters. (Vandenberg to Marshall, June 6, 1951, GCMRL/G. C. Marshall Papers [Secretary of Defense, Number Indexed, M200-7-15].)

Also around this time, Marshall offered his condolences to the Dawes family following the death of Charles Dawes on April 23. Marshall wrote to Dawes's son Dana that he had "lost a rare friendship—one which I have enjoyed for over thirty-five years. [See pp. 230–31.] Your father lived a long and fruitful life and his accomplishments in the fields of business and government have earned for him a high position in history." He also sent a telegram to Dawes's widow, Caro Blymyer Dawes, to offer Mrs. Marshall's and his "deepest sympathy and affection," and he later wrote to her that he regretted that he could not attend the funeral on April 25 in Evanston, Illinois. He hoped Mrs. Dawes had been comforted "by the knowledge of the wonderful example you have given of a devoted, loyal and most helpful wife." Mrs. Dawes replied on June 30 that she appreciated Marshall's letter and added that "Charlie went just the way he would have chosen. Going in to his office every day, no long illness." (Dana Dawes to Marshall, telegram, April 23, 1951; Marshall to Dana Dawes, April 24, 1951; Marshall to Caro Dawes, May 21, 1951, and telegram, n.d.; and Caro Dawes to Marshall, June 30, 1951, ibid., [M200-5-18].)

291

MEMORANDUM TO THE SECRETARY OF THE ARMY (FOR THE JUDGE ADVOCATE GENERAL[1]) — April 30, 1951, Washington, DC

Restricted

As a matter of urgency, I would like to get a flash opinion from the Judge Advocate General as how best to meet immediately, without having to wait for legislative action which must be taken, the serious situation we are in regarding men disabled by service in Korea. The following quotation from General [Carl R.] Gray [Jr.], Administrator of the Veterans Administration, illustrates the problem and its serious reactions:

"At present the Veterans Administration has received requests from Walter Reed Hospital for the designation of Veterans Administration Hospital for three military patients *who are amputees*. These men have appeared before the Physical Evaluation Board of the hospital and it is evident from the information provided that they will be retired for physical disability, probably within a period of 30 to 60 days."

(Now this is the important part of the quotation)

"They all served in the Korean situation; however, they have not served *during the period of war* and must, therefore, be considered at the time of retirement as persons retired for physical disability *from peacetime service*. As such, they have no entitlement to hospitalization from the Veterans Administration unless they file a claim for compensation and, being found entitled thereto, elect to take compensation from the Veterans Administration in lieu of a like portion of their retirement pay."[2]

The procedure now available is long drawn out and very complicated and would awaken a storm of protest if the plight of these men became public. The issue as I see it is can we get a position regarding the Korean struggle that will cover all the participants as participating in a war and at the same time not embarrass politically the government otherwise.

I am further informed that the same situation may arise on re-employment rights in civilian industry and probably in other matters.

Please treat this as a matter of urgency.[3]

GCMRL/G. C. Marshall Papers (Secretary of Defense, Number Indexed, M200-7-36)

1. Major General Ernest M. Brannon had been the US Army Judge Advocate General since January 27, 1950.

2. The editors have been unable to determine the source document for this quotation.

Since "military service in Korea was technically peacetime service" because there was never a formal declaration of war, veterans of the Korean conflict tended to receive fewer benefits than veterans of World War II. Korea veterans "could receive full wartime rates of disability compensation when their disabilities resulted directly from armed conflict or were received while engaged in extrahazardous service. Otherwise, reduced peacetime rates were payable for service-connected disabilities, and they could go to a VA [Veterans Administration] hospital for service-connected disabilities; get prosthetic appliances, special help if they lost their sight or the use of their legs, and a few other benefits." (Robinson E. Adkins, *Medical Care of Veterans* [Washington: GPO, 1967], 231.)

3. News broke on May 9 that a twenty-one-year-old marine who had fought in Korea was denied treatment for possible throat cancer at the VA hospital in Tucson, Arizona, for the reasons outlined by General Gray in the document above. The following day Truman forwarded to Congress draft legislation that "would extend certain benefits to persons who shall have served in the Armed Forces on or after June 27, 1950." A compromise bill passed both chambers that same evening, and Truman signed it into law the next day. (Adkins, *Medical Care of Veterans*, 231; *Public Papers, 1951*, 277; "Benefits for Korean Veterans Voted After Hospital Bars an Ex-Marine," *New York Times*, May 11, 1951, p. 1; "Congress Votes Medical Care By VA for Korean War Troops," *Washington Post*, May 11, 1951, p. 1.)

292

To Dean G. Acheson — May 1, 1951
Top Secret — Washington, DC

Dear Mr. Secretary: On 2 February 1951 the President approved NSC 72/4, "United States Policy Toward Spain" and directed its implementation by all appropriate executive departments and agencies of the United States Government under your coordination. Shortly thereafter I requested that the Joint Chiefs of Staff provide me with their views concerning the proposals which should be recommended by this department in implementation of NSC 72/4.[1]

In response to this request, the Joint Chiefs of Staff have recommended that Admiral Carney, the Commander-in-Chief, U. S. Naval Forces Eastern Atlantic and Mediterranean, conduct initial military discussions of an exploratory nature with Spanish military authorities. The Joint Chiefs of Staff have recommended the immediate issuance of the attached directive to Admiral Carney. This directive will not be implemented by Admiral Carney until he is informed that the requisite political arrangements have been concluded.[2]

In recognition of the urgency to develop the military potentialities of Spain's strategic geographic position for the common defense of the NAT area, I have approved the immediate issuance of this directive by the Joint Chiefs of Staff, and I consider that we should proceed without delay in arranging for the conduct of these military discussions. I request that you notify me at such time as the requisite political arrangements have been concluded in order that I may inform the JCS that Admiral Carney may be instructed to implement the directive.[3]

I am aware that in proceeding on a bilateral basis we risk complications with the United Kingdom and France. The Assistance of this department is available in your consideration of such placating measures as may be required to satisfy the legitimate interests of our allies. In this respect, this department does not at this time view with favor the initiation of exploratory military discussions of a strategic nature with military representatives of the United Kingdom and France regarding the relation of Spain to Western Europe as suggested in Mr. Matthews' letter of 16 March 1951 to General Burns. From a military viewpoint, such discussions would be premature, and further, would delay Admiral Carney's visit to Spain.[4]

Admiral Carney's directive contains a list of U. S. military requirements in Spain which supplement those contained in the enclosure to the letter from the Secretary of Defense to you, dated 19 May 1949. For convenience, an extract of that document insofar as it pertains to military rights in Spanish territory is enclosed.[5] Faithfully yours,

G. C. Marshall

NA/RG 330, CD 092 (Spain)

1. See pp. 356–57. Marshall had requested the views of the JCS on NSC 72/4 on February 7. (Marshall to JCS, memorandum, February 7, 1951, NA/RG 330, CD 092 [Spain].)
2. The JCS reported these views in an April 24 memorandum to Marshall. The directive to Admiral Carney listed three urgent matters: "Long term rights . . . in Spain and her ter-

ritories" for bases; "Naval anchorage rights" at critical ports; and long term rights, among others, to "occupy, . . . expand, . . . [and] maintain" airfield and port facilities at several other specific locations. (Bradley to Marshall, memorandum and appendix, April 24, 1951, ibid.)

3. Marshall authorized the JCS "to issue immediately your proposed directive" to Carney but insisted that it not "be implemented" until Acheson responded regarding the completion of the "political arrangements" necessary for Carney to initiate these talks. (Marshall to JCS, memorandum, May 1, 1951, enclosure in Lalor and Carns to JCS, May 3, 1951, NA/RG 218, Geographic File, 092 [Spain].)

4. Matthews had speculated that conversations with the British and French, which might include discussing the strategic value of Spain and its role in joint defense, "should increase understanding of the United States position." He had requested the views of the Defense Department as to whether or not such "military talks would be advisable." (*FRUS, 1951*, 4: 810.)

5. This enclosure differentiated between normal peacetime rights and those during times of war for use of bases. Acheson replied on May 16 that he disagreed with Marshall and recommended "further discussions with the British and French" to avoid splitting "completely with them over this issue" and endangering "important NATO relationships." (Enclosure to Marshall to Acheson, May 1, 1951; Acheson to Marshall, May 16, 1951, NA/RG 218, Geographic File, 092 [Spain]; *FRUS, 1951*, 4: 816–17.)

Marshall forwarded Acheson's response to the JCS on May 23 and requested "the basis of a reply to Secretary Acheson." Before the JCS formulated a response for Marshall, however, they conceded to the State Department and agreed to discuss this policy with the British and French before beginning "direct conversations" with the Spanish government. NSC 72/4 was subsequently revised and approved on June 27, 1951, as NSC 72/6, which included an explicit requirement for the US to discuss its Spanish policy with the British and French, with the goal of "agreeing on a common policy," if possible. (Marshall to JCS, memorandum, May 23, 1951; enclosure in Lalor and Carns to JCS, May 24, 1951, NA/RG 218, Geographic File, 092 [Spain]; *FRUS, 1951*, 4: 819–22.)

Admiral Sherman and Assistant Secretary of State Perkins met with British and French military officials on June 21 and 22 to discuss US "policy and objectives" with regard to Spain, which included bilateral discussions beginning in mid-July between Spanish Generalissimo Francisco Franco and Admiral Sherman, "or another high-ranking officer," along with US Ambassador to Spain Stanton Griffis. Despite continued British and French opposition to this plan, Sherman departed for Spain on July 15, with the understanding he had agreed to with Truman, Acheson, Marshall, and Bradley that he would "confine initial discussions of the base program to exploratory discussion of rights to stage aircraft through Spanish fields, overfly Spain, and generally make use of Spanish air facilities, and to anchorage rights for naval vessels." (*FRUS, 1951*, 4: 825–29; Lovett to Acheson, July 13, 1951, enclosure to Kreps to JCS, memorandum, July 13, 1951, NA/RG 218, Geographic File, 092 [Spain].) See pp. 587n1 and 595–96.

Marshall was simultaneously in discussions with Portuguese Minister of National Defense Fernando dos Santos Costa to secure base rights in the Azores Islands to fulfill NATO defense requirements. The US and Portuguese governments signed an agreement on September 6, 1951. (Marshall to Santos Costa, February 9 and May 11, 1951; Santos Costa to Marshall, March 25, 1951; Marshall to Acheson, July 16, 1951, NA/RG 330, CD 092.2 [Portugal]; *FRUS, 1951*, 4: 771–72.)

293

To Harry S. Truman — May 1, 1951
Top Secret — Washington, DC

Dear Mr. President: The Joint Chiefs of Staff have advised me that the Soviet capability to mount amphibious and airborne attacks against Japan, in conjunction with the present lack of defending ground forces, constitutes a grave and immediate threat to the security of Japan. I strongly concur in their estimate of the gravity of this threat.

There is now in existence a Japanese National Police Reserve [JNPR] of 75,000 men organized into four partly equipped divisions. In view of the precarious security situation, the Commander-in-Chief, Far East, has urgently requested sufficient arms to equip these units as full combat divisions. Accordingly, the Joint Chiefs of Staff have recommended that the Department of the Army be authorized, as a matter of urgency, to furnish full equipment, including heavy armament, for the existing four divisions of the Japanese National Police Reserve.[1]

The Secretary of State, however, has pointed out several serious political considerations which weigh against the provision of heavy armament to Japanese forces at this time.[2] These considerations may, I believe, be summarized as follows:

(1) Such action would violate decisions of the Far Eastern Commission which are, in effect, international obligations of the United States.

(2) It would jeopardize support both in Japan itself and among our allies for a Japanese Peace Treaty of the type which the United States is seeking. Such a treaty would itself be the best means to remove existing restrictions on Japanese rearmament and to obtain maximum Japanese support for the cause of the free world.

(3) It might isolate the United States from its allies and make it difficult for us to obtain international support for counter-action in the event of a localized Soviet attack on Japan.

(4) It might have adverse effects on the possibility of any degree of success of a meeting of the Council of Foreign Ministers.[3]

In view of these considerations, the Departments of State and Defense have agreed to recommend your approval for the establishment, from U.S. Army stocks, of a "Special Far East Command Reserve", which would be available as a stockpile of equipment for the four JNPR divisions, but which would not be placed in the hands of the Japanese without specific prior agreement by the Department of State or approval at the highest governmental level.

I further recommend, on the advice of the Joint Chiefs of Staff and with the concurrence of the Secretary of State, that you authorize the Department of the Army to undertake planning and budgeting for material sufficient fully to equip an overall total of ten JNPR divisions by July 1, 1952.

This recommendation means that the Department of the Army would have authority to plan and budget a program to equip an overall total of ten JNPR divisions, but the decision to stockpile such equipment for an additional six divisions will be made by appropriate military authority at a later date, and in view of the then existing situation. The authority immediately to ship heavy armament for the four existing JNPR divisions will cause some extension of the period during which Army units in the United States must train with a 50% allowance of major critical items of equipment, and may also result in some delays in MDAP deliveries.[4]

With great respect, Faithfully yours,

GCMRL/G. C. Marshall Collection (Harry S. Truman)

1. In the wake of the North Korean invasion and subsequent movement of US forces stationed in Japan to the Korean peninsula, as well as domestic unrest within Japan, MacArthur in a July 8, 1950, letter to Prime Minister Shigeru Yoshida had authorized the Japanese government to establish a national police reserve of up to seventy-five thousand men and a maritime security force of eight thousand men. (*FRUS, 1950*, 6: 1251; James, *Years of MacArthur*, 3: 242.)

On February 9, 1951, the JCS reported to Marshall "that the gravity of the current threat to the security of Japan (which is expected to become particularly acute by early May) makes it urgent to ship immediately to General MacArthur the equipment" he had requested on January 3, 1951, to arm this national police reserve. The chiefs consequently recommended that Marshall request presidential authorization for the army to dispatch a reply to MacArthur and request "funds to support a program for equipping up to ten" JNPR divisions "in a manner similar to that recommended by General MacArthur in the case of the four" JNPR divisions currently in existence. Due to "the international and domestic political implications" of these recommendations, however, the JCS suggested that Marshall "discuss this matter with the Secretary of State and the President" and "that this program hereafter be referred to wherever possible as the 'Special Far East Command (FECOM) Reserve' program." Marshall concurred and forwarded the JCS memorandum to Acheson on February 15 for his views. (*FRUS, 1951*, 6: 884–85.)

2. Marshall accurately summarized in the ensuing four points and subsequent paragraph the March 1 response of Acting Secretary of State James Webb to his February 15 letter. Marshall accepted these suggestions in an April 20 letter to Acheson and enclosed a draft of the above letter to Truman that Acheson approved on April 30. (*FRUS, 1951*, 6: 898–900, 1001–2.)

3. The anticipated Council of Foreign Ministers meeting did not occur.

4. Truman approved this plan on May 3. (Truman to Marshall, May 3, 1951, GCMRL/G. C. Marshall Collection [Harry S. Truman].) See pp. 582–83.

294

Meeting with Israeli Prime Minister David Ben-Gurion
May 4, 1951 Washington, DC

ON MAY 4, Marshall met with visiting Israeli Prime Minister and Defense Minister David Ben-Gurion at 10:00 a.m. Following up on previous conversations and correspondence with Marshall, Lovett, and other officials regarding Israel's military needs (see pp. 298–99 and 329–30), Ben-Gurion first thanked Marshall for his assistance in obtaining military training for his officers in the United States and then went into a lengthy explanation of Israel's defense capabilities and needs in light of the threats posed by both the Arab states and the Soviet Union. He informed Marshall of a recent and "very agreeable talk" he had with General Sir Brian Robertson about British defense plans in the Middle East and Israel's role in those plans. Robertson had defined a defense line Britain proposed to hold in the event of war running "from the mountains between Iran and Iraq and from the Turkish mountains up to the Black Sea." He could not state the exact part Israel would be expected to play in Middle East defense, but it would "certainly be expected to back up this line of defense," and he envisaged immediate use of Israeli port facilities and transit rights for troops and supplies. Ben-Gurion emphasized to Marshall "the importance of knowing how Israel fitted in to this plan and what, if any, plan had been developed between the United States and Great Britain." In this regard, he "imagined" the area would be defended by "a small British force, the Israeli Army and an American force." Ben-Gurion "made a special point" of emphasizing US interest in the survival of Israel and explained Israeli mobilization strength as well as additional expected manpower available for military-related industry. He requested US assistance in building up such industry as well as equipment to bring the Israeli Army up to US standards. (Memorandum of Conversation, "Visit of Israel Prime Minister David Ben-Gurion," May 4, 1951, NA/RG 330, CD Memorandum of Conversation.)

Marshall then responded that his part in obtaining additional training for Israeli officers had been "very small," that he was "very interested" in the discussions Ben-Gurion had with Robertson, and that he "certainly shared" Ben-Gurion's belief that Israeli forces would be "useful" once built up to defend the Middle East in case of a Soviet invasion. "Much discussion remained," however, "to determine exactly what part" Israeli forces would play in that defense. Marshall also questioned Ben-Gurion on both available manpower and Israel's relations with Greece and Turkey, whose membership in NATO Marshall and the JCS had recently supported (see pp. 485–86). He mentioned the problems he was having with Congress over UMT (see pp. 369–71, 409–13, 423–26, and 481–84) and stated that without it the nation could not afford the very large army it imagined, thereby casting some doubt on Ben-Gurion's belief that US forces would be committed to defense of the Middle East. He was also "very sympathetic to the needs of Israel but told the Prime Minister that our commitments placed a great demand on the resources and funds allowed by Congress. Nevertheless, the request of Israel would be considered." Marshall then ended the conversation with a "special point" that he hoped would not "seem impertinent. He felt it extremely important that the border incidents that continued to occur with their neighbors should be controlled and prevented"—a reference in particular to recent hostilities along the border with Syria. As secretary of defense he felt this was "the most important contribution that Israel could make to the stability and the future defense of the area." (Ibid.) ★

295

TO GENERAL OF THE ARMY DWIGHT D. EISENHOWER — May 7, 1951
Top Secret US Eyes Only — Washington, DC

Dear General Eisenhower: I enclose a memorandum by the Joint Chiefs of Staff concerning the method by which the Standing Group nations should pass military judgment on the German proposals for rearmament. As you know, that judgment is but a step toward later agreement on a governmental basis.[1]

It is quite evident that we should not wish to embarrass the French by seeking an agreement with the German military authorities prior to the time the French are able to give equal assent at Bonn and in Paris. At the same time the political aspects of a German contribution are of increasing complexity and may delay practical military programming to an extent detrimental to United States policy objectives. I am therefore of the opinion that military agreement as to a logical and forceful German military program should be achieved between the Occupying Powers and Germany in a steadfast, orderly manner.[2]

I am forwarding the enclosed memorandum to you, before acting upon it, to determine your advice on how we might best proceed. If you desire to take cognizance of this problem we would, from the United States point of view, adapt our action to conform with your recommendations. It is my feeling that we should seek to have a comprehensive German proposal at an early date.[3] Faithfully yours,

NA/RG 330, CD 091.7 (Europe)

1. As a result of the agreements at the December 1950 NATO defense ministers meeting in Brussels, the Allied high commissioners and representatives of the West German government had been meeting since January 1951 in Bonn to discuss "the military aspects of a German contribution" to European defense. Simultaneously, representatives of the continental European members of NATO, joined by observers from the US, UK, and Canada, were meeting in Paris to develop plans for a European defense force. (Condit, *Test of War*, 384–86; Robert L. Beisner, *Dean Acheson: A Life in the Cold War* [New York: Oxford University Press, 2006], 373.) See pp. 167–68, 218–20, 303–4n1, and 386–89.

Colonel Beebe reported to Marshall on May 4 that Bonn talks were "practically on dead center" and would soon require "judgment by the Occupying Powers." This was being stalled due to "over-emphasis of the political uncertainties developing from the Paris discussions on the European Army, the French elections and the Council of Foreign Ministers." In order to promote the Defense Department's aim to gain approval of German participation in European defense, Beebe requested that Marshall use this May 7 letter to "obtain the personal views of General Eisenhower as to whether he wishes to enter these proceedings at this time." (Beebe for Burns to Marshall, memorandum, May 4, 1951, NA/RG 330, CD 091.7 [Europe].)

The JCS had recommended to Marshall on April 16 that the members of the NATO Standing Group represent "the Chiefs of Staff of the occupying powers . . . for the purpose of considering the military aspects of the German proposal." They also suggested that the "German proposal" be "simultaneously considered by the Allied High Commissioners" in order to expedite a decision. Bradley detailed a suggested process for the collection of military reaction to German rearmament, including debate and agreement on the "'single package' proposal" among the representatives of the chiefs of staff; resolution of any discrepancies beyond the purview of the military representatives at "the governmental level or, if necessary," in NATO; and initiation by the secretary of defense of "necessary action on the governmental level" on the final report. (Bradley to Marshall, memorandum, April 16, 1951, attached to Lalor to US representative to Standing Group, June 13, 1951, NA/RG 218, Geographic File, 092 [Germany, Sec. 7].)

2. At this time Marshall also participated in planning for the establishment of a "German Guerilla Warfare Organization." In addition to Marshall, Acheson, the JCS, Walter Bedell Smith, Eisenhower, and US High Commissioner for Germany John J. McCloy were involved in the effort to create such an organization. (Marshall to Acheson, May 5, 1951, NA/RG 330, CD 092.3 [NATO Council of Ministers].)

3. Eisenhower replied on May 18 that he shared Marshall's opinions. He also concurred with the April 16 JCS proposals, although in order to remain neutral in "the politi-

cal aspects" surrounding the questions of "unit size and level of integration," Eisenhower requested that Marshall forward to him the JCS recommendations "informally . . . for my comment on a 'U.S. Eyes Only' basis before the U.S. position is presented to the members of the Standing Group." (Eisenhower to Marshall, May 18, 1951, NA/RG 330, CD 091.7 [Europe].)

On June 5, Lovett, as acting secretary of defense, replied to Eisenhower that Marshall, prior to his departure that morning for West Point, St. Louis, and then the Far East (see pp. 544–51), had asked Lovett to inform Eisenhower that the JCS would solicit his comments on the US position "prior to their final action." On June 11, Lovett forwarded to the JCS the department's and Eisenhower's agreement to the process suggested in their April 16 memorandum. (Lovett to Eisenhower, June 5, 1951, NA/RG 330, CD 091.7 [Europe]; Lovett to JCS, memorandum, June 11, 1951, NA/RG 218, Geographic File, 092 [Germany, Sec. 7].)

The Bonn Report, issued on June 6, set the strength of the German armed forces at no more than "20% of forces assigned SACEUR and the hypothetical total strength of 100,000 for 1951 and 250,000 by end of 1952" made up of divisions as opposed to brigades or combat teams within the larger European defense framework. (Beebe to Carter, memorandum and attachments, June 13, 1951, NA/RG 330, CD 091.7 [Europe].)

On June 29, Marshall forwarded to SHAPE the "broad acceptance" by the JCS "of the principle of a European Army" provided that "SACEUR would be authorized to deploy and assign these units without regard to their European Army origin" and that "German units of division size, could be assigned to British, American or French sectors of command." (Marshall to Eisenhower, radio no. DEF-95320, June 29, 1951, NA/RG 218, Geographic File, 092 [Germany, Sec. 8].) See pp. 563–65 and 583–85.

ON APRIL 25, the Senate unanimously voted to have its Armed Services and Foreign Relations Committees conduct joint hearings regarding MacArthur's relief, with Armed Services Committee Chairman Russell presiding, rather than an earlier proposal by Russell to have Marshall, followed by MacArthur, testify in executive session before the Senate Armed Services Committee on April 18. (Marshall to Russell, April 13 and 16, 1951, and Marshall to MacArthur, April 14, 1951, GCMRL/G. C. Marshall Papers [Secretary of Defense, Number Indexed, M200-2-29]; *MSFE*, 3568–71.) Democrats rejected a Republican proposal for open hearings broadcast over radio and television, opting instead for closed hearings with the issuance each day of transcripts that had been censored to protect classified information. Those censored sections were declassified in the mid-1970s.

The hearings were to cover the entire situation in the Far East as well as the MacArthur relief, and Russell and his colleagues soon requested a large number of classified documents covering these matters. On April 26, Carter informed Lovett that Marshall had told him "at considerable length and deep conviction" that the Defense Department needed to furnish "as much of the pertinent information, both in advance and during the hearings, as we can appropriately provide without really grave and serious endangerment of our national security. . . . He anticipated a reluctance on the part of the military to release this information to the Committee, and he said that this reaction was completely understandable but that under the circumstances he hoped they would handle the problem on the basis of 'maximum amount of what we can say' rather than 'minimum amount of what we may be forced to say.'" (Carter to Lovett, memorandum, April 26, 1951,

GCMRL/G. C. Marshall Papers [Secretary of Defense, Chronological, Director, Executive Office (Marshall S. Carter), 1950–1952].) On April 27, Marshall sent Russell an interim reply and promised to send on May 1 as many of the documents as possible that Russell had requested by that date. On May 1, he also informed Russell that the JCS would "furnish as much information as possible without endangering our national security"; that they had prepared an attached chronological record of their actions relative to Korean operations to provide background information; but that war plans, operational plans or directives, and JCS minutes "cannot be made available under any circumstances without grave danger to our national security, or without endangering the lives of our troops and the troops of our Allies." Furthermore, as per previous oral discussions between Russell and members of Marshall's staff, if necessary, the Defense Department would, "within the framework outlined above, make the basic documents available for inspection by a subcommittee to be named by you." (Marshall to Russell, April 27 and May 1, 1951, GCMRL/G. C. Marshall Papers [Secretary of Defense, Selected].)

MacArthur testified first, from May 3 to 5. Marshall testified next, from May 7 to 14, and was accompanied each day by OSD General Counsel Larkin. At Truman's direction, Marshall had met in late April with Acheson, Harriman, and the JCS to prepare his testimony. (Carter to Bradley, memorandum, April 23, 1951, ibid.) On Saturday, May 5, Marshall met in his office separately with Lovett, Bradley, Vandenberg, and Leva, and on Sunday afternoon first with Lovett, then Leva and Larkin, followed by Bradley. He also received advice on his opening statement and ensuing testimony from Bernard Baruch, who had met with Marshall Carter "for approximately two hours." Carter produced a five-page personal and confidential memorandum for Marshall containing Baruch's suggestions. Baruch urged Marshall "to be sure and keep your guard up, because this MacArthur affair was a strictly political business and knowing the Administration as well as he does he said the politicos will sacrifice anybody and anything to meet their ends." He believed that "Part of the present Republican attitude is an attempt to unseat you as Secretary of Defense, in addition to Acheson as Secretary of State, all with a view to embarrassing the Administration." He recommended that Marshall testify "with the greatest frankness" and not "hold back on anything" that the committee would later "be able to squeeze out of you." Marshall wrote to thank Baruch for his advice on May 3 and spoke with him by telephone the following day. In his May 3 letter, Marshall confessed that "All of this business is most unpalatable and there are not only wheels within wheels but ulterior purposes behind almost every action and question. However, I am somewhat accustomed to this but I can't claim to enjoy it." (Carter to Marshall, memorandum, and Marshall to Baruch, May 3, 1951, GCMRL/G. C. Marshall Papers [Secretary of Defense, Selected, MacArthur].)

In all, twenty-six senators from the two committees asked questions in order of their seniority, resulting in a great deal of duplication of questions and answers. Taking place over seven days, Marshall's testimony lasted nearly twenty-eight hours and took up more than four hundred pages of the published hearings (eleven hundred pages of transcript according to *U.S. News and World Report*) as well as many pages of classified material. ("Senator Russell, the Man Who Heard 2 Million Words, Thinks MacArthur Inquiry Did Some Good, Some Harm," *U.S. News and World Report*, June 29, 1951, p. 35.)

In his previous testimony as well as his April 19 address to Congress (see pp. 487–88), MacArthur had called for expanded air reconnaissance and bombing of Manchuria, intensification of the economic blockade against China, a naval blockade of the China coast, and the use of Chinese Nationalist troops. Citing the JCS memorandum that Collins and Vandenberg had delivered to him in January (see pp. 330–31), MacArthur claimed that the Joint Chiefs agreed with him but had been overruled by civilian authorities, including Marshall.

Reproduced below is Marshall's opening statement on his first day of testimony, followed by summaries of the ensuing questions and replies. The editors have determined that the letters Marshall wrote during the time of his testimony be included in this volume following the entire text of the hearings summary in order to provide continuity to the testimony. ★

296

Statement before the Senate Committee on Armed Services and the Committee on Foreign Relations[1] — May 7, 1951, Washington, DC

Testimony of Secretary of Defense George C. Marshall,
Accompanied by Felix Larkin, General Counsel

Secretary MARSHALL. I have a brief statement to make, but first I would like to observe that it is a very distressing necessity, a very distressing occasion, that compels me to appear here this morning and in effect in almost direct opposition to a great many of the views and actions of General MacArthur.

He is a brother Army officer, a man for whom I have tremendous respect as to his military capabilities and military performances and from all I can learn, as to his administration of Japan.[2]

I am here primarily to answer whatever questions you and the members of the committees may care to ask me.

However, I think it may be helpful if, at the outset, I make a brief preliminary statement which I think will clarify some of the issues raised in the course of your hearings last week.

BASIC DISAGREEMENT BETWEEN ADMINISTRATION AND MACARTHUR

From the very beginning of the Korean conflict, down to the present moment, there has been no disagreement between the President, the Secretary of Defense, and the Joint Chiefs of Staff that I am aware of.

There have been, however, and continue to be basic differences of judgment between General MacArthur, on the one hand, and the President, the Secretary of Defense, and the Joint Chiefs of Staff, on the other hand.

In his testimony last week, General MacArthur indicated that, in his understanding, there had been at least two instances in which the Joint Chiefs of Staff had been overruled by the Secretary of Defense or by higher authority.

One of these instances related to the views expressed by the Joint Chiefs of Staff with respect to the disposition of Formosa and the seating of the Communist Chinese Government in the United Nations.

RELATIONSHIP OF FORMOSA AND THE SEATING OF COMMUNIST CHINA IN THE UN TO KOREAN SETTLEMENT

In his testimony of May 4, General MacArthur suggested that I, as Secretary of Defense, had overruled the Joint Chiefs of Staff in their opposition to turning Formosa over to Communist China and to seating Communist China in the United Nations.

At the time I became Secretary of Defense last September, the established policy of the United States was to deny Formosa to Communist China and to oppose the seating of the Communist Chinese in the United Nations.

There has been no deviation from that policy whatsoever. At no time have I entertained the opinion that there should be any deviation. These two issues were to be excluded from any armistice terms.

When the time comes for the negotiation of a settlement of the conflict in Korea, the questions of Formosa and the seating of the Chinese Communists in the United Nations will undoubtedly be raised by other parties to the discussion.

The position which the United States has taken in the United Nations in connection with such negotiations is that this Government will not oppose discussion of these questions. In such discussions, however, I am confident that the United States will continue to adhere to its present position, namely, that it will oppose any settlement of the Korean conflict which would reward the aggressor in any manner whatever, and it will oppose the attempt of any nation or regime to shoot its way into the United Nations.

JCS MEMORANDUM OF JANUARY 12, 1951

The second instance referred to by General MacArthur, of a supposed overruling or veto of the views of the Joint Chiefs of Staff, relates to the courses of action proposed by the Joint Chiefs of Staff in a memorandum addressed by them to the Secretary of Defense under date of January 12, 1951. Of 16 courses of action enumerated in the memorandum, the following 4 were quoted by General MacArthur in his testimony of May 3:

> Continue and intensify now an economic blockade of trade with China.
>
> Prepare now to impose a naval blockade of China and place it into effect as soon as our position in Korea is stabilized, or when we have evacuated Korea, and depending upon circumstances then obtaining.
>
> Remove now restrictions on air reconnaissance of China coastal areas and of Manchuria.
>
> Remove now the restrictions on operations of the Chinese Nationalist forces and give such logistic support to those forces as will contribute to effective operations against the Communists.

At the time this memorandum was prepared, we were faced with the very real possibility of having to evacuate our forces from Korea. The proposals advanced by the Joint Chiefs of Staff, which I have just quoted, were put forward as tentative courses of action to be pursued if and when this possibility came closer to reality.

I transmitted this memorandum to the National Security Council for its consideration. At about this time, however, the situation in Korea began to show signs of improvement.

General Collins who, with General Vandenberg, had left for Korea to obtain a first-hand view of the situation, reported back from Tokyo on January 17, stating that he had just returned from Korea where he had found that the Eighth Army was in good shape and was improving daily.[3]

Thereafter, the situation of our forces in Korea continued to improve and during the latter half of January the enemy forces remained on the defensive. Throughout February and March our forces maintained the initiative against the enemy.

As the result of this change in the military situation from that which prevailed during the early part of January, it became unnecessary to put into effect all of the courses of action outlined in the Joint Chiefs' memorandum of January 12.[4]

None of these proposed courses of action were vetoed or disapproved by me or by any higher authority. Action with respect to most of them was considered inadvisable in view of the radical change in the situation which originally had given rise to them.

BASIC DIFFERENCES ON EXTENSION OF CONFLICT

Now, as to the basic differences of judgment which exist between General MacArthur on the one hand, and the Joint Chiefs of Staff, the Secretary of Defense, and the President, on the other hand.

Our objective in Korea continues to be the defeat of the aggression and the restoration of peace. We have persistently sought to confine the conflict to Korea and to prevent its spreading into a third world war. In this effort, we stand allied with the great majority of our fellow-members of the United Nations. Our efforts have succeeded in thwarting the aggressors, in Korea, and in stemming the tide of aggression in southeast Asia and elsewhere throughout the world. Our efforts in Korea have given us some sorely needed time and impetus to accelerate the building of our defenses and those of our allies against the threatened onslaught of Soviet imperialism.

General MacArthur, on the other hand, would have us, on our own initiative, carry the conflict beyond Korea against the mainland of Communist China, both from the sea and from the air. He would have us accept the risk of involvement not only in an extension of the war with Red China, but in all-out war with the Soviet Union. He would have us do this even at the expense of losing our allies and wrecking the coalition of free peoples throughout the world. He would have us do this even though the effect of such action might expose Western Europe to attack by the millions of Soviet troops poised in Middle and Eastern Europe.[5]

This fundamental divergence is one of judgment as to the proper course of action to be followed by the United States. This divergence arises from the inherent difference between the position of a field commander, whose mission is limited to a particular area and a particular antagonist, and the position of the Joint Chiefs of Staff, the Secretary of Defense, and the President, who are responsible for the total security of the United States, and who, to achieve and maintain this security, must weigh our interests and objectives in one part of the globe with those in other areas of the world so as to attain the best over-all balance.

PUBLIC VOICING OF THE DISAGREEMENT

It is their responsibility to determine where the main threat to our security lies, where we must fight holding actions, and where and how we must gain time to grow stronger. On the other hand, the responsibilities and the courses of action assigned to a theater commander necessarily apply to his own immediate area of responsibility. It is completely understandable and, in fact, at times commendable that a theater commander should become so wholly wrapped up in his own aims and responsibilities that some of the directives received by him from higher authority are not those that he would have written for himself. There is nothing new about this sort of thing in our military history. What is new, and what has brought about the necessity for General MacArthur's removal, is the wholly unprecedented situation of a local theater commander publicly expressing his displeasure at and his disagreement with the foreign and military policy of the United States.

It became apparent that General MacArthur had grown so far out of sympathy with the established policies of the United States that there was grave doubt as to whether he could any longer be permitted to exercise the authority in making decisions that normal command functions would assign to a theater commander. In this situation, there was no other recourse but to relieve him.

IMPORTANCE OF CASUALTIES IN KOREA

As to the question of the specific campaign in Korea, as to the casualties that are daily occurring there, with our troops, and those of our allies, no one, I believe, is more conscious of them than I am.

I realize, though, that the commander on the spot, who actually witnesses the casualties, is even more impressed by what is going on.

However, during some very painful years, I had a daily question of casualties from all over the world, and it is an agonizing procedure, so I can fully understand the reaction of a commander in General MacArthur's position, to the struggle in Korea, unless he could clearly see an early and victorious way out.

But there are many other considerations that this Government has to take into account; and it becomes the hard duty of those responsible to consider what is the wisest course to follow in such matters.

What our troops have done has really been magnificent. Thank goodness, a few of them are now coming back and they will return in much larger numbers beginning the end of this month; but we have small choice at the moment in the matter; and what we can do is appreciate to the full the heroism, the endurance, and the skillful fighting that those men are doing for us.

Now, gentlemen, I am ready to answer any questions you may wish to ask.

MSFE, 321–26.

1. Prior to Marshall's opening statement, Russell introduced Marshall, whose "eminent career as a military leader and as an able administrator is known to all American citizens." He briefly summarized Marshall's previous service, noting that his name had "become synonymous with integrity and devotion, throughout the land, to duty," and that when he thought of Marshall, "I like to recall some words I read a few years ago. They went something like this: 'Most men are the slaves of their ambitions. General Marshall is the slave of his duties.'" Russell encouraged Marshall to "speak fully and freely and to rely upon the methods that we have devised for the protection of this record to delete from the transcript any information that might aid our enemies." Russell administered the oath to Marshall, who then began with his opening statement. (*MSFE*, 321–22.)

2. Larkin stated in a 1972 oral history interview that he and Frank C. Nash, Marshall's representative on the NSC senior staff, had prepared an opening statement at Marshall's request. After reviewing and approving their draft with minor changes earlier in the morning of May 7, Marshall informed Larkin and Nash that he intended to begin his testimony "with something of my own." The result was his inclusion of these two opening paragraphs. ("Oral History Interview with Felix E. Larkin," September 18 and October 23, 1972, HSTL/Oral History Interviews.)

3. See pp. 330–31.

4. MacArthur had first cited this January 12 JCS memorandum during his April 19 address to a joint session of Congress (see pp. 487–88). In response Marshall and the Joint Chiefs had proposed to Truman on April 20 a press release similar to this statement by Marshall regarding the memorandum, but the statement released to the press on April 21 merely stated that "Operations in the Far East are being carried out in accordance with the views of the Joint Chiefs of Staff. . . . An analysis of the basic differences which exist between the Joint Chiefs of Staff and General MacArthur will be presented" to the congressional committees. Both the Marshall memorandum to Truman and the final press release as well as additional supporting documents are attached to an April 24 memorandum by Carter detailing the convoluted history of these documents. (Carter memorandum for record, April 24, 1951, and attachments, GCMRL/G. C. Marshall Papers [Secretary of Defense, Selected].)

5. "The big question is are we going to go alone in the world without friends or go along with the United Nations," Marshall had asserted in this regard during an April 20 cabinet meeting. "MacArthur's failure to mention United Nations [in his April 19 speech to Congress] was prompted by his realization that it would complicate his logic. The General has been out of the country so long that he is completely out of touch with domestic problems." Marshall went on to note that it would be "hard to meet MacArthur's statements without wrecking the morale of Chiang's forces on Formosa," a problem he resolved by keeping classified his ensuing testimony on why those forces should not be used as MacArthur had proposed. ("Cabinet Meeting, Friday, April 20, 1951," HSTL/Matthew J. Connelly Papers [Notes on Cabinet Meetings II].) See the next editorial summary.

297

Senate Testimony on the Military Situation in the Far East
May 7–14, 1951 Washington, DC

Monday, May 7, 1951

FOLLOWING Marshall's opening statement (see previous document), Senator Russell as chair began the questioning by asking Marshall about the role of the UN in the limitations placed on MacArthur. Marshall explained UN opposition to so-called "hot pursuit" of enemy aircraft across the Yalu River. In classified testimony he also explained that a directive had already been written and approved by Truman authorizing MacArthur to bomb air fields and depots in Manchuria and the Shantung province in central China in the event of a "massive air attack" by the Chinese, that Acheson had already advised the allies of this fact, and that MacArthur had previously been authorized to "take air action in response to any action against us outside of Korea." (*MSFE*, 326–28; Senate Committee on Armed Services and Committee on Foreign Relations, "Hearings: Inquiry into the Military Situation in the Far East and the Facts Surrounding the Relief of General of the Army Douglas MacArthur from His Assignment in that Area," declassified transcripts, 82d Cong., 1st sess., NA/RG 46, Records of the Senate Foreign Relations Committee [hereafter MSFE declassified transcripts], 807–8.)

Discussion then turned to the courses of action, proposed by the JCS on January 12, that MacArthur had cited as evidence of the JCS being overruled and that Marshall had previously explained in his opening statement. Marshall now emphasized that these proposals had been drawn up when "We were at our lowest point" and in response to MacArthur's January 10 warnings that troop morale was low, that the Chinese counteroffensive and "limitations and conditions" placed upon him made the US military position in Korea "untenable," and that he could not simultaneously hold Korea and defend Japan (see pp. 323–24 and 330–31). When Generals Collins and Vandenberg had contradicted MacArthur's gloomy assessment after a visit with General Ridgway, however, many of the proposed measures "were held in abeyance" at the recommendation of the JCS "as being unwise measures to take in view of the fact that we had greatly improved our situation in Korea"; consequently the memorandum never received NSC approval. (*MSFE*, 329–30, and classified testimony deleted from 330 [MSFE declassified transcripts, 820].) On request Marshall then read fifteen of the sixteen points in the memorandum, some in open session and some classified, and in response to a question he said that twelve or thirteen of them had now been put into effect. He also pointed out that MacArthur had in the summer of 1950 advised against accepting Chiang Kai-shek's offer of thirty-three thousand troops "because of their ineffectiveness and lack of logistic support," that he reversed his position in late November, but that the JCS disagreed in light of a report by members of MacArthur's own staff regarding the inadequate training and equipment of the Nationalist Chinese soldiers as well as the fact that sending them to Korea would weaken Formosan defenses. (*MSFE*, 333–34, 337, and classified testimony deleted from 334 [MSFE declassified transcripts, 829–31].)

MacArthur had not violated any of his or Truman's orders or directives relating "to the conduct of the campaign," Marshall stated in response to another question from Russell, but "In relations to public statements, he has." (*MSFE*, 341.) He then provided examples of MacArthur's violations of Truman's December 5 directive (received in Tokyo on December 6 and referred to as the December 6 directive in the hearings) regarding the prior clearance of public statements, with emphasis on the March 24 public statement that led to abandonment of the effort to begin armistice negotiations and the Martin letter that resulted in the decision to relieve MacArthur immediately. (See pp. 282–83, 459–60 and 478–81) Marshall explained the meetings from April 6 to 10 and the original plans to have Pace inform MacArthur of his relief. He also reiterated his agreement with JCS and administration policies regarding defense of Formosa and opposition to the seating of Communist China in the UN. "At no time have I entertained the opinion that there should be any deviation from that policy, that these two issues were to be excluded from the armistice terms," he asserted. Along with the JCS, he was opposed "to any attempt of a nation or regime to shoot its way into the United Nations." Could the Chinese be "driven out of Korea and Korea pacified" without implementing MacArthur's recommendations, Russell asked? Marshall doubted they could be driven out even with the implementation of those recommendations. "Wait a minute," Russell asked after Marshall's classified comments on JCS fear of vulnerability to Chinese retaliatory bombing from Manchuria, "do you mean to say in your opinion that there is doubt even if we do bomb them whether they could be driven from there?" "Yes, sir," Marshall responded. How then, Russell asked, would the Korean conflict ever end? "The best possibility," Marshall replied, again in classified testimony, was to continue to attack the Chinese "and inflict such tremendous losses on them in proportion to what has occurred in the past two weeks that we have broken the power of their trained armies." They would consequently be willing to negotiate. MacArthur's recommendations, Marshall and the JCS agreed, would not end the war but would risk "the loss of our allies, the loss of continuation and development of collective action, collective defense, and the hazard of entering into a general war," while jeopardizing NATO and the defense of Western Europe "very, very seriously." Furthermore, no blockade of the China coast could affect the Chinese "seriously" because the bulk of their supplies came from the neighboring Soviet Union. (*MSFE*, 351–54, and classified testimony from those pages [MSFE declassified transcripts, 876–84, quote on 878].) After brief discussion of the refusal to allow MacArthur to bomb Rashin in North Korea near the Soviet border (see p. 407) and Marshall's agreement to review MacArthur's testimony on this matter to see if it could be released, the hearings adjourned at 1:10 p.m. until 10:00 a.m. the following day.

Tuesday, May 8, 1951

Following Marshall's first day of testimony, President Truman gave his own response to MacArthur in a forceful address the evening of May 7 to the conference of the Civil Defense Administration. In that address he emphasized the fact that Korea was part of a global struggle and that expanding the conflict in the Far East would not end it or save American lives. Instead it would play into the Kremlin's hands by leaving Europe exposed to the Red Army as well as deprive the United States of European allies and perhaps wreck the UN and the concept of collective security (*Public Papers, 1951*, 265–69). "That was a fine speech you made last night," Marshall wrote Truman on May 8 while sending birthday greetings to the president. "I wish I could do equally well before the committees of Congress this morning. However, I will do my best. It probably will be a rather warm affair." (Marshall to Truman, May 8, 1951, GCMRL/G. C. Marshall Papers [Secretary of Defense, Selected].)

Marshall testified before the two committees for a second time on May 8, from 10:00 a.m. to 1:10 p.m. Russell continued his questioning by asking Marshall to clarify the restrictions placed upon MacArthur in Korea. Marshall explained both the restrictions and the reasons for them, noting again (partially in classified testimony) the fear of Communist retaliation against vulnerable US/UN targets in Korea, the attitude of allies and the UN, and the "considerable" ground and air forces the Soviets had in the area and could use should they decide to retaliate against a US air attack on Manchuria. Reading from a prepared text, he also clarified what the UN had and had not authorized in Korea, while emphasizing (again in classified testimony) that Washington "had made clear to the United Nations that in the event that extensive enemy air action in Korea" occurred, "appropriate and retaliatory measures would have to be taken, including hot pursuit and the bombing of enemy air bases in Manchuria." He also reiterated the choices that he had said on May 7 the US faced in Korea and his support for continuation of the policy "to inflict the greatest number of casualties we could in order to break down not only the morale but the trained fabric of the Chinese Armies" so as to bring them to the negotiating table. He put Korea into the larger context of the cold war and containment policy, stating that "For the last five years our supreme policy has been to curb Communist aggression and, if possible, to avoid another world war in doing so." He also compared Korea to other and lengthier cold war crises, such as Berlin and Greece, that had appeared to be stalemates at the time but turned out not to be. (*MSFE*, 359–67, and classified testimony for those pages [MSFE declassified transcripts, 902–3, 910, 917, 921–22, quote on 910].)

Marshall then explained, as he had on the previous day, the hazards of MacArthur's proposals. Bombing China would not have a major impact on the Chinese war effort. As for using Chinese Nationalist forces in Korea or on the Chinese mainland, he cited a September report from officers sent to Formosa from MacArthur's own headquarters that had concluded "their condition of training . . . was so low that they could not be depended upon to defend the island." Such extension of the war would not only run the risk of a world war "but would not lead to a quick decision." In addition, Soviet intervention that MacArthur had claimed to be a remote possibility Marshall rated "a very real possibility," as they had furnished the Chinese with their aircraft and might not be willing to "stand by and see this crushed." Soviet intervention meant a world war, Marshall warned. "You do not believe then," Russell asked, "that the war could be limited to the Far East, but would spread to Europe and all other places of the world?" "That is our view of the matter," Marshall responded. Withdrawal from Korea, on the other hand, would have "tragic" consequences; affect Indochina, Thailand, Indonesia, and the Philippines; and have a "very depressing effect on all of those people who have been looking to us for leadership and as an example." The best option remained to stay in Korea and inflict maximum losses on Chinese forces. (*MSFE*, 66, 198,

220, 368–71, and classified testimony for those pages [MSFE declassified transcripts, 928, 930–31, 934, quotes on 928].)

Senator Styles Bridges (R-NH) began his questioning by asking if Marshall approved the method by which MacArthur had been relieved. Marshall referred back to and repeated his testimony on this from the previous day, adding now that there had also been discussion during the April 6 to 10 meetings as to whether to retain MacArthur in his role as Allied occupation commander in Japan but that it had been rejected because it would have "put Ridgway in an almost impossible position" and created "divided authority." In response to another question by Bridges regarding suppression of the Wedemeyer Report, Marshall again asserted, as he had during his September confirmation hearings (see p. 162), that he personally suppressed it, because it had recommended Korea and Manchuria be put under a UN trusteeship that would have included the USSR. Furthermore, "at the time we were heavily involved" with Congress and the UN regarding Greece, and "it was thought inadvisable to release" the report for publication. Marshall also added that he had requested the report, had proposed sending Wedemeyer, and "had him write his own directive." Was Korea of strategic importance, Bridges asked? Yes, Marshall replied, provided "we can afford, and find it possible to maintain it," for "it is not absolutely vital." Wouldn't the United States "have been better off today, possibly not at war in Korea," had Wedemeyer's advice regarding Korea been taken? "I wouldn't answer that in the direct fashion you apparently would like me to do," Marshall replied, "because, if we take every advice that we get, we would never arrive anywhere. There have to be modifications in all of these matters." Did Marshall think Russia possessed the atomic bomb? "I assume they have," he replied, but "it will be a tedious and difficult development" for them. Had he been consulted on the decision to enter the Korean War? "No, sir," nor did he know who had made the decision. Shouldn't MacArthur have been supported in the Far East to the same extent Eisenhower was in Europe? "I do not think the comparison is quite a fair one," Marshall replied. He had "great regard" for MacArthur's military abilities and had "played a very large part in his various assignments, promotions, and decorations; but when it comes to the point of the commander not recognizing—being unwilling to recognize—the decisions of his Government, that is quite another matter." (*MSFE*, 371–77.)

In response to additional questions from Bridges, Marshall first made clear his belief that the Chinese Communists were indeed "Marxist Communists, and so stated in my presence, and insisted, in my presence, that they were. . . . There was never any doubt in my mind." As for the apparent contradiction between his plan to inflict heavy casualties on the Chinese as a way to bring them to the negotiating table and China's nearly limitless manpower as well as his previously expressed belief that "human life was very cheap or considered very cheap in China," Marshall clarified that trained Chinese forces were limited "and that it is the trained force that we are tearing down." Hadn't Congressman Martin been "entitled to get a frank reply" to his letter from MacArthur? "No, sir," Marshall replied, not in public when he was "in total disagreement" with administration policy. (Ibid.,

377–80.) When Bridges asked later that day if this would apply to Eisenhower's statements as well, Marshall replied affirmatively. (Ibid., 387–88.) He also cited examples from his own career with Franklin Roosevelt and that of Pershing with Woodrow Wilson when each of them had disagreed with the president but kept silent in public as opposed to former Army Chief of Staff General Leonard Wood, who had not and who as a result was "denied service" during World War I. What would Marshall have done, Bridges asked, if a difference with Roosevelt "had become an absolute difference of opinion, where you thought the best interests of the country were not being served by the President or the administration?" "I probably would have resigned as chief of staff," Marshall responded. (Ibid., 380–81, 389–91, quotes on 390–91.)

Hadn't the JCS and Defense Department consistently favored a policy regarding China and the Far East "more positive than the Department of State," Bridges asked? Not really, Marshall in effect asserted. While the JCS had been concerned about State's position regarding Formosa, a "firm decision" had been reached that it was "under no circumstances" to come under Communist control. The JCS had been "just as firm," however, "that we must not commit our strength in relation to Formosa and other points in China, in a manner which we could not afford." In Korea, policy had always been not to recognize the Communist government in the north; few troops were available for the Philippines; and while the JCS had favored equipment and training if requested for anti-Communist forces in French Indochina, the JCS had insisted that "under no circumstances should we commit ourselves to troop action in Indo-china," Marshall asserted in classified testimony. He also emphasized how limited in size American forces had been before the Korean War. "When you judge decisions," he stated, "you have to judge them in the light of what there was available to do it." Marshall also did not know of any occasion where Truman had sided with the State Department over the Defense Department. Indeed, during Marshall's tenure as secretary of defense it had been "common procedure" for him, Acheson, and their principal subordinates to meet with the JCS and reach agreement before bringing a matter to Truman's attention. "As a matter of fact, we practically didn't take anything to him that we could not resolve, and I found that with discussion we could resolve practically everything that came up." (Ibid., 381–84, and classified from 382 [MSFE declassified transcripts, 961].)

Marshall admitted that the buildup of NATO forces in Europe ran the risk of triggering a Soviet military move and world war before the buildup was completed, but the "hazards were inescapable. . . . We had no choice, literally no choice whatever there. I don't think the same is true in Korea." (*MSFE*, 385.)

Senator Walter F. George (D-GA) also questioned Marshall extensively on his 1945–46 mission to China, after which Marshall reiterated that Manchuria would be bombed if US troops were threatened by a major Chinese air offensive, and on whether he would feel differently about MacArthur's recommendations if assured of no Soviet intervention. (Ibid., 393–403, and classified from 399, 400, and 402 [MSFE declassified transcripts, 1008–11, 1017].)

Wednesday, May 9, 1951

Marshall's testimony continued on May 9 from 10:00 a.m. to 1:15 p.m. with a series of sharp exchanges between him and Senator Alexander Wiley (R-WI), who noted that Marshall had been a colonel when MacArthur was a four-star general and that the defense secretary had never been a theater commander. The exchanges concerned whether the Martin letter constituted sufficient grounds to relieve MacArthur (see pp. 478–81), the role of UN allies in the relief and other decisions by the administration, the method of relief, and the right of a field commander to disagree with civilian authority. Both the specific questions and Marshall's answers often repeated what had been said on May 8, with Marshall again emphasizing the difference between a private and a public disagreement and the fact that "there can only be one voice" in foreign policy. "I don't mean by that that you don't debate them up here," he clarified, "but you cannot have two voices." (*MSFE*, 407–27, quote on 427.) Also repeated by and to Senators Saltonstall and H. Alexander Smith (R-NJ) were questions and answers regarding policy on Formosa, Marshall's China mission, the impact of MacArthur's March 24 statement (see pp. 459–60), possible endings to the Korean War, and the bombing of Rashin (see p. 407), with Marshall twice noting that MacArthur had been relieved for "an accumulation of things" rather than just the March 24 statement or the Martin letter. (Ibid., 445.) On numerous questions both on this day and throughout his testimony, Marshall suggested that the JCS be asked when they testified.

Thursday, May 10, 1951

Marshall testified on May 10 from 10:05 a.m. to 1:12 p.m., with Senator Smith continuing his questioning from the previous day and focusing this time on Marshall's 1945–46 China mission, Wedemeyer's mission in 1947, and Marshall's China policy as secretary of state. The situation in China at that time, Marshall asserted, "was such that we would literally have to take over control of the country in order to insure that the [Nationalist] armies functioned with efficiency." At that time "we had one and a third divisions in the United States." Wedemeyer had estimated that approximately ten thousand personnel would be needed in China. "In view of our general world situation, our own military weakness, the global reaction to this situation, and my own knowledge out of that brief contact of mine in China," Marshall concluded, "we could not afford to commit this Government to such a procedure." (Ibid., 465.) Once again Marshall was asked questions he had previously answered, with Russell consequently requesting that his colleagues "cull out" questions that had already been asked and answered, but for the remainder of his testimony repetition of previously asked and answered questions continued, albeit with some new ones added and some novel twists given to older ones. (Ibid., 471.) Senator Wayne Morse read a series of MacArthur's statements and asked if they complied with Truman's December 6 directive (see pp. 280–81); Marshall responded that he did not think any of them did. Senator Lyndon Johnson then shifted the questioning to military preparedness and the pending UMT bill (see pp. 325–29, 338–47, 369–71, 409–13, 423–26, and 481–84), with Marshall bluntly stating that he was not satisfied with the present mobilization effort and that the nation was not prepared for the global war that could result from the measures MacArthur was advocating. He emphasized in this regard that bombing Manchuria would bring the 1950 Sino-Soviet Treaty into effect and trigger a global war, as would a naval blockade that included Port Arthur, which had been under Soviet control since the end of World War II. Additional leading questions from Morse and Senator Theodore Green (D-RI) enabled Marshall to reiterate this point and note that it would increase rather than reduce US casualties as MacArthur had claimed. In classified testimony responding to a question from Senator Bourke Hickenlooper (R-IA), Marshall also reiterated that the Communists could bomb UN bases in retaliation for bombing their Manchurian bases and inflict more damage than UN forces could on them. "Our hazards were greater than their dispersed hazards," he emphasized, and the JCS believed "there has not been sufficient material harm to the forces involved to justify the tremendous hazard that may flow" from bombing their bases in Manchuria. (Ibid., 495, and deletion from that page [MSFE declassified transcripts, 1272].)

Friday, May 11, 1951

On May 11, Marshall testified from 10:05 a.m. to 1:15 p.m. and then from 2:30 to 5:05 p.m. (See photo #10.) He again made clear in classified testimony, this time after informal conversations with two members of the JCS, that UN forces were gaining more than they were losing by not bombing Manchuria, especially in light of the vulnerability of Pusan to Communist retaliatory air attack. (Ibid., 501, and deletion from that page [MSFE declassified transcripts, 1300–1302].) MacArthur's reply to Martin he labeled "an expression of views in one way or another practically in complete disagreement with the Commander in Chief," while the March 24 statement had "brought to a halt" Truman's efforts to obtain an armistice (*MSFE*, 513). In lengthy questioning, Senator William Knowland (R-CA) once again asked about the April 6–10 meetings that resulted in MacArthur's relief and JCS recommendations regarding Formosa and the seating of Communist China in the UN, with Marshall once again denying that he had countermanded their recommendations on these matters. In the afternoon session, Knowland focused on US-China policy during and after World War II, lecturing more than questioning on such matters as Lend-Lease aid, the Yalta Conference, Marshall's 1945–46 mission, the murder of US military intelligence officer and missionary Captain John Birch in August 1945 by Chinese Communists, the end of the war against Japan, the State Department's China "White Paper," and the Wedemeyer Report, with Marshall once again repeating the reasons he had previously given for its suppression. Was it "the unanimous judgment of the top command of this Government that our Nation's security is best furthered and best protected by the policy we are pursuing in the Far East," Senator Brien McMahon (D-CT) countered for the Democrats after pointing out that Patrick Hurley, Marshall's Republican predecessor as ambassador to China, had spoken favorably of the Communists? "Exactly that, sir," Marshall responded. (Ibid., 573.)

Saturday, May 12, 1951

The pattern of repetitious questions and speeches by senators continued throughout Marshall's Saturday, May 12, testimony, which lasted from 10:02 a.m. to 1:35 p.m. and again from 2:30 to 5:33 p.m. Senator Harry P. Cain (R-WA) did ask a few new questions, such as whether there were any Communists in the US Army and why the Allied military contribution in Korea was so small, with Marshall responding in classified testimony that the JCS preferred NATO members to strengthen their still-weak forces in Europe first. Wasn't the failure of a non-NATO member such as India to contribute troops in Korea "a real disappointment," asked Senator Henry Cabot Lodge Jr.? "It was to me," Marshall replied. (Ibid., 606, 622, and deletions from those pages [MSFE declassified transcripts, 1575–81, 1620–12].) Marshall was also questioned on casualty rates, and when asked what kind of war Korea was, he responded that it was "a limited war which I hope will remain limited." (*MSFE*, 610.) He questioned what he labeled MacArthur's "overemphasis" on the importance of Formosa as the first and only line of defense short of the West Coast, but admitted "it would be a highly dangerous business for the United States to have Formosa pass into unfriendly hands." (Ibid., 616.) Once again he was questioned on the use of Chinese Nationalist troops in Korea, and once again he noted in classified testimony their inadequate training and the need to use them to defend Formosa. He also noted in open testimony that the fighting in Korea "had a very direct relationship" to the fighting in Indochina, and that Chinese losses of trained troops in Korea "probably restrained action by the Communist Chinese forces on the Indochina frontier." (Ibid., 622.) He also revealed in extensive classified testimony to Lodge that Soviet pilots and communication personnel had been operating MIG fighters; that Soviet personnel were also involved in the antiaircraft systems around the North Korean capital of Pyongyang and in the laying of mines; and that Japan as well as airfields, ground transportation, and the port of Pusan in South Korea were all vulnerable to air attack. (Ibid., 624, deletion from that page [MSFE declassified transcripts, 1626–30].) He also noted again the importance of passing the UMT bill in order to obtain adequate ground forces. Had the United States demobilized "too much and too rapidly at the end of World War II," Lodge asked? "Oh yes, sir," Marshall replied, though "the important thing was to firmly set up a system that had some chance of enduring, and the failure to do that was the most serious error of all." UMT was the heart of such a system. "I am talking at considerable length," Marshall admitted, "but I feel very strongly about it and I am almost absolutely certain I am right. I apologize for my emphasis." (*MSFE*, 626–28.)

In the afternoon session, Marshall agreed with Senator J. William Fulbright (D-AR) that he did not view the present struggle "as sort of a crusade against communism everywhere and in any form," but rather against the "power of the Russian state"; that unconditional surrender was not the only way to terminate a war; and that full-scale war with Russia was not "inevitable," though it was "a very dangerous possibility." (Ibid., 642–43, 646.) He responded very sharply to a reported comment by General Courtney Whitney, MacArthur's military adviser and counsel during the former commander's earlier testimony before the joint Senate committees, that Truman's January 13 letter to MacArthur had been designed "to make the Eighth Army a scapegoat," something that Marshall said would "almost be treasonable." Senator John Sparkman (D-AL) agreed, but noted he was quoting Whitney. "I didn't select that aide, you know," Marshall tartly replied, and then refused to discuss it further. (Ibid., 656.) The Chinese Communists, he declared in response to another question from Sparkman, were "operating not only in conjunction with but literally under the direction of the Soviet Union." The Nationalists had lost mainland China, he asserted to Senator Russell Long (D-LA), primarily because of "very ineffective leadership and . . . a great deal of ineptitude" in regard to military operations, while substantial additional US aid would not have changed the result. US military advisers "would have been helpful," he admitted, "but what was basically lacking was the support of the army by the people, meaning the men in the army themselves had acquired a feeling of resentment toward the Government or uncertainty as to the Government which so weakened their willingness to fight that along with the incapacity of leadership their effectiveness was greatly limited." He agreed with Long that Russia's aim "is to have us bled white in Korea. There is no question about that in my mind—to have us more completely engaged there than we can afford to be, in view of the situation, the vulnerability of Western Europe." (Ibid., 659–62, 669.) Marshall also revealed in response to questioning by Senator Guy Gillette (D-IA) that MacArthur had refused numerous requests to return to the United States from 1945 to 1950, including one from him on September 17, 1945, one from Truman in 1946, and three from members of the House and Senate in 1948 and 1949. (Ibid., 675–76.)

"I think you have made a wonderful contribution in the manner in which you have cleared up many of these things that many of us were wondering about," Sparkman had previously told Marshall. "I think you have given us background and perspective that otherwise we might not have had." (Ibid., 652.) Now as the afternoon session ended, Russell offered his own praise. "Your recollection as to details and as to dates of all these various transactions has been perfectly astonishing to me," as had been Marshall's "almost infinite" patience in light of the repetitious nature of the questions asked. The hearings would be "a rich treasure house for the historian when he goes to analyze and to write the history of this period in our Nation's history." He thanked Marshall for his cooperation but then stated that it would be necessary for Marshall to return on Monday morning, May 14, for additional questioning. In the meantime he asked his colleagues once again to avoid "going over the same ground again and again." "You wish me to be here" Monday morning, Marshall asked? "I'm afraid I must ask you to be here," Russell replied. "I will be here," Marshall confirmed. Russell in turn made clear to his colleagues that Marshall would have to leave Monday afternoon for the event in his honor at VMI (see pp. 518–23). (Ibid., 678–79.)

Monday, May 14, 1951

In this second round of questioning from 10:00 a.m. to 1:09 p.m., Marshall once again had to answer questions by Bridges, Smith, and others regarding the bombing of Manchuria, the Yalta conference, the JCS January 12 memorandum and Truman's January 13 message to MacArthur, the way MacArthur was recalled, Formosa, aid to Chiang Kai-shek, and the difference in treatment accorded to Europe. He disagreed with Bridges that withdrawal of US aid had caused Chiang's defeat, noting that as secretary of state he had requested and received from Congress large sums for the Nationalists. They had misused all they had been given by attempting "a military impossibility for them, and they had wrecked themselves on that basis together with the character of leadership that was involved"—despite their superiority in equipment and numbers. In response to Bridges's claim that the 80th Congress had "possessed some foresight" on aid to China as compared to the State Department, Marshall noted once again that he had requested $575 million but received only $400 million—a fact "which would have some bearing on that particular question." (Ibid., 688–89.) Johnson asked if Marshall knew "of any responsible or respected high military man now in the Department of Defense that feels our policy is unwise?" "None has been brought to my attention," Marshall replied. Johnson also gave Marshall an opportunity to emphasize once again the importance of prompt action on the UMT bill. "I have talked about that so often," he admitted, "I almost give offense by talking about it again." Had any Defense Department proposal been given "more adequate consideration" than UMT, Johnson asked? None Marshall could think of, save perhaps "the question of what an officer can and should talk about before a committee, and what he should not, if anything"—a rejoinder that brought forth laughter from the committee members. (Ibid., 704–7.) Russell concluded the session by once again thanking Marshall, noting he had given "a remarkable exhibition of stamina, both physical and mental. . . . It has been a very grueling experience, I know, and it is one that would have tested the fire of any man. Throughout it all, you have handled yourself as a soldier would—as the soldier we know you to be." He and Connally also congratulated Marshall on the honors he was about to receive at VMI. (Ibid., 722–23.)

The OSD official history concluded that "Marshall's seven days of testifying were long, tiring, and repetitious because he was asked the same questions over and over," but that he "effectively countered MacArthur's call for victory at any cost and set the stage for the Joint Chiefs, Acheson, and others who had yet to testify." (Condit, *Test of War*, 108.)

"I am very much impressed with your testimony," William Spencer had written Marshall on May 11. "You have handled things to perfection—with character, courage, and with conviction. I cannot imagine a tougher assignment and my hat is off to you." (Spencer to Marshall, May 11, 1951, GCMRL/G. C. Marshall Papers [Secretary of Defense, Number Indexed, M200-13-36].) Others who wrote echoed these sentiments and/or sent press clippings that did so. Marshall thanked each of them for their "support and confidence." (See, for example, Clem to Marshall, May 9, 1951; Marshall to Clem, May 15, 1951; Marshall to Spencer, May 16, 1951; Brougher to Marshall, May 18, 1951; and Marshall to Brougher, May 22, 1951, ibid; and Kean to Marshall, May 15, 1951, and Marshall to Kean, May 22, 1951, ibid., [M214-8-23].) See also pp. 529–30. ★

298

TO WILLIAM LANGER May 11, 1951[1]
Washington, DC

Dear Senator Langer: I have your letter of April 29, quoting a letter you received from a group of reservists who have been recalled to active duty.[2]

Essentially, reservists recalled to active duty will be required to serve for a period of twenty-one months under present law, or until the expiration of their current enlistment as it was extended for one year. However, we have now been able to issue plans for the releasing of reservists on active duty that I hope will allow us to return these men to civilian life prior to the time that their term of duty would expire. In order that you may have readily at hand a copy of a press release setting forth our plans for the release of reservists, I am enclosing one.[3]

Your correspondent's reference to a rotation program and his question as to its effect on him can be best answered by sending you copies of press releases that explain the rotation program for the Services.[4]

I am not enclosing a press release explaining the rotation program for the Navy since that Service does not have a formal rotation program, but returns men to the United States when ships undergo overhaul.[5] Faithfully yours,

NA/RG 330, SD 326.02

1. This and the next document written by Marshall during the Senate hearings on General MacArthur's relief are included here out of chronological order from Marshall's testimony in order to provide continuity in the hearings. (See the previous three documents.)

2. Senator Langer (R-ND) informed Marshall on April 29 that "a group of reservists who have been recalled to active duty" had asked for information on policies regarding inactive reserve forces and rotation plans. Langer requested information from Marshall "as to the general rules and policy of the present reserve program" in order to respond to this inquiry. (Langer to Marshall, April 29, 1951, NA/RG 330, SD 326.02.)

Marshall had approved a report of the Defense Department's Civilian Components Policy Board in April 1951 that addressed reserve policy. The board recommended new classifications of ready, standby, and retired for reservists as well as new standards for pay and promotions and the creation of a Reserve Forces Policy Board to direct the development of these systems. Marshall subsequently requested that the service secretaries prepare more detailed plans for implementation in each branch to be presented to Congress. In June, Marshall abolished the Civilian Components Policy Board and reestablished it as the Reserve Forces Policy Board under Anna Rosenberg. (Press release, "Secretary of Defense Announces New Reserve Policies," and attachments, April 18, 1951, NA/RG 330, SD 040 [Manpower & Personnel, 1951]; Condit, *Test of War*, 489, 492.) See pp. 609–10.

3. This press release was not attached in the Marshall Papers. The Defense Department announced on April 18 that it would begin to release reserve forces in Korea beginning in June. ("Reserve Releases Will Start in June; Draft Cut for May," *New York Times*, April 19, 1951, p. 1.)

4. These press releases were not attached in the Marshall Papers either. See pp. 436–37, 463, and 488–89.
5. This press release was also not attached in the Marshall Papers.

299

Memorandum for All Personnel of the Defense Department

May 14, 1951
Washington, DC

During the recent months considerable progress has been made in the development of civil defense planning throughout the United States. In line with this effort, all Government agencies are developing emergency plans for carrying out their operations in case of an hostile attack upon the Nation's Capital. It is extremely important that the operations of the Department of Defense continue with the least amount of disruption possible.

In the event of an attack which might destroy our facilities for operating at our present headquarters, we must be prepared to operate at locations removed from Washington. Such alternate locations have been selected.[1] For a short period following an attack, only the most vital functions would be performed at such alternate locations. It is, however, essential that our total functions be reconstituted as soon as possible. With this thought in mind, some of you already have received and many others will be receiving notice of the role you are to perform in case of attack. The attached card, in addition to giving you information for your protection, also lists the steps to take after an attack to ensure that your services will be available when required.[2]

I would like to emphasize that these steps are similar to those currently carried out in many other places in the United States and represent precautionary measures desirable in view of the continued tension in the world situation.

GCMarshall

GCMRL/G. C. Marshall Papers (Speeches Binder #13)

1. While the Defense Department press release announcing these plans insisted that the specific location of "the alternate headquarters" would remain classified, the *New York Times* reported that there were rumors it "would be established at Camp Ritchie in Western Maryland," located about seventy miles north of Washington. The camp had been used during World War II by the army and the Office of Strategic Services (OSS), the predecessor to the CIA, as a training site for intelligence officers, but the land on which it was situated had reverted to the state of Maryland following the war. The federal government had been in the process of reacquiring the camp from the Maryland National Guard since the summer of 1950 for the development of a "'supplemental communications installation,'" but a massive construction project in Raven Rock Mountain near Camp Ritchie that had begun earlier in 1951 fueled speculation that it would serve as a substitute Pentagon in the event of an attack. (Press release, "Emergency Headquarters Planning Announced by Defense Department," GCMRL/G. C. Marshall Papers [Speeches Binder #13]; "Pentagon Orders New Center for Communications," *Washington Post*, July 27, 1950, p. 1; "Sites Are Chosen As 'War Pentagon,'" *New York Times*, May 15, 1951, p. 21; "141,000 Here Told Where to Go If Pentagon Is Air Attacked," *Washington Post*, May 15, 1951, p. 1; "U.S. Acquires Camp Ritchie as Radio Base," *Washington Post*, June 2, 1951, p. 4; "'2d Pentagon' Almost Ready, Army Indicates," *Washington Post*, October 27, 1951, p. 3.)

Rather than an alternate Pentagon, CIA Director Smith wrote to Marshall on May 23 to request that the CIA be allowed to use Camp Ritchie "as a training base for covert operations." Marshall directed Secretary Pace to assign an officer to consider Smith's request, although the editors have not located any additional correspondence on the CIA's use of Camp Ritchie. (Marshall to Pace, memorandum, May 23, 1951, GCMRL/G. C. Marshall Papers [Secretary of Defense, Chronological, Director, Executive Office (Marshall S. Carter), 1950–1952].)

2. The attached card directed Defense Department employees first to "Help save lives by rendering aid to others in every way possible," then as "soon as possible, try to report to your regular post of duty." If that post had been "destroyed," they were to report to one of twenty designated "assembly points" around Washington, northern Virginia, and the Maryland suburbs, "within 48 hours for registration." "KEEP THIS CARD WITH YOU AT ALL TIMES," the card concluded. ("Instructions for Procedure in an Emergency Issued to Department of Defense Personnel," GCMRL/G. C. Marshall Papers [Speeches Binder #13].)

JOHN CAMP (VMI, 1905), president of the Virginia Military Institute Foundation, on December 1, 1950, had invited alumni "to attend the ceremonies at V. M. I. on May 15, 1951, honoring General George C. Marshall, '01, for his fifty years of service to the nation." This ceremony would include "the dedication of the new arch to be called the 'George C. Marshall Arch.'" This third arch was the entry to a new portion of the barracks constructed after World War II and used for the first time in the 1949–50 academic year. The other two arches in the old barracks were named for George Washington and General Thomas "Stonewall" Jackson, a professor at VMI prior to the outbreak of the Civil War who is buried in Lexington, Virginia. The celebration would also take place in conjunction with VMI's annual New Market Day ceremony, which commemorates the participation of 257 VMI cadets under the command of General John C. Breckinridge in the Battle of New Market on May 15, 1864, during which fifty-seven cadets were wounded and ten killed. (Camp to VMI alumni, December 1, 1950, GCMRL/G. C. Marshall Papers [Pentagon Office, Selected]; Marshall Day program, n.d., GCMRL/G. C. Marshall Papers [Secretary of Defense, Number Indexed, M214-8-23].) Marshall declined all invitations to attend other events on the days surrounding the VMI celebration, asserting that he could not "justifiably absent myself from the office" for any time longer than was required to attend the VMI event. (Adams to Marshall, January 29, 1951, and Marshall to Adams, February 1, 1951, ibid., [M214-7-42].)

In response to a request from Superintendent Marshall that he wear his army uniform to the festivities, Secretary Marshall replied on April 30 that he did not "think it would be appropriate, in my present position, to wear my uniform and shall plan to wear the customary business suit." He would also "inspect the guard of honor," witness the corps of cadets march in review, and participate in "trooping the line." (R. J. Marshall to Marshall, April 25, 1951, and Marshall to R. J. Marshall, April 30, 1951, ibid., [M214-8-23].)

Numerous distinguished guests as well as friends and family members attended the ceremony, including members of Congress and the Defense Department;

Virginia Governor John Battle; Bernard Baruch, who was invited to give the keynote address; Mrs. Marshall; Marie and Mary Bovard, family friends from Greensburg, Pennsylvania; the Winns and Pendletons; Virginia Stettinius; and Margaret Emerson. (See pp. 465–66.) The Marshalls had originally planned to drive from Leesburg to Lexington with Emerson on May 14, so that Marshall could provide a tour of the Civil War battlefields in the Shenandoah Valley, although his engagement logs indicate that he flew from Washington to Roanoke on May 14 instead. Marshall would attend a dinner that evening, and he wrote to Emerson that following the ceremonies on May 15, they would drive to nearby Natural Bridge, a unique geological formation, for lunch, and then fly back to Washington from either Lynchburg or Roanoke as his "time schedule is getting rather tight." ("VMI Honors Marshall," *VMI Cadet*, May 15, 1951, p. 1; Marshall to McCarthy, May 16, 1951, GCMRL/Frank McCarthy Papers [Additions, Box 1]; Marshall to Emerson, April 18 and 23, 1951, GCMRL/G. C. Marshall Papers [Secretary of Defense, Number Indexed, M200-7-47].)

"It was a perfect day in every respect," Marshall wrote to Frank McCarthy after the event. It began with the honor guard reporting to him, followed by "a reception of several hundred people." He then received the Virginia Distinguished Service Medal from Governor Battle, "trooped the line," and reviewed "the Corps of Cadets on parade. That was followed by the New Market Day ceremony at the conclusion of which my party returned to the Superintendent's quarters where we had a chance to freshen up before the dedication of the arch a half-hour later." There "were about eight thousand people in attendance." (Marshall to McCarthy, May 16, 1951, GCMRL/Frank McCarthy Papers [Additions, Box 1].)

In the keynote address, Baruch declared Marshall "VMI's most illustrious graduate" and praised him as "a living example of the tradition of the civilian soldier which Washington began," and "the very prototype of the soldier-statesman." He told anecdotes about Marshall as army chief of staff and called him "a warm friend; a fine fishing and hunting companion." Underlying his entire being, Baruch concluded, was a sense of duty that led him to accept any position offered to him. Baruch believed that the example of General Robert E. Lee (USMA, 1829), who chose to fulfill his "*duty* to the young men of the South" after the Civil War by becoming president of then Washington College, now Washington and Lee University, from 1865 until his death in 1870, etched "an indelible portrait of the man we honor here today." (Address by Baruch at VMI, May 15, 1951, GCMRL/G. C. Marshall Papers [Secretary of Defense, Speeches and Statements, Others Than Marshall].)

Following Baruch's address, Marshall delivered his remarks. See photo #11. ★

300

REMARKS AT THE MARSHALL DAY CEREMONY AT THE VIRGINIA MILITARY INSTITUTE[1]

May 15, 1951
Lexington, Virginia

Mr. Superintendent, Your Excellency, Mr. Baruch, Members of the Corps of Cadets, Ladies and Gentlemen. I think it will be evident to all of you that it would be utterly impossible for me to find the appropriate words to express my appreciation, my gratitude, for the honor and distinction that have been paid me today. So I will not undertake to do it, other than what I have just said, lest I fail to give you the impression of how deeply I am affected. It has been a great thing for me to come back here in any event, and particularly under these circumstances.

I had a meeting of my classmates last night; we're all getting along a little bit, and, of course, we went back into our recollections of those great days of our youth and our first cadet days here.[2] And in these memories, my mind turned then, and more today, with all these references that have occurred here, to what a great change in American history was initiated at that time.

As has already been said, I entered the Corps of Cadets in September of 1897. That's a good many years ago, some 53, I believe—or 54. But the following May 1 there occurred the Battle of Manila Bay, the sinking of the Spanish fleet by Admiral Dewey, and for the first time the United States stepped into the international picture.[3] At that period, there was not a single ambassador accredited to the United States. We were recognized in the world largely as a country of Indians and buffalo, crude and remarkable manners, and the sudden wealth of a few.

Actually, the first step in our international development began with that May day—the first of May, '98. We were enthused over the victory, we magnified the Spanish fleet, and we were still more excited as summer approached, in June, and the campaign in Cuba was undertaken. And when we came back in the fall, we were approaching another affair. The Philippine Spanish defense had collapsed in August and the Philippine insurrection was about to develop—which it did the fourth of February, 1899. In the fighting that started there, there were started to a large extent—a larger extent than heretofore, because there had been no war—the feats of our graduates. The most distinguished, the former superintendent who is sitting here on our platform, General Kilbourne, who came out of that brief campaign in the Philippines with the highest decoration of our country, the Medal of Honor. Another of our graduates gained notice in the country because of his locating the whereabouts of the missing insurgent leader, Emilio Aguinaldo. He was the adjutant when I came here; now his name leaped up in the press and we were very much impressed.[4]

We had other men there, and then we came out of that and into the first World War.

I sailed for France in the First Division on the first convoy, and in that group were a great many—a very large number—of second lieutenants from the Virginia Military Institute. As a matter of fact, one Marine Regiment attached to our division had a junior officer corps almost entirely of graduates of the Institute.

And it went on from there in a constantly developing evidence of something that came out of this place that was of great value. I'm not talking about tactics, I'm not talking about strategy; I am talking about character, I am talking about dependability, and the acceptance of responsibility with whatever crisis the crisis might demand.

Then we passed into this last war, and there I don't need to enumerate what happened—the number of men who reached highly conspicious positions all throughout our armed forces efforts from this institution.

I was saying to the Governor last night that I thought the greatest product of this institution was not engineering of one kind or another. It was not these other courses that are offered here, but it was the development of character, of integrity and of responsibility to constituted authority. And that is one of the most valuable contributions that can be made.

I remember so well the first anniversary of the Battle of New Market. The previous fall when I was an entirely new cadet—which meant a great many things—the Corps had gone to New Market for the dedication of a monument, and I literally recollected nothing of that affair. The truth was, I had to carry two undergraduates' guns, including my own, and I was totally unfamiliar with the geography of the battlefield. But the following May 15, that is 53 years ago, the Corps was marched over into that corner of what is now the parade ground, and was then a little vale of an acreage of woodland surrounded by a little fence, and there were buried these boys whose remains are where you saw the celebration this morning. . . . Very simple graves . . . no other graves there that I recall, in this little vale here, which is now the parade ground. And we marched over there under those trees and lined up facing those graves. I believe something was said, but I have remembered more distinctly their names being called and certain members of the Corps reporting that they died on the Field of Honor; but there were the graves right in front of you, just as they'd been at the time and as they had continued through the years. And I also remember that Mrs. Stonewall Jackson was present at that ceremony, and it made a profound impression on me that I have never forgotten.[5]

I could look out the window of my room at that time and see five or six cannon balls still sticking in the wall, where they had come to no friendly purpose.[6] However, another May 15—and my room was right up there where that ivy is, on that face of the barracks—I spoke of, it was tougher then; we had to be here for parade that night and we were allowed the freedom of the midday roll call for mess; that was the extent of the concessions of the period. And there was no motion picture theater, there were no automobiles. There was literally no place to go until we decided on House Mountain over there. I don't know how far it is, but it seemed at the time about thirty miles away.[7] Anyway, one of the classmates of mine who was with me at the time was here last night, and my other classmate who was my roommate here for four years—Nicholson of New Orleans—we decided we'd do something with that day. So we started and marched, or walked to House Mountain. I don't recall that we got anything to eat—my friend, Johnson,[8] thinks we did get something to eat—but, anyway, we went to the top of the mountain. I think we were the only cadets up to the time of the development of the automobile that ever did see the top of that mountain. It was a gorgeous display of wild azaleas, a solid mass. Of course, the view of the countryside was pretty wonderful.

And my thinking went back there, thinking of the fact that that had been a Hessian prison camp at the foot of that mountain. So that was one way to spend May 15. And then, of course, there were others.

But all of these memories came back to me when I talked to these friends—some of them I had not seen for many years. And I thought of how we formed out here on the parade ground at our final formation, and then had separated and gone literally to every part of the world. And it was intensely interesting to think over what happened in these years in this country—to this country, I mean—what a tremendous development has taken place, and how confused, as they often say, the public is. You can't move at that speed without some confusion, and you certainly can't move at that speed with a free press without considerable confusion. Now understand me, I am in no way reflecting on a free press. That's a vital necessity of this country, but it touches your vitals every now and then.

I mustn't talk any longer. It has been a wonderful day to me. I am as deeply appreciative as it is possible for a human being to be. And I think whatever comes to me to do again—or further, I should say—I'll take my inspiration from this day. Thank you very much.[9]

GCMRL/G. C. Marshall Papers (Secretary of Defense, Speeches and Statements)

1. See the previous editorial note and photo #11.
2. The *VMI Cadet* reported on May 15 that "Seventeen of forty graduates of the class, which entered the Institute in 1897 with one hundred and twenty-two members, will be present" at the dedication. ("'01 Reunion To Celebrate Anniversary," *VMI Cadet*, May 15, 1951, p. 1.)
3. See p. 107n3.
4. On February 5, 1899, the day after hostilities began between the US and Philippine independence forces, then First Lieutenant Charles E. Kilbourne (VMI, 1894), an officer in the Signal Corps, climbed a telegraph pole near Manila while under enemy fire to reestablish a broken line of communication. He received the Medal of Honor in 1905 for his bravery, rose to the rank of major general, and served as superintendent of VMI from 1937 to 1946. In February 1901, First Lieutenant James D. Taylor (VMI, 1898) acquired and passed along to his superiors documents containing the location of the headquarters of Emilio Aguinaldo, the leader of the Philippine independence movement. This intelligence played a crucial role in the capture of Aguinaldo on March 23, 1901.
5. The *Lexington Gazette* reported on May 18, 1898, that the entire corps of cadets had traveled to the New Market battlefield on May 12 to participate in the unveiling of a monument to the ten fallen cadets. ("The Newmarket Monument," *Lexington Gazette*, May 18, 1898, p. 3.)
6. The barracks were bombarded on June 12, 1864, by Union troops under the command of General David Hunter (USMA, 1822), who occupied Lexington from June 11 to 14, 1864.
7. The straight-line distance between the VMI barracks and House Mountain is approximately seven miles, and the distance by contemporary automobile roads approximately 8.5 to 13.5 miles, depending on whether one is approaching the front or the back side of the mountain.
8. Although there were currently two living members of Marshall's class with the last

name Johnson, Marshall was in all likelihood referring to Reverend James V. Johnson, pastor of Westminster Presbyterian Church in Miami, Florida, who was photographed at this time with Marshall and two other members of the VMI class of 1901. ("Marshall at Class Reunion," *St. Louis Post Dispatch*, May 15, 1951, attached to Kean to Marshall, May 15, 1951, GCMRL/G. C. Marshall Papers [Secretary of Defense, Number Indexed, M214-8-23].)

9. The Marshalls and Margaret Emerson proceeded from VMI to a luncheon with special guests in nearby Natural Bridge before driving to Roanoke, Virginia, to fly back to Washington. (Marshall to Roller, April 20, 1951, and memorandum to George, May 14, 1951, ibid.)

Marshall received several tributes from dignitaries on the occasion of this celebration. One came from President Truman, who praised Marshall as "a public servant of great character and strong moral fibre, a soldier of outstanding ability, a strategist of the highest order, and a man of action." (Truman to R. J. Marshall, May 14, 1951, ibid.)

Marshall later sent a "movie reel" of the event to his VMI roommate Leonard K. Nicholson, who planned to screen the film for VMI alumni in New Orleans. Nicholson also thought he would "invite the 'Minks' alumni," a term used to refer to students of Washington and Lee University, "and keep my fingers crossed so that the party does not break up in a riot as we had after the last time V.M.I. and W. & L. played football." Marshall responded that he doubted "that the film will give cause for a brawl as it runs but 8 1/2 minutes, and I think that the 'Minks' will be pleased since W & L was given some billing." He also sent copies of these reels to VMI Superintendent Marshall for possible use by the alumni associations. (Marshall to Nicholson, July 16 and 23, 1951; Marshall to R. J. Marshall, July 16, 1951; and Nicholson to Marshall, July 18, 1951, ibid.)

301

To Dean G. Acheson — May 18, 1951

Top Secret — Washington, DC

Dear Mr. Secretary: I wish to call your attention most urgently to some very serious aspects of the planning for transfer of certain non-military functions from SCAP to State Department authorities which was the subject of a recent exchange of letters between Deputy Under Secretary Matthews and General James H. Burns (27 April and 11 May, respectively).[1]

The Joint Chiefs of Staff and General Ridgway are seriously concerned over certain military implications of this planning. This concern I am having brought to your attention by separate hand since it involves very sensitive considerations.[2]

In view of this concern, which I share, I recommend as strongly as I can that (1) the present powers and authority of the United States military commander in Japan should not be abridged in any way at this time, (2) that the planning proposed by the Department of State on any eventual transfer of non-military functions of SCAP should be confined to an American "eyes only" basis and that, explicitly, no Japanese officials be informed in any manner whatsoever of such planning; (3) that such planning should be strictly confined at this stage, and until future developments permit, to U.S. government agencies in Washington; and (4) that any plans developed by the Department of State and Defense not be implemented in any degree or manner at least until after the termination of hostilities in Korea, and then only after consultation between our two Departments.

I realize that the letter of 27 April from Deputy Under Secretary Matthews has indicated that the proposals therein referred only to planning or recommendations and not to actual implementation of such transfer, and were without prejudice to the question of the Japanese Peace Treaty.[3]

However, it would relieve the Joint Chiefs of Staff, General Ridgway, and myself, of considerable anxiety if you would reaffirm the above stipulation in the 27 April letter and if you would also inform me of your concurrence with the above four numbered points.[4] Faithfully yours,

NA/RG 330, CD 387 (Japan)

1. H. Freeman Matthews had informed Burns on April 27 that with the completion of a Japanese peace treaty, which would end US military occupation and restore full diplomatic relations (see pp. 324–25, 427–29, and 494–46), "certain non-military functions . . . now performed by the Department of the Army will become the responsibility of the Department of State." Matthews therefore recommended that the State and Defense Departments send representatives to Tokyo to begin to discuss plans "in connection with the establishment of the American Embassy" and the transfer of these responsibilities. Burns replied on May 11 that only "the broadest planning" should take place at this time, and he thus declined to send a Defense Department representative to Tokyo. (Matthews to Burns, April 27, 1951, and Burns to Marshall, May 11, 1951, NA/RG 330, CD 387 [Japan].)

2. Ridgway had informed Marshall on May 6 of his opposition to any transfer of authority, "regardless of the conclusion or ratification of a Japanese Peace Treaty," until "the menace of potential Soviet surprise attack shall have materially abated." (Ridgway to Marshall, telegram, May 6, 1951, ibid.) Marshall replied on May 8 that he was unaware of the status of the discussions in Washinton and was asking the JCS for their views. Marshall believed Ridgway's logic was "compelling" but reminded him "that this is an off hand comment until I have been fully briefed." (Marshall to Ridgway, quoted in Carter to Vogt, memorandum, May 9, 1951, GCMRL/G. C. Marshall Papers [Secretary of Defense, Chronological, Director, Executive Office (Marshall S. Carter), 1950–1952].)

On May 14, Bradley reported to Marshall that the JCS agreed with Ridgway's assessment and warned that a "surprise attack against Japan" by the Soviet Union "constitutes the most serious single threat to the United States over-all security position in the Far East." Therefore the military commander must retain full authority to resist any such attack, and any transfer of authority should wait "at least until after the termination of hostilities in Korea" and any planning for an eventual transfer "should be conducted on an American 'eyes only' basis" at least until the Korean conflict had ended. (Bradley to Marshall, memorandum, May 14, 1951, NA/RG 330, CD 387 [Japan]. For the differing views of other military and civilian Defense Department officials, see Young to Carter, memoranda, May 17 and 18, 1951, ibid.)

3. In his April 27 letter, Matthews assured Burns that the State Department was considering the views of the JCS on the Japanese Peace Treaty negotiations as transmitted in Marshall's April 19 letter to Acheson and that his recommendations on a transfer of power from SCAP were "without prejudice to the question of the date the treaty comes into effect." Kenneth Young confirmed this with U. Alexis Johnson on May 16. (Matthews to Burns, April 27, 1951, and Young memorandum for the record, May 16, 1961, ibid.) For Marshall's April 19 letter to Acheson and the attached views of the JCS, see *FRUS, 1951*, 6: 989–93.

4. Acheson replied on May 22 and assured Marshall that the "only purpose" of Matthews's April 27 letter was to begin "planning between our two Departments" on these issues. Any mention by State Department officials regarding the transfer of any other non-military functions between the signing and coming into effect of the treaty was "purely exploratory" and only to obtain the opinions of the Defense Department and Ridgway. Acheson concluded by concurring with the four recommendations Marshall had made in his May 18 letter. (Acheson to Marshall, May 22, 1951, ibid.)

302

To Mrs. Franklin D. Roosevelt — May 18, 1951
Personal — Washington, DC

Dear Mrs. Roosevelt: I have your letter of April 27 and appreciate your writing me of your conversation with Dr. Ruegger and also the one which you recently had in London.[1]

I met Dr. Ruegger for the first time in May of last year when he came over here in connection with the work of the International Committee, and also gave a luncheon in his honor at the Sulgrave Club. I found him to be a very energetic individual and from a first and brief contact feel confident in his ability. As to Chou-en-lai not being a true Communist, in China he insisted to me personally and on another occasion to Mrs. Marshall that he was a true Marxist Communist. In my conversations with Chou, I found him to be one of the ablest negotiators with whom I had come in contact. He was very agreeable, clever and inscrutable in the sense that one could never quite tell what were his objectives or intentions of the moment.[2]

Am glad to report that Mrs. Marshall and I are feeling extremely well and are now comfortably situated in our summer quarters at Leesburg. We continue to marvel at your energy and the great contribution you continue to make to the country and the United Nations.

With warm personal regards. Faithfully yours,

GCMRL/G. C. Marshall Papers (Secretary of Defense, Number Indexed, M200-14-2)

1. Roosevelt informed Marshall in her April 27 letter that Paul Ruegger had spoken with her at a dinner and "said many fine things about his devotion to you." Ruegger told her about his recent trip to Peking, during which he met with Chou En-lai, whom he did not think "is a communist, certainly not a communist in the Russian sense." Roosevelt thought that Ruegger "felt that with proper handling something might be done to straighten out the present difficulties between China and the outside world." (Roosevelt to Marshall, April 27, 1951, GCMRL/G. C. Marshall Papers [Secretary of Defense, Number Indexed, M200-14-2].)

She also enclosed "a report of a conversation" she had in London with Lord Elibank, Colonel Arthur Murray, a former assistant military attaché in Washington and former member of the House of Commons. (Ibid.)

2. Marshall met Ruegger on May 29–30, 1950. See pp. 93–94.

Marshall met extensively with Chou En-lai during his 1945–46 mission to China. (See *Papers of GCM*, 5: 369–776 passim.) See also pp. 9 and 14.

303

Remarks at the National Armed Forces Day Banquet[1] — May 18, 1951
Washington, DC

In referring to the Armed Forces I will content myself with the statement that we have unity, coordination, cooperation and a state of generous mutual understanding. It only remains for this to become a habit of thought and action rather than a mere compliance with the law, and I think that habit is rapidly crystallizing.

I do not want to make a speech tonight but rather to read to you a special message which I have just sent to General Ridgway, the Commander of our American forces in Korea.

Here is the message:

"On this anniversary of Armed Forces Day, in the midst of the great battle in which your forces are now engaged, my thoughts and those of every American are with the men of your command.

"The deadly efficiency of the fighting men under your leadership is conclusive evidence of their high morale and courage. The North Korean army has been destroyed and the Chinese Communist armies have been dealt terrific blows. All Americans are proud of this inspiring record.

"But when troops are as deeply engaged in fighting as yours, they have little time to appreciate the far reaching results of their fighting.

"Therefore, we here at home want your men to know that we realize how much they are contributing to the global fight against Communist aggression.

"Less than a year ago the Communist forces were threatening to engulf the whole of the Far East. The prestige of Red China was at its peak. Its armies were exhilarated by a series of victories over the Chinese Nationalist troops. The entire Chinese mainland had been overrun. An invasion of Formosa was in preparation. Indo-China and Malaya were in grave danger.[2]

"Today, however, the prestige and armies of Red China have been seriously damaged. The situation in Indo-China and Malaya has improved. Japan has been reinforced, Formosa has been made more secure. The defense system of the entire Pacific has been invigorated.

"Here at home the stand of the troops in Korea has given us the inspiration and the time to mobilize on an impressive scale. In nine months the strength of our armed forces has been more than doubled. A tremendous effort is being made in the production of munitions. We are now well on the way towards building the kind of defense required for our own security and the peace of the world.

"Our decision to go into Korea and the determination of your forces to hold in Korea against all odds, have had another most important result. Last June the North Atlantic Treaty Organization, the great alliance of twelve of the free countries of the west, was only a paper promise. There was no certainty that its aims would ever be consummated. It had no real teeth, for the members of this alliance were not yet sufficiently confident of each other. The European members, directly in the path of the Soviet armies in case of war, were not absolutely certain as to the determination of the United States.

"The hostile invasion of Korea was probably the most critical test this country has ever faced. But we met this challenge. That decision gave new life to the United Nations, to the North Atlantic Treaty Organization, and to the entire free world. The decision to resist, however, is only a small part of the story, for it was the courageous action of the troops in the field that gave real meaning to this decision.

"The will to fight, demonstrated so compellingly by our men in Korea, is contagious. Today it is not too much to say that your soldiers and sailors, your airmen and marines and your gallant allies have dissipated the defeatism of a year ago. The lights are going up again all over the free world and they are growing brighter day by day.

"So, on this anniversary of Armed Forces Day, I say to you and your courageous men: You are fighting to great purpose because you have a great purpose to fight for. May God bless you and protect you in the great battle now in progress."[3]

GCMRL/G. C. Marshall Papers (Secretary of Defense, Speeches and Statements)

1. Louis Johnson first announced the creation of Armed Forces Day in August 1949 to replace separate days of remembrance for the individual services in light of the progress made in the unification of the armed services. President Truman declared that the new day would first be celebrated on May 20, 1950. The 1951 celebration was to take place on May 19, with a banquet hosted by the Air Force Association, the Military Order of World Wars, and the Navy League to take place the preceding evening at the Hotel Statler. Marshall indicated to C. J. George on February 16 that he would attend the 1951 banquet and review the following day's parade. On May 9, George informed Marshall that while he had not been invited to speak at the banquet, Truman in accepting an invitation to attend had "indicated that General Marshall would do the talking," though "no such information . . . was passed on to anyone in your office." Truman did speak to this gathering as well. (Roberts to Marshall, memorandum, February 16, 1951; and George to Marshall, memoranda, February 16 and May 9, 1951, GCMRL/G. C. Marshall Papers [Secretary of Defense, Number Indexed, M214-11-48]; "The Texts of Truman and Marshall Addresses to Troops Overseas," *New York Times*, May 19, 1951, p. 4.)

2. While France was fighting the Communist-led Viet Minh in Indochina, Britain was fighting a Communist guerrilla insurrection in its southeast Asian colony of Malaya.

3. This message, cable DEF-45837, is in GCMRL/G. C. Marshall Papers (Secretary of Defense, Number Indexed, M214-11-48). Marshall also recorded a statement "for television and newsreel" on April 3 in which he invited Americans "to visit the military installations nearest to you which will be open to the public on Armed Forces Day, May 19th, and become better acquainted with your own military forces." (Statement for Armed Forces Day, May 19, 1951, GCMRL/G. C. Marshall Papers [Secretary of Defense, Speeches and Statements].)

304

MEMORANDUM FOR GENERAL WADE H. HAISLIP

May 21, 1951
Washington, DC

I have been thinking some more regarding this promotion business for the Eighth Army and I have the following observations to make.

There seem to be regulations regarding promotions in the company and field grades that are not suitable to the character of service being rendered by the Eighth Army, particularly in the light of the publicity and criticism of employment of that army, etc. I am referring specifically to the regulations which govern the question of vacancies. As I understand it, a certain number of vacancies, ~~usually~~ in the grade of lieutenant colonel for example, are credited to a division and that number cannot be exceeded though the combat units lack full complement of that grade because staff or supply units may fill up the number. As to this, I think the promotions should be within the discretion of the Army and higher commander, meaning that the Army commander could recommend the promotions without regard to the present regulation and the supreme commander could confirm it for action here or actually make it there.

I do not think we should endeavor to have a promotion policy that will move evenly clear around the world and thereby restrict prompt recognition of great valor and leadership in this critical situation in Korea, especially considering the fact that we are sending no reserves to that Army and they are meeting and throwing back overwhelming hordes. In my experience I find always a desire, and in peacetime conditions a very proper reaction, to establish a routine that is in terms of uniformity, and to consider to too great an extent the factor of possible injustice to one man in Europe now or in Washington against the man recognized in Korea.[1]

There is another factor involved in this matter of morale and stimulation and that is the detailed amount of paper work that is required to permit an award, particularly of the Distinguished Service Cross. I feel that the division commander should have the right to make these awards on the basis of the literature concerning them being prepared later. What we want is the morale ~~fact~~ effect and we don't get ~~them~~ that by delaying a month or two for the arduous preparation of papers by people who are under terrific combat conditions.[2]

All of these factors are virtually old stuff with me. They came up in the first World War where I saw quite a number of the young men of the First Division killed before they received their Distinguished Service Crosses which had been won by outstanding feats and where I saw a great injustice in promotion of those heavily engaged in very dangerous situations in order to, you might say protect the interests of some officer far distant from the combat. From Washington, in the last war, I tried to take measures that would avoid this by giving division commanders considerable authority. But I think this situation in Korea is extraordinarily special one in our history and we should clear away the details in every way we can and trust to the leaders we have over there as we do trust the lives of our men to those leaders.[3]

GCMRL/G. C. Marshall Papers (Secretary of Defense, Number Indexed, M200-13-30)

1. Marshall was also concerned at this time with the promotions of general officers. MacArthur had submitted to Marshall on April 6 a list of officers for whom he recommended promotion to the next highest rank: Lieutenant Generals Stratemeyer and Ridgway; Vice Admiral C. Turner Joy (USNA, 1916), commander of US Naval Forces in the Far East; Major Generals William M. Hoge (USMA, 1916), commander of IX Corps; Leven C. Allen, chief of staff of the Eighth Army; Doyle O. Hickey, acting chief of staff at the Far East Command (FEC) under MacArthur and chief of staff under Ridgway; and Brigadier General Edwin K. Wright, operations officer in the FEC. Marshall did not act on this list prior to MacArthur's relief (see pp. 478–81). He asked Ridgway on April 26 for his "recommendations regarding promotions" of Hoge, Allen, Hickey, and Wright, while recognizing that "the midst of a great battle is not the time to discuss general promotions." Ridgway replied the following day to "warmly endorse recommended temporary promotions to Lieutenant General" of Hoge, Allen, and Hickey, while recommending "further personal observation" of Wright "prior to submitting my views." (MacArthur to Marshall, radio no.

DA-IN 18878, April 6, 1951; Marshall to Ridgway radio no. SVC-899, April 26, 1951; Ridgway to Marshall, radio no. SVC-2160 JC, April 27, 1951, GCMRL/G. C. Marshall Papers [Secretary of Defense, Categorical, Memoranda, Marshall S. Carter, 1950–1951].)

Marshall replied further to Ridgway on May 21 in a "personal, confidential and eyes only" message that he thought "Hoge's and Hickey's nominations for Lieutenant General will probably go forward today." Marshall added that he "would like to get someone on the list who has conspicuous service prior to or in this recent battle," such as Brigadier General John H. Michaelis (USMA, 1936), former commander of the Twenty-seventh Infantry Regiment and assistant commander of the Twenty-fifth Infantry Division who had gained a reputation for his bravery on the battlefield. Michaelis had been promoted to brigadier general in February 1951 and left Korea to join General Eisenhower's staff at SHAPE as deputy assistant chief of staff for organization and training in mid-May 1951. If Ridgway had "any such names, I suggest that you recommend them directly to the Chief of Staff concerned, and I will do my best to put them through the administrative machinery." The editors have not located any response from General Ridgway. (Carter to F. W. Marshall, memorandum, May 21, 1951, GCMRL/G. C. Marshall Papers [Secretary of Defense, Chronological, Director, Executive Office (Marshall S. Carter), 1950–1952].) The *New York Times* reported on May 23 that Truman recommended Generals Hoge and Hickey for promotion to lieutenant general on May 22. ("Named for Promotion in Army," *New York Times*, May 23, 1951, p. 5.)

2. See p. 471.

3. Haislip sent a message to Ridgway around May 23 on the issue of promotions which the editors have been unable to locate. Marshall added to this message that "As to promotions as an immediate recognition of leadership in current action the Secretary had in mind company and field grades more than that of brigadier general." (Carter to Beishline, memorandum, May 23, 1951, GCMRL/G. C. Marshall Papers [Secretary of Defense, Chronological, Director, Executive Office (Marshall S. Carter), 1950–1952].) See pp. 626–27.

305

TO GENERAL CHARLES KILBOURNE

May 22, 1951
Washington, DC

My dear Kilbourne: Many thanks for your letter of May 18th. It was good to see you at Lexington last week and to spend such a pleasant and memorable day among old friends. I was quite overwhelmed by the honor paid me by the Institute and agree with you that the whole affair was executed to perfection. It was a great day in my life and shall long be remembered.[1]

As for your rebuttal on my behalf to comments by columnists, frankly I must remain out of the picture entirely. Even though I appreciate the thought which prompted your taking up the cudgel for me, I do not want to put myself in the position of endorsing such replies but prefer to remain ignorant of the matter. You do as you wish.[2]

Mrs. Marshall and I send you and Mrs. Kilbourne our warm regards. Faithfully yours,

GCMRL/G. C. Marshall Papers (Secretary of Defense, Number Indexed, M200-13-36)

1. In his May 18 letter, Kilbourne wrote that he appreciated Marshall's comments about his service during his remarks at the Marshall Day ceremony at VMI on May 15. (Kilbourne to Marshall, May 18, 1950 [*1951*], GCMRL/G. C. Marshall Papers [Secretary of Defense, Number Indexed, M200-13-36].) Kilbourne had been on the stage with Marshall

during the dedication of the Marshall Arch at VMI, and Marshall mentioned Kilbourne's receiving the Medal of Honor during the Philippine-American War. See pp. 520 and 522n4.

2. Also in his May 18 letter, Kilbourne enclosed a draft letter to the editor of the *Richmond News Leader* in response to two columns in the paper's May 17 issue. If Marshall preferred, however, he would "keep it silent about these columnists" and dispose of the letter. In the first column, George Sokolsky had attacked Marshall for his behavior at the 1945 Yalta Conference and in China as well as his testimony at the MacArthur hearings (see pp. 499–516). In the second, David Lawrence accused the Joint Chiefs of acquiescing in Truman's demand to relieve MacArthur without offering any dissent out of fear of discipline. Kilbourne in his draft response challenged the validity of each of Sokolsky's specific charges and asked Lawrence to consider "that no man reaches the four star grade who lacks the courage to stand up to his convictions let the chips fall where they may." He labeled both columns "one-sided attempts to shake confidence, not only among our own people, but also among our allies," and he thought they gave "'aid and comfort' to the enemies of democracy." (Ibid.; George Sokolsky, "Marshall Judgment Wasn't Infallible," and David Lawrence, "Truth on MacArthur Case Slowly Appears," *Richmond News Leader*, May 17, 1951, pp. 11–12.)

306

To Charles S. Murphy — May 22, 1951
Washington, DC

Dear Murphy: I have, rather hastily I admit, gone over the first draft of the foreign aid message that you sent me yesterday afternoon. Others have also looked it over.[1]

My own frank reaction is it is entirely too long, it covers too many subjects and therefore offers unnecessarily opportunities for controversy which might well be avoided. I think the message has to be viewed in the light of the hearings now in progress on the Hill. Therefore, a very concise statement seems more appropriate at this time.

I have not attempted specific cuts since a process of condensation will necessarily have to affect a rearrangement of subjects.

I am sorry not to be more helpful but the time limit is so short that I feel that a general suggestion might be more helpful to you than the detail involved in a detailed re-draft.[2] Faithfully yours,

GCMRL/G. C. Marshall Papers (Secretary of Defense, Number Indexed, M200-14-11)

1. Murphy, special counsel to the president, had sent Marshall a draft of Truman's foreign aid message on May 21. He admitted that it was "still rather rough in certain places," but he requested Marshall's "comments by the end of the day or the first thing in the morning, so that we can spend tomorrow smoothing out the style and form. The President tentatively expects to send the message up Wednesday afternoon," May 23. The attached draft was thirty-five pages long, although the copy in the Marshall Papers does not contain pages one through nine. (Murphy to Marshall and attachment, May 21, 1951, GCMRL/G. C. Marshall Papers [Secretary of Defense, Number Indexed, M200-14-11].)

2. On March 23, 1951, Colonel George A. Lincoln (USMA, 1929), Marshall's senior strategist in the War Department during World War II and a professor on the faculty at West Point following the war, had been appointed a special assistant to Marshall "responsible for assisting in the interdepartmental coordination of the Foreign Aid Program for presentation to the Congress." (Lovett to service secretaries, JCS, assistant secretaries

of defense, chairmen of boards, councils, and committees, and directors of OSD offices, memorandum, March 23, 1951, NA/RG 330, SD 091.3.) Lincoln informed Marshall on May 23 that "In spite of your letter to Mr. Murphy," the draft of the presidential message remained "lengthy." While Lincoln was meeting with Murphy on May 22, Truman entered and asked if the message had been reduced to six pages. Lincoln noted that Truman said he had spoken with Marshall about this, likely during their 12:30 p.m. meeting that day. Lincoln estimated that he could only succeed in holding the message to its current length, although he hoped Murphy would recognize the benefit "of using only the introductory section thereto" or Truman would adopt Marshall's view. (Lincoln to Marshall, memorandum and attachment, May 23, 1951, ibid.)

In his final message, delivered on May 24, Truman requested an appropriation in fiscal year 1952 of $8.5 billion in aid, $6.25 billion of which would be military equipment and $2.25 billion of economic aid in grants. Over 81 percent of this total would be allocated to Europe, approximately 6 percent to the Middle East and northern Africa, 9 percent to Asia, less than 1 percent to Latin America, and the remainder to administrative costs. ("Text of President Truman's Message to Congress Asking $8,500,000,000 Aid to Allies," *New York Times*, May 25, 1951, p. 4; *Public Papers, 1951*, 302–13.) See pp. 569–77 and 597–603.

307

To Mrs. John B. Wilson — May 23, 1951, Washington, DC

Dear Rose: What has become of you? In my times of trial you usually come forward with a morale boost.

And also I have just taken on your mayor as an Assistant Secretary. Are you mad about that?[1]

I am feeling fine, but pretty busy. However, my first hoeing, transplanting and similar first garden chores have stimulated me tremendously.

With my love, Rosie,[2] Affectionately,

GCM

GCMRL/J. Page Wilson Collection; H

1. Daniel K. Edwards, mayor of Durham, North Carolina, and a member of the Red Cross Board of Governors, had succeeded Marx Leva as assistant secretary of defense for legal and legislative affairs on May 1. ("Leva Resigns Post as Marshall Aide," *New York Times*, April 13, 1951, p. 12.)

2. In her memoir, Rose Wilson recalled that "At the time of the MacArthur fiasco," she "had intended to hold off writing my godfather until I had simmered down and could write a calm letter, but I heard from him first." (Rose Page Wilson, *Remembered* [Englewood Cliffs, NJ: Prentice-Hall Inc., 1968], 353.)

Rose Wilson replied on June 4 that she tried "to think of MacArthur with restraint and reason but I hate his guts and always have since childhood. I once remarked disparagingly about him and you very sternly cut me off so I've practiced saying nothing about him that I possibly can help. . . . Oh Brother!," she lamented. "I wish he would hurry up and fade away." She reassured Marshall, "You are wonderful, you are brilliant, you are a great patriot and I love you." (Wilson to Marshall, June 4, 1951, GCMRL/G. C. Marshall Papers [Secretary of Defense, Number Indexed, M200-6-31].)

Wilson later confessed in her memoir that Marshall had "rarely referred to me in a letter as 'Rosie,' and indeed, even orally, had used this appellation of my childhood quite seldom in recent years." She was glad she had written Marshall "a letter true to form" rather than "a more restrained one, for the letter amused him." (Wilson, *Remembered*, 353.) See pp. 553–54.

308

To Frederick D. Eddy

May 24, 1951
Washington, DC

My dear Mr. Eddy: Thanks for your letter of April 30 and for your pleasant comments regarding the visit Mrs. Marshall and I paid Hood College the other day.[1]

I was much interested in your resume of educational factors involved in our present role of world leadership. You can and do state the fundamental bases regarding this matter much better than I can. However, as I tried, in a rather ineffective manner, to make clear the other day, my point is that in the actual educational procedures along these lines, especially those which relate to historical developments and examples, that the manner of teaching fails to impress upon the student's mind a real picture of the events and the conditions surrounding these events.

To take an immediate example, we have so much talk about liberties and yet I think I am reasonably correct in saying that very few understand really what it means,—what are these liberties and what it means to have them denied you. They have never lived in fear of their life and for their family and their property because of a single statement from some person evilly inclined towards them. When it comes to other peoples of the world, probably most of the good and fair students can give you statistics regarding them and yet have little or no realization as to the meaning of the traditions of those people, as to their points of view and what they have undergone and the vast differences between them and their situation and we in ours. How you make these pictures so that they penetrate the student's mind is, I think, one of the important factors to be developed in education along this line. But I am making a very poor presentation of the matter in this letter. If I had more time I might do better. Faithfully yours,

GCMRL/G. C. Marshall Papers (Secretary of Defense, Number Indexed, M214-8-34)

1. Marshall had spoken at the all-female Hood College in Frederick, Maryland, on April 21. He encouraged the students to recognize and reflect upon the "many blessings and advantages in our country," such as freedom of worship, press, and assembly, which are taken "as a matter of course." After they learn "to appreciate fully what America really means" and understand the "haven of freedom this country presents to the rest of the world," Marshall asked the students to consider "the problem of what you personally should do to see that the United States of America continues a great democracy and a bulwark of freedom." (Remarks at Hood College, April 21, 1951, GCMRL/G. C. Marshall Papers [Secretary of Defense, Speeches and Statements].)

In planning for this speech, Marshall was "especially gratified" by a request from the college that it honor Mrs. Marshall, who had attended the all-female Hollins College in Roanoke, Virginia, by surprising her with an honorary doctorate following his speech. (Truxal to Marshall, February 20, 1951, and Marshall to Truxal, February 24, 1951, GCMRL/G. C. Marshall Papers [Secretary of Defense, Number Indexed, M214-8-34].)

Eddy, chairman of Hood College's Department of Modern and Classical Languages, had written on April 30 to ask for Marshall's opinion on "the study of foreign languages and literatures" and the role such study could have in the education of "citizens of the world" needed for the US to "discharge its world responsibilities." (Eddy to Marshall, April 30, 1951, ibid.)

309

Remarks at the Industrial Public Relations Orientation Conference
May 25, 1951 Washington, DC

MARSHALL delivered welcoming remarks to a group of "about 90 of the public relations directors of America's largest industries" who had been invited to the Pentagon to receive "a first-hand briefing on military policy and mobilization." (Fritchey to Marshall, memorandum and attachments, May 24, 1951, GCMRL/G. C. Marshall Papers [Secretary of Defense, Number Indexed, M200-3-28].) He began by discussing the "great strain" that the United States had faced "for the last five years" and the "unswerving position" taken "to contain and subvert as far as possible the communist endeavor to spread." He mentioned in this regard the post–World War II conflicts in Iran, Trieste, and Greece. (See pp. 41–42, 132–34, and 304–6, and *Papers of GCM*, 6: 55–600 passim.) Each of these had been deemed a "stalemate" or "unprofitable," Marshall noted, but the record showed that each had actually been "a great victory. We saved Greece from the communist overrunning, which means, in effect, we saved Italy and Turkey to a large extent. But more particularly it led us into the development of the first great serious crack in the communistic front": the expulsion of Yugoslavia from the Cominform, the Soviet-dominated Communist Information Bureau, on June 28, 1948, after Marshal Tito (Josip Broz) broke with Stalin. (Transcript of Remarks at the Industrial Public Relations Orientation Conference, May 25, 1951, NA/RG 330, SD 337.)

The same was true of the Berlin blockade in 1948, which "was a very dangerous situation." Early recommendations were "that we should crash through" or "fix up a tank column and go straight through," which Marshall thought "would walk right into an unalienable conflict." The "simple" solution of the airlift "was not simple at the time" and "required us to get our strength from this part and that part of the world." The British were also hesitant about the practicality of continuing the airlift through the winter. Then Secretary of State Marshall had spoken with General Clay, after which Marshall assured British Foreign Minister Ernest Bevin that doing so "was entirely practicable," and the United States was "going to do it whether they did or not. That was that." The British then supported a continuation of the airlift. Yet again, the Berlin blockade was called a "stalemate," but the success after eighteen months "was a great victory psychologically and actually, and we didn't get into war doing it." (Ibid. See also *Papers of GCM*, 6: 489–587 passim.)

In the midst of "semi-political battles," the Korean War was "another so-called stalemate." Marshall rejected that accusation. The state of the war had been grim in the summer and fall of 1950, he admitted, but the Communist forces now had "a profound tragedy on their hands." Regarding reports about UN casualty rates in Korea, Marshall reminded the attendees that such figures, which he said currently stood at 145,000, included "a man with a tooth ache, ear ache, stomach ache, or what not," which allows for much "distortion." During the occupation of Korea, prior to the outbreak of war, the casualty rate for American troops there "was six per cent." Since the North Korean invasion, "it has been nine and one-half per cent." That increase "only includes 132 deaths all together," however, "over a considerable period of time." Marshall cautioned about "misrepresentation" of such statistics in order "to prove a point." The "twisting and perverting part is too bad as to the battle itself." (Ibid.)

Generals Ridgway and Van Fleet, Marshall affirmed, were running "one of the best conducted affairs . . . that I have ever seen followed out in my military experience." Their recent successes gave "every reason to be proud of what those men have done. Some parts of it are almost unbelievable," such as a recent casualty report that indicated "enemy casualties running up to somewhere between fifty and seventy thousand" as opposed to 132 US/UN deaths over a five-day period. (Ibid.)

Marshall discouraged criticism of "the South Korean forces in the way you normally might" in light of their collapses, failures, and high casualty rates. Despite these heavy losses, "the individual Korean soldier I think has proved he is a real fighter. The trouble is they lack leadership," which cannot be created quickly, "and their unwillingness to have our fellows take that leadership control has been one of the great difficulties." Marshall was confident that the actions of Van Fleet to improve the performance of the Korean troops would prevent such a "disastrous result in the future." Marshall also praised MacArthur's early decision to "put 30,000 South Koreans in the ranks of our forward divisions," even though they only received "two to three weeks' training." Marshall remained convinced that the efforts to reform military education in Korea would provide qualified leaders for the Korean military in the future, although he admitted "that's a long procedure." (Ibid.)

Marshall also praised the "phenomenal" contributions of the air force and navy in the war. Air force pilots were easily "directed on their targets by the ground troops, radar, and things of that sort." The navy was able to put its gunfire "as much as 15 to 20 miles ashore" on both sides of the Korean peninsula "and pinpointed on the targets." (Ibid.)

Marshall then turned to the progress regarding manpower since the outbreak of the Korean War. At the outbreak of the war, the US "had no resources at all in the way of trained men, so we had to come in this country and cannibalize practically all our units." Finally by March 1951 "we received enough basically trained men" and "caught up with our debts," which allowed for the rotation of troops abroad to return to the United States. (See pp. 436–37, 440–41, 463, 488–89, and 516–17.) "Now the problem is reversed. The problem over there is how rapidly they can accept this without too greatly weakening the efficiency of the divisions." (Ibid.)

Part and parcel of the effort to avoid such problems in the future was the UMT bill currently being considered by Congress. (See pp. 325–29, 338–47, 369–71, 409–13, 423–26, 481–84, 551–53, and 558–59.) Marshall cited a Gallup poll released that day indicating 60 percent support for the UMT bill. ("Universal Military Training Program Has Strong Support," *Washington Post*, May 25, 1951, p. 27.) Marshall had been a proponent of UMT "for 30 years and it involves what

I feel—and I am speaking I think conservatively—is a monumentally historic decision because if we are going in the future of ups and downs, it's going to be all downs finally, and you can't do this thing financially unless you have some system like I am now describing." Marshall could think of no other system that would provide for an adequate supply of manpower "except a large standing army, and I know—I am certain, there is no doubt in my mind whatever—you can't maintain a large standing army in this country," due to cost and lack of public support. "No one has ever offered any substitute" for UMT, Marshall pointed out, "only objections. I think the time for that is washed out." He added that the current bill had received support of women's clubs, labor organizations, and education groups. (See pp. 291, 334n3, 350–54, and 393–97.) Now was the time to act on this matter "of vital importance." (Ibid.) ★

310

Memorandum for the Service Secretaries and the Joint Chiefs of Staff

May 26, 1951
[Leesburg, Virginia]

SUBJECT: Protection of Moral Standards

It is in the national interest that personnel serving in the armed forces be protected in the realization and development of moral, spiritual, and religious values consistent with the religious beliefs of the individuals concerned. To this end, it is the duty of commanding officers in every echelon to develop to the highest possible degree the conditions and influences calculated to promote the health, morals, and spiritual welfare of the personnel under their command.[1]

This traditional responsibility of command is of especial importance at this time when the Congress is preparing to broaden the base of inductions into the armed services. The people of this country have made it plain to both houses of Congress that they are determined that adequate effort be made both in military installations and in adjacent communities to safeguard the moral welfare of members of the armed forces. The Department of Defense, sharing this determination, directs that increased efforts of commanding officers be directed to insure the accomplishment of this objective.[2]

GCMRL/G. C. Marshall Papers (Secretary of Defense, Number Indexed, M200-3-26)

1. Marshall had long been wary of morale problems facing US troops and their families. In a December 1950 statement for the United Defense Fund (see p. 364n1), Marshall stated that "A sense of loneliness and confusion is usually the first reaction of the young man new to the military service," which makes him "liable more to temptation than might be the case at home." In addition, an enlarged military would create "strains and stresses that tear at the fabric of our American life" on the home front. Without adequate preparation and unified moral and financial support for the soldiers on duty and their families at home, Marshall feared, these conditions would lead to "a rise in juvenile delinquency." (Statement for the United Defense Fund, December 30, 1950, GCMRL/G. C. Marshall Papers [Secretary of Defense, Number Indexed, M214-6-2].)

On March 8, Marshall had informed the service secretaries that he was "very much troubled" about the "extraordinarily difficult problem in morale" of troops in the four divisions that were being sent to Europe, who would have "no occupation other than training" while stationed "far from home" with "no war" to fight. (See pp. 380–86 and 472–74.) He feared that the US was "going to have a larger collection of troubles than we ever dreamt of" and could not "merely leave it to our officials over there to handle." Consequently, he requested that the service secretaries give "very careful preliminary consideration" to this matter in order to develop "a comprehensive plan . . . for the guidance of our commanders who will have the immediate responsibility in the field." (Marshall to service secretaries, memorandum, March 8, 1951, GCMRL/G. C. Marshall Papers [Secretary of Defense, Number Indexed, M200-10-34].) "I'm sorry I cannot give you any ideas," Marshall admitted in a dictated but unsent earlier draft of this memorandum, "because I am at a loss to know just how to meet this." (Draft of Marshall to service secretaries, memorandum, March 7, 1951, GCMRL/G. C. Marshall Papers [Secretary of Defense, Memoranda, Marshall S. Carter, 1950–1951].)

Secretary Pace replied on April 23 that the army had been concerned about such problems since 1948 and that plans developed since then had "been a progressive coordinated staff accomplishment." He enclosed a four-page summary of "the general tenor of increased planning" to combat low morale. (Pace to Marshall and attachment, April 23, 1951, NA/RG 330, CD 330.11.)

2. Marshall rewrote the prose of this directive from earlier drafts written by his staff before signing it by, for example, adding that this memorandum "be disseminated to all commanding officers in every echelon, and that appropriate service procedures be established and promulgated to effect adherence to this policy." (Carter to the JCS and service secretaries, memorandum, May 26, 1951, GCMRL/G. C. Marshall Papers [Secretary of Defense, Number Indexed, M200-3-26].) See pp. 325–29, 338–47, 369–71, 409–13, 423–26, 481–84, 551–53, and 558–59.

311

Senate Testimony on the Defense Production Act of 1951

May 29, 1951 Washington, DC

MARSHALL testified before the Senate Banking and Currency Committee on May 29, 1951, in support of a two-year extension of an amended and strengthened Defense Production Act, which Truman had initially signed on September 8, 1950, and which had granted the government the authority to ensure priority of orders deemed necessary for national defense and to enact price and wage stabilization measures to combat inflation through June 30, 1951. (Harry S. Truman, *Public Papers of the Presidents of the United States: Harry S. Truman, 1950* [Washington: GPO, 1966], 626–31; *Public Papers, 1951*, 244–54.) In his opening statement, Marshall insisted that the act was critical to the US "plan for national security," which included "a rapid build-up to a minimum level of safety" and "the maintenance thereafter of a level of mobilization and a capacity for immediate large expansion." Marshall believed the reasons for renewal of the Defense Production Act were "more compelling than the reasons for its original enactment," as the "full impact" of the "defense mobilization effort" on the national economy would not reach its peak "until the calendar year 1952 and the winter of 1953." Letting the act's provisions lapse at the end of June would lead to "confusion" for military planners, who envisioned providing "materiel for the equivalent of 24 active divisions" and, "on short notice, for 21 National Guard divisions" in the army, "equipping 95 wings for the Air Force," and preparing "1,161 combat vessels by July 1, 1952, for the Navy and Naval Air requirements." (Senate Committee on Banking and Currency, *Hearings . . . on S. 1397, A Bill to Amend the Defense Production Act of 1950, and for Other Purposes*, 82d Cong., 1st sess., 787–90.)

While private investment had been of great help in some areas, it was very difficult to justify such investment in the production of "things urgently needed in the defense effort but for which there is little or no long-term civilian demand." The passage of the revised Defense Production Act currently under consideration would allow the government to "close that gap by providing authority for the expansion of facilities by means similar to those carried out by the Defense Plant Corporation," which had been established in 1940 as a subsidiary of the Reconstruction Finance Corporation to speed US production capabilities for military equipment. "It is difficult to prophesy exactly where and when" certain defense needs "may arise, yet the authority and the means through which to meet them should be provided." (Ibid., 790.)

Controlling inflation and "attaining some reasonable stability in prices" was also of great concern to the Defense Department, as "Substantial rises in prices have the effect on our procurement program of reducing the end amount to be delivered to us." Inflation had critically reduced the actual purchasing power of the Defense Department's budgeted funds, while "anticipated price decreases" per unit due to "increased volume of procurement" had not materialized. Marshall bluntly estimated that "the cost of inflation to the Department of Defense during the past year has been roughly the equivalent of the 20% increase in the wholesale price index. Thus, approximately 7 billion dollars out of the 35 billion authorized for procurement of hard and soft goods and military construction for the Department of Defense during fiscal 1951 can be regarded as the cost of inflation." If inflation was not checked, the situation would only deteriorate. The Defense Department, "as the largest single purchaser in our economy, has a vital stake in the sufficiency of our stabilization efforts to meet the challenge that will be presented in the near future by our accelerated production and procurement program. The loss of guns, tanks, and planes to a creeping inflation is just as damaging to national security as if they had been destroyed in battle or captured by a more visible and concrete enemy. In either case, it is the nation that suffers." Marshall concluded that this amended bill was the only method the Defense Department could see that would allow it to meet its current targets while retaining the authority to make adjustments that fit "the need as it arises in the unforeseeable future." (Ibid., 790–92.) Marshall also delivered at least part of his prepared opening statement in executive session before the House Banking and Currency Committee on June 14.

Following his prepared statement, Marshall began a lengthy question-and-answer session, much of which dealt with complaints about the way requested appropriations were presented, the methods by which the Defense Department should award and oversee government contracts, and efforts to control inflation. Munitions Board Chairman John Small, Major General Kirke B. Lawton, deputy army chief signal officer, and Major General William O. Reeder, deputy assistant army chief of staff for logistics, as well as Marshall, answered many of the questions asked by the committee members. (Ibid., 792–828.)

Senator Homer E. Capehart (R-IN) cited the example of "a special type of radio set that has gone from $4,597 to $20,185" to question the efficiency of the Defense Department's contract procedures. Marshall attributed the increase to unanticipated differences between pre-production cost estimates and the actual cost after the item was manufactured. General Lawton did admit that many of the bids for new products were negotiated instead of open, but he asserted that such a policy was the only practical one and was also necessary for the continued production of materiel to meet defense needs. Senator Capehart suggested a statutory requirement that producers subcontract a certain percentage of each order to "small manufacturers" in order to improve efficiency and reduce costs. Marshall informed Capehart that he had issued a directive to the military departments on December 18, 1950, to ensure "equitable distribution of procurement contracts among the maximum number of competent suppliers" unless there was a definite need to concentrate "contracts with a few leader suppliers." In addition, the departments should make the "fullest possible use of small business concerns." Marshall concluded that he could not quite see "How you would draw up the provision" to require a certain portion of subcontracting or "how you would state it in terms of a directive in a legal way." He later agreed with Senator Blair Moody (D-MI) that "The broader the base" of businesses used to fulfill contracts, "the better we are off, of course, in the future." The situation in the fall of 1950, however, required the Defense Department to "move with the greatest possible speed, because our deficiencies were so great and so serious." He admitted that this was not the most cost-efficient procedure but was necessary at the time. To legislate such requirements, though, Marshall stated, was not "a practical proposition, and I would imagine we would get into delays, if not almost an impossible situation." (Ibid., 799–802, 805, 807–8, 823–24.)

The session then moved onto the question of rent and price control and the costs of inflation. When Senator Benton asked whether or not Marshall was "increasingly convinced you have to have Federal power in addition to local control," Marshall replied, "I am very much of that opinion. We had a very sad time during the war [World War II] not in connection with manufacturing so much as we had with the camps, when the rents went up to the prohibitive figures, and with most distressing types of quarters involved." Regarding the price of meat, which had increased 31 percent over the previous year, Marshall asserted that meat "is essential to any American boy, by habit," though "Vegetarians may testify otherwise." In response to Benton's suggestion that rations be switched from beef to a less expensive substitute protein, such as eggs or chicken, Marshall joked, "I am not interested in mutiny," to laughter from those in attendance. He recalled a similar issue regarding substitution during his time with the Civilian Conservation Corps in the Pacific Northwest. His subordinates from the southeastern US, particularly Georgia and Alabama, "objected violently to the Coca-Cola" that was available

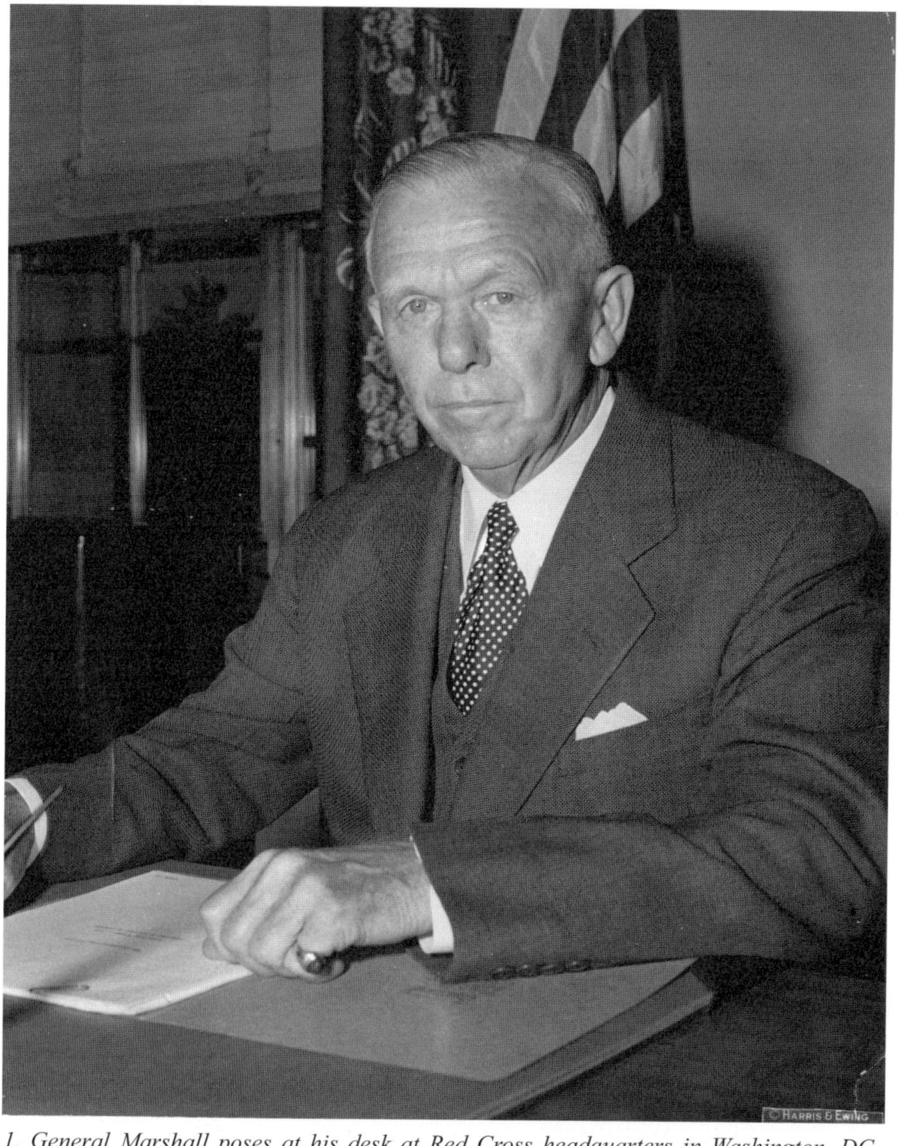

1. General Marshall poses at his desk at Red Cross headquarters in Washington, DC, on September 13, 1950, the day after President Truman nominated him to succeed Louis Johnson as secretary of defense. (See pp. 155–56.) From late September to early December 1950, Marshall served simultaneously as president of the Red Cross and secretary of defense. (See pp. 220–22, 247–51, and 283–84.)

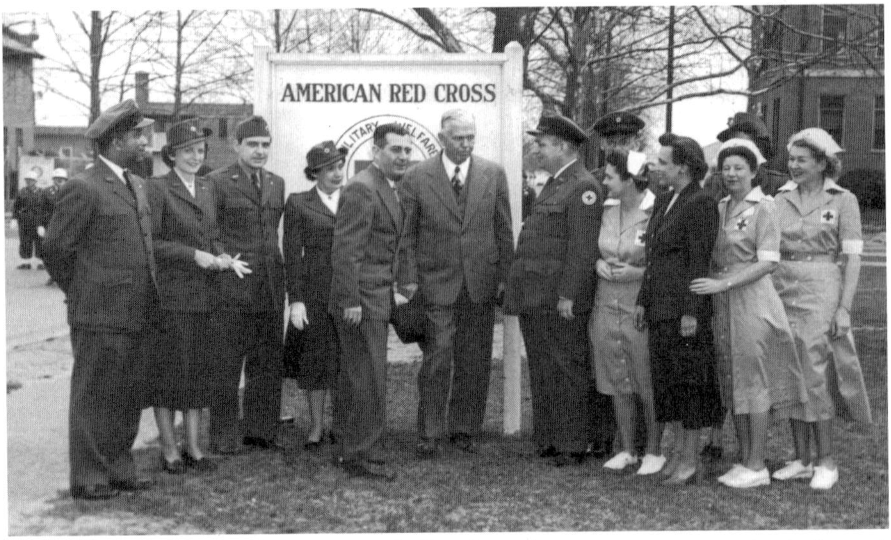

2. As president of the Red Cross, Marshall undertook two cross-country trips to inspect Red Cross facilities, one in October 1949 and the other from January to March 1950. (See pp. 19–21 and 47–48.) During one of these trips, an attentive Marshall (at center) meets with members of the field director's staff and Red Cross volunteers at Fort Bragg, North Carolina. George Brinkly, chairman of the local Red Cross chapter, and Dick Hart, Red Cross field director, are on Marshall's right and left, respectively.

3. Standing behind a podium with an array of flags of countries participating in the European Recovery Program—commonly known as the Marshall Plan—Marshall speaks to a gathering of several hundred employees of the plan's implementing organization, the Economic Cooperation Administration. The event took place on April 3, 1950, in the Hotel Statler in Washington, DC, to celebrate the second anniversary of congressional approval of the Economic Cooperation Act of 1948. (See pp. 74–76.) Several ECA officials and members of Congress sit on either side of Marshall.

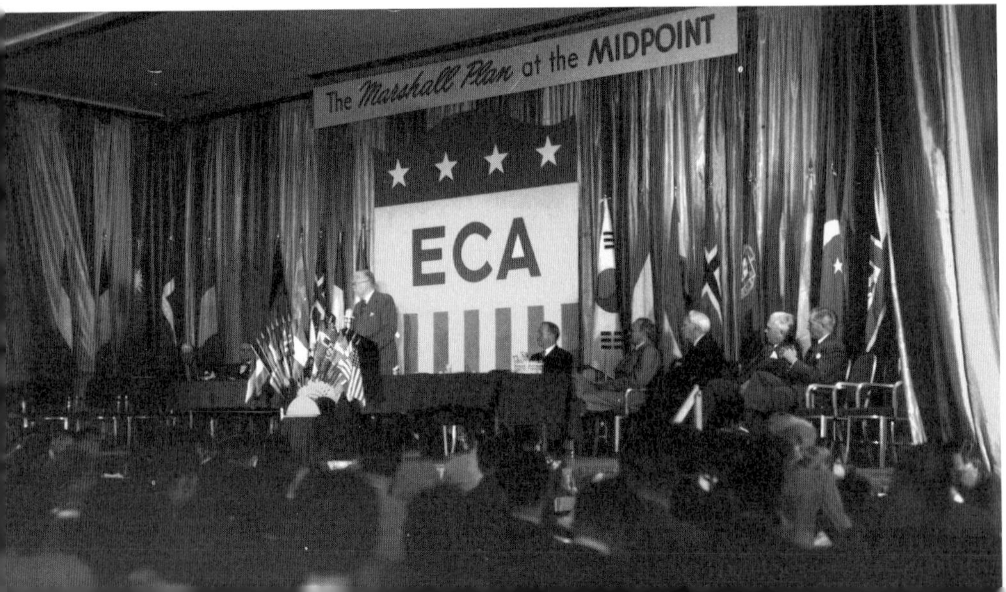

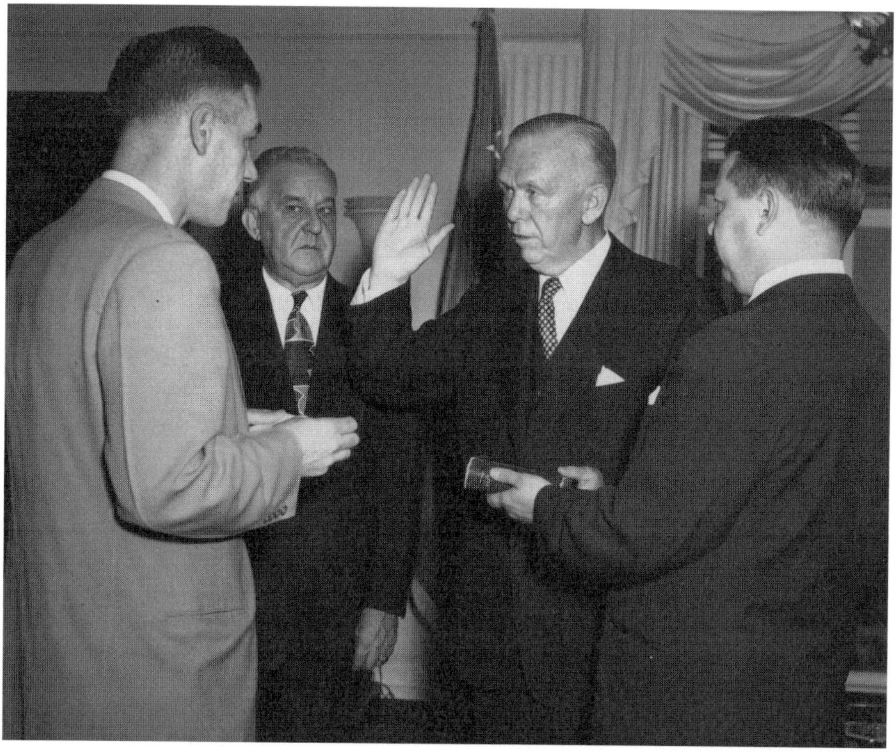

4. After enduring a somewhat contentious confirmation hearing (see pp. 155–56 and 160–63), Marshall takes the oath of office as secretary of defense on September 21, 1950. His longtime aide Major C. J. George holds the Bible, which Marshall also grips with his left hand, as General Counsel in the Office of the Secretary of Defense Felix E. Larkin administers the oath and Deputy Secretary of Defense Stephen T. Early witnesses the ceremony. Upon his resignation in August 1951, Larkin would ask for an inscribed copy of this photograph from Marshall. (See pp. 605–6.) Marshall's office as secretary of defense was the same one used by Secretary of War Henry L. Stimson during World War II. (See p. 163.)

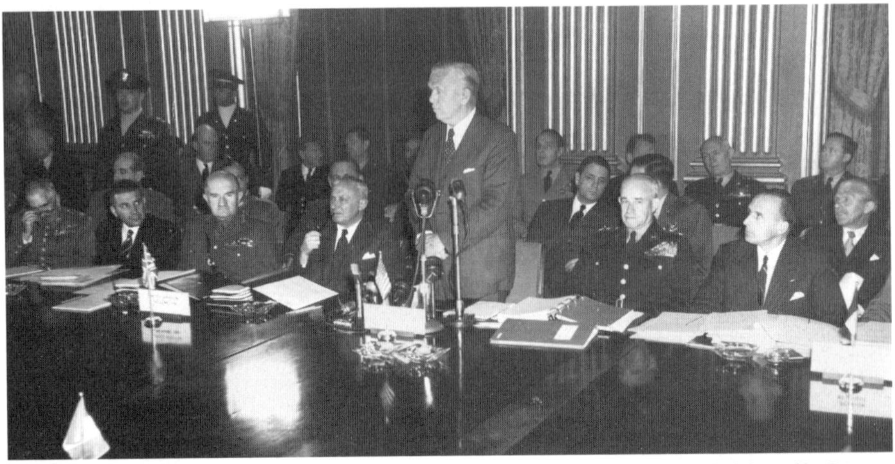

5. As chairman of the fourth meeting of the NATO defense ministers held at the Pentagon, Secretary Marshall delivers opening remarks on October 28, 1950, during which he argues for German rearmament within a NATO defense force. (See pp. 218–20.) Seated to Marshall's right are Lieutenant Colonel Fernando dos Santos Costa, Portuguese minister of defense; British Field Marshal Sir William Slim, chief of the Imperial General Staff; and Emanuel Shinwell, British minister of defense. To Marshall's left are General of the Army Omar N. Bradley, chairman of the US Joint Chiefs of Staff; and Colonel E. V. G. A. deGreef, Belgian minister of defense.

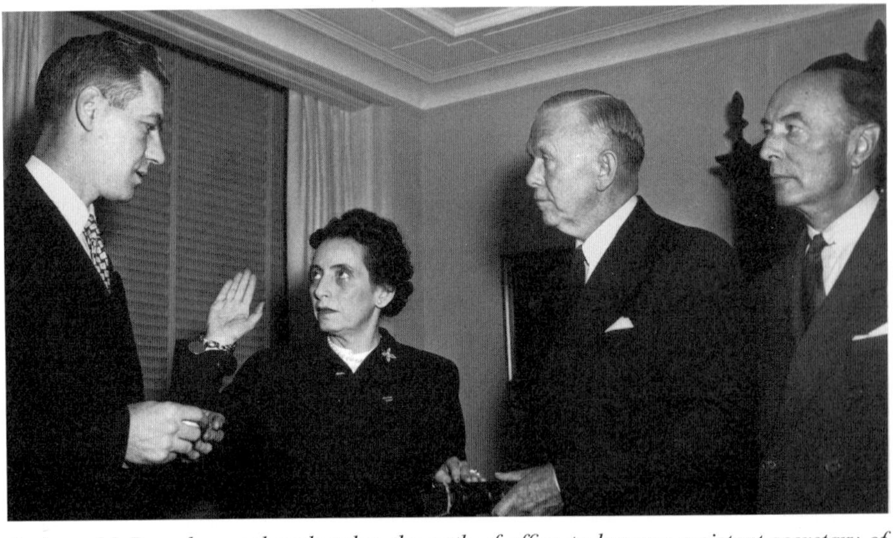

6. Anna M. Rosenberg solemnly takes the oath of office to become assistant secretary of defense for manpower and personnel on November 15, 1950, as Marshall holds the same Bible he used to be sworn in as secretary of defense. General Counsel Larkin administers the oath in Marshall's Pentagon office, and new Deputy Secretary of Defense Robert A. Lovett looks on. Rosenberg served on a recess appointment until her confirmation in December 1950 after hearings filled with controversy. (See pp. 206–7, 232–33, and 296–97.)

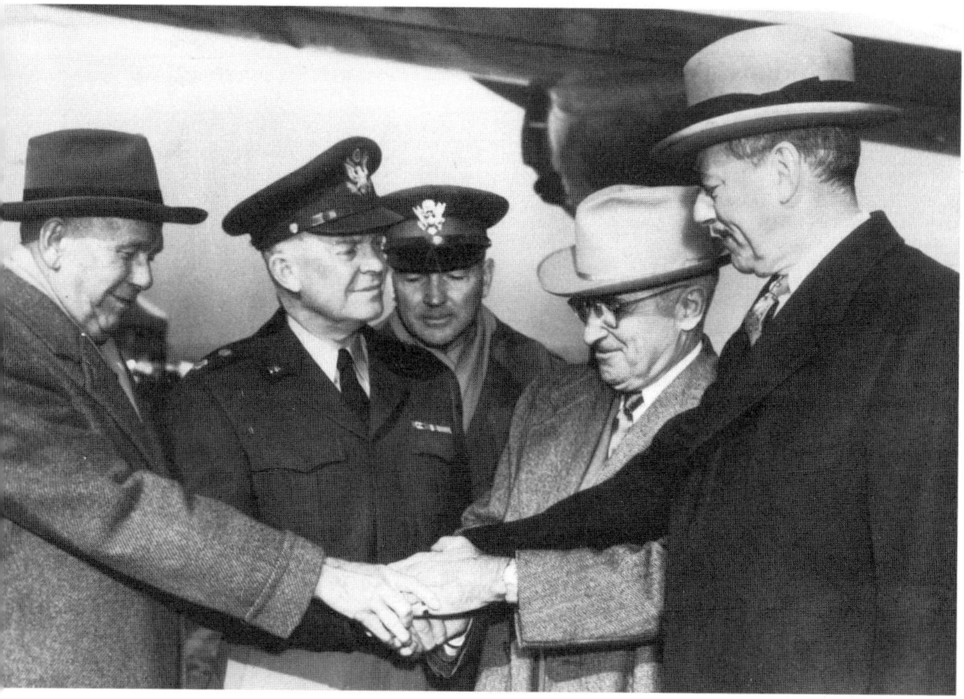

7. Prior to his departure for an inspection tour of NATO countries in Europe, recently appointed Supreme Allied Commander, Europe General of the Army Dwight D. Eisenhower (second from left) shakes hands with Secretary Marshall, President Harry S. Truman, and Secretary of State Dean G. Acheson. The photo was taken at the behest of the press covering the sendoff at the Military Air Transport Service field in Washington, DC, on January 6, 1951. (See p. 304n2.) The editors have been unable to identify the man standing behind Eisenhower.

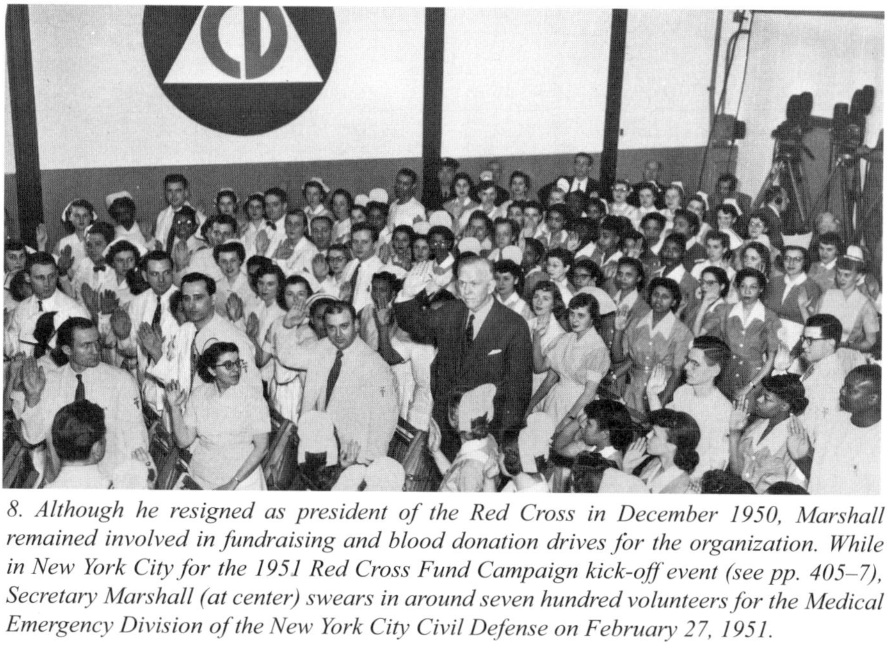

8. Although he resigned as president of the Red Cross in December 1950, Marshall remained involved in fundraising and blood donation drives for the organization. While in New York City for the 1951 Red Cross Fund Campaign kick-off event (see pp. 405–7), Secretary Marshall (at center) swears in around seven hundred volunteers for the Medical Emergency Division of the New York City Civil Defense on February 27, 1951.

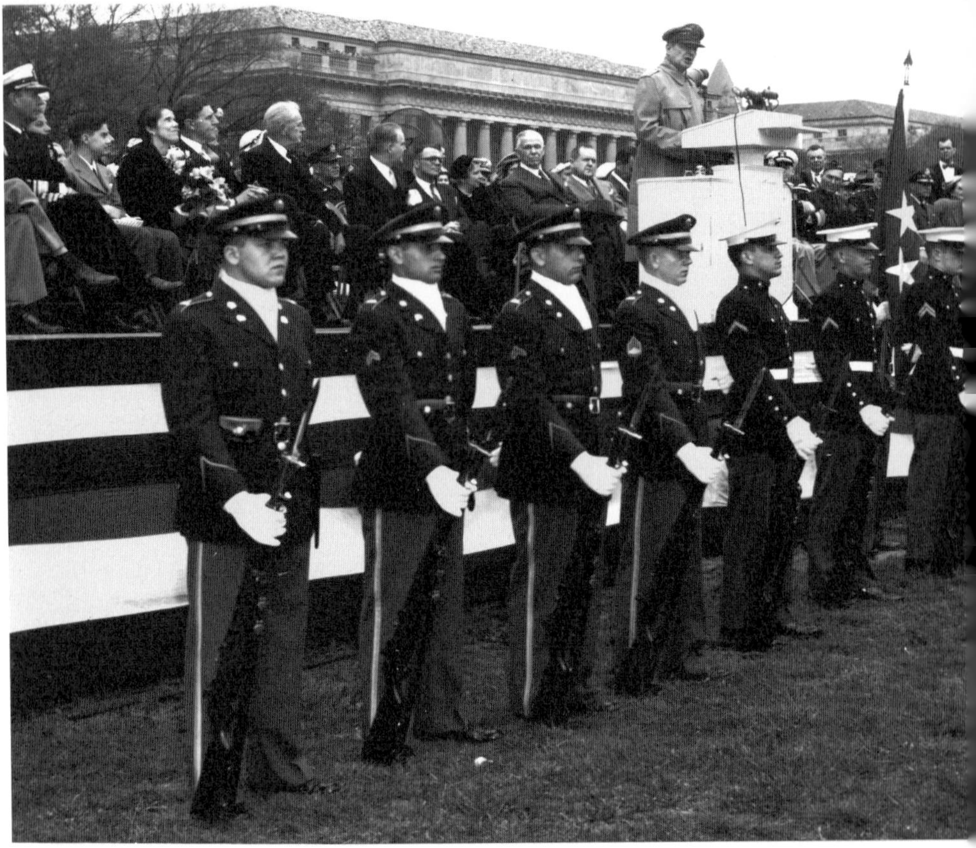

9. On April 19, 1951, a crowd estimated at 250,000 people gathered on the Washington Monument grounds in Washington, DC, to hear General of the Army Douglas MacArthur after he returned to United States for the first time in fourteen years. Here, MacArthur stands at the podium and Secretary Marshall, looking toward the camera, sits behind him. General Courtney Whitney, MacArthur's aide, sits to Marshall's left, and MacArthur's son, Arthur, and wife, Jean, clutching a large bouquet, sit second and third from the left. Earlier that day MacArthur had addressed a joint session of Congress. (See pp. 487–88 and 499–501.)

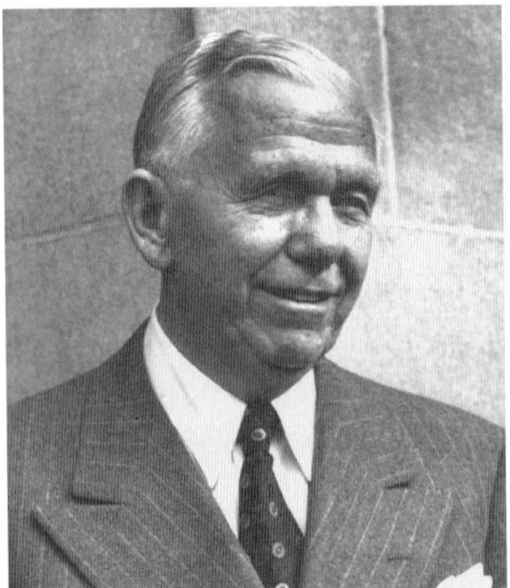

10. Secretary Marshall manages to smile at the press as he emerges from the Senate office building on May 11, during his fifth full day of testimony before the Senate Armed Services and Foreign Relations Committees investigating the reasons that General MacArthur was relieved of all his commands on April 11, 1951, (see pp. 478–81), as well as the entire military situation in the Far East. (See pp. 505–16.)

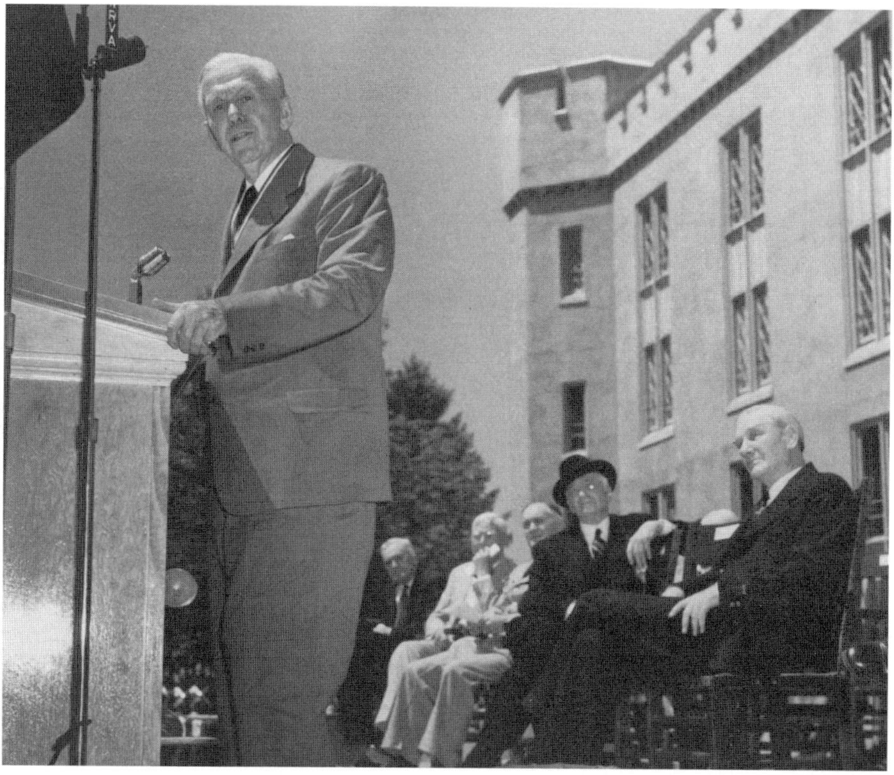

11. Secretary Marshall reminisces during the dedication ceremony of the Marshall Arch at his alma mater, the Virginia Military Institute, in Lexington, Virginia, on May 15, 1951. Seated on the platform from left to right are James S. Easley, former president of the VMI Board of Visitors; Ernest A. Sale, current president of the VMI Board of Visitors and Marshall's successor in that position; Lieutenant General Richard J. Marshall, VMI superintendent; financier Bernard M. Baruch, who delivered the keynote address at the ceremony; and Virginia Governor John S. Battle. (See pp. 518–23.)

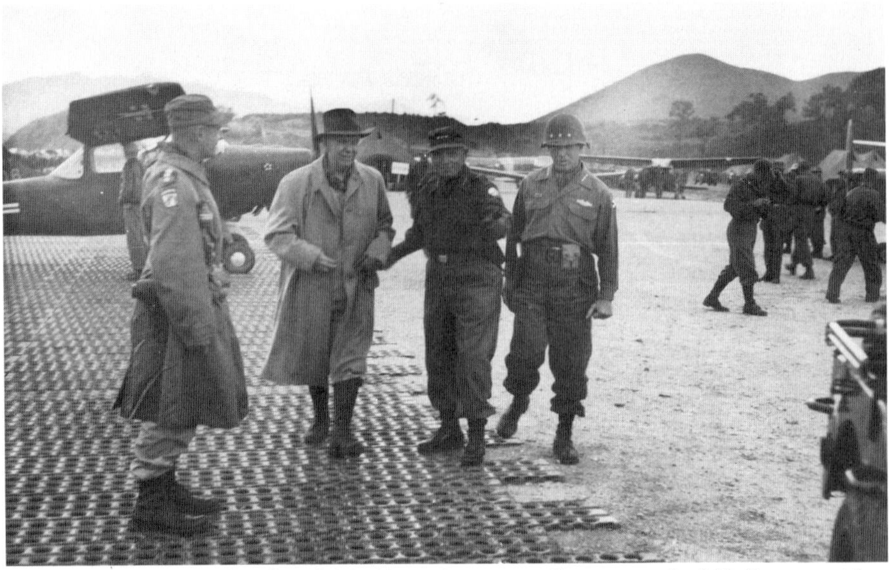

12. Lieutenant General Edward M. Almond, commanding general of X Corps, guides Secretary Marshall with General Matthew B. Ridgway (to Marshall's right) and Lieutenant General James A. Van Fleet, commanding general of the Eighth Army (on Almond's left), as they prepare to leave for X Corps headquarters in Hongchon, Korea, on June 8, 1951. (See pp. 548–50.) Marshall enjoyed using a light liaison airplane to travel around the front lines in Korea so much that he began to commute between Washington and Leesburg on a similar aircraft for the remainder of his tenure as secretary of defense.

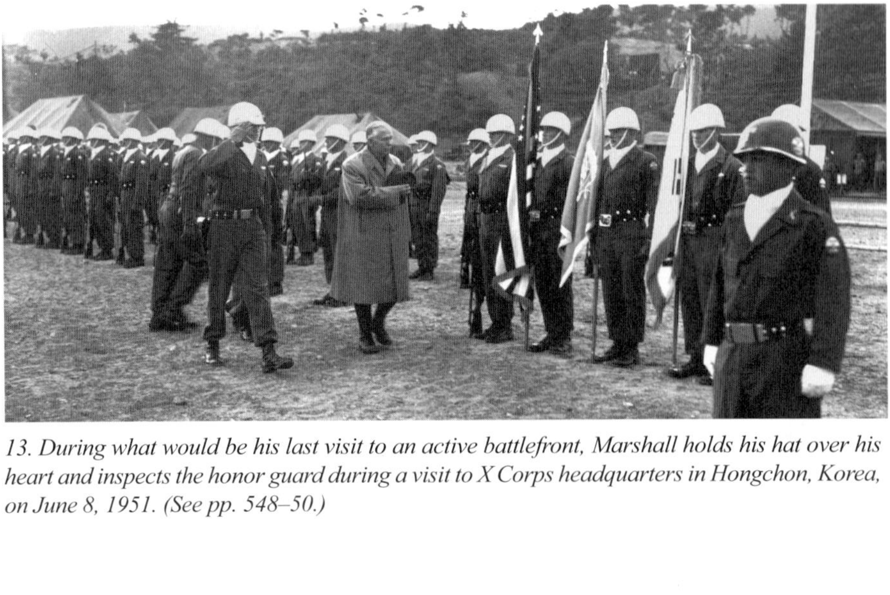

13. During what would be his last visit to an active battlefront, Marshall holds his hat over his heart and inspects the honor guard during a visit to X Corps headquarters in Hongchon, Korea, on June 8, 1951. (See pp. 548–50.)

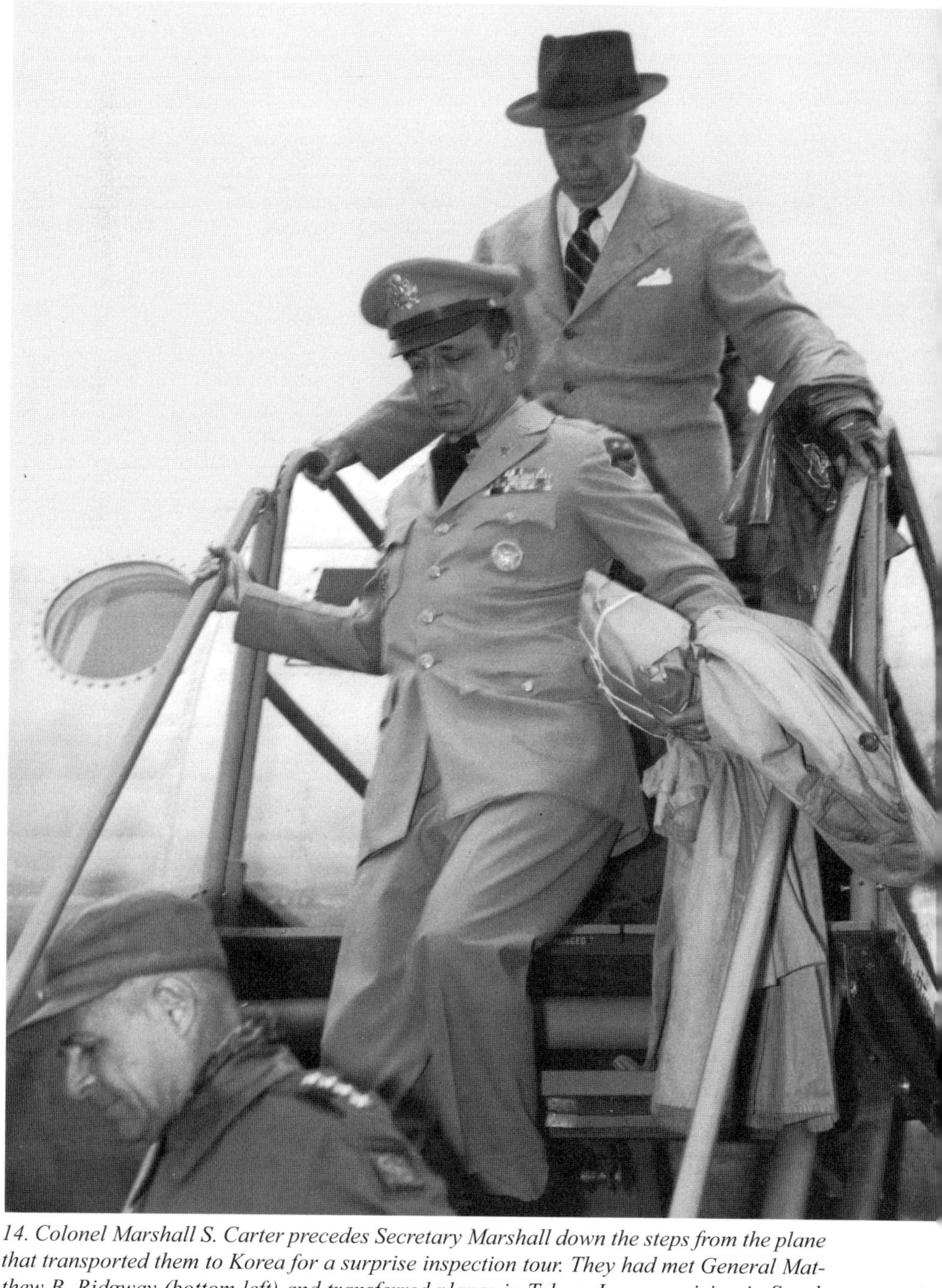

14. Colonel Marshall S. Carter precedes Secretary Marshall down the steps from the plane that transported them to Korea for a surprise inspection tour. They had met General Matthew B. Ridgway (bottom left) and transferred planes in Tokyo, Japan, arriving in Seoul, Korea, on June 8, 1951. (See pp. 548–50.)

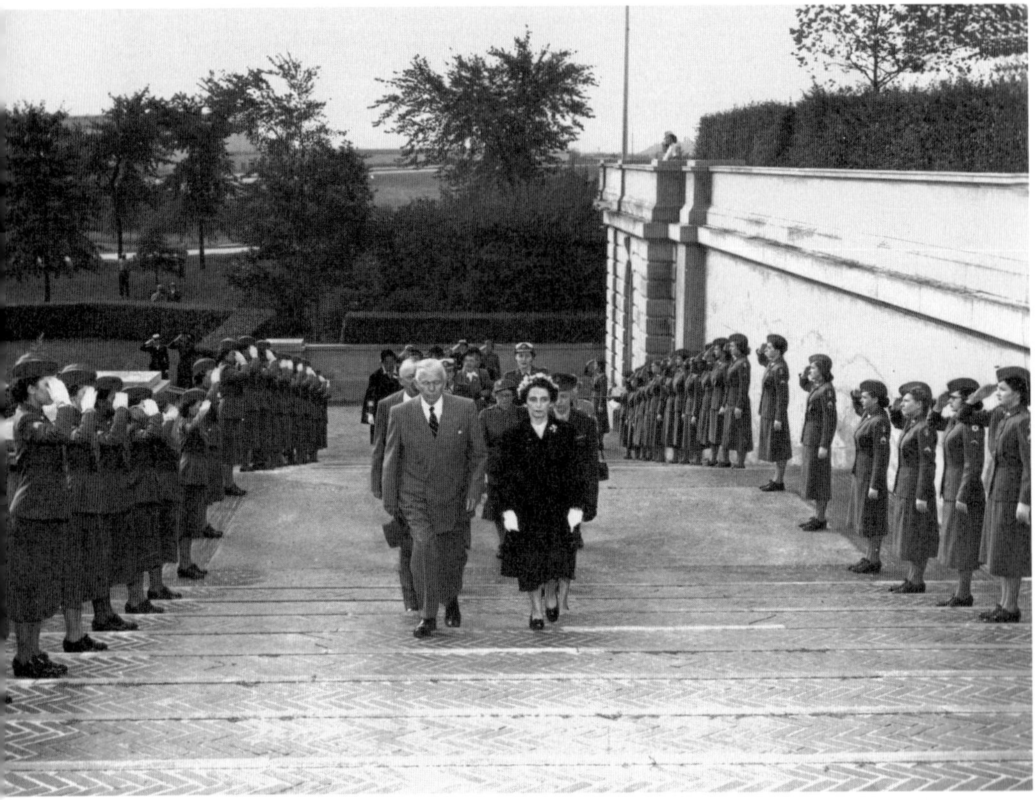

15. Marshall and Assistant Secretary of Defense Rosenberg lead a procession of Defense Department officials, members of the Defense Advisory Committee on Women in the Services, and leaders of the women's services, flanked by saluting members of the women's services, up the steps of the river entrance of the Pentagon to open the first meeting of the committee on September 17, 1951, five days after his resignation as secretary of defense. *(See pp. 639–47.)*

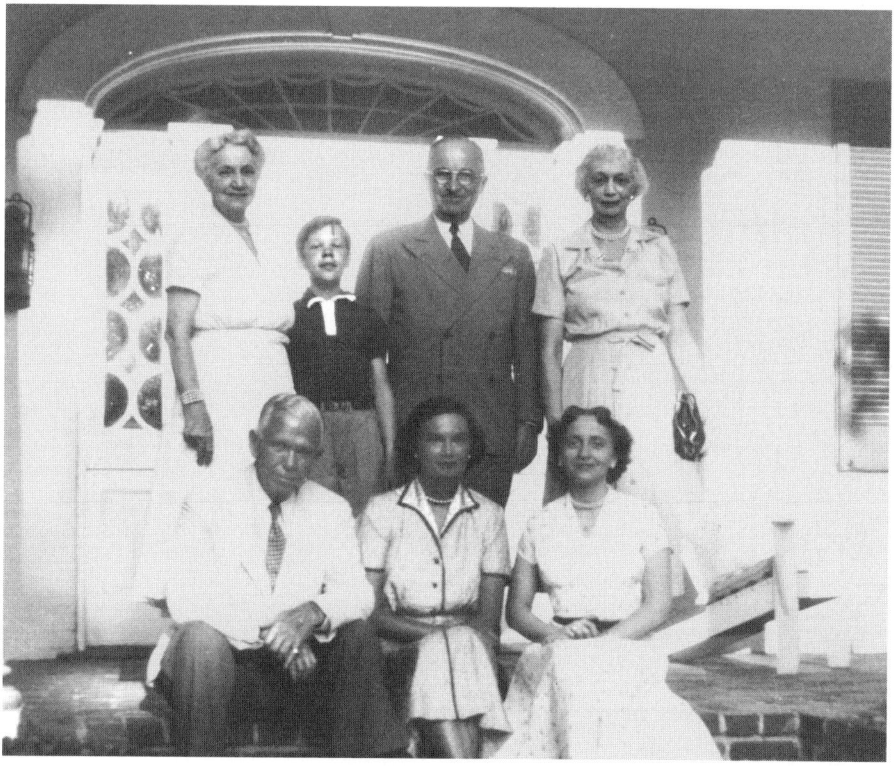

16. President Truman visits the Marshalls' Leesburg home for the last time, probably following the death of Katherine Marshall's son Clifton in May 1952. (See p. 698.) Seated from left: Marshall; Mary Lee, Clifton Brown's fiancée; and Margaret Truman, the president's daughter. Standing: Katherine Marshall; Tupper Brown, only child of Katherine Marshall's other deceased son, Allen; Truman; and Helen Lee, Mary's mother.

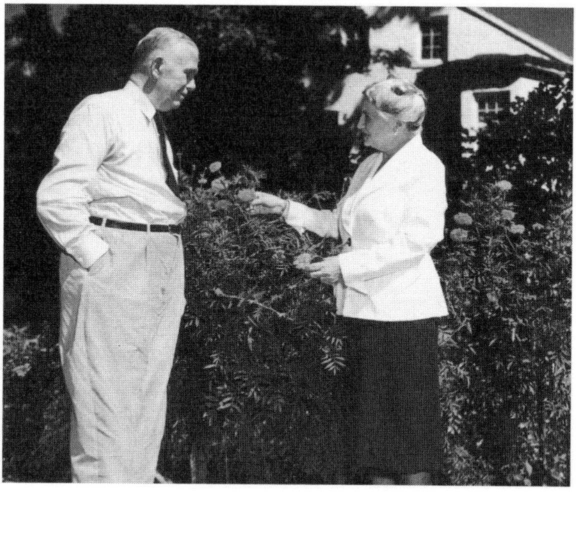

17. Three days after resigning as secretary of defense (see p. 637), newly retired General Marshall, an avid gardener looking forward to "just plain loafing," and Katherine Marshall admire the fruits of their labor on September 15, 1951, at Dodona Manor, their Leesburg, Virginia, home.

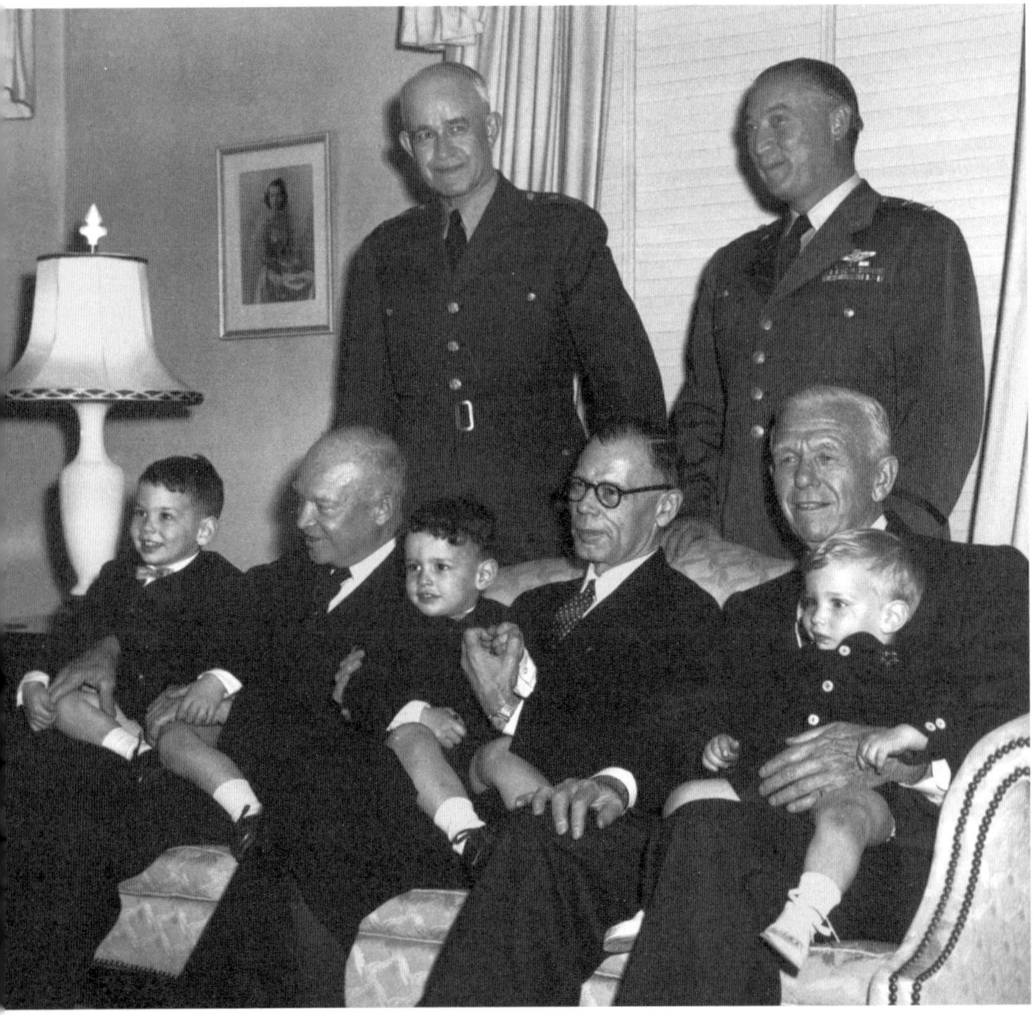

18. An impressive group of generals meet their godsons and namesakes, all children of Louis and Idella Marx, in General of the Army Omar N. Bradley's quarters at Fort Myer, Virginia, on April 6, 1953. Standing are Bradley and US Air Force Lieutenant General Emmett O'Donnell. Seated are President Dwight D. Eisenhower, holding Spencer Bedell Marx; Undersecretary of State Walter Bedell Smith, holding Emmett Dwight Marx; and Marshall, holding Bradley Marshall Marx. (See pp. 746–47.)

19. Although feeling far from well, Marshall tries to relax on the deck of the Italian liner Andrea Doria *in December 1953 en route to Naples, Italy, on the first leg of his trip to Oslo, Norway, to receive the Nobel Peace Prize. This photograph was provided by his shipmate Elizabeth Stetson Barry. (See pp. 805–6.)*

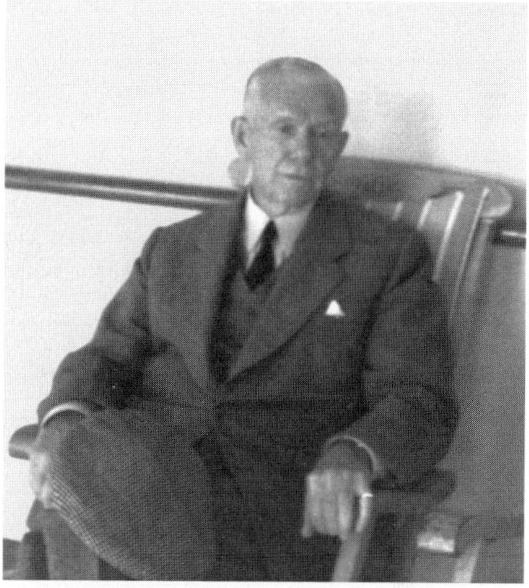

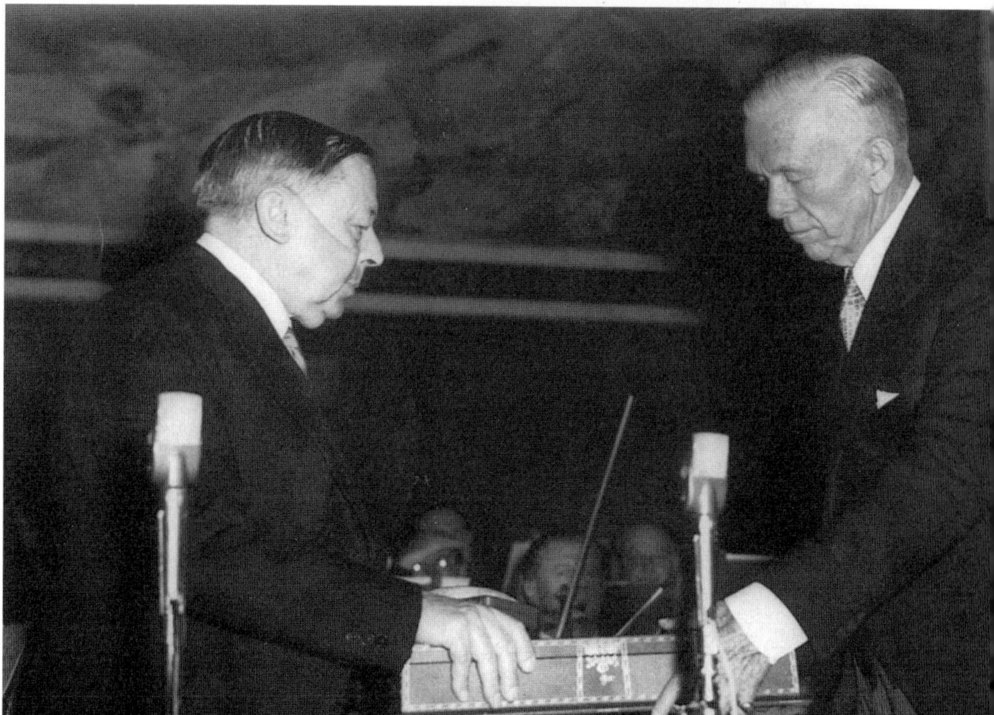

20. Gunnar Jahn, chairman of the Norwegian Nobel Committee, presents Marshall with the medal and citation for the Nobel Peace Prize in the Oslo University Auditorium on December 10, 1953. (See p. 809.)

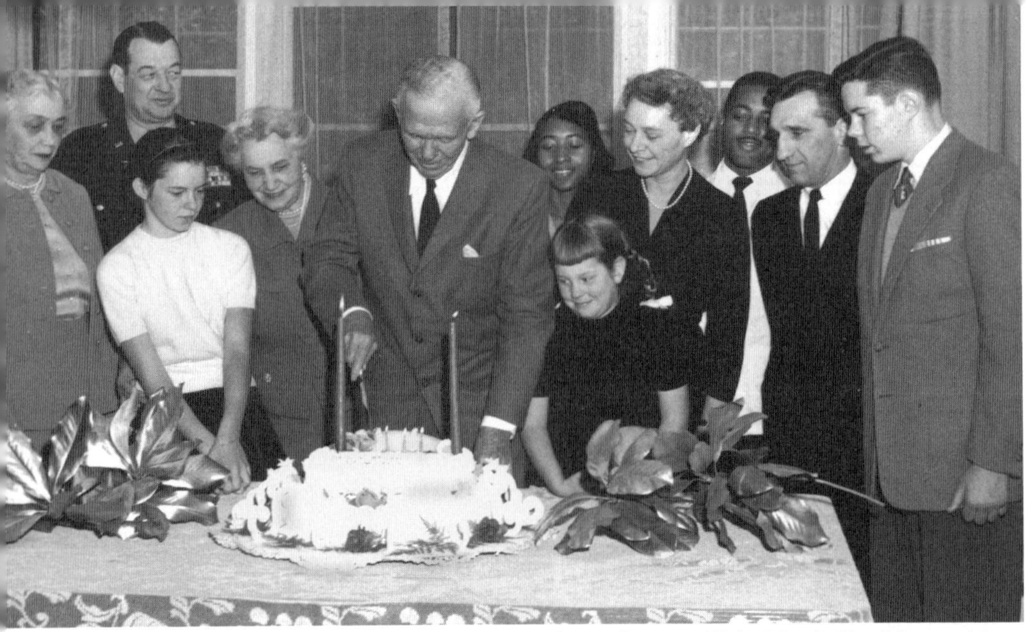

21. Cutting into a cake provided by the Pinehurst Country Club, Marshall celebrates his seventy-fifth birthday on December 31, 1955, with family and friends at Liscombe Lodge, the Marshalls' bungalow in Pinehurst. Joining the celebration (left to right), are Helen Lee, Colonel James Winn, Katherine Tupper "Kitty" Winn, Katherine Marshall, General Marshall, Julia Ray, Ellene Westmoreland Winn, Molly Winn, Floyd Ray, Sergeant William J. Heffner, and James J. Winn Jr. (See p. 913n1.)

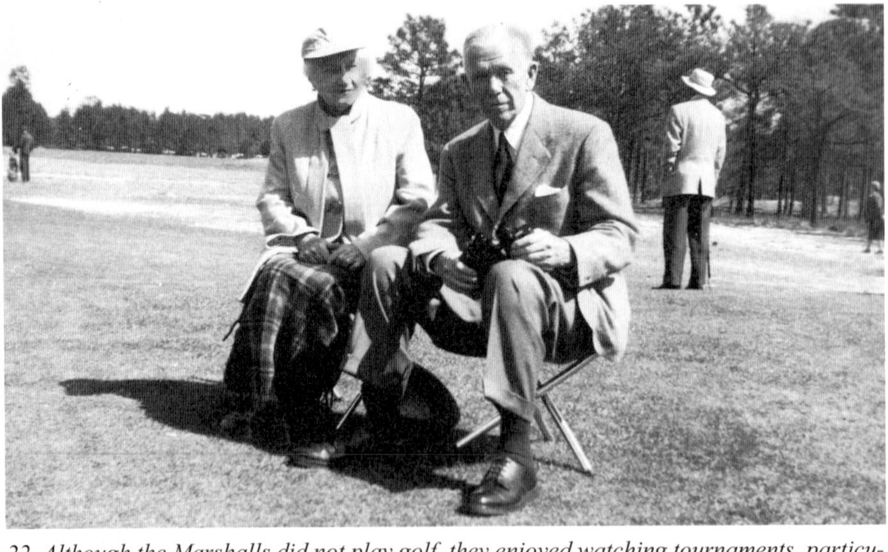

22. Although the Marshalls did not play golf, they enjoyed watching tournaments, particularly at the famous Pinehurst Country Club, where they view the North-South Open in this undated photograph. In retirement, they usually spent late autumn through early spring at their North Carolina residence.

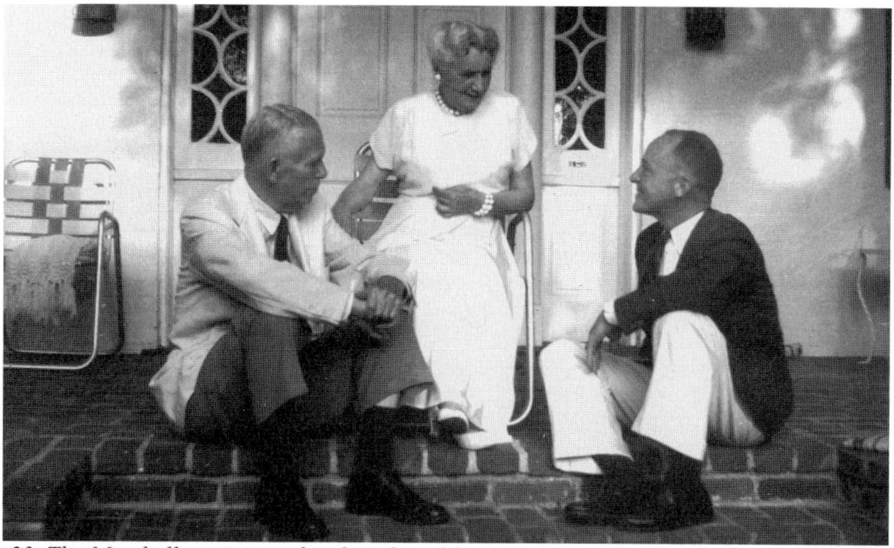

23. The Marshalls maintained a close friendship with World War II aide Frank McCarthy, even after he moved to California to work in the film industry. During a visit in July 1956, to discuss the formation of the George C. Marshall Research Foundation, McCarthy chats with the Marshalls on the porch of Dodona Manor. *See p. 950.*

24. In May 1955, Katherine Marshall donned a fur stole to welcome longtime friend Bernard Baruch and his nurse and companion, Elizabeth "Hampton" Navarro (left), as they arrive in Pinehurst, North Carolina. Marshall, looking thin and older than his age after numerous lengthy bouts of serious illness, looks on.

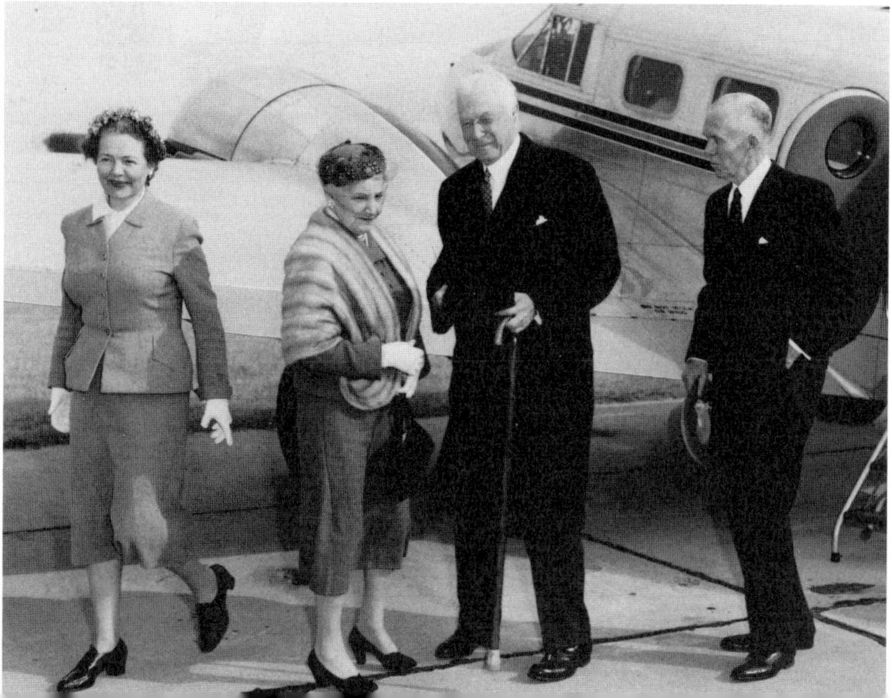

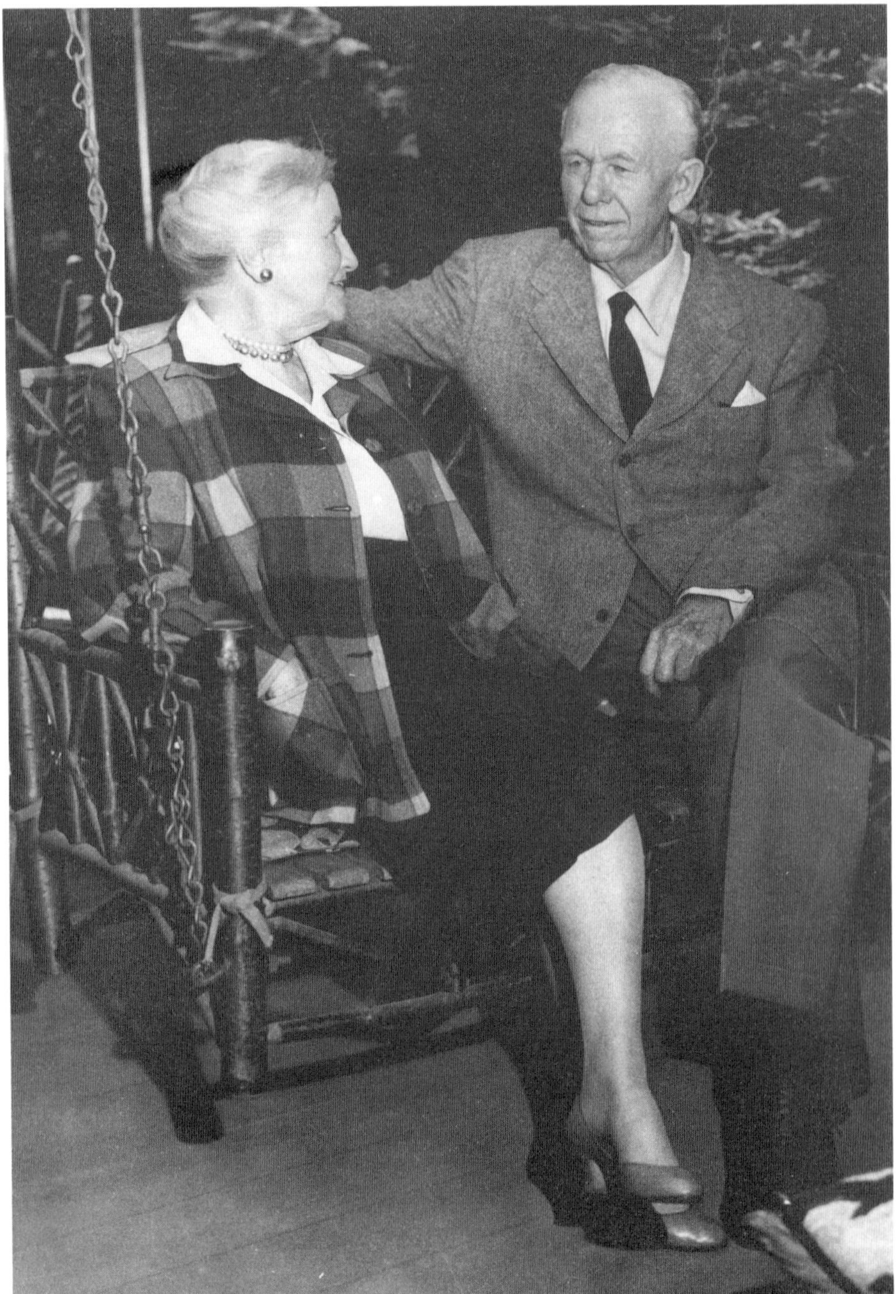

25. The Marshalls relax on the porch swing of their cottage during a vacation in Eagles Mere, Pennsylvania, in August 1955. Marshall later recalled Eagles Mere as the place "we enjoyed more than any locale visited in a long while." See pp. 892–93.

in the northwestern section of the country. Marshall "became so irritated with this grousing, Coca-Cola was Coca-Cola to me, so I finally sent a few bottles to the lab, Atlanta headquarters of Coca-Cola, and found the water they were using was different than that they used in Georgia." He "had a crisis on my hands, and I was receiving letters from Senators and Representatives with regard to northwestern Coca-Cola for southeastern boys. When you get into meat, there you would have a much larger issue." (Ibid., 810–11, 823.)

Marshall went on to insist that price controls were necessary, because if prices continued to increase, "the effect on the defense program gradually approaches the point of being disastrous, because the money ceases to buy the desired quantities of materiel." He ended this response with a more emphatic tone: "that this present struggle that we are engaged in, cold or hot war, or whatever you wish to call it, takes many forms from the standpoint of our opponents. One is to embarrass us as much in an economic way as they possibly can. It is conceivable they might play their hand purely on the basis, one way or another, unless we do it ourselves, of getting to the point where we might, say, break our backs economically. That is one way for the Soviets to win." It was precisely because of this concern for the nation's economy that Marshall was such a strong supporter of UMT. (See pp. 551–53 and 558–59.) Without UMT, "I thought we were doomed to a financial impossibility, and we couldn't hope for the continuance of appropriations that would be necessary to maintain the power that we must have in the coming years. I think economically the same thing applies." (Ibid., 822–23.) ★

312

TO GENERAL OF THE ARMY DWIGHT D. EISENHOWER — May 31, 1951
Top Secret — Washington, DC

Dear Eisenhower: Your letter of 12 May was of considerable interest, and I have had the delays you mentioned looked into carefully. A full report is attached for your information. While Dutch and Belgian hesitations and last minute changes have unquestionably contributed to the delays, it also appears that our own people haven't always acted in the most expeditious manner possible. Their attention has been called to the possible results, and I feel certain that future requests will be handled in such a way as to leave no room for excuses by country authorities or to doubt U. S. intentions. There is, of course, some delay inherent in necessary security checks and in the present highly involved procedure required to provide U. S. specifications and technical information to foreign nations. This has been under study for some time and our draft of the Mutual Security Program legislation, which has been cleared by the Bureau of the Budget, provides for more expeditious handling of such matters. If the Congress acts favorably, a considerable speed-up should be possible in future cases.[1]

I have long shared your concern that there should be one individual charged with expediting all aspects of the Mutual Defense Assistance Program, and on 11

January I appointed Major General James H. Burns my Assistant for International Security Affairs. Through him, and still within my own office, the direct responsibility for the expeditious and efficient implementation of the program rests with Major General Stanley L. Scott, Director of the Office of Military Assistance. Both Burns and Scott have these matters under constant study, and I believe generally the program has gone forward in a satisfactory manner.[2]

I have recently had the three Services go thoroughly into the matter of expediting delivery of equipment furnished under MDAP and give me a forecast of their expectations for the future. Stenographic copies of these presentations are attached for your information, and I believe you will agree, after studying them, that our foreign military assistance program is being attacked with vigor.[3]

I am very glad to get your reaction about the Italian military establishment, as well as that of Montgomery. It is interesting to note that both your and Montgomery's feelings agree with the impression gained by Admiral Sherman during his tour of duty in the Mediterranean. It would appear that with proper integration and strategic guidance you may have something on your south flank which will prove to be of value. The Montgomery inclosure was shown to Averell Harriman and has been destroyed.[4] Faithfully yours,

NA/RG 330, CD 370.21 (SHAPE)

1. Following an inspection tour of Belgium, the Netherlands, Germany, Denmark, and Norway, Eisenhower had on May 12 sent Marshall a three-page letter in which he reported complaints regarding delays in US fulfillment of requests and orders from other countries through MDAP. While perhaps "unavoidable," these delays were creating "a bad impression." (Eisenhower to Marshall, May 12, 1951, GCMRL/G. C. Marshall Papers [Secretary of Defense, Selected]; see also *Papers of DDE*, 12: 276–79.)

The attached report to which Marshall is referring attributed the complaints about delays to the need to conduct thorough analysis of the requests and impatience on the part of some of those requesting assistance. (Marshall to Eisenhower, enclosure 1, June 1 [*May 31*], 1951, DDEL/Dwight D. Eisenhower Papers [Pre-Presidential Files, Principal Files, Name Series, Marshall, George C.].) See pp. 569–77 and 597–603.

2. In his May 12 letter, Eisenhower reported that his concerns about these delays were shared by a group of American civilians currently in Europe, a number of whom thought someone in the Munitions Board office should be assigned to expedite requests. (Eisenhower to Marshall, May 12, 1951, GCMRL/G. C. Marshall Papers [Secretary of Defense, Selected].)

In the preparation of Marshall's response to Eisenhower, William van Atten, vice chairman for international programs for the Munitions Board, noted that his office existed to expedite requests as Eisenhower had mentioned and to support US interests "in the Defense Production Board in London." (Van Atten to Burns, memorandum, May 22, 1951, NA/RG 330, CD 370.21 [SHAPE].)

3. Copies of these extensive transcripts, dated May 9, 10, and 11, 1951, are attached to Marshall to Eisenhower, June 1 [*May 31*], 1951, DDEL/Dwight D. Eisenhower Papers (Pre-Presidential Files, Principal Files, Name Series, Marshall, George C.).

4. Eisenhower had in his letter also praised "the élan and spirit of all the troops" he saw on a recent trip to Italy, a sentiment shared by his deputy, Field Marshal Montgomery, who had also visited the country. Eisenhower forwarded with this letter a copy of Montgomery's lengthy top-secret report and of his response to Montgomery "as an example that we are making progress—that things are not stagnated at dead-center." He requested that Marshall show Montgomery's report to Averell Harriman, after which it should be "destroyed." (Eisenhower to Marshall, May 12, 1951, GCMRL/G. C. Marshall Papers [Secretary of

Defense, Selected]; Montgomery to Eisenhower, May 4, 1951, and Eisenhower to Montgomery, May 5, 1951, DDEL/Dwight D. Eisenhower Papers [Pre-Presidential Files, Principal Files, Name Series, Montgomery, Bernard].) Admiral Sherman reported to General Bradley on May 22 that he concurred with Montgomery's comments about the Italians. (Sherman to Bradley, memorandum, May 22, 1951, NA/RG 330, CD 370.21 [SHAPE].)

This paragraph of Marshall's response came from a JCS memorandum to Marshall Carter. (Matthews to Carter, memorandum, May 22, 1951, ibid.)

313

Graduation Remarks at the US Naval Academy, the US Military Academy, and Washington University

June 1, 5, and 6, 1951
Annapolis, Maryland; West Point, New York; and St. Louis, Missouri

IN THE SPRING OF 1951, Marshall accepted invitations to speak at commencement ceremonies at the US Naval Academy in Annapolis, Maryland, on June 1; the US Military Academy in West Point, New York, on June 5; and Washington University in St. Louis, Missouri, on June 6. C. J. George noted that Marshall had declined "some 28 similar invitations." (Hill to Marshall, February 20, 1951, and Marshall to Hill, March 5, 1951, GCMRL/G. C. Marshall Papers [Secretary of Defense, Number Indexed, M214-9-18]; Irving to Marshall, March 23, 1951, and Marshall to Irving, April 13, 1951, ibid., [M214-11-8]; George to Marshall, memorandum, April 24, 1951, Compton to Marshall, May 11, 1951, and Marshall to Compton, May 21, 1951, ibid., [M214-13-4].) Marshall deemed the Washington University speech "the most important because it will be my first offering in the Middle West. I am only going there because Dr. Compton is head of the institution and I and the military owe him a great deal." (Marshall to Ginsburgh, memorandum, April 30, 1951, ibid., [M214-13-4].) Washington University Chancellor Arthur Compton was a Nobel Prize–winning physicist who had played a major role in the development of the atomic bomb as leader of the Metallurgical Laboratory at the University of Chicago that produced the first nuclear chain reaction. See pp. 955–56.

On April 30, Marshall asked General Ginsburgh to present some ideas "as to what subjects I should touch on in each of these three addresses." Marshall told Ginsburgh that he intended to mention his experiences on navy ships and "unity in the services" during the Annapolis speech. He would also emphasize the importance of "professional development," which was crucial to the development of "an intimate understanding of national policy in relation to armed forces." At West Point, he would also discuss professional education but warn the graduates that there were still many officers who completed these advanced courses yet "still arrived in the War Department with little appreciation of the practical manner in which the staff had to operate." (Ibid.)

Other Defense Department staff members offered their own suggestions for Marshall's remarks at West Point. In a conversation with Marshall Carter, Lieutenant General Charles Herron suggested that Marshall use this speech to "give West Pointers an indication that it was a responsibility of theirs as regular army officers to bring along and push ahead outstanding officers from other schools or from civil life." Herron thought the graduates would be inspired to know that Marshall had been able to advance to the positions in the army that he did only with the assistance of "West Pointers." Carter, a 1931 West Point graduate himself, believed that Herron's suggestions would reinforce "the belief that West Pointers consider themselves in a class by themselves." Carter rejected this claim and told Marshall he resented "even more the implication that West Pointers, as such, had anything to do with 'pulling you along.'" (Carter to Marshall, memorandum, May 28, 1951, GCMRL/G. C. Marshall Papers [Secretary of Defense, Categorical, Memoranda, Marshall S. Carter, 1950–1951].)

In each of these speeches, Marshall deviated significantly from his prepared statements, which are available in GCMRL/G. C. Marshall Papers (Secretary of Defense, Speeches and Statements). In order to provide an accurate account of what Marshall actually said, the editors have used transcripts of recordings of the speeches as the source texts.

Friday, June 1, 1951

In Annapolis, Marshall spoke at 11:00 a.m. before a crowd of approximately seventy-five hundred people, including Vice Admiral Harry W. Hill (USNA, 1911), superintendent of the Naval Academy; Admirals Sherman and Fechteler; Secretary Matthews; Undersecretary of the Navy Dan A. Kimball; and Assistant Defense Secretary McNeil. ("Marshall Hails Training Bill Gain," *New York Times*, June 2, 1951, p. 29.) As he had suggested to General Ginsburgh, Marshall began by recounting his experiences and contact with the navy throughout his career. (For the anecdotes Marshall recalled, see *Papers of GCM*, 1: 110, 715–20, and 4: 58, 187–90; Marshall, *Memoirs*, 9, 14–15; and Forrest C. Pogue, *George C. Marshall*, vol. 3, *Organizer of Victory, 1943–1945* [New York: Viking, 1973], 301–2.) Through these experiences, his involvement with the navy as a member of the JCS and Combined Chiefs of Staff during World War II, and his tenure as secretary of defense, Marshall had "acquired not only a great respect, but a great admiration" for the navy and its officers, and he "had feelings of great assurance because of my profound respect for the naval views of the present Chief of Naval Operations." Turning to the Korean War, Marshall believed "that in time, as to leadership, as to courage and skill of the men concerned, as to the handling of reserves and limited reserves, as to the final blow giving a demonstration of active defense, that fighting will be considered a classic in military history." He noted that in Korea, "With almost no opportunity to refresh either the outer or inner man, . . . the ground problem" was "exceedingly difficult." He praised the "tremendous impression the ship gunners have been making on the land forces," particularly the accuracy of bombardments throughout the "narrow peninsula, with our Navy on all sides but the northern border and being able to sail very close in shore along the east coast" and land sixteen-inch shells "with pinpoint accuracy as much as 15 miles inland."

This, Marshall said, "made a profound impression on all of the troops because there could be nothing more comforting during a difficult period than the explosion of the 16-inch shell." The "present effectiveness" of "coordination and cooperation in Korea" between the army and navy was unprecedented. (Transcript of remarks at the US Naval Academy, June 1, 1951, GCMRL/G. C. Marshall Papers [Secretary of Defense, Speeches and Statements].)

Marshall believed that the present world situation constituted "the most dangerous threat to our national existence which has ever occurred in the lifetime of this country. What I mean is that there are so many approaches beginning with another world tragedy and down through the successive steps of political conquest of countries through connivance and propaganda and terrorism methods of that sort of people, and of their armies, with the spread of disunity." Even within the United States, Marshall warned of "devious, but always very clever ways of stirring up in our minds all sorts of feelings" through "skillful propaganda" and the threat of "defeat through economic means." The "economic structure that we have in our democratic process," he warned, was "susceptible to great weakness because of the periods of indifference on the part of our public and representatives." In crisis situations, "probably the most difficult phase" was "if we are lulled into a feeling of complete peace, profound peace, for which we all hope and pray, and our military posture is so weak that we present a vital weakness to the Communist aggression and we fail in our world leadership." Adequate preparation of the American military required, in addition to the "efficiency" of its officers and the continuous improvement of its weapons, the ability "to endure through a long period of public indifference." Marshall did not think the graduates would "understand this" yet, as "tremendous appropriations are obtainable" during the height of a crisis, but he recalled that after World War II "it was more difficult to get a dime than it had been before to get a dollar and we were cut down, stripped down until we had almost nothing left." The nature of the American military up to that point had been going "From this peak of getting all the money you need to the valley of literally nothing at all. The test of your organization is that valley." (Ibid.)

Marshall admitted that he was discussing "this in some detail" because of the ongoing debate on the conference committee's report on the UMT bill, which had been produced on May 28. (See pp. 481–84, 551–53, and 558–59.) "For thirty years," Marshall had been a vocal proponent of UMT, which he believed was "the only conceivable method by which we can maintain a respectable military posture in the world for enduring periods of time," yet despite overwhelming support for the program following World War II, it had not passed Congress at that time. Marshall speculated that "public reaction of indifference" and the hesitance of the services to "entertain anything that introduced a new factor which would demand money" were the culprits. He credited the support of the services as a major reason why the 1951 bill had progressed as far as it had. Marshall supposed the midshipmen had "heard that money makes the major go." In the debate over UMT, "money was the really controlling factor," and that would continue to be the case "the more closely we approach that period of profound peace, for which we all hope and pray." He concluded by charging the graduates as "a selected part of the young manhood of this country who must be responsible for the future of the country and I think will be basically responsible for general peace in the world." (Ibid.)

Tuesday, June 5, 1951

Marshall spoke at 10:00 a.m. before approximately fifty-five hundred people at West Point, including Major General Frederick A. Irving (USMA, 1917), superintendent of the academy since January 1951; General Vandenberg; and Assistant Secretary Rosenberg. ("Marshall Speaks at Cadet Exercises," *New York Times*, June 6, 1951, p. 5.) Marshall first called the cadets' attention to "the tremendous changes that have occurred since you entered the Academy in 1947. We had just completed a rather tumultuous demobilization of an armed force which had reached a peak of power unprecedented in the world, and then as always after a war we rapidly descended to a position of virtually military impotence." He reminded them that when he became secretary of state, "there was but one and a third divisions on active duty in the entire United States to back up our foreign policy" and all of Western Europe was experiencing "the depths of despair" in the aftermath of World War II. The economic rehabilitation of Western Europe since 1947 had "been truly remarkable" and was having "a vast effect on the whole democratic setup of the European continent." Despite the economic successes, Marshall added, it quickly became apparent "that we would have to undertake the rehabilitation of the military power of Western Europe" as well, "something that we had hoped would never be necessary following the victory on VJ-Day in this new world into which we all felt we were then entering." There was still "a long way to go for our friends in those democracies before that rehabilitation can reach sufficient strength, and we have a long way to go to recover from our too rapid demobilization." (Transcript of remarks at the US Military Academy, June 5, 1951, GCMRL/G. C. Marshall Papers [Secretary of Defense, Speeches and Statements].)

Realization of this lack of preparation became "a tragic dilemma" at the outbreak of the Korean War, when the US had "very few divisional units" and "absolutely no available trained reserves." There were so few troops available that MacArthur "took a very courageous decision and integrated some 30,000" South Koreans with little training "into the ranks of the four divisions we then had in the Far East." Not until March 1951—eight months into the conflict— was the US military able "to catch up with the situation" and send units to Korea at "full strength with American manpower." (See pp. 440–41.) Marshall asked the cadets to "reflect in your own minds the enormity" of "the fact that our military system was so ill-adapted to any such emergency." The rotation policies established by the services (see pp. 436–37, 516–17, and 550–51) were crucial to allow reservists who were called to duty under the "partial mobilization" to return home to "their normal life as rapidly as possible." These policies were also important to allow World War II veterans who had been recalled to active duty and "were being penalized again" for their prior service to return home. Marshall added that the UMT bill, on which Congress was nearing a final vote, was critical to "getting a stable system" so that the US "can continue on into the future without collapsing at each relaxation of our population." (Ibid.) See pp. 551–53 and 558–59.

Thanks to, the "magnificent leadership" of all officers "from the top down to the squad leaders," and their "very remarkable, coordinated, cooperative, aggressive performance," Marshall believed that the recent battlefield successes in Korea (see p. 534) would "be considered a classic in military history." It had been "a complete demonstration in the most perfect form of coordinated operations between the Navy and the Air and the Army. It has been a lesson to us all, and it is something that none of you should ever forget." Marshall consequently asked the graduating cadets "to make a real effort to learn all you can, not in the abstract, but in the concrete, of the other arms of the services, because that is a very essential factor in an efficient team, and also because if you reach an outstanding position, you, yourself, some day, will be called upon to coordinate all three services in their activities. It is very important that you should understand not only your own but the other arms of the general armed forces." (Ibid.)

Marshall cautioned the graduates about the challenges facing the military in a democracy, which he admitted would be "exceedingly difficult at times." Nevertheless, "we are in a democracy and I ask you never to forget that you are an officer in an army of a democracy, and only by your generous understanding of the position that an officer holds in a great democracy such as ours will lead you to a successful career." Marshall recalled that "the political climate" at the time had prevented his own admission to West Point, but despite this obstacle, he "succeeded in getting in the Army." (See *Papers of GCM*, 1: 7–8, and Forrest C. Pogue, *George C. Marshall*, vol. 1, *Education of a General, 1880–1939* [New York: Viking, 1963], 39–42.) Examples of criticisms of the military throughout US history made it "very necessary that you understand the workings of a democracy as applied to our military forces." One particular example Marshall noted were "open comments" made in 1920 by Charles W. Eliot, president emeritus of Harvard, who said, according to the *New York Times*, "that West Point was all that an educational institution should not be" given "the inefficiency and failure of its graduates" during World War I and that "'no nation should be allowed to maintain an army of the kind called regular, that is, an army all of whose officers are men who have embraced for life the profession of soldier." The American concept of "a great citizen army," Marshall added, naturally leads to "antagonisms, frictions, and certainly a cloud of misrepresentations." (Ibid.; "Change West Point, Dr. Eliot Advises," *New York Times*, May 9, 1920, p. 19.)

Marshall concluded by expressing his "greatest admiration for the Military Academy," which was enhanced "by the fact that though I was not a graduate, I found throughout my entire service, particularly as I neared the top, that my strongest supporters, my strongest helpers, my closest friends were graduates of the Military Academy, and usually those in a high position." In addition, his assistants throughout his career "have been largely from the graduates of West Point, and very prominent, outstanding men at the time." He had "deep" gratitude and admiration for West Point, "but all of it goes back to an understanding of what it is to be an officer of the military forces in the Army of a great democracy." (Transcript of remarks at the US Military Academy, June 5, 1951, GCMRL/G. C. Marshall Papers [Secretary of Defense, Speeches and Statements].) See pp. 565–66.

Wednesday, June 6, 1951

Marshall flew directly from West Point to St. Louis, Missouri, where he delivered remarks the next day at Washington University to nearly nineteen hundred graduates, a full gymnasium of guests, and an additional fifteen hundred people sitting in overflow seats outside, where large television screens had been installed to broadcast the speech. ("Marshall Voices Korea Peace Hope," *New York Times*, June 7, 1951, p. 5.) He began by encouraging the students to pursue "sober thinking" and "a solid foundation of facts" in these "critical days." Only by doing so would they be able "to form a reasonable judgment as to what was the most appropriate action at the time." He went on to recount the changes in world affairs since the "much too rapid—almost tumultuous demobilization" of the US military after World War II, which sank the United States "into a position of military impotence at a time when virtually by acclamation, saving for the Soviets, we were accorded the responsibility of leadership for the world." The European Recovery Program, the conclusion of Iran Crisis of 1946, the status of Trieste, the successful assistance to Greece during its civil war, the subsequent break between Yugoslavia and the Soviet Union, and the Berlin blockade and airlift presented "a remarkable record to-date, a record of unusually difficult and dangerous situations, met each in turn by courageous decisions and so far with the avoidance of general war." (Remarks at Washington University's Graduation Ceremony, June 6, 1951, Washington University in St. Louis Archives/University Records [Commencement Collection, Audio-Visual Media].) For more on the preceding Iran and Trieste crises Marshall mentioned, see p. 533.

Turning to Korea, Marshall praised "the amazing performance of our heavily outnumbered troops in striking a deadly blow at Communist prestige in Asia" since its "peak" in the fall of 1950. He warned that despite "terrific—almost unbelievable—losses" by the enemy in recent weeks, "We have not seen the end in Korea. No man can predict exactly what that will be. But it is becoming more and more apparent that without fatally sapping our military resources we have posed a terrific problem for the hostile regime in China." Marshall hoped that "our opponents" would soon "come to realize that war is not a profitable business and that world disputes should be settled by peaceful negotiations and the establishment of a reputation for good faith as to all commitments." (Ibid. See also p. 534.)

Marshall then discussed in some detail what he labeled "one of the most remarkable military campaigns in history," that of Missouri lawyer Alexander William Doniphan and his regiment of Missouri Volunteers during the Mexican-American War of 1846–48. He described their difficult marches "across the plains" and into Mexico, and he cited these men as "a perfect example of American qualities and leadership, of initiative and individual competence at their best, and apparently with a complete absence of recriminations and complaints because of lack of food, lack of pay, and lack of public appreciation." After a lengthy exposition of Doniphan's experiences, Marshall apologized for going "into the details of military history in this matter." He did so, however, because he believed the qualities presented by Doniphan and his men were ones that needed to be cultivated today, as they were "inherent, I think, in our quality of citizenship. Yet they are very apt to be lost in the luxuries, excitements, and diversions of our too-complex civilization and extraordinarily high standards of living." (Ibid. Marshall had previously written an article recounting Doniphan's story, which is very similar to the language he used in these remarks. See George C. Marshall, "Epic March of Americans," *Illinois Guardsman* 3, no. 1 [December 1935]: 14–16.)

Marshall concluded by reiterating his support for UMT, as Congress was nearing the conclusion of its debate on the bill. (See pp. 551–53 and 558–59.) This plan, Marshall asserted, would "be an enduring system to maintain this country in the position of leadership in which it finds itself in the world today." The United States could not afford the "long delays" it took to build up its military after the outbreak of the Korean War, and Marshall was convinced that the new law would "work to make us, with a minimum of appropriations, so powerful in the world that our peaceful intentions can be made effective for all countries." (Ibid.) ★

314

To Colonel James Winn

June 4, 1951
Washington, DC

Dear Jim: I received the mortgage papers and am sending them down to Colonel Hawes at Pinehurst to have a record made there.[1]

The provisions are satisfactory to us but we had intended that the rates should be 1%. Also, as to the due date in 1956, that we can accept as a mere matter of form and extension of the mortgage continued thereafter.

I am off tonight or tomorrow morning for West Point and tomorrow afternoon from there to St. Louis. These, I think, are the last speaking dates I have, for which I am duly thankful.[2]

Katherine and I flew from Washington to Annapolis on Friday in a Navy duck and from there to Leesburg, the latter trip taking us only forty minutes.[3] We had a very pleasant weekend though it was extremely hot except in our house. We both got up about 7:00 A.M. each morning and did our garden work before 10:00. During the remainder of the day it was too hot for pleasure outside of the house.

With my love to you all.[4] Affectionately,

GCMRL/G. C. Marshall Papers (Secretary of Defense, Number Indexed, M200-4-17)

1. See pp. 349–50. On June 1, Winn had sent Marshall a "note for $10,000^{\underline{00}}$ as indenture on the house in Pinehurst," less than a half mile from the Marshalls' home there. In the attached promissory note, dated January 15, 1951, and notarized on June 1, the Winns

agreed to pay Marshall "the principal sum of Ten Thousand and No/100 Dollars . . . with interest thereon from January 15, 1951 at the rate of two per centum (2%) per annum, said principal to be due and payable on January 15, 1956." (Winn to Marshall, June 1, 1951, and attachments, GCMRL/G. C. Marshall Papers [Secretary of Defense, Categorical, Winn Mortgage, 1951]; H.) Major George forwarded these attachments to Colonel George P. Hawes, a realtor in Pinehurst, North Carolina, on June 5.

2. See the previous editorial summary.

3. See the previous editorial summary.

4. In a letter to Frank McCarthy, Katherine Marshall expressed her happiness "that Molly has bought a house at Pinehurst just a block down from us." As the Winns lived at Fort Monroe, Virginia, they had rented the house in Pinehurst "until they can live in it." (Marshall to McCarthy, July 15, 1951, GCMRL/Frank McCarthy Papers [Additions, Box 1].)

AFTER delivering his commencement address at Washington University (see pp. 546–47), Marshall secretly flew to the Far East for a visit to Korea. According to the official OSD history, "He wanted particularly to greet and encourage Ridgway who, according to Marshall Carter, was probably 'the single officer in the whole military establishment that the secretary most admired.'" The trip had been planned "sometime ago," Marshall admitted during a press conference in Tokyo, but he had waited until certain that his presence in Washington would no longer be needed in regard to the UMT bill or the 1951–52 budget discussions. (Condit, *Test of War*, 114; "Marshall Pays Surprise Visit to Korea Front," June 8, 1951, GCMRL/Vertical File.) See next document and pp. 558–59.

Marshall was accompanied by Marshall Carter (see photo #14), who later stated in an oral history interview that "General Marshall thought, and I agreed with him, that it was necessary for him to go to Korea. Now, General MacArthur had been relieved, General Ridgway was in command in Japan, and the problem was how to get to Korea without anyone knowing about it, so he could visit Korea and get out without any press involved or anything else." (Interview with Marshall S. Carter by Mr. James F. Schnabel and Dr. Walter S. Poole, March 19, 1973, GCMRL/Pogue Research Materials [Box 1], p. 10.) Ridgway recalled that he received a top secret message "about a week" before the trip stating that "General Marshall will fly out to Tokyo . . . and there will be no publicity given whatever until he gets off the plane in Korea." (GCMRL/Oral History Collection, Tape 21, interview with Ridgway, February 26, 1959, pp. 34–35.) According to Carter, Marshall swapped planes in St. Louis with a general who was returning from Japan so that the press would incorrectly conclude that Marshall was returning to Washington. (Marshall Carter interview, p. 10.) Following the plane swap in St. Louis, Marshall and Carter stopped in Tacoma, Washington, and the Aleutian Islands in Alaska before landing at Yokota AFB, headquarters of FEAF, near Tokyo, Japan, at 9:00 a.m. on Friday, June 8, local time. Ridgway met them there, and they "immediately" boarded Ridgway's plane to fly to Seoul. Once they arrived at Seoul, they "transferred into light aircraft" to fly up for "a tour of the front line units." (Ibid.; Ridgway interview, p. 35.)

Marshall had previously paid a brief visit to Korea and Japan during a 1914 leave from his second tour of duty in the Philippines to examine Manchurian battlefields of the Russo-Japanese War of 1904–5. This 1951 visit was also brief, and it was to be his last to an active battlefront. (*Papers of GCM*, 1: 85–92; Pogue, *Education*, 124–25; Pogue, *Statesman*, 488.) The weather, Ridgway recalled, was "foul" with "lots of turbulence" during their flight in the small plane to the front line. Ridgway suggested that they transfer to jeeps rather than continue in a light aircraft, but Marshall asked if Ridgway would continue using the planes if Marshall were not there. When Ridgway replied affirmatively, Marshall insisted on flying. James Quirk, Ridgway's special adviser on public relations, had been on the flight and told his wife that the pilots "shuddered" at Marshall's insistence that they keep flying but they "agreed that if the Old Man could do it so could they. It was so dangerous it was silly but Generals are like that." (Ridgway interview, p. 35; Rory Quirk, *Wars and Peace: The Memoir of an American Family* [Novato, CA: Presidio Press, 1999], 195–96.) Marshall enjoyed the performance and convenience of these small aircraft so much that upon his return to the United States, according to the *New York Herald Tribune*, he began to commute between Washington and Leesburg in a similar army plane a few times a week. Marshall later reported to Lewis Douglas that this trip "takes about twenty-five minutes from door to door." ("Marshall: A Man Who's in a Hurry," *New York Herald Tribune*, August 5, 1951, GCMRL/G. C. Marshall Papers [Secretary of Defense, Scrapbooks and Scrapbook Materials]; Marshall to Douglas, September 6, 1951, GCMRL/G. C. Marshall Papers [Secretary of Defense, Number Indexed, M200-10-36].)

In Korea, Marshall met with Van Fleet; Lieutenant General Frank W. Milburn (USMA, 1914), commanding general of I Corps; and "several division commanders" in "a green camouflaged Army tent on the western front" for approximately forty-five minutes, according to a press report, while "Fighter planes droned overhead" and "The thunder of artillery echoed." He also flew to meet with IX Corps commander General William Hoge and X Corps commander General Edward Almond at their respective headquarters. Marshall later revealed that he had met with "all corps commanders, most division commanders and all but two of the commanders of foreign units" present in Korea at that time. Marshall then moved from the front to Eighth Army headquarters where he met with Van Fleet; Lieutenant General Chung Il Kwon, chief of staff of the South Korean Army; and Brigadier General Garrison H. Davidson, acting chief of staff of the United States Military Advisory Group to the Korean Army, on the plane while it sat on the runway. Marshall held an "informal press conference" before departing for Tokyo, where he arrived at 11:30 p.m. (Commanding General's Journal, June 8, 1951, GCMRL/James A. Van Fleet Papers [Korea, 1951–1953, Eighth United States Army, Commanding General's Journal]; "Korean Visit Just Routine, Marshall Says," *Washington Post*, June 9, 1951, pp. 1, 3; "Bradley Discusses Korea Cease-Fire in Talks in London," *New York Times*, June 9, 1951, pp. 1, 2.) See photos #12 and 13.

Due to the secrecy around the plans for Marshall's visit and his conferences with high-ranking army officers at the front, the press speculated that the purpose of the trip was to deliver a new directive to Ridgway and to discuss the coming possibility of cease-fire negotiations. Following his return to Tokyo, Marshall asserted to the press that his visit "had 'no connection whatsoever' with any current peace moves"; his trip "was 'purely military,'" and he "carried no new directives on fighting the Korean war." When asked if he knew of "any new peace efforts," Marshall replied: "'I don't know. I think you should ask Mao Tse-tung and Chou En-lai.'" As with the Greek civil war and the Berlin blockade, he rejected the notion that the Korean War was a stalemate. (See *Papers of GCM*, 6: 344–600 passim.) "'Whenever we start something and don't finish it the same afternoon,' he replied with a laugh, 'in our country that's a stalemate.'" Instead, Marshall dubbed the Korean War a "'military classic,'" because of the ability of the UN forces to counterattack successfully against the Chinese offensives in the spring and to diminish Communist morale and prestige. ("Korean Visit Just Routine, Marshall Says," *Washington Post*, June 9, 1951, pp. 1, 3; "Bradley Discusses Korea Cease-Fire in Talks in London," *New York Times*, June 9, 1951, pp. 1, 2.)

Marshall held conversations with Ridgway in Tokyo on June 9, 10, and 11, although the editors have been unable to locate records of these meetings. He attended church services with the Ridgways on Sunday, June 10, and then spent the afternoon at their home at the American embassy. He was scheduled to have additional conferences on June 11 with Lieutenant General Otto P. Weyland, commander of FEAF, and "possibly" Vice Admiral C. Turner Joy (USNA, 1916), commander of US naval forces in the Far East. ("Marshall Sees Top Officers In Far East," *Washington Post*, June 11, 1951, p. 1.) Apparently Marshall also inquired as to whether he should visit Formosa while in the Far East, for Lovett informed him during the trip that the State Department saw "no, repeat no, point in your going to Formosa." (Lovett to Ridgway for Marshall, cable, n.d., GCMRL/G. C. Marshall Papers [Secretary of Defense, Chronological, Secretaries, Carlson].)

Before returning to the US, Marshall held another hour-long press conference in Tokyo, in which he stated that the Communists, despite their heavy losses, were still striving to expel the US forces from Korea "to be in a better position to attack Japan." While he did not believe the Korean War would continue for years, Marshall reiterated that the US was planning "for a long period" of tension. He again denied rumors that his trip was related to potential peace talks, stating instead that its purpose "was to see the Eighth Army and to study rotation plans," and announcing that by summer's end fifty thousand fresh troops would be available every month. He also informed the press that he had only briefly "discussed" the Japanese Peace Treaty. In response to a question "about American plans and the Chinese conception of the war," Marshall became "almost explosive" and expressed his frustration that "'We tell the whole world everything we have and plan,'" yet "'nobody on the other side tells us about anything. I wish they would.'" Despite prodding, Marshall, with a "somewhat testy" attitude, concluded the press conference by declining to offer any comment on a recent telegram from General MacArthur to Senator Knowland that criticized Marshall's 1945–46 China mission as "one of the greatest blunders in American diplomatic history for which the free world is now paying in blood and disaster and will in all probability continue to do so indefinitely." ("Knowland and MacArthur Letters," *New York Times*, June 10, 1951, p. 68; "Marshall Says Foe Has Eyes on Japan," *New York Times*, June 11, 1951, pp. 1, 5; "Marshall Says Too Much Talk Is Hurting U.S.," *New York Herald Tribune*, June 12, 1951.)

Marshall and Carter departed for the United States at 3:00 p.m. on June 11. At 6:30 a.m. (still on June 11 due to the International Date Line), they stopped in Naknek, Alaska, a popular fishing destination, where they spent "about five hours" fishing for trout. They each caught "one about 4 1/2 pounds," Carter reported to Ridgway's wife, Penny. They departed Naknek at 3:30 p.m. and after stopping in Anchorage, Alaska, they arrived at National Airport in Washington at 11:33 a.m. on June 12. Upon landing Marshall praised the "high" morale of the Eighth Army, which was likely "'the most ably trained Army we ever had.'" He then went immediately to the Pentagon for a brief meeting with Lovett and Rosenberg before heading to the White House to meet with President Truman. As Lovett and Fritchey had recommended, Marshall met with the press at 3:00 p.m. and "most willingly discussed" questions regarding "troop morale" and "the rotation scheme," although he now stated that there would be available "as many as 25,000 soldiers" per month to rotate, rather than fifty thousand as he had announced during his final press conference in Tokyo. He praised "the coordination," strength, and leadership of the UN forces and again declined to say he had discussed "possible cease-fire negotiations" while in the Far East. When asked "about reaction in the Orient to the removal" of General MacArthur, Marshall "replied that on the whole it had been very peaceful out there, even though a war was in progress." ("Marshall Asserts Foe is Badly Hurt," *New York Times*, June 13, 1951, p. 3; "Marshall Calls 8th Best Trained Army," *Washington Post*, June 13, 1951, p. 4; Carter to Penny Ridgway, June 15, 1951, GCMRL/Marshall S. Carter Papers [Department of Defense, Correspondence]; George to commanding officer, Airways and Air Communications Service, cable, June 11, 1951, GCMRL/G. C. Marshall Papers [Secretary of Defense, Chronological, Secretaries, Carlson].)

While Marshall was in Tokyo, Congress passed the conference committee's version of the UMT bill. Marshall wanted to be sure to recruit his preferred choices for the National Security Training Commission, the creation of which the bill mandated to devise a more specific plan for the implementation of UMT. ★

315

To Major C. J. George — June 9, 1951

Confidential — [Tokyo, Japan]

Deliver following personal message to Assistant Secretary, Ann Rosenberg: "Congratulations to you very personally on the final passage of the manpower bill.[1] Also question as to how you made out on selection of civilian committee and also the hope that you are taking a weekend rest.[2] G. C. Marshall."

NA/RG 330, Office of the Assistant Secretary of Defense for Manpower and Personnel (201, Rosenberg, Anna)

1. A conference committee chaired by Senator Russell that had convened in April to reconcile differences between the House and Senate versions of the UMST bill issued its compromise bill on May 28. (See pp. 481–84.) It passed the Senate by voice vote on June 1 and the House by a vote of 339–41 on June 7 and was then forwarded to Truman for his signature. The bill extended the current Selective Service provisions, which were set to expire in July 1951, until 1955. It also lowered the minimum draft age for Selective Service from nineteen to eighteen and six months, though all men between nineteen and twenty-six would have to be drafted before anyone between eighteen and six months and nineteen could be inducted into service. In addition, those inducted would serve for twenty-four months, increased from the twenty-one months that had been required previously. Physical and mental standards were lowered to allow the induction of some men who had been classified as draft-ineligible, and the 2-percent cap on women in the armed services was suspended until 1954. This bill also approved the concept of UMT beginning with six months of military training for all men over the age of eighteen. Those who received deferments on their training would be liable to complete the training before they turned thirty-five. All trained men would then be required to serve eight years in the reserves, assuming they were not called to active duty in that time. The bill capped the size of the military at five million men. Before any program of UMT would be instituted, however, a National Security Training Commission, consisting of three civilian and two military members appointed by the president and confirmed by the Senate, would need to be established. This commission was charged with presenting to Congress within four months a detailed plan for the implementation of UMT that had received the approval of the secretary of defense. Each chamber would then vote on whether the plan should be enacted. Even if a plan was developed quickly, it would not be put into practice until either the president or Congress determined that there was no current need for the active military service of these trained men. ("U.M.T. Plan is Set in Draft Extension," *New York Times*, May 29, 1951, p. 1; "Draft Compromise Passed By Senate," *New York Times*, June 2, 1951, p. 1; "Draft-UMT Bill Sent To Truman by House," *Washington Post*, June 8, 1951, p. 3.)

2. Marshall was intensely interested in having Baruch, who had been a vocal supporter of the UMST bill, as one of the three civilians on the commission; Marshall asked George from Tokyo on June 9 (see the previous editorial note) to send Baruch a message urging that he accept the request, which would come through Anna Rosenberg. George replied later that day that Rosenberg was "delighted and extremely grateful" for Marshall's message and that he had delivered the message to Baruch. He also reported that Truman had spoken with Rosenberg "on the telephone. He said your trip was a ten strike and will have great effect." (George to Baruch, telegram, June 9, 1951, GCMRL/G. C. Marshall Papers [Secretary of Defense, Chronological, Secretaries, Ackerman]; George to Ridgway, cables, June 9, 1951, ibid., [Carlson]; "U.M.T. Bill Urgent, Baruch Declares," *New York Times*, April 9, 1951, p. 4.)

George informed Marshall on June 10 that Truman would ask James W. Wadsworth to chair the commission and that Rosenberg had not yet been able to reach Baruch. On the following day, while Marshall was flying back from Tokyo to Washington via the Aleutian Islands, George informed him that Baruch was "reluctant to accept the post" and that Rosenberg would share more about his response upon Marshall's return. (George to Ridgway, cable, June 10, 1951, and George to commanding officer, Adak AFB, Aleutian Islands, Alaska, cable, June 11, 1951, GCMRL/G. C. Marshall Papers [Secretary of Defense, Chronological, Secretaries, Carlson].)

On June 11, Rosenberg drafted a memorandum for Marshall informing him that at his request, she had submitted the names of the Defense Department's preferred committee members to Truman and had also spoken with Truman on this topic. After receiving Marshall's telegram, Rosenberg mentioned to Baruch that "the Chairman was the only one who would have to devote full time," so "he needn't worry about be [*being*] able to serve just limited time. . . . From that moment on he didn't feel that we needed him and that he would be just one of many on the 'Wadsworth Committee.'" Later that day Baruch informed her by telegram that he had sent Marshall a telegram stating he could not serve on the commission because of his planned travel to Europe. (Rosenberg to Marshall, memorandum, June 11, 1951, NA/RG 330, Office of the Assistant Secretary of Defense for Manpower and Personnel [Chronological File (Nov 50–Dec 51)]; George to Marshall, memorandum, June 12, 1951, GCMRL/G. C. Marshall Papers [Secretary of Defense, Chronological, Secretaries, Carlson].) See pp. 558–59, 609–10, and 679–80. ★

316

To Mrs. John B. Wilson

June 12, 1951
Washington, DC

Dear Rose: Many thanks for your letter of June 4th. As usual, you were very generous with your superlatives and emphatic support of my activities. I must say that I am glad to have you "on my side."[1]

Daniel Edwards has had a rather vigorous but quick indoctrination on the aims and functions of the Defense Department and is grasping his responsibilities in an admirable fashion. He seems to have all four wheels on the track and developing fine contacts on Capitol Hill.[2]

The daily crises of a mother of young boys are not to be sneezed at; however, I did find your presentation of the problems in general rather amusing and imagine that you, too, have many a laugh over their scrapes.[3]

Don't you believe that I was bored with the script you sent me! On the contrary, I was and am interested in your activities in connection with my favorite humanitarian organization.[4]

The day at V.M.I. on the 15th was perfect in all respects. I am sorry that you were omitted from the guest list, but it was not intentional. Dick Marshall, at the Institute, handled all the arrangements. I was just their honored by-stander.[5]

I have just returned, as you are probably aware, from a round of speaking engagements and a fast and furious trip to Korea, which was interesting, informative, and tiring. Mrs. Marshall took advantage of my absence to visit her daughter, Molly, and her family at Fort Monroe over the week-end.[6]

Thanks again for your letter. Give our regards to John, and love to the children, and I long to see you again. Affectionately,

I landed here at 11:30 this A.M. Just completed a press conference.[7]

GCMRL/J. Page Wilson Collection

1. See p. 531n2.
2. See p. 531n1.
3. Rose had reported in her June 4 letter that her "boys are big and strong and full of beans. They had a marvellous time at the farm feeding pigs, milking, riding the hay wagon; Page even plowed and worked tobacco. The only altercation was the day I found them both, and Tom was just four in April, astride the rooftop of the cabin. I got them down but it was touch and go for a while. Page was the best in his class this year. . . . Tom can charm a bird out of a tree and continues to be exasperating. I never worry about him much but rather, what awful thing he'll do next to what neighbor. He just doesn't give a damn about nothing." (Wilson to Marshall, June 4, 1951, GCMRL/G. C. Marshall Papers [Secretary of

Defense, Number Indexed, M200-6-31].)

4. Rose had written that year's report for her local Red Cross chapter and offered to send a copy to Marshall. She had also written "a lot of speeches and radio script during the drive; I sent you one but I think it bored you." (Ibid.)

5. Rose had also expressed her hope on June 4 that Marshall "had a good time at VMI. I wish you'd invited me, you know me a lot better than you do Edna and Bill [Pawley], I felt real bad." (Ibid.) See pp. 518–23.

6. See pp. 541–51.

7. This was added by Marshall's hand before it was sent.

317

MEMORANDUM FOR GENERAL OF THE ARMY OMAR N. BRADLEY — June 14, 1951
Confidential — Washington, DC

Subject: Cooperation and Coordination with the CIA

I get the impression that there is a very considerable reluctance, if not opposition, on the part of the services generally towards furthering the plans of General Smith of the CIA in the development of personnel to carry out a rather elaborate program of tasks. I realize that there are complications involved in this matter but the impression I get, correctly or incorrectly, is there is too little of a desire to cooperate in what to me is a very important function.[1]

I have not talked to General Smith in regard to this but he will probably call on me in regard to the long delays already in reaching decisions as to his various requests. I would like to have the view of the Chiefs of Staff in regard to this general phase of the matter.[2]

GCMRL/G. C. Marshall Papers (Secretary of Defense, Chronological, Secretaries, Ackerman)

1. See pp. 253–55 and 484–85. Smith had written to Marshall on March 5 and to Anna Rosenberg on April 30 to request JCS and DOD approval of a plan that would allow the armed forces to assign 150 "candidates" annually to the CIA "after their military service." In his April 30 letter to Rosenberg, Smith reported that in response to his March 5 letter, General Bradley had replied that the JCS had "certain reservations on this program because of budgetary considerations." Smith suggested a two-year trial period for this plan to Bradley. Considering the "extremely pressing" need for personnel in the CIA, he requested "an early decision" on what he deemed a "perfectly innocuous" program. (Smith to Rosenberg, April 30, 1951, NA/RG 330, CD 350.3.) The editors have been unable to locate Smith's March 5 letter to Marshall.

General Vandenberg reported to Marshall on May 16 that the JCS had considered Smith's proposal and determined that up to two hundred individuals could be trained each year for the CIA on a reimbursable basis as long as they were not ROTC graduates given the shortage of such individuals to meet service requirements. He attached a draft letter for Marshall's signature informing Smith of this decision. (Vandenberg to Marshall, memorandum and attachment, May 16, 1951, ibid.) Smith apparently received a copy of Vandenberg's proposed letter, and he urged Rosenberg on May 23 to support the acceptance of "this small project . . . without such restrictive conditions," reminding her that "after all, we *are* co-belligerents." (Smith to Rosenberg, memorandum, May 23, 1951, ibid.)

2. Bradley reported on June 15 that the JCS maintained their earlier views that due to the lack of surplus ROTC graduates, the CIA should be responsible for procuring person-

nel from other sources. If the CIA continued to "desire ROTC graduates," the JCS would be open to discussions about expanding the ROTC program, assuming such action would be financially supported by the CIA. (Bradley to Marshall, memorandum and attachment, June 15, 1951, ibid.)

Marshall replied to Bradley on June 22 that this response was "a prime example of the instances mentioned in my memorandum to you of June 14." He pointed out that the ROTC would produce approximately twelve thousand graduates each year and that the CIA request for two hundred of them would constitute "approximately 1.7% of our total intake and to my way of thinking is a nickel and dime proposition. After re-reading the two pleas from Smith, I am constrained to make the following comment on the JCS response 'The mountain labored and came forth with a mouse.' I think the time has come for some broad gauge consideration of this problem, but more particularly of our relationships with CIA. It should not be necessary to point out that I give every appearance of being completely dissatisfied with our actions in this regard to date." (Marshall to Bradley, June 22, 1951, ibid.)

Nevertheless Marshall agreed after meeting with the JCS on June 22 to sign and send the draft memorandum. He attached a handwritten note to Smith, however, stating that in light of his "long talk" with the JCS, they were "disposed to do all in their power to help you. Two of them had never seen the request for 600 [*200*]." Smith replied on July 5 that he appreciated "The proffered cooperation of the Services in training Agency career personnel" and was "grateful for your support in this matter." (Marshall to Smith, June 23, 1951, NA/RG 330, SD 040 [Central Intelligence Agency].)

ON JUNE 14, Senator McCarthy delivered a blistering attack on Marshall on the Senate floor. This was not his first assault on Marshall (see p. 84n2), but it was the lengthiest by far as well as the most vicious, with one journalist labeling it "one of the most bitter that ever has been made on a cabinet officer." While never actually using the word "treason," McCarthy in effect accused Marshall of just that by claiming he had made common cause with Stalin since World War II and was, along with Acheson, the leader of "a conspiracy so immense and an infamy so black as to dwarf any previous such venture in the history of man." Tiring after approximately three hours of speaking to a by-now nearly empty Senate chamber, McCarthy inserted the entire speech of almost sixty thousand words, drawn from what he deemed "statements from sources 'friendly' to Marshall," into the *Congressional Record* and later had it published as a book entitled *America's Retreat from Victory: The Story of George Catlett Marshall* (New York: Devin-Adair Company, 1951). For more on this speech see Pogue, *Statesman*, 488–90, and Thomas C. Reeves, *The Life and Times of Joe McCarthy: A Biography* (New York: Stein and Day, 1982), 371–74. ("Marshall Leads Red Plot, McCarthy Says," *Washington Post*, June 15, 1951, p. 21.)

Democratic Senate leaders maintained that McCarthy's speech "was not 'worthy of comment,'" and during its delivery the Defense Department sent to members of the press in the Senate gallery quotes that praised Marshall from the same books McCarthy had quoted in his speech. ("Marshall U.S. Foe, M'Carthy Charges," *New York Times*, June 15, 1951, p. 3; "Marshall Leads Red Plot, McCarthy Says," *Washington Post*, June 15, 1951, p. 21.) Hanson K. Baldwin (USNA, 1924), military editor of the *New York Times*, and author of *Great Mistakes of the War* (New York: Harper & Brothers, 1949), one of the books McCarthy used in his attack, wrote to assure Marshall that he did not "associate myself in any way" with McCarthy's "vitriolic attack. I have made an earnest attempt to be objective and fair—to criticize when I felt criticism was justified—but I have never believed and could never endorse the McCarthy methods." Marshall replied that he had "always regarded you as a highly respected member of your profession and it would have never occurred to me to associate you with any attack similar to which you wrote me about." (Baldwin to Marshall, July 10, 1951, and Marshall to Baldwin, July 16, 1951, GCMRL/G. C. Marshall Papers [Secretary of Defense, Number Indexed, M200-15-10].) See pp. 653, 721–22, and 852–55.

Marshall carefully avoided responding to or commenting on this or any other political attack, typically making only indirect references to recent events in his correspondence, as in the next document. ★

318

To Colonel Ralph D. Mershon June 18, 1951
Washington, DC

Dear Mershon: Your mangoes arrived in Leesburg Saturday in excellent condition. Mrs. Marshall and I were very appreciative, but what I really do appreciate very much is the fact that you still have me in mind. The other day I started to dictate a note to you to find out how you were doing as I had not heard from you or of you for a long time. I put the question now. And I do hope you are in excellent health.[1]

I had a pretty strenuous high speed trip to Korea but fortunately was able to include some successful rainbow trout fishing in the Aleutians on my way back home. And I have just had a very restful weekend, so I am back here in the game which is pretty strenuous because it is so highly political and viciously so.[2]

With warm regards and our thanks again. Faithfully yours,

GCMRL/G. C. Marshall Papers (Secretary of Defense, Number Indexed, M212-5-13)

1. Mershon, an eighty-four-year-old alumnus of The Ohio State University and a longtime friend of Marshall who was now in retirement in Florida, had been active in drafting legislation for the ROTC provision in the National Defense Act of 1916. From 1929 to 1936, Marshall had been a member of the board of the Civilian Military Education Fund, financed since its creation in 1928 "by the Ralph D. Mershon Fund in the New York Community Trust." The fund's goals were to improve civilian-military relations and to promote civilian military and reserve officer training. (Hayes to Marshall, June 25, 1951, GCMRL/G. C. Marshall Papers [Secretary of Defense, Number Indexed, M200-16-26]. See also *Papers of GCM*, 1: 386–87, 514, and 4: 586–87.)

As the New York Community Trust began to conclude the activites of the Civilian Military Educational Fund, Marshall wrote to the trust's director, Ralph Hayes, that "The Mershon Fund was most helpful in the efforts toward the enactment of the Universal Military Training Law." Marshall added in a statement requested by Hayes that Mershon and the Civilian Military Educational Fund had been "a strong voice for adequate national defense and universal military training," and "the nation owes Colonel Mershon a debt of gratitude for his generous and continuing contributions to keep the effort alive through a long period of years." (Marshall to Hayes, July 9, 1951, ibid.; Statement on the Mershon Fund, n.d.,

GCMRL/G. C. Marshall Papers [Secretary of Defense, Speeches and Statements].)

2. See the previous editorial note and pp. 548–51. Drew Pearson, who wrote the syndicated *Washington Merry-Go-Round* column and hosted a radio show, had attacked McCarthy in his June 17 broadcast for using "'the safety of his senatorial immunity'" to throw "'60,000 words of oral mud at Marshall.'" Edmund Coles informed Marshall of Pearson's defense, and Marshall replied that he had read a transcript of Pearson's remarks. "He is usually generous in his remarks of me," Marshall stated, "but now and then he takes me to task; however, in this business one must take the bitter with the sweet." (*Congressional Record* 97, pt. 5, 82d Cong., 1st sess., 6815; Coles to Marshall, June 18, 1951, and Marshall to Coles, June 20, 1951, GCMRL/G. C. Marshall Papers [Secretary of Defense, Number Indexed, M200-2-11].)

Marshall also thanked several members of Congress, including House Majority Leader John McCormack, who defended him in response to McCarthy's attack. (Marshall to McCormack, Marshall to Robertson, Marshall to Bolling, Marshall to Hays, and Marshall to Mitchell, June 22, 1951, GCMRL/G. C. Marshall Papers [Secretary of Defense, Chronological, Secretaries, Carlson]; Marshall to Jackson, June 27, 1951, ibid., [Hawkins]; Marshall to Shelley, Marshall to Mansfield, and Marshall to McCormack, June 28, 1951, GCMRL/G. C. Marshall Papers Secretary of Defense, Number Indexed, M200-15-10].)

319

To Lieutenant General James A. Van Fleet — June 18, 1951
Washington, DC

Dear Van Fleet: I should have written you earlier but I returned to Washington to find myself in a terrifically busy period for the following four days. Now, having just returned from a quiet weekend at Leesburg, I must take the time to tell you how much I appreciated the courtesies you showed me and the efforts you made to facilitate my visit to the Eighth Army. I realized that I was taking your time at a very critical period of your responsibility. I was duly appreciative.[1]

There is little I can say in regard to you and your Eighth Army other than my admiration for the magnificent job you are both doing. As you know, you have my complete confidence in the difficult business of fighting. I can only hope that a way out will soon be found. There seem to be some signs behind the scenes that the Chinese Communist regime is deeply troubled and considering ways and means of escaping from the tragic dilemma in which they find themselves. I hope these signs have a solid foundation but of course you never can tell.

I am calling up Mrs. Van Fleet to tell her how I found you because I know she will be interested in every small item of information regarding your welfare and your job.[2]

With warm regards and again my thanks. Faithfully yours,

GCMRL/James A. Van Fleet Papers (Korea, Personal Correspondence, Alphabetical)

1. See pp. 548–51.

2. Marshall spoke with Van Fleet's wife, Helen, on June 18. (Ackerman to Marshall, memorandum, n.d., GCMRL/G. C. Marshall Papers [Secretary of Defense, Number Indexed, M200-15-15].)

320

Statement on the Enactment of the Universal Military Training and Service Law of 1951

June 19, 1951
Washington, DC

The signing by the President a few minutes ago of the Universal Military Training and Service law represents a step of historic significance. It will enable us to face the uncertainties of an explosive international situation with the knowledge that we can be strong militarily without having to imperil our security economically, no matter how long the present world tension may continue. And it will permit us thereafter to continue strong militarily in keeping with our great purpose of promoting the peace of the world.[1]

My visit to the Far East battle area has left me more firmly convinced than ever that our best hope today for restoring peace lies in convincing the communist forces of Russia and her satellites that they cannot win.[2] By establishing this enduring base under the structure of our defense, we serve notice on the world that we are prepared to continue strong in all the elements of our great power—our armed forces, our industries, our farms, our scientific laboratories and our educational system.

The law does not contain all the provisions the Defense Department would have desired, but I am confident that Congress will enact the necessary supporting legislation to carry into actual effect the historic principles unified in the bill. The objective of a universally shared obligation for the defense of our country on a basis that we can support is now within our grasp, for the first time since George Washington began the pursuit of this goal a century and a half ago.[3]

GCMRL/G. C. Marshall Papers (Secretary of Defense, Speeches and Statements)

1. See pp. 551–53. Prior to the signing of the Universal Military Training and Service Bill (commonly referred to as UMST), Marshall had attended and spoken at the graduation exercises of the National War College at 10:00 a.m. The editors have been unable to locate a transcript of Marshall's remarks, but according to the *Washington Post*, Marshall "told members of the National War College graduating class that he had worked 30 years to bring about UMT and felt confident Congress would follow through with the further legislative action necessary to make it a fact." He urged "the graduates to give the program their 'unlimited support.'" ("Draft-UMT Bill Signed; Commission Appointed," *Washington Post*, June 20, 1951, pp. 1, 12.)

Marshall departed the Pentagon at noon along with Secretary Rosenberg to witness the signing of the UMST bill into law at the White House. "I should think that you would, and rightfully so, mark this day down in your little black book as one of high compliment and personal pleasure," Marshall wrote to Rosenberg that day. "I think it is a very fine coincidence that you should celebrate your birthday and on the same day to witness the signing into law of the Universal Military Training and Service Bill to which you gave so much effort, time, and an unlimited amount of patience. Mrs. Marshall, if she knew of my writing, would join me in heartiest congratulations on this special occasion." (Marshall to Rosenberg, June 19, 1951, GCMRL/G. C. Marshall Papers [Secretary of Defense, Number Indexed, M200-15-33].)

2. See pp. 548–51.

3. Marshall recorded this statement at 3:03 p.m.

After signing the law, Truman submitted to the Senate for confirmation the names of his nominees for the five-member National Security Training Commission: James Wadsworth;

Will Clayton; Karl T. Compton, president of MIT from 1930 to 1948 and chairman of Truman's Advisory Commission on Universal Training in 1946 and 1947; Admiral Thomas C. Kinkaid (USNA, 1908), commander of the Allied naval forces and the Seventh Fleet in the southwest Pacific during World War II; and Lieutenant General Raymond S. McLain, commander of the Forty-fifth Infantry Division artillery, the Ninetieth Infantry Division, and the XIX Corps during World War II. The Senate confirmed their nominations on June 29. ("Draft-U.M.T. Bill Signed by Truman," *New York Times*, June 20, 1951, pp. 1, 5; "Senate Confirms U.M.T. Board of 5," *New York Times*, June 30, 1951, p. 15.) See pp. 552–53n2.

Marshall wrote to Truman on June 20 to apologize "for walking out of your office yesterday and leaving behind the pen you had so graciously given me a few minutes earlier." He was "embarrassed especially because the entire meeting was a favor by you to a request of mine because I knew you had not originally been so disposed." Truman replied the following day that he understood "very well why the pen was on the radio set, because I knew that you had to make a statement to the press outside the office. Personally, I didn't see anything unusual in my calling you and giving you the pen. I am most happy that you left it because I don't know of any letter I have ever received that I appreciated more." (Marshall to Truman, June 20, 1951, and Truman to Marshall, June 21, 1951, GCMRL/G. C. Marshall Papers [Secretary of Defense, Number Indexed, M212-5-36].) See pp. 609–10, 679–80, and 877–78.

321

To Brien McMahon — June 20, 1951

Secret — Washington, DC

Dear Senator McMahon: Thanks for your letter of 2 May 1951 informing me of the resolution approved that date by the Joint Committee on Atomic Energy.[1]

I join heartily with the committee in its anxiety to avoid the crystallization of any issue which might ultimately lead to strong differences of opinion or to the absence of mutual cooperation. The suggestion that informal consultation might assist in ironing out the matter is particularly appealing.

In order to have an informal discussion of some of the factors surrounding this problem, could you, and several of your associates have lunch with me in my office sometime during the next ten days? If agreeable to you I will have my aide call your office to arrange a mutually convenient time and date.[2] Faithfully yours,

GCMRL/G. C. Marshall Papers (Secretary of Defense, Chronological, Secretaries, Ackerman)

1. The editors have not located McMahon's May 2 letter, but according to a record of Marshall's correspondence with McMahon created by Robert LeBaron, this letter indicated "that informal consultation, if necessary, might assist in orienting the thinking of the Joint Congressional Committee with respect to the views expressed in" Marshall's April 2 letter (see pp. 468–69). The resolution in question urged expansion of the Atomic Energy Commission's production facilities. On June 15, the JCS proposed a response for Marshall, although it was edited before being sent. (Robert LeBaron, "Log of Significant Events re JCS Proposed Response to Senator McMahon's Letter of 2 May 1951," June 19, 1951; and Bradley to Marshall, memorandum and attachment, June 15, 1951, NA/RG 330, CD 471.6; Hewlett and Duncan, *Forging the Atomic Shield*, 547.)

2. "There are some personal cross currents that have confused the primary problem," LeBaron warned Marshall on June 19, "and it might be well for me to stand by when you

meet with Sen. McMahon to make certain that secondary matters not related to the main issue are not brought into discussion and confused with the main question." LeBaron also offered to brief Marshall "on these personal elements" if so desired. (LeBaron to Marshall, memorandum, June 19, 1951, NA/RG 330, CD 471.6.)

The luncheon meeting took place on July 5, with Lovett, LeBaron, Representative Charles Melvin Price (D-IL), and William Borden, executive director of the Joint Congressional Committee on Atomic Energy, as well as Marshall and McMahon in attendance. "Both Lovett and Marshall spoke enthusiastically," the official history of the Atomic Energy Commission noted, "of the tremendous impact large numbers of nuclear weapons would have on military strategy." (Hewlett and Duncan, *Forging the Atomic Shield*, 548.) According to the official OSD history, "Marshall and Lovett agreed that some expansion, particularly of lightweight, tactical atomic weapons, might be useful; the Joint Chiefs also seemed interested." (Condit, *Test of War*, 469–70.) See pp. 616–17.

322

To General Matthew B. Ridgway — June 22, 1951
Washington, DC

Dear Ridgway: I returned here to a very strenuous four days, commencing with a congressional hearing the day I got in. In the circumstances I find I confused my writing to Mrs. Ridgway with the thought that I had written to you. Therefore I submit my thanks to you now with apologies for the long delay.[1]

You two did so much for my comfort that I cannot adequately thank you, but also I was deeply appreciative of the extreme care you took in making the arrangements for my visit to Korea and in looking after my interests in a very personal manner.

It is not necessary for me to tell you again what a magnificent job I think you did as commander of the Eighth Army and are now doing in your present position. I have every confidence in your sound judgment and in your courageous leadership. You have many great problems on your hands but at least I think you have a more healthy atmosphere in which to work than one lives in here in Washington these days.

With affectionate regards and my thanks again.[2] Faithfully yours,

P.S. I think I addressed Mrs. Ridgway with a surplus "e" in her name. Tell her that is a compliment and not a display of ignorance.

GCMRL/G. C. Marshall Papers (Secretary of Defense, Number Indexed, M200-7-7)

1. See pp. 537 and 548–51.

Marshall had upon his return from Korea sent Mrs. Ridgway a handwritten note of thanks that Marshall Carter enclosed with his own June 15 letter to her. Marshall used a draft letter that George had composed "as a guide" according to his secretary Mildred Carlson. (Marshall to Penny Ridgway, June 13, 1951, with Carlson note, GCMRL/G. C. Marshall Papers [Secretary of Defense, Number Indexed, M200-7-9]; Carter to Penny Ridgway, June 15, 1951, GCMRL/Marshall S. Carter Papers [Department of Defense, Correspondence].)

2. Katherine Marshall also wrote to Ridgway on June 30 to thank him for some photographs of Marshall's trip. She added that she prayed for Ridgway's "strength and wisdom to carry through . . . to a brilliant and successful end." Ridgway replied on July 9 to express his appreciation for all of the letters received from the Marshalls. (Katherine Marshall to

Ridgway, June 30, 1951, and Ridgway to Katherine Marshall, July 9, 1951, USAMHI/Matthew B. Ridgway Collection [Series 2: Correspondence, Subseries 1: Official Correspondence, CINCFE, L–M].)

323

To Albert P. Morano

June 22, 1951
Washington, DC

My dear Mr. Morano: I have your letter of June 12th reporting on your inspection of Camp Pickett last week. I appreciate your intense interest in the Division and am passing your letter to Secretary Pace so that he might know of your findings, and have requested that he take whatever action is deemed appropriate.[1]

There is one point, however, I would like to make clear. General Collins informs me that all National Guard divisions that have been called into active service have received identical directives, missions, and instructions, and your comment on "confusion" due to the 43rd's mission not being "clearly defined" is the first that has come to our attention. All such divisions have had approximately equal numbers of inductees assigned to them for training. All such divisions have been required to prepare themselves for combat duty. All such divisions have had at times service functions to perform. It is essential that these divisions be organized and commanded with such flexibility that they can assume any or all of these three functions with minimum dislocation of morale. It should be, in fact, this very flexibility that prevents a properly trained unit from going stale.[2]

Your attitude in the matter and your desire to be of help are appreciated. Faithfully yours,

GCMRL/G. C. Marshall Papers (Secretary of Defense, Number Indexed, M200-14-44)

1. Representative Morano (R-CT) had previously written to Marshall to express concern about "reports concerning the morale, living conditions and training conditions and training of the 43rd Division," which consisted of National Guardsmen from Connecticut, Vermont, and Rhode Island as well as draftees added to fill the ranks and was training at Camp Pickett, near Blackstone, Virginia. He sent similar letters to Senator Russell and Representative Vinson. ("Morano to Make Own Study Of Conditions at Camp Pickett," *Washington Post*, June 6, 1951, p. B2; "Guard Unit Held Abused," *New York Times*, June 4, 1951, p. 26.) See p. 293.

Morano's letter stemmed from a report in the June 4, 1951, issue of *Time* magazine which stated that the division was not combat ready, was experiencing very low morale, had not received all of the necessary equipment from the Defense Department, despite having arrived at Camp Pickett in September 1950, and had been dubbed the "crybaby division" by Pentagon officials. ("The Troubled 43rd," *Time* 57, no. 23 [June 4, 1951]: 25.)

Marshall replied on June 4 that he was referring the letter to Pace with directions to respond directly to Morano, while he would "personally follow through" to see that proper action was taken. Marshall added that the division had undergone the highest "degree of inspection . . . that I have ever heard of in my Army career," but this additional scrutiny had not revealed anything "that would justify" Morano's "unfavorable comments." Marshall suggested that Morano visit Camp Pickett to assess the problems in person. (Marshall to Morano, June 4, 1951, GCMRL/G. C. Marshall Papers [Secretary of Defense, Number Indexed, M200-14-44].)

Representative Winston Prouty (R-VT) also wrote to Marshall to complain about this issue, and Lovett replied in Marshall's absence. (Prouty to Marshall, June 5, 1951, quoted from *Congressional Record* 97, pt. 5, 82d Cong., 1st sess., 6626; Lovett to Prouty, June 7, 1951, GCMRL/G. C. Marshall Papers [Secretary of Defense, Number Indexed, M200-14-44].)

In a lengthy June 12 letter and report to Marshall following his inspection of Camp Pickett, Morano found "no basis" for the division to be called the "'Cry Baby Division'" and believed that any complaints about conditions at the camp "were perfectly justified." Much of the problem resulted from "*confusion*" about the division's role as "a combat unit, a service unit or a training unit," a clarification of which by the Pentagon would improve "the efficiency and the morale" of the division. (Morano to Marshall, June 12, 1951, NA/RG 330, SD 330.14.)

2. General Taylor reported to General Collins on June 20 that Marshall should clarify in his response to Morano that the "primary mission" of army reserve forces within the continental United States was "'to be trained, equipped, and maintained in a state of readiness for immediate use in an offensive or defensive role.'" (Taylor to Collins, June 20, 1951, ibid.)

324

To Frank McCarthy | June 22, 1951
Washington, DC

Dear Frank: I witnessed a showing of your movie, DECISION BEFORE DAWN, which you played such an important part in producing. I enjoyed it thoroughly and am only sorry that Katherine was not there to see it. Our Signal Corps people made the arrangements and there were only about five or six people in the projection room when it was run off. Incidentally, Joe Abbate was one of them.[1]

I thought the film was exciting and cleverly done and thought the young actor they called "Happy" turned in a superb performance.[2] I can well understand now the amount of detail which was involved, and the many hours you must have worked in perfecting the arrangements and in the actual filming of the picture.

Your picture was preceded by a very clever, short movie which ran approximately nine minutes on the Lexington affair. This film took in Washington and Lee, Jackson's Tomb, the Institute, my old room, the New Market Day celebration, and the dedication ceremony. Mr. Baruch was the feature player, and I had a small part![3]

Katherine has been spending all of her time at Leesburg, but came up Wednesday afternoon to be here to attend the dinner which President Truman gave in honor of the President of Ecuador. Last night we went to a dinner at the Army-Navy Country Club which Colonel Byroade gave for John McCloy, who is back here for a business visit. Tonight we go to the Statler Hotel for a dinner given by the President of Ecuador, reciprocating President Truman's party.[4]

The week so far has been pretty strenuous and I will have to remain in town for a meeting Saturday morning, but hope to leave immediately afterwards for the country. I have just learned from George that two beetles were seen on the grape arbor, so my work in the garden is pretty well cut out.

I hope that you are well and enjoying your activities on the west coast. I was pleased to see your name in large letters on the screen and it looks like you have made an excellent start in what should be a very interesting career.[5]

With love from us both, Affectionately,

GCMRL/G. C. Marshall Papers (Secretary of Defense, Number Indexed, M200-2-14)

1. Marshall had seen the film at 2:25 p.m. on June 18 at the Pentagon. The film did not premiere until December 21. See pp. 183–84n3 and 365. Abbate was Marshall's barber.

2. Oskar Werner played Corporal Karl "Happy" Maurer, a captured German soldier who volunteers to go behind German lines to provide intelligence on troop movements to the Allies.

3. See pp. 518–23.

4. Marshall had on June 14 received the invitation to attend Truman's June 20 dinner for the president of Ecuador and replied that he was already committed to address the Business Advisory Council that evening but could easily cancel that engagement if so desired. "I always attach particular importance to any engagement I have with you," Truman responded on the following day, "but it seems to me that the public's interest would be better served if you kept the previous engagement." Marshall nevertheless cancelled dinner with the Business Advisory Council to attend the White House dinner on June 20 after meeting with the Council for a luncheon earlier that day. (Marshall to Truman, June 14, 1951, and Truman to Marshall, June 15, 1951, GCMRL/G. C. Marshall Collection [Harry S. Truman]; "President Truman Honors Galo Plaza at State Dinner," *New York Times*, June 21, 1951, p. B5; Marshall to Business Advisory Council dinner committee, June 28, 1951, GCMRL/G. C. Marshall Papers [Secretary of Defense, Number Indexed, M214-13-29].) Henry A. Byroade was director of German affairs in the State Department.

5. *Decision Before Dawn* was nominated for an Academy Award in the best picture category in 1952. It lost to *An American in Paris*.

McCarthy replied on July 2 that he was "delighted to know that you saw DECISION BEFORE DAWN, and I am really thankful to you for taking time out of your busy day to look at it." He told Marshall that he had seen "newsreel coverage" of the Marshall Day ceremony and regretted that he could not attend in person. McCarthy added that he hoped to be in Washington "for some research in the State Department within the next two weeks or so." (McCarthy to Marshall, July 2, 1951, ibid., [M200-2-14].) Marshall met with McCarthy at 4:05 p.m. on July 9.

325

Memorandum for General of the Army Omar N. Bradley — June 26, 1951
Top Secret — Washington, DC

I enclose a statement concerning plans for United States forces in defense of Western Europe and the Joint Chiefs of Staff position on North Atlantic Treaty Organization (NATO) force levels, which was approved by the President on 25 June 1951. This approval was given after consideration of the major factors involved and therefore constitutes the initial United States position on the matter.[1]

I also enclose a letter from the Chairman, International Security Affairs Committee, Mr. Thomas D. Cabot, dated 26 June, 1951, which constitutes the best available reply to your request of 28 May 1951, for an economic and financial evaluation of the proposed United States position on forces for the Medium Term Defense Plan. I am forwarding this report to you for consideration by the Joint Chiefs of Staff. The tenor of the report shows the advisability of reviewing the distribution by country of the "Gap", both at this time and as negotiations proceed, but I leave to your judgment the desirability of modifications to your proposal.[2]

I approve the proposals made in the last three paragraphs of Mr. Cabot's letter and request that the Joint Chiefs of Staff instruct the United States Representative to the Standing Group accordingly. I desire that you keep me informed on this action and that we work closely with other United States Representatives in NATO on the various aspects of the problem.

In order to put substance into the ensuing negotiations with the European nations concerning defense levels, the President has approved the principles embodied in the enclosed public statement to be made to the United States Congress as to the outlook on continued United States aid.[3]

NA/RG 330, CD 091.7 (Europe)

1. At their October 1950 meeting (see pp. 218–20), the NATO defense ministers had approved a revised Medium Term Defense Plan (MTDP) which, according to the OSD official history, "projected a military buildup sufficient to deter an attack or, if one occurred, to permit establishment of a strong European defense line," with a July 1, 1954, target date. Despite agreeing to this plan in principle, many of the European governments were concerned about the funds needed to meet these goals. Having further reviewed the MTDP following the December 1950 Brussels defense ministers meeting (see pp. 303–4n1), the Standing Group realized the emergence of a growing "gap" between total military forces required to fulfill NATO defense plans and the forces that the allies could reasonably provide. The Standing Group thus requested that each NATO country evaluate its manpower potential in an effort to eliminate this gap. The JCS provided Marshall on May 28, 1951, with "a tentative force list for 1954" to be reviewed by the interdepartmental International Security Affairs Committee (ISAC), led by Thomas Cabot, in light of that committee's study of European production and mobilization capabilities, as the JCS believed "that a final position could not be derived purely from military considerations." (Condit, *Test of War*, 369–71; Poole, *History of JCS*, 4: 125–27.)

On June 21, Marshall met with Acheson, Bradley, and other representatives from the State, Defense, and Treasury Departments, the ECA, Bureau of the Budget, and the White House to discuss the ISAC's conclusions. During this meeting Marshall "emphasized that we are buying European manpower in place of U.S. manpower. The European people have real economic problems resulting from the war. They have lost great numbers of men and they have a difficult Communist vote problem. In helping them solve these problems and get ahead with the defense effort with U.S. assistance, we are defending the U.S. It is essential that we not mislead the Congress on possible costs and we must make clear that they will be as heavy or heavier thereafter." He also thought "we should restate more positively what our plan is and what commitments we have. The divisions required for 1952 are all committed. We can and should explain to Congress that we have yet to secure commitments, and are now going after them for those required by 1954. We must, by this course, back Eisenhower, or frankly give up supporting him." Marshall also accentuated "the need for making clear that the problem of the Europeans in terms of standard of living is wholly different from the U.S. situation. A five-percent cut to the Europeans is the difference between white bread and black bread on the table; for us it is the difference between having radios and televisions, etc. It is also essential to make clear what a great loss to U.S. security the loss of the industrial potential of the Ruhr and of Eastern France would be." General Bradley was also "reluctant to press the Europeans for too much now." (*FRUS, 1951*, 3: 197, 201–2.)

The group reached no new conclusions at this meeting but agreed to send Truman a statement of the JCS proposal for increased US military contributions to NATO through the period of the MTDP, which Marshall did on June 23. According to this statement, "The general extent of the United States obligation" through fiscal year 1954 would include "a total of 13 United States divisions by 90 days after the opening of any hostilities" in

Europe, six of which would "be stationed in Europe by the end of 1951," thus satisfying "our present commitments to General Eisenhower." The other seven divisions would be sent to Europe within ninety days of the beginning of hostilities with the Soviets, with the decision as to whether they should be dispatched before hostilities commenced to be decided "as the situation develops." By this plan, the US would contribute approximately 13 percent of NATO's ground forces. The JCS also recommended that the US offer to NATO "a total of 22 wings" from the air force (15 percent of total NATO air strength), an increase of fourteen wings from what had been approved previously, and "39 additional small naval vessels above the 470 United States vessels, all types, now obligated" (25 percent of total NATO naval strength). "The bulk of the NATO forces are supplied by our Allies under the Medium Term Defense Plan," this statement concluded. Truman approved the statement orally during a June 25 meeting at Blair House and in writing on June 27. (Condit, *Test of War*, 371–72; Poole, *History of JCS*, 4: 127–28; Beebe to Conway, June 26, 1951, and Conway to Beebe, June 27, 1951, and attached statement, "United States Forces in Defense of Western Europe," NA/RG 330, CD 091.7 [Europe].) See pp. 497–99.

2. The editors have been unable to locate Cabot's letter, but according to a summary by General Burns, it enclosed "an ECA estimate that Europe will be unable to pay for the forces that we are proposing they should raise." In light of this, Cabot suggested that the JCS might, in the words of the official JCS history, "soften the impact" of its proposal by informing the Standing Group "that non-military factors might legitimately lessen the commitments expected from particular countries." Marshall agreed with this suggestion. (Burns to Marshall, memorandum, June 26, 1951, NA/RG 330, CD 091.7 [Europe]; Poole, *History of JCS*, 4: 128. See also Cabot's June 25 letter to Marshall in *FRUS, 1951*, 4: 205–7, which deals with the same issues.) The lengthy and detailed ECA estimate included a country-by-country analysis and concluded that "if the forces Gap is made up by the European countries, the economic cost of the Gap will in all probability have to be made up by U.S. economic and military aid." ("Economic Analysis of the Allocation of the MTDP Gap to European Countries," June 23, 1951, NA/RG 59, Decimal File, 1950–54 [740.5/6-2551].)

3. This statement is not attached to the version of the document available at the Marshall Library, but Marshall was in all likelihood referring to a statement Truman approved to provide "guidance to witnesses" during the forthcoming congressional hearings on the Mutual Security Program with "respect to US aid to NATO partners in FY 1953 and FY 1954." Acheson forwarded to Spofford on June 26 a copy of this statement, which said that US appropriations for military assistance to NATO in fiscal years 1953 and 1954 would need to be "'as large as those requested for the current fiscal year, and maybe larger.'" Only after the completion of "'the build-up of North Atlantic Treaty forces'" under the MTDP can "'the amount of aid . . . be substantially reduced.'" (*FRUS, 1951*, 3: 210–11.) See pp. 569–77 and 597–603.

The JCS "provided the Standing Group with somewhat altered recommendations on tentative forces" in late July, including Cabot's suggestion mentioned in n2 above. (Condit, *Test of War*, 372; Poole, *History of JCS*, 4: 128.)

326

To John J. Scanlon

June 27, 1951
Washington, DC

My dear Mr. Scanlon: Thank you for your letter of June 13th enclosing a copy of your editorial which was to appear in THE SPECTATOR, in conjunction with the Convention of the American Legion at Roselle Park. I appreciate your generous comments regarding my career, and this evidence of support and confidence.[1]

While you were very complimentary to me, I was greatly disturbed by your comments about the United States Military Academy. I have the greatest admiration for it and think it to be one of the finest schools in the world. Frankly, I found throughout my entire service, particularly as I neared the top in the Army, that my strongest helpers and closest friends were graduates of the Academy. Today, three alumni of the Academy are members of the Joint Chiefs of Staff. I am sorry that you so freely and publicly criticized the Academy, as I strongly feel that you are not justified in saying the things about it that you did.

I have attempted to be utterly frank in what I had to say in the matter and hope you will understand the sincerity of my remarks.

With my thanks again for what you had to say about me personally, Faithfully yours,

GCMRL/G. C. Marshall Papers (Secretary of Defense, Number Indexed, M204-2-34)

1. John J. Scanlon, editor of the Roselle, New Jersey, *Spectator*, had sent Marshall on June 13 an editorial he had written, entitled "The Marshall Story," that would be published in the following day's issue, which he hoped would "bring the truth to our readers" and serve "as a tribute to a great American." He offered to publish any comments Marshall might wish to make. The editorial called Marshall "a man who perhaps travelled the hardest road to the top ever traversed by an American citizen," as he "never attended that imposing citadel on the Jersey side of the Hudson River," West Point. "There was no short cut to the goal he had set for himself, no loving mother to stay at West Point during her son's four years of matriculation," a reference to MacArthur's experience. "Today's anti-Marshall campaign by the 'West Point clique,'" he continued, "does not phase [*faze*] the general one iota." (Scanlon to Marshall, June 13, 1951, and attachment, GCMRL/G. C. Marshall Papers [Secretary of Defense, Number Indexed, M204-2-34].)

Marshall Carter noted that in response, Marshall had said to use a copy of his recent speech at West Point (see pp. 544–46) and "blast this fellow." Carter and George drafted two replies to Scanlon for Marshall's signature, one giving "him both barrels" and the other more subdued. Marshall "bought the 21 gun barrage." The editors have only located the version of Marshall's reply as it was sent to Scanlon and have been unable to determine if these comments were published in the *Spectator*. (Carter memorandum, n.d.; George to Marshall, memorandum, n.d., ibid.; George to Carter, June 29, 1951, GCMRL/G. C. Marshall Papers [Secretary of Defense, Chronological, Secretaries, Hawkins].)

327

Memorandum for the Deputy Secretary — June 28, 1951
Top Secret — Washington, DC

Subject: Public and Congressional Reaction to the Effect of Malik Proposals[1]

In NSC discussions yesterday of the problem of meeting the inevitable public and legislative relaxation due to the possibility of a cease-fire in Korea, I made the following statement which I quote for your information and consideration:

"It seems to me the psychological advantages are not all against us because if we do secure a satisfactory cease-fire agreement in Korea, it will go to prove our policies in the matter of that campaign were correct. That is a positive advantage.

"On the other hand, mere speeches, articles and columns will not suffice to offset the dangerous reaction which is almost bound to follow a cease-fire agreement.

"In thinking this over, it seems to me that we should make some motion immediately after a Korean agreement, if we get one, which would indicate the necessity for a further build up of our strength. Off-hand, my first thought is that we might ask of Congress an increase in airplane production. This to indicate that apparently there is some justification for not only the continued urgency of our military build up but the necessity for an immediate increase in our present program."[2]

Mr. Wilson [ODM director], to my surprise, voiced enthusiastic approval and thought we would have to go along with a similar increase in electronics—which I suppose would be the case. He went so far as to state he would like to see 100% increase because he felt that while it gave him more reassurance, it would precipitate the institution of cut backs and necessary control procedures which up to the present time they have been avoiding, and would get the defense mobilization procedure on a sounder basis.

I have just been told that inquiries are already coming into the various draft boards asking whether or not it is desired that the individual report in view of the peace talks. General Hershey's office reports that large numbers of these inquiries are being received there. Furthermore, we are receiving similar inquiries from reservists who are under call.

I would like you to think this over and let me have your views at the next Armed Forces Policy Council meeting.

GCMRL/G. C. Marshall Papers (Secretary of Defense, Selected, MacArthur)

1. Coincident with the failure of the fifth Chinese offensive in Korea, planning began for secret Soviet-American discussions regarding the possibility of an armistice in Korea. On the evening of June 23, Soviet UN representative Jacob Malik publicly proposed in a UN radio broadcast a "peaceful settlement of the Korean question," with a "first step" being the start of discussions "for a cease-fire and an armistice providing for the mutual withdrawal of forces from the thirty-eighth parallel." (*FRUS, 1951*, 7: 421–22, 460–62, 483–86, 507–511, 546–47, quotes on 546–47.) See pp. 592–95.

It is unclear whether Marshall ever sent this memorandum to Lovett, even though he extensively edited the draft, as the word "Cancel" is written in the left margin next to the second paragraph in the quote. The editors have been unable to determine whether that referred to just the paragraph or the entire memorandum. Either way the memorandum clearly expresses his thoughts on the matter.

2. The NSC meeting took place on June 27 at 3:30 p.m. and covered numerous topics in addition to Korea. According to Acheson, "There was considerable discussion of the Malik proposals, with no decision being reached. The general conclusion was that truce proposals should be most seriously pursued." ("Notes from Secretary of State Dean Acheson Regarding National Security Council Meeting, June 27, 1951," HSTL/Dean G. Acheson Papers [Secretary of State File, Memoranda of Conversations File, 1949–1953].)

328

To Dean G. Acheson — June 28, 1951
Secret — Washington, DC

Dear Mr. Secretary: Reference is made to the draft Japanese peace treaty received on 15 June 1951 from Mr. John Foster Dulles, special representative of the

President in relation to Japanese peace treaty matters. The Joint Chiefs of Staff have considered this draft peace treaty. Their views and comments, which have my general concurrence, are forwarded herewith.[1]

With regard to paragraphs 3 to 8, inclusive, of the Joint Chiefs of Staff comments, it is my understanding, based on a conference with Mr. Dulles, that the recommendations made by the Joint Chiefs of Staff have been under discussion between our two Departments and will present no difficulty for incorporation into the treaty.[2]

On the question of signature of the treaty by Communist China, raised in paragraph 9 of the Joint Chiefs of Staff memorandum, it is my understanding that China will not be permitted to sign this treaty. I should appreciate your confirmation of this.[3]

The first sentence of paragraph 10 of the memorandum indicates clearly that the Joint Chiefs of Staff would object to this treaty coming into force as between Japan and any of the allied powers until after the date of its ratification by the United States. As a result of my discussion with Mr. Dulles, I am aware of the difficulty which this point of view raises and I recognize that it may not be practicable to give the United States such unlimited control over the actions of its sovereign allies, as this sentence would seem to call for. In view, however, of serious objection raised by the Joint Chiefs of Staff, I suggest that the matter be brought to the attention of the President at the earliest possible date for resolution.[4] Faithfully yours,

NA/RG 330, CD 387 (Japan)

1. See pp. 485–87. Dulles had forwarded to Marshall on June 15 a copy of the draft Japanese Peace Treaty that he and Herbert Morrison, Bevin's successor as British foreign minister, had agreed to the previous day in London. Dulles informed Marshall that it would be discussed with other concerned powers as soon as it received formal US and British approval, and he requested "a prompt expression of any comments you may care to make." (Dulles to Marshall, June 15, 1951, NA/RG 330, CD 387 [Japan]. For the text of the June 14 draft, see *FRUS, 1951*, 6: 1119–33. See also ibid., 989–92 and 1019–21.)

2. Bradley offered the comments of the JCS in a four-page memorandum to Marshall on June 26. Paragraphs three through eight of this memorandum discussed the need for US ratification of the treaty before termination of the state of war; the sole authority of the United States to control certain former Japanese islands at least until the UN took "favorable action" on a US request for a strategic trusteeship over the islands; a clarification of language to ensure that sovereignty over any such islands as well as Formosa and several others could not revert to Communist China; distinctions between Allied forces of occupation and those stationed in Japan due to mutual security arrangements; Japan's obligation to recognize all treaties with Allied nations but not between the USSR and Soviet bloc countries, including Communist China; and Japan's right to refuse any negotiations with Communist China. (Bradley to Marshall, memorandum, June 26, 1951, NA/RG 330, CD 387 [Japan].) For the full memorandum, see *FRUS, 1951*, 6: 1156–59.

3. Paragraph nine expressed the concern of the JCS that some language in the draft treaty would entitle Communist China to "qualify as an Allied Power and thus be accorded all the rights and benefits of an Allied Power accruing to the signators." Acheson confirmed later on June 28 that "China will not be permitted to sign this Treaty." (Bradley to Marshall, memorandum, June 26, 1951, and Acheson to Marshall, June 28, 1951, ibid.)

4. Paragraph ten reiterated the opinion of the JCS that the treaty should be revised to affirm that it must not come into force until it was ratified by the United States, no matter

the action of the other signatories. In addition, if the treaty was "to become effective prior to the completion of hostilities in the Far East," it should contain a provision allowing the United States to continue to base troops in Japan "whether or not under United Nations aegis." (Bradley to Marshall, memorandum, June 26, 1951, ibid.) The current draft stated that should the US not ratify the treaty within nine months following its ratification by Japan, any Allied country that had ratified it during that period could "bring the Treaty into force between itself and Japan." (*FRUS, 1951*, 6: 1131.) Also being negotiated at this time was a security treaty with Australia and New Zealand, a draft of which Dulles had sent to Marshall on June 27 following consideration of previous JCS objections. (Dulles to Marshall, June 27, 1951, NA/RG 330, CD 387 [Japan]. See pp. 485–87 and *FRUS, 1951*, 6: 207, 989–92.)

Acheson replied to Marshall later on June 28, stating that he concurred that the JCS recommendations could all be accommodated, "except in relation to Paragraph 10." As Marshall had suggested, Acheson then sent Truman a memorandum on this matter, in which he argued for retention of the present language on the grounds that it "will give us veto over the treaty coming into force in any respect until about July 1, 1952," that this veto had been obtained "only with great difficulty," and that attempting to secure a "perpetual" veto would fail and would contradict actions by the United States to "vigorously and repeatedly" condemn the Soviet Union's effort to obtain such a veto. Regarding the JCS concerns about future access to bases in Japan, Acheson believed the existing arrangement would be "fully protected." Should "hostilities persist into next year," Acheson "assumed that the other Allied Powers" would cooperate to prevent any enactment of the treaty provisions "which would embarrass our common effort." Acheson thus recommended that the entire June 14 draft be circulated to the governments of the other Allied nations "with minor textual modifications" to address the JCS concerns that did "not involve security or important substantive considerations." (Acheson to Marshall, and Acheson to Truman, memorandum, June 28, 1951, ibid.)

Following a cabinet meeting on June 29, Truman discussed this issue with Acheson, Bradley, and Lovett, who represented Marshall while the latter was testifying before the House Foreign Affairs Committee (see next two documents). During this conversation, Acheson and Bradley reiterated their points outlined in their earlier respective memorandums, and Lovett relayed the sentiment of Marshall that the State Department's opinion should "be pretty nearly controlling" on this matter. Marshall, according to Lovett, believed the State Department and Dulles "had accomplished a great deal by having" the other nations "waive their rights for nine months after the Japanese ratification" and suspected that "an attempt to renegotiate this" might "do harm." Truman verbally approved Acheson's recommendation to proceed with the June 14 draft language at the conclusion of this June 29 meeting and in writing on July 3. (*FRUS, 1951*, 6: 1161, 1163–64.)

329

STATEMENT BEFORE THE HOUSE FOREIGN AFFAIRS COMMITTEE ON THE MUTUAL SECURITY PROGRAM — June 29, 1951, Washington, DC

Three years ago, as Secretary of State, I appeared before the Congress in support of a plan to assist the countries of Europe to recover from the devastating effects of a major war.[1]

These countries had emerged from the war with disrupted economies and war-weary populations. Congress, in recognizing the fact that this situation endangered the establishment of a lasting peace, enacted into law the Economic Cooperation Act of 1948.

As the reviving economies of Europe diminished the threat of internal subversion, the fear of external aggression became the great menace to the stability of our common effort.

The Mutual Defense Assistance Act of 1949 was a recognition of the existence of the disruptive element of aggressive force. Now in 1951 our goal continues to be a free world of nations with strong and healthy economies.[2]

I am here today in support of a Mutual Security Program which integrates our programs of military and economic assistance as a bulwark against the threat of these aggressive forces.

There are in the world two great centers of power and influence. One of these is the family of the free nations. The other is the Soviet-controlled group. The United States is the keystone of the free world, and must be the leader in resisting the Soviet threat.

The strength of a nation does not depend alone on its armies, ships, and planes; it is also measured by its qualities for leadership, by its resources and industries, by the determination of its people, and by the strength of its friends and allies.

We are now engaged in building up our military and materiel strength, and as part of that effort we are assisting other nations in preparations for their own defense, those nations whose strength will contribute to our security.

The security of the United States rests on our own strength and on our unity with the other friendly nations. To develop unity this government has joined in regional arrangements through the North Atlantic Treaty and the Rio Pact.[3]

It would be quite unwise for us to rely solely on our own strength. The most effective and least costly means of insuring the security of the United States is through collective security. Less than two years ago the Congress, by passing the Mutual Defense Assistance Act and ratifying the North Atlantic Treaty, recognized this factor and formally endorsed the concept of collective security.

This has seen its greatest realization in the development of the North Atlantic Treaty Organization. The other free nations of the world are receiving our assistance to organize their defenses. This is a project of self interest for this country, of the highest and most pressing urgency.

Our experience with the administration of military assistance to free nations since 1949 has been encouraging. The free world is stronger today because of such military assistance and the strength will grow.

I am not implying that we have solved all problems of mutual defense or that they will be solved completely in the next year, but I do believe that the results already attained justify further American investment in a Mutual Security Program.

I have stressed the world "mutual" because this must be basically a program of partnership. The nations that have been given assistance have joined with us in collective security measurements.

They are raising, training, and organizing troops to support mutual security. They lack certain items of military equipment that they cannot produce or cannot produce in time to meet planned mobilization schedules.

Our assistance basically consists therefore in furnishing them with certain matériel and equipment and of helping them to develop their own organization, training, and production facilities so that they can more readily take care of themselves. In other words, we propose to help them to help themselves.

The extent of the mutual assistance already given the free nations since the enactment of the Mutual Defense Assistance Program in 1949 and through May 1951 has been significant.

There has been shipped more than 1,400,000 measurement tons of equipment, exclusive of aircraft and naval vessels delivered under their own power, as follows:

Eight hundred and ninety thousand tons to the countries of Western Europe; 380,000 tons to the Middle East, and 160,000 tons to the Far East. The major items of equipment already transferred include more than 4,300 tanks and combat vehicles, 2,750 major artillery pieces, 18,000 general purpose vehicles, 850 aircraft, and more than 175 naval vessels and small craft.

Boxed and crated equipment included small arms, mortars, recoilless rifles, bazookas, electronic equipment, and millions of rounds of ammunition. This equipment is valued at more than one billion dollars.

To insure proper use of the equipment and to provide a nucleus of instructors for improved training within their military establishments, our armed forces schools in this country and abroad are training, or have already graduated, as a part of the military assistance program, more than 12,000 foreign students.

With the aid of the military items already furnished, the nations concerned have now laid the foundation for their more effective defense. There should be a continuous growth of real strength as deliveries of military equipment are increased.

The campaign in Indochina offers an excellent example of the practical effect of such deliveries. In January, the Communist Viet Minh troops, equipped and trained by the Soviets and their satellites, were driving in full force against Hanoi, the capital of Tonkin.

The timely arrival permitted the use by the Franco-Vietnamese troops of planes, artillery, and napalm bombs supplied under the Mutual Defense Assistance Program in halting the Communist attack less than 20 miles from its objective. Some of the equipment was landed in Indochina less than two weeks before the battle.[4]

While the courageous conduct of the French and Vietnam troops was responsible for this military success, the timely military aid may well have provided the needed margin for victory.

That victory has served Vietnam as a tonic. Since then it has steadily increased its armed forces. It has greatly expanded its training programs. It has pledged 55 percent of its revenue to national defense.

While Vietnam is the most dramatic example of the impact of United States aid in stemming the aggressive aims of the Kremlin, the result of such support in Greece, Turkey, and the Philippines has been far reaching.[5]

A crucial test of the success of the Mutual Security Program must be met in Western Europe. Military assistance to these nations offers the best prospect for the success of our collective security efforts.

The North Atlantic Treaty Organization has been in existence less than 2 years.

The members have agreed to concentrate on the creation of balanced collective forces for the NATO area as a whole rather than attempt to build up in each country the forces deemed necessary for its own independent defense.

The acceptance of the principle involving difficult and often unpopular departures from national traditions demonstrated a willingness to rely on others for tasks vital to a nation's own defense.

The North Atlantic Treaty Organization has recently improved the machinery of its operations. It has taken affirmative steps to mobilize defense efforts. The military committee, its standing group and subordinate command headquarters have been established and are operating.

General Bradley, who represents the United States on the military committee, will discuss this subject with you.[6]

The recommendations of the military committee as to the forces to be provided by each member country have been approved by the Defense Ministers and received governmental agreement as the desired objective.[7]

The Defense Ministers have recommended to their respective countries the adoption of basic principles for effective training and mobilization procedures and measures for the maintenance of sufficient trained military manpower. The establishment of an integrated defense force has been approved and is in process of organization under the leadership of General Eisenhower.[8]

The organization of the military procurement and production of the NATO nations is being pressed so as to secure the maximum production at least cost and in the shortest time possible.

All of the NATO countries (in Western Europe), except Iceland which has no army, have compulsory military service. Since the signing of the Treaty, five have extended their training periods.

All of them have tightened the conditions for exemption from military service. Since the receipt of equipment from the United States, the quality of training among all of them has improved. Morale has improved. The confidence and the determination of our Treaty partners has grown considerably in the past year. An added sense of urgency has been developed among them.

The United States has taken more positive steps to meet the dangers of our times than have the governments of Europe. I regret to report that some, for one reason or another, have not seemed to do all that they could do. They have their problems, of course, but so do we, I make this comment because we should not build up in any one country a false sense of security in the belief that present efforts are adequate.

In the Near East, in response to request for aid, we have entered on a grant basis into bilateral mutual defense assistance agreements with Greece, Turkey and Iran.[9] Improved conditions in Greece and Turkey today are in great measure the result of such assistance.

We are continuing our mutual assistance to these three countries to enable them to maintain internal security and to increase their capability to resist external aggression.

The maintenance of stable conditions in this area is just as important as the development of military strength. Economic stability and military security taken together are the most dependable antidotes to communism.

In Asia, we are proceeding along similar lines. In Formosa we are strengthening its military defenses and have increased both the size and the scope of our military assistance advisory group to that island. In Indochina and in the Philippine Islands our military assistance continues to support successfully operations against the spread and influence of aggressive communism.[10]

In the Western Hemisphere the need for cooperative defense has become increasingly clear to our American neighbors. Under existing legislation, we have been providing them with military equipment on a reimbursable basis. We have assisted Canada in her rearmament program. We have also made considerable progress in the standardization of equipment among the nations of the Western Hemisphere.[11]

At their meeting in Washington earlier this year, the Foreign Ministers of the American Republics charged the Inter-American Defense Board with preparing as vigorously as possible the military planning for their common defense.[12]

That task is now being rapidly carried forward. To assure a more active role in the defense of the Western Hemisphere by the Latin American Republics a plan of grant aid will have to be undertaken.

The full program should associate the military and strategic resources of the other American Republics with those of the United States and assure the delivery of essential strategic materials and the accomplishment of hemisphere defense tasks.

I have dwelt largely upon the military assistance aspects of the Mutual Security Program. Now I wish to emphasize the great importance of its economic features. Under the Economic Cooperation Act of 1948 the free nations of the world have made a remarkable economic and spiritual recovery.

Now when they are in a position to reap the advantages of their renaissance, they find themselves, just as we find ourselves, in a position where we must strain our economy to become sufficiently strong in a military way to deter, and if necessary to resist, aggression.

The need for prompt rearmament and the importance of giving economic support to the defense of the free nations make it essential that economic assistance be continued by the United States.

Economic aid in varying size for the individual nations will be required for the following general purposes:

1. To support rearmament programs among nations which might become impoverished if they had to depend solely on themselves.

2. To enable some nations to produce their own munitions, especially in Europe where armament facilities can be adapted to produce modern equipment. Such production could relieve the United States ultimately of a continuing grant-aid program.

3. To assist in the financing and building of civil facilities required to meet

military plans, such as communications, airfields, and harbors.

4. To strengthen the underdeveloped areas of extremely low standards of living, low standards of literacy, poor conditions of sanitation and health and high death rates. There a large part of the world's natural resources are found and there the Communists are trying to exploit the impoverished situation to their advantage. It is the tradition of the United States to aid the aspirations of people to improve their lot. This is the time when American self-interest and the welfare of the peoples in the undeveloped areas become a common cause which can be advanced by a judicious distribution of our economic assistance.

In urging these measures of foreign aid, the Defense Department is keenly aware of the cost involved and especially that this cost must be added to the funds required for the defense of this country and its interests overseas.

Foreign aid will represent about 15 percent of our total defense budget. We consider the investment necessary because we believe that it will strengthen the security of America and of the free nations.

The duration of the military assistance program must depend on future events. All things being equal, and I realize that things will not remain static, I feel that the requirement for funds for our Military Assistance Program will be at least the same level in fiscal year 1953 and in fiscal year 1954 as is being requested for this fiscal year.

Thereafter most of the European countries should be in full production, their initial rearmament well under way, with general financial capabilities to maintain such a level of defense, so that their requirements for military end items from the U.S. can be substantially reduced.

The requirements of each of the nations participating in this Mutual Security Program have been examined carefully in the light of our own plans and resources, and the capabilities of each nation to help itself. The program is designed to keep war from our shores, to discourage attack on ourselves and our friends, and to support the principles of freedom which are our heritage.

In brief, I believe that the Mutual Security Program, which will be presented to you by other witnesses in more detail, should be authorized by the Congress of the United States.

I would like to add more informally, Mr. Chairman, an expression of my feeling that this program is integrated with our general program, specifically our recent budget request of the Congress for some $60,000,000,000. All of these matters have been considered together. At the present time I consider the foreign aid program of major importance to be done as quickly as it can be managed. It has tremendous importance—tremendous significance—and a great psychological influence on what happens in the world among our friends.[13]

House Committee on Foreign Affairs, *Hearings . . . on H.R. 5020 and H.R. 5113, The Mutual Security Program*, 82d Cong., 1st sess., 81–86.

1. See *Papers of GCM*, 6: 309–28.
2. See ibid., 741–43.
3. See ibid., 203–5, 681–82, 705, 717.

4. See pp. 194–203, 320–22, and 357–60. See also Fredrik Logevall, *Embers of War: The Fall of an Empire and the Making of America's Vietnam* (New York: Random House, 2012), 260–71, and *History of the Joint Chiefs of Staff: The Joint Chiefs of Staff and the First Indochina War, 1947–1954* (Washington: Office of Joint History, Office of the Chairman of the Joint Chiefs of Staff, 2004), 70–71.
5. See *Papers of GCM*, 6: 67–68, 391–96.
6. Bradley testified before this committee on July 13. (House Committee on Foreign Affairs, *Hearings . . . on H.R. 5020 and H.R. 5113*, 285–316.)
7. See pp. 563–65.
8. See pp. 497–99.
9. The US and Iran had signed a mutual defense assistance agreement on May 23, 1950. (*FRUS, 1950*, 5: 551–52; "U.S. Agrees to Give Arms Aid to Iran," *New York Times*, May 24, 1950, p. 7.)
10. See pp. 300–303, 306–7, 426–27, 429–31, 438–39, and 486–87.
11. See pp. 434–35.
12. See pp. 414–17.
13. This final paragraph was not included in Marshall's reading copy of his statement, which can be found in GCMRL/G. C. Marshall Papers (Secretary of Defense, Speeches and Statements). See the next editorial summary.

330

House Testimony on the Mutual Security Act of 1951
June 29 and July 2, 1951 Washington, DC

Friday, June 29, 1951

FOLLOWING Marshall's prepared statement (see previous document), Committee Chairman James P. Richards (D-SC) began the question-and-answer session by asking "from the standpoint of security, how does this proposal compare with the $60,000,000,000 budget request in importance?" Marshall replied that in his view, the funding for the Mutual Security Program was "the more important at the moment," but he clarified that "Both programs are part and parcel of the general plan, and they could have been put in a one-budget approach to the Congress." Proposing the two bills separately removed the "difficulty in making clear the various issues involved, and just what portion was foreign aid, and what portion was" the regular budget. "This particular bill will create a very impressive reaction all over the world among our friends," he continued. "It is exceedingly important that they have the earliest possible assurance that we are going ahead with the general build-up plans. This is a part of these plans. . . . The $60,000,000,000 bill is in part for arms for our men. This bill is for arms for their men." In response to concerns about his statement that some European countries had not been producing materiel as rapidly as the US hoped, Marshall reminded the committee that "we should bear in mind we are dealing with nations that have been under the aggressor's heel for years, and have had their wrecked economy to recover, and their spirit and their courage to revive. Their picture is quite different from ours in the human reactions." (House Committee on Foreign Affairs, *Hearings . . . on H. R. 5020 and H. R. 5113*, 86–87.)

Several members of the committee, including Frances Bolton (R-OH), wondered "upon what basis you feel that the United States can stand the impact" of the cost of the combined Defense Department budget and the Mutual Security Program in addition to the "many other expenditures that have to be met." Marshall confessed that "we have a limited choice unless we resign ourselves to a tragic situation." It was precisely because of fiscal concerns, Marshall added, that he had been such a strong supporter of "a very definite date of termination" for the European Recovery Program and the establishment of universal military training, without which "we could never have an enduring system of defense, for we would be wrecked financially." In response to a question from Representative Laurie Battle (D-AL), Marshall reiterated that "we cannot go on with this business indefinitely," and he hoped that by the end of fiscal year 1954 "we will have been able to arrange things so that the provisions as to raw materials and matter of that sort will be taken care of" by the European countries rather than by the United States. Several representatives questioned Marshall on European versus Asian commitments. "Is it not a fact that this is the pay-off vote on the big debate?," Representative Jacob Javits asked. (See pp. 333–34, 380–86, 431–32, 455–56, and 472–74.) "In other words, we are asked to decide whether we are to go it alone or have allies, and the Mutual Security Program represents saying that that we want Allies?" "That is correct sir," Marshall responded. Questions also arose as to the need for a program of this magnitude should negotiations on a cease-fire agreement in Korea begin (see pp. 566–67 and 592–95), which led Marshall to caution the committee members that "aside from the tragedy of the casualties, Korea is an incident, and the world picture requires us not only to continue to build up our strength, but I think in some respects to increase the effort." (Ibid., 88–95.)

The committee members were called to floor votes at 11:25 a.m., so Marshall agreed to appear before the committee again at 10:00 a.m. on Monday, July 2, to conclude the hearing.

Monday, July 2, 1951

The second day of testimony focused on topics similar to the first. Representative B. Carroll Reece (R-TN) asked "if the Defense Department has taken into account the impact this whole program will have on the entire strength of the United States, that is, how far we can go without exhausting our economic resources to the point where Russia might feel that we are ripe for them by subversion or otherwise move in for the kill, so to speak?" After repeating that "the Defense Department has taken that into most careful and continuous consideration," Marshall reminded the committee that during his congressional testimonies "last November and December I personally was under considerable attack for not asking for enough for our defense, and not viewing the situation as seriously as it, in their opinion, really was." (See pp. 276–78 and 291–93.) He believed that "the record proves that I am very much aware of the consideration you have just been talking about. I am deeply concerned that what we do is along the lines that we can maintain." Indeed, he had previously been attacked for "leaning too much towards matters of economics and not sufficiently along the line of a more rapid build-up of our military position." In response to another of Reece's questions regarding the percentage of the national budget designated for defense in the United States versus other NATO countries, Marshall defended those countries by recalling that the situation in Europe "is quite different from ours, in that they are recovering from a devastating experience, both as to personnel and as to their installations of one kind or another in their countries. Just as they are beginning to lift themselves out of that depression, there is imposed on them the necessity for building up a very heavy charge against their economies for purely military purposes. So they are in quite a critical state." He went on in response to another question to support the admission of Greece, Turkey, and Spain into NATO (see p. 486), and then argued with Bolton over congressional versus executive responsibility for the too rapid demobilization at the end of World War II. He also assured the committee that the requested appropriations for the program were "in no way . . . a padded figure. It has been pared down as much as we felt it could be done, and still accomplish our purpose." This expenditure was necessary as "a display to the world of a determination to go through with our plans. . . . I would like to see nothing done that would in any way seem to reduce our effort to build up our strength at the present time. I would rather be inclined to think we should make some motion to increase it further, though I dislike thinking of that in terms of budget. However, there should be no doubt in the world's mind that we are determined to be strong enough to stand up in this present crisis in the world's history." (Ibid., 104–7, 109–12, 114, 116.)

Long a critic of Marshall's China policies, Representative Walter Judd asked whether Marshall believed "that the independence of Asia is essential to the independence and security of Europe?" While the loss of Asia would have an "adverse effect" on the defense of Europe, Marshall replied, "I do not think it would be fatal" to that defense. He reiterated his previously expressed belief "that we should not become involved in fighting on the mainland of Asia" and added that "we should not lessen our efforts for the defense of Europe because of the Pacific." After some additional questioning the committee adjourned at 11:58 a.m. (Ibid., 118–24.) For Marshall's Senate testimony on this bill, see pp. 597–603. ★

331

Remarks on Independence Day[1]

July 4, 1951
Leesburg, Virginia

Every American old enough to talk and think celebrates this day with wide and sometimes wild acclaim. The young are enthusiastic. They feel proud to be Americans. The older of us reflect more on what this day means in the history of our nation and of the world.

We celebrate the day but we must do more than that in this critical period of our history. The duties of citizenship should be foremost in our minds. Long before the Declaration of Independence was proclaimed there was a general acceptance of the principle that the first duty of a citizen was to be prepared to serve in the defense of his country. This was recognized by the tradition of the English Common Law. Our first settlers carried that obligation to these shores. At the time of the signing of the Declaration of Independence every one of the thirteen colonies required of every able bodied male citizen military service in an emergency and military training in peacetime.

Gradually during the following 175 years that principle—that ideal of Universal Military Training in peacetime was lost. As a result of our failure to maintain the traditions of those early colonial days, thousands of Americans died in Europe, and Africa, in the Far East and in the islands of the Pacific.

Fortunately, Congress a few weeks ago laid the legal foundations for such a system of peacetime training. So I think today we can look into the future with more assurance than has been possible in the past. The thing for us to remember is that our ancestors who founded this country for us took their duties of citizenship seriously in thought and sacrifice. It is of equal importance—maybe of more importance that we do the same today.[2]

GCMRL/G. C. Marshall Papers (Secretary of Defense, Speeches and Statements)

1. Marshall flew from Washington to Newport News, Virginia, and traveled by car from there to Williamsburg on July 3 to deliver remarks at the opening performance of *The Common Glory* on the campus of the College of William and Mary. He and Mrs. Marshall drove to Fort Monroe on the morning of July 4 to visit with the Winns before flying home, where Marshall delivered this statement live at 10:15 p.m. from radio personality Arthur Godfrey's home studio, located just outside Leesburg. The broadcast, which celebrated the 175th anniversary of the signing of the Declaration of Independence, also included US Supreme Court Chief Justice Fred Vinson, actor Gregory Peck, and others. (Marshall to Molly Winn, July 5, 1951, GCMRL/G. C. Marshall Papers [Secretary of Defense, Number Indexed, M200-4-17]. For General Ginsburgh's notes on Marshall's remarks in Williamsburg, see ibid., [214-13-2].)

2. See pp. 551–53 and 558–59.

While Marshall's former brother-in-law, Edmund Coles, wrote that he and his wife had enjoyed Marshall's "crystal clear" comments, Marshall replied that Mrs. Marshall "thought it was very poor, that I was in too serious a vein." (Coles to Marshall, July 5, 1951, and Marshall to Coles, July 9, 1951, ibid., [M200-2-11].)

332

To Thomas H. White — July 6, 1951
Washington, DC

Dear White: Your letter of July 3rd came as a pleasant surprise and recalled many pleasant memories of our trip to Honolulu. I see Pryor and Trippe occasionally but missed Admiral Towers who was in the building the other day.[1]

Mrs. Marshall and I are looking forward to receiving the Norwegian Elkhound puppy and the brochure which you inclosed has added considerably to our interest in this breed. Your enthusiasm assures me that we will derive much pleasure from the puppy. We appreciate your offer of assistance and if any unusual traits are noticed I will certainly write you.[2]

Mrs. Marshall and I spent the holiday by witnessing the drama, "The Common Glory," at Williamsburg the evening of the 3rd, spending the night there, and flying up to Leesburg the following afternoon. On the evening of the Fourth I participated in the Declaration of Independence program by broadcasting from Arthur Godfrey's house near Leesburg.[3] We have not as yet decided what our plans will be for a summer vacation. We had thought about going to Nantucket or Fire Island but there is much indecision on our part since it is very difficult for me, with matters here at the Pentagon, to make any definite plans. For the past few days Mrs. Marshall has been suffering from an attack of shingles of the eyes—a most unpleasant ailment which crops up every now and then. Otherwise we are both in the best of health and look forward to a vacation to escape the heat of Washington and Leesburg, particularly the former.[4]

Thanks again for the information on the puppy and offer of assistance.

With warm regards to you both in which Mrs. Marshall joins me, Faithfully yours,

GCMRL/G. C. Marshall Papers (Secretary of Defense, Number Indexed, M212-3-28)

1. An industrialist from Cleveland, White had served with Marshall on the Pan American World Airways Board of Directors, which had met in Honolulu, Hawaii, on February 21, 1950. Samuel F. Pryor and Admiral John H. Towers (USNA, 1906) were vice presidents of Pan American.

2. George had informed Marshall on June 7 that "the Norwegian children" were collecting money "toward the presentation of a Norwegian elkhound (which is the counterpart of our American eagle) to you." Norwegian schools were conducting an essay contest on the topic of NATO, and the winner would "come to America with the dog and present it to you." The *Washington Post* reported this on June 28. (George to Marshall, memorandum, June 7, 1951, GCMRL/G. C. Marshall Papers [Secretary of Defense, Number Indexed, M212-3-28]; "Norway Pupils to Give Elkhound to Marshall," *Washington Post*, June 28, 1951, p. B14.)

White, who served as secretary-treasurer of the Norwegian Elkhound Association of America and owned a kennel, had sent a brochure about the breed to Marshall on July 3 and offered his assistance if the Marshalls needed anything "to help you with the puppy." (White to Marshall, July 3, 1951, GCMRL/G. C. Marshall Papers [Secretary of Defense, Number Indexed, M212-3-28].)

Arnt Natland, the eighteen-year-old Norwegian high school student who won the essay contest, presented the four-month old puppy, named Nato, to Marshall on July 11 in front of the Pentagon. During the presentation, according to the press, Marshall praised "the dog for his faultless behavior during the presentation ceremony" and added, "'If all the rest of the world were as well-behaved as this young fellow there would be less trouble in the world.'" In a memorandum preparing Marshall for the presentation, George suggested that Marshall "mention that Mr. White . . . heard about the gift to you and provided you with information on how to care for the puppy." (George to Marshall, memorandum, July 11, 1951, ibid.; "Marshall Pats His 'Tip' From Norway," *New York Times*, July 12, 1951, p. 14; "Then the Dog-Gone Dog Had To Go and Show Up Marshall," *Washington Times-Herald*, July 12, 1951, GCMRL/G. C. Marshall Papers [Secretary of Defense, Scrapbooks and Scrapbook Materials].) See also pp. 628–29 and 662–63.

3. See the previous document.

4. See pp. 603–4.

333

Memorandum for the President
Secret

July 6, 1951
Washington, DC

It is desirable at this time to alert two National Guard Divisions for shipment to Europe. The first of the four divisions for this service is now in Europe. An armored division is now in process of shipment. Two more divisions remain to go to make up the original four.[1]

The terms of the Senate Resolution regarding troops to Europe call for certification of the Chiefs of Staff and Secretary of Defense to the Senate, justifying the necessity for such a movement. Under the terms of the Resolution, the original four divisions have already been covered. The question at the present time is whether or not we should go through the form of certification regarding the last two of the four. The members of Congress from whose states these National Guard Divisions come have already been or will be notified. Two members of the Senate Committee concerned, Lodge of Massachusetts and Smith of New Jersey, inquired of the Defense Department regarding the certification of these remaining two divisions. They are being personally informed of the status of the matter and of the fact that the Resolution definitely does not require certification with respect to these particular divisions.[2]

Your direction is desired as to whether we go through the form of certification or content ourselves by informal notification. It is the unanimous opinion in the Department that no certification is required.[3]

NA/RG 330, CD 371 (Europe)

1. The Fourth Infantry Division and Second Armored Division along with two National Guard divisions had been designated for service in Europe in April 1951. The two National Guard divisions were the Twenty-eighth Infantry from Pennsylvania and the Forty-third Infantry from Connecticut, Rhode Island, and Vermont. See pp. 293, 431–32, 472–74, and 561–62.

2. See pp. 333–34, 380–86, 419–22, 431–32, 462, and 472–74.

3. "General Marshall took this to the White House and obtained approval this date," a July 6 memorandum attached to this document stated. The president's signature is at the bottom of the memorandum. According to Truman's engagement log at the Truman Library, Marshall met with the president "off the record" from 10:50 to 10:55 a.m. and attended a cabinet meeting at 11:00 a.m.

334

To Dean G. Acheson
Top Secret

July 9, 1951
Washington, DC

Dear Mr. Secretary: I refer to your letter of March 15, 1951 requesting reconsideration of the availability of military assistance for denial and conservation plans established under NSC 26/2 and specifically regarding the earmarking of a small military contingent for this purpose.[1]

The Joint Chiefs of Staff have reconsidered the availability of military assistance for denial and conservation plans established under NSC 26/2. They find that although forces are being augmented to support NSC 68, world conditions are worsening and global requirements are increasing. They realize that under certain circumstances a force such as the battalion of Marines now in the Mediterranean might be available for this mission. On the other hand, there might be many missions which would have a higher priority.[2]

I therefore consider that the earmarking of a military contingent for the specific use in connection with NSC 26/2 should not be done in advance. The Joint Chiefs of Staff are of the opinion that the sending of a force to Saudi Arabia must be decided at the time in view of the over-all situation confronting us.[3] Faithfully yours,

NA/RG 330, CD 386.1

1. NSC 26/2, which was approved on January 10, 1949, had established plans for the US and UK to destroy "oil facilities in the Middle East in the event of imminent capture" by the Soviet Union. The Defense Department assigned a marine battalion in the Mediterranean to implement "denial and conservation tasks" in the Saudi Arabian oil fields in the event of a Soviet invasion, but the battalion was withdrawn prior to April 1950. The State Department expressed concern in September 1950 about the lack of military support to fulfill NSC 26/2. In light of buildup of the military projected under NSC 68, Acheson hadreiterated this earlier concern and requested on March 15, 1951, that the Defense Department "reconsider" and "earmark a small military contingent" to fulfill NSC 26/2 "as a matter of priority." (Acheson to Marshall, March 15, 1951, NA/RG 330, CD 386.1; *FRUS, 1950*, 5: 72–73.)

2. Marshall had forwarded Acheson's letter to the JCS on March 21 for their review and informed the secretary of state he had done so. Carter notified Marshall on June 19 that the JCS reported "that such earmarking was *not warranted*," because it would not be the most effective use of forces as "'world conditions are worsening and global requirements are increasing.'" According to Carter, Lovett was not averse to assigning personnel to the task rather than specific units to meet Acheson's request. Carter agreed, adding that it could be accomplished "by assigning such a mission to the commander of our Mediterranean forces, along with his other missions." Using Carter's memorandum as a guide, Marshall informed Bradley on June 19 that he agreed with the JCS decision about designating a unit, but he asked them to consider Carter's suggestion of assigning the mission to "an appropriate Mediterranean commander" in order to "satisfy the immediate concern of the State Department." The JCS did not support this recommendation, believing that the decisions on assigning troops to Saudi Arabia in the event of an emergency must be made "at the time in view of the over-all situation confronting us." (Marshall to JCS, memorandum, March 21, 1951; Marshall to Acheson, March 21, 1951; Carter to Marshall, memorandum, June 19, 1951; Marshall to Bradley, June 19, 1951; and Bradley to Marshall, memorandum, July 3, 1951, NA/RG 330, CD 386.1.)

3. US officials in Saudi Arabia recommended on August 14 that the Saudi government be informed "in a most general way of denial and evacuation plans," but the State and Defense Departments decided against this or any other disclosure indicating "that the Western powers might abandon the area." (*FRUS, 1950–1955, The Intelligence Community, 1950–1955* [Washington: GPO, 2007], 243–45, quotes on 245.)

335

To Dean G. Acheson July 13, 1951
Top Secret Washington, DC

Dear Mr. Secretary: The Supreme Commander for the Allied Powers has advised the Department of Defense that progress in bringing the Japanese National Police Reserve to a state of combat effectiveness for the defense of Japan is severely restricted by the lack of qualified officers. As you know, former Japanese "career officers" are barred from holding office by a policy decision of the Far Eastern Commission [FEC]. In order to meet this situation, General Ridgway has proposed certain measures which would permit the "de-purging" of a limited number of former Japanese officers. I am inclosing copies of cables from SCAP to the Department of the Army in which the reasons and justifications for these proposals are set forth in full.[1]

SCAP has proposed, first, to permit the de-purging, on an individual basis, of officers below the rank of General or Admiral who can be shown to have been opponents of Japanese totalitarianism and expansionism. He has been advised that the Department of State and the Department of the Army have no objection to a broad interpretation of the pertinent FEC directive in this respect.[2]

Second, SCAP has proposed to effect the blanket de-purging of several thousand junior officers through an administrative interpretation of the term "career officers", as used in the FEC directive, which would exclude from the category of "career officers" those commissioned on or after 7 July 1937, the date when Japan first became engaged in major hostilities. This would be a logical extension of SCAP's previous action in which he excluded from the category of "career officers" those commissioned after 7 December 1941.

Assistant Secretary of State Rusk, in a letter of June 22, 1951, to Assistant Secretary of the Army Johnson, has expressed the opinion that the latter proposal might appear to undermine a decision of the Far Eastern Commission and, hence, might adversely affect General Ridgway's international position as SCAP. For this reason, he suggested that the de-purging of military officers be administered on a case-by-case basis so that those officers commissioned after 7 July 1937 who actually intended to make a career of the military service would remain under the purge. This would require provision for the hearing of evidence in each individual case.[3]

This suggestion has been fully considered. General Ridgway has stated that the procedure suggested by the Department of State would (1) release fewer persons, (2) impose an added administrative burden on both the Japanese Government and his headquarters, and (3) so delay the actual release of persons as to vitiate its value as an interim measure.

The Joint Chiefs of Staff have advised me that, in view of the urgent need to provide an immediate source of competent officers for the Japanese National Police Reserve, they consider that it is vitally important for the United States to concur in SCAP's proposal with the least practicable delay. I concur with the views of the Joint Chiefs of Staff as to the necessity for this action. I also wish to express my agreement with General Ridgway in his view that the proposed definition of "career officers" is not inconsistent with the spirit and intent of the FEC decision.

Accordingly, I hope that you may be able to indicate your concurrence in this proposal as soon as possible.[4] Faithfully yours,

NA/RG 330, CD 092 (Japan)

1. Following Truman's May 3 approval of Marshall's request that the US stockpile materiel for the Japanese National Police Reserve (see pp. 494–96), Marshall asked the JCS on May 10 to report "on the present status and estimated capabilities" of the JNPR. After receiving messages from Ridgway on May 23 and June 4, Bradley informed Marshall on July 11 that while "the current capability of the JNPR is limited to quelling internal disorders, by late summer this force should be capable of tactical employment in battalion size units." He also noted Ridgway's estimate that "the four existing JNPR divisions can attain a fair level of combat effectiveness approximately 11 months after necessary equipment (including heavy armament) is released to the Japanese, provided he can recruit qualified officers into this force." One of the major problems that had to be resolved before the JNPR program could be "fully implemented" was obtaining the State Department's acceptance of Ridgway's proposal that he be allowed to depurge former Japanese career officers "commissioned on or after" July 7, 1937. (Bradley to Marshall, memorandum, July 2, 1951, with attached May 23 and June 4 cables from Ridgway; and Bradley to Marshall, memorandum, July 11, 1951, NA/RG 330, CD 092 [Japan].)

2. See *FRUS, 1951*, 6: 1140n5.

3. See *FRUS, 1951*, 6: 1138–41.

4. Acheson's response is not in the Marshall Papers, but by mid-August, Ridgway had depurged over five thousand former officers and was intending to depurge around thirty thousand more by the end of that month. (*FRUS, 1951*, 6: 1328–29n2.) See pp. 610–11.

336

Conversation on a European Defense Force
July 16, 1951 Washington, DC

ON JULY 16, Marshall met at the Pentagon with Acheson; Lovett; Bradley; Frank Nash, designated as General Burns's successor as assistant to the secretary of defense for international security affairs (see pp. 607–8n3); Colonel Beebe; Phillip Jessup; and H. Freeman Matthews to discuss a July 12 memorandum drafted by Acheson and Jessup entitled "German Rearmament and Problems of the Defense of Europe." (For the text of this memorandum, see *FRUS, 1951*, 3: 827–32.) See pp. 497–99 and 596–97.

In response to a question from Marshall about the level of dedication of European countries to "the objectives of NATO," Acheson replied that there was "a hesitancy, and even resentment," in Europe because of what the US believed they should be able to contribute. A European defense force, Acheson continued, would "promote a greater sense of purpose and accomplishment" among the European countries. In the ensuing discussion, Lovett added that there was a need for "more real action" regarding Germany in order to confirm to Congress the urgency "for continued United States support of Europe's defenses," particularly if the cease-fire talks in Korea led to reduced defense budgets throughout

NATO countries. (*FRUS, 1951*, 3: 820–21, 827–32, 836–38, 847–48; memorandum of conversation, "United States Position on European Defense Force," July 16, 1951, NA/RG 218, Geographic File, 092 [Western Europe], Sec. 86.) See pp. 566–67 and 592–603.

After expressing his concurrence with the JCS and Eisenhower that immediate German rearmament within NATO was mandatory and should not await full agreement on a European defense force (see pp. 619–21), Marshall suggested that the United States pursue an agreement with first France and Great Britain and then West Germany to authorize the latter's immediate rearmament within a NATO framework and to begin consultations on the long-term development of a European defense force. These European forces would not have an "immediate operational military significance," but the United States would not "stand in the way of the development" of such an organization. Acheson replied that the United States needed "to go farther" and express "real support to the French concept" of a European defense force rather than "merely 'not standing in the way.'" He offered "a three-part objective," including "restoration of sovereignty to the German Federal Republic," a "plan for initiating German rearmament and training," and "Agreement on a plan for the European Defense Force without necessity for implementation of all details." At Marshall's suggestion, the State Department drafted a memorandum in order to secure Truman's and the NSC's approval for the implementation of Acheson's objective. The Defense Department received the draft on July 20 and reported no major objections by July 25. (*FRUS, 1951*, 3: 836–38, 847–48; memorandum of conversation, "United States Position on European Defense Force," July 16, 1951, NA/RG 218, Geographic File, 092 [Western Europe], Sec. 86; unsent draft of Marshall to Acheson, July 16, 1951, GCMRL/G. C. Marshall Papers [Secretary of Defense, Chronological, Director, Executive Office (Marshall S. Carter), 1950–1952].)

The final memorandum, entitled "Definition of United States Policy on Problems of the Defense of Europe and the German Contribution," was signed by Acheson and Lovett as acting secretary of defense while Marshall was on vacation (see pp. 603–4) and was presented to Truman on July 30. In order to break "the stalemate" between Germany and France over stipulations for German rearmament as well as to promote "more general Continental European arrangements," they recommended a process to follow Acheson's three-point objective outlined during the July 16 meeting. The memorandum indicated that US support of a European Defense Force within NATO "would be contingent upon" that issue "being treated simultaneously" with the establishment of German units and the restoration of German sovereignty. Acheson and Lovett reminded Truman that he had received Eisenhower's views on this matter and had agreed to Eisenhower's request to send an observer to the Paris Conference on the European Defense. (See *FRUS, 1951*, 3: 838–39, 842–43.) They recommended that the US "make known in the clearest terms" to all concerned countries that it "supports the concept and will be prepared to assist in its execution and implementation provided that certain conditions are met." These included arrangements to ensure that the

European Defense Force would "participate in the common defense of Europe, not simply for the support of individual national aspirations"; a structure "based on the idea of European contingents which could be disposed of by the Supreme Allied Commander of Europe in accordance with military necessity"; German contribution at an early date, notwithstanding the conclusion of any necessary "political arrangements"; and the delegation of relevant "administrative machinery" to NATO. Achieving such plans would require that the US and other NATO countries "move broadly and decisively in creating a new status for Germany," which would shift from "a defeated enemy . . . to a partner who is freely contributing to our mutual defense." This would require "abolishing the unilaterally-imposed Occupation Statute and replacing it with a negotiated agreement or agreements" as well as substituting "Ambassadors for High Commissioners." The Allied Powers would only retain "supreme authority" regarding "the right to station troops in Germany and to protect their security"; Berlin; "the unification of Germany and a subsequent peace settlement"; and "territorial questions." Germany should also be "admitted as a full member" of NATO. (Memorandum from Acheson and Lovett for Truman, July 30, 1951, NA/RG 330, CD 091.7 [Europe].) See p. 388n3.

Acheson delivered this memorandum to Truman at a noon meeting on July 30, during which the president initialed his approval. It was forwarded to the NSC, and following its concurrence, Truman officially approved the memorandum on August 2. It became NSC 115. (*FRUS, 1951*, 3: 848–52.) ★

337

To General of the Army Dwight D. Eisenhower — July 16, 1951
Washington, DC

Dear Eisenhower: Six of the Congressmen who visited you in connection with the Mutual Security Program were my guests for lunch on Monday. They are the last of the group to meet with me, the other twelve having been here on two earlier occasions.[1]

These men were very favorably impressed with what they saw and heard in the NATO countries they visited, and particularly with what they learned in your Headquarters. They have a very clear idea of the magnitude of the problems facing you and are very laudatory in their descriptions of the way you are going about things.

I invited their comments both on what they had seen and heard and what they expect or hope for the future of the military and economic aid programs. They were very frank, and at the same time very well informed and realistic. This, undoubtedly, is a result of their having visited Europe, and was reflected in their attitude and questions during the hearings on the Mutual Security Program. As you know, I testified on 29 June and 2 July. The hearings were obviously expedited and conducted on a basis of common understanding in a manner that would not have been possible had the Committee not visited Europe.[2]

I know you will be pleased that the trip had such beneficial results, particularly since you are now entertaining a group of Senators and may be faced with further visits by Congressional parties. The importance of the Mutual Security Program is something that I regard as equal to that of our own defense budget. Obviously, the Congress must come to the same opinion, or we may face the possibility of restricted authorizations and reduced appropriations for military and economic assistance.[3]

These Congressional visits undoubtedly are a burden on you and your Headquarters, but considering the benefits that followed from the House visit, I hope you will feel they are worth the effort. My thanks for what you have done and are doing for the visiting members of the Senate and House groups.[4] Faithfully yours,

GCMarshall

DDEL/Dwight D. Eisenhower Papers (Pre-Presidential Files, Principal File, Name Series)

1. As part of the deliberations on the Mutual Security Act, a group of eighteen members of the House Foreign Affairs, Armed Services, and Appropriations Committees led by James Edwards had met in mid-June with NATO, ECA, and other US aid and military organization leaders, including Eisenhower, on June 9 and 18 in Paris. (*Papers of DDE*, 12: 333–35, 346, 348, 433–34.) On July 10, Marshall had forwarded to Eisenhower the confidential report of one of the congressional representatives, by which time Eisenhower was meeting with a similar group from the Senate Foreign Relations Committee. See n3. (Marshall to Eisenhower, July 10, 1951, DDEL/Dwight D. Eisenhower Papers [Pre-Presidential Files, Principal File, Name Series, Box 80, Marshall, George C.].)

According to Marshall's engagement logs, only three members of the committee had lunch with him on Monday, July 9: Norris Cotton (R-NH), James Richards, and Walter Judd. Robert Chiperfield (R-IL), Lawrence Smith (R-WI), and John Rooney (D-NY) sent regrets. Marshall had lunch with the following six committee members on June 21: Edward de Graffenried (D-AL), Robert Sikes (D-FL), Richard Wigglesworth (R-MA), Overton Brooks, Dewey Short, and W. Sterling Cole. On June 25, Marshall had lunch with Thomas Gordon (D-IL), Christian Herter (R-MA), J. Vaughn Gary (D-VA), Frederick Coudert (R-NY), Mike Mansfield, and Laurie Battle.

Assistant Secretary Daniel Edwards had recommended that Marshall sign this letter to Eisenhower. Due to "some newspaper comment he has seen, General Eisenhower has some doubt about the success of the Congressional trip. It is felt by the people over there that encouragement from you would be helpful." (Edwards to Marshall, memorandum, July 13, 1951, NA/RG 330, SD 032.1.)

2. See pp. 569–77.

3. Nine members of the Senate Foreign Relations Committee's Subcommittee on US Foreign Aid to Europe had arrived in Europe on July 7 to tour and evaluate US economic and military aid facilities and programs. They remained abroad until July 23.

4. Eisenhower thanked Marshall on July 21 for his letter. He hoped that the results of the senators' visit "will be as good as you feel they were in the first instance," although he reported that "one or two" senators "seem to be somewhat hostile. We shall do our best. . . . Sometimes this process seems like an attempt to empty the ocean with a teaspoon, but we still remain hopeful." Eisenhower concluded with a handwritten postscript that "The Senators just left *apparently* in a very fine frame of mind." (Eisenhower to Marshall, June 21, 1951, ibid.; *Papers of DDE*, 12: 433–34.) See pp. 592 and 597–603.

338

To Queen Frederica of the Hellenes July 16, 1951
Washington, DC

Your Majesty: Prior to your recent letter of June 8 you had written me a note expressing your views on command in the Eastern Mediterranean. I delayed answering the early note until I could give you definite news in the matter. A final decision has not yet been reached but Admiral Sherman is now in Europe and I think his visit will precipitate the decision, and I hope it will be to your satisfaction.[1]

I felt much disturbed for His Majesty and you over the affair Papagos. Your letter of June 8 therefore was an illuminating description. In this morning's New York Times I saw the supposed record of an interview of His Majesty with the General. It seems to bear out your description of his reactions. I do hope you will be spared any further embarrassment and related crises, though the interview reported in the press this morning does not encourage that hope.[2]

You referred to Van Fleet's performance in Korea. He did a masterful job during the two Communist offensives, which I now think inflicted on them more serious damage than we had at first supposed. They now appear to have been badly crippled. I think his instant and deeply penetrating counter-offensive which was launched while the Communists were still pursuing their most successful penetration—that on the Eastern front against South Korean divisions, was an astonishing and demoralizing surprise to them.[3]

I saw Van Fleet in Korea, in fact flew—in a tiny plane, all along the front with him and Ridgway, and found him in excellent shape. I talked, incidentally, at some length with the Commander of your Greek unit which has been doing a fine job.[4]

Mrs. Marshall is down in the country forty miles from here, at our Leesburg, Virginia, home to escape the torrid heat of Washington—92 degrees the past few days with high humidity. I have to be here in town from Monday to Friday, as commuting that distance is too much of an effort, so we only have weekends together. I thought we had finished with that business of separations, but such is not yet the case, nor finished with frequent tiring appearances before Congressional committees. In that connection, I had to hurry back from Korea to appear before a committee for some four hours the same day I returned.[5]

With warm regards to His Majesty and yourself, believe me, with great respect, Faithfully yours,

GCMRL/G. C. Marshall Papers (Pentagon Office, Selected)

1. Frederica had written to Marshall on April 15 to offer her "honest opinion" as well as that of her husband and "the whole of Greece" that they "would very much like to see an American in the position of Supreme Commander" in the Mediterranean. (Frederica to Marshall, April 15, 1951, quoted in Lilika S. Papanicolaou, *Frederica, Queen of the Hellenes: Mission of a Modern Queen* [San Gwann, Malta: Publishers Enterprises Group Ltd., 1994], 409–10; Frederica to Marshall, n.d., GCMRL/G. C. Marshall Papers [Retirement, General].) Admiral Sherman had departed for Europe on July 15 to discuss US base rights in Spain with Generalissimo Francisco Franco. See pp. 439–40, 493–94, and 595–96.

2. In her lengthy June 8 letter to Marshall, Frederica explained the May 30 resignation

of Field Marshal Papagos as commander in chief of the Greek armed forces and described the response of Greek officials and the public as well as the unsuccessful efforts of King Paul to prevent the resignation. She also praised the efforts of John Peurifoy, US ambassador to Greece, who had only increased Greece's "confidence in American unselfish leadership." (Frederica to Marshall, June 8, 1951, quoted in Papanicolaou, *Frederica*, 411–14.) The editors have been unable to locate any relevant articles from the July 16, 1951, edition of the *New York Times*.

Marshall had given Acheson a copy of Frederica's June 8 letter. (Acheson to Marshall, July 2, 1951, GCMRL/G. C. Marshall Papers [Pentagon Office, Selected].)

3. In her April 15 letter to Marshall, Frederica had noted the "pride" she and King Paul felt at Van Fleet's appointment in Korea. "How happy our soldiers will be to serve under him." (Frederica to Marshall, April 15, 1951, quoted in Papanicolaou, *Frederica*, 410; Frederica to Marshall, n.d., GCMRL/G. C. Marshall Papers [Retirement, General].) See pp. 133–34 and 480.

Marshall is referring to the fifth and sixth Chinese offensives and the Eighth Army's counteroffensives in late April and mid-May 1951, respectively. See p. 534; Millett, *The War for Korea*, 2: 426–35, 441–52; and Spencer C. Tucker, *Encyclopedia of the Korean War: A Political, Social, and Military History*, 2d ed., vol. 1, *A–L* (Santa Barbara, CA: ABC-CLIO, 2010), 162–64.

4. Frederica had commented in her June 8 letter that she could "imagine that you well enjoyed your trip to Korea. A visit to the Front is always a great compensation for the troubles one has with people who do nothing but talk" constantly "with nonsensical details." (Frederica to Marshall, June 8, 1951, quoted in Papanicolaou, *Frederica*, 414.) See pp. 548–51.

5. Frederica had reported that she was enjoying reading an autographed copy of Katherine Marshall's "excellent book." (Frederica to Marshall, June 8, 1951, quoted in Papanicolaou, *Frederica*, 414; Katherine T. Marshall, *Together: Annals of an Army Wife* [New York: Tupper and Love Inc., 1946].)

Marshall had testified before the House Banking and Currency Committee on June 14. (See p. 537.)

339

House Testimony on Defense Department Appropriations

July 18, 1951 Washington, DC

DUE TO Marshall's testimony on General MacArthur's relief (see pp. 505–16), Lovett and Bradley had initially appeared before the House Subcommittee on Department of Defense Appropriations regarding the department's fiscal year 1952 budget on May 7, with the understanding that Marshall would testify at a later date. Marshall did so on July 18, accompanied by Bradley. The subcommittee's chairman, George H. Mahon (D-TX), began by criticizing the military for not conserving "manpower and dollars as well as they should," and he requested that Marshall inform the committee promptly if the Defense Department decided to reduce its appropriation request in light of the ongoing armistice negotiations in Korea (see pp. 592–94). Marshall responded that he saw "no reduction" in the Defense Department appropriation request; indeed, the department might have to ask "Congress for certain increases, particularly for 1953 and 1954." Except "for the tragedy of the casualties," Marshall regarded the Korean War "as an incident in the world situation," and he was "deeply concerned at this talk about the trap or the clever procedure that may be facing us in Korea; because I think the trap and the cleverness are entirely on the part of the Soviet Government, addressed to the world situation." He thought it was "most distressing that by a single speech," referring to Malik's address (see pp. 566–67), "they, the Soviets, could develop an attitude of relaxation, of a let-down in our defense program on the part of the American people. It is tragic that we should be so susceptible to propaganda, that a single speech would create a state of mind that can very seriously react to our disadvantage in the world picture." (House Committee on Appropriations, *Department of Defense Appropriations for 1952*, 82d Cong., 1st sess., 195–96.)

Marshall reminded the committee that the Defense Department had "tried very hard in the preparation" of the 1952 budget request "to go through it with extreme care, to eliminate the unnecessary, and to make certain that the estimates are on a very solid basis." When asked about the true Soviet intentions in Korea, Marshall warned that they would not be known for "quite a period of time," and that "a correct conclusion" on what those intentions were must be made "in view of our past experiences" with the Soviet Union's "previous record of frustration, disruption and complete ignoring at times of even the minor relationships in international procedure." Whatever their intention, "the important thing now is that we appear before the world as determined, implacably determined, to get ourselves in such a strong position that the Kremlin will not dare to upset the peace of the world." This determination was "imperative" and would be a more effective deterrent than any weapon system, including atomic weapons. "We should not suspend our efforts merely at the call of the Soviet Government." Simultaneously, however, the US "must do this tremendous business in an orderly manner" in order to prevent becoming vulnerable "if we over-extended ourselves," as Marshall had cautioned during his testimony on supplemental budget requests in late 1950 (see pp. 276–78 and 291–93). While specific amounts and policies could be debated, Marshall insisted "we must be able and determined to build up the strength and not be wobbling back and forth at every dictation of the Kremlin." Whatever decisions were reached regarding an armistice in Korea, the need for manpower and materiel would not be reduced. The "main effect of the cessation of hostilities, aside from the terrific casualty lists, would be to make it possible for us to proceed in a more orderly manner toward building up our over-all program." (Ibid., 197–98.)

After Marshall concluded his lengthy answer to Mahon's opening statement and questions, Mahon continued by asking Marshall if he believed that the military should not shrink below 3.5 million men and production of military materiel should continue at the current pace "regardless of developments in Korea." Marshall reiterated his "firm" conviction that Congress "should proceed along the basis which has been presented to you." Mahon went on to ask whether the Defense Department could save money by using more trained military personnel rather than civilian employees. Marshall reminded the subcommittee that the department "had scheduled, I think, 50,000 less civilians than the budget provides for." Should the situation improve sufficiently in Korea to allow a significant number of American troops to return home, Marshall added, Congress might "want to consider" the question of employing trained soldiers over civilian employees. He did think that these trained and experienced troops would "have an important place" in "conducting the training" provided for in the recently signed UMT law. (Ibid., 199–201.) See pp. 558–59.

In response to another question from Mahon, Marshall stated that "the likelihood of a major war" at that time was "just about the same as 2 or 3 months ago. There has been a constant build-up in the Soviets and their satellites, of their military strength. Unfortunately we do not know a great deal about it." The threat of an all-out war, Marshall continued, was "continuing, and, from the viewpoint of the enemy's build-up, it is increasing." He declined to estimate when Congress would know about the timeline for a cease-fire in Korea, citing the "frustrating" conferences in which he had been participating and the stubbornness of the Communists regarding an agenda for armistice discussions, although he did not think such a timetable would be decided "during the next 6 weeks." Marshall urged the subcommittee to act on the appropriations bill "before any armistice comes to a final decision, because I think it will help us very much in getting the decision that we want. In other words, this bill is a declaration of determined intent, and that is the most helpful factor we can emphasize at the present time." Representative Harry Sheppard (D-CA) asked if Marshall agreed "that if this particular overture of peace was deliberately planned for strategic purposes, to lull us into a state of apathy, as it were, that the speedy enactment of this appropriation bill as a preparedness measure, would have a salutary effect." Marshall responded affirmatively and added that "the most tragic fact is that in the way of public reaction we are so easily led by the nose. I do not think we ought to admit any such docile and dangerous tendency as that." (Ibid., 201–2.) ★

340

To Herbert H. Lehman and Hubert H. Humphrey — July 20, 1951
Washington, DC

Dear Senator Lehman and Senator Humphrey: I have delayed replying to your joint letter in order that I might be able to furnish you in some detail the present status of Army plans for the integration of Negro personnel.[1]

For the past several months the Department of the Army has been conducting an intensive study in Korea directed toward improved employment of Negro manpower, particularly in combat units. Comments and recommendations were obtained from commanders concerned and the opinions of several hundred personnel, both white and Negro, were compiled from written questionnaires and personal interviews. The following planned action is based upon the findings of this study.

Far East Command has been directed to inactivate the Negro 24th Infantry Regiment and to replace it with an integrated infantry regiment. Further, general integration has been ordered in the Eighth Army in Korea and in units in Japan of both combat and service type, excepting only the 40th and 45th Infantry Divisions. This integration will be phased over a three-month period with a target date of 30 September for completion. Integration within the 40th and 45th Infantry Divisions will follow at a later date and will be accomplished through the normal flow of replacements.[2]

Secretary Pace, General Collins and General Ridgway are giving the above plan their full support. They ask that you consider this information confidential until a public statement is released on the subject by Far East Command about August 1st. They propose to give equally careful consideration to other areas. The Department of the Army is hopeful that it will be able to carry forward the principle of integration in a planned and orderly manner.[3] Faithfully yours,

NA/RG 330, SD 291.2

1. Senators Lehman (D-NY) and Humphrey (D-MN) had written to Marshall on June 25 after reading in the May 28 edition of the *New York Times* an excerpt of an interview with General MacArthur that later appeared in full in the June 2 issue of the *Pittsburgh Courier*, a weekly African-American newspaper. When asked by Stanley Roberts, the *Courier*'s Washington bureau chief, about the state of integration in the Far East Command, MacArthur declared that he had "'one criticism of Negro troops. . . . They didn't send me enough of them!'" MacArthur insisted that he "'did not create Negro (jim-crow) units in the United States armed forces. They were created in Washington and sent to me. . . . I don't believe that any theatre commander in American war history accepted and integrated the number of Negro troops that I did." ("M'Arthur Assails 'Jim Crow' in Army," *New York Times*, May 28, 1951, p. 3; "MacArthur Talks!," *Pittsburgh Courier*, June 2, 1951, pp. 1, 4, quotes on p. 4; "MacArthur Feared Race War," *Pittsburgh Courier*, June 9, 1951, pp. 1, 5.)

Despite ongoing conversations and progress, Lehman and Humphrey wrote to urge Marshall to support the rapid abolition of segregation in the armed forces, and they asked him for a report on "what further steps are contemplated toward the achievement of the desired goals." (Lehman and Humphrey to Marshall, June 25, 1951, NA/RG 330, 291.2.)

James C. Evans wrote to Osgood Roberts that this joint letter was part of an effort by the *Pittsburgh Courier* "to secure a rejoinder to" MacArthur's statements. Evans later reported that Stanley Roberts "came to the Pentagon on 22 June to seek an interview with the Secretary of Defense to get a response to the quotation" from MacArthur. "After an extended discussion," Clayton Fritchey recommended that the request be declined. (Evans to Roberts, memorandum, June 27, 1951, and Evans supplementary notes, July 2, 1951, ibid.) See pp. 466–67, 469–70, and 474–75.

2. See pp. 474–75n1 and MacGregor, *Integration of the Armed Forces*, 442–47.

3. The Defense Department made this announcement on July 26 and declared that it hoped to reach full integration in the Far East Command within six months. ("Army to End Segregation in Asia Command, Closing History of Its Last Negro Regiment," *New York Times*, July 27, 1951, p. 2.)

Lehman replied on July 28 that he "was much gratified at the news that the 24th Infantry Regiment was to be replaced with an integrated Infantry Regiment and that further integration will follow at a later date through a normal flow of replacements." He thanked Marshall for his cooperation and attached a copy of a statement he had given to the press praising the plans for full integration of the Far East Command. (Lehman to Marshall, July 28, 1951, and attachment, NA/RG 330, SD 291.2; "Army Race Action Lauded," *New York Times*, July 28, 1951, p. 2.)

341

To General of the Army Dwight D. Eisenhower — July 21, 1951
Radio No. JCS-96929. *Top Secret* — Washington, DC
From Marshall Personal for Eisenhower. Noforn.

Chairman Richards, House Foreign Affairs Committee, has expressed deep concern of himself and others favorably disposed to MDAP that hearings are coming to close in discouraging atmosphere. He has advised State and Defense Departments that he considers it essential that record contain effective testimony dealing with prospects, requirements, and atmosphere in Europe from your viewpoint. He considers General Gruenther ideal witness to meet Committees needs, and states Committee will see him any time if you can make him available for a single appearance. I agree with importance of getting such testimony in record and recommend your favorable consideration of chairman's request which may, in addition to primary purpose, serve to reduce constant request for your presence. With General Gruenther's testimony in record, believe we could successfully withstand pressures from other committees which will later deal with MDAP program. Please advise whether you agree, and if so how promptly Gruenther can be made available. End[1]

GCMRL/G. C. Marshall Papers (Secretary of Defense, Chronological, Director, Executive Office [Marshall S. Carter], 1950–1952)

1. Eisenhower cabled on July 23 that after the recent visit of the House Foreign Affairs, Armed Services, and Appropriations Committees delegation (see pp. 585–86), he was "somewhat astonished" that the congressmen required the additional testimony of one of his representatives. "Nevertheless," Eisenhower ensured Marshall, he would make Gruenther, his chief of staff at SHAPE, available. (Eisenhower to Marshall, cable, July 23, 1951, DDEL/Dwight D. Eisenhower Papers [Pre-Presidential Files, Principal File, Name Series, Box 80, Marshall, George C.]; *Papers of DDE*, 12: 436–37.) Eisenhower admitted in a further reply to Marshall on July 25 that Gruenther was not the most qualified individual to present the details about "MDAP programs at country and regional levels." He therefore suggested that either Major General Abram Franklin Kibler (VMI, 1912), the director of the Joint US Military Advisory Group for Europe, or General Handy as the US military representative for Mutual Defense Assistance in Europe as well as commander in chief of US forces in Europe, testify before Gruenther. (Eisenhower to Marshall, cable no. SH-20912, July 25, 1951, in *Papers of DDE*, 12: 438–39.)

Between July 28 and August 2, Generals Gruenther and Kibler both testified before the House and Senate committees, with Kibler submitting a report from General Handy. (*Papers of DDE*, 12: 436–39; House Committee on Foreign Affairs, *Hearings . . . on H.R. 5020 and H.R. 5113*, 1344–85, 1505–52; Senate Committee on Foreign Relations and Committee on Armed Services, *Hearings . . . on S. 1762, Mutual Security Act of 1951*, 82d Cong., 1st sess., 207–32, 235–316.) See pp. 569–77 and 597–603.

When KOREAN armistice negotiations formally began at Kaesong on July 10, 1951 (see pp. 566–67), the North Koreans and Chinese insisted the agenda include recognition of the 38th parallel as the military demarcation line between the opposing armies and the withdrawal from the peninsula of all foreign forces. Marshall strongly supported the JCS position that these were political issues and that present negotiations should be limited to purely military matters concerning the establishment of a military armistice, with political matters to be discussed only later. On July 13, he asked Acheson in a memorandum to issue a public statement to this effect, a draft of which he attached, "not only for the information of our public but for its effect on the Chinese negotiators." Acheson did so on July 19, by which time the North Koreans and Chinese had dropped their demand that the 38th parallel issue be included on the armistice negotiations agenda but not the one regarding withdrawal of all foreign forces. Consequently, Acheson announced on July 19 that UN truce negotiators would not accept their demand that foreign troops withdraw from Korea prior to the beginning of armistice talks, and that UN forces would not leave the Korean peninsula "until a genuine peace has been firmly established and the Korean people have assurance that they can work out their future free from the fear of aggression." (Marshall to Acheson, July 13, 1951, NA/RG 330, CD 092 [Korea]; *FRUS, 1951*, 7: 688–91, 706; "Acheson's Statement," *New York Times*, July 20, 1951, p. 2; Condit, *Test of War*, 120–21; Schnabel and Watson, *History of JCS*, 3, pt. 2: 10–11.)

On the previous day, July 18, Marshall had sent Truman "without comment" the recommendations of the JCS on courses of action in Korea if the armistice talks failed, which called for expanded operations to "increase military pressure" on the enemy, but not action that would lead to a "general war" with China. On July 19, Truman responded that he had read the JCS recommendations and wanted to discuss them with Marshall and Acheson. (Bradley to Marshall, memorandum, July 13, 1951; Marshall to Truman, July 18, 1951; and Truman to Marshall, July 19, 1951, NA/RG 330, CD 092 [Korea]; *FRUS, 1951*, 7: 667–68; Schnabel and Watson, *History of JCS*, 3, pt. 2: 35–36.)

In the days prior to Acheson's July 19 statement, the JCS had exchanged a series of messages with Ridgway regarding the inclusion of political matters on the agenda for the military armistice talks, particularly that of removing all foreign troops from Korea. At Ridgway's request, and with the consent of Truman, Acheson, and Marshall, the JCS approved a statement on July 16 to be delivered by Ridgway or Admiral Joy, who led the UN negotiating team, asserting that the armistice negotiators would not "become a transmittal agency through which political questions can be raised by commanders who we consider are not entitled to raise them on a governmental level." In light of this exchange and a memorandum from Kenneth Young reporting that "State planning on what happens if ceasefire succeeds is not very far along," Marshall forwarded to Acheson on July 20 the belief of the JCS, which he shared, in "'the importance of making all necessary preparations now to start the political and diplomatic settlement immediately upon an armistice being implemented'" and their concern "'as to the dangerous effect of any delay in pursuing negotiations on a governmental level leading to final settlement of the Korean problem.'" Consequently, Marshall requested "assurances from you that preparations for the political and diplomatic settlement of the Korean problem are now under way for implementation immediately upon the arrangement of an armistice" and that the State Department "would keep the

Defense Department informed of the terms and the time for the negotiations of the political and diplomatic settlement." Acheson replied on July 27 that the State Department concurred with Marshall's letter, that it was "regularly consulting with all of the Governments participating in the military action in Korea," and that it would keep the Defense Department "informed of plans in this regard." He reminded Marshall "that a final political settlement of the Korean problem will require agreement by the Communists, an agreement which will be difficult to achieve," and as such, "it is of the utmost importance that any armistice arrangement be acceptable to us over an extended period of time, in the event no progress is made, despite our efforts, in reaching an agreement on political and territorial questions." (Young to Burns, memorandum, July 17, 1951; Marshall to Acheson, July 20, 1951; and Acheson to Marshall, July 27, 1951, NA/RG 330, CD 092 [Korea]; *FRUS, 1951*, 7: 681–82, 687–88, 706–7, 737–38; Schnabel and Watson, *History of JCS*, 3, pt. 2: 13–14.) For the ensuing State Department position paper on August 18, 1951, and the response of Marshall and the JCS on September 4, 1951, see *FRUS, 1951*, 7: 831–35 and 877–79.

At Acheson's request, Marshall also addressed the armistice negotiations during his July 24 press conference. ★

342

REMARKS AT A PRESS CONFERENCE
July 24, 1951 Washington, DC

ON JULY 20, Marshall informed Lovett, Fritchey, Bradley, and either Ginsburgh or Frank Nash that he had spoken at that morning's cabinet meeting with Acheson, who desired that Marshall or Bradley make "a public statement within the next five days" regarding "Fundamentals of an Armistice." Acheson "had in mind making clear to the public and incidentally to the Chinese that an armistice imposed on us the necessity for determining on a secure position (not an arbitrary line) an arrangement guaranteeing us against hostile preparations, etc." Marshall asked for advice as to "Just how this might be staged" and requested that Ginsburgh or Nash begin to prepare a statement "while the matter of execution is being determined." (Carter crossed out Ginsburgh's name on this memorandum and replaced it with Nash's. Marshall to Lovett, Bradley, Ginsburgh [*Nash*], and Fritchey, memorandum, July 20, 1951, NA/RG 330, CD 092 [Korea].)

The resulting statement, which Marshall read at the beginning of his July 24 press conference, stated that Ridgway was "trying to accomplish . . . a suitable *military armistice*," not "a political settlement. It is essential that the two matters be kept entirely separate and distinct." Only after "an acceptable armistice" was "obtained" could "discussion of the political questions" begin among the governments involved. Any armistice arrangement, Marshall continued, must contain "agreement upon a military line which will be defensible in the event of any renewal of hostilities; there must be agreement not to reinforce the troops now in

Korea; there must be provision for adequate supervision and actual inspection by representatives of both sides to insure against any preparations for a surprise attack and as continuing evidence of good faith; there must be a satisfactory agreement regarding prisoners of war. There are basic conditions to an armistice and agreement with respect to them must precede a later effort to reach a final settlement of the Korean question." Marshall added that he was referring particularly to "the Communists' insistence that withdrawal of all foreign troops from Korea be made a firm part of the armistice agenda," a point which Acheson had insisted was "not suitable" for talks concerning a military armistice. Such a withdrawal "will naturally follow a satisfactory peace settlement" and would "pose no problem if the Communists are sincere in wanting to work out with us a real settlement of the Korean conflict." While the "long-range objective of the United Nations in Korea" was a free and unified nation, maintaining a presence of UN forces in Korea was "the only assurance we have of meeting the threat of renewed aggression if the peace talks should break down." Marshall also noted the continuing "necessity for caution," as the current disagreements had "been only on the adoption of an agenda. The real points to be settled have not yet been discussed." After reading this prepared statement, Marshall told the press that he was "not going to make any other comments about Korea." (Transcript of remarks at a press conference, July 24, 1951, GCMRL/G. C. Marshall Papers [Secretary of Defense, Speeches and Statements].) See frontispiece photograph.

The press then asked Marshall about reports of "possible inter-service friction" due to the air force's desire to expand beyond the ninety-five wings that had been authorized. Marshall responded that "an increase of the Air arm" was being discussed, but a decision would not be made until October. "I see no great complications unless they are stirred up in the press!" Marshall commented that "present production plans" provide "planes for, I think, 195 groups or wings." When one reporter asked Marshall to clarify that number, as it was "a new figure to us," Marshall replied that he was referring to "Production capacity in the plants which we can keep going along with the present 95-wing program." (The transcript of this press conference indicated at this point that Marshall's reference was revised from 195 to 180 groups.) Marshall indicated that the expansion of the air force would likely not follow a "balanced-force concept," with a complementary increase in supporting ground and naval units, because "other factors are involved." While "certain phases" of that concept remained applicable, current needs and "commitments like those in Western Europe" were "additional" and could not be met under a balanced force model. He also noted the difficulty in budgeting for the buildup, because "you can't draw a sharp line" in production when some items "carry over" into a new fiscal year. (Ibid. See also "Armed Forces Reported Split on Proposed Air Power Rise," *New York Times*, July 24, 1951, pp. 1, 13, and Condit, *Test of War*, 255 and 259.)

The questions then turned to the death of Admiral Sherman, who had died of a heart attack on July 22 in Naples, Italy, as he was preparing to return to the US after holding a series of positive discussions with Generalissimo Francisco Franco regarding US base rights in Spain (see pp. 493–94 and 587n1) and touring NATO countries. Upon learning of Sherman's death, Marshall released a statement that he felt "the deep personal loss of a close associate and friend for whom I had the highest respect and admiration. The Department of Defense, and the United States Navy in particular, has lost an outstanding leader. He was a great personality, and his death is a definite and serious loss to the nation at this critical time." (Statements on the Death of Admiral Forrest Sherman, July 22, 1951, GCMRL/G. C. Marshall Papers [Speeches Binder #14].) He added during this press conference that Sherman's career had "been most remarkable. He's had a tremendously heavy responsibility, both within the Navy, considering the conditions at the time he came in, and in connection with the Chiefs of Staff." Marshall thought Sherman's death was "a little evidence" of the "burden" and "very great" strain placed on the chiefs of staff. Rather than effecting "a change in the unification law" as one reporter suggested, Marshall insisted that this "indicates the desirability of a change in the world in not having so many crises a day! We run, it seems to me, about five a morning. I get in here at eight o'clock, or about eight-fifteen, and it's just one crisis after another, it seems to me, from that time on. Very peaceful!" (Transcript of remarks at a press conference, July 24, 1951, GCMRL/G. C. Marshall Papers [Secretary of Defense, Speeches and Statements].) Marshall would attend the arrival of Sherman's body in Washington on July 25 and his funeral at Arlington National Cemetery on July 27. Immediately prior to the funeral, Marshall wrote to Admiral Byrd that "many of the senior officers of the Navy, including Nimitz," were in Washington for the service, which had allowed Dan Kimball, the new secretary of the navy, "to consult with them" regarding Sherman's successor. "No decision has yet been arrived at." (Marshall to Byrd, July 27, 1951, GCMRL/G. C. Marshall Papers [Secretary of Defense, Number Indexed, M200-12-5].) See p. 621n4.

Shifting to manpower policies, Marshall would not estimate whether the Defense Department would need to ask for an increase in the manpower ceiling, which had been set at five million men in amendments to the Selective Service Act in June 1951. He noted his desire and belief that the UMST bill and the subsequent report by the National Security Training Commission could "be put into operation at a considerable period earlier than is anticipated, and I think it is very important that it should be." (See pp. 551–53 and 558–59.) He later clarified that he hoped a "small beginning" could occur "within a year" before expanding to "an all-over affair," although there were "a great many factors" involved, such as the requirement for an additional act of Congress and the urgent need to use available manpower to rotate troops from Korea. (Transcript of remarks at a press conference, July 24, 1951, GCMRL/G. C. Marshall Papers [Secretary of Defense, Speeches and Statements].)

Regarding Europe, Marshall declined to comment on a report by a group of senators who had recently visited General Eisenhower, which stated that Eisenhower was now supporting a unified European army. Marshall was having lunch with many of those senators on July 25, "so I'll probably hear it direct from them in more detail." (See pp. 497–99, 583–85, and 586n3, and "Eisenhower Said to Seek 1-Flag Army," *Washington Post*, July 24, 1951, pp. 1, 5.) Reports from Eisenhower and the JCS indicated that some European NATO countries "have done a surprising amount" to support mutual defense, "particularly in their budget buildups and particularly in their increasing the length of service periods," but that many were still lagging in production. All of the reports "indicate that we're at a very critical period. We're at a time where we apparently can go forward, we think, to great success, or we can go into reverse in a very fatal manner." It was a "tremulous moment, . . . so that's one reason that we are very much concerned to see that" present plans and production authorizations were "not cut and that we go ahead because it may mean, psychologically, a great reverse, whereas, at the moment, I think we can develop a tremendous feeling of encouragement and of desire to do among those nations." (Ibid.) See pp. 569–77 and the next two documents.

The press conference ended on a lighter note when one reporter asked "How is NATO getting on?" and Marshall joked in return "Are you talking about the dog or Western Europe?" (See pp. 578–79) Marshall added that the dog had "taken over the place. He tore a hole in Mrs. Marshall's skirt yesterday and had a little plug out of a pair of flannel trousers of mine. He's doing very well. He's a very cute dog, very well behaved, except in spots! . . . We've allowed him to run loose all over the place. He hasn't gone off the premises yet. I wouldn't be surprised if, as a result of his residence down there, he may find a much more interested and friendly disposition toward the NATO organization around Leesburg than elsewhere!" (Ibid.) ★

343

Statement to the Senate Foreign Relations and Armed Services Committees on the Mutual Security Program[1]

July 27, 1951
Washington, DC

In the years that have passed since 1945 we and other free nations have been faced with the growing threat of Soviet tyranny and oppression. The Soviet campaign operates through internal subversion and by direct military attack. It aims at dominating the free world by force or by any other means.

Recognizing this threat, Congress enacted the programs for military aid to Greece and Turkey in 1947, the Economic Cooperation Act in 1948, the North Atlantic Treaty and the Mutual Defense Assistance Act in 1949, and last year's amendments to that Act.[2]

Thus, the United States has been playing a leading part in reviving the devastated economies of Western Europe and eliminating the breeding grounds of communism. The will to resist Soviet aggression and subversion has been stimulated.

The program of economic assistance has largely achieved its major objectives. The more recent program for helping Europe to rearm is now gaining real momentum.

The strength of a nation does not depend alone on its armies, ships, and planes; it is measured as well by its qualities of leadership, by its resources and industries, by the determination of its people, and by the strength of its friends and allies. Although we, as a nation are strong and have great resources it would be unwise for us to rely solely upon our own strength. The most effective and least costly means of insuring peace is through mutual aid and collective security arrangements with our allies.

In the North Atlantic Treaty Organization we have joined in such collective arrangements with Canada and ten European nations. The combined allied contributions in troops, Army-Navy-Air Force, to General Eisenhower and the Atlantic Naval Command constitute a substantial force. This force has a mobilization potential greater than our own presently authorized strength. Our allies plan to contribute approximately 85% of the manpower for this combined force. They are providing for their own forces all the facilities, pay, individual equipment, administrative and housekeeping supplies, and as much of the major arms and equipment as they can produce in time to meet scheduled plans. They are contributing the land, the bases, and certain logistic facilities that we require in their territories. They have increased their training program, their lengths of military service, and their defense budgets.

We in this country are strengthening our forces and increasing our industrial capacity. We are assisting our allies by providing (a) major items of military equipment that they cannot produce in time, (b) support for their own production of military equipment, (c) general economic aid in selected areas to keep nations from becoming impoverished by their defense efforts, and (d) technical assistance to under-developed areas.

The total cost of this program for Fiscal '52 is $8.5 billion. It includes our total foreign aid program, military, economic, and technical. Military aid totals $6.2 billion; economic aid and technical assistance total $2.3 billion.[3]

The major portion of these funds is intended to aid in the highly important task of raising, equipping and training the troops required to make General Eisenhower's command an effective defensive force. The funds that are being requested for the NATO area are in the amount required to make operative those forces committed for 1952. This estimate of funds required has been developed to provide only the essential minimum requirements. Any delay in the appropriation of these funds will mean that General Eisenhower will not have the trained and equipped forces on which he is basing his plans. It is essential that we, having placed this responsibility on him, provide him the means of accomplishing this mission. It is the security of the United States as well as our allies that is at stake.

As the requirements for the Fiscal Year 1952 military aid programs were developed, they were integrated with the requirements for our own military services, in order to determine the feasibility of the combined production schedule. This schedule has been reviewed by the Munitions Board and the Office of Defense Mobilization, and has been determined to be altogether feasible.

The Army, Navy, and Air Force technical personnel who will procure these items of military equipment have assured me that, barring unforeseen changes in present conditions, the funds can and must be obligated in Fiscal Year 1952 in order to produce the equipment in time to meet NATO mobilization schedules.

Our plans are based on maximum self-help by our allies. But in estimating the maximum of which they are capable, we must recognize that we are working with countries that were devastated by war. . . . [4]

It is urgent that we take effective measures now for the security of the free world, of which the United States is the heart. The proposed military aid program will be about 10 percent of our own military budget for Fiscal 1952. This is not a high proportion when we consider the additional forces in men and organizations that it will make effective for collective security.

As to the duration and extent of military assistance programs, it is impossible to make a reliable forecast. However, based on estimates of requirements under present plans and a reasonable expansion of military production by our allies, the requirements for military assistance funds in Fiscal Years 1953 and 1954 will be at least as large as the amount we are requesting for this year. By then, progress in rearmament and in developing European military production will have reached the point where requirements for military equipment from the United States can be reduced.

I strongly endorse the Mutual Security Program in its entirety as a sound and workable plan for meeting the communist challenge on every front. It is the best investment that can be made in the collective security of the free world.[5]

GCMRL/G. C. Marshall Papers (Secretary of Defense, Speeches and Statements)

1. Marshall had lunch on July 25 with several members of the Senate Foreign Relations Committee who had just returned from an inspection tour in Europe (see pp. 585–86, 592, and 596–97). On July 26, Marshall Carter wrote to Major George that despite a "fine" luncheon, "it appears that the Secretary will have to testify before that group tomorrow; however, I don't believe it is anything that will put a kink in his vacation plans." (Carter to George, July 26, 1951, GCMRL/G. C. Marshall Papers [Secretary of Defense, Chronological, Secretaries, Carlson].) For Marshall's earlier testimony on this bill before the House committee, which was similar to this Senate appearance, see pp. 569–77.

2. See pp. 99–101 and *Papers of GCM*, 6: 67–68, 309–28, 391–96, 681–82, 699–705, 713–17, and 741–43.

3. Acheson had announced in his July 26 testimony on this bill before the Senate committee that it would cost around $25 billion over three years for the US to equip its allies adequately with military equipment. ("Cost of 25 Billions for Aid to Allies Is Set by Acheson," *New York Times*, July 27, 1951, p. 1.)

4. Marshall at this point listed the concerns and needs of several countries and regions that would be participating in the Mutual Security Program, such as France, Norway, Italy, Greece, Turkey, Iran, Indochina, the Philippines, Canada, and Latin America. He also discussed "the deliveries of military equipment under the present Mutual Defense Assistance Act" and the need for continued and expanded deliveries in the coming years as well as the importance of training manpower in all participating countries.

5. See the next editorial summary.

344

Senate Testimony on the Mutual Security Program
July 27, 1951 Washington, DC

AFTER COMPLETING his prepared statement (see previous document), the secretary of defense first took questions from Senator Connally, the committee chairman, who asked Marshall to comment on recent reports "that the program as proposed now by the administration, by you, might be spread over 2 years." Marshall responded by reading a letter he had signed and sent to Representative James Richards that morning, in which he reminded Richards that "these funds are carefully calculated as one element in a complex plan to bring about a certain result. The alternative is a change in the basic aims which we had when we agreed to the appointment of General Eisenhower as Supreme Allied Commander in Europe" and "would imply almost complete renunciation of our current objectives in other parts of the world." He added that altering the time frame would set back General Eisenhower "by a considerable number of divisions," which "would be a very serious thing." Marshall responded later to a question by Senator H. Alexander Smith that "You have to have, I think, the authority to negotiate on a dependable basis." Marshall also agreed with several senators that any improvement in the situation in Korea would be no reason to reduce military aid to other countries through the Mutual Security Program. He reiterated his shock at the American reaction to Malik's cease-fire statement (see pp. 566–67 and 592–95), which was "a very sad admission to have to make that our people would react in any such manner" to the statement of "one man, representative of such a government" whose "ethics, standards, dependability, and good faith" were widely recognized to be suspect. "I like gentle people," Marshall remarked, "but I would like the American public to get a little more hard-boiled." Indeed, "If one is logical there is more reason than ever to prepare." (Senate Committee on Foreign Relations and Committee on Armed Services, *Hearings . . . on S. 1762*, 40–42, 58, 60.)

Marshall continued by affirming the statement of Senator Theodore Green that "these plans contemplate not only our defense in time of war but also the probability of preventing war itself." Marshall added "that the best deterrent to war is preparedness and that's what we are striving to do—to be prepared and to develop an effective basis of collective security." Senator Green wondered if "the arguments of those who are opposed to the full implementation of this program are those that are helping to bring about a war," to which Marshall replied "that many are involved in that argument without fully realizing what they are doing." His own experience "in the many struggles in which I have been engaged, has been that if things are delayed too much then you are involved in stupendous sums which makes these present requirements seem trivial." By supporting such aid programs and standing up to Communist aggression in Korea, "We have established before the world that we mean what we say. We announce a principle and we will stand behind it." Such conviction "has reduced the fear" of the European countries "that they are left to stand alone and be submerged." In response to Green's ensuing question regarding the effect on the US should Europe "fall," Marshall warned that "there would be built up, under the Soviets' domination, a productive power that would exceed ours, which would very markedly change our position in the world. We would have the Atlantic dominated on the far side by governments hostile to our purpose. That would extend into the Mediterranean. Our whole position would be one of isolation which we could only successfully defend by a tremendous military build-up." In addition, "We would be affected economically in other ways than those I just referred to. It would put us in an extremely perilous position, I feel, and our national existence would be threatened." (Ibid., 43–45.)

Senator Alexander Wiley then shifted to a more technical series of questions and asked Marshall "whether the executive branch of Government has done everything it could to get efficiency into procurement." Marshall confessed that he did not "know that we have done everything we could," but he assured Wiley that "we have been doing it every day in a very searching way to insure that it was not only all wool and a yard wide, but to find improvements in methods and procedures to reduce costs and expedite production. . . . I think the general integrity of the individuals concerned in the defense military production is on a very high level." Marshall echoed his recent testimony on the Defense Production Act (see pp. 536–39) on the need "to control this inflationary development" in order to protect both the defense program and the US economy. Wiley also asked Marshall for specific figures for "the over-all contribution of our allies in Europe over a similar period" as the US would be providing in military aid to them. Marshall replied that he could not provide "the exact figures" as they had not been made public, but he reported that "in 1952 our allies will have about two million and a half men on active service. We will have, I think, about 340,000 in ground forces and some fifty or sixty thousand in the Air Forces." (Ibid., 46–48.) For more on this statement, see the penultimate paragraph of this editorial summary, pp. 602–3 below.

After Wiley and Senator Guy Gillette had asked a series of questions regarding the defense contributions of the other NATO members and the amount being requested for military as opposed to economic and technical aid, Gillette expressed his concern "that it is possible to press the American people too far economically." Marshall retorted that he "was under considerable attack in November and December because I wasn't asking for enough, in the way of a charge against the American economy." (See pp. 276–78 and 291–93.) Gillette asserted that Marshall "got no attack from me," and Marshall replied that he was "stating a fact, and my reason was just the question that you are putting there, that I thought that for us to go out into much more expensive terms, into a major mobilization at that time, which was being pressed and argued and demanded, would put us in a very dangerous position economically and militarily. In the first place, we couldn't do what was demanded at that rate level, and in the next place we would get out on the end of a plank, as it were, which could very easily be sawed off against us, and we would be defeated economically rather than militarily. I have been very conscious of that, and I have taken quite a beating in regard to it, so I am aware of the economic factors." Indeed, they were "a dominating consideration in my mind." In discussing aid to the Middle East and North Africa as opposed to Europe, he noted that "The problem is, and the military problem very particularly is, how you allocate, and you just can't do it all. I have lived in that struggle for the last 10 years, almost." (Ibid., 48–55.)

Senator H. Alexander Smith asked Marshall if it was "a fair question to ask you whether probably in 1954," the year through which both Marshall and Acheson had testified the same elevated levels of military aid would be required, "we will see the end of this phase of our operation?" Marshall believed that "you should definitely see the end of the phase of what I might call the capital build-up. Just how we are going to work out the replacement and maintenance factor remains to be determined." He refused to say, however, when the Europeans might be able to defend themselves without large numbers of US troops. Despite any progress that would be made in defense spending, arms, manpower, and many other areas, Marshall stated to Senator Bourke Hickenlooper, "we are inevitably confronted with a considerable period of tension, high tension; that whatever agreements we might develop, starting, we will say, with the question of Korea, we never could let up until good faith has been established. How long it takes to do that, in what ways they demonstrate good faith, is something else. And of course a good bit depends on what we know about them, their affairs, their military build-up, and their military potential." The implementation of universal military training in the United States, Marshall continued, was "the only economical way that I could see that we could face the future," and the aid for the Europeans being requested was of "vital, critical importance." He predicted that the Soviets would "outwait us, outsit us in this thing, as they do so often in conferences. That is, it is their aim to do that." He thought, however, that "they will have increasing troubles—as this thing goes along, and we get ourselves in a very firm, strong collective position which will do more to break down this menace than anything else." He admitted "that reduction of expenses doesn't reduce the tension in a sense, but it makes it more possible to endure it, because if you have a taxpayer in despair on the one hand and the tension staring you in the face on the other, you have an almost impossible situation." (Ibid., 56, 59–60, 64–66.)

Marshall's statement at this hearing that the United States would have approximately three hundred forty thousand ground forces and fifty to sixty thousand air forces in Europe (see p. 601 above) appeared to contradict his February 15, 1951, testimony at an earlier Senate hearing that six US divisions totaling about one hundred thousand troops would be required for the NATO defense force. (See pp. 380–86.) Senator Smith commented after the hearings that it was "'difficult for me to understand how six divisions of about 20,000 men each could total 400,000. I don't want to charge bad faith too soon,'" so he recommended waiting to hear General Collins's testimony later that week before criticizing Marshall's statement too harshly. According to the Associated Press, "highest defense officials at the Pentagon told reporters, after hours of frantic checking and double-checking, that they were unable to explain or clarify the basis for General Marshall's statement" and suspected that Marshall may "have made a slip of the tongue." These officials affirmed "that so far as they knew, there was no change in present plans to limit the number of United States troops in Europe to about 200,000." ("Marshall Prefers Cutting U.S. Arms to Saving on Allies," *New York Times*, July 28, 1951, pp. 1, 4; "Marshall Says 400,000 Men For Europe Estimate Is Correct," *Washington Post*, July 29, 1951, p. M1; "Troop Issue Spurs Shift of Aid Bill," *New York Times*, July 30, 1951, pp. 1, 10.) On July 28, Marshall clarified in letters to Richards and Connally that the 340,000 figure included all "the necessary 'combat support' and 'logistic support' troops to maintain supply and support these six divisions in combat readiness, the necessary corps and army headquarters troops, the necessary antiaircraft units for the protection of both ground and air units, and also includes our forces in Austria and Trieste." These forces were necessary to maintain the six divisions "both in combat readiness and in combat itself," and the number per combat division was "less than that required in Europe for the support of our combat divisions in World War II." (Marshall to Richards, July 28, 1951, GCMRL/G. C. Marshall Papers [Secretary of Defense, Number Indexed, M200-17-17].)

On the same date that Marshall provided this testimony, the NSC senior staff circulated a status report on the NSC 68/4 rearmament programs that warned the Western powers were "already in a period of acute danger," and that the programs should be "achieved at the earliest practicable date." (See pp. 300–301.) While Marshall was on vacation (see next editorial note), the JCS informed him that they agreed, the NSC adopted the report after emendation as NSC 114/1, and Truman immediately approved its conclusions and directed that they be implemented. (Poole, *History of JCS*, 4: 46–49.) ★

ON SATURDAY, July 28, Marshall began a month-long vacation by flying from Leesburg to Mitchel Field, Long Island, where he and Katherine Marshall were driven to Margaret Emerson's house. Then on Monday, July 30, the Marshalls flew from Mitchel Field to Camp Edwards, Massachusetts, and drove to Waquoit on Cape Cod, where they stayed with General Frank and Frances McCoy in the cottage of Harold Dodds, who was on vacation in Great Britain. They also spent time with visitors such as Bernard Baruch and his son; Hayden Harris, an old friend and neighbor from Leesburg, and his wife; and for a weekend on Naushon Island, Massachusetts, with W. Cameron Forbes, former governor general of the Philippines and ambassador to Japan, who had invited them to stay with him before Marshall had completed his plans with the McCoys. (Marshall to Emerson, July 24, 1951, GCMRL/G. C. Marshall Papers [Secretary of Defense, Number Indexed, M200-7-47]; Marshall to McCoy, July 16, 1951, ibid., [M200-7-27]; Marshall to McCoy, July 24, 1951, ibid., [M217-4-9]; Forbes to Marshall, June 25 and July 16, 1951, and Marshall to Forbes, July 26, 1951, ibid., [M200-16-44]; George to Heffner, memorandum, July 21, 1951, GCMRL/G. C. Marshall Papers [Secretary of Defense, Chronological, Secretaries, Carlson]; Katherine Marshall to George, August 9, 1951, GCMRL/Katherine T. Marshall Correspondence Collection [C. J. George]; Marshall to Huntington Harris, August 10, 1951, NA/RG 330, SD 091 [China].) For the Dodds's previous stay at the Marshalls' home in Pinehurst, see pp. 236–37.

"We are having the most restful and delightful" vacation, Katherine Marshall wrote to C. J. George on August 9. "We are very lazy and fish, canoe and bathe when we feel like it—or just sit in the sun on the beaches. Cape Cod is lovely with many pretty drives." (Katherine Marshall to George, August 9, 1951, GCMRL/ Katherine T. Marshall Correspondence Collection [C. J. George].) "We have been having a pleasant time and the weather, for the most part, has been good," Marshall wrote to an old friend on August 18. "However, the past several days have been a little dismal—showers and overcast. I have been out fishing several times but have nothing to brag about. Actually, I am so lazy that it takes a little while to develop enough energy to go out on the water." (Marshall to Ayres, August 18, 1951, GCMRL/G. C. Marshall Papers [Secretary of Defense, Number Indexed, M200-13-9].) See pp. 672–73.

While Marshall was on Cape Cod, Marshall Carter, who had been promoted to the permanent rank of brigadier general on July 27, established a courier service from Washington to Camp Edwards, where the commanding general had agreed to provide Marshall with secretarial assistance to take dictations of his responses to the mail he received. Carter had been promoted to the temporary rank of brigadier general effective April 8, 1947, during the Moscow Conference of Foreign Ministers until reverting to his permanent rank of colonel on August 28, 1949. He remarked to Lewis Douglas on July 28, 1951, that his "star was given back to me by a benevolent Congress, a loyal President, and a reluctant Secretary of Defense at 7:00 P. M. last night." (*Papers of GCM*, 6: 142; Witsell to Carter, August 24, 1949, GCMRL/Marshall S. Carter Papers [Central File, Selected Correspondence, Promotions–Congratulations]; Carter to Douglas, July 28, 1951, GCMRL/ Marshall S. Carter Papers [Defense Department, Correspondence].) ★

345

TO COLONEL JAMES H. VAN HORN

August 15, 1951
Cape Cod, Massachusetts

Dear Van Horn: I have your letter of August 5th in which you express your views on the General Crawford and West Point incidents. It would be inappropriate for me to interject myself into the administrative affairs of the Department of the Army, unless I was convinced that there was a serious failure on the part of the officials in acting to the best interests of the national defense.[1]

Incidentally, your letter was forwarded to me here on Cape Cod where Mrs. Marshall and I are enjoying a brief vacation. I hope all goes well with you.

With warm regards,[2] Faithfully yours,

GCMRL/G. C. Marshall Papers (Secretary of Defense, Number Indexed, M200-17-46)

1. Van Horn was a retired signal corps officer who had known Marshall since 1912, first

at Fort Leavenworth and then in the Philippines and in France in 1918–19. (Van Horn to Pogue, October 10, 1960, GCMRL/Vertical File [Philippines, 1913–1916, Misc.]. For their 1938 correspondence, see *Papers of GCM*, 1: 595–96.)

In the summer of 1951, the army faced a series of scandals. Brigadier General David J. Crawford, commanding general of the Ordnance Tank–Automotive Center in Detroit, Michigan, was accused of misusing government materials and accepting improper gifts from defense contractors. He was relieved of his command on July 29, and the Associated Press reported on August 1 that he was being transferred to US Army headquarters in Heidelberg, Germany, with his specific position to be determined by General Handy. ("Tank Chief Admits Free Hotel Suite," *New York Times*, July 24, 1951, p. 15; "Warrants Are Issued for Two in Detroit Arsenal Scandal," *Washington Post*, August 1, 1951, p. 6.)

Marshall Carter recalled that during Marshall's trip to deliver the commencement address at West Point in June 1951 (see pp. 544–46), General John K. Waters (USMA, 1931), the commandant of cadets at West Point, informed Carter privately that "All hell is going to break loose" surrounding accusations of cheating by ninety cadets, many of whom played on the football team. Carter replied that he was going to keep General Marshall "the hell out of it." On August 3, the press reported that the army would be discharging the ninety cadets. Carter later recalled that "General Marshall refused to see anybody about it, write anybody about it, or even take it up with anybody," including West Point head football coach Earl Blaik. (Interview with Marshall S. Carter by Mr. James F. Schnabel and Dr. Walter S. Poole, March 19, 1973, GCMRL/Pogue Research Materials [Box 1], p. 19; "West Point Ousts 90 Cadets for Cheating in Classroom; Football Players Involved" and "Texts of Expulsion Statements," *New York Times*, August 4, 1951, pp. 1, 5.)

Van Horn wrote to Marshall on August 5 to complain that Crawford had been treated too leniently, especially in light of the harsher actions taken at West Point. He thought a response from Marshall "that further action in this case can be expected would be most reassuring to many of your contemporaries." (Van Horn to Marshall, August 5, 1951, GCMRL/G. C. Marshall Papers [Secretary of Defense, Number Indexed, M200-17-46].)

2. After further investigation, the army announced on August 30 that Crawford would become a special assistant to the commanding general at Aberdeen Proving Ground in Maryland. Secretary Pace demoted Crawford to the rank of colonel and ordered him to the joint military mission in Turkey in January 1952. ("Suspended General Gets Aberdeen Post," *New York Times*, August 31, 1951, p. 11; "Crawford Reduced to Colonel's Rank; Is Sent to Turkey," *Washington Post*, January 9, 1952, p. 1.)

346

To Felix E. Larkin

August 22, 1951
[Cape Cod, Massachusetts]

Dear Larkin: It is with regret that I accept your resignation as General Counsel for the Department of Defense to be effective August 31, 1951.[1]

Since your appointment almost four years ago you have played a major, and in many instances, a principal role in a large number of unification measures. Your foresight and planning have brought about such Department-wide improvements as a Uniform Code of Military Justice, a single-package public works program, and a highly efficient Legislative Conference. Through your negotiations with the Attorney General, the Department of Defense has been able to negotiate lower freight rates, in many cases with sizable annual savings.

Over and above these Department-wide accomplishments, you deserve special commendation for the outstanding work you have done as counsel to me and my predecessors on important matters concerning the Congress. But more particularly you have my genuine appreciation for the service you rendered me in connection with my many appearances before the various committees of the Congress.[2]

Although most reluctant to see you leave, I am aware of and sympathetic with the personal considerations which motivate your resignation at this time. The Department has been fortunate to have had your services over the past four years, and I hope we may continue to call upon you from time to time for advice and counsel.

With every good wish for your future and with warmest regards to Mrs. Larkin and you, believe me,[3] Faithfully yours,

NA/RG 330, CD 201.22

1. Larkin reminded Marshall on August 17 that they had agreed "some time ago" that he would resign as general counsel on August 31. He described his four years at the Defense Department as "a most rewarding experience" but confessed that he had stayed "much longer than my original plan." He would become an executive with W. R. Grace & Company, at that time a ship operation firm in New York. (Larkin to Marshall, August 17, 1951, GCMRL/G. C. Marshall Papers [Secretary of Defense, Number Indexed, M211-1-21]; "Larkin, Fighter for Unification, Resigns As Defense Department General Counsel," *New York Times*, August 23, 1951, p. 10.)

2. In addition to Marshall's other congressional testimonies, Larkin was instrumental in the secretary's preparation for and performance during the MSFE investigation in May 1951, drafting Marshall's opening statement with Nash and accompanying Marshall each day of the hearings (see pp. 499–505). Marshall had also given Larkin "absolute control" in securing the confirmation of Anna Rosenberg as assistant secretary of defense in late 1950. ("Oral History Interview with Felix E. Larkin," September 18 and October 23, 1972, HSTL/Oral History Interviews. See pp. 206–7, 232–33, 262–63, and 296–97.)

3. This letter was drafted in Washington while Marshall was on vacation (see pp. 603–4), but Marshall approved of the letter over the telephone. (Carter to Lovett, memorandum, n.d., GCMRL/G. C. Marshall Papers [Secretary of Defense, Number Indexed, M211-1-21].) At Larkin's request, Marshall inscribed a photograph of his swearing-in as secretary of defense, which Larkin had administered (see photo #4), using the following language suggested by C. J. George: "While you got me into this job you didn't stick around long enough to get me out." (George to Marshall, memorandum, August 27, 1951, GCMRL/G. C. Marshall Papers [Secretary of Defense, Categorical, Memoranda, Marshall S. Carter, 1950–1951].) After Marshall resigned as secretary of defense (see pp. 629–30), Larkin wrote on September 21 that he wondered whether the inscription "was prophetic or you did not need my help." Marshall replied that when he inscribed the photograph, he "had in mind the [resignation] letter I was submitting to the President the next day, with which you are now acquainted." (Larkin to Marshall, September 21, 1951, and Marshall to Larkin, September 27, 1951, GCMRL/G. C. Marshall Papers [Secretary of Defense, Number Indexed, M200-19-24].) Marshall presented Larkin with the Department of Defense's highest civilian honor at that time, the Certificate of Appreciation, on August 31 at the Pentagon.

Also around this time, Marshall accepted the resignation of General James Burns, who resigned as his assistant for international security affairs. Frank C. Nash, a forty-year-old former special assistant to the secretary of the navy for international security affairs and current deputy US representative in the UN Commission for Conventional Armaments, was sworn in to succeed Burns on August 28. (Marshall to Acheson, July 11, 1951, NA/RG 330, SD 040 [International Security]; Marshall to Burns, July 27, 1951, NA/RG 330, CD 201.22; "New Defense Aide Sworn In," *New York Times*, August 29, 1951, p. 14.)

347

Remarks at the Seventy-second Canadian National Exhibition
August 24, 1951 Toronto, Canada

ON FRIDAY morning, August 24, the Marshalls ended their vacation on Cape Cod by flying from Camp Edwards to Toronto where Marshall was to open the Canadian National Exhibition. He had been officially invited to do so by Canadian Ambassador to the US Humphrey Hume Wrong on June 25, and on July 10, he accepted the invitation, which also included "taking the salute" at the Warriors' Day Parade of veterans on Saturday, August 25. At Marshall's request for advice on topics he should "accentuate" in his remarks, US Ambassador to Canada Stanley Woodward recommended on August 9 that Marshall should address "the need of keeping up our defenses" rather than conceding to the "temptation to relax." Woodward also invited the Marshalls to fly back to Ottawa with him after the August 25 events and stay at the embassy that evening and the next day, a Sunday, before returning to Washington. (Woodward to Marshall, July 3 and August 9, 1951; and Marshall to Woodward, July 10 and 23, 1951, GCMRL/G. C. Marshall Papers [Secretary of Defense, Number Indexed, M214-14-47].)

Richard C. Berkinshaw, the president of the Canadian National Exhibition, expressed his hope to Marshall on August 3 that Mrs. Marshall would accompany Marshall and attend a women's luncheon while Marshall attended the directors' luncheon before his address, and that they would both attend a dinner in their honor the evening of August 24. Marshall replied affirmatively on August 8. (Berkinshaw to Marshall, August 3, 1951, and Marshall to Berkinshaw, August 8, 1951, ibid.)

On August 22, C. J. George sent Marshall a lengthy and detailed itinerary, which called for the Marshalls' arrival in Toronto at 11:00 a.m. on August 24 followed by a brief stop at their hotel. They then moved to the exhibition grounds, where Marshall inspected a guard of honor, met distinguished guests in the general manager's office, and proceeded to their separate luncheons. The opening ceremonies began at 2:30 p.m. with a welcoming address by Berkinshaw. Canadian Defense Minister Brooke Claxton then introduced Marshall, whose address was broadcast on both Canadian and US radio networks. (George to Marshall, memorandum, August 22, 1951, ibid.)

Marshall began by recalling his previous visits to Canada, including accompanying General Pershing to Montreal, where Pershing received an honorary degree from McGill University in 1922. Marshall stopped in Montreal with the other American chiefs of staff en route to the August 1943 Quebec Conference and presumably during the 1944 Quebec Conference, and he also received an honorary degree from McGill University in 1947. ("McGill University to Honor Pershing," *New York Times*, April 14, 1922, p. 12; *Papers of GCM*, 6: 222–23; Pogue, *Organizer*, 244.) During his 1947 visit, Marshall was "chided for appearing entirely too serious" during the celebration. Having come to Canada directly from a meeting of the UN General Assembly in New York (see *Papers of GCM*, 6: 212–18), Marshall was convinced that "it was a serious occasion." Now, four years later, Marshall felt the world situation was "even more serious." (Remarks to the Canadian National Exhibition, August 24, 1951, GCMRL/G. C. Marshall Papers [Secretary of Defense, Speeches and Statements].)

In order to provide context for the exhibition, which exemplified "well-being and human happiness and all the things that we would have in our civilization in our countries," Marshall summarized "the course of events" since the end of World War II. After the "joy at the end of the fighting" had faded, "we quickly became aware of the chaotic situation with famine in the various lands, in Europe and in Asia, and at the same time we became aware of the fact that" the Soviet Union had "quite evidently ceased to be an ally and threatened all that we had fought for." This "despair . . . reached its peak in the summer of 1947 with the frustrating results of the Moscow Conference" coupled with the growing famine in Western Europe. The successful efforts "for rehabilitating the economy of Europe as well as Japan" then followed. (See *Papers of GCM*, 6: 122–739 passim.) The "constant opposition" to US policies made it clear, however, that in addition to promoting economic recovery, the US and its allies needed to rearm themselves. Marshall praised the "very great progress" made in strengthening the UN and NATO, particularly thanks to the "very conspicuous part" played by Canadians. In Korea, Canada's contributions had been "significant," with the shipment of "three destroyers, . . . a squadron of transport planes," and "a very gallant brigade of ground troops." Marshall believed that the Korean War proved "the futility of expecting sincerity in the effort to obtain peace from the Soviet Government, if that be needed after its grasp of power and control of other countries since 1945." (Ibid.)

Marshall expressed his pleasure with the "constantly growing working accord" between the US and Canada, which he had witnessed since its infancy prior to World War II. The citizens of the two countries "must play a leading part in meeting this present crisis which threatens most directly the countries of Western Europe," which is why mutual defense plans between the countries was so important. (See pp. 203, 398–400, and 434–35.) The two countries had "been spared the destructive effects of a great war. In other words, we owe it to the free world to do our best to make it secure and to find some basis for a permanent peace." The US, Marshall added, was doing its part by developing "a very great strength in a very short time," critical elements of which were "a tremendous reserve of trained men" and a reliable production and manufacturing program. The US and Canada, who shared "thousands of miles of frontier" for "a long period of years" without requiring the construction of "any fortifications," represented "an ideal of international relationships where they are based fundamentally on good will and good faith." Marshall ended his speech by officially declaring open the Canadian National Exhibition. (Remarks to the Canadian National Exhibition, August 24, 1951, GCMRL/G. C. Marshall Papers [Secretary of Defense, Speeches and Statements].)

Woodward later wrote to Truman that Marshall's speech was a "masterpiece," which he delivered without notes before a crowd of around ten thousand people. After his remarks, Marshall gave a brief radio interview in Berkinshaw's office, and he spoke briefly at the Warriors' Day Parade on August 25. (Graling to Woodward, memorandum, August 16, 1951, and Woodward to Truman, August 27, 1951, GCMRL/G. C. Marshall Papers [Secretary of Defense, Number Indexed, M214-14-47]; transcript of radio interview, August 8 [*24*], 1951, and "Suggestions for Warriors' Day Address by the Secretary of Defense," August 25, 1951, GCMRL/G. C. Marshall Papers [Secretary of Defense, Speeches and Statements].)

Woodward assured Truman that embassy officials gave Marshall "what 'protection' we could in an effort to get him back to you in Washington alive," which was "not an easy task" given the "enthusiasm" of the Canadian people surrounding Marshall's visit. The Marshalls flew to Ottawa with Woodward and his family and "spent a quiet Sunday at the Embassy" before returning to the US later on August 26. Marshall admitted to Truman that he "found the Toronto affair more strenuous than that, I think, of any trip I have taken in a long time, but the people were so genuinely friendly that I felt repaid for the effort." (Woodward to Truman, August 27, 1951, and Marshall to Truman, September 5, 1951, GCMRL/G. C. Marshall Papers [Secretary of Defense, Number Indexed, M214-14-47].) Woodward also informed Marshall Carter that Marshall's visit played a part in convincing the Canadian cabinet to commit to sending the Canadian Twenty-seventh Brigade to Europe. (Woodward to Carter, August 30, 1951, GCMRL/G. C. Marshall Papers [Secretary of Defense, Memoranda, Marshall S. Carter, 1950–1951 (Classified File #2)].) ★

348

To James W. Wadsworth

August 25, 1951
[Toronto, Canada]

Dear Senator Wadsworth: I have your letter of August 3 and I look forward to discussing its contents, in detail, with you upon my return to Washington late this month.[1]

In the meantime, I want to give you this assurance. The Department of Defense is not planning, and has not planned, to use universal military training in combination with reserve obligation as a substitute for the draft.

As I have told you, we are planning to institute universal military training at an early date. However, we are not planning to institute it on a scale so large that those who have completed their six months in the National Security Training Corps will immediately thereafter be required to give service as reserves. Faithfully yours,

NA/RG 330, CD 353

1. Wadsworth had written to Marshall on August 3 to convey the concern of the members of the National Security Training Commission regarding an "impression" of some

members of Congress that the Defense Department was planning to immediately place eighteen-year-olds in "extended active service as reserves" following six months of training in the National Security Training Corps. Wadsworth warned Marshall "that such a procedure would be regarded" by even "the warmest friends of UMT . . . as a basic subversion of Congressional intent," which indicated that UMT would not be implemented until "the international situation permitted a rather significant reduction in the size of our standing forces." If the Defense Department was "planning to use UMT in combination with obligations placed upon reservists" to serve "as a substitute for the draft," the congressmen had told Wadsworth that there would be "little or no chance for Congressional approval" of the commission's recommendations. He added that the commission believed UMT must first be implemented "upon a small scale." (Wadsworth to Marshall, August 3, 1951, NA/RG 330, CD 353.) See pp. 551–53 and 558–59.

Anna Rosenberg, who was touring US military facilities and studying manpower issues in Europe at the time Wadsworth sent his letter, received word of these concerns and asked her office to assure Wadsworth that the Defense Department would comply with the "spirit and intent" of the law and would consult with Congress before finalizing any plans. She suggested that Marshall wait to respond to Wadsworth until she returned to Washington on August 17. (Rosenberg to Dabney, cable, S-1882, August 6, 1951; Carter to Marshall, memorandum, August 7, 1951, ibid.) On August 30, Marshall met with Wadsworth and the other members of the National Security Training Commission; Townsend Hoopes, executive director of the commission; Anna Rosenberg and her special assistant, Charles Tyroler; General Collins; and Brigadier General John A. Dabney, director of the Military Policy Division of the Office of Personnel Policy under Rosenberg.

This controversy coincided with a related one regarding a bill to restructure the reserve system. (Condit, *Test of War*, 492; "House Maps Revision of Military Reserve," *New York Times*, July 2, 1951, p. 13; "Standard Policies on Reserves Asked," *New York Times*, July 3, 1951, p. 4.) See p. 516n1.

349

To Harry S. Truman — August 28, 1951
Top Secret — Washington, DC

Dear Mr. President: The Joint Chiefs of Staff have recommended that I obtain your approval on the following policy respecting the arming of Japanese-manned ships. Current policy decisions of the Far Eastern Commission prohibit the arming of coastal patrol ships that are Japanese-manned. The Joint Chiefs of Staff have now informed me that the depletion of the occupation forces in Japan has created a situation in which the internal security of the islands and the security of the occupation forces may be seriously threatened.[1]

Consequently, the Departments of State and Defense have re-evaluated the political and military aspects of this new situation and have jointly agreed to a new policy which will permit the Supreme Commander for the Allied Powers (SCAP) to utilize Japanese forces adequately armed for defense and the maintenance of internal security. This new policy, which I recommend for your approval, is as follows:

"In view of the radically changed conditions and the increased need to insure the security of Japan, the Supreme Commander for the Allied Powers is authorized to establish a Japanese-manned coastal security force, organized and equipped along normal coast guard lines, composed of vessels with appropriate armament and speed, and under SCAP operational control, to be operated in waters contiguous to the Japanese islands."

This represents the appropriate interim policy statement for the period between the signing of the Treaty of Peace with Japan and the coming into effect of the Treaty. When Japan regains her sovereignty and the right to provide for her own defense, a new United States policy, in connection with the Japanese security forces, will be appropriate.[2]

It is the understanding of the Departments of State and Defense that the coastal security force established by SCAP would be placed under the direct operational control of American officers, and that the vessels would carry armament appropriate for coast guard craft. The Secretary of State has concurred in this proposed policy statement on the understanding, which the Joint Chiefs of Staff and I confirm, that this coastal security force will be organized along normal coast guard lines; the armament and speed of the vessels will be that of normal coast guard character; the force will, in general, be constituted so as to provide no valid basis for an assumption that it is in fact the nucleus of a revived Japanese navy; and that no action will be taken looking toward the reestablishment of a Japanese navy without approval at the highest levels of this Government.

The Secretary of State has recommended, and the Joint Chiefs of Staff and I have concurred, that the proposed statement of policy be presented to you for approval with the understanding that it will not be implemented until after the signing of the Treaty of Peace with Japan. The Secretary of State has informed me that, if this proposed policy meets with your approval, he will inform certain friendly members of the Far Eastern Commission of the implementation of this action at the appropriate time.[3]

With great respect, Faithfully yours,

GCMarshall

NA/RG 330, CD 092 (Japan)

1. See pp. 494–96 and 582–83. The JCS had first proposed the arming of Japanese ships in mid-April, and after informal State-Defense consultations, Marshall on April 26 had formally referred the matter to Acheson. On July 20, Acheson suggested the wording included in the above letter to Truman in light of the "serious legal and political problems" leading up to the signing of the Japanese Peace Treaty. Marshall forwarded this proposal to the JCS, who on August 22 agreed that Acheson's proposal was "the appropriate interim policy statement" for the period between the signing of the Japanese peace treaty and its "coming into effect." Upon implementation of this policy the chiefs intended to approve the transfer to Ridgway "on a loan basis . . . 10 Patrol Frigates (PFs) and 50 Landing Ships Support Large (LSSLs) to meet his requirements for naval patrol-type craft," provided Congress appropriated the necessary funds, which Marshall had previously authorized the navy to request. (Acheson to Marshall, July 20, 1951; Kreps to JCS, memorandum, July 27, 1951; Vandenberg to Marshall, memorandum, August 22, 1951; and Nash to Marshall, memorandum, August 31, 1951, NA/RG 330, CD 092 [Japan].)

2. See pp. 324–25, 427–29, 567–69, and 623–24.

3. Truman marked his approval on this letter on August 29. Marshall so informed Acheson on September 4 and also shared that he had requested that the JCS "take appropriate action to implement this policy, at the appropriate time." (Marshall to Acheson, September 4, 1951, ibid.)

350

REMARKS FOR THE RED CROSS BLOOD CAMPAIGN PROGRAM[1] August 28, 1951
Washington, DC

GEN. MARSHALL: As Secretary of Defense, I feel a personal obligation to every parent in America who has a son or daughter in the Armed Forces. I will carry out this obligation so far as possible in a military way. But in a personal way, I cannot fulfill this obligation without the genuine assistance of our people. I am referring to the urgent need for blood plasma. Reserve supplies have been completely exhausted. The military needs for whole blood from which plasma can be processed have been set at 300,000 pints per month—for every month between now and next July. Present donations fall far below this figure . . . in June only 50,000 pints. In July the offers dwindled to 36,000. Even after we manage to reach this quota of 300,000 pints per month, a *continuing* effort is imperative. Donations must continue indefinitely, so that our country will never again be in the position of having our available supplies of whole blood and plasma totally exhausted.

If every qualified American will donate a sufficient amount of blood during this period to meet the necessities of our Armed Forces—more of our wounded fighting men will live to return home. It is imperative that plasma be available for immediate use at the front and wherever our forces are stationed, at home or overseas. The instruments of war can be manufactured . . . human blood cannot be. Our field commanders consider plasma just as essential to the combat efficiency of our troops as food and ammunition.

As Secretary of Defense, I appeal to you for your support in this matter of such great and immediate importance. I appeal to your generosity and nobility of spirit. We must not hazard the lives of our men and women by the lack of blood.[2]

******

You have heard General Bradley speak of the Armed Forces' need for 2,800,000 pints of blood, and the statement that the military would provide one-half of that quantity. In the Armed Forces, at the present time, there are well over 5 million members who will provide 1,400,000 pints of blood for this program. In the United States, there are well over 150 million people, and all that is being asked of them is that they provide the necessary other half. There are fifty times as many civilians as there are soldiers, but these civilians are not being asked to give fifty times as much . . . nor ten times as much . . . or even twice as much. All that we ask is that you—the American public—match the contributions made by the members of the Services, pint for pint.[3]

******

GEN. MARSHALL: The need for an adequate blood supply, and an adequate reserve supply, for the care of our wounded men will never diminish. For every man who received an emergency transfusion of plasma on the battlefield, the need for whole blood to be used in further transfusions later in the hospitals is increased just that much more. Plasma can sustain the life of a wounded man until he can receive the needed medical attention in the hospital, but that demands whole blood.

It is almost impossible to estimate accurately the number of casualties who might be evacuated, yet it is essential that an adequate supply of blood be available upon their arrival at the hospital. More blood is needed during the course of the hospital operations than at the time the man is wounded.

Blood is being given by patriotic citizens all over our country, but in far from sufficient quantity. The lack of just one pint of blood could mean the life of an American soldier, sailor, airman or Marine. Do your part to help in this effort.

******

GEN. MARSHALL: Before our program ends, there is an important thought I would like to leave with you. Please call your Red Cross Chapter or Blood Donor Center, and make an appointment to donate your pint of blood. If every American whose blood meets the tests will give three pints of blood before next summer, our immediate problem will be solved. It must be done in a systematic manner. Red Cross and Blood Donor Centers can accommodate only a certain number of people at any one time, so—please call them before you report to the Center—and then, most important of all, please keep your appointment. Remember—you can't transfuse a promise.

GCMRL/G. C. Marshall Papers (Secretary of Defense, Speeches and Statements)

1. Acting Secretary of Defense Lovett had issued a directive on August 2 announcing the creation of the Armed Forces Blood Donor Program, effective September 10, to coordinate and encourage the procurement of blood with the Red Cross for the US military. (Douglas B. Kendrick, *Blood Program in World War II*, Medical Department, United States Army [Washington: Office of the Surgeon General, Department of the Army, 1964], 734.) Marshall and Bradley recorded this broadcast at 5:55 p.m. on August 28 at the Pentagon. It aired on radio and television stations across all major networks on September 10 as the official launch of the blood donor campaign. Reproduced here is the draft of the prepared remarks as revised by Marshall. A full draft transcript of the broadcast, including General Bradley's statements which are located at each of the lines of asterisks within Marshall's remarks above, is available in GCMRL/G. C. Marshall Papers (Secretary of Defense, Speeches and Statements).

Following this broadcast Marshall sent letters of thanks to several industrial and labor leaders for their "quick response to my statement on the critical need of blood." (Marshall to Ferguson, et al., September 12, 1951, GCMRL/G. C. Marshall Papers [Secretary of Defense, Number Indexed, M200-19-19].)

2. The transcript noted that Marshall introduced Bradley at this point only in the recording used on the radio.

3. According to the transcript, this paragraph was used only in the radio broadcast.

351

To Harry S. Truman

August 29, 1951
Washington, DC

Dear Mr. President: Attached are the following papers:

Memoranda for the Secretary of Defense from the Joint Chiefs of Staff, dated respectively 16 July, 15 August and 16 August, 1951.[1]

Copy of Mr. Lovett's reply to the Joint Chiefs of Staff, dated 18 August 1951.[2]

The usual budgetary screening and justifications will, of course, be followed routinely by the Department of Defense. The attached papers establish authorization for the increased armed forces required by the Joint Chiefs of Staff.

I have approved this procedure and request your approval of the memorandum to the Joint Chiefs of Staff dated 18 August 1951.[3]

With great respect, Faithfully yours,

GCMRL/G. C. Marshall Papers (Secretary of Defense, Selected)

1. These three papers all dealt with force requirements for FY 1952 and revealed a serious split within the JCS between Vandenberg and his colleagues over the extent to which the air force should be expanded as opposed to the army and navy in light of the perceived Soviet military threat and need to accelerate the US military buildup as enunciated in NSC 68/4 and NSC 114/1. In their July 16 memorandum, the JCS reported to Marshall that they had "been unable to agree as to what these forces should be or on a common approach to the problem." On August 7, with Marshall on vacation (see pp. 603–4), Lovett directed the Joint Chiefs to "narrow their area of disagreement" or ask Marshall to resolve the dispute. The JCS responses on August 15 and 16 revealed greater accord than in July but continued disagreement. (Condit, *Test of War*, 248 and 261–66; and Poole, *History of JCS*, 4: 46–52; "Decision on J.C.S. 1800/154, A Note by the Secretaries on Augmentation of FY 1952 Forces and Guidance for Service Programs and Budget Through FY 1952," July 16, 1951, and enclosures; and Lalor and Carns to JCS, "JCS 1800/159, Interim Force Requirements for FY 1952 to Support Objectives of NSC 68/4," August 15, 1951, and enclosures, in Paul S. Kesaris, ed., *Records of the Joint Chiefs of Staff*, pt. 2, *1946–1953*, *Strategic Issues*, section 2, *Postwar Requirements for Military Forces* [Frederick, MD: University Publications of America, 1981], microfilm reel IV, items 0863 and 0876.)

2. Lovett apparently consulted with Marshall on Cape Cod by telephone, for in this August 18 reply to the JCS, he informed them that Marshall had "considered the basic conclusions" in their papers and "has directed me to advise you of the general comments he will make when forwarding your memoranda to the President." Marshall agreed to army and navy expansion but only to the "principle of an increase in Air Force combat strength," and he offered no approval "at this time of any specific number of types of units" or any increase in personnel beyond currently approved levels. Rather than present these recommendations in this August 29 memorandum to Truman, however, Marshall apparently let Lovett's August 18 reply speak for itself. (Lovett to JCS, memorandum, August 18, 1951, enclosure to Lalor and Carns to JCS, note on "J.C.S. 1800/160, Interim Force Requirements for FY 1952 to Support Objectives for NSC 68/4," August 22, 1951, in ibid., item 0881.)

3. Marshall met with Truman off the record at 3:25 p.m. on August 29, before a meeting of the NSC that afternoon. Truman approved the conclusions in this Lovett memorandum on the same day and soon thereafter increased army, navy, and marine strength, to a total of more than 3.7 million men. (Carter to JCS, memorandum, August 30, 1951, GCMRL/G. C. Marshall Papers [Secretary of Defense, Chronological, Director, Executive Office (Marshall S. Carter), 1950–1952]; Condit, *Test of War*, 266–67.)

352

MEMORANDUM FOR ROBERT A. LOVETT

August 29, 1951
Washington, DC

I am sure you will remember the attached directive which I received from Mr. Stimson, and my compliance therewith.[1]

As Secretary of Defense, I direct that during the period between Thursday, September 6th, and the late afternoon of Monday, September 10th, you absent yourself from the Pentagon and go far afield for your own pleasure and divertissement.

During this period you are to be under the exclusive control and direction of Mrs. Lovett. Any additional time she should impose on you is authorized in advance.

If Mr. Stimson could issue such a directive and get away with it, I think I have a sound precedent for this action.

You have no recourse but to comply.[2]

GCMRL/G. C. Marshall Papers (Secretary of Defense, Chronological, Secretaries, Hawkins)

1. The attached directive over Stimson's signature stated the order of the president that Chief of Staff Marshall should visit Charlotte, North Carolina, from October 11 to 19, 1940, to report on "the comparative skill and valor of the football teams of Davidson and Virginia Military Institute." During this time, Marshall "shall be under the exclusive control and direction of Mrs. Marshall," and "the War Department shall be relegated to the tender mercies of the Secretary of War, the Assistant Secretary of War, and the Deputy Chief of Staff, General Bryden." VMI defeated Davidson 13–7 on October 12.

2. The Lovetts spent this time at their new home in Locust Valley on Long Island, New York. (See p. 620.) After succeeding Marshall as secretary of defense on September 12 (see pp. 629–32), Lovett wrote to Marshall, "I knew I'd miss you but I never dreamed how much; this is, I find, a very lonely job. Lots of things in the training you have given me are now becoming apparent to me and I just wanted to let you know, by George's pouch, how grateful I am to you for the countless intangible bits of armor you bequeathed me." Marshall replied to this letter, but the editors have been unable to locate this response. (Lovett to Marshall, September 20, 1951, GCMRL/G. C. Marshall Papers [Secretary of Defense, Number Indexed, M200-19-37]; H.)

353

To John F. Shelley — August 29, 1951, Washington, DC

Dear Mr. Shelley: This is in reply to your letter of 18 June regarding modification of the Department of Defense policy in respect to the assignment of sole surviving sons.[1]

In response to your request a complete restudy of this policy has been conducted with the net effect of adding two new categories to those previously listed.[2]

A copy of the new directive is attached for your information. You will note that it no longer is restricted to sole surviving sons but now applies to sole remaining sons. This change came about by the addition of the father to the category of persons to be considered, and the addition of a sub-category to over 100% physically or mentally disabled cases.[3]

I have formally suggested to the Secretaries of the military departments that wherever military considerations permit, leniency in the administrative handling of this policy be exercised.[4] Faithfully yours,

NA/RG 330, OASD (M&P), 210.3 Rosenberg

1. See pp. 295–96. Representative Shelley (D-CA) had written to Marshall on June 7 to share the situation of a married couple in his district with two sons, one in the army and the other disabled due to "a mental disease" from service during World War II. The army had denied their request that the son presently in service be given a noncombat assignment, because their situation did not qualify under the existing sole surviving sons policy. Shelley strongly urged modification of this policy "to take in cases of this kind." Marshall replied on June 13 that he had referred Shelley's letter to Pace for a response, but Shelley wrote on June 18 to clarify that his June 7 letter had been "properly addressed" to Marshall in order to encourage a revision of the entire policy, not only action "in the particular case I outlined." (Shelley to Marshall, June 7 and 18, 1951; and Marshall to Shelley, June 13, 1951, NA/RG 330, OASD [M&P], 210.3, Rosenberg.)

2. According to a memorandum to Admiral John McCrea, an initial review by the Defense Department indicated that the navy, marine corps, and air force were "lenient" in such cases, but the army was much more "strict" due to the large number and varied nature of the cases. The army would endeavor to fulfill these "hardship" requests should "circumstances allow." (Schumm to McCrea, memorandum, July 2, 1951, NA/RG 330, OASD [M&P], 210.3, Rosenberg.)

3. The attached directive, numbered 110.06-2, "Administrative Handling of Sole Remaining Sons," stated that a sole surviving son whose situations met one of the requirements, or the parent of such a son, could request assignment to noncombat duty, and those qualified who were currently serving in combat could ask to be reassigned. Marshall made clear that "This directive shall not be interpreted to mean that subject individuals will not be assigned to overseas commands, but rather that they will be assigned to appropriate areas as designated by the major commanders concerned." (Directive 110.06-2, "Administrative Handling of Sole Remaining Sons," August 27, 1951, ibid.)

4. Marshall did so in a memorandum to the service secretaries. (Marshall to service secretaries, memorandum, August 27, 1951, ibid.)

354

To Brien McMahon — September 4, 1951
Confidential — Washington, DC

Dear Senator McMahon: With reference to your letter of 21 August 1951 and the accompanying memorandum commenting on tactical uses of atomic weapons, I have given the memorandum a careful reading, and have requested supplemental information on the subject including the views of the Joint Chiefs of Staff.[1]

As soon as possible I shall let you know further regarding the questions raised.[2] Faithfully yours,

GCMRL/G. C. Marshall Papers (Secretary of Defense, Chronological, Secretaries, Ackerman)

1. The editors have been unable to obtain a copy of McMahon's August 21 letter, but the accompanying document was in all likelihood a lengthy memorandum from J. Kenneth Mansfield, chief of special projects of the Joint Congressional Committee on Atomic Energy, calling for much greater emphasis on research, development, and use of tactical nuclear weapons. (*FRUS, 1951*, 1: 158–63.) See pp. 468–69 and 559–60.

Throughout this time period McMahon had continued to press for expansion of the US atomic weapons program (see ibid., 772; Hewlett and Duncan, *Forging the Atomic Shield*, 546–49, 556–61; Condit, *Test of War*, 470). Simultaneously, discussions were taking place regarding Anglo-American-Canadian collaboration on atomic weapons. (Marshall to Eisenhower, July 5, 1951, GCMRL/G. C. Marshall Papers [Secretary of Defense, Number Indexed, M200-3-6]; *Papers of DDE*, 13: 1561–62.)

2. McMahon joined Marshall and others for lunch on September 6, two days after Marshall sent him this letter. Referring to the September 4 letter and/or comments made during this lunch, McMahon stated at a September 26 dinner speech in Washington that Marshall had assured him that US military planners, including Eisenhower and the JCS, were closely studying "the potentialities of future improved weapons in defending Western Europe." (*Congressional Record* 97, pt. 15, 82d Cong., 1st sess., A5936–38.)

355

To Henry Cabot Lodge Jr. — September 5, 1951, Washington, DC

Dear Lodge: Thank you for your letter of August 22nd in which you quote excerpts from a letter which you received from Father Murphy regarding missionaries and other civilians who are prisoners of the Communists in Korea.[1] I understand Father Murphy's and your concern for these unfortunate people, and we here in the Department of Defense are doing everything possible in their behalf. Most confidentially, there are two complicating factors, and I would appreciate your not repeating them but I give them to you for your information only:

(1) the difficulty in making a distinction, for purposes of negotiation, between the few United States and European nationals involved and the many thousands of South Koreans who are technically in the same category; and
(2) the US-UN position that the truce talks are limited to purely military subjects.[2]

While the State Department is responsible for the protection of our people in foreign countries, we here are cooperating to the fullest.

I am sorry to learn of the death of Fathers Collier and Reilly, and that seven others of the St. Columban's Foreign Mission Society are still missing. I am hopeful that something good may come of these cease-fire talks and at which time I am sure that questions other than purely military subjects will be discussed.[3]

Many thanks for your interest in this matter of great importance, and with warm regards.[4] Faithfully yours,

NA/RG 330, CD 383.6

1. Lodge had written on August 22 to share a letter he had received from Father Thomas L. Murphy, associate editor of *The Far East* magazine published by the Roman Catholic St. Columban's Foreign Mission Society, commonly known as the Columban Fathers. Murphy had written Lodge with a "strong request" that UN negotiators at the ongoing armistice talks in Korea consider civilian prisoners and missionaries as well as military personnel in discussions relating to prisoners of war. The Columban Fathers, Murphy noted, had suffered two confirmed deaths in the Korean War—Fathers Anthony Collier and Patrick Reilly—and seven other members of the society were still missing, two of them American and five Irish. Lodge urged Marshall's "personal attention" in the matter. (Lodge to Marshall, August 22, 1951, NA/RG 330, CD 383.6.)

2. According to a September 6 memorandum from a Defense Department aide to Colonel G. V. Underwood Jr., assistant director of EXOS, the Department of the Army and the State Department "do not object to the inclusion of the classified information in sub-paragraphs (1) and (2) of the attached letter to Senator Lodge. They would object, however, to inclusion of similar information in letters to other members of Congress who are less

reliable than Senator Lodge from the standpoint of security." (Mitchell to Underwood, memorandum, September 6, 1951, ibid.)

3. The same memorandum quoted in n2 stated that Robert McClurkin, deputy director of the Office of Northeast Asian Affairs in the State Department, had recommended deletion of this sentence or at least clarification within the sentence "that non-military subjects will be discussed only *after* successful conclusion of the cease-fire talks." Carter approved sending the letter to Lodge "as written in spite of State's bleat." (Mitchell to Underwood, memorandum, and routing slip, September 6, 1951, ibid.)

4. Marshall had received a similar letter from Representative Carl T. Curtis (R-NE) on August 22. Marshall replied on September 6 to assure Curtis that the Defense Department was "doing everything possible in their behalf." (Marshall to Curtis, September 6, 1951, GCMRL/G. C. Marshall Papers [Secretary of Defense, Number Indexed, M200-19-2].)

356

MEMORANDUM FOR FREDERICK J. LAWTON — September 6, 1951
Confidential — Washington, DC

My dear Lawton: I spoke to the President the other day in regard to the proposal of your agency that there would be no new funds for construction in FY 1953 budget for the Battle Monuments Commission. I did not go into the amounts requested or any details though I had that data with me. I merely stated to the President what is my firm conviction, that he cannot afford politically to have a series of uncompleted cemeteries abroad with others completed and thousands of visitors going over there each year to visit the grave of their sons or husbands—and this number is increasing rapidly each year.[1]

I am sending you this memorandum because I understand that two of your people called at the office of the Battle Monuments Commission to get figures in the matter. Of course you have to have these. But I also found out in talking to the officials in charge there (General North, the head of the working level of the Commission is in Europe) that they made no mention whatever of what is the determining factor in this matter, in my opinion, and apparently in the opinion of the President.[2]

GCMRL/G. C. Marshall Papers (Secretary of Defense, Categorical, Organizations, American Battle Monuments Commission, 1950–1951)

1. Elmer B. Staats, acting director of the Bureau of the Budget, had written to Marshall on June 26 that the anticipated FY 1953 budget request would not "allow the inclusion of additional funds for the construction program." Recognizing the disruption of activities this would have on the ABMC as well as the negative public relations effect, North "strongly" urged Marshall to discuss the matter with Truman in person. Leslie L. Biffle, a member of the ABMC since 1941 and a close confidant of President Truman, concurred. Carter noted in an undated memorandum that Marshall had spoken with Truman, "who said he would immediately dictate a note to Lawton." (Staats to Marshall, June 26, 1951; North to ABMC members, memorandum, July 18, 1951; North to Marshall, July 19, 1951; George to Marshall, memorandum, August 8, 1951; Carter to George, memorandum, n.d., GCMRL/G. C. Marshall Papers [Secretary of Defense, Categorical, Organizations, American Battle Monuments Commission, 1950–1951].)

In an effort to obtain funds in the event that the Bureau of the Budget did not approve any appropriations, Marshall asked Treasury Secretary Snyder on August 28 what "foreign currencies might be available to the Commission," as the ABMC had been directed in its FY 1952 appropriations to use such currency "'available to the credit of the Treasury'" to reduce costs when possible. Marshall estimated to Snyder that the ABMC would require $7.9 million in FY 1953. (Marshall to Snyder, August 28, 1951, ibid.) See pp. 289–90 and 435–36.

2. On September 25, Marshall forwarded to Truman and Lawton copies of a five-page report that House Appropriations Committee member Fred E. Busbey (R-IL) had sent to a committee colleague after a tour of European and North African cemeteries. He thought the incomplete World War II cemeteries would give a "sickening feeling" to any relative who had "come to visit a soldier's grave." Busbey wrote that Congress "should do everything within our power" to ensure this work was completed quickly. (Busbey to Phillips, August 18, 1951; and Marshall to Truman, and Marshall to Lawton, September 25, 1951, ibid.)

Truman advised Marshall on October 3 that "the House Appropriation Committee has left us out on most of the things" relating to the ABMC. He added that he was working with the Bureau of the Budget to get ABMC funding in the FY 1953 appropriations bill. Marshall replied on October 9 that he appreciated Truman's assistance and reiterated their mutual hope "that something constructive can be accomplished" in regard to the funding. The ABMC received five hundred thousand dollars for construction expenses in FY 1953 in addition to up to $4.5 million in foreign currencies currently held by the US Treasury. (Truman to Marshall, October 3, 1951, and Marshall to Truman, October 9, 1951, GCMRL/G. C. Marshall Papers [Secretary of Defense, Number Indexed, M208-1-27]; *Independent Offices Appropriation Act of 1953*, Public Law 455, 82d Cong., 2d sess. [June 3, 1952], 4–6.)

357

To General of the Army Dwight D. Eisenhower — September 6, 1951
Top Secret — Washington, DC

Dear Eisenhower: Your letter of August 3rd reached the office while I was on leave with Mrs. Marshall on Cape Cod. It was particularly interesting to me in connection with the "European Army" discussions here. The authorization you gave Carter for limited circulation of your views in that connection was most helpful. However, your entire letter was shown to Lovett, and to Bradley who read it to the Joint Chiefs. Upon my return I sent the letter over to the President and he had a copy made for his file. He was intensely interested in your views.[1]

Your Colonel Wood is leaving at noon today and I hope to send this letter via him. He will tell you that the money for French participation in the maneuvers has been made available.[2]

I can understand your concern in not receiving a reply from the President to your message of 17 July. The situation at the moment is that the President is still thinking the matter over and while he has indicated a desire to talk to Acheson and me about it, has thus far not brought it up again. Unless you are desirous of making the trip, we think it preferable not to reopen the matter from this end, but rather to wait for some indication of the President's wishes.[3]

The other evening I had an introductory dinner for Admiral Fechteler and the President attended. Anna Rosenberg gave us an impassioned and highly amusing account of her trip. She is most enthusiastic about the leadership and morale of the troops, and in particular the fine showing the dependents are making on the countryside. I do not have to tell you how refreshing her viewpoint is to all of us.[4]

I had two hours with Sarnoff shortly after his return, and in addition have read the complete transcript of his press conference. I agree with you that he is down to earth and that his impressions and convictions are comprehensive.[5]

Lovett is leaving today for a short week, or a long weekend, at his new house in Locust Valley. He is a tower of strength to me. The Hill has been unusually demanding this year in the way of calling our top people as witnesses, and Lovett has absorbed most of it at terrific cost to his equanimity. How he takes it, and retains his sense of humor is beyond my understanding.[6]

Your informal reports of your troubles and points of view are particularly helpful to Bradley, Lovett and myself, and, I think, to the President.[7]

Mrs. Marshall joins me in warmest personal regards to you both. Faithfully yours,

GCMRL/G. C. Marshall Papers (Secretary of Defense, Selected)

1. Eisenhower had sent Marshall a five-page letter on August 3 on "the European defense problem," leaving Marshall to decide "whether or not" to show Truman "such a rambling combination of fact, opinion, and assumption." The letter addressed the numerous problems caused by West European disunity and Eisenhower's decision to shift his position and support a European army, which he believed was the best "immediate" method "of developing, on a basis acceptable to other European countries, the German strength that is vital to us." He suggested that Marshall meet with David Sarnoff, who had just spent at least four weeks in Europe, to hear his "comprehensive" and "accurate" thoughts on these "vast subjects." Eisenhower concluded that he had spoken with Anna Rosenberg for "a couple of hours, after which she tackled the staff. Her approach to difficult questions is refreshing—and sound!" (Eisenhower to Marshall, August 3, 1951, GCMRL/G. C. Marshall Papers [Secretary of Defense, Selected]; *Papers of DDE*, 12: 399–400, 457–63.) See pp. 497–99, 583–85, and 610n1.

Carter had cabled Eisenhower on August 14 that Marshall was away (see pp. 604–5) but that his August 3 letter had been shown to Lovett and Bradley. He requested permission to show the portion of the letter containing Eisenhower's changed position on the European army on a "'read only' basis" to Admiral Wright and Colonel Beebe as well as Acheson, Cabot, Matthews, Perkins, and Byroade in the State Department. Marshall sent Eisenhower's letter to Truman on August 27 and requested that the White House return it to him. (Carter to Eisenhower, radio no. DEF-98861, August 14, 1951, GCMRL/G. C. Marshall Papers [Secretary of Defense, Chronological, Director, Executive Office (Marshall S. Carter), 1950–1952]; Marshall to Truman, August 27, 1951, GCMRL/G. C. Marshall Papers [Chronological, Secretaries, Ackerman].)

2. Colonel Robert J. Wood was secretary of the General Staff at SHAPE.

Joint air and ground exercises were scheduled to take place in late September in the Rhine River valley to assess the performance of NATO troops under a unified command. ("1,000 Planes Will Test Defenses Of Eisenhower's Central Command," *New York Times*, September 28, 1951, p. 6.)

3. Truman had sent a message to Eisenhower that he desired to meet with him in the United States. Eisenhower misunderstood Truman's request and thought that the president wanted to meet with him secretly. He replied in a top secret message to Truman through Marshall on July 17 that he would "comply with any plan you may decide to approve," but he was hesitant to hold "a meeting on clandestine basis" as such an event "would inevitably become known." Eisenhower suggested a September meeting to avoid involving himself in congressional hearings on the military aid bill. (See pp. 569–77, 592, and 597–603.) Truman wrote Marshall on July 19 that he wanted to meet with Eisenhower in mid-August and asked him to think about this proposal before their next conversation. The president

replied to Eisenhower on July 20 that he did not expect "to hold a secret meeting" but only wanted to discuss reports that SHAPE was not getting adequate support from the NATO governments. Eisenhower responded on July 26 that he would "plan a trip to Washington for late September or thereabouts," and he clarified to Marshall on September 8 that Truman had already responded to his July 17 message. Truman and Eisenhower did not meet until November 5. (Eisenhower to Marshall, July 17 and September 8, 1951, and Truman to Marshall, July 19, 1951, GCMRL/G. C. Marshall Papers [Secretary of Defense, Selected]; *Papers of DDE*, 12: 426–28, 442–43, 528–29, 560–61.)

4. Admiral Fechteler had been appointed chief of naval operations following the death of Admiral Sherman in July 1951. (See pp. 595–96.) At Lovett's suggestion, Marshall hosted a dinner in Fechteler's honor on August 28 at the Pentagon. (George to Lovett, memorandum, August 15, 1951, GCMRL/G. C. Marshall Papers [Secretary of Defense, Number Indexed, M206-1-38]; memorandum for Marshall, August 28, 1951, GCMRL/G. C. Marshall Papers [Secretary of Defense, Chronological, Secretaries, Ackerman].)

5. Marshall met with Sarnoff on August 29. Upon his return to the United States, Sarnoff had praised the rebuilding of Europe through the ERP but added that Europe would only become "free, strong and self sustaining . . . 'through a federated or United States of Europe.'" ("Sarnoff Holds Aid to Europe is Vital," *New York Times*, August 14, 1951, p. 12; *Papers of DDE*, 12: 462n11.)

6. See p. 615.

7. Eisenhower replied on September 8 that he was "hopeful" that the September meeting of the North Atlantic Council ministers in Ottawa would "be useful in encouraging" NATO countries to build "enthusiasm and support for the whole project." He was also "delighted that Bob Lovett seems to retain his strength in order to have the greatest of usefulness to you. He has always been, of course, one of my favorites." (Eisenhower to Marshall, September 8, 1951, GCMRL/G. C. Marshall Papers [Secretary of Defense, Selected]; *Papers of DDE*, 12: 528–29.) See pp. 649–50.

358

To Henry Cabot Lodge Jr. — September 7, 1951
Secret — Washington, DC

Dear Lodge: I have delayed my reply to your letter of August 1 pending the return of Mrs. Rosenberg in order that I might have the benefit of her investigations in Europe regarding the Volunteer Freedom Corps with all of its implications. While over there she discussed the subject at length with General Eisenhower and the other commanders and got the benefit of their reasoning and recommendations.[1]

After lengthy discussions with Mrs. Rosenberg, Secretary Pace, and General J. Lawton Collins, I came to the conclusion that because of changed conditions since we first discussed the project, manpower from Iron Curtain countries can be employed better within the NATO framework than in the United States Army. Not only does this appear at this particular time to be the more desirable approach; the House Foreign Affairs Committee and the Senate Foreign Relations and Armed Services Committees in reporting out the Mutual Security bill appear by their action to hold to the same view. Section 101(a)(1) of this bill as reported out in the Senate authorizes the use of "not to exceed $100,000,000 of such appropriation for any selected persons who are residing in or escapees from the Soviet Union, Poland, Czechoslovakia, Hungary, Rumania, Bulgaria, Albania, Lithuania, Latvia, and Estonia, or the Communist dominated areas of Germany and Austria, and any other countries absorbed by the Soviet Union either to form such persons into elements of the military forces supporting the North Atlantic Treaty Organization or for other purposes, when it is similarly determined by the President that such assistance will contribute to the defense of the North Atlantic area and to the security of the United States."[2]

I suppose that on your recent visit to Europe you were informed concerning the present status of labor service units in the European Command. There are at present a total of 151 such organizations composed of Germans, Poles, Latvians, Lithuanians and Albanians.

I am in agreement with you as to reasons for the lack of progress being made to implement P. L. 597 (81st Congress). Initially the Army sought to carry out the legislative intent by establishing such high standards as to make the measure largely unworkable. These standards have since been eased by lowering the requirements that personnel be able to speak English, have certain vocational skills, and be of officer caliber. The recruiting which has naturally been slow because of the Counter Intelligence Corps clearance required in each case is now showing more progress, and the first packet of recruits is expected to arrive in the United States during the month of September. After essential processing at Camp Kilmer [in New Jersey] they will be assigned to training divisions throughout the United States. Those with certain skills may be assigned for further schooling. The men who need additional training in English will be retained at Camp Kilmer until they have progressed sufficiently to be assigned to a duty station.

With the lowering of the standards mentioned above I believe we should now push our recruiting program and General Handy has been so directed.

I might mention that the Army has considered translating the AFQ [Armed Forces Qualification] Test as suggested by you. To a certain extent this is possible, but since our present requirements for personnel are limited to European peoples from other than Germany and the ERP and NATO countries it has not been entirely feasible. This is due to the large number of dialects involved in the Iron Curtain countries. Hundreds of tests would be required as well as a sizable training program for the administrators of the tests. At the moment we are successfully employing a non-language test for those persons who do not read. It is conducted entirely in pantomime and has already proven to be quite satisfactory.

The Army has assigned to its Assistant Secretary for Manpower and Reserve Forces the responsibility for assuring that this program is carried on vigorously and to its fullest advantage.[3]

As you know, I have been keenly desirous of making far greater progress in building up a foreign element force that would eventually lessen the manpower pressure on us and materially reduce the expense of maintaining the necessary U. S. Forces abroad. Mrs. Rosenberg and I have both labored to that end but I now find difficulties that make progress at this time impracticable beyond the measures I have described above. Faithfully yours,

NA/RG 330, CD 342.18

1. Lodge had previously sponsored several pieces of legislation that would authorize the US military to enlist anticommunist foreigners, including deserters from Soviet-controlled countries. In June 1950, Truman signed into law one of these bills allowing the army to enlist up to twenty-five hundred such men as potential commissioned and noncommissioned officers, who would agree to serve for five years, receive the same pay and benefits as Americans in the army, and be eligible for citizenship if honorably discharged. In January 1951, Lodge also reintroduced another bill that would establish a Volunteer Freedom Corps of up to two hundred fifty thousand men interested only in wartime service who would serve abroad and would not have the same privileges or status as those in the first bill. In addition, during the Senate debate on the UMT bill (see pp. 325–29 and 369–71), Lodge had convinced Lyndon Johnson's subcommittee to add an amendment that would allow the army to enlist up to one hundred twenty-five thousand "carefully screened aliens" over the first five years of UMT. On March 12, he proposed to Marshall another method of obtaining such individuals, this time via the proposed European army and creation of three elite international combat teams under Eisenhower's direct authority. ("Enlisting of 125,000 Aliens Is Authorized; Pentagon-Guard Row Over Recruits Ended," *Washington Post*, February 10, 1951, p. 1; "Army Accepts Iron Curtain Aliens Abroad," *Washington Post*, March 25, 1951, p. M3; *Congressional Record* 97, pt. 1, 82d Cong., 1st sess., 90–92; Lodge to Marshall, March 12, 1951, NA/RG 330, CD 342.18.)

Marshall had expressed support for Lodge's Volunteer Freedom Corps proposal and met with him on at least two occasions (April 13 and July 9) to discuss the bill. Extensive correspondence and negotiation ensued among the two of them, Collins, Rosenberg, Eisenhower, Bradley, and the JCS, as well as Acheson and State Department officials regarding the terms of a new bill that would establish such a program. (See NA/RG 330, CD 342.18; George to Marshall, memorandum, July 6, 1951, and Marshall to Eisenhower, cable, July 9, 1951, GCMRL/G. C. Marshall Papers [Secretary of Defense, Chronological, Secretaries, Carlson].) On August 1, Lodge wrote to Marshall after a visit to Europe, where he assessed the implementation of the law regarding "the enlistment of aliens in the U.S. Army" and studied "the prospects" for "the Volunteer Freedom Corps legislation." There was "a big enough pool in Europe from which to draw these soldiers," he wrote, but few applications for the US Army and no admissions due to the army's "unreasonably rigid requirements." (Lodge to Marshall, August 1, 1951, NA/RG 330, CD 342.18.)

Marshall received this letter while on vacation (see pp. 603–4) and requested that Carter send copies to Rosenberg, Collins, and Pace "on a personal and confidential basis" for them to review and discuss with Marshall once he returned to Washington. Pace wrote to Marshall on August 20 stating that he had investigated the progress based on Lodge's bill and found the results to be "substantially in accord" with Lodge's letter. The remainder of his memorandum generally formed the basis for the final five paragraphs of Marshall's response to Lodge. (Carter to Rosenberg, Collins, and Pace, memorandum, August 13, 1951; and Pace to Marshall, memorandum, August 20, 1951, ibid.)

2. See the previous document and pp. 497–99 and 583–85.

3. This was likely Karl R. Bendetsen, assistant secretary of the army for general management.

359

To General Matthew B. Ridgway — September 8, 1951
Radio No. DEF-20357. — Leesburg, Virginia

On the occasion of the signing of Japanese Peace Treaty I want you to know immediately of my deep satisfaction in the great achievements of the occupation under the command of General MacArthur and under your command.[1]

The peace conference and the signing of the treaty by so many governments were made possible today largely because of the success of the occupation in helping to restore Japan in so short a time to a place of trust and equality among the nations of the world.[2]

NA/RG 330, SD 092.2

1. The Japanese Peace Treaty was signed the morning of September 8 in the San Francisco Opera House. (See pp. 324–25, 427–29, 523–24, and 567–69.) As the JCS had insisted, a US-Japan Security Treaty was signed later that same day, this time at the Presidio. These treaties had been preceded by the US-Philippine Mutual Defense Treaty, signed at the State Department in Washington on August 30, and the Australia–New Zealand–United States (ANZUS) Security Treaty signed in San Francisco on September 1. Marshall and Bradley attended the signing of the Philippine treaty.

Marshall also sent the following message to General MacArthur on September 8: "I can appreciate the satisfaction with which you received the news of the signing of the Japanese Peace Treaty today in San Francisco. Without the achievements of the occupation during your command the endorsement of the treaty by so many governments would not have been possible." Marshall Carter drafted these messages to Ridgway and MacArthur, which Marshall approved over the telephone. (Marshall to MacArthur, cable, DEF-20358, September 8, 1951, and Carter memorandum for the file, n.d., NA/RG 330, SD 092.2 [1951].) On September 12, Marshall also sent congratulatory messages to Acheson and Dulles (see pp. 632–33).

2. Forty-nine governments signed the treaty.

360

Conversation with French Minister of Finance and Economic Affairs René Mayer

September 10, 1951 Washington, DC

RENÉ MAYER was in Washington for the annual meeting of the Board of Governors of the International Bank for Reconstruction and Development (World Bank) from September 10 to 14, 1951. (*FRUS, 1951*, 4: 427n1.) In addition to Marshall and Mayer, Jean Dariden, the minister counselor at the French Embassy; European Economic Cooperation (EEC) Secretary General Thierry de Clermont-Tonnerre; Nash; Beebe; and Colonel Andrew Samuels, executive officer in the Office of Foreign Military Affairs, attended this one-hour meeting that began at 10:30 a.m.

Mayer addressed "the serious condition in France due to the dollar shortage." There was "great need in France for raw materials, chiefly coking coal which must be purchased outside the country." France was unable to purchase "sufficient coal from Germany or England and must now buy great quantities of coking coal from the United States." As such purchases required payment in dollars and did not produce items available for export, "a serious dollar shortage results." Mayer also "talked at length about the need for additional aid to Indochina," as France could not afford to increase its financial contributions in the region above current levels. He noted that "Approximately 30 per cent of France's gross national product is being utilized for military purposes in France and Indochina." Mayer believed "U.S. aid to Indochina has been insufficient and too slow." (See pp.

187–88, 194–203, 320–22, 331–32, 357–60, 572, and 599n4.) He was gratified by the participation of the Associated States of Laos, Cambodia, and Vietnam "in the recent San Francisco conference to sign the Peace Treaty with Japan," which was "a strong indication" that those countries were "oriented strongly to the West" rather than to Communist nations. (Memorandum of conversation, September 10, 1951, NA/RG 330, CD Memorandum of Conversation.) See previous document.

Marshall replied "that he had a fair understanding of these French problems." While the "dollar shortage" was "not in his field of responsibility as Secretary of Defense," Marshall assured Mayer that he would be sure "to see that this matter was given serious study" by a board chaired by ODM Director Charles Wilson, of which Marshall was also a member. Regarding aid to Indochina, Marshall "explained in detail the time lag between appropriations and delivery of end-items," a process that usually takes about nine months, "which means that appropriations made last November are just now realizing deliveries in Indochina." Marshall then turned to "a subject which Mr. Mayer himself did not mention"—France's "lack of trained officers, non-commissioned officers, and cadres for both the Indochina forces and France's European Army." (See pp. 167–68, 187–88, 194–203, 218–20, 348–49, 357–60, 497–99, 583–85, and 619–21.) The "lack of well trained replacements" was a "critical problem" for French forces in Korea. He also emphasized the infrastructure needs to support troops sent to Europe. Congress had approved sending four divisions to Europe (see pp. 472–74), but "one unit planned for Europe was already sent to Korea" because there were "inadequate facilities available in Europe to receive these units." To alleviate this problem, Marshall gave Mayer a table "with a list of countries participating in the Central Europe Infrastructure Program for 1951 showing proposed percentages and amounts of money that each country should contribute." Mayer wanted to discuss this information with Charles Spofford and other US officials "within the next few days and hoped that tripartite agreement could be obtained." Marshall's proposed breakdown by percentages and millions of dollars had the United States contributing 35 percent ($83.44 million); Britain, 20 percent ($47.6 million); France, 26 percent ($61.88 million); Belgium, 9 percent ($21.28 million); Netherlands and Canada, 4.7 percent each ($11.2 million each); and Luxembourg, 0.6 percent ($1.4 million). (Ibid.)

On the same day that this meeting took place, Marshall forwarded to Acheson the comments of the JCS, with which he concurred, on a State Department position paper regarding Indochina for use at the September 10–14 meetings in Washington with the British and French foreign ministers preceding the NATO Council meeting in Ottawa. While the chiefs agreed with most of the sections "having military implications," including a statement that the US was "not in a position to promise military intervention" in Indochina "in the event of an overt Chinese Communist aggression," they objected to the statement that "any such decision in such an event would depend upon the circumstances at the time." They feared this might mislead the French into believing that US forces "might be committed to Indochina under such circumstances as overt Chinese Communist aggression."

(Marshall to Acheson, September 10, 1951, NA/RG 330, CD 092.3 [NATO].) A few days later, however, in preparation for talks with the visiting General de Lattre regarding aid to the French in Indochina, the chiefs concluded, in what constituted a modification of past policy, that the US should, if necessary, "take military action short of the actual employment of ground forces in Indochina to prevent the fall of that country to Communism." These might include a blockade of the China coast along with air and naval action against "selected targets held by Communist China," possibly with the participation of Nationalist Chinese forces. (*The Joint Chiefs of Staff and the First Indochina War, 1947–1954*, 79–80.)

At his first meeting with French Foreign Minister Schuman on September 11, Acheson noted that Mayer's statements on French financial and Indochina problems the previous day "had made a deep impression upon " Marshall, who was "examining all possible ways" with ECA Director Foster to provide additional military aid to the French in Indochina (*FRUS, 1951*, 3: 1250). Marshall hosted a luncheon for Schuman that day as well, and following his resignation (see pp. 629–32), he cohosted another luncheon with Lovett for General de Lattre on September 14. Lovett also had a follow-up conversation with Mayer on September 13. (*FRUS, 1951*, 4: 426–28.) ★

361

MEMORANDUM FOR ANNA ROSENBERG — September 10, 1951, Washington, DC

Reference our conversation on the attached letter to the Bureau of the Budget concerning a proposed executive order providing for the suspension of certain provisions of the officer personnel act pertaining to regular army officers.[1]

I wish you would inform Secretary Pace and General Collins of my general reaction to this proposed executive order, in so far as it applies to the retention on active duty of older officers whose service would normally require mandatory retirement. I have already spoken to General Hull about ways and means for vitalizing the Army, particularly as to recognition by promotion of younger officers.[2]

I have always fought for a promotion system which would create incentive in younger officers, increase the morale of younger officers and provide recognition promotions for outstanding services. I think the present officer personnel act, if wisely applied, will accomplish these things.[3]

It seems to me that the Army has been top heavy in older officers, many of whom have passed the point of useful efficiency. Only by continued induction into the senior ranks of younger, well-qualified officers (and I refer most specifically to temporary grades of Brigadier and Major General) can the Army provide the continuity and the life spark required for vitalization.

If I understand the problem, the Army desires authority now to retain on active duty about 975 officers who would normally be retired in June of 1953, two years hence. The reasons for requesting a decision now are not particularly compelling to me. I would much rather see the Army immediately appoint a board of general officers to determine on a "selection-in" basis rather than on a "selection-out" basis those officers included in the 975 who would, because of their unique qualifications, be desired for retention. I would anticipate that this number would not exceed 10% of the total, and that the board could complete its work within several months.

In any event I deplore any premature action which will place a stultifying effect on the promotion system in the Army, particularly as it refers to our younger, more virile officers. I wish you would ride close herd on this proposition to insure that maximum effort is expended to vitalize the Army along the lines indicated above.

GCMRL/G. C. Marshall Papers (Secretary of Defense, Chronological, Secretaries, Hawkins)

1. While the editors have not located the letter from the Bureau of the Budget or the proposed executive order, Truman had issued an executive order on June 30, 1951, which suspended the regulations in the Officer Personnel Act of 1947 concerning limits on the number of junior officers serving in the navy and marine corps "for the duration of the national emergency" proclaimed by Truman on December 16, 1950. (Executive Order no. 10,266, *Federal Register* 16 [July 1951]: 6420.) See p. 300.

2. General Hull had been appointed vice army chief of staff on July 31.

3. For Marshall's earlier expressions of his views on promotions, see pp. 527–29; Pogue, *Ordeal*, 91–101, and *Organizer*, 89–91; and throughout volumes 2–5 of the *Papers of GCM.*

362

To General Matthew B. Ridgway — September 11, 1951, Washington, DC

Dear Ridgway: Thanks for your letter of the 30th in regard to having some influential women take a look at Korea. I have talked it over with Lovett, the Chiefs of Staff, and Mrs. Rosenberg and we have come to the conclusion that it would not be wise to make such a move at this time.[1]

We have been under continual pressure here to send all sorts of groups to overseas areas, including Korea. Labor and industry, veterans organizations, and numerous senators and congressmen (including some congressional committees) have indicated desires to make such an inspection trip. It seems to us that if we send one we will be pretty well forced into the position of having to send all, and we question whether this would be desirable, particularly at this stage of the campaign.

You are having a tough time, with your interrupted negotiations, a growing battle, and I suppose many other difficulties which I am not aware of. You seem to take it all calmly, which is very impressive to the general public.[2]

With most affectionate regards to your Penny and yourself, Faithfully yours,

GCMRL/G. C. Marshall Papers (Secretary of Defense, Number Indexed, M200-7-9)

1. Ridgway had written Marshall on August 30 to ask if he thought there was "any merit" in bringing some "carefully selected members of the great womens clubs" to Korea so they could witness the conditions of the war. He suspected they might have a "very great" influence on "public opinion upon their return" and suggested that a visit in October to provide the "best weather." (Ridgway to Marshall, August 30, 1951, NA/RG 330, SD 092 [Korea].) See pp. 639–47.

Rosenberg and the JCS agreed that this idea was "ill-advised . . . at this time." Rosenberg also warned that such a visit "might result in a plea for disarmament" and "would highlight" demands "from servicemen that their dependents be permitted to go to Korea." Marshall formulated his response to Ridgway in light of this memorandum from Rosenberg. (Rosenberg to Marshall, memorandum, September 10, 1951, ibid.)

2. See pp. 566–67 and 592–95. The Battle of Bloody Ridge had taken place in the second half of August and ended on September 5, to be followed on September 13 by the month-long Battle of Heartbreak Ridge and the resumption of armistice negotiations at Panmunjom. Ridgway would later label the fighting in these battles "perhaps the bloodiest to date and the most strenuous." (Tucker, *Encyclopedia of the Korean War*, 1: 87–88, 305–7; Matthew B. Ridgway, *The Korean War* [New York: Doubleday, 1967], 186.)

363

To Thomas H. White — September 11, 1951
Personal and Confidential — Washington, DC

My dear Mr. White: At the time the Norwegian elkhound was presented to me you wrote a very nice letter telling me of your interest in the breed and also that you were the owner of a kennel. Mrs. Marshall and I were most appreciative of your offer of assistance with the dog, and for that reason I am now writing you.[1]

We are extremely fond of Nato (which he was christened before he left Norway and the name he still carries), but now find that it is not possible to give him the care that he deserves, the reason being that we spend our winters at Pinehurst, North Carolina, where there are no accommodations for the dog. Secondly, we want to be most careful of his care during the five months which we are in residence in the south and as I, of course, only have the opportunity of spending week-ends there Mrs. Marshall is alone except for a maid. I am sure you will understand that this creates somewhat of a problem and in this connection I offer you the dog for your permanent possession, or whatever appropriate disposition you wish to make of him.

Mrs. Marshall and I are very reluctant to give Nato up but in fairness to the dog I think it best that we do so. I would appreciate having your reaction to this proposal and also that you keep the matter on a confidential basis as I certainly don't want to do anything that would embarrass or offend those who were so generous in making him available to me.[2]

I am sending you the register and other allied papers on Nato for your information.[3] Faithfully yours,

GCMRL/G. C. Marshall Papers (Secretary of Defense, Correspondence, Selected)

1. See pp. 578–79.

2. On Katherine Marshall's instruction, C. J. George sent a separate letter to clarify that the public should have no "knowledge of the dog's disposition" which would be "most

embarrassing to General Marshall." Thus the Marshalls should be indicated as the owners when appropriate. If White did accept custody of the dog, the Marshalls would tell the press that it had "been placed in the kennels because of their frequent traveling." (George to White, September 11, 1951, GCMRL/G. C. Marshall Papers [Secretary of Defense, Selected].)

White asked George on September 20 if Marshall desired to keep the dog now that he was retired (see the next editorial note). George responded negatively on September 27, adding that the Marshalls' frequent travels would make "the problem of caring for the dog . . . greater than before." (White to George, September 20, 1951, and George to White, September 27, 1951, ibid.)

3. See pp. 662–63.

IN LATE AUGUST or early September, Marshall had submitted to President Truman his letter of resignation as secretary of defense, dated September 1 but to take effect September 12, along with a draft letter for Truman's use to accept his resignation and a draft press release. "With deep regret," Marshall began his resignation letter, "I feel I must terminate my active daily service in the government, and therefore submit my resignation as Secretary of Defense to be effective within the next two weeks.

"Our original understanding prior to my appointment was that I would serve only until 30 June 1951—that time has now been extended more than two months.

"As I explained to you personally, I do this with deep regret, but as you well know I will always be available for whatever temporary service you may desire of me.

"Meanwhile I assure you of my loyal devotion to you and the national Government." (Marshall to Truman, memorandum, n.d., and attached September 1, 1951, memorandum, GCMRL/G. C. Marshall Papers [Secretary of Defense, Chronological, Secretaries, Carlson].)

The draft press release announcing that Truman had accepted the resignation noted that Marshall had previously agreed to serve until June 30, 1951, but "on that date so much legislation of great importance to the Armed Services was still largely in a state of hearings before Committees of Congress that the General agreed to carry on until the end of the summer, specifically until the Commission to recommend to the Congress the basic policies to govern the Universal Military Training had completed its report, which it has now done." It also announced that Truman was on that day forwarding to the Senate his nomination of Lovett to succeed Marshall. (Draft White House Press release, September 1, 1951, attached to Marshall to Truman, memorandum, n.d., ibid.)

Marshall departed the Pentagon at 12:20 p.m. on Tuesday, September 11, for a 12:30 p.m. meeting at the White House with the president, during which Truman accepted the resignation to be announced at 11:00 a.m. the following day. Truman used Marshall's draft letter accepting the resignation in its entirety but added four additional paragraphs:

"In again accepting your resignation from a position of high responsibility I realize how many times previously you have sought to retire to private life. But one time after another you have responded to the call to public service.

"To all of these offices you have brought great talent and wisdom. In fact, no man ever has given his country more distinguished and patriotic service than have you.

"On behalf of our country I want to thank you for all you have done. On my own behalf, I want to tell you of my deep personal appreciation for the wise counsel and the unwavering support you have given me in these trying days.

"You have earned your retirement many fold and I wish you many good years at Leesburg." (Truman to Marshall, September 11, 1951, GCMRL/G. C. Marshall Collection [Harry S. Truman].)

On the morning of September 12, Marshall sent a series of letters and telegrams of appreciation to numerous individuals with whom he had worked (see pp. 632–33) and met individually with Anna Rosenberg, Robert Lovett (twice), Clayton Fritchey, and General Bradley prior to a 10:00 a.m. meeting of the Armed Forces Policy Council, attended by Lovett, the service secretaries, the JCS, Carter, and Colonel Carey A. Randall, Lovett's executive and secretary of the group. According to notes of this meeting taken by Carter, Marshall informed the council that he would cease to be secretary of defense at 11:00 a.m. and asked them to be "careful of leaks to intimates." He went on to explain the reasons for the timing of his decision, noting the absence of any "good time" to resign, as there were "always crises" with which to contend. He stated that he had initially agreed to serve for six months, which Truman extended to June 30, but the state of various legislative proposals critical to the Defense Department was "such a mess" at that time that Marshall "did not bring up" the question of his resignation. In addition, Acheson was "perturbed" about the status of the Japanese Peace Treaty negotiations and had requested that Marshall delay his resignation until September 15. With the signing of the treaty having taken place on September 8 (see p. 624n2), the date for Marshall's resignation was set for September 12. Marshall insisted that he was "leaving for personal reasons—very personal" and thanked the members of the Armed Forces Policy Council "for all you've done," commenting on the "heavy progress" that had been made over the previous year with "fundamentals ironed out" and "things looking up a little." He complimented their "competence, efficiency, integrity & loyalty," calling them the "best staff [he had] ever known." (Marshall Carter notes, September 12, 1951, GCMRL/G. C. Marshall Papers [Secretary of Defense, Categorical, Memoranda, Marshall S. Carter, 1950–1951]; H.)

Following this meeting, Marshall held a staff meeting at 10:10 a.m. and then proceeded to hold a press conference at 10:19 a.m. ★

364

DRAFT OF INFORMAL REMARKS TO THE PRESS

September 12, 1951
Washington, DC

I have asked you to come here so I could personally and quite privately tell you of my resignation effective today upon announcement by the White House at 11 a.m. I trust you all implicitly to keep the fact of my resignation to yourselves until the official White House announcement has been made.[1]

My reasons for leaving government service at this time are purely personal, and I think will be readily understandable. But so there can be no mistake or misinterpretation of my action, I want you to know in a very personal way of my thoughts at this time.

More than fifty years have elapsed since I graduated from VMI in June, 1901. Since that time, and with literally no break at all up to the present, I have been in continuous, daily, uninterrupted service to the government, in one job or another. It has seemed to me for some time that 50 years of government service is just about as much as should be expected of one man—don't misunderstand me, I'm not complaining—I'm merely stating the fact of the matter.

It was with that thought in mind, and I might say that I have had those 50 years staring me in the face for some considerable time, that it was agreed with the President originally that I would serve as Secretary of Defense until June 30th. Actually so much was going on in the Defense Department, particularly as to legislation and future plans, that it did not seem either propitious or appropriate to resign at that time.

I suppose there is never an appropriate time for such action. Certainly the operations of the Defense Department are of a daily and continuing nature. Legislation is always being prepared for, or supported before, the Congress. Crises occur with their usual frequency, if not abroad on an international scale, then surely within the country on domestic matters. The problems are great and will continue so for many years—most certainly throughout the indefinite period of tension we now face.

Several important factors led me to the conclusion that the middle of September would be as appropriate a time as any to ask the President to accept my resignation. In the first place, the Department of Defense had done all it could do toward obtaining its required appropriations. The Japanese Peace Treaty would shortly be signed. The Commission on Universal Military Training had virtually completed its report. The Reserve Forces Bill had been presented to the Congress. Other programs of equal importance appeared to be well-launched.

But over and above all these immediate factors, and what was the compelling factor to me, is the continuity of purpose—the unity of effort—being constantly displayed by Bob Lovett, the three Service Secretaries, the Joint Chiefs of Staff, my own Assistant Secretaries, and the Defense Department staffs in general. Certainly the manner in which basic decisions are made, and basic disagreements are resolved, all with high integrity—as well as intensity—is a tower of strength to the country at this time.

As I have said before—my reasons for leaving now are purely personal, based entirely on the fact that now appears to be as appropriate a time as any to wind up 50 years of uninterrupted daily service to the government. I leave with very real regret, and with high devotion to the President and to the government.[2]

GCMRL/G. C. Marshall Papers (Secretary of Defense, Number Indexed, M200-3-28)

1. The editors have been unable to locate a transcript of Marshall's remarks to the press, but from quotes the press attributed to him the following day, he appears to have used both this draft and the notes described below.

In his notes preparing Marshall's remarks, Carter had recommended that Marshall indicate only off the record that he had agreed to stay in office through the signing of the Japanese Peace Treaty at Acheson's request and that his decision to leave was "influenced by Mrs. M's health." (Marshall later informed Erskine Wood that Mrs. Marshall's health was not among the "'personal reasons' for my leaving the Pentagon.") He also suggested that Marshall praise the Pentagon press corps while giving them some advance notice and "time to reflect" before the announcement was released. (Marshall Carter notes, September 12, 1951, GCMRL/G. C. Marshall Papers [Secretary of Defense, Categorical, Memoranda, Marshall S. Carter, 1950–1951]; H; Marshall to Wood, September 20, 1951, GCMRL/G. C. Marshall Papers [Secretary of Defense, Number Indexed, M200-19-24].)

A sheet of notes prepared by Marshall's staff attached to these draft remarks reproduced above encouraged Marshall to stress his "50 years in daily government service, without appreciable break"; his high regard for the "Unanimity of purpose, high integrity and resolve, close cooperation of effort" of Lovett and the rest of his staff; and his "completed, continued, real devotion to President, the government, etc.," and gratitude "for having had opportunity so to serve." The notes concluded that Marshall should deflect any "Attempts to tie your resignation in with MacArthur, McCarthy, China, Eisenhower candidacy, flat feet, or disagreement with President." ("Statements and Cliches to Avoid in Your Remarks, Things [Questions Possibly] to be Alert for, and Points to Stress," September 12, 1951, ibid., [M200-3-28].)

The press reported that Marshall "took the unusual step of calling into his office the reporters who normally cover the Pentagon. . . . Two dozen reporters filed into the long room and "sat down in a circle with him." Anna Rosenberg was also present. ("Gen. Marshall Resigns; Post Goes to Lovett," *New York Herald Tribune*, September 13, 1951, GCMRL/G. C. Marshall Papers [Secretary of Defense, Scrapbooks and Scrapbook Materials].)

2. The White House issued a press release announcing Truman's acceptance of Marshall's resignation and his nominations of Lovett as Marshall's successor and ECA Administrator William C. Foster as Lovett's successor as deputy secretary. (Press release, September 11, 1951, GCMRL/G. C. Marshall Papers [Secretary of Defense, Number Indexed, M200-19-24].)

IN LIKELY his "last official act" as secretary of defense on September 12, Marshall congratulated Acheson for his "splendid leadership" at the Japanese Peace Treaty conference. While "the task that we face in the Pacific may still not be easy," Marshall continued, "I believe that great strides have been made in the ultimate desires of the great and free nations of the world." Acheson replied the following day that Marshall's presence "in the last year of grave peril to our country . . . steadied all of our vital actions and decisions. . . . I shall not try to put into words how deeply your letter touched my heart, nor what courage and resolution it gives me to face the problems still ahead." Marshall wrote a similar letter to John Foster Dulles, who replied that he attached "the utmost value to words of commendation from you," and that he treasured "our associations of the past." General Bradley conveyed his "deep sense of loss" following Marshall's resignation and his "indebtedness for your guidance and for the inspiration and the leadership you have given me over the years in the performance of my duties." Marshall responded that he would "miss greatly our daily association" and hoped to have "the opportunity of dropping in occasionally for a brief chat" during his less frequent trips to Washington. In a later letter to Felix Larkin, Marshall reassured him that "Bob Lovett is hard at work, and, as a superb helmsman, I know he will keep this ship headed into the wind and on an even keel." (Marshall to Acheson, September 12, 1951, GCMRL/G. C. Marshall Papers [Secretary of Defense, Number Indexed, M214-16-35]; Acheson to Marshall and Bradley to Marshall, September 13, 1951; Marshall to Bradley, September 20, 1951; and Marshall to Larkin, September 27, 1951, ibid., [M200-19-24]; Dulles to Marshall, September 12, 1951, ibid., [M200-3-9].) Marshall also wrote to Generals Eisenhower (see pp. 649n1) and Ridgway. ★

365

To General Matthew B. Ridgway | September 12, 1951
Radio No. DEF-21295. | Washington, DC
From General Marshall for General Ridgway

You probably have already heard through the radio of my resignation as Secretary of Defense which becomes effective this morning. I cannot leave the office without expressing my appreciation for the superb job you are doing under most trying and difficult circumstances. You have shown exceptional judgment and demonstrated magnificent battle leadership for which we all in the United Nations must be deeply grateful.[1]

GCMRL/G. C. Marshall Papers (Secretary of Defense, Number Indexed, M211-1-24)

1. See pp. 629–32. Ridgway replied the next day that Marshall's "consummate thoughtfulness touches me deeply and your message of appreciation will be cherished by us both as long as we live." (Ridgway to Marshall, cable no. Z-36967, September 13, 1951, GCMRL/G. C. Marshall Papers [Secretary of Defense, Number Indexed, M200-19-24].) See also pp. 649–50.

I Have Sown Some Seeds

September 12, 1951–October 16, 1959

I have done my best, and I hope I have sown some seeds which may bring forth good fruit.

—Nobel Peace Prize Lecture
December 11, 1953

IN THE DAYS and weeks following the announcement that he had resigned as secretary of defense, Marshall maintained an extensive correspondence with family, friends, and colleagues in which he reported his feelings about his retirement. (Many of these letters are filed in GCMRL/G. C. Marshall Papers [Secretary of Defense, Number Indexed, M200-19-24].) Marshall shared with Madge Pendleton that "Katherine and I are busily making plans for the future and it is a wonderful feeling to know that we can now move leisurely." He wrote more informally to his longtime friend General Claude "Flap" Adams about Mrs. Marshall: "I am at her command these days and we have countless long-delayed plans to execute. It's wonderful!" In addition, Marshall informed Erskine Wood that he and Mrs. Marshall were anticipating being able to "move leisurely without the ever-present possibility of interruption." He confessed to Felix Larkin that his plans "include travel and sport, but primarily just plain loafing." (Marshall to Pendleton and Marshall to Wood, September 20, 1951, and Marshall to Larkin, September 27, 1951, ibid.; Marshall to Adams, September 14, 1951, ibid., [M214-14-43].)

Robert E. Sherwood, a Pulitzer Prize–winning playwright and author of *Roosevelt and Hopkins: An Intimate History* (New York: Harper & Brothers, 1948), who had been a speechwriter for President Roosevelt and overseas director of the Office of War Information, requested Marshall's confirmation of a story he had written for the London *Evening Standard*, which contributed to the attitude Marshall adopted in his retirement. According to the story, Marshall, who had taken to flying between Leesburg and Washington after his return from Korea (see pp. 548–52), landed at Leesburg "One Sunday last winter," and by the time he walked to the front door, "the telephone was ringing" to tell him to return to Washington. Marshall was "compelled to say good-bye to his wife almost before he had time to say hello. Mrs. Marshall smiled. This was an old story to her. 'Do drop in again some Sunday,' she said to her husband, 'when you can stay a little longer.'" Marshall replied to Sherwood that this story was "sufficiently correct to illustrate our situation at the time. My most irritating difficulty was the fact that Leesburg was on Standard Time so as not to confuse the numerous dairy herds, and Washington on Daylight Saving Time. So in order to reach my desk around 8:00 A.M. I had to leave home about 6:15 A.M.!!" (Sherwood to Marshall, September 25, 1951, and Marshall to Sherwood, September 27, 1951, ibid., [M219-2-19]; "So General Marshall can go home to his wife," London *Evening Standard*, September 14, 1951, GCMRL/© Marshall-Winn Collection [Secretary of Defense, Clippings].) ★

366

To Frank McCarthy

September 12 [*13*], 1951
Washington, DC

Dear Frank: News has, no doubt, already reached you by radio or newspaper of my resignation this morning as Secretary of Defense. This has been a very busy day, beginning at Leesburg where I left this morning at a few minutes before 6:00

Standard Time, arriving at my desk a few minutes after 8:00 local time. There was the usual raft of papers to be reckoned with and at 10:00 I had a meeting with the Armed Forces Policy Council, in my old office, which consists of the service secretaries and Joint Chiefs of Staff, where I made known to them my resignation. While I was sitting at the table telling them about it my immediate staff was being assembled in my new office and I told them of my departure. This was immediately followed by a press conference at 10:30. I was walking on soft ground for a little better than an hour, as the announcement was to be made by The President from the White House at 11:00 o'clock. Fortunately, there was no leak, and naturally this amazed me somewhat.[1]

I appreciate your telling me of your non-paying job with the State Department, and while I have not heard from the FBI regarding your appointment I will be prepared to see their agent when he calls.[2]

Thanks for telling me about your new picture, "The Facts of Life". I will look forward to seeing it when it is released. I think the American public can stand a lot more of the light type of film, because there are too many serious problems confronting the people of the world.[3]

I didn't read previously of Mr. Zanuck's gambling experience but noticed in the paper the other morning that King Farouk's vacation expenses amounted to something like $86,000![4]

Thanks for telling me about Capra's new picture. It is good to know that he is back on top, and I will always be appreciative for the work he did for us during the last war.[5]

I was interested in your comments about the Japanese Peace Treaty Conference. In my opinion, Mr. Acheson did an outstanding job; actually, such a job that many of his severest critics commended him highly.[6]

Katherine and I are going to take things easy for a while and look forward to this fall at Pinehurst. She said that she was going to take up riding again, and now I will have a partner when I hit the bridle path.

Mrs. Lacy has not been well; as a matter of fact, she has been in Doctors Hospital undergoing treatment but expects to be discharged soon. Molly and the children spent the month of August at Leesburg while we were vacationing on Cape Cod with the McCoys, and when we write her we will convey your regards.[7]

With love from us both, Affectionately,

Leesburg, Sept. 13th. Your telegram reached me last evening here in peace and idleness. K is now on the lawn waiting for me to rest up with a bit of pruning.[8]

GCMRL/Frank McCarthy Papers (Additions, Box 1)

1. See pp. 630–33.

2. McCarthy had written a two-page letter to Marshall on September 10, which began by sharing that "Some months ago the State Department asked me to fill out certain papers which would lead to my appointment as a consultant on film matters. This would mean nothing except an occasional brief visit to Washington, without compensation." As part of this process, the FBI was contacting his previous employers. He informed Marshall of this so that if the FBI had "approached you, you will know what it's all about. If I had known they were going to question my previous employers, I should certainly have asked your

permission before submitting your name." (McCarthy to Marshall, September 10, 1951, GCMRL/G. C. Marshall Papers [Secretary of Defense, Number Indexed, M200-2-14].)

3. McCarthy reported that his film *Decision Before Dawn* had "opened in London with success," and that he was currently "working on the manuscript of my new comedy, THE FACTS OF LIFE. This story is as light as DECISION BEFORE DAWN is heavy, a film which can be produced very inexpensively. It is designed only for laughs." (Ibid.) See also pp. 563–64.

4. McCarthy wrote in his September 10 letter that Darryl Zanuck, who had recently returned from a lengthy trip to Europe, told him that "the accounts of his gambling with King Farouk are greatly exaggerated." King Farouk of Egypt was on a three-month honeymoon cruise touring southern European casinos. (Ibid.; "Farouk Leaves for Egypt," *New York Times*, September 11, 1951, p. 8; "King Farouk Returns Home," *New York Times*, September 16, 1951, p. 37.)

5. McCarthy shared that he had "not seen Frank Capra for a long time, but at last he has a hit, a Bing Crosby picture called HERE COMES THE GROOM. This is his first major success since the war, and it is good to see him back on top at last." (McCarthy to Marshall, September 10, 1951, GCMRL/G. C. Marshall Papers [Secretary of Defense, Number Indexed, M200-2-14].) Capra had directed the *Why We Fight* series of films during World War II. See *Papers of GCM*, 3: 411, 449–50, 538–39; 4: 424–25, 506–7, 614–15; 5: 212–13, 223–24; and 6: 726.

6. McCarthy praised "Mr. Acheson's victory" at the Japanese Peace Treaty conference and commented on the "fickle quality of public opinion" in light of the signing of the treaty, with some of his "Republican friends who have never had a word" for Acheson "except in condemnation and who have always stood at the pole opposite his," now pulling "at least 90 degrees in his direction." (Ibid.) See p. 625.

7. McCarthy concluded his September 10 letter with a handwritten note: "In the meanwhile, affectionate regards to you, Mrs. Marshall, Clifton, the Lacys, and the Winns when you write." (Ibid.) See pp. 604–5.

8. Although this letter is dated September 12, 1951, Marshall added this postscript on September 13 before sending it. Upon receiving news of Marshall's resignation, McCarthy had sent a telegram to the Marshalls at Leesburg stating that "This is one of the most selfishly happy days of my life because I know you both will now have the relief from high responsibility so often anticipated and so fully deserved." (McCarthy to Marshall, telegram, September 12, 1951, ibid., [M200-19-24].)

367

Transcript of Welcoming Address to the Defense Advisory Committee on Women in the Services[1] — September 17, 1951, Washington, DC

GENERAL MARSHALL: Thank you very much.

I want to say good morning here again and tell you at the start that, as you know, of course, I'm speaking—I don't mean to call this overrated or what—but I am not Secretary of Defense, but I did invite you and you did accept most graciously and to a degree I have never known before. I think out of fifty invitations forty-nine accepted. And again something unique here, in addition to the distinguished character of your group, which I don't think has ever been exceeded in any gathering that I know of in this country, you're all on time! So that this is a very remarkable affair, really. Whether or not it has partly a great deal to do with Mrs. Rosenberg or not, I don't know. She's pretty hard to dodge and duck.

Now, seriously, when I was Secretary, I thought, and Mrs. Rosenberg thought, it was very important that we have a really outstanding group of the women of this country to do two things, to know what we were doing and give us their comments, their observations, and their continuous suggestions and learn at first-hand and close up how we were proceeding in this matter and what were the fundamental purposes involved in the work of the Defense Department at this time.

Now, I would like first to talk about some things rather apart from the question of sex! We're facing a very difficult future, I'll say, in the immediate future, but you can't tell whether it's a year or two or five or ten, but it's quite evident that our success in doing that will depend on the organization that we have and on the fundamentals on which it is based. By that, I mean it must be some system, some setup, that will have a fair chance to endure against the fluctuations of public opinion.

I might go back a little bit to tell you of some of the lessons we've had this year that apply to what I am just about to say and what I've been referring to, and I'll tell you that, when Mr. Lovett and I came into this picture at the end of last September, the first appropriations had just been made following the Korean affair—to be accurate, I think on the 27th of September we got an authorization of $22 billion.[2] Well, people sort of feel that, if you get an appropriation of $22 billion, you write a lot of speeches about it, you've had a lot of arguments about it and now you've got it—all right, but it's a long, long time before anything results from that. It takes you months to accomplish the contracts for such a vast sum of money. The minimum time for production involved in that is about eight months. Well, if your contracts begin to have effect, say, the end of October, then you have to count eight months from the end of October to see the first items coming in, and, of course, for others that are what we call "long lead," it will be a year and a half, possibly. So that was the situation in which Mr. Lovett and I came into the Defense Department, and Mrs. Rosenberg. Then, we were immediately under the necessity of getting ready for another appropriation. The first was a rush affair. It was done in a hurry. It takes you months and months and months to build up these things, so that we had to start immediately on filling this out and evening it up, and that appropriation which actually passed on the 6th of January was for $17 billion.

Now, I want to explain a little bit what happened in that interval between the $22 billion and the $17 billion which wasn't money. We found ourselves faced with almost united opposition of the Congress. Now, I just said the other day that I thought Congress's action was rather remarkable, that they had gone through an extremely difficult period with large sums of money and had given us pretty much what we had asked for. But at this particular time, when Mr. Lovett and I started in here, we found ourselves faced with almost united opposition in the Congress, from the people, within the Government, which reached such a degree that, as I recall, in early December, they were calling for my retirement. They met the argument that I had a long experience in this thing and I knew something about it by saying that that didn't count any longer, that the senility crept up and I didn't know what I was talking about. Well, I had good reason for having it creep up under the pressure! But this was a most remarkable thing because they were all insisting we do about three times more than we were asking for. They wanted us to call out all the National Guard. They wanted to talk about 100 divisions. They were what I consider afflicted with an emotional "numbers racket." I had been forced into this thing in the summer of 1940, forced into a mobilization of the National Guard, etc., much more rapidly than we could efficiently accommodate it and I was determined I was never going to have that happen again.[3] But I was in the curious position of being, what was much criticized, a soldier in a civilian office, and yet I was being criticized because I was not asking for as much as they thought was necessary, that I didn't see the great menace that was in front of us. Well, I saw the menace all right. The question was how you efficiently met it.

The same applied to materiel factors and, when we went into the procedure of that, which Mr. Lovett handled in a very marvelous fashion, what we were insisting particularly on was that we have facilities rather than items. Of course, we had to have immediate items for the immediate need of Korea and the divisions that we were getting into active service, but what we were after were facilities which take, again, eight to nine months to put into place, sometimes longer. An assembly line isn't just a line which you designate on the floor. It's got all sorts of jigs and dies and very elaborate machinery which takes a long time to produce because it has to be produced for a particular item and particular standards, and what we wanted was the capacity, the power, to produce tremendous quantities quickly. If you didn't have that, you were eight or nine months behind if we blossomed unfortunately and tragically to a full war.

Well, that was not satisfying. They wanted numbers. They wanted numbers of planes. They wanted numbers of this. They wanted numbers of that.

But on top of this and the reason I am going into this is it was an emotional reaction and we were in the curious position of being attacked because we had not realized the true menace that we were faced with and we should do all these other things.

Now, as a matter of fact, if we had done some of these things like calling out all the National Guard and everything, we couldn't have equipped them. We didn't have the stuff. We didn't have the accommodations. We would have been bitterly criticized for not having adequate accommodations. We would have been bitterly criticized for not having the adequate materiel and the troops of each state would have all their political power coming in. We wouldn't have had time to do what we had to do immediately for Korea and for the forces that we were sending over to Europe.

Well, we succeeded in resisting that, but it was a very curious thing. And one of the attacks that was most pointed that struck General Bradley in particular and me was that we dared to talk about the fluctuations of public opinion. I had gone through some very terrifying experiences with that, and the ups and downs that you encounter, and you must encounter, particularly in a young democracy like ours, and I was bitterly criticized by some of the groups of editors of the most telling publications in this country for daring to refer to that. I "shouldn't consider economics, the effect of these vast appropriations on the economy of the country." That wasn't my role. Mine was "purely military," and these attacks were very severe and very pointed. As I say, they went to the point of recommending my retirement.

Now, Mr. Lovett and I, before these Appropriations Committees, before the Armed Forces Committees, resisted this and succeeded in getting done the things that we proposed and not a lot of other stuff that would have harassed us and made it unduly difficult. But I had said that I was certain, if there was not a full war, that by the fall of '52, by '52, we would suffer a public reaction; it would be very damaging because it would instantly affect all the appropriations before the Congress and I thought that it might come even as early as September of '51. Well, I doubt if I have ever been so inaccurate. It came in February '51. The combination of the crime investigation and the new use of television and Ridgway's success in Korea just wrecked us and we ran into a complete letdown. Now, then, we were before the Congress and everything we were putting in for was being attacked as too much. In a brief period of weeks, we suffered a complete reversal.[4]

Then there was another one that came to me. This was the most humiliating experience that I have had in connection with the American public. One man, and not a top man, in the Soviet Union made a speech and he knocked a dent right square in the middle of our whole defense program—one man and not a top man—Malik. I thought the public reaction from that was one of the most humiliating experiences that I had ever gone through with the American public. Nothing the President said or I said or Lovett said or a number of Senators said or a number of leading people said affected this practically at all. We battled with that for about a month and a half or two months to stay this letdown on all sides, and it was a bitter battle in order to maintain ourselves. The fact that we would get a reaction from the public on the speech of one man from a discredited government so far as honor and integrity is concerned beat anything that I had ever experienced.[5]

I had gone through the terrific demobilization which was carried out after I left as Chief of Staff but was started while I was Chief of Staff. I had met the surge of Congressional reaction that demand persisted and listened to no other excuses of any kind. They tried to say, "Now, that was an order or something that did this thing." Of course it was an order that did it, but it did it under the compelling pressure of public opinion and the members of Congress, and yet that was what we were so criticized for, that we would refer a thing like that in time of great danger. I had gone through it. I had seen it with General Pershing when we came back from the first war where they took, from the spring of 1919 to the end of November in 1919, hearings of everybody important connected with the first war and then debated the question and, finally, in June 1920, June 4th, they passed a very creditable act.[6] It left out the Universal Military Training part. That was scotched, but otherwise it was a very respectable defense act. That was a long debate right after the war, but still after months and months and a year or more of investigation and debate and everything, they wrecked that within two years completely. It started out we were going to have 285,000 in the Army and we ended up I think it was with 18,000 about eighteen months or two years later, and that included everything. That included chauffeurs, the men in the depots. You could have put all the troops in the Brooklyn baseball park and yet that was done in that short time after a very fine act under the leadership of Senator Rogers [*Wadsworth*], now Representative Rogers [*Wadsworth*], recently resigned.[7]

I had gone through these things and I had seen them and the point I am leading up to is this—whatever we do has got to have a sound basis in the line of an enduring policy, one that we think can endure these fluctuations of public opinion. If this tension continues, and anybody that analyzes it recognizes it is going to continue, everybody gets tired. Everybody gets tired. You might say, "Well, that's a little far-fetched in this troubled world," and just remember that we saved the Army completely. There would have been no Army there left. About three or four months before Pearl Harbor, by one vote, the National Guard was going to be sent home; all the Selective Service men were going to be sent home. That meant there would have been no regular Army because there weren't over fifteen per cent regular soldiers in any uniform, and yet that was done with a full war in Europe with a complete occupation of the Continent and we saved ourselves by one vote in the House.

I have gone through these things and gone through them so they come down to the present day. What I am deeply concerned with is that we have a fundamental policy that has a chance of enduring, that can ride through these turmoils and sudden sweeps of public opinion.

Now, that means, of course, we've got to find the most economical way of doing a very expensive thing, and this Universal Military Training is the fundamental policy at the basis of that, and I know of no other one that meets it, because what we're working for is to put in the ranks of these Reserve units, more particularly the National Guard units, trained men. They can't train them themselves.[8] They can't possibly do that on an hour a week. The man would be so old he couldn't fight by the time they got him trained on that basis, but, if we can fill their ranks with men that have had the fundamental individual what we call basic training while they're home, about their own business, then we have transformed this whole setup and we have a tremendous power, a great immediate potential, not a remote potential, and I must explain there that the divisions that had been called in last September had just now, this September, qualified for field service—a year—and yet look at the tragedy of Korea.

We had a great difficulty here with the Senate. For the moment we've gotten by. The bill has not yet—oh, I think it has passed, but they were imposing restrictions on us there that would have tied up a great many of our ships, would have grounded our planes, in the business of calling in men from the Reserves and forcing us to return. Well, you can't take a man off the street and give him this training that he has to have. And we were confronted with a great emergency. They have to have crews for planes, not six months from now, but next week, in Korea. They have to have ships taken out of mothballs, put to sea, not six months, but the next week. The only way in the world we could do it was to take the men that we had in training from the Reserves, which is the basis of our military system, our military policy, as a citizen Army. Well, this was because the war didn't spread all over the place and these men were taken from their business, from their families. We ran up a great service and still have it. The battle hasn't been settled up on the Hill yet to have these men immediately returned, which would just wreck us completely. Now, we can get most of them out. We can get all the men out by December. A great many are going out right now. The officer part takes a little longer. It takes, from the time he goes in, seventeen months as the minimum we think we can do it in without just spoiling ourselves literally.

But the reaction doesn't take consideration of that. It's the momentary reaction of the constituent to the Congressman and what he insists upon being done regardless of what happens at some other place, and then we're responsible for what happens at some other place. All of these things come into public reactions so we're trying to build a system that will endure. We won't have large numbers of troops in uniform in this country day in and day out. The country would never accept that, and the cost is enormous. The cost is beyond our capacity to meet, I would feel, beyond a rather brief period, but the people would never accept these men and the men would never accept it.

We've got a problem in Europe. I'm not advertising it publicly, but those men go over there. They're enthusiastic. They're seeing a new country. They're getting settled down and, following the American habit, in two months they all want to come home and you've got quite a problem on your hands to meet that. You can't meet it by Cook tours. We're dealing now with the Ford Foundation and all to try to get into the educational thing and do something very fine for them, but it's got to be done on a military basis or they won't do it. They'll all take photography or something like that. We want to make a real educational thing and they can either take that or drill. They can take their chance—drill or that, and I think we can educate a great many under these conditions! I don't know whether that will be the harsh policy of my successor, but that's what I was going to do![9]

So what we would like you to look at in particular, beyond the question of the WAVES [US Navy's Women Accepted for Volunteer Emergency Service program] and the WACS and other organizations of women, is how we're trying to set this thing up as an enduring thing that will not wreck us economically. We can be defeated economically in a sense more easily than we can be militarily.

And I'll give you one more example of this business. I wasn't Secretary of Defense at the time this affair developed in Korea, the end of June last, a year ago, but they had no trained Reserve of any kind! The units themselves were at about sixty per cent of strength though it happened to be in Japan close at hand, so that they could be sent over but, if you send a sixty per cent unit, it is not only that much under strength, but the wastage of a campaign strikes it within two weeks, even if it didn't fight, in sickness, this, and that, and the other, detachments you can't avoid, and the only way you could get them was cannibalizing units in this country, in Panama, in Hawaii, in Germany, in Austria, in Trieste, all over the world. We just ripped everything we had apart, and we sent practically all of the private soldiers and about fifty per cent of the non-commissioned officers, and it was not until March that we were turning out basically trained men that could meet this requirement and could give us our first small group for the business of rotation.

Now, rotation was vital because those men were just fighting in desperate battle and it was desperate, outnumbered ten to one.[10] They had no prospect at all of getting back. The only prospect they could see was death or being wounded. Now we are running 40,000 men a month, individuals, trained individuals, basically trained. That's the business we did. The whole string of divisions is what a Reserve we have of basically trained men, and by October we'll be coming out with fifty thousand men a month. We've only been sending forty thousand here in the last two months and we won't continue that number right away because we have other things to do back here, and the men are flowing back out there after they leave. After the time is absorbed in their transfer, they'll go in units over here and form a tremendously valuable training guard. But for those long months of that desperate fighting in Korea with these swarms of enemy we had nothing except as we cannibalized every unit. Then, when we had to take some men out of the National Guard, we got a terrific political repercussion. We had almost no regular troops at all. They'd been literally destroyed. Yet, at the same moment, we were having to build complete new divisions to go to Europe. Only it was a desperate dilemma. We were bankrupt. We were in debt so deep that we thought we'd never get out, but we finally, in March, for the first time, had enough men.[11] We got twelve thousand in March, and in April we got about twenty-five thousand, that is, individuals that had been trained at least four months. When you say four months, that isn't exact either because you've got the time of processing the man, of getting him there, of giving him leave at the end of this thing to go home. If you don't send him home to his wife or his mother, you are in deep trouble right away. All of that is time-consuming. Then the buildup came in. But here we were still struggling with these divisions that we'd brought in, in September, and were not ready for field service until September. Well, the world doesn't permit of any such procedures as that. There's no time. We talk about a push-button war, but there's nothing push-button about a thing that takes twelve months. I don't know what that is. That's an "oxen team" procedure in comparison with the other.

Now we've got a system, we think, that will meet this dilemma, that will enable us to do these things without a bankruptcy procedure financially, and it's the only way in the world I know, and I think it's the most democratic way, and I think as a sideline it's a very excellent thing for the young men of America.

Now, we want you to see this. We want you, as far as you can—I say "we"—I'm just talking "as was" and not "as is"! We want you to be thoroughly familiar with it because you're the most influential group of women I have ever seen gathered together. When you come to the women's contribution, that will be brought so close to you that I won't take your time now, but it's vastly important because we're up against a manpower limitation now and it will become more limiting as we go along, so we've got to find the best way of doing all these things and any suggestions you have after you've looked at it a little bit and studied over it a little bit will be of great importance to us and your influence outside when you understand this can be far-reaching in its effect and most helpful.

I am awfully glad that it is my privilege to invite you here and I leave you in much better hands. Thank you very much.[12]

GCMRL/G. C. Marshall Papers (Retirement, Speeches, Statements, and Writings)

1. See pp. 361–63 and 402–4. Anna Rosenberg informed the service secretaries on April 17, 1951, that "General Marshall has decided to establish a Defense Advisory Committee on Womanpower Policies" and asked for recommendations for committee members. On June 12, Marshall invited approximately fifty women to join this committee, now officially known as the Defense Advisory Committee on Women in the Services, which would report to Secretary Rosenberg. The Defense Department announced on August 11 the formation of the forty-eight-member committee, which would hold its first meeting in Washington from September 16 to 19. Following Marshall's resignation (see pp. 630–32), Rosenberg informed the committee members that Marshall would still speak at the upcoming conference because of his "deep and continuing interest" in its work. (Rosenberg to Pace and Matthews, memoranda, April 17, 1951; Marshall to Lee, June 12, 1951, and attachment; Rosenberg to members of the Defense Advisory Committee on Women in the Services, radio no. DA-21692, September 13, 1951, NA/RG 330, SD 334 [Defense Advisory Committee on Womanpower Policies]; press release and attachment, August 11, 1951, GCMRL/G. C. Marshall Papers [Secretary of Defense, Number Indexed, M201-2-47]; Marshall to members of the Defense Advisory Committee on Women in the Services, telegram, August 17, 1951, GCMRL/G. C. Marshall Papers [Secretary of Defense, Chronological, Secretaries, Hawkins].) See photo #15.

Prior to Marshall's remarks, Lovett spoke to the group and expressed his gratitude for having had the "privilege" to serve twice under Marshall's "magnificent towering leadership." He went on to hope that in the future, "the General will not take on any more jobs! If he does, I'll be heartbroken if he doesn't ask me to come along with him."

Marshall delivered similar remarks to the Drexel Institute in Philadelphia, Pennsylvania, on October 30, 1951, and on November 6, he forwarded excerpts from that speech for a statement on UMT to be published in the November 17 issue of *Army–Navy–Air Force Journal* (GCMRL/G. C. Marshall Papers [Retirement, Speeches, Statements, and Writings]; ibid., [Secretary of Defense, Number Indexed, M200-18-39]).

2. In addition to the $13.278 billion basic budget appropriation for FY 1951 signed on September 6, 1950, the Defense Department received an $11.729 billion supplemental appropriation on September 27, 1950, bringing the department's total authorization to around $25 billion. (Doris M. Condit, *History of the Office of the Secretary of Defense*, vol. 2, *The Test of War, 1950–1953* [Washington: Historical Office, OSD, 1988], 224, 227.)

3. See *Papers of GCM*, 2: 230–35, 263–64, 267, 284, 310–11.

4. See pp. 407–13 and 440–41. Senator Estes Kefauver (D-TN) had chaired a special committee to investigate organized crime. It held televised hearings across the country, the most notorious being the March 1951 session in New York, during which mob boss Frank Costello testified.

5. See pp. 566–67 and 592–95.

6. Marshall is referring to the National Defense Act of 1920.

7. See *Papers of GCM*, 1: 193–94. James Wadsworth, chairman of the National Security Training Commission, had served as a senator from New York from 1915 to 1927 and as a representative from 1933 to 1951.

8. See pp. 552–53, 558–59, and 609–10.

9. For more on Marshall's concerns about the morale of American troops stationed in Europe, see pp. 535–36. For more on educational programs available for members of the military in 1951, see p. 397n4.

The *New York Times* had published a series of articles from May 14 to 19, 1951, exposing the inadequacy of education and information programs provided to members of the armed forces. In light of these reports, the Ford Foundation began a nationwide study of the offered programs. It resolved in October 1952 to sponsor and direct the improvement and dissemination of these resources. ("Ford Fund Backing An Education Plan for Armed Forces," *New York Times*, October 26, 1952, pp. 1, 4.)

10. See pp. 436–37, 463, and 488–89.

11. See pp. 440–41.

12. Following the conclusion of the conference on September 19, the committee reported to Rosenberg that it believed "an immediate and urgent need" existed "for a minimum of 72,000 additional women in uniform within the next few months," with "a short-term recruiting program to start November 11." (Report to the Assistant Secretary of Defense Anna M. Rosenberg from the Defense Advisory Committee on Women in the Services, n.d. [September 19, 1951?], NA/RG 330, SD 334 [Defense Advisory Committee on Women in the Services].)

368

TO STANLEY M. RINEHART JR.

September 17, 1951
[Washington, DC]

Dear Mr. Rinehart: Thank you for your letter of September 13th and the nice things you wrote about me. Shortly after moving into the Pentagon this last time and the beginning of mobilization plans, many members of Congress chided me for not ordering enough towards the defense effort. Quite a contrast to happenings during the early stages of the last war![1]

Bob Lovett is ideally suited for the job. I know of no one who is more capable, and in all of our service together he was a tower of strength to me.[2]

I would like to visit Eaton's Ranch again, but have no thought as to when this might be.[3]

I have definitely and flatly stated a number of times that I would not write my memoirs. There is no change in this decision and there is no prospect of a change. I do not know who gave you the information about the Tupper and Love organization. No such commitment has ever been made or even discussed.[4]

With my thanks again for your generous sentiments. Faithfully yours,

GCMRL/G. C. Marshall Papers (Secretary of Defense, Number Indexed, M200-19-22)

1. Rinehart, president of the publishing house Rinehart and Company, had written to Marshall on September 13 to express his "feeling of loss when I read in the papers that you were about to retire, but you have certainly earned and need a rest. And the country can never express the gratitude it feels to you for what you have done through all of these difficult years." (See pp. 630–32,) He recalled Marshall telling him at the Pentagon "on the day the draft bill first went through before World War II that if a Congressional committee could ever prove that you had ordered too much you would be the happiest man in the world. Time has certainly proven you right." (Rinehart to Marshall, September 13, 1951, GCMRL/G. C. Marshall Papers [Secretary of Defense, Number Indexed, M200-19-22].) According to Marshall's engagement records as army chief of staff, he met with Rinehart, then president of Farrar & Rinehart Publishers, briefly on Thursday, July 25, 1940, at 2:15 p.m.

2. Rinehart added that he had "known Bob Lovett for a number of years and feel sure that he can carry on in the grand tradition which you established." (Ibid.)

3. Rinehart hoped that Marshall "will have time now to go out to Eaton's Ranch again." (Ibid.) For more on Marshall's 1929 visit to Eaton's Ranch, Wyoming, see *Papers of GCM*, 1: 343–46, 352, 358.

4. Rinehart had written to Marshall in September 1945 that he had "heard, on what seems

to be good authority, that you have been keeping a Diary for a good many years" and asked if there was "any possibility of its being published." One of Marshall's assistants replied on September 20, 1945, that Marshall had "never kept a diary." (Rinehart to Marshall, September 10, 1945, and Davenport to Rinehart, September 20, 1945, GCMRL/G. C. Marshall Papers [Pentagon Office, General].) Rinehart persisted in this 1951 correspondence, writing that he knew "that the public is sincerely hoping that you will do your own personal story for it should certainly supersede in interest any that have been published. You told me that if you ever did it would be published by Tupper & Love of Atlanta, Georgia," which had published Katherine Marshall's memoir, *Together: Annals of an Army Wife*, in 1946. Rinehart suspected that the firm "would agree that a book of such importance as yours would be really ought to be distributed by a publishing house with a reputation for coverage throughout the country." (Rinehart to Marshall, September 13, 1951, GCMRL/G. C. Marshall Papers [Secretary of Defense, Number Indexed, M200-19-22].)

For more on Marshall's refusal to accept invitations to write his memoirs or publish his papers, see the next document and pp. 161, 843–44, 878–80, 896–97, 916–17, and 931–32. See also *Papers of GCM*, 6: 638, 661, 663, and 743.

369

TO LUTHER H. EVANS

September 24, 1951
[Leesburg, Virginia]

Dear Mr. Evans: I have your letter of September 20th and appreciate your generous sentiments and expression of good will on the occasion of my departure from the Defense post.[1]

With regard to my papers, as I explained several times to General Palmer, there is little in them of historical interest. I refrained throughout the war and as Secretary of State from expressing views on national or international affairs in personal or semi-official correspondence. I did this because of the inevitable hazards regarding publicity and, as to my military correspondence, to avoid any chance of confusion in the minds of the recipients between what I wrote and the campaign directives from the Operations Section over my signature. For example, Eisenhower wrote me frequently and at considerable length but I seldom if ever replied using personal correspondence. His letters are in the official files. The answers are a part of the subsequent directives.

I will consider the matter further but I see little of historical interest involved, and have the impression that my actions were few, far between, and relatively colorless.[2] Faithfully yours,

GCMRL/G. C. Marshall Papers (Secretary of Defense, Number Indexed, M200-19-24)

1. Librarian of Congress Evans had written on September 20 that Marshall's "withdrawal from public life saddens your fellow-countrymen who have found pride and assurance in your service. Certainly you must carry with you a profound sense of satisfaction in their appreciation of your accomplishments in their behalf." (Evans to Marshall, September 20, 1951, GCMRL/G. C. Marshall Papers [Secretary of Defense, Number Indexed, M200-19-34].) See pp. 629–32.

2. Evans continued his letter by saying that Americans have had, and will "continue to have, need for your example and experience," and he thus urged Marshall "to consider the ultimate and most appropriate disposition of your personal papers." He hoped Marshall would allow him to explain the "compelling" reasons why he should consider the Library

of Congress. (Ibid.)

Marshall handwrote the preceding two paragraphs on an American Red Cross notepad. (GCMRL/Mildred K. Carlson Collection [Letters].)

Evans replied on October 5: "Forgive me if I demur from your opinion; your actions were neither 'few,' nor 'far between,' nor 'relatively colorless.'" (Evans to Marshall, October 5, 1951, GCMRL/G. C. Marshall Papers [Secretary of Defense, Number Indexed, M200-19-34].)

For more on Marshall's refusal to accept invitations to write his memoirs or publish his papers, see previous document and pp. 161, 843–44, 878–80, 896–97, 916–17, and 931–32. For documents relating to the establishment of the George C. Marshall Research Foundation, see pp. 862–64, 897–99, and 902–3. See also *Papers of GCM*, 6: 638, 661, 663, and 743.

370

To General of the Army Dwight D. Eisenhower — September 24, 1951 [Leesburg, Virginia]

Dear Eisenhower: I have your letter of September 15th and appreciate, realizing the tremendous job you have, your writing me so soon after my departure from the Pentagon. It is difficult for me to express the feeling of appreciation I have for your appraisement of my service. We have been over many difficult roads together in our search for peace, and I hope and pray that the goal will soon be reached. While I sit and read of what's happening in the world, my thoughts will often be with you in the difficult task you have undertaken. Great progress has been made, and I am sure will continue to be made under your leadership.[1]

Mrs. Marshall and I have many plans, including traveling, fishing, and just plain loafing. She is grateful for your generous thought of her.

With great respect for your judgment, and with warmest regards. Please remember Mrs. Marshall and me to Mrs. Eisenhower. Faithfully yours,

GCMRL/G. C. Marshall Papers (Secretary of Defense, Number Indexed, M200-19-24)

1. Eisenhower had cabled Marshall on the day of his resignation (see pp. 629–32) to "join all the other millions in thanking you for what you have done for your country. May good fortune and happiness follow you and yours all your days." (Eisenhower to Marshall, radio, September 12, 1951, GCMRL/G. C. Marshall Papers [Secretary of Defense, Number Indexed, M200-19-24].) Marshall also wrote to Eisenhower on September 12 that he could "not leave this office without expressing to you my tremendous appreciation for the job you have done and are doing in Europe. I am sorry I did not have the opportunity to see you in your new headquarters and I want to make certain that you are aware of my very deep personal appreciation. You are rendering a great service to this country and to the world in a manner that wins the approbation of everybody without exception." (Marshall to Eisenhower, radio no. DEF-21296, September 12, 1951, ibid., [M211-1-23].) Eisenhower replied to Marshall's message on September 15 that upon receiving Marshall's cable, his "mind flashed back over the hundred incidents of our personal association since I joined you in the War Department in December, 1941. I am sure that throughout all that time you have never been in doubt as to the depth and sincerity of my respect and esteem; I hope that you are equally aware of the amount of inspiration I have drawn from your unselfish devotion to our country, with never an indication of desire on your part to count the personal cost. I most fervently hope that you and Mrs. Marshall will have many more years together, all of them made happier by the knowledge that throughout a long career you have been

concerned only with service, never with personal gain." (Eisenhower to Marshall, radio, September 15, 1951, ibid., [M200-19-24]; *Papers of DDE*, 12: 541.)

371

To Harry S. Truman

September 27, 1951
Leesburg, Virginia

My dear Mr. President: I have just received your long hand note tendering me a renewal of the job of head of the Red Cross. I appreciate your recalling your comment at the time of my resignation and offering to carry it out. Actually Mrs. Marshall and I think it best for me to hold off from jobs of daily requirements, so I must decline your generous and thoughtful offer. I am having a fine time doing little or nothing for the present and Mrs. Marshall appears greatly relaxed. She sends you her thanks and love.[1] Faithfully yours,

GCMRL/G. C. Marshall Collection (Harry S. Truman); H

1. Truman had sent a longhand note the day prior reminding Marshall that "When you resigned from the Red Cross to become Secretary of Defense we made an agreement with Mr. Roland Harriman that, if you wanted it you should be President of the Red Cross again. I am ready to carry out that agreement whenever you say the word." (Truman to Marshall, September 26, 1951, GCMRL/G. C. Marshall Papers [Retirement, General]; H.) See pp. 220–22, 247–51, and 283–84.

372

Speech to the Governors' Conference
October 1, 1951 Gatlinburg, Tennessee

MARSHALL had addressed the Governors' Conference on several occasions throughout his career and had hosted the conference's executive committee at the Pentagon while secretary of defense. (See pp. 377–79 and *Papers of GCM*, 6: 172–76.) On September 5, he accepted the conference's invitation to address its gathering in Gatlinburg, Tennessee, on October 1. (Bane to Marshall, July 5 and 18, and September 4, 1951; Marshall to Bane, July 9 and September 5, 1951, GCMRL/G. C. Marshall Papers [Retirement, General].) The Marshalls flew from Leesburg to Knoxville, Tennessee, on September 30 and traveled to the Greystone Lodge in Gatlinburg, where General Marshall participated in a 10:00 a.m. round-table discussion on emergency problems chaired by Governor Adlai Stevenson. (GCMRL/G. C. Marshall Papers [Secretary of Defense, Chronological, Secretaries, Carlson].)

Marshall's speech to the conference the next day mirrored his remarks to the Defense Advisory Committee on Women in the Services to a large extent. (See pp. 639–47.) He began by providing "a little sketch of the base of the problem" facing the United States "so far as the Defense Department is now and was concerned." At the outbreak of the Korean War, US forces in Japan "were all under strength," and "there were no" substantial "trained reserves in this country." He reminded the governors that "it was not until March of 1951 that we caught up with ourselves and, in a sense, got out of debt." (See pp. 440–41.) A critical task at the outbreak of war, Marshall noted, was "to build up basically trained reserves" while providing sufficient immediate manpower to fight in Korea. That required the Defense Department "to cannibalize units" from "every place we could find trained men" around the world. Later in his speech, Marshall admitted that this need had a direct effect on the additional divisions that were being sent to Europe to support NATO, as the US "had to draw on them in the middle of their training, take the men out to Korea." (Speech to the Governors' Conference, October 1, 1951, GCMRL/G. C. Marshall Papers [Retirement, Speeches, Statements, and Writings].) See pp. 472–74.

Marshall then discussed the general confusion about the "large appropriations" for the Defense Department that Congress had made following the North Korean invasion: $11.729 billion on September 27, 1950, and $16.795 billion on January 6, 1951. (See pp. 276–78, 291–93, and 646n2, and Condit, *Test of War*, 223–42.) He reminded the governors that those funds did not produce "immediately available results." Marshall estimated that it took approximately eight months after funds were authorized to "get any result in the form of material" and up to eighteen months to realize "a great portion of the needed material." Proper handling of the appropriations also "requires a great deal of tedious labor, a great deal of time-consuming procedure. . . . Then to that you must add the many months required for productions, for shipment, for delivery." It was not until the summer of 1951 "that we began to get the first products, except as to personnel, transportation and food." (Ibid.)

Despite the initial delays in providing adequate manpower to Korea, which required the extension of the Selective Service Act of 1948 in June 1950 (see p. 325) and left some National Guard units without proper training before being ordered abroad, Marshall praised the implementation of a rotation scheme for members of the US military fighting in Korea beginning in the spring of 1951. This plan "was absolutely essential to maintain the morale of the force that had gone through the exhausting and terrific experience of inadequate numbers, inadequate materiel, overwhelming numbers of the enemy." Following "a month's rest," the rotated men "were assigned to the various new units and put into the training camps to help instruct recruits." (See pp. 436–37, 516–17, and 551–52.) Marshall also lauded the unanimity among all of the countries fighting on behalf of the UN in Korea and stated that the US Army there "has reached a degree of excellence in coordination, in cooperation, in the ability to bring great firepower to bear without spreading the command so as to present weak points to an aggressive enemy, that have never been exceeded in any army." In light of the upcoming Armistice Day ceremonies on November 11, Marshall asked the governors for their "cooperation" in promoting the Defense Department's efforts to recruit more "women in the forces of the Navy, the Army, and the Air Force." (Ibid.) See pp. 639–47.

Marshall then addressed "the recently enacted" universal military training law, which had required "a long and difficult siege" to earn congressional approval.

(See pp. 551–53 and 558–59.) The National Security Training Commission had "reached a conclusion regarding the regulations the law requires them to propose; the general terms of policy have been drawn up and are quite acceptable to the Defense Department. The issue is now before Congress for final action." Marshall reiterated his belief that a program of UMT that would "build up the quality of our reserve forces" was critical "to conserve manpower" and "to avoid an economic crisis" during the "long period of strain until we can credit good faith on the part of the Communists." The National Security Training Commission's proposals, particularly the notion of training "young men" for this reserve program, had received widespread support from education leaders and organized labor, which was "a very unusual state of affairs." Once UMT was established, "The factor of safety for this country and the factor of safety in maintaining the peace in the world will be greatly increased." Marshall added that his former colleagues in the Defense Department were "all deeply concerned to see that this arrangement becomes effective at an early date, so that it can be put into being as soon as possible." Marshall remained adamant in his support of UMT in spite of the opinions of some officers in the Defense Department who opposed it. "I am certain that they are wrong, seriously wrong, and I think I know full well what I am talking about." Although the Defense Department had not been considering UMT when Marshall took office in September 1950, his "own decision then was that I wouldn't have anything to do with any procedure that was not based on the proposition of universal military training; that we get that issue settled. We have gotten the basic law; the next problem of its detailed confirmation ought to be very simple." (Ibid.) See pp. 679–80.

Marshall returned to a discussion of the Defense Department budget and materiel procurement regarding the $60 billion appropriation bill pending approval by Congress. While there was "no great argument about the amounts," there were several potentially crippling amendments that would derail many of the Defense Department's efforts. One such amendment was a restriction on the length of the tour of duty of inactive reservists who had served in World War II. While this limit was manageable for most enlisted men, it was "virtually impossible" for officers, particularly in the navy and air force. "A very important result would be a check on our rotation in respect to officers who are counting on us to keep our word that we are not going to have any man serve a second winter in Korea." Marshall admitted that "Congress is under unusually heavy pressure—and I imagine you gentlemen have also been—because the family, the mother or the wife, are naturally desperately anxious to have their man released." Marshall concluded with praise for Lovett as his successor as secretary of defense, particularly relating to the pending appropriations bill. The first proposed budget came to Lovett with a total of "$104 billion. When he got through with it, it was down to $60 billion." Marshall thought "the job done by Bob Lovett has been superb. I know of no one who has conserved the interests of the government and at the same time promoted the interests of national defense more than he has in connection with these appropriations bills." (Ibid.) The final appropriation approved by Congress and signed by Truman on October 18, 1951, was $55.5 billion. (Condit, *Test of War*, 258.)

After completing his prepared remarks, Marshall welcomed "any questions." For a transcript of the question-and-answer session as well as a slightly edited version of Marshall's opening remarks, see *Proceedings of the Governors' Conference, 1951* (Chicago: Governors' Conference, 1952), 12–19 and 28–44.

Following his appearance before the Governors' Conference, the Marshalls flew from Gatlinburg back to Knoxville accompanied by their friends Claude "Flap" and Ruth Adams. They arrived at 4:00 p.m., fished that afternoon, and spent the night at the Adams's home in Humboldt, Tennessee, before returning to Leesburg on October 2. ★

373

TO WILLIAM BENTON

October 4, 1951
[Leesburg, Virginia]

Dear Benton: Thanks for your letter of September 29th and a copy of the testimony which you recently made before the congressional committee.[1] I appreciate your support and thought of me.

As to your request for suggestions or comments, the next time I talk with you I will give you my views on the matter.

Mrs. Marshall and I are enjoying ourselves very much and looking forward to much leisure and the opportunity of enjoying the pleasures that our present circumstances offer.

With warm regards, Faithfully yours,

GCMRL/G. C. Marshall Papers (Secretary of Defense, Number Indexed, M200-15-10)

1. Senator Benton had appeared before the Senate Subcommittee on Privileges and Elections on September 28, 1951, for more than two hours to present, under oath, ten "case studies" to substantiate his resolution to expel Senator Joseph McCarthy. The next day he sent Marshall a copy of his testimony and called his attention to "case number 3," which dealt with McCarthy's "vicious and scurrilous attack" on Marshall in June 1951. (Benton to Marshall, September 29, 1951, GCMRL/G. C. Marshall Papers [Secretary of Defense, Number Indexed, M200-15-10].) See pp. 557 and 721.

374

TO MRS. JOHN B. WILSON

[October 5, 1951]
Leesburg, Virginia
Friday noon

Dear Rose: I have just received and read your note of the 2^{d}. Thanks for your comments on my retirement, But, most of all congratulations on your new prospects.[1] That's grand, wonderful. You are an ideal mother I'm absolutely sure, and the larger the family the better you'l be. I hope its a girl this time, one with two older brothers would make a perfect set up. I am just in from Tenn. and off in an hour for N. Y. C. Some day soon I can settle down. But the Carnegie Corporation wants me to go New Zealand, Australia and So. Africa[2] Love,

GCM

GCMRL/J. Page Wilson Collection; H

1. Rose Wilson had written to tell her godfather that she was "simply delighted" with the news of his resignation and revealed that "to my amazement, I discovered that by February, we will have another baby. After the initial shock, John and I are pleased in spite of our advanced years!" (Wilson to Marshall, October 13 [*2*], 1951, GCMRL/G. C. Marshall Collection [Rose Page Wilson].) See p. 695n3.

2. See p. 669n4.

375

OUTLINE OF TALK AT FREEDOM HOUSE DINNER[1] October 7, 1951
New York, New York

Historians offer much evidence that there is a man for every important occasion, perhaps because the very severity of the situation automatically eliminates mediocrity and concentrates attention on the commanding figures in the field concerned. So, when the postwar economy of Europe was drifting into a swampy breeding ground for communism, there appeared the man to meet that world dilemma. Whatever may have been the forces we have to thank for the selection of Paul Hoffman, they were in rare conjunction when they lifted him into the direction of our economic assistance to Western Europe.

I do not want to embarrass Mr. Hoffman with praise, but when I say he was the man for that occasion it is merely the statement of a simple fact. He won a decision of such magnitude that it belongs to the whole of history—a decision which could not have been won by any plan, no matter how well conceived, nor by American dollars, no matter how high they might have been heaped, without leadership and administration of the highest order in an enterprise which was a unique combination of big business, big government, and critical international relations.

In the Europe he sought to help, he faced an economic jungle, a lush growth of trade barriers, cartels, inefficient production, conflicting ideologies, and national jealousies, the world overshadowed by dark fears, poverty, and tragic surroundings.

At home, Mr. Hoffman was beset by the doubtings of legislators on the one hand, and by considerable portion of the American public by those who regarded the Economic Cooperation Administration as a mere relief program to subsidize American surpluses.

Convincing integrity, superlative salesmanship, and truly international economic statesmanship were the personal resources he drew on to meet these issues. Under the magic of his direction new factories, shipyards, power plants, homes, and flourishing farmlands had pushed up through the rubble of war. He had convinced doubters that money spent strengthening the economy of Europe was to yield great returns in the fight for security and freedom.

All of this has been better said or written many times. We have heard much of the story here tonight. But what I most wish to emphasize is a quality all too rare in American official life that makes him, in my opinion, not only as a great economic leader and a great administrator but as one who was utterly selfless and purely objective in his every action. No matter how sound a plan and legislative authorization, its principal difficulties usually flow from the character of the principal individual in his dealing with the situation, in his relations with other governmental agencies, with the Congress and especially with reference to the credits or criticisms he receives from the public and the press.

My friend, you rose above these human frailties. You had the courage of honesty in your devotion to the great purpose of your mission. As Secretary of State I found a rare satisfaction in my official dealings with you.

You gave one of the finest examples of an efficient and selfless public official. May this Country be blessed with more and more men of your character.

It is these reasons, much more than my friendship for you, that commanded me to accept the invitation of Freedom House to present this award—with the citation for "imagination, leadership, and unselfish public service for world peace and freedom".[2]

GCMRL/G. C. Marshall Papers (Retirement, Speeches, Statements, and Writings)

1. A diverse bipartisan group of prominent Americans had established Freedom House in New York City in 1941 to encourage the spread of democracy around the world. Marshall had received the organization's annual Freedom House Award in 1947. (See *Papers of GCM*, 6: 232–33.) Paul Hoffman, former ECA director and current president of the Ford Foundation in Pasadena, California, was selected to receive the 1951 award following a dinner in the Waldorf-Astoria Hotel, which would be broadcast by NBC. In a July 30, 1951, letter to Marshall reconfirming his participation in the ceremony for Hoffman, Pulitzer Prize–winning journalist Herbert Bayard Swope, who was to preside over the event, had stressed the need to use this opportunity "to show that a general can be of great importance to the so-called civilian activities of our government. It would be singularly fitting for the executive of the Marshall Plan to be honored by the creator of that plan." (Swope to Marshall, July 30, 1951, and Field to Marshall, September 19, 1951, GCMRL/G. C. Marshall Papers [Secretary of Defense, Number Indexed, M214-11-11].)

Hoffman had written to Marshall that "coming from you the award will have much added value." He also felt "deeply indebted" to Marshall "for having taken on the great responsibilities for the Department of Defense when you did. It was the climactic act of our 'greatest living American.'" (Hoffman to Marshall, September 27, 1951, ibid.) Marshall replied on October 3 that it would be "a great pleasure for me to have the opportunity of presenting you with the Freedom House award. You certainly deserve it for your great contribution to the free peoples of the world." (Marshall to Hoffman, October 3, 1951, HSTL/Paul G. Hoffman Papers [Eminent Personages, Marshall].)

2. "The fact that you really believe what you said about me last evening touched me very deeply and almost made me speechless," Hoffman wrote to Marshall on October 8. He told Marshall he would show a transcript of Marshall's remarks to his grandchildren "on every possible occasion in an effort to impress them." Hoffman also expressed regrets that he had not seen Katherine Marshall during the event and extended an invitation to visit in California. "It is easy to convince people of one's sincerity when it is so genuinely believed to be true," Marshall responded on October 11. "Mrs. Marshall appreciated your message

and was very sorry that she missed talking to you. We shall keep very much in mind your open invitation to us to visit Mrs. Hoffman and you this winter. At the moment our plans vaguely include a couple of months abroad, but we will let you know if the opportunity presents itself for a visit with you." (Hoffman to Marshall, October 8, 1951; Marshall to Hoffman, October 11, 1951, GCMRL/G. C. Marshall Papers [Retirement, General].) See p. 721n4.

376

To Adolf A. Berle Jr.[1]

October 10, 1951
[Leesburg, Virginia]

Dear Berle: I have your letter of October 2nd in which you suggest, at the request of the Board of Directors of the International Refugee Committee, that I take on the Chairmanship of this year's Iron Curtain Refugee campaign. I appreciate your outlining the scope of the program, and telling me of the support to be expected.

I am sorry that I do not feel free to accept. I have already refused a number of more or less similar invitations, giving as my reason the fact that I must get some relaxation from the responsibilities necessarily involved.[2] The acceptance of your invitation would compromise me directly and I am accurate in stating that I must free myself for a considerable time from responsibilities of this nature.

Please make my compliments to Mrs. Berle.[3] Faithfully yours,

GCMRL/G. C. Marshall Papers (Secretary of Defense, Selected)

1. Berle, a prominent author and scholar of corporate law, had served on the Columbia Law School faculty since 1927. He had been a member of Franklin D. Roosevelt's "brain trust" and was influential in shaping New Deal legislation to reform banking, the stock market, the bankruptcy system, and railroads. From 1938 to 1944 Berle had served as assistant secretary of state for Latin American affairs.

2. The next day Marshall sent a similar letter to Eleanor Roosevelt on the same subject. (Marshall to Eleanor Roosevelt, October 11, 1951, GCMRL/G. C. Marshall Papers [Retirement, General].)

3. Berle had married Beatrice Bishop in 1927.

377

To Mrs. Lago

October 15, 1951
[Leesburg, Virginia]

My dear Mrs. Lago: Since my retirement as Secretary of Defense I have received letters from several of the girls in your class in which they told me that they were writing at your suggestion. I appreciate very much your thinking of me in this way and was impressed with the serious and thoughtful letters which your students wrote.

One of the girls asked for advice to the class on how to become better citizens.[1] Below is a quote from a speech which I made some time ago, and I wish you would tell your class that it is my advice to them for successful living.

"A philosopher, I am told, was asked what he thought boys should be taught. He replied simply, 'Those things which they will use when men' (this, of course, applies to girls as well). Certainly the fundamental duties or obligations of successful living are involved in this alleged reply. The progress and welfare of our great nation depend almost entirely on our youth of today. A sound body and strong character are essential in the development of an entire generation which will soon assume its responsibilities to community and country. Now is the time to prepare for the roles you will play in the days to come."[2]

Please express to your class my sincere appreciation for the nice things they said about me, and my thanks to you also for your thought of me. I have taken the liberty of sending, under separate cover, an autographed picture for your classroom. Faithfully yours,

GCMRL/G. C. Marshall Papers (Secretary of Defense, Chronological, Secretaries, Carlson)

1. "We have been reading about you and your retirement and our teacher has been telling us about your great work," wrote Linda J. Betts, one of the eight girls in Mrs. Lago's seventh grade class at the Cleveland School in Skokie, Illinois, who had written to Marshall. "I think you could tell us because you are such a good citizen." (Cleveland School, September 24, 1951, GCMRL/G. C. Marshall Papers [Retirement, General].)

2. See pp. 393 and 397n2.

378

Remarks at the Red Cross Building Dedication Ceremony[1]

October 24, 1951
Washington, DC

There is little I can add to what has just been said, or probably will be said by the President, with reference to the importance of the Red Cross here at home in Washington and also nationally and internationally.[2] That importance is greatly emphasized by the critical character of the times in which we live.

The immediate problem of the blood banks is especially serious and must be met without delay. While I was with the Red Cross Headquarters this particular problem consumed the major portion of my time, and when I moved over to the Defense Department I there found myself faced with the urgency of securing supplies of whole blood for the army in Korea, and reserves of plasma for the entire military force and the civil defense set-up.

It is regrettable that the public contributions lag so seriously—apparently until the emergency is on us ~~and~~ but then for many of the victims the offerings of the individual citizen will be too late. Wounded fighting men or injured civilians will find it difficult to explain the failure of their fellow citizens to make this personal offering—actually from the heart—to save life. But I am certain that there is no citizen who would not do his full part if he could be brought to realize the tragedy of his failure to do so.

Shortly before my resignation as Secretary of Defense I made an appeal on the radio and by television for blood donors to meet the tremendous deficiency that was then facing us. I was gratified to receive from the leading labor organizations and the heads of great industries an immediate response promising complete cooperation toward obtaining three ~~personal contributions each by~~ offerings of blood before June 30th from individuals in their ranks. If a similar coordinated effort were made by every organization—business, patriotic, and religious—we would have the typical American response to those in need.[3]

There are a great many Red Cross activities that are large in the local and national interest. The Greater Washington Chapter has been conspicuous in regard to these and particularly in the hospital service—which is a ~~tremendously~~ heavy burden in this vicinity. This fine building is significant of the importance of the Red Cross organization to the District of Columbia and the surrounding countryside. It is in keeping with the vital importance of the work to be done. Further, it also releases the old headquarters to the over-crowded national headquarters, which will be a material contribution towards the efficiency of the whole.

I hope that the ceremonies today will focus interest on the activities and necessities of the whole Red Cross effort.

GCMRL/G. C. Marshall Papers (Secretary of Defense, Chronological, Secretaries, Carlson)

1. "We felt the exercises would not be complete unless you and Mrs. Marshall were present," John Clifford Folger had written to Marshall on October 12. Marshall responded that they were "looking forward" to the event. "I will always continue to have a great interest" in the work of the Red Cross, "on an inactive basis." (Folger to Marshall, October 12, 1951, and Marshall to Folger, October 17, 1951, GCMRL/G. C. Marshall Papers [Retirement, General].)

2. E. Roland Harriman spoke before Marshall at the dedication of the new headquarters for the District of Columbia chapter, and President Truman followed. "General Marshall has broken many a precedent and I am sure he will break many more before he leaves this world," Truman said. The president departed from his prepared text "to pay a tribute" to Marshall "who has been criticized by Sen. McCarthy," the *Washington Post* reported, declaring: "General Marshall is my ideal of a great public servant." ("D.C. Residents 'Among Finest' in Country, Truman Says at Red Cross Building Rites," *Washington Post*, October 25, 1951, p. B1.)

3. See pp. 612–13.

379

Remarks to United Nations Korean War Veterans[1] — October 24, 1951
Washington, DC

Mr. Chairman and veterans of the fighting in Korea, ladies and gentlemen: Today is the sixth anniversary of the ratification of the United Nations Charter for which you men have actually been fighting and risking your lives to support. We honor you for your courage and sacrifices in the field. We honor the countries you represent so courageously.[2] We join with you and all the free world in this bitter and costly effort to secure the peace of justice we all hope and pray for.

In Article One of the U.N. Charter the peoples of the several nations state their purpose in making this covenant, the maintenance of international peace and security, the development of friendly relations among nations, the achievement of international cooperation, and in promoting respect for the fundamental freedoms. The struggle in Korea is the great test of that charter. Do we actually commit ourselves, our lives and our resources to the struggle for a peaceful world? Korea is proof positive that we do.

Your presence here tonight, the representatives of your comrades in arms who are daily and hourly enduring great hardships and dangers, risking their lives in the greatest demonstration the world has yet seen of a determined effort to bring peace and security to all and especially to our children and our children's children. We long for peace. We pray for peace, but you men fought for peace against an utterly ruthless enemy.

Your visit to this country with your presence here tonight is unique in all that it suggests. The representatives of our countries have been gathered together for some years discussing, appealing and negotiating to create a solid front in this troubled world of ours to guarantee the peace. But you men have stood forth with life itself as the hazard to make good our promises and purposes, to give small nations confidence that they can guard their freedom with the assurance that the larger and more powerful nations will stand beside them in facing the effort of any aggressor to overwhelm them and take over their governments.

Your presence here is therefore of great historic importance. It should hearten the entire free world. Nothing quite like it has ever happened before.

I am sorry that the meaning of my words cannot reach many of you. There is so much I would like to say to you in appreciation of what you and your companions have done for the good of the world, for my people and your people. There is so much that is fine, exalted in your contribution that I would like to refer to. But we must trust to the spirit of the moment to interpret our thoughts, to emphasize our unity. You inspire our confidence. You have our heartfelt thanks. God bless you and protect you.

GCMRL/G. C. Marshall Papers (Secretary of Defense, Selected)

1. While still secretary of defense, Marshall had asked Ridgway on August 31 for his opinion of a suggestion by the State Department that as Far East commander he be asked by the UN to select from his forces two representatives from each country fighting in Korea as well as two from each of the four US services for participation in UN Day ceremonies in Washington and Lake Success, New York, to be followed by a tour of major US cities. On September 7, Marshall submitted to Acheson a formal proposal that the Defense Department was "prepared to plan, finance and execute such a tour," one that would end in San Francisco, the UN's "birthplace." (Marshall to Ridgway, radio no. DEF-80457, August 31, 1951, GCMRL/G. C. Marshall Papers [Secretary of Defense, Chronological, Secretaries, Ackerman]; Marshall to Acheson, September 7, 1951, GCMRL/G. C. Marshall Papers [Secretary of Defense, Number Indexed, M200-19-5].)

Marshall spoke at approximately 8:25 p.m. at a dinner which the veterans attended in the Mayflower Hotel hosted by the Washington Board of Trade. This was the final event for them in a very full day that had included a ceremony and meeting with Truman at the White House and another at the Capitol, during which Acheson addressed them. ("D.C. Extends Hearty, Busy Welcome to U.N. Servicemen," *Washington Post*, October 25, 1951, p. 1.) Clayton Fritchey had suggested that Marshall attend the dinner and speak briefly, which "should have a great effect on the public and should also be instrumental in the blood donor program, defense bond program, and our defense effort as a whole." (George to Marshall, memorandum, October 12, 1951, GCMRL/G. C. Marshall Papers [Secretary of Defense, Categorical, Organizations, United Nations Veterans, 1951].)

2. The *New York Times* reported that the forty-eight veterans represented nineteen nations. "Few of them speak more than a smattering of English." ("Fighting Men of 19 Nations Pay U.S. Visit From Korea," *New York Times*, October 24, 1951, p. B1.)

380

TO ROBERT E. SHERWOOD — October 30, 1951
Leesburg, Virginia

My dear Sherwood: I have read your confidential letter of October 29*th*. I must reply from memory if I am to get this to you before your dead line.[1] I should refresh my memory on the cables involved and the Joint Chief's comments regarding them made to Mr. Roosevelt.[2]

My general impressions are these regarding that period and the Cairo Conference in particular: He was emphatically and persistently intent on a landing on Rhodes the entire time we were engaged in that conference.[3] The problem of troops and their relation to or effect on the Italian Campaign and the Normandy or Overlord build up was one phase of the discussion. The assignment of 26 or 27 LSTs [landing ship, tank] was the other. I am of the same opinion today as I was then regarding inadvisability of involving our~~self~~ selves in the uncertainties of the conquest of Rhodes, with the necessities for Burma to be considered, the continuation of the Italian Campaign without delaying the movement of troops to England for Overlord—the availability of ocean transport for the movement at that certain time being an important factor and the state of the weather for the movement of LSTs to England.

As to Overlord and *especially* Anvil the record is clear.[4]

Decided issue could be taken in these matters. The Cairo Conference for these reasons was one of the two most difficult we had. Whether or not you cite the points you suggested is not questionable as to the facts. It is more a question of advisability of which you are the best judge.[5] Hastily yours,

Harvard, Houghton Library/Robert E. Sherwood Papers; H

1. Sherwood had written to Marshall on October 29 to request "a few words" about events in 1943 and 1944 preceding the Normandy invasion, in preparation for a review, due November 6, of Winston Churchill's *Closing the Ring* (Boston: Houghton Mifflin Company, 1951), the fifth volume in Churchill's *The Second World War*. "This new Churchill book contains far more controversial material than any of its predecessors," Sherwood wrote to Marshall, noting that "in a lot of it" Churchill "is very much on the defensive," particularly when claiming "enthusiasm for OVERLORD" while never denying his efforts "to delay it, if not cancel it altogether." (Sherwood to Marshall, October 29, 1951, GCMRL/G. C. Marshall Papers [Pentagon Office, General].)

2. In his letter, Sherwood had recounted exchanges of cables between Roosevelt and Churchill in which "Mr. Churchill was begging for troops from Eisenhower's command in England [*Italy*] to be diverted to the eastern Mediterranean for the taking of Rhodes and other islands in the Dodecanese," but Roosevelt replied to each appeal "in the negative. The decision was left to Eisenhower and he decided the troops could not be spared." Simul-

taneously, Sherwood had continued, "two British divisions were about to be sent from Italy to the U.K. for OVERLORD." Churchill protested against this move to Roosevelt, declaring that "every man was so desperately needed" in Italy and pouring "forth all of his eloquence against any weakening of Eisenhower's Command." Sherwood thus asked if Marshall thought he "would be right in citing this, in my review as an example of Mr. Churchill's extraordinary ability to reverse himself completely?" (Ibid.)

3. For more on the November 1943 Cairo Conference, see *Papers of GCM*, 4: 191–96.

4. ANVIL was the code name for the invasion of southern France in the summer of 1944.

5. "Thank you very much indeed for your prompt and helpful reply to my letter," Sherwood responded on November 3. "I am sorry that I put you to all this trouble, but I was anxious to be exceptionally careful in my review of the Churchill book." (Sherwood to Marshall, November 3, 1951, GCMRL/G. C. Marshall Papers [Secretary of Defense, Number Indexed, M219-2-19].) Sherwood did include this controversy in his review. (Robert E. Sherwood, "On the Threshold of Allied Triumph," *New York Times*, November 25, 1951, p. 244.)

381

To Stanton Griffis

November 1, 1951
[Washington, DC]

Dear Griffis: It was good to hear from you, although distressing to know that you recently found it necessary to come home for a physical check-up.[1] I do hope that you now have whatever it was completely under control. I suppose a word of caution would fall on deaf ears, but nevertheless I wish you would not overdo yourself in any way. If, as you hope, this is your last post, you should try to leave it in good health so you can enjoy your retirement as much as I hope to enjoy mine after commitments made while still at Defense are fulfilled. Mrs. Marshall and I are very happy with our new circumstances, and hope that it will be a permanent arrangement.

Many thanks for your invitation to visit you in Spain and take a shot at the partridge, but I do not believe such a trip is in the books for us; however, and most confidentially, we have in mind a trip to the Central Pacific area, "down under", and South Africa beginning sometime after the turn of the new year.[2] Thanks also for your generous gift.[3] The previous remembrance was greatly enjoyed by us and those close friends who were on hand when the cork was out.

The matter of pensions has been of concern to me for some time, and recently Mrs. Rosenberg spoke at length before a congressional committee on the inadequacy of the amounts now authorized. I do not know at the moment what the outcome will be, but should I learn something definite I will drop you a line.[4]

Mrs. Marshall joins me in warm regards and sincere thanks for your generous thought of us. Faithfully yours,

GCMRL/G. C. Marshall Papers (Retirement, General)

1. Ambassador Griffis had returned to New York for treatment the previous month after three months of illness in Madrid. (Griffis to Marshall, October 24, 1951, GCMRL/G. C. Marshall Papers [Retirement, General].) He had also served the Truman administration as ambassador to Poland, Egypt, and Argentina.

2. See pp. 668–69.

3. "The purpose of this letter," Griffis had explained on October 24, "is to tell you that there is wonderful partridge shooting in Spain now with the idea that if you like to shoot, you and Mrs. Marshall might pay us a visit," adding that he was sending "from my old New Canaan homestead a little more of that old bourbon that I think you liked. It will help you to relax." (Ibid.)

4. While in Washington, Griffis reported, he "had a few minutes with Bob Lovett protesting against the iniquitous military retirement laws of our country," which had left the widow of his friend Admiral Forrest P. Sherman "with a pension of $75 a month. . . . It is a terrible thing that the wife of a man who has become head of the Navy should have about the same treatment as a second class seaman's widow." (Ibid.) See pp. 595–96.

382

To Gordon Gray[1] November 2, 1951
Personal and Confidential [Washington, DC]

Dear Gray: Reference your letter of October 29th in which you request my opinion as to the suitability of Samuel L. A. Marshall as your successor as Director of the Psychological Strategy Board, I have only seen the man once but I have been familiar with his writing activities for some years. He appeared to be unusually well informed, an especially able reporter of what he had seen—Korea in particular, straightforward, pleasant personality, in touch with many leading figures in the Pentagon. If the facts you can ascertain regarding his background are satisfactory, I think he would be an excellent man.[2]

I'm very sorry you have had such a frustrating time. It was bound to happen somewhat in a job of that character in this country in these particular times.[3]

With warm regards, Faithfully yours,

GCMRL/G. C. Marshall Papers (Retirement, General)

1. "As you perhaps know, my Trustees imposed a terminal point on my current service in Washington as of January 1, 1952," Gray had written to Marshall on October 29. (Gray to Marshall, October 29, 1951, GCMRL/G. C. Marshall Papers [Retirement, General].) Gray was on a leave of absence from the presidency of the University of North Carolina, serving since July 18 as the first director of the Psychological Strategy Board, which reported to the National Security Council.

2. Samuel Lyman Atwood Marshall (better known as S. L. A. Marshall) was a military historian who had served in the Historical Division of the General Staff of the Army from 1943 to 1946. University of Washington President Raymond B. Allen succeeded Gray as director of the Psychological Strategy Board in May 1952.

3. "I have never tackled an assignment which presented greater problems," Gray had confided to Marshall. "I might also say that a stranger to Washington might well find himself pretty well carved up in a hurry." (Ibid.)

383

To Windsor T. White II November 16, 1951
Personal and Confidential [Washington, DC[1]]

Dear Mr. White: I appreciate your returning the papers on Nato. He has been placed in the hands of a dog specialist, who happens to be the brother of my orderly, and has a 500 acre plot to ramble over.[2]

I cannot express my feelings and emotions regarding the tragedy that befell your family.[3] Faithfully yours,

GCMRL/G. C. Marshall Papers (Secretary of Defense, Chronological, Secretaries, Carlson)

1. The Marshalls had moved to their winter home in Pinehurst, North Carolina, on November 12 but this letter was typed on his Pentagon office stationery.

2. See pp. 578–79 and 628–29. Sergeant Heffner's brother John reported to C. J. George the following year that "Nato makes his home at the Monastery Stables in Fairmount Park in Philadelphia." (Heffner to George, April 14, 1952, GCMRL/G. C. Marshall Papers [Retirement, General].)

3. "I am back in town now and would be glad to arrange to drop over to Leesburg to see General and Mrs. Marshall and Nato," Thomas H. White had written to C. J. George on October 18. On October 26, White was piloting his Beechcraft Bonanza private plane from his home in Ohio when it crashed into the Potomac River near National Airport, killing White, his wife, and his daughter. The *New York Times* reported that the Whites were "on the way to keep a luncheon appointment" with Marshall. (White to George, October 18, 1951, GCMRL/G. C. Marshall Papers [Secretary of Defense, Chronological, Secretaries, Carlson]; "Industrialist Flying to See Marshall Killed as Plane Crashes in Potomac," *New York Times*, October 27, 1951, p. 1.)

"I can't tell you how much my brothers and I appreciate you having attended the funeral services for my Mother and Father," Windsor T. White II had written to Marshall. "I am returning the papers of Nato which were furnished my Father, and I hope you will be able to make satisfactory disposition of the dog." (White to Marshall, n.d., GCMRL/G. C. Marshall Papers [Secretary of Defense, Chronological, Secretaries, Carlson].)

384

TO QUEEN FREDERICA OF THE HELLENES — December 1, 1951
Pinehurst, North Carolina

Your Majesty: This very informal note carries Xmas greetings and every good wish for the new year to Your Majesties and the children from Mrs. Marshall and me. We sincerely hope that all of you are in good health and happy and that your ~~country and~~ people are enjoying the fruits of success and a feeling of greater security.

We are both well and enjoying very much the restful period following my resignation as Secretary of Defense. We are here in our winter home, with occasional game shooting trips to Georgia and South Carolina. It is possible that we will spend two months at Cuernavaca in Mexico this winter, but we haven't quite made up our minds.[1]

I have purposely waited ~~until~~ for the change to be effected before writing to express my regret at the failure and embarassment following the detail of General Frederick to Greece. Quite evidently since I had last seen him a serious change ~~it~~ had occurred, very possibly the reaction of a daring, restless fighting man to the boredom of peace time conditions, for which most of us pray.[2] He was selected for the detail~~ed~~ to Greece before I came into office, but I felt that an unusually fine choice had been made and wrote to you accordingly.[3] I'm very sorry over the result.

In Korea last June I talked with the Commander of your Greek troops.[4] He gave a very fine account of his people which was emphatically concurred in by both General Ridgway and Van Fleet.

With our very best wishes, Faithfully yours

GCMRL/G. C. Marshall Papers (Secretary of Defense, Number Indexed, M219-1-27); H

1. See pp. 669n1 and 676–78.

2. Major General Robert T. Frederick (USMA, 1928) had been selected in March to head the Joint US Military Advisory and Planning Group (JUSMAPG) in Greece and slated to arrive there in early May 1951. ("Army Shifts 2 Commands," *New York Times*, March 24, 1951, p. 3; Carter to Marshall, memorandum, March 8, 1951, GCMRL/G. C. Marshall Papers [Pentagon Office, Selected].) On July 21, Frederick had cabled General Collins: "Senate Foreign Relations Committee recently here registered complaint with Ambassador about me. Am unable to learn grounds of complaint." (Frederick to Collins, cable, July 21, 1951, NA/RG 319 [Chief of Staff, Secretary, General Staff, Security Classified General, 1951–1952].) Four days later, Frederick cabled General Hull suggesting that his "military briefing may not have satisfied senators," and recommended that "an inspector general come here as soon as possible so you may have an impartial report on my administration this mission and can determine whether I should continue here." Frederick also acknowledged that "I have been ill since arrival here." (Frederick to Hull, cable, July 25, 1951, ibid.) "I am presently all right," he wrote to Deputy Chief of Staff General Maxwell Taylor on August 7, but "the doctors who treated me last fall and winter said that it would be one and one-half years to two years, at least, before I fully recovered from the illness and that I could expect it to flare up from time to time during that period. It is apparent to me, and it is also the opinion of the medical officers here, that I should not attempt to go through next summer here or in any place with a similar climate." He also reported that "at our meeting this morning the Ambassador told me that he was annoyed by a letter he had received from a friend in Washington who had written that an Army officer in the Pentagon recently returned from Greece had stated to him a malicious allegation against me. The Ambassador told me that he is replying to his friend saying that the allegation is absolutely false and to so inform the officer who made it." (Frederick to Taylor, August 7, 1951, ibid.)

Queen Frederica apparently sent a "card of Holiday greetings and New Year's wishes," in response to Marshall's letter; however, her next letter to him was dated May 7, 1952. She admitted that she "had a very bad conscience" that she had not written more promptly after receiving Marshall's December 1 letter. "General Frederick" she observed, "never fell foul with us. We liked him very much. If he had a few failings they never became apparent to us, and after all, a brave man like him is allowed to have some kind of weakness." (Lilika S. Papanicolaou, *Frederica, Queen of the Hellenes: Mission of a Modern Queen* [Malta: Publishers Enterprises Group, 1994], 418, 421.)

3. Marshall had written to Queen Frederica on March 13 that he felt about General Frederick "very much as I did regarding General Van Fleet." Marshall had praised Frederick's service and bravery during World War II, and he concluded that Frederick was "a very able man and I am certain his advice would be sound and his help invaluable." (Marshall to Frederica, March 13, 1951, GCMRL/G. C. Marshall Papers [Pentagon Office, Selected].) Frederica replied the following month that she and King Paul were "delighted to receive General Frederick whom you so highly recommend. Your confidence in him is enough to give him ours." (Frederica to Marshall, April 15, 1951, GCMRL/G. C. Marshall Papers [Retirement, General]; Papanicolaou, *Frederica*, 409–19.) For more on Frederick, see pp. 675 and 708.

4. See pp. 548–49. The Greek battalion commander was Lieutenant Colonel Dionyssios G. Arbouzis.

385

Address to the Council of World Affairs[1] December 3, 1951
Cleveland, Ohio

By way of introduction I wish to say that Newton Baker has been a great admiration of my life. I did not come in contact with him personally, except momentarily during the St. Mihiel battle, until my return from France in the fall of 1919.[2] Thereafter, until he retired from office as Secretary of War, I saw him frequently and talked with him at some length.

To me Mr. Baker possessed an amazingly clear comprehension of the full meaning of momentous events. I never met Mr. [President Woodrow] Wilson, but I did have opportunities to meet and listen to most of the leading figures of the First World War—Lloyd George, Lord Milner, Clemenceau, Winston Churchill, Foch, and most of the top military leaders of that day.[3] Of all of these, Mr. Baker's judgment and vision made the most profound impression on my mind.

I never knew a man who could present a problem or review a situation in such concise and simple terms as he. I frankly admit to the feeling that his thinking seemed about ten years ahead of mine in regard to nations and peoples and the great sociological factors of humane life. And this was emphasized by his command of English which was second to none in clarity and I have heard the Honorable Winston Churchill at his best.

In a speech in the Fall of 1927 Mr. Baker made several comments, interesting to us today, with relation to the problems of that decade. The First World War, he said, 'finally determined that the democratic rather than the autocratic principle should govern the modern world'. Later he remarked that 'when the guns ceased firing, no doubt many of us thought that the world had learned its lesson and would usher in immediately an era of freedom and justice as sweet and as wholesome as the silence of No-Man's-Land'. And he added that those of us who had early expectations of this change were beginning to be disillusioned.

What a spectacle the world has had since that remark, and, correspondingly, how dire is our need of men of his extraordinary vision, of completely unselfish purpose, men to find a way to lead us into better understanding amongst men and peoples.

What I particularly admired about Mr. Baker was the selflessness with which he pursued his tasks, his genuinely modest demeanor and his simplicity of character. It was a great privilege to hear him outline a situation and proceed with the clear-cut instructions he wishes to have carried out.

Newton Baker came to the War Department at a critical moment. The proposal of his predecessor for a new concept for our national defense system had failed to secure the approval of President Wilson and he immediately resigned. The Mayor of Cleveland stepped into the national picture, little known to the general public.[4] His known views seemed rather at odds with the thinking and working processes of the General Staff. Yet, I do not think there has ever been a man who worked in more complete harmony with the personnel of the War Department, who received more of wholehearted support from its officers and accorded them more complete and able support in all of their endeavours. His view of the so-called military attitude or brain is best expressed in a line taken from his defense of West Point against the criticism of that institution leveled at its graduates by Doctor Eliot of Harvard.[5] In summarizing the qualities developed and fostered in its men by the Military Academy, Mr. Baker said that it turned them out 'with that cultured restraint which is essential to intercourse among gentlemen'. Of course there have been exceptions in the matter of cultured restraint, but usually in the case of extraordinarily able battle leaders conspicuous in each of our wars.

Throughout his war service he took many very courageous decisions and he firmly supported his officers through every difficulty in which they became involved. Never did he seek to excuse himself from the dilemma. Always he accepted full responsibility for the failure or the embarrassing explosion or expose. Mr. Baker was in every characteristic a strong man, a brilliant man, a modest man and a great gentleman.

Later on when a slurring reference was made to his services in a write-up in the Encyclopedia Britannica, General Pershing was in Europe, so I drew up a proposed reply for him stating in strong terms his unequivocal admiration for Mr. Baker's leadership and support throughout the war. Upon his return to this country General Pershing accepted my draft without alteration, I believe, because I was familiar with his view of the man, with the added emphasis that he had worked intimately with him throughout the war years and immediately thereafter.

It is a matter of wonder to me what Mr. Baker would think, would recommend as our course in these troubled times. You may be sure it would be logical, but I am even more certain that it would include a vision into the future far more penetrating than that of ordinary men. He understood democracy, he knew his history, he understood men and his brain functioned smoothly through brilliant channels. Above all he had the courage of his convictions and could not be swayed by passing public emotional reactions. I think his conclusions would be somewhat along the line of the final paragraph of a statement regarding Foreign Affairs made by him in 1933 on the subject of 'The New Spirit and its Critics'.

'The world is cursed by its common fears. It is made better by its great faiths. The new spirit is the evidence of such a fighting faith. The agencies it has so far devised have in them the seeds of growth. Lawyers with their doubts and statesmen with their policies may encumber this spirit and delay its achievements. Its progress by trial and error may be slow and its course may sometimes seem to be inviting new perils. Some of the steps it eagerly takes may have to be retraced and fresh starts made, but if this is ever to be a world in which nations, like civilized men, are governed by moral restraints, and from which licensed war for the private objectives of ambitious states will disappear, it must be fought for in this spirit. Those who share this faith and work in this hope have no apology to make to their own or future generations.'[6]

GCMRL/G. C. Marshall Papers (Secretary of Defense, Number Indexed, M200-3-28)

1. On August 10, Shepherd L. Witman, executive director of the Council on World

Affairs, had invited Marshall to deliver the Newton D. Baker Memorial Lecture on the anniversary of Baker's birth, noting that "the advice of such a distinguished successor" would be an "appropriate and valuable tribute" to the former secretary of war. Marshall had replied that his schedule was "quite unpredictable" but that he "would like to make a tentative acceptance." Witman had renewed the invitation on September 18, adding his "appreciation as an individual citizen for the services which you have so ably rendered to our country." (Witman to Marshall, August 10, 1951; Marshall to Witman, August 20, 1951; Witman to Marshall, September 18, 1951, GCMRL/G. C. Marshall Papers [Secretary of Defense, Number Indexed, M200-3-28].)

Marshall delivered his speech at 1:00 p.m. following a luncheon meeting held at the Hotel Carter. Marshall's address was open to the public. (Memorandum for General Marshall, November 23, 1951, ibid.) "I admired him beyond any other man that I have ever known," Marshall pronounced later, calling Baker's "the greatest mind that I came into contact with in my lifetime." (*George C. Marshall Interviews and Reminiscences for Forrest C. Pogue*, 3rd ed. [Lexington, VA: George C. Marshall Research Foundation, 1996], 269.) See also *Papers of GCM*, 1: 364, 385.

2. See George C. Marshall, *Memoirs of My Services in the World War 1917–1918* (Boston: Houghton Mifflin Company, 1976), 137–47, for more on the battle of St. Mihiel; for Marshall's encounters there with Baker, see 145 and 148.

3. David Lloyd George was Great Britain's prime minister from December 7, 1916, to October 22, 1922; Viscount Alfred Milner served under him as secretary of state for war from April 18, 1918, to January 10, 1919. Georges Clemenceau served as prime minister of France from November 16, 1917, to January 20, 1920. Marshal Ferdinand Foch, who had commanded French troops throughout the war, had been named supreme commander of the Allied Armies in early 1918. Winston Churchill, who later became British prime minister, had served in numerous capacities during World War I, including minister of munitions and first lord of the Admiralty. For more on Marshall's World War I associations, see Marshall, *Memoirs*.

4. Secretary of War Lindley M. Garrison had resigned in 1916 over President Wilson's unwillingness to continue to support his plan to create a large federal reserve force, the so-called Continental Army, instead of relying on the state-controlled National Guard. He was succeeded by Newton D. Baker, who had been mayor of Cleveland, Ohio, from 1911 to 1915.

5. See p. 545.

6. Newton D. Baker, "The 'New Spirit' and Its Critics," *Foreign Affairs* 12 (October 1933): 1–19.

386

TO HARRISON WALKER BUSBY

December 4, 1951
Pinehurst, North Carolina

Dear Busby: Thanks for your letter of November 21st. I was very interested in your comments regarding education as related to the Armed Forces.[1] I recall the good work that you did, and apparently are continuing to do, to help the young men in the C.C.C. [Civilian Conservation Corps] when I ran that organization in Oregon and Washington so many years ago, and know that your counsel and guidance has helped many boys in overcoming their educational handicaps as well as their social and moral misconceptions.[2]

Mrs. Marshall and I are enjoying this old-but-new business of retirement, but this time we hope it is a permanent arrangement. We like our place at Leesburg and have only just closed the house there for the winter and moved to a warm-er climate where we will escape the damp cold of Washington. We find it very pleasant during the winter here in North Carolina and are happy that our present circumstances permit us to move about freely as we wish. It is very good to anticipate the restful days ahead.

I know Mrs. Busby and you will be glad when you can retire to your home in Lake Grove.[3] As a matter of fact, I know of no section of the country that can beat the Pacific Northwest for beauty and inspiration, not to mention the fishing!

Thanks for writing me as you did. Mrs. Marshall and I send you both our very best regards and hope that you have a happy holiday season. Faithfully yours,

GCMRL/G. C. Marshall Papers (Secretary of Defense, Number Indexed, M200-19-24)

1. Busby, an education counselor at the Colorado State Reformatory in Buena Vista, Colorado, had written to Marshall on November 21 to congratulate him on his retirement. (See pp. 629–32.) "I was startled this morning when I heard, over the radio, that the armed forces were to cut down on education. We have so many illiterates here that it is astounding to hear that education is to be curtailed. To me this means another step toward a nation of morons." (Busby to Marshall, November 21, 1951, GCMRL/G. C. Marshall Papers [Secretary of Defense, Number Indexed, M200-19-24].)

2. Marshall had been commanding officer of the Fifth Brigade of the Third Division, Vancouver Barracks, from October 1936 to June 1938. See Forrest C. Pogue, *George C. Marshall*, vol. 1, *Education of a General, 1880–1939* (New York: Viking, 1963), 307–11. "Only today I received a letter from one of our C.C.C. boys who has not forgotten what we tried to do for him," Busby wrote. He is now with Bethlehem Steel and is working on Government contracts. He claims that I helped him, which, of course makes me feel proud." (Ibid.)

3. Busby had mentioned that he and his wife had purchased "a little place" in Lake Grove, a suburb or Portland, Oregon. (Ibid.)

387

To Mrs. John B. Wilson — December 5, 1951
Pinehurst, North Carolina

Dear Rose: This carries our Xmas greetings to your family along with all my best wishes for you in the New Year.

We came down here November 12th, but aside from getting settled have been away a good bit. First for a week Thanksgiving time for a shooting spree on Pickney [*Pinckney*] Island off Savannah.[1] Got my limit of turkey, daily limit in pheasants—4, but not so good on quail. Since then I have been out to Cleveland, Ohio and we are off Xmas week for quail shooting with Baruch in So. Carolina.[2] We may spend 2 months at Cuernavaca near Mexico City.[3] The Carnegie Corporation wants us to do a good will tour through New Z, Australia, and So. Africa, but we think not.[4] I have just been invited to be the guest of the government in New Z including all the celebrated fishing I can manage.[5]

I am beginning to relax, though I have had so many hold over engagements involving travel that, in addition to getting the fall outside work done on our place at Leesburg I have been far to busy.[6] But I feel fine and they tell me I look all right?

My love to you Rosie, Affectionately,

G.C.M.

GCMRL/J. Page Wilson Collection; H

1. The Marshalls had spent the holiday on Pinckney Island, which Marshall misspelled in this and several subsequent letters, with James Bruce, who had been US ambassador to Argentina during much of Marshall's tenure as secretary of state, and his wife, Ellen Bruce. Bruce had invited the Marshalls in September 1951 to the opening of the South Carolina shooting season and offered to have them picked up at Pinehurst on the morning of November 22. He had also invited Bernard Baruch to join them. Marshall accepted the invitation and offer for transportation on September 29. (Bruce to Marshall, September 12, 1951, and Marshall to Bruce, September 20, 1951, GCMRL/G. C. Marshall Papers [Secretary of Defense, Number Indexed, M200-19-24]; Bruce to Marshall, September 17 and 25, 1951, and Marshall to Bruce, September 21 and 29, 1951, ibid., [M214-17-35].)

Marshall had boasted to David Rockefeller on November 30 that he and Mrs. Marshall "had a grand holiday over Thanksgiving, on a shoot in South Carolina with the James Bruces. I came home with several quail, a couple of turkey, and even some pheasant—a shoot I would call a thumping success!" He reported more modestly to Marion C. "John" Tarapata on November 28 that he "met with mild success on this jaunt and brought home enough birds for a good meal." (Marshall to Rockefeller, November 30, 1951, and Marshall to Tarapata, November 28, 1951, GCMRL/G. C. Marshall Papers [Retirement, General].)

2. See p. 43n2.

3. See pp. 676–78.

4. Marshall had been a trustee of the Carnegie Corporation, a philanthropic trust fund established by steel magnate Andrew Carnegie, from 1946 until he resigned in person at the board's November 14, 1950, meeting. Following Marshall's resignation as secretary of defense (see pp. 629–32), the Carnegie Corporation repeated an earlier invitation for the Marshalls to visit Australia, New Zealand, and South Africa at the corporation's expense. Marshall never made a "definite reply" to the corporation, and the Marshalls never went forward with plans for this trip. (Dollard to Marshall, September 28, 1951, and George to Marshall, memorandum, December 10, 1951, GCMRL/G. C. Marshall Papers [Retirement, General].)

5. US Ambassador to New Zealand Robert M. Scotten, on behalf of Prime Minister Sidney Holland, had also invited the Marshalls to visit New Zealand. Holland had visited Washington the previous February and thought Marshall would like to "try out the wonderful fishing in the New Zealand streams." Marshall had sent his regrets to Holland on December 4. (Scotten to Webb, October 29, 1951; Marshall to Holland, December 4, 1951, GCMRL/G. C. Marshall Papers [Secretary of Defense, Secretary of Defense, Selected].) See pp. 374–76.

6. In a letter written to Major George the same day, Katherine Marshall had listed numerous recent expenses including having the Leesburg house painted and grounds seeded. "My bank account is so low I do not see how I will get through the expense of Christmas," she fretted. (Katherine Marshall to George, December 5, 1951, GCMRL/Katherine T. Marshall Collection, File 2.)

MARSHALL composed variations on his handwritten Christmas greetings to Rose Page Wilson and sent them to many friends during December. He told President Truman on December 12 that he and Mrs. Marshall had "been trying to relax and loaf while settling things in the house and grounds and getting ready for Xmas." (Marshall to Truman, December 12, 1951, GCMRL/G. C. Marshall Collection [Truman]; H.) "It seems strange to me to be free of responsibilities, free to sleep late, read late and do much as I please—tho my mail continues very heavy—now about fifty letters a day with many pressing invitations to do this or that," he disclosed to Matthew Ridgway on December 14. He explained that "until a couple of weeks ago it was running about 150 letters a day, and for some weeks after my resignation it ran up to 500 and even a thousand a day." (Marshall to Ridgway, December 14, 1951, USAMHI/Matthew B. Ridgway Collection [Series 2: Correspondence, Subseries 1: Official Correspondence, CINCFE, L–M]; H.) He admitted to his childhood friend Catharine Lindsey Armstrong on December 18 that "it is particularly pleasant to get up about 9-30 a.m. instead of leaving Leesburg for Washington at 6[15] a.m." (Marshall to Armstrong, December 18, 1951, GCMRL/G. C. Marshall Collection [Armstrong]; H.) ★

388

Memorandum of Conversation with Winston Churchill[1] January 17, 1952
Top Secret Washington, DC

There were present at lunch Mr. Churchill's daughter, Sarah with her husband, his son-in-law (Mary's husband), a lady member of Parliament, Lord Cherwell, Lord Makins (?) and Miss Margaret Truman.[2]

Mr. Churchill and I sat apart from the others before and after lunch.

He was first interested, in his remarks, as to what impression he had made on the Congress and the public. My replies were tactful and of no interest.[3] He spent some time expressing a desire for me to return to public office. He spoke in most sincere and complimentary terms of Mr. Lovett.[4] That was about all of any degree of importance before lunch.

After lunch he brought up the question of the Atlantic Naval Command and put forward his view of the feasibility of having two commands with a central group such as the Standing Committee to iron out differences, most of which he thought would never occur. I did not express any opinion.

He referred to the rifle question and said he thought a satisfactory agreement had been reached. I made no comment.

He then, in utmost confidence as he termed it, spoke of Eisenhower's strong indorsement of Gruenther as his successor.[5] He asked me my opinion of Gruenther as an officer: I described his past service during the War and when I referred to my belief that he was an immensely able officer— brainy, Mr. Churchill responded, "Yes he thought so too". He referred to the fact that Gruenther had had no battle command experience but remarked that of course Montgomery could be there to supply that necessity. He referred to Ridgway in most complimentary terms but assumed that he could not be released from his present post.

In commenting on Eisenhower's recent political statement he remarked that overseas the opinion undoubtedly was that Eisenhower as President would be even more influential in strengthening Western Europe than in his present position.[6]

As a matter of fact the Prime Minister was far more interested in the possible reactions to his speech than to other matters that I had expected him to bring up.[7]

GCMRL/G. C. Marshall Papers (Retirement, General)

1. Winston Churchill had become prime minister of Great Britain again on October 26, 1951. "I hope Churchill's visit does not suck me into Washington, tho there are rumors that I will be sent for," Marshall had confided to Frank McCarthy on December 20. (Marshall to McCarthy, December 20, 1951, GCMRL/Frank McCarthy Papers [Additions, Box 1]; H.) On January 2, Marshall was informed by Ambassador Franks that Churchill did indeed wish to see and speak with him during his forthcoming visit to the United States. Franks proposed that Marshall join him, Lady Franks, and Churchill for lunch at the British Embassy after the prime minister's January 17 address to a joint session of Congress. Marshall accepted the invitation on January 8. (Franks to Marshall, January 2, 1952; Marshall to Franks, January 8, 1952, GCMRL/G. C. Marshall Papers [Retirement, General].) Two days later he informed Ismay that he hoped to see him as well but that he intended to fly up to Washington from Pinehurst for the lunch on January 17 and then fly back "immediately. If I hang around here I will be before Congress in about 20 minutes on some of these hearings on the military, foreign aid, and similar legislation." Ismay responded on January 14 that he was leaving Washington the next day but added, in a handwritten postscript, "I am so glad that you are seeing Mr. Churchill. He will be delighted." (Marshall to Ismay, January 10, 1952; Ismay to Marshall, January 14, 1952, ibid.)

2. Sarah Churchill was married to photographer Anthony Beauchamp. Mary Spencer-Churchill was married to Conservative politician Christopher Soames. Lady Priscilla Buchan Tweedsmuir was the Conservative member of Parliament and held a seat on the Council of Europe from 1950 to 1953. Physicist Frederick Lindemann, Lord Cherwell, who had been Churchill's leading scientific adviser during World War II, was the paymaster-general of Great Britain from 1951 to 1953. Sir Roger Makins was British undersecretary of state from 1948 to 1952.

3. Churchill's personal physician, Charles Wilson, Lord Moran, who also attended the luncheon, noted in his diary that Churchill was "deeply touched" that Marshall was waiting for him at the embassy after the speech and Churchill "hurried to take both his hands," as Marshall declared, "'It was a great success, Prime Minister.'" Marshall, Moran continued, "knew that every speaker, when he is back in his seat, has the same craving; he wants to know, in Mr. Churchill's words, if he has hit the target. They could now talk of other things." (Charles Wilson Moran, *Churchill Taken from the Diaries of Lord Moran: The Struggle for Survival 1940–1965* [Boston: Houghton Mifflin Company, 1966], 392.)

4. Churchill had met Lovett at a meeting with the Joint Chiefs of Staff on January 6. The two met again the following day at the White House in meetings attended by the entire British delegation, President Truman, Acheson, and Snyder, among others. (HSTL/Appointment Diary for January 7, 1952.)

5. See pp. 592, 787n1, and *Papers of GCM*, 5: 303n2.

6. Eisenhower had issued a statement on January 7 implying that while he "would not seek nomination to political office," he would "respond to a clear-cut call to political duty," suggesting that he would accept if he was selected as the 1952 Republican nominee for president. ("Text of Eisenhower Statement," *New York Times*, January 8, 1952, p. 15; *Papers of DDE*, 13: 856n2 [Document 583].)

7. "I would like to have seen you on this brief visit of mine but I thought it best to keep out of Washington so far as I could," Marshall wrote to Acheson while in Washington on January 17. "I declined your dinner for tonight in order to keep out of the picture as much as possible and I am sorry that they tagged me for this luncheon, as I felt I could not decline because of past intimate relations." Acheson replied, "I fully comprehend your desire to remain in the background," and added that he was "glad, though, that you were able to talk with Mr. Churchill over an informal lunch." (Marshall to Acheson, January 17, 1952; Acheson to Marshall, January 23, 1952, GCMRL/G. C. Marshall Papers [Retirement, General].)

389

To Samuel "Corty" Slaymaker IV — January 20, 1952
Pinehurst, North Carolina

Dear Corty: I was not quite certain whether you were well enough known at Princeton for a letter to reach you addressed to the Honorable Corty FPE, meaning Fisherman par Excellence.[1] So I am sending this up to Washington to have Mrs. McCoy send it on properly addressed.[2] Your Xmas card was our prize display. I think we received nearly a thousand but your's took the cake. A small friend of ours rooting through the pile found your's and immediately insisted on going home to try and make one himself and then go fishing on a nearbye lake.[3]

Your letter with the pictures, the hooks and the tarpon came this morning, with your love and is very much appreciated.[4] It pleases me very much to learn in this way that you haven't forgotten me.

We are going fishing Monday for bass and brimm [*bream*] on a nearbye lake. Down in So. Carolina Xmas time on a tidal stream in from the ocean, three of us caught 34 1 1/2 to 2 1/2 pound "spots" in a half hour.

We are going to Cuernavaca, Mexico January 31st to spend the month of February.[5] We will fly down. I flew 350 miles up to Washington Thursday morning and flew back here the same evening.[6] I am looking for a good picture to send you of me, or a fish or something more exciting.[7] With my love,

GCMarshall

GCMRL/G. C. Marshall Collection (Slaymaker); H

1. Marshall had met "Corty" Slaymaker while vacationing on Cape Cod. (See pp. 603–4.) "Corty and General Marshall became great friends," recalled John Gunn, who had been a guest at a nearby home at the same time. "They fished together a number of times, and on one deep sea expedition, Corty was the only member of the party to catch anything, he being about 7 years old at the time." (Gunn to Royster Lyle, May 5, 1965, GCMRL/G. C. Marshall Collection [Slaymaker].)

2. Marshall sent this letter in care of Frances McCoy.

3. "I was surprised and delighted to get your Xmas card," Marshall had written on December 14, after receiving Slaymaker's first note. "Dear General, Why not come every year?" Slaymaker had responded. (Marshall to Slaymaker, December 14, 1951, and Slaymaker to Marshall, n.d., GCMRL/G. C. Marshall Papers [Retirement, General].)

In a postscript on Marshall's initial longhand letter to Slaymaker, Marshall had inquired, "Any recent contracts for hauling seaweed?" (Marshall to Slaymaker, December 14, 1951, ibid.) Gunn recalled that while on Cape Cod, "for recreation, the General was repairing the driveway to the Dodds house, hauling up seaweed in a wheelbarrow, for ballast. He hired Corty as his assistant, paying him 10¢ an hour to sit on top of the wheelbarrow loaded with seaweed so that the seaweed would not fall off in transit." (Gunn to Royster Lyle, May 5, 1965, GCMRL/G. C. Marshall Collection [Slaymaker].)

4. Slaymaker's next letter had included three nautically themed pictures and "fish hooks 4 small bait." (Slaymaker to Marshall, n.d., GCMRL/G. C. Marshall Papers [Retirement, General].)

5. See p. 678.

6. See previous document.

7. Marshall wrote to Slaymaker again the following year in response to another "beautiful Christmas card." (Marshall to Slaymaker, January 8, 1953, GCMRL/G. C. Marshall Collection [Slaymaker].) "I am very much pleased that you still have me in mind, and I

might add that I have never had any luck with fish since we separated," Marshall admitted. (Ibid.)

390

To Mrs. John B. Wilson

January 21, 1952
Pinehurst, North Carolina

Dear Rose: I saw Tom Morgan at the BAC meeting January 9th and he told me something of how you were getting along—as I understand it your expected date is early in February.[1] I pray that all goes well with you and I suppose it will as you have had good experience.

We leave by air for Mexico City February 1st to spend the month at Cuernavaca, and possibly a week at Acupulco.[2]

Then in March I have three dates in a row, one at Lawrenceville School in New Jersey, one at Wellesley and one in New York to receive the award of the Four Freedoms issue whatever that is.[3] I have put it off for three years and now I must come across. Tell me what line to take with the young women at Wellesly.

On my birthday I received a second hand copy of a book I had been talking about, published long ago, which was a great favorite of Lily's, and of mine.[4] Alexander Woolcott in recent years referred to it as one of the most appealing tales ever written.[5] I am sending it on to you to read to the children. I think they will like it and I am sure you will. Keep it for me, they are hard to locate now, and I will pick it up when I drive up to call on you and the baby.[6] With my love and my prayers for you, Rosie,

G.C.M.

GCMRL/J. Page Wilson Collection; H

1. Thomas A. Morgan, a member of the Commerce Department's Business Advisory Council, was chairman of the Sperry Corporation and married to Rose Page Wilson's older sister, Celeste. For more on Wilson's pregnancy, see pp. 653–54.
2. See p. 678.
3. Marshall was scheduled to give the Forum Lecture at Lawrenceville preparatory school in Lawrenceville, New Jersey, on March 12 and a speech at Wellesley College in Massachusetts on March 13, and had agreed to receive the Four Freedoms Award in New York on March 14. See pp. 681–89.
4. "The book is *Timothy's Quest*, one of Kate Douglas Wiggin's first stories, published in 1890," clarified Wilson in her memoir. "It is a sunny, whimsical little tale, spiced with a gentle humor, about the adventures of two small orphans. I can easily understand why *Timothy's Quest* appealed to Lieutenant Marshall and his bride—Colonel Marshall being particularly sensitive to children, Lily being tender-hearted and sentimental, and both of them longing for children of their own." (Rose Page Wilson, *General Marshall Remembered* [Englewood Cliffs, NJ: Prentice-Hall, Inc., 1968], 359–60.)
5. Alexander Woolcott was a noted American literary critic.
6. Wilson reported that Marshall "was never able to make the trip." (Ibid.)

391

To Frank McCarthy

January 30, 1952
Washington, DC

Dear Frank: I believe you may be acquainted with Comte de Marenches, who I think is better known as Alexander de Marenches, the son of General Pershing's French Aide with whom I had almost daily contact during World War I and whose friendship I enjoyed until his death several years ago. Incidentally, Alexander's mother is an American and for the moment I fail to recall her maiden name.[1]

de Marenches during the War was in the French Army and assigned to General Eisenhower's headquarters. He is an exceptionally fine man and for his services was awarded the Legion of Merit and Bronze Star. Since the War he has held the position as adviser to General Juin and in the past year I have seen him on two different occasions.[2] In this particular position he was not on active duty or employed by the civil service. The expenses which he incurred have had to come from his mother's savings and he now feels that he must secure gainful employment. I did not hear from him directly on this matter but he had a conversation with Major George in which he expressed a desire to become associated with an American firm which had offices in France.

I know him well and believe he would be an asset because of his connections and unusual knowledge of public and World affairs.

The thought occurred to me, because of your planned European film commitments, that de Marenches, if there is a position available, could be very useful to you.[3] My purpose in writing you is to just let you know of his interest and to tell you something about him.

Mrs. Marshall and I are now in Washington. Unfortunately Clifton has developed a tumor or cyst on his lung and is being operated on at George Washington Hospital on Friday. We had definite plans to leave here Friday, February 1st for Mexico but naturally had to postpone our departure indefinitely. However, we hope he will respond favorably and if so should be able to leave the latter part of next week.[4] With affectionate regards,

GCMRL/G. C. Marshall Papers (Retirement, General)

1. Alexandre de Marenches was the son of Captain Charles-Constant-Marie de Marenches and Margaret Clark de Lestrade, a US citizen.

2. Eisenhower had awarded de Marenches the Legion of Merit for "exceptionally meritorious service from June 1944 to May 1945" as aide-de-camp to General Alphonse Juin and personal liaison among Juin, Eisenhower, and his senior staff at SHAEF. (Order and Citation for Legion of Merit, June 4, 1947, GCMRL/G. C. Marshall Papers [Secretary of Defense, Number Indexed, M200-14-36].) In June 1951 de Marenches became head of Juin's Paris staff in the general's new position as commander in chief of the Allied Army Forces in Central Europe for NATO. Secretary of Defense Marshall had met with de Marenches at 2:15 p.m. on October 20, 1950, and had lunch with him on January 30, 1951, when he accompanied General Juin during the visit of Prime Minister Pleven. See pp. 357–60.

3. "My own productions will not take me at all to France," McCarthy responded from London on February 9. "I have written, however, to both our continental production office and our European Distribution office and asked the head of each of them to have de

Marenches in for interview. I am sure they will do this, regardless of their present personnel situations. Both offices are in Paris, and both can at least know about him." (McCarthy to Marshall, February 9, 1952, GCMRL/G. C. Marshall Papers [Retirement, General].)

4. "I was distressed to hear of Clifton's illness and operation," McCarthy wrote. "The irony of it is that I was in Washington for one day, Friday January 31, the day of the operation, and had no idea any of you were there. I hope soon to hear that the operation was a success and that Clifton came through well." (Ibid.) See pp. 694–95 and 697–98.

392

To Queen Frederica of the Hellenes

February 1, 1952
Washington, DC

Your Majesty: Mrs. Marshall and I were greatly appreciative of the card of Holiday greetings and New Year's wishes from His Majesty and yourself.[1] It is a great compliment for us to feel that you still have us in mind.

I am taking the liberty of sending you a photograph to indicate my state of health and state of mind these days.

I wrote you a longhand note a month or two ago describing what had been happening to us and expressing my regret over mis-endorsement of a certain officer and I hope you find the present arrangements entirely satisfactory.[2]

Having in mind your earnest recommendation regarding command arrangements, I hope your Majesty and you are satisfied with the final decision in the matter.[3]

Most confidentially, with regard to your Army leadership, when I took over as Chief of Staff of our Army in 1939 and 1940 I picked up Eisenhower and Bradley (now Chairman of our Chiefs of Staff and of our NATO organization) as Lt. Colonels, and Collins (now Chief of Staff of the Army) and Smith (Eisenhower's Chief of Staff in the War) as Majors and they were comparatively young for their then rank. Smith is now the head of our Central Intelligence Agency. Ridgway in Japan and Korea, was incidentally a Major in 1940 and Lt. General at the finish. Apropos of these comments I must admit the military departments find it very difficult in these so called peaceful days to reach down to the younger generations with any purpose of overslaughing their seniors.

With warm regards to His Majesty and yourself and with great respect, Faithfully yours,

GCMRL/G. C. Marshall Papers (Retirement, General)

1. See pp. 663–64n2.
2. See pp. 664n2 and 708.
3. See pp. 587–88. "We are delighted to know that things have turned out so well about Admiral Carney and us. Let us hope nothing will upset that apple-cart," Frederica wrote in her May 7, 1952, letter, referring to Admiral Robert B. Carney, who was appointed commander in chief of NATO Forces in Southern Europe on June 18, 1951. (See pp. 439–40n1.) He was responsible for the fleets of five countries and the armed forces of Italy, Turkey, and Greece. "Carney suits us to the ground and we had a very happy reunion when he was here a short time ago," she continued. (Papanicolaou, *Frederica*, 421.) Greece and Turkey officially joined NATO on February 18, 1952. (See p. 486.)

393

To Robert M. Schuman

February 1, 1952
Washington, DC

Dear Schuman: This note is to carry my congratulations to you on your remarkable achievement in regard to the Schuman Plan, and to express the earnest hope that the French Government and the World will have you at the helm throughout the New Year.[1]

Mrs. Marshall and I have been wintering in our cottage at Pinehurst, North Carolina and we are in Washington now for a few days due to the illness of her son.[2] Our place in Leesburg that you knew has been closed since early November and we will not return there until about May 1st.

I had a very interesting discussion with Churchill.[3] He had me up for lunch and a long talk on the day he addressed our Congress. I flew up in the morning and flew back the same afternoon, the political climate in Washington is not particularly healthy for me these days.

With affectionate regards and many most agreeable memories of our service together.[4] Faithfully yours,

GCMRL/G. C. Marshall Papers (Retirement, General)

1. See p. 203n4. Belgium, France, Italy, Luxembourg, the Netherlands, and West Germany signed the Treaty of Paris on April 18, 1951, forming the basis of the European Coal and Steel Community. The signatories were in the process of ratifying the treaty, which would go into effect on July 23, 1952.
2. See pp. 674–75 and the next document.
3. See pp. 670–72.
4. "The letter that you were kind enough to write to me and that I received on my departure for London and Lisbon moved me deeply," Schuman responded, in longhand, on March 4. The North Atlantic Council had met in Lisbon, Portugal, on February 20, 1952, to consider a coordinated analysis of NATO's defense plans, among other issues. "That you wrote to me about the political climate prevailing in Washington at the beginning of the last month, was for me of a great help, although it did not surprise me. I hope that after the result of the Lisbon conference that climate has happily improved, in spite of our governmental crisis," adding, "Once more personal contacts and sincere explanations have greatly clarified a troubled situation." (Schuman to Marshall, March 4, 1952, GCMRL/G. C. Marshall Papers [Retirement, General].) French President Vincent Auriol had accepted the resignation of Prime Minister Rene Pleven's cabinet on January 7, 1952. ("Pleven's Cabinet Falls in France; Long Crisis Likely," *New York Times*, January 8, 1952, pp. 1, 4.) For more on Marshall's interactions with Schuman, see *Papers of GCM*, 6: 500–625 passim.

394

To Bernard M. Baruch

February 7, 1952
Washington, DC

Dear Baruch: Katherine and I are leaving ~~Friday~~ Saturday morning for Cuernavaca, flying on the American line and should reach Mexico City at 5:30 in the evening.[1]

We came up to Washington last week because of the fact that Clifton was in the hospital here with a pending operation, which actually occurred on Friday. Fortunately his apartment which we took is directly across the street from the hospital.[2]

He had a serious operation, removing a tumor from his chest cavity, and suffered considerable pain for the first thirty-six hours but since then has come out of it very rapidly and is now walking around the ward.[3] Katherine had given up our Mexico trip but the Doctor insisted that we should go to reduce Clifton's worry over our giving up the trip and the suspicion that we were staying because of the seriousness of his condition, regarding which he is not fully aware.[4]

Clifton expects to go down to stay with a friend of his mother's at Palm Beach in about ten days after they have made some progress with X-Ray treatment, and if there is nothing unusual we will be at Cuernavaca for about four weeks.[5]

I do not know whether you are at Little Hobcaw or in New York, so I will send a carbon to Hobcaw, and the original to New York.[6]

I had an interesting meeting with Churchill but not a very serious discussion as he was more or less completely absorbed in the possible reactions to his speech an hour before to the Congress.[7] In referring to you, he said that he thought you felt that he was not doing enough. I knew pretty well what he was referring to and I talked to him about the vast importance of his taking the lead on the Continent.

Katherine knew I was writing and she sends you her love.

With affectionate regards to you and Hampton.[8] Faithfully yours,

GCMRL/G. C. Marshall Papers (Retirement, General)

1. See the next editorial note. "Friday" was crossed out and "Saturday" is handwritten above on the file copy of this letter.

2. Clifton Brown's surgery had been performed on February 1 at George Washington University Hospital in Washington, DC. Marshall wrote to Lady Mary Burghley that day that he and Mrs. Marshall had arrived in Washington "en route supposedly yesterday to Mexico," but they "had to halt all our plans until we can know the result" of Clifton's surgery. He added that while staying at Clifton Brown's apartment they were "existing on light housekeeping, Mrs. Marshall being the housekeeper, which is a good thing for her because it keeps her busy." (Marshall to Burghley, February 1, 1951, GCMRL/G. C. Marshall Papers [Retirement, General].) A column in the *Washington Star* reported that the Marshalls' presence in Brown's apartment "has electrified . . . the entire neighborhood." The apartment building's tenants appreciated "the Marshalls' gentle ways," and "Women who have ridden in the elevator with Mrs. Marshall report with possessive pride that she carries her groceries home in a bag just like the rest of them." (Betty Beale, "Gen. and Mrs. Marshall Are Favorites in Apartment Where Currently Residing," *Washington Star*, February 10, 1952.)

3. "He has gotten through the operation wonderfully well and is on the mend," Katherine Marshall wrote to Jeanette and Tom Watson on February 8, adding that they would leave for Mexico the following morning because the surgeon "tells us that Clifton should be able to take up his regular life in anywhere from six to eight weeks." (Katherine Marshall to Watsons, February 8, 1952, GCMRL/G. C. Marshall Papers [Retirement, General].) Thomas Watson was the president of International Business Machines, where Clifton Brown was employed in the Washington office.

4. "My heart is very heavy going on this trip now," Katherine Marshall confided on February 8 to Madame Chiang Kai-shek. "The Doctor feels if we stay it will alarm and perhaps worry Clifton more than if we should go ahead with our plans." (Katherine Marshall to Madame Chiang, February 8, 1952, ibid.)

5. See pp. 674–75. Brown planned to recuperate with General and Mrs. Ralph Robert-

son in West Palm Beach, Florida. (Katherine Marshall to Watsons, February 8, 1952, ibid.) The Marshalls had visited Ann and Ralph Robertson in Palm Beach, Florida, in 1949. See *Papers of GCM*, 6: 675n1. For more on Clifton Brown's condition, see pp. 694–95 and 697–98.

6. See p. 318n1.

7. See pp. 670–71.

8. Hampton Baruch was apparently a special name for Elizabeth Navarro. See p. 318n2.

FOLLOWING the recommendation of Clifton Brown's doctor (see previous document), the Marshalls departed on February 9 from Washington for almost a month's vacation in Cuernavaca, Mexico. Marshall reported to C. J. George on February 15 that they had a "pleasant and uneventful" trip to Mexico and were "very comfortable here." As they were the guests of Brigadier General Alberto Salinas-Carranza, the Mexican military attaché in Washington, the Marshalls received the attention of "servants, guards, waiters, 2 aides, [and] female nurse," as well as "all food." The Marshalls were enjoying the "perfect" climate in Cuernavaca and the ability to do "nothing but loaf," although Marshall added that he and Mrs. Marshall were looking forward to "some pleasant all day trips." Mexico's English-language newspaper, *The News*, reported on February 29 that the Marshalls' "desire for undisturbed rest has been meticulously observed" and that they "have known the full warmth of Mexican hospitality." According to this article, "General Marshall, reading one or two books daily, almost exhausted the Bellavista Patio Bookshop's supply of appropriate rental titles for one who reads history for diversion," and "Mrs. Marshall finds great pleasure in discovering the typical Mexican 'handcraft gadgets' in the street puestos as well as in shopping for Cuernavaca clothes." The paper also noted that the Marshalls had visited Cortes Palace, where "the only other persons there were three tourists" from Marshall's hometown of Uniontown, Pennsylvania. "The General recalled that he once rode a bicycle 6 miles to visit the mother of one of the young ladies present." ("Marshalls Will Leave Lasting Impression Here," *The News*, February 29, 1952, p. 11A.) In a later summary of the vacation to Admiral Stark, Marshall wrote that Cuernavaca was "really a remarkable place to spend a vacation." (Marshall to Stark, March 10, 1952, GCMRL/G. C. Marshall Papers [Retirement, General].) See also p. 884n1.

The Marshalls were scheduled to depart Cuernavaca in the early morning hours of March 4 to arrive in Washington at 8:10 a.m., but mechanical difficulties on their plane and the time required for a replacement plane to arrive from Dallas led to a five-hour delay in their departure. Marshall later thanked Brigadier General Charles Sabin Ferrin, military attaché at the US embassy in Mexico City, for "coming down to the airfield at such an ungodly hour and for his hospitality during this delay. After landing in Washington at 1:30 p.m. with "only a 300 foot clearance," the Marshalls flew to Pinehurst, where they arrived "rested and relaxed." (Marshall to Ferrin, March 4, 1952, and Marshall to Stark, March 10, 1952, ibid.) ★

395

To Major C. J. George

March 5, 1952
Pinehurst, North Carolina

Dear George: On thinking it over it seems to me the best arrangement on the 12th would be for me to fly direct to field near Lawrenceville and have the small plane pick me up the morning of the 13th just in time to get me to Wellesly.[1] Then, on arriving in New York to land at Mitchell Field.[2] There (N.Y.C.) if you can get a car I might come by rail to Washington going direct from dinner to car, spending a few hours in the Pentagon and fly back here. See if this will ~~wror~~ work out.

My remaining piece of baggage should now be at the Mat terminal from San Antonio.[3] Hold it until I fly again from Washington.

We had a smooth flight down yesterday and found beautifully clear weather here.

I see Anna had her greatest disappointment.[4] We are headed I fear for another ghastly repetition of disasterous results and vast expenditures ~~ar~~ as a consequence.[5] Hastily,

GCM

GCMRL/G. C. Marshall Collection (George); H

1. In a November 26, 1951, letter to Lawrenceville School faculty member Lewis Perry Jr., Marshall had requested a change in the timing of the Forum lecture he had agreed to give in Lawrenceville, New Jersey, shifting the date to March 12, 1952, so that he could segue with a speech he was scheduled to give at Wellesley College on March 13 and the Four Freedoms Foundation's Award ceremony in New York City on March 14, "in order to avoid making an extra trip up that way, possibly in bad weather." (Marshall to Perry, November 26, 1951, GCMRL/G. C. Marshall Papers [Retirement, General].) See pp. 680–89.

2. Mitchel Air Force Base was located on Long Island.

3. The MATS terminal closest to Washington, DC, was Andrews Air Force Base.

4. As assistant secretary of defense for manpower and personnel, Rosenberg had led the 1951 campaign for universal military training in Congress and had remained one of its most ardent supporters. (See pp. 232–33 and 325–26.) As required by the UMST bill that she had played a major role in getting passed in June 1951, the National Security Training Commission was established to study the issue of UMT further and draft legislation to outline a plan for its implementation, which Congress would consider in its next session (see pp. 551–53, 558–59, 609–10). On October 29, 1951, this commission issued its report, which recommended a "limited" initial implementation of UMT for sixty thousand men. It also stated that up to eight hundred thousand men could be trained per year under a "fully implemented program," which would be enacted at the discretion of the president and only after world conditions had improved. (National Security Training Commission, *Universal Military Training: Foundation of Enduring National Strength* [Washington: GPO, 1951], quote on 74.) The House and Senate Armed Services Committees began to consider this legislation in January 1952, and the hearings exposed confusion and disagreement among UMT supporters as to what should be included in the bill. (James M. Gerhardt, *The Draft and Public Policy: Issues in Military Manpower Procurement, 1945–1970* [Columbus: The Ohio State University Press, 1971], 170–71; "Early U.M.T. 'Test' Favored By Pentagon," *New York Times*, January 18, 1952, p. 9.) The House and Senate committees passed distinct versions of the bill in February 1952, each with its own restrictions on the authorities of the president and Defense Department to implement UMT. Through a series of parliamentary maneuvers, opponents of UMT in the House were able to get the bill recommitted to the

Armed Services Committee. Chair Carl Vinson stated that his committee would not take any further action on the bill during its current session, and the Senate took no action on the floor on its own version of the bill. (Gerhardt, *Draft and Public Policy*, 171–73; Condit, *Test of War*, 491; George Q. Flynn, *The Draft, 1940–1973* [Lawrence: University Press of Kansas, 1993], 124; "U.M.T. Is Shelved in House, 236–162, As Coalition Wins," *New York Times*, March 5, 1952, pp. 1, 10.)

5. The following day Marshall wrote more handwritten instructions to George, and enclosed his speech for Lawrenceville and Wellesley. "Have this typed up for my Lawrenceville Academy talk. Then send me by air mail (not special delivery) the two talks, one for Lawrenceville and one for Wellesly in time to reach me Monday if possible. To play safe give my pilot a copy of each so that if this slow mail fails to reach me in time I will have the carbons." (Marshall to George, March 6, 1952, GCMRL/G. C. Marshall Collection [George]; H.)

THE MARSHALLS departed Pinehurst on March 12 from nearby Southern Pines Airport for Lawrenceville, New Jersey, where Marshall would address the Lawrenceville School that evening; and the following day for Wellesley, Massachusetts, where Marshall would give a nearly identical speech at Wellesley College. (See next document.) Marshall then continued on to New York City, where he was to receive the Four Freedoms Foundation Award at a formal dinner. See pp. 687–89.

"In connection with any publicity with General Marshall's talk at Lawrenceville," George had advised Lewis Perry Jr. on March 6, "he wishes me to say that if you desired to have this publicized outside the College he would have to modify to a considerable degree what he intends to say because naturally he has to be very conservative or cautious in statements that are going to be widely broadcast. On the other hand, if it is your desire to have him talk as effectively as he can to your students and the faculty, that can only be arranged if a general broadcast and wide publicity is curtailed." George continued, "He has no secrets to confide but in these political days he would have to be so ultra-conservative in his comments he feels it would be of very little interest to your students." (George to Perry, March 6, 1952, GCMRL/G. C. Marshall Papers [Retirement, General].) George informed Marshall on March 11 that Perry had "not invited any members of the news or radio media to the Forum. They prefer to have it in the form of a lecture to the students and faculty only." (Memorandum for General Marshall, March 11, 1952, GCMRL/G. C. Marshall Papers [Retirement, Chronological].)

Perry and Lawrenceville School Headmaster Allan Vanderhoef Heely greeted the Marshalls at the Mercer County, New Jersey, airport. They joined "the older boys" for tea and the Heelys, who also provided overnight accommodations, for an informal dinner. (For Marshall's speech at the Lawrenceville School, see GCMRL/G. C. Marshall Papers [Retirement, Speeches, Statements, and Writings].) The following day Army Captain Leffler flew the Marshalls to the Norwood, Massachusetts, airport near Wellesley College, where they were met by an army vehicle, which drove them to the president's home. (Ibid.) ★

396

Remarks at Wellesley College[1]

March 13, 1952
Wellesley, Massachusetts

I have been wondering what I might talk about this evening that would be most interesting to you young women, and possibly helpful. I have been influenced by the fact that you will not only soon take your places among those with the right to cast a vote, but by virtue of your education will possess a considerable power to influence others. Your degree of education will be much better than most and our immediate future will certainly be the day of the younger generation in public affairs.

I suppose you would be much interested in a discussion of the Korean struggle and its possible outcome or of the Far Eastern question in general; possibly Western Europe and the Middle East complication, or the Communist problem, but I have come to the conclusion that in the long run it would be more profitable to discuss something of the problems of cause and effect in relation to high governmental decisions.[2]

It is extremely difficult today for the citizen to comprehend the real facts concerning our great international problems, and even more difficult to understand the manner in which the decisions are arrived at. Our tremendous and sometimes flashy press, the overwhelming ranks of columnists and commentators, the widely reported speeches in Congress and of administration leaders, the television, the radio, the newsreels, the mixture of all of these tend to confuse rather than orient the general public, except in particular instances.

Probably the commentators exert the most immediate influence, next the columnists. In one case it is often the voice of the man that appeals rather than the logic and sound basis for his comments, or for the columnist it may be largely his art of presentation. The principal trouble seems to be that listeners or readers too frequently devote themselves to one or two favorites particularly those who make it their business to put forward popular or exciting appeal. It runs a little like the reactions to our press where the majority of people admittedly are much more interested in the scandals, the murders and other unfortunate excitements than in the less spectacular news reports and editorials.

In view of these conditions I think it might be helpful to describe something of how great governmental decisions are arrived at, utilizing my own experiences over the past fourteen years which cover the most critical period of our history up to the present time. But first let me make the point, that, for example in military matters the logical decision from a purely technical or military standpoint is usually very simple to arrive at. It is the pressures, the influence of many subsidiary factors that present the problem of decision.

Let us take probably the most far reaching and bitterly contested decision of the last war, the decision for the cross channel invasion of Normandy and the advance across the lowlands of Northern Europe and the Rhine towards Berlin. On a map or a blueprint, as it were, it seemed completely logical to make the great thrust in the manner indicated. But there were those that favored the advance against Central Europe from the Mediterranean, others thought the drive should be launched across the Western rather than the Northern coast of France. Still others strongly favored the great effort being made first in the Pacific. Added to the complication resulting from these pressures was the extremely critical time factor. To stage a colossal effort like the channel crossing followed by the drive east across France and the Rhine, required at least a year and a half for the assembly of the forces in England and it was always a desperate question as to whether or not we would be able to secure the materiel and the vast amount of shipping in time. For evident reasons of tide and weather the invasion had to be in the late spring or summer otherwise a delay of another year must intervene, which made the consideration of the time factor dominant for this operation. There was another factor of almost equal importance and that was the fact, in view of the necessarily long period of preparation that leaders of State, Mr. Roosevelt and Mr. Churchill in this instance, had to meet the insistent public demand for action. Yet such action, meaning other military efforts here and there, would always threaten to absorb, so much of troops, materiel and particularly shipping that the concentration for the main effort would be fatally delayed. In war one can never tell how prolonged a particular struggle will be however careful the planning estimates. In this particular case the reactions from the Pacific with its fierce island campaigns and resulting casualties, and the popular appeal of subsidiary operations in the Mediterranean, developed pressures which seriously threatened the concentration in England for the invasion of Normandy. Ocean shipping became a most critical matter. The turn around to England was the shortest haul and therefore more troops, equipment and supplies could be moved in a given time. Yet, except for the air forces there was no battle being fed from England at that time. Shipping to the Mediterranean took longer than to England and much longer to the Southwest Pacific and shipping was always in short supply and continued to suffer heavily from submarine attack. Then there was the landing craft, the famous LST's. There were more arguments regarding the allotment of these craft than over any other subject, for they were the initial basis of any landing operation.

During Mr. Churchill's recent visit we were discussing the fact that in the famous Cairo Conference in December 1943 more time and bitter differences of opinion related to disposal of 27 LST's than to all the great subjects of the Conference combined.[3]

In the face of these many conflicting pressures we stood by our conclusion that the fundamental operation to precipitate the end of the war lay in the build up of the forces and means for invading Normandy. And please keep this in mind—the public could not be informed of either the details or the reasons. Columnists, commentators, newspapers and magazines could discuss and illustrate to prove that this or that plan would be the best plan, but our procedures had to be completely secret, no explanation or defense was possible. Special pleaders to the White House or the Congress or the press were only a little less numerous than starlings in the summertime. It almost seemed a miracle to me that we survived these difficulties and eventually had our way. Yet because of public impatience it did become necessary to carry out other operations to some of which we were strongly opposed because of possible limiting effect on the concentration in England.

Take another example, this time concerning appropriations to implement this or that policy. I will risk this statement, that, if the appropriations of the billions first given us in the summer and fall of 1940 had been authorized in the early fall of 1939, the war having started on September 1st of that year, I feel certain that the fighting would have ended at least six months earlier, possibly even a year or more earlier. That would have meant the saving of millions of casualties and tens of billions of funds. Then what prevented such action?

In the first place the majority of Congress had not yet been convinced of the necessity, and the majority of the public fully supported that attitude. In other words no matter how necessary Mr. Roosevelt felt these appropriations to be, in his opinion it was politically impossible to secure them. Even he seemed at times to his impatient military leaders to be far too slow in pressing for their acceptance. This was undoubtedly because as our great civil leader he was under terrific political pressure of both parties to move exceedingly slow.

Considering the hundreds of billions that were finally appropriated certain early approaches to this problem today seem almost ridiculous by comparison. For instance in the late fall of 1939 the White House had authorized the Bureau of the Budget to approve my recommendation for a certain 26 million dollars. I am talking of millions, not billions as is usually the case today, just 26 millions. Congress declined to authorize this appropriation. Later on in the early spring when Hitler suddenly invaded Denmark and Norway I immediately requested authority to renew the appeal to Congress for this small amount of money. The President, just landing at Miami on returning from a cruise in the Caribbean, notified me that he approved but 18 millions of the 26 millions, omitting the remaining 8 millions which were largely for detectors against possible air raids from Japanese carriers off the Pacific coast. I was instructed to call on the Secretary of the Treasury to discuss the matter and there found that it was not for discussion of the disapproved 8 millions but whether or not I should even be permitted to ask for the 18 millions. I quickly convinced the Secretary that the situation was incredibly dangerous and he suggested that we see the President together, which we did that afternoon. After a heated argument and much discussion concerning the mounting debt and an increasingly strong political opposition, I came away with authority to ask not for 26 millions but over 700 millions, the first of the great military war appropriations. Three weeks later, following the fall of France, I secured authority to ask for about 800 additional millions.[4]

I must not bore you, or confuse you, with figures but they are essential to explain the procedures. Here was the President of the United States at a time when he was being severely criticized politically for demanding increased military appropriations, faced with an issue that directly affected the security and the eventual freedom of our Country.

In current discussions or criticisms of why this or that was done or not done the public is seldom reminded of what its own state of mind was and what the conditions were at the time of the incident. For example, particularly in connection with our unpreparedness at the outbreak of fighting in Korea, there has been a great deal of comment on the lack of essential materiel and more particularly on the lack of available troops to meet the crisis in June and July of 1950. When I became Chief of Staff in the summer of 1939 we possessed just 15 of the famous flying fortresses, the great [B-17] bombers of that day and we lacked sufficient funds properly to maintain even that small number. By way of contrast, the last weeks I was Chief of Staff in the fall of 1945 we had reached the point where I was called upon to concur in an order for the scuttling of 2700 of these same flying fortresses because of obsolescence. Now the difference between 15 with a lack of sufficient funds to maintain them and 2700 we could afford to abandon represents a considerable bracket which well illustrates the degree to which our public opinion shifts from complete indifference to national necessities for security to prodigal support at the last minute when it threatens to be too late.

Shortly before I left the office of Chief of Staff, the popular demand for the rapid demobilization of the armed forces had reached such a peak of power that we were compelled to dissipate all that we had so hurriedly built up and at such tremendous cost and this in the face of a huge Russian Army. There was not time even to protect or ship home the huge dumps of arms and supplies in the Pacific and in relatively a few months they were taken over by the jungle. This demobilization continued its wasteful and dangerous pace until when I, as Secretary of State, was involved in conference with the Soviets in Moscow we had only one and one-third divisions of troops in the entire United States and Alaska and these were at low strength. That means but four regiments of infantry with supporting artillery. There were not enough men to guard the airstrip at Fairbanks in Alaska against a parachute attack from nearby Siberia, yet I was receiving radio messages from patriotic Americans to "give them Hell", meaning the Soviets.[5]

Very much the same reaction occurred in the early months of the fighting in Korea. We were utterly unprepared and while the critical debate related mostly to air power, the fact was we completely lacked any trained reserves for the ground troops which had to fight the main battle. You may remember that the fighting started the last week in June and that the Selective Service or draft act was not re-enacted until September. Therefore, the first trained men as a result of this act did not begin to be available until February.[6]

Meanwhile our men in Korea had to face overwhelming numbers fighting with complete savagery and utter disregard of human life. The divisions that we drew from the National Guard in September of that year were not fully trained for combat until a year later. The divisions we sent to Europe had to be created from the ground up. You may have followed the tremendous debate which was launched regarding the question of sending divisions to Europe and the fear expressed by many that the President might send large numbers. The truth was that at that time we had no divisions immediately available to go to Europe and it was not until seven months later that we were able to complete the four that were scheduled for that assignment.[7]

In this connection I should explain that invariably the argument is put forward that the public has not been kept well enough informed, otherwise they would not react as they did. There are two factors concerned with this: (1), that if you tell your enemy everything he has you at a frightful disadvantage to be weighed in human lives if not in the ultimate victory and it is with the greatest difficulty that we learn anything regarding his numbers and plans. Short shrift is given any who talks. And (2), most of those in the important positions in Congress know the facts but that sometimes does not deter them from fathering the idea that the public should be better informed and therefore the fault is that of the administration, or more specifically, the Pentagon. All of these reactions and difficulties are a part of the processes of democracy which we are fighting so hard to preserve. But it is very difficult at times to maintain the free processes without literally defeating ourselves in the field of action or before the World. Yet it must be done.

An educated public opinion is the only method I know of to protect us against such dangerous and wasteful procedures. Dangerous in the reckless dispersal of any military power we may possess and wasteful in the vast sums that are required when haste is necessary to re-establish our military position before the World. And I think it is young women like yourselves who can do more than any other group to protect us against such hazardous and illogical procedures in the future. And beside that your lives and your future are directly concerned.

While I was Secretary of State and out of the country a great deal of the time at lengthy conferences in Latin America and England and Europe, I had little time for public appearances at home. Yet I invariably arranged to meet any groups of young people who came to Washington as they frequently do, groups of high school students selected for excellence and furnished the trip by various organizations usually veterans. My reason was this: I felt that if they could get a sound start as citizens of the leading democracy in this troubled world of ours they would probably do more permanently to influence public opinion than almost any other group. My counsel to them was to go after the facts and avoid the special and partisan pleadings. And also to avoid expressing youthful opinions, though this was rather asking for a miracle of restraint. I explained that if at the family dinner table they could bring out the real facts concerning this or that question it would very definitely influence their parents' opinions and they in time would spread the word in that community. On the other hand if the young people became strongly opinionative resulting from the influence of this or that person or group they would merely antagonize their elders. I hope some followed my suggestion. If they did, I am certain it will not only make more stable citizens of them but in the end will exert a profound influence in their communities.

I would have you remember that the spectacular or exciting, the super-critical, the hasty advocacy of this or that is seldom the part of wisdom. When we come to world affairs, emotions, partisanship and ignorance of the characteristics or history of the peoples involved are bad medicine. And remember also that we are new, extremely youthful in matters of World leadership. In a way we have been forced into a position which other nations, like the British for example, have been hundreds of years in reaching and that in close physical contact with the other nations involved. We are thousands of miles distant from the Far East and several thousand of miles distant from the nations of Europe and the Mediterranean. We have so much to learn as a people and so little time in which to learn it and yet here we are in a position of World leadership such as no other nation has ever approached. We have to act and learn at the same time, which means that the public must learn to judge in these grave matters and not to plunge suddenly into violent acclaim or bitter criticism.

In the midst of all these complications we are also in the midst of a World revolution. The benighted people, the little people of the earth have begun to realize how tragic their situation is, how unfair. The Communists seize this growing revolt as a spring board, or surf board for their own purposes. They use it. We largely ignored it through the years, with all our kindly and generous feelings toward our fellow men. Much of our present trouble springs from this source. We can't buy our way out, though we can help. We must not spread ourselves thinly over the troubled areas of the World. We, in effect, must put our finger in the dike at one place while we first accomplish great things at another, though each region has its special pleaders in our midst. One great trouble during the war was the public and Congressional pressure to do everything at once, which would have meant doing nothing effectively anywhere and very probably being defeated by an enemy who concentrated.

So you see there is much to learn about each situation, so many facts and factors to be considered. Fortunately for the present we are far removed from the distressing scenes of trouble, but they present a wonderful field for you young women in which to play a great part in the leadership of our country through these difficult years.[8]

GCMRL/G. C. Marshall Papers (Retirement, Speeches, Statements, and Writings)

1. Marshall had submitted a "first draft" for this speech to Anna Rosenberg with an undated note. "Please let me have your completely frank reaction," he urged. (Marshall to Rosenberg, n.d., GCMRL/G. C. Marshall Papers [Retirement, General].) See n2 and n5 below. The two opening paragraphs were delivered only at Wellesley College. The remainder of the speech virtually duplicates the address Marshall had given the previous day at the Lawrenceville School (see previous editorial note). Only the version delivered at Wellesley is included here.

2. "The theme that we are charged with the individual and collective responsibility, particularly in terms of national and international affairs, to reach reasonable conclusions based on careful thinking and reliable facts is a theme with which we all need closer acquaintance," Rosenberg had responded. "Particularly in view of the audience, I don't think you could have picked a better topic." She continued, "the girls might be currently more excited about the Korean situation, but your discussion of the subject you have chosen can have a much greater value to these embryonic citizens." Rosenberg closed with a compliment: "I think the speech accomplishes just what you set out to do, and I believe that its dissemination across the nation can have great benefit in addition to its value to the key audience at Wellesley." (Rosenberg to Marshall, n.d., ibid.)

3. See pp. 670–72, *Papers of GCM*, 4: 191–96, and Forrest C. Pogue, *George C. Marshall*, vol. 3, *Organizer of Victory, 1943–1945* (New York: Viking, 1973), 305–9, 317–18.

4. See *Papers of GCM*, 2: 209–11, and Forrest C. Pogue, *George C. Marshall*, vol. 2, *Ordeal and Hope, 1939–1942* (New York: Viking, 1965), 29–32.

5. Rosenberg suggested that at this point in the speech Marshall "might return briefly to the subject of our 'Korea day' unpreparedness in order to clinch your point as to the dangerous situation into which we had gotten ourselves as the result of the stampede of public opinion in favor of pell-mell demobilization and disarmament." (Ibid.) As a result, the following three paragraphs were inserted into the draft speech.

6. See pp. 325–26.

7. See pp. 333–34, 380–86, and 472–74.

8. "I speak for our whole academic community in expressing our appreciation of your visit with us yesterday," wrote Charles Kerby-Miller, chairman of the lecture committee at Wellesley. Marshall's comments "to the larger audience" and those "to the smaller groups with whom you talked made a profound impression. And your presence on our campus and in our midst was a most meaningful and moving experience." (Kerby-Miller to Marshall, March 14, 1952, ibid.)

397

REMARKS AT THE FOUR FREEDOMS FOUNDATION DINNER[1] — March 14, 1952
New York, New York

After all that has been said tonight, together with the high compliment and honor of this citation I find myself lacking in suitable words to express my truly great appreciation.[2] By this gathering and this award I have been paid a tribute that would tremendously appeal to any man, and I am very grateful.

The caption of the award refers to the Four Freedoms. I was in President Roosevelt's party at Argentia, New Foundland that August day in 1941 when the great principle of the Four Freedoms was given to the world.[3] Your Chairman tonight was a principal at that meeting of Mr. Roosevelt with Mr. Churchill while I was merely involved in military discussions with the British Chiefs of Staff.[4]

What great events in World History had their beginnings there, what storms and agonizing stresses were soon to develop, and what a long bitter road we would labor along for the next four years. We anticipated most of our difficulties but we were unable to visualize them in their enormity, as to the casualties to be suffered and the billions to be expended.

News of one happening at that very moment shocked us all and I think it would not be amiss for me to refer to it here tonight particularly in the light of a recent action of the House of Representatives concerning the security of the nation.[5] While the principle of the Four Freedoms was being discussed at Argentia the House of Representatives saved the Army by a margin of only one single vote from complete disintegration.[6] We had been struggling through tremendous difficulties with shelter, lack of equipment, vicious attacks on the morale of the soldiers and heavily built of pressures to return them to their homes. There would have been virtually no organized military force left in this country if this last had been done, as the tiny regular forces have been milked now of all their trained men for instructors and their ranks were filled with Selective Service men: When one thinks of the Japanese calculated attack but three months distant and our forced entry into that world holocaust, this dissolution of the hastily reorganized military forces would have been I think the greatest national tragedy in our history and a world tragedy probably of equal proportions. The Four Freedoms would have become merely a remote dream.

Yet today we struggle with many of the same influences which may lead us into another disaster. We never seem to learn no matter how bitter and costly the lesson.

The turbulence of difficulties and crises following the victory in 1945 leave most of our people in a state of confusion and political recriminations which seem common to all democracies. My mind turns back to a quite similar period in Great Britain following the termination of the protracted Napoleonic wars. Napoleon dominated most of Europe as did the Nazis. When his regime fell with the astounding victory at Waterloo, all England relaxed and turned to peaceful affairs at home. These rapidly deteriorated into one of the grimmest of British battles, all in effect the outcome of the desperate war years. The feeling of a great victory turned sour with the violent political and economic struggle that so quickly followed the military triumph.

And so it goes. Maybe we learn something from the past but certainly not clearly, not definitely. There always seem to be too many conflicting and disturbing factors for a calm appraisement, too much special pleading, too much of violent prejudice. The hope persists that always we will come out on top, but these past survivals have been protected by the Monroe Doctrine and two great oceans.[7] Today with the whole world necessary as our field the task is far more difficult. It certainly requires more of unity. The title of this meeting and organization provides an exalted text for our efforts—the Four Freedoms.

GCMRL/G. C. Marshall Papers (Retirement, Speeches, Statements, and Writings)

1. See p. 679n1. Emil K. Ellis, chairman of the program committee of the Four Freedoms Foundation had cabled Marshall on September 26, 1951, that the foundation had "awarded you a special citation for outstanding service in the cause of achieving freedom for all people throughout the world," and mentioned that the founders of the foundation included former Vice President Alben W. Barkley, Eleanor Roosevelt, Judge Robert Patterson, political scientist and diplomat Ralph Bunche, and Secretary of Labor Maurice J. Tobin. Ellis had also noted that Barkley, Roosevelt, and Bunche were previous recipients of the Four Freedoms Award. (Ellis to Marshall, telegram, September 26, 1951, GCMRL/G. C. Marshall Papers [Retirement, General].) The Four Freedoms Foundation was incorporated in 1951 to advance the objectives championed by President Franklin Roosevelt in his 1941 State of the Union message: freedom of speech, freedom of worship, freedom from want, and freedom from fear.

Marshall received another letter from Ellis on January 17 indicating that Secretary of State Acheson had been invited to make the principal address at the dinner. "I just wanted to tell you that I will thoroughly and sympathetically understand if you regret because I think it is rather an imposition on you, particularly when you are so heavily engaged," Marshall wrote to Acheson the same day. "Your note is typical of your generous and understanding nature," Acheson responded on January 23, adding that he had "regretfully declined" because of prior commitments. (Ellis to Marshall and Marshall to Acheson, January 17, 1952, and Acheson to Marshall, January 23, 1952, ibid.) The formal dinner took place at 8:00 p.m. at the Waldorf-Astoria Hotel in New York City; Marshall's remarks began at 9:00 p.m.

2. "General Marshall received a plaque bearing a citation hailing him for his 'outstanding service as a soldier, statesman, and diplomat in the cause of the four freedoms—the basic rights of human beings everywhere'," the *New York Times* reported the next day,

adding that a letter from President Truman was also read. "Soldier, statesman, and diplomat, General Marshall in peace no less than in war has rendered high service to his country whenever duty called," Truman declared. "It is fitting also that he should receive through all of his days the plaudits of the nation he served so heroically and with such selfless devotion." ("Pace Calls for a Citizens Unit to Give Faith in Government," *New York Times*, March 15, 1952, p. 1.)

3. Marshall is referring to the announcement of the Atlantic Charter at the conclusion of the August 1941 Atlantic Conference. See *Papers of GCM*, 2: 586–88.

4. Judge Robert P. Patterson was to have presided at the Four Freedoms event; however, he had been killed in a plane crash on January 22. Although Patterson had been undersecretary of war at the time, he did not attend the Atlantic Conference. Former New York Supreme Court Justice Ferdinand Pecora succeeded Patterson as co-chairman of the dinner. It is unclear to whom "your chairman tonight" refers.

5. See p. 679n4.

6. See p. 268n9.

7. The Monroe Doctrine, declared in President James Monroe's 1823 Annual Message to Congress, asserted that while the United States would not interfere in existing European colonies in North and South America, it would consider any attempts by the European nations to acquire new colonies in the Western Hemisphere as acts of aggression.

398

To Harry S. Truman

March 15, 1952
Washington, DC

My dear Mr. President: I had expected to see you on my return from Mexico but found you had left for Key West, therefore there has been a delay in transmitting to you a message from President Aleman.[1]

Mr. Aleman treated me very graciously and in a very complimentary manner. In the first place he directed that practically everybody in the home that had been turned over to us by an old friend should be replaced by the Army, chefs, assistant chefs, waiters, trained nurse, G-4 [logistics], guards, automobiles, etc. Then to save me from any effort in driving the forty-five miles over the mountains to Mexico City to pay my respects to him, he came down to Cuernavaca to see me, drove down one evening and left immediately after our meeting. There he charged me with a message to you to the general effect first of his regards and high esteem and then most emphatically the assurance that whatever was the lead of the United States, Mexico would be right along with us, that you could depend on that.[2]

I feel negligent in not getting this personal message from the President of Mexico to you at an earlier moment but as I stated above I thought I was going to see you personally.

I do hope you are getting some rest in the balmy climate of Key West. We had a perfectly delightful time at Cuernavaca. I have never been quite so pleasantly lazy in my life.[3]

With warmest regards to you. Affectionately,

G.C. Marshall

GCMRL/G. C. Marshall Papers (Retirement, Chronological)

1. President Truman was in residence at the Little White House in Key West, Florida,

from March 7 to 27, 1952. Miguel Alemán Valdés served as president of Mexico from December 1, 1946, to November 30, 1952.

2. "I certainly did appreciate your letter of the fifteenth regarding your visit with the President of Mexico. He is a very able man, I think, and the very fact that he took care of you as he did shows that he appreciates a great man when he sees one," Truman responded on March 18. "I was most happy to have his assurances that Mexico would be with us in case of trouble." (Truman to Marshall, March 18, 1952, GCMRL/G. C. Marshall Papers [Retirement, General].)

3. "I hope you had a most satisfactory rest," Truman rejoined. "I am trying to get one myself and I am being rather successful at it." (Ibid.)

399

TO ROY P. JOHNSON[1]

March 17, 1952
Pinehurst, North Carolina

My dear Mr. Johnson: I have just received your letter of March 13th regarding Colonel Steele, and I am very glad to comply with your request.[2] But I must ask your indulgence for saying it in this informal way. I have no office, secretary or aide here and I find it much easier in writing lengthy letters, etc., to use this soft paper at full length.

I first met Colonel Steele in the fall of 1906 at the Commandant General Staff School at Fort Leavenworth, Kansas—an old frontier post from which the military convoys and guard escorts started westward in the early days.

He was the professor of military history and delivered a series of lectures which are or were in fact the contents of the very well known book Steeles American Campaigns.[3] I much admired Colonel Steele who was then a major of cavalry. I remained at Leavenworth three more years, one in the Staff College and two as an instructor.[4] During this time I came to know him intimately and Mrs. Steel also, and developed an affectionate regard for both of them.

On my return from France with General Pershing in 1919 I saw something again of Colonel Steele in Washington. And in later years we exchanged letters several times. Once during our Italian Campaign in 1943 he wrote to me in a spirit of a critical discussion of the progress of that campaign. My reply was the only discussion I ever indulged in outside of my official channels and contacts during the war.[5] I had such a high regard for Colonel Steele personally and as a military strategist, that I made this single exception: Several years ago I had a search made of my files in an endeavor to find his letter and the carbon of my detailed reply and his acknowledgement, but was unsuccessful in locating the papers. Perhaps his file will reveal them. The discussion I think was quite interesting, and possibly instructive.

Colonel Steele's book of American Campaigns is the standard work on the subject.[6] It stands in very high regard among military students, even though, as he states, he did not make the effort, necessarily a prodigious effort, to include a consideration of the voluminous official records of the ~~Rebellion~~ Civil War—the fighting from 1861 to 1865.

In 1944 or possibly 45, General Henry H. Arnold and I were pheasant shooting near Bismark, N. D. Colonel Steele called me on the telephone from Fargo inviting me to stop over for a visit. Unfortunately I had engagements which preventing me from doing so, much to my regret. I am very sorry to learn that he is in the hospital and will write to him immediately.[7]

I hope these comments satisfy your requirements.[8] Faithfully yours,

G.C. Marshall

State Historical Society of North Dakota; H

1. Roy P. Johnson was a staff writer for the *Fargo Forum* newspaper in Fargo, North Dakota.

2. Johnson had written to Marshall because Lieutenant Colonel Matthew F. Steele (USMA, 1883) "is a patient in St. Luke's hospital in Fargo and since he is approaching his 91st year there is a probability that he may not survive much longer. For this reason, we are preparing his biography for use in the event he dies." Steele, Johnson recalled, had "once told me that during the period 1903–08 he was a lecturer in the General Service and Staff College at Fort Leavenworth, Kans, and on a subsequent occasion he added that you had been one of the officers who heard some of his lectures." As a result, Johnson had contacted Marshall "with the request that you send me some comment on him to be included in his biography with the provision that it be used for that purpose unless you specify otherwise. It would be of interest if you mention some of the other students who gained prominence who also were in Steele's classes." (Johnson to Marshall, March 13, 1952, GCMRL/G. C. Marshall Papers [Retirement, General].)

3. Matthew Forney Steele, *American Campaigns*, 2 vols. (Washington: B. S. Adams, 1909).

4. See *Papers of GCM*, 1: 36–50 passim.

5. See *Papers of GCM*, 4: 144–45.

6. See ibid., 145n1.

7. Marshall wrote to Steele later that same day to send his "sympathy with my very sincere prayers for your quick recovery. He also reported that during his vacation in Mexico (see pp. 676–78), two Americans had "sent me their copies of your American Campaigns." (Marshall to Steele, March 17, 1952, USAMHI/Matthew F. Steele Papers; H.)

8. "I appreciate your kindness in taking time to answer my query," Johnson replied on March 21. Johnson explained that "the colonel has now reached the state where his memory has failed and his eye sight is very dim." As a result Johnson wondered whether Marshall "would be willing to make an effort to recall" his 1943 exchange with Steele. "I realize this is asking a great deal, yet I do not like to see this highly interesting exchange lost." (Johnson to Marshall, March 21, 1952, GCMRL/G. C. Marshall Papers [Retirement, General].) On March 27, C. J. George wrote to Johnson to advise him that Marshall "does not think it wise nor practicable for him to attempt to recall the details of Colonel Steele's letter to him during the Italian Campaign nor the details of his reply," adding that Marshall "would appreciate your letting him know should anything happen to Colonel Steele." (George to Johnson, March 27, 1952, ibid.)

400

Draft of Letter to Rex Stout[1] n.d., 1952

[Pinehurst, North Carolina?]

Dear Mr. Stout: I have given careful consideration to the request made in your letter of March 31, and have decided that any comments I could make now on World Government would not serve the purpose you have in mind.[2]

I believe that our hopes for harmony among nations at this time lie in the United Nations; that that organization is the surest foundation for permanent peace and security throughout the world.[3] A world government may develop from it, but now it is within its framework that nations are facing their problems side-by-side and by so doing are developing a habit of cooperation. When this habit has grown strong enough we will have international order based on peace with justice and freedom. Faithfully yours,

GCMRL/G. C. Marshall Papers (Retirement, General)

1. A writer of popular detective fiction, Stout had written to Marshall on March 31, 1952, in his capacity as chairman of Writers Board for World Government.

2. "We do believe that you recognize the necessity for international cooperation for peace by our country and the desirability of effecting that cooperation through a strengthened United Nations," Stout had written, requesting that Marshall submit "250 to 300 words" on the subject, which the committee would offer "for publication in American newspapers." (Stout to Marshall, March 31, 1952, GCMRL/G. C. Marshall Papers [Retirement, General].)

3. See *Papers of GCM*, 6: 212–18.

401

To General Walter Bedell Smith[1] — April 7, 1952, New York, New York

Dear Mr. Smith: We are honored to serve a great American humanitarian effort to aid several thousand Chinese intellectual leaders in British Hong Kong who have escaped the Communist dominated mainland. Among these are more than 2,000 graduates of American colleges and universities. They include some of the leading educators, engineers, administrators and other professional people who have chosen to take their stand with the Free World.

Our Survey Mission has just returned from Hong Kong to report on the tragic situation among our Chinese friends there and to outline a program of action to relieve these great human needs. They will report to a group of leading citizens at dinner at the Hotel Plaza, Fifth Avenue and 59th Street, New York City, on Monday, April 28th at seven o'clock. We will be greatly honored to have with us as speakers on this occasion Dr. Hu Shih, former Chinese Ambassador to the United States and one of the great intellectual leaders of our time, and Mr. Dean Rusk, formerly Assistant Secretary of State and now President of the Rockefeller Foundation.[2]

It is a source of pride to us as Americans that within the wholesome diversity of opinion fostered by our free institutions we have preserved the willingness to work together when overwhelming human tragedy strikes our friends. The association in this work of the undersigned, who have differed in the past on American policy in the Far East, is an earnest of our determination to act unitedly to help our Chinese friends who stand with us against Communist tyranny.

We will be happy to receive your acceptance of this invitation to serve as a member of the Committee of Sponsors for this dinner launching our campaign, and to receive your reservation for the dinner. It will be a great pleasure to meet with you on the evening of April 28th in this demonstration of concern for the fate of our Chinese friends.[3] Sincerely yours,

Walter H. Judd G. C. Marshall

DDEL/W. B. Smith Papers (Personal)

1. This letter was sent on Aid Refugee Chinese Intellectuals, Inc. letterhead. Prominent banker W. Randolph Burgess, former Massachusetts Institute of Technology President Karl T. Compton, and *Time* magazine editor and publisher Henry R. Luce comprised the dinner committee with Congressman Judd and Marshall.

2. Hu Shih was chancellor of Peking University between 1946 and 1948.

3. An April 12 memorandum to Smith noted that he planned to be in New York for a meeting on April 29 and pointed out that "General Marshall is on the Dinner Committee." Smith responded that the occasion was "a fine enterprise but I should not be identified with things like this no matter how meritorious they are. Decline on this basis," Smith handwrote on the memo. (DR to Smith, memorandum, April 12, 1952, DDEL/W. B. Smith Papers [Personal].)

The same letter was sent to President Truman. "I wish you would examine the situation," Truman wrote to his administrative assistant, David Lloyd. "I don't believe I want to get mixed up with it but I hate to refuse General Marshall anything he asks." (Truman to Lloyd, memorandum, April 12, 1952, GCMRL/G. C. Marshall Collection [Truman].) Truman did not attend the dinner.

"I am glad to be able to report the great success of our campaign-opening dinner," Judd wrote on May 12 to Marshall, who was unable to attend the event because of his stepson's illness. Marshall responded that he was "relieved and delighted with your success." (Judd to Marshall, May 12, 1952; Marshall to Judd, May 15, 1952, GCMRL/G. C. Marshall Papers [Retirement, General].) The following January Marshall thanked Judd for sending a report about the activities of the organization's Hong Kong and Taiwan offices. Marshall considered the report "impressive" and expressed an interest in meeting its author "in order to have him explain to me some of his views regarding cooperation in the proposed program." (Marshall to Judd, January 12, 1953, ibid.) See pp. 799–800.

402

To General James A. Van Fleet April 15, 1952
[Washington, DC]

Dear Van Fleet: You have my profound sympathy in the matter of your son.[1] I do hope it works out in the end with his return to the family unscathed.

I hardly know what to tell you, except to express my admiration for the manner in which you have carried yourself through this distressing business. Your position has made it very difficult for you, and your attitude has been altogether splendid.

With warmest regards and all my prayers and hopes for the future, I am, Faithfully yours,[2]

G. C. M.

GCMRL/G. C. Marshall Papers (Retirement, General)

1. Captain James A. Van Fleet Jr. had been shot down during a night bombing raid over Korea and was missing in action.

2. "I greatly appreciate your beautiful message of sympathy and hope," Van Fleet replied. "I gain strength in the knowledge that Jim, Jr., was performing his duty as he

clearly and correctly saw it—the same as thousands of other American casualties in Korea. He would have been unhappy otherwise." (Van Fleet to Marshall, May 5, 1952, GCMRL/G. C. Marshall Papers [Retirement, General].)

Marshall sent a copy of his letter to Helen Moore Van Fleet. "I have sent the foregoing to your husband. There is little I can add to it for you. I know you are all courageous, and I think your faith will carry you through the uncertainties of this period." (Marshall to Helen Van Fleet, April 15, 1952, ibid.) Captain Van Fleet was declared presumed dead in 1954. ("James A. Van Fleet, Leader in Korean War, Dies at 100," *New York Times*, September 24, 1992, p. D24.)

403

TO MRS. JOHN B. WILSON | April 21, 1952
Pinehurst, North Carolina

Dear Rose: I have been planning to have you and John—and the children if they can manage it, come down during the big North and South Amateur Golf tournament. Now so much of the unexpected has developed that, aside from your possibilities, I am so uncertain as to dates that I am writing this description of the situation so that when I do telephone you will have this "background" information.

Katherine was going into the hospital for a thorough examination as soon as we returned to ~~Pinehurst~~ Leesburg about May 1st. However, Clifton took such a serious turn ~~from~~ for the worse on his return from convalescing at Palm Beach that he was taken to the Walter Reed and is in a most serious state, painful and probably fatal.[1] Katherine therefore went up to Washington last Monday (I took her) and entered the hospital herself. She has had a week of exhausting tests, 36 Xrays I believe, but is comforted by the fact that she is in touch with Clifton. She transfers to the Hostess House there today.

I returned here Tuesday because a Charlotte firm were going to work on a big job of reconstruction in the Cottage due to termite destruction ($2000 worth!) So I have to be here. That makes the house a noisy place and later it will be a smelly place when they treat the surroundings with the poison.[2]

I have my sergeant orderly here and a cook, so except for the noise I am well established.

Unless I am called to Washington I would like to have you and John come down for the finals in the Golf tournament Saturday—36 holes commencing at 10 am.

You might come down Friday evening rather than early Saturday. If you came Saturday we could take care of the kids.[3]

I will telephone later in the week when I know more of my situation.[4] Love—
GCM

GCMRL/J. Page Wilson Collection; H

1. See pp. 674–75 and 676–78. C. J. George had informed Frank McCarthy on April 9 that Clifton Brown had been "suffering with a severe pain in his back, nausea, and profuse sweats at night," and his surgeon thus recommended that he be admitted to Walter Reed Army Hospital. George added that Mrs. Marshall would undergo "observation and treatment" at the hospital. "Nothing serious, but she felt that this would be a good time for

a check-up while Clifton is there." (George to McCarthy, April 9, 1952, GCMRL/G. C. Marshall Papers [Retirement, General].)

2. Marshall had written sarcastically to Frances McCoy on April 14 that he would return "to Pinehurst tomorrow for a pleasant social engagement with the termite hunters. I don't know who owns the cottage now, the termites or the Marshalls." (Marshall to McCoy, April 14, 1952, GCMRL/G. C. Marshall Papers [Retirement, General].)

3. Rose Page and John Wilson had three children: John Page; Thomas Morgan; and Celeste Rose, who was born on January 29, 1952. See p. 653–54.

4. Marshall attempted to call on April 24 "without success." (Wilson later recalled that she was in Florida with her husband when Marshall called. See Wilson, *Remembered*, 360.) He wrote the following day that his "invitation has to be canceled for Saturday. Clifton has sunk into a coma and his death is expected any day." Marshall was planning to "fly up to-morrow unless I hear more encouraging news." Marshall confided to Rose that it was "pretty sad for he [Clifton] is not old, has a fine job and (most confidentially) was engaged to marry Mary Lee," the great granddaughter of General Robert E. Lee. Mary Lee had been with Clifton "at Palm Beach while he was convalescing and flew up to Washington with him where he collapsed again and was returned to the hospital." (Marshall to Wilson, April 25, 1952, GCMRL/J. Page Wilson Collection; H.)

"I just wrote to Mrs. Marshall about Clifton," Wilson replied on July 25. "Honest to goodness, it's just so hard on her—both boys. It wakes me up at night—it just doesn't seem fair. There's no use in my keeping on writing about it but I'm so *damn* sorry." (Wilson to Marshall, July 25, 1952, GCMRL/G. C. Marshall Papers [Retirement, General].) See pp. 697–98.

404

Memorandum for the Secretary of the General Staff

April 30, 1952
Washington, DC

There is established in my office a GS [General Service]-7 position as administrative assistant and secretary to me.[1] I believe your office originally approved this position at GS-8, but reduced it to GS-7 when Mrs. Mildred Carlson could not qualify for a two-grade increase. Mrs. Carlson has resigned and I have asked my Aide, Major C. J. George, to recruit a replacement.

Major George serves in the dual capacity of Assistant Executive of the Defense Department for Secretary Lovett and Aide to me. At the time the secretarial position was established, it was anticipated that Major George would spend approximately half of his time supervising the day-to-day operation of my office and that the assignment of a secretary and administrative assistant at the GS-7 or GS-8 level would provide competent coverage. However, the heavy pressure of Major George's duties with Secretary Lovett and his lengthy absences from the country with Secretary Lovett have made it especially important that I have an administrative assistant and secretary of the highest caliber—a person upon whom I can depend to transact my business with the highest officials of the Government, with Congress, and with persons of importance in civil life.

Accordingly, it is my intent to assign additional responsibilities to the person selected.[2] I would appreciate having the position now established at GS-7 reallocated to GS-10 and am attaching a revised position description.[3]

GCMRL/G. C. Marshall Papers (Retirement, General)

1. Marshall's Pentagon office was located in room 2E664. Much of his correspondence was handled there by C. J. George and Mary Louise Spilman. Marshall explained in a 1953 letter to a correspondent that he often sent letters "to my office in Washington to be typed and mailed, as I want to keep a record of our correspondence, which is not convenient for me if I indulge in longhand letters." (Marshall to Owens, March 10, 1953, GCMRL/G. C. Marshall Papers [Retirement, General].) See Forrest C. Pogue, *George C. Marshall*, vol. 4, *Statesman, 1945–1959* (New York: Viking, 1987), 500.

2. Spilman, "who for four years was secretary to Felix Larkin, the General Counsel of the Department of Defense, and who is now serving as your secretary, has held the grade of GS-8 since March 5, 1950," George had written to Marshall in a separate memo, dated April 25. "I feel she is qualified and over-due for this promotion and, therefore, recommend that you sign the attached memorandum." (GCMRL/G. C. Marshall Papers [Retirement, General].)

3. Notation at the bottom of this memorandum indicates that it was originally prepared by the personnel office in the Office of the Secretary of Defense, revised by George, and "revised by GCMarshall." (Ibid.)

405

To Mrs. James Wadsworth[1] May 1, 1952
Washington, DC

Dear Mrs. Wadsworth: I just learned, in a telephone conversation with Mildred Bliss, of Wadsworth's serious illness.[2] I send you my deepest sympathy and to him, through you, my sympathy and devotion. I was dreadfully sorry to learn of this happening.

We are going through much the same experience with Mrs. Marshall's eldest boy, who is at the Walter Reed Hospital and not expected to live.[3] I brought her up from Pinehurst on the 14th and she has been staying at the Hostess House ever since.

I had to return to Pinehurst while some work was done on our place, and just flew in yesterday.[4] Faithfully yours,

GCMRL/G. C. Marshall Papers (Retirement, General)

1. James Wolcott Wadsworth was married to Alice Hay Wadsworth.

2. According to the *New York Times*, Wadsworth had undergone a "major abdominal surgery" in September 1951. Mildred Bliss sent a telegram to Marshall on April 29 informing him that Wadsworth was in the hospital again, adding that the situation was "hopeless and temporarily stationary." Wadsworth died on June 21, and Marshall attended his June 25 funeral at the Washington National Cathedral. ("J. W. Wadsworth Seriously Ill," *New York Times*, March 25, 1952, p. 12; "James Wadsworth, Ex-Senator, 74, Dies," *New York Times*, June 22, 1952, p. 1; "Notables Attend Wadsworth Rites," *New York Times*, June 26, 1952, p. 29; Bliss to Marshall, telegram, April 29, 1952, GCMRL/G. C. Marshall Papers [Retirement, General].)

3. The next day Marshall wrote to James W. Wickenden, headmaster of Tabor Academy in Marion, Massachusetts, that there were "no chances for recovery" for Clifton Brown. (Marshall to Wickenden, May 2, 1952, GCMRL/G. C. Marshall Papers [Retirement, Chronological].) See pp. 697–98.

4. See p. 695n2.

406

To Frank McCarthy May 6, 1952
Washington, DC

Dear Frank: Thanks for your letter of April 26 and the enclosures.[1] At the time I received your letter, I was dictating a note to Irving Berlin thanking him for the four tickets he made available to me for the Washington premiere of CALL ME MADAM.[2] I mentioned to him that you had sent me a copy of his song WHAT CAN YOU DO WITH A GENERAL and that I hoped soon to hear the words put to music.[3]

I am sorry that I missed you, but Katherine told me how delighted she was to see you.[4] I gave her your message, but there is little that any of us can do for Clifton, except try to keep his spirits up. This is the one thing that seems to amaze everyone, since he is very optimistic and determined to get well.[5]

George has made the necessary contacts with regard to the proceeds from THIS IS THE ARMY and, as soon as all the information is available, I will write Berlin as you suggest.[6]

You seem to have your hands full with your movie business and political effort.[7] I hope you will not push yourself too hard. There is just so much that the human body can stand, even a young one.

Katherine joins me in affectionate regards. Faithfully yours,

GCMRL/Frank McCarthy Collection

1. In his letter, McCarthy had given Marshall an account of his recent one-day trip to Washington. (McCarthy to Marshall, April 26, 1952, GCMRL/G. C. Marshall Papers [Retirement, General].)

2. Marshall wrote to songwriter and composer Irving Berlin that he and Mrs. Marshall were "delighted with the show. The spontaneity, gayety, and wit of the performance were far above par." (Marshall to Berlin, May 6, 1952, ibid.) The Washington *Evening Star* reported that Clifton Brown's fiancée, Mary Lee, and her mother, Helen, attended the performance with the Marshalls. ("Senators and Socialites at Opening," *Evening Star*, May 6, 1952.) See p. 695n4.

3. McCarthy also related that "The other day Irving Berlin sang me a song he has written for a new movie. I thought you might get a laugh out of it, so I asked Irving to send me a copy of the lyrics." (McCarthy to Marshall, April 26, 1952, GCMRL/G. C. Marshall Papers [Retirement, General].) "What Can You Do with a General?" would be sung by Bing Crosby in the 1954 movie *White Christmas*.

4. "I had time to go out to Walter Reed for a little visit with Mrs. Marshall and Molly [Winn] Monday afternoon," McCarthy wrote, adding that Mrs. Marshall's "morale seemed good. When I told her I was going to call you, she said I should tell you she was getting along fine." (Ibid.)

5. "I wish there were something I could do to cheer her in her present worry about Clifton," McCarthy added. (Ibid.) See next editorial note.

6. Berlin had mentioned to McCarthy that he had never seen an accounting of how the money earned by *This Is the Army*, Berlin's 1942 Broadway musical and 1943 motion picture, which Marshall had authorized, was used. Proceeds of almost $10 million had benefitted Army Emergency Relief. McCarthy suggested that Marshall "ask Major George to have the appropriate agency in the Department of Defense make up some sort of report" for Marshall to send to Berlin. (Ibid.)

Two days later, C. J. George wrote to Berlin on Marshall's behalf, clarifying that "the money received is deposited in the General Welfare Fund and is used for loans or, if the situation necessitates, an outright grant." The Korean War had led the organization to spend "well over $1,200,000 last year." (Marshall to Berlin, May 8, 1952, GCMRL/G. C. Marshall Papers [Retirement, Chronological].) Berlin replied that he appreciated the response and was "particularly happy to know that it is of use in the present Korean situation." (Berlin to Marshall, May 21, 1952, GCMRL/G. C. Marshall Papers [Retirement, General].)

7. McCarthy had gone to Washington "at the request of the Messrs. Zanuck, Goldwyn, and Warner . . . to attend a meeting of the State Finance Chairman of the Eisenhower drive. We are trying to raise funds for the campaign here and I am the fourth member of the committee." (McCarthy to Marshall, April 26, 1952, ibid.) Darryl Zanuck, Samuel Goldwyn, and Jack Warner were Hollywood movie studio executives. See p. 671n6.

CLIFTON S. BROWN died on May 11, never having recovered from an operation on his lung in February. He was thirty-eight years old, and a lieutenant colonel in the army reserves at the time of his death. Services were held at the Fort Myer, Virginia, chapel on May 13, with interment in Arlington National Cemetery. For background on Clifton Brown's illness, see pp. 674–75, 676–78, and 694–95.

On May 19, Marshall wrote to Major General Paul H. Streit, commanding general at the Walter Reed Army Medical Center, to express Mrs. Marshall's and his "deep appreciation for the many kindnesses you and the members of your staff showed her son. We know that he received the finest of care and the best of treatment." (Marshall to Streit, May 19, 1952, GCMRL/© Marshall-Winn Collection.) Similar letters, drafted by C. J. George on the Marshalls' behalf, were sent to the attending physicians and Major General Wallace H. Graham, President Truman's personal physician, who had kept the president informed of Clifton Brown's condition. Mary Louise Spilman composed and sent letters to the five nurses who had cared for Clifton Brown. "We feel so helpless in the presence of advanced cancer such as Mrs. Marshall's son had," Streit responded on May 23, "our treatment of course was only palliative." (Streit to Marshall, May 23, 1952, ibid.) The Marshalls received and General Marshall acknowledged 245 letters and cards of condolence on the death of Clifton Brown. ★

407

To Harry S. Truman — May 29, 1952
Leesburg, Virginia

Dear Mr. President. We will be delighted if Margaret and you—and of course Mrs. Truman if she has not yet gone west, will drop in Sunday morning next—and stay to lunch. The last time you would not break bread with us. Please arrange to do so this time.[1]

Mrs. Marshall is delighted with the prospect.[2] With great respect, Faithfully yours,

G. C. Marshall

GCMRL/G. C. Marshall Collection (Truman); H

1. Truman had written to Marshall on May 9 that he and his daughter, Margaret, "were about to drive down to your place last Sunday," but he "thought on account of Mrs. Marshall's son being ill you would probably be with him." (See previous editorial note.) Marshall apologized for the delay in his reply on May 21 and admitted that Clifton's death "and a bout which I am now fighting against the flu have left many things undone." He assured Truman that the president would be welcome at Leesburg anytime, especially "while the spring blooming is at its best." (Truman to Marshall, May 9, 1952, and Marshall to Truman, May 21, 1952, GCMRL/G. C. Marshall Papers [Retirement, General].)

Truman wrote on May 26 that he hoped "you have recovered from the flu." He wondered if he and his daughter could "organize a Sunday morning drive so as not to interfere with your plans or Mrs. Marshall's we may do what we have done in the past—take a drive to Leesburg and stop in and see General and Mrs. Marshall." (Truman to Marshall, May 26, 1952, GCMRL/G. C. Marshall Collection [Truman].)

2. "I did not receive your note until nearly noon yesterday and I was working my head off on a safety speech to be delivered this morning," Truman responded in longhand on June 2, explaining why he had not kept the June 1 date proposed by the Marshalls. "I hope you and Mrs. Marshall will give us a 'rain check.'" (Truman to Marshall, June 2, 1952, GCMRL/G. C. Marshall Papers [Retirement, General]; H.) See photo #16.

The president also mentioned that he "had quite a meeting with Ike yesterday. I'm not so sure he is happy over his decision." (Ibid.) General Eisenhower had retired from active service on May 31. Secretary of Defense Lovett, General Bradley, and Secretary of the Army Pace also attended the June 1 White House meeting with Truman and Eisenhower. See p. 671n6.

408

Recorded Remarks for the Congress of European American Associations[1] — June 3, 1952 [Leesburg, Virginia?]

I regret that it has not been possible for me to be present, in person, with you at this Conference of the Congress of European-American Associations.

The leadership of such statesmen as your illustrious speaker today, Dr. Spaak, guarantees a growing appreciation of the mutual dependency of nations.[2] The Council of Europe, the North Atlantic Treaty Council, the European Defense Council, and the Organization of European Economic Cooperation under the Schuman Plan are impressive evidences of this.[3] It is further exemplified by the common desire of the West to negotiate a peace treaty for Austria; to terminate the state of war with Germany and to welcome Germany into the European community.

However, no such endeavors can be effective without full appreciation of the spiritual values that unite us in the New World with the older civilization which you represent.

The European community is conscious of the variety of national characteristics it includes. The proximity of your nations and their related histories provide a common understanding.

On the other hand, the United States, because of its geographic location, its youth, its unusually rapid development, has not yet sufficiently enjoyed the benefits of intimate associations such as the nations of Europe have experienced. We are a nation whose blood lines stem principally from the Old World, but it is not generally realized, I think, that we have developed a spiritual and cultural pattern of our own creation which has been confined largely to the North American continent.

Undoubtedly the average, educated European is intimately acquainted with the cultural history of France or the religious upheavals so significant in the past history of the Netherlands, for example. Unfortunately, such intimate knowledge, which makes for understanding and mutual appreciation, is not general in Europe in regard to the United States of America. Today, when modern communications have shrunk distances, it is very important that we do what we can to promote such understanding. In this task, the Congress of European-American Associations is playing a very important role.

One more comment I would make regarding mutual understandings among our peoples, or the lack of such understandings. I ask you to keep in mind that millions of the citizens of my country have spent many months, years as a matter of fact, in the British Isles and Western Europe. They have lived intimately with your people on the farms and in the towns and the cities. In this matter, for evident reasons, there has not been a corresponding exchange. In other words, while you know much of each other, you know far less of the American and his way of life than he does of you.[4]

In the letter inviting me to attend this meeting, you referred to the accomplishments for the program which was commonly referred to as the Marshall Plan. I appreciate your comments and assure you that Americans were motivated in their endorsement, their authorization of the plan by a keen sense of mutual responsibility and moral obligation. It was not merely a question of economics. It represented far more than that.

It is my belief that no plan, economic or political, can be effective unless it is strongly influenced by spiritual and moral considerations. In the political debates over financial authorizations these are often lost sight of, seemingly ignored. But they constitute the fundamental basis for the plan.

Too frequently, because of political emphasis in public debates upon the material things, it would seem that those material advantages are the goal rather than the *means*; that they are the master rather than the servant. It might seem that on our side of the Atlantic we place too much faith in physical strength and too little in the fundamental, moral and spiritual values which are necessary to such successes.

Those who have an intimate knowledge of the American people know that this is not the case.

You are dedicating your efforts to a wider dissemination of such knowledge. In a broader sense, you are working for the brotherhood of man.

I fully realize the great, the world importance of your endeavor. I wish that I could join with you in person today.[5]

GCMRL/G. C. Marshall Papers (Retirement, General)

1. "Ever since you made your world resounding speech from Harvard University which culminated in the birth of the now famous Marshall Plan, it has been the most fervent and

universal wish of the grateful peoples of Europe to acclaim the man, who by his foresight and sagacity lifted our war ravaged continent from the brink of economic chaos and anarchy, which loomed as a dark and constant threat, during those first perilous and difficult post-war years," began a long letter from Hans Fr. Nielsen, president, and J. G. van Heurck, secretary general, of the Congress of European American Associations. (Nielsen and van Heurck to Marshall, February 25, 1952, GCMRL/G. C. Marshall Papers [Retirement, General].) Fifteen associations representing twelve European countries had met in London on September 22 and 23, 1951, to adopt the charter of the Congress of European American Associations. (Congress of European American Associations, London Assembly, ibid.) The letter continued with an invitation for "a European tour" by the Marshalls to coincide with the first annual meeting of the congress, to be held in Oslo, Norway, from June 25 to 27, 1952. (Nielsen and van Heurck to Marshall, February 25, 1952, ibid.) "Unfortunately, I cannot see my way clear to accept the obligations such a program would entail," Marshall had responded on April 4. (Marshall to Nielsen and Heurck, April 4, 1952, ibid.)

On April 16, C. J. George contacted the Office of the Secretary of State to explain that Marshall had been asked to record remarks to be played at the meeting in Oslo. If the State Department agreed Marshall should "comply," C. J. George asked if the department would "be good enough to develop a talk." Public relations adviser for the British Commonwealth and Northern Europe Robert Donhauser forwarded a draft statement on May 9. Marshall recorded his heavily edited version of the remarks on June 3. (George to Asbjornson, April 16, 1952; Donhauser to George, May 9, 1952, ibid.)

2. Former prime minister of Belgium and honorary president of American Belgian Associations Paul-Henri Spaak gave an address titled "The Relations between U.S.A. and Western Europe."

3. See p. 676.

4. Marshall had explored a similar theme in a 1948 speech to the Association France–États Unis. See *Papers of GCM*, 6: 610–12.

5. "Your voice came exceedingly well over the loud-speakers," Frank Darvall, vice president of the Congress of European American Associations and director-general of the English-Speaking Union (ESU) of the British Commonwealth, reported on July 1, "and both what you had to say, and the way you said it, made a deep impression." Marshall replied that he was glad his words "were received sympathetically." (Darvall to Marshall, July 1, and Marshall to Darvall, July 9, 1952, ibid.)

409

Remarks at the 200th Birthday Celebration of Winchester, Virginia[1] — June 6, 1952, Winchester, Virginia

It seems to me I should make some mention on this memorial day of my previous connection with things Southern and of Virginia and Winchester in particular.

In 1897, I first came to know Winchester. A Kentucky aunt had nursed and married a Union Colonel. He promoted a job for my father in the iron, coal and coke development in West Pennsylvania.[2] Though all the other members of my family were born in Kentucky, I appeared north of Mason's and Dixon's line and lived my boyhood there. At 16 I moved on Winchester enroute to Lexington and the Virginia Military Institute. During a summer visit to springs in Virginia, Colonel Charles Marshall, one-time aide to General Lee, had persuaded my parents in favor of the Virginia Military Institute, to which my older brother preceded me. He had been born in Kentucky, so he fared well there, but I was received as a damn Yankee and was more or less hazed and baited for my entire four years.

Twice a year I changed cars and railroads in Winchester. I first changed from the Baltimore & Ohio in Martinsburg to the Norfolk & Western. Then I changed here back to the B. & O. to Strasburg; again transferred there to the Southern Railway; and finally changed back to the B. & O. in Harrisonburg for Lexington, where I always wound up with a heavy coating of cinders after hours of screenless day coaches, and coal-burning locomotives.

But, to get back to Winchester. There was a two or three hour delay here, and I always spent it on the veranda of the old Taylor House. There was a hack to and from the depot. But no taxis, no buses, no encouragement to see the town. I knew no one in Winchester, and strange to say, I never found any intimates from Winchester during my four years at the Virginia Military Institute.

So, twice a year I shuttled back and forth, with the Taylor House veranda as my way station. I am inclined to think that I must have lacked imagination or initiative to make so little of those opportunities. But each year I did become increasingly aware of the historic significance of this community and the Valley; of Washington during his days of command at Cumberland, responsible for protection against the Indians along the length of the Shenandoah Valley; of Jackson and his world famous campaigns; and a long list of great events of those Civil War days.

Then, strange to say, I faced a crisis here in my military career, and I am going to take you into my confidence and tell you what a close call I had in your town and on what little things one's future sometimes depends.

Forty-four years ago I came East from the Staff College at Fort Leavenworth, Kansas, with members of that year's class. We were supplied Army mounts at Manassas and our tentage and mess were managed for us by a troop of cavalry from Washington. It was a military-historical ride, and we crossed Fauquier County through Front Royal to Middletown, thence south to Strasburg and Tom's Brook, and north again to Winchester—on through Berryville and Charlestown to Harper's Ferry, across the Potomac into Happy Valley, Maryland, back east over Crampton Gap, and back westward again via Frederick over Turner's Gap to Antietam—then to Williamsport and Hagerstown, and across Monterey Gap and down through Cashtown, of great historic significance to Gettysburg.[3] There were no paved roads in those days, and we had a wonderful ride through fertile and beautiful country, crossing five mountain ranges.

When our agreeable expedition reached Winchester, we camped on the fairgrounds and were given a day to rest the horses. One member of the group had many friends here, and he delivered an invitation from some unknown and unnamed young ladies for a basket picnic—we each to furnish the horse and buggy the young lady to provide the basket supper. Our rendezvous was on Apple Pie Ridge, as I recall, and it was a perfect setting for a moonlight night. We returned to town about midnight and had an impromptu dance at someone's house, my recollection being confined to the old grandmother who got up and dressed and came down to provide the music.

When we reached the fairgrounds, there was a delay in the arrival of the colored boys to take over the buggies, so some genius suggested that we occupy our time with a battery drill, buggies for caissons. We carried out the idea at a gallop with many loud commands. The caissons were certainly rolling along, when our commanding officer, a brilliant but very serious-minded type, appeared in his pajamas and called a halt. We subsided instantly and took our reproof.

Today, you honor not only those who sacrificed themselves to our future, but particularly, you honor those men who with their women and even with their children, gave all that they had in defense of the Southern ideal. Half fed, half clothed and half equipped at times, they made a name, a reputation for the South of courage and gallantry, which all of you enjoy and profit today because of how they lived and fought some 90 years ago. Winchester was constantly in the midst of the struggle because of its geographical location, its importance in those days, and its closeness to the Potomac River.

Your kinsmen saw the Federal forces coming and going, largely going for the first three years of the war. They saw their beautiful valley devastated, and they lived through the long, lean years of the slow recovery period.

Pride in the courage and sacrifice of its sons—pride in the great military victories of the early years of the war—enormous and ever-continuing; pride in the courage, quiet brilliance and superb Christian example of its great leader, General Lee—upheld the country. But what a tremendous change and effect would have followed from a national policy not dedicated largely to revenge.

The commercial development of the North was so rapid, so multitudinous, as it were, that the people of the North found little occasion to brood over the South. The war, in general, had touched no more than the extreme southern edges of the North. Whatever the loss of men and the consequent disruption of families, the North had no land and home scars to serve as daily reminders. A small Indian fight on the western frontier aroused and seemed to hold more interest than the colossal struggles of the Civil War.

Try and think out what would have been the situation today in our country if a policy of restoration, of help and assistance had governed the days immediately following that terrible War Between the States. It is both fascinating and tragically depressing to surmise on the result of such a policy. Western Germany, a national suicide of destruction, material and governmental, is well out of the woods—as a matter of fact, far ahead in production—within 6 years, in spite of every Soviet effort to prevent this. Italy and Japan are well on their way to a fine recovery, not to mention the recovery of the Western European States, Greece, and Africa.

Many here at home strongly disagreed with the course we followed in these matters, but, when I see the measure of these few years abroad and think of the half-century and more of the desperate struggle of our own people in the Southland, I can but bitterly regret the past procedures and thank God for our present efforts.

"Marshall Makes Luncheon Talk on City's 200th Anniversary," *Winchester Evening Star*, June 6, 1952, pp. 1, 3.

1. The *Washington Post* reported that more than three hundred people gathered in the local armory to hear Marshall give the luncheon address at Winchester, Virginia's bicenten-

nial celebration on June 6. ("General Marshall Talks on South at Winchester," *Washington Post*, June 7, 1952.) The complete speech is not in the Marshall Papers. The text reproduced here was excerpted in the *Winchester Evening Star*.

2. Marshall's father's sister Elizabeth had married Colonel John Ewing and was living near Pittsburgh in 1869. (Pogue, *Education*, 9–10.)

3. The Cashtown Inn functioned as Confederate General A. P. Hill's headquarters from June 29 through the morning of July 1, 1863.

410

TO HARRY CLIFTON BYRD[1]

June 18, 1952
[Leesburg, Virginia]

Dear Dr. Byrd: I am taking the liberty of approaching you with regard to the possibility of a scholarship at American University for a young Chinese in whom I am much interested.

His name is James H. C. Lo, and he is 30 years of age. He was in charge of the Embassy where I lived for a part of a year in China in 1946, having the entire care of the staff and housekeeping and everything of that nature. He also had charge of my summer place in the mountains. He was concerned with arrangements involving a great many people, many more than we would think of in this country.

Lo has been a student at the Washington Missionary College in Takoma Park for two years. He has pursued a course in business administration. His subjects include the following: Business Law, Principles of Accounting, Intermediate Accounting, Fundamentals of Education, Economic Geography, Medical Air, Health and Hygiene, and a Bible course.

He managed to escape from China—where, of course, there would have been a price on his head because of his service to me—to Hongkong and finally succeeded, through the help of several people, including Mrs. Marshall and myself, to get transportation across the Pacific and the Continent for this course at the Washington Missionary College.

He has done exceptionally well there considering that he has to work exceedingly hard to make his tuition. By very industrious application in the Bakery last summer and this summer in the Hospital at Takoma Park, he manages to get along.

In China, he was appointed by representatives of the Generalissimo and not by me.

He hopes to develop himself for hotel work, as he has a considerable ability along this line, particularly as to personality.

He is a handsome fellow and absolutely dependable. For example, after he had been in this country a year, he sent us a check to repay us for the money we had put forward for his transportation over here. When we returned the check to him, he insisted upon re-submitting it and said that he could make his way and preferred to have it on that basis. Incidentally, the first year he spent at the Missionary College, he won a so-called scholarship financed by the District Rotary Clubs.

I can speak of him in the highest terms as a man of great promise, once given the opportunity.

If there is any possibility of his obtaining such a scholarship, I hope you will consider him carefully.[2] Faithfully yours,

GCMRL/G. C. Marshall Papers (Retirement, General)

1. Harry Clifton Byrd was president of the University of Maryland from 1935 to 1954.
2. Byrd responded on June 29 that "it would be a pleasure to help" Lo "if possible. Probably the best procedure would be to suggest that he drop by the office here at College Park to talk with me, sometime, at his convenience." (Byrd to Marshall, June 29, 1952, GCMRL/G. C. Marshall Papers [Retirement, General].) Marshall sent identical letters on June 25 to Reverend J. Hunter Guthrie, S.J., and Cloyd Heck Marvin, presidents of Georgetown and George Washington Universities respectively, and James J. Robbins, acting president of American University. All three institutions are in Washington, DC.

American University Provost Donald Derby notified James Lo on August 27 that he had been awarded a scholarship from funds "made available by the Missionary Emergency Fund which is interested in assisting students of strong Christian principles and motivation." (Derby to Lo, August 27, 1952, ibid.) Lo attended but did not complete his studies at American University. See p. 871–72.

411

TO LEWIS CARTER BURWELL JR.

June 18, 1952
Washington, DC

Dear Burwell: I have your letter of June 9 concerning General Andrews, and I shall commence by saying that I am *not* to be quoted.[1]

I made General Andrews G-3 in the War Department, put him in command in the Caribbean, and sent him as our senior at Cairo as part of an educational experience. He was, of course, a possibility for command in Europe, but that assignment to England was too far in advance of the time of decision. He was practically a certainty for command of our Air in Europe. British Air command, at the start, in France was a certainty, and American overall command later on a certainty. A Britisher had to be in Tedder's place, Deputy to Eisenhower.

My best to that nice wife of yours. Her beautiful geraniums are on our terrace, where we have most of our meals.[2] Faithfully yours,

GCMRL/G. C. Marshall Papers (Retirement, General)

1. Burwell, who lived in Pinehurst and was associated with Resort Airline Inc., had written to Marshall on behalf of his "close friend," former air force Colonel Ramsay Potts, who had "served as chief of staff of the strategic bombing survey to Germany and Japan. He has recently been serving as a consultant to General [Hoyt] Vandenberg." Potts, Burwell explained, had agreed to write two articles for an air force magazine and had requested that Burwell pose Potts's questions to Marshall concerning Lieutenant General Frank Andrews (USMA, 1906), who had been "put in command of the European Theater of Operations." According to Potts, "General Andrews was being mentioned in some circles as a contender for the position of overall commander of invasion forces and I believe, was very highly regarded by General Marshall." Andrews had been killed in a crash in Iceland in early 1943, but Potts wondered whether there was "any possibility" that Andrews "would have been given the job of commanding invasion forces against Normandy in place of General Eisenhower, and failing this, is there any possibility that he would have been the overall air commander in place of Tedder or Leigh Mallory, or failing this, overall U. S. Air Commander?" (Burwell to Marshall, June 9, 1952, GCMRL/G. C. Marshall Papers

[Retirement, General].) Andrews was one of the founders of the US Army Air Corps and had served on Marshall's general staff from 1939 until Marshall sent him to Panama in November 1940. In 1941 he became commander of the Caribbean Defense Command, and in January 1943 he took Eisenhower's place as commander of all US troops in the European Theater of Operations. For more on Andrews's May 3, 1943, death, see *Papers of GCM*, 3: 678. Air Chief Marshal Sir Trafford Leigh-Mallory, commander in chief of the Allied Expeditionary Air Force and air commander for the Allied invasion of Normandy, had been killed in a November 1944 crash en route to Ceylon.

2. Edith Branson Burwell was Lewis Burwell's wife.

412

To Clarence Cannon[1]

June 20, 1952
[Leesburg, Virginia]

Dear Mr. Chairman: Just the other day, a special meeting of the American Battle Monuments Commission was called by me to discuss current matters of interest and, particularly, the appropriations bill for the Commission now before Congress.

The meeting brought out that the appropriations requested were submitted to the Senate, rather than in the normal procedure to the House, and, pursuing this point, I found that this was not done purposely, but rather as a matter of timing.[2] It seems that the staff at the Commission were pressed for time and the request for funds was not finalized in time to be included in the House Bill and, to avoid being left out completely, it was immediately sent to the Senate. I am sorry that this happened, and, unfortunately, neither I nor the other members of the Commission were aware of these circumstances.

I am in complete accord with the request for appropriations, including that part which concerns the matter of dedication ceremonies. I hope that you will give generous consideration to including the funds for the ceremonies and that you will act favorably upon the bill.

The work of the Commission abroad is moving forward as rapidly as time and funds will permit. It has been the hope of the Commission that our cemetery at Suresnes, France, could be dedicated in September of this year.[3] I think it is important that we dedicate, as soon after completion as possible, these monuments to our war dead, particularly since many pilgrimages are scheduled for this coming Fall.[4]

I will appreciate every consideration you can give to the efforts of the Commission. You have my genuine thanks for this kindness, as well as the many others over the years which also involved us. Faithfully yours,

GCMRL/G. C. Marshall Papers (American Battle Monuments Commission)

1. Representative Clarence Cannon was chairman of the House Committee on Appropriations. "After the discussion with Mr. Cannon's secretary yesterday there appeared a fair prospect of getting the desired appropriation for the dedication ceremonies," Marshall had written in a note to C. J. George on June 18. "The secretary felt it would be highly desirable for me to write a note to the Chairman" of the Appropriations Committee, which controlled the ABMC's budget, "not detailed proposals but intelligent reference to the situation." Marshall then requested that George "draft such a letter and telephone it to me." (Marshall

to George, June 18, 1952, GCMRL/G. C. Marshall Papers [American Battle Monuments Commission].)

2. The ABMC budget had been briefly discussed in the Senate on June 18, 1952. (HJ Res. 483, *Congressional Record* 98, pt. 6, 82d Cong., 2d sess., 7451.)

3. Suresnes Cemetery is located five miles west of the center of Paris. See pp. 726–27.

4. "I am still waiting to hear what action the Congress will take with respect to the funds for a dedication ceremony," General North had written to Marshall on May 27 from France. "But meanwhile we are starting to make tentative plans." (North to Marshall, May 27, 1952, GCMRL/G. C. Marshall Papers [American Battle Monuments Commission].)

SECURING FUNDING for the American Battle Monuments Commission remained a concern for several weeks, as did managing personality conflicts between staff members and commissioners. General North wrote to Lieutenant Colonel Charles B. Shaw, officer in charge of the ABMC in Washington, about the budget on June 20 and to Marshall on June 23, when North indicated he wanted to discourage involvement of commissioners other than Marshall during preparations for the dedication of the memorial to American dead at Suresnes on September 13. (See pp. 722–23.) North cited potential problems with "division of authority and responsibility" and expressed concern about "demands upon our limited personnel and transportation" when his staff was already extremely busy. (North to Shaw, June 20, 1952, and North to Marshall, June 23, 1952, GCMRL/G. C. Marshall Papers [American Battle Monuments Commission].) ABMC Commissioner Harold A. Keats of Fort Lauderdale, Florida, who had been head of AMVETS volunteer veterans' organization in 1948 and 1949 and was AMVETS liaison officer to the White House from 1949 to 1952, had apparently championed the appropriation bill and was interested in helping with preparations in France. On July 7, Marshall sent a memorandum to C. J. George stressing that the introduction and "follow up on the legislation (no direct advisement of committee members of the House)" had been "poorly managed." Marshall credited Keats with saving the appropriation bill, "if it has been saved." Marshall concluded that "Shaw seems to have been legislatively asleep and now North has become extremely jealous of power." (Marshall to George, memorandum, July 7, 1952, ibid.; H.) See previous document.

On July 11, Marshall wrote to Keats to express his "appreciation for the job you did in connection with the matter of appropriations. It was on your initiative—and I consider you responsible—that what appeared to be a lost cause was rectified." (Marshall to Keats, July 11, 1952, ibid.) He also encouraged Keats, who was due to leave for France on September 1, to support General North. "I think you can be of great assistance in making the dedication a success; however, General North, who has been in Europe for several months, has already accomplished a great deal of the preliminary work. Therefore, it is important that there be no confusion in arrangements, in keeping with the Committee's program. You should not only cooperate with him, but accept his leadership in the implementation of the program." (Ibid.) See pp. 724–28. ★

413

To Queen Frederica of the Hellenes

June 25, 1952
[Leesburg, Virginia]

Your Majesty: I was very much pleased and interested to receive your letter, and immensely gratified and flattered by your observation regarding me, personally, and my services. I won't elaborate on this last other than to comment on the great pride I feel in the knowledge of your good opinion of me.[1]

I have delayed writing this letter waiting for a photograph to be finished, one in colors, that I wish to send you. It has not yet been completed, but I will probably get it off next week. I am taking the liberty of sending you two, one of me alone and one, most informal, of Mrs. Marshall and myself.

We were delighted and deeply appreciative to receive the two photographs of you, both of which are excellent, and the informal one charming.

I am a little puzzled by the serious part of your letter in that you are careful to state that the fact of your writing as frankly as you did to me must be carefully guarded, because I do not know exactly how to make profitable use of the information you recited. However, I think I may find a satisfactory procedure. Certainly, your situation is very complicated, as well as serious.[2]

I was relieved to find that the General Frederick incident had not embarrassed His Majesty or you, though it may be you were being merely kind in what you had to say about the affair.[3]

Mrs. Marshall has not been too well this Spring, suffering from a severe pain in her back. A complete hospital examination revealed nothing wrong in any respect other than as a result of pressure, and she was given a supporting harness, I suppose you would call it. This proved, at first, too tight and did more harm than good, but now, with a refitting, she is getting along very much better.[4] Incidentally, she has had an extremely hard time. Her oldest and remaining son (the other boy was killed in Italy) died from cancer four weeks ago.[5] Her brother was operated on for a possibly malignant tumor the day after her son's death.[6] Now her son-in-law, a Colonel in the Army, has just been operated on for a back injury due to polo, which has been threatening his retirement for the last four years. He is under orders for Korea, and Mrs. Marshall's only daughter, his wife, is engaged in packing up their household things, and she chose this moment to fall over something and sprain her ankle, so she is on crutches.

This is quite a list of calamities, but, gradually, things seem to be working out.

I see that you went to Turkey and the press reports a very successful visit.[7] We are spending August at Santa Barbara, California, and then are due in Paris September 13 for the dedication of the first of the World War II American Military Cemeteries.[8] I am the Chairman of our Battle Monuments Commission and, therefore, have to be present on that occasion. Also, I will probably have to make an inspection tour of all of the cemeteries in England, France, Belgium, Luxembourg, Germany, Italy, and Africa that are under construction at this time.

With warmest regards from Mrs. Marshall and me to you and His Majesty, and with great respect, Faithfully yours,

GCMRL/G. C. Marshall Papers (Retirement, General)

1. Frederica had expressed in a May 7, 1952, letter to Marshall her "high opinion and esteem" for Marshall and former South African Prime Minister Field Marshal Jan Christian Smuts, who had died in 1950. (Papanicolaou, *Frederica*, 420.) See *Papers of GCM*, 6: 662.

2. Frederica had emphasized to Marshall that the letter she had sent on May 7, in which she had written at length about internal politics in Greece, should not "fall into the wrong hands." (Ibid.)

3. See also pp. 664n2 and 675.

4. "Modern orthopedic appliances seem to have good effect on many ailments," Marshall had written to his friend Leonard Nicholson on May 21, confiding that Mrs. Marshall "had to be fitted with one and is now more comfortable than she has been in years." (Marshall to Nicholson, May 21, 1952, GCMRL/G. C. Marshall Papers [Retirement, General].)

5. See pp. 697–98 and *Papers of GCM*, 4: 468.

6. Tristam Tupper was Katherine Tupper Marshall's brother. His company had published her memoir, *Together: Annals of an Army Wife*. See *Papers of GCM*, 5: 667–68.

7. "King Paul and Queen Frederika of Greece ended a triumphal week-long state visit to Turkey today," the *New York Times* had reported in June. ("Greek King Ends Visit to Turkey," *New York Times*, June 16, 1952, p. 3.)

8. When he died, Clifton Brown had been engaged to Mary Lee, whose mother, Mrs. George Bolling Lee, had invited the Marshalls to visit her in August in Santa Barbara. See pp. 695n4, 718–19, 725, and 727–28.

414

TO CHESTER WILMOT[1]

July 7, 1952
[Leesburg, Virginia]

My dear Wilmot: I must apologize for my long delay in thanking you for the copy of your book.[2] I purposely would have delayed answering until I read the book, but, in addition, so many other things intervened that I have not even completed reading it yet. After I saw you, we had a death in the family—Mrs. Marshall's remaining son—and she and I were, in turn, staying at the hospital for three weeks or more until his death.[3] Then, I had three speeches and trips to make, and a great deal to do here on the place.[4] With an acute local labor shortage and a long delay in getting started on the spring clean-up and planting, I have ranked a little better than a manual laborer.

I will address myself to your questions now (I have numbered them for convenience in reference):[5]

[*1. Do you agree with the view that the Allies should never have invaded North Africa but should have concentrated on carrying out ROUNDUP in 1943?*]

(1) Very hard to answer in view of the now known fact that Russia survived the fall, the winter saved Moscow, and the miracle of Stalingrad completely reversed a desperate situation: In July 1942, the destruction of the Russian Army, unless the pressure was eased in some way, was commonly accepted as inevitable. As the Russian situation developed, it was far better that we did not attempt the desperate effort involved in the Sledgehammer operation.[6]

[*2. Do you feel now that the Allies made a mistake in not being militarily prepared to take advantage of the political opportunity created by the overthrow of Mussolini?*][7]

(2) I don't understand the question.

[*3. Was your opposition to operations in the Balkans based wholly on military grounds, or were you influenced by the fear that Mr. Churchill would involve the United States in a political venture that was no concern of the United States?*][8]

(3) Both—the mountainous country and dispersion of effort, and the political implications.

[*4. Did you feel that Mr. Churchill's advocacy of operations in the Balkans was actuated by a desire to forestall the Russians in this area? If so, when did this desire become evident to you?*]

(4) Yes.

[*5. Was this question ever raised in the Combined Chiefs of Staff or in your conversations with Mr. Churchill?*]

(5) If you mean the political factors, I don't recall such a Combined Staff discussion.

[*6. When Mr. Churchill proposed that General Eisenhower's armies should drive on to Berlin was this question decided entirely on military grounds by the Joint Chiefs of Staff, or was it determined in consultation with the president and the State Department?*]

(6) As I recall, it was dealt with in a general discussion with the President. I think Mr. Churchill advocated ignoring the previously agreed areas (a London agreement). The Joint Chiefs of Staff were opposed to this as a breach of faith based on suspicion. It meant, we thought, greatly increased American losses unless we virtually threw the Russians down and made a separate surrender deal with the Germans. The Churchill suspicion seems to have been entirely correct.

[*7. Do you think now that you were right to insist that "the single objective should be quick and complete victory"?*]

(7) Yes.

[*8. When the question arose of American forces advancing into Prague, was this matter referred to the Combined Chiefs of Staff or was it decided entirely by General Eisenhower in the field?*]

(8) I don't recall.

I would add this general comment to your discussion re logistics in connection with the movement of troops from Italy to France: I think you were reaching your conclusions more by a slide rule technique than is acceptable in solving situations in war.

With apologies for my long delay in acknowledging your letter and the book, Faithfully yours,

GCMRL/G. C. Marshall Papers (Retirement, General)

1. Australian-born journalist Chester Wilmot had recently published a military history of World War II, entitled *The Struggle for Europe*, that was highly critical of US wartime strategy and policy vis-à-vis its British and Soviet allies. On April 26, he wrote to Marshall in Pinehurst, while visiting the US Air Force Ground School near Southern Pines, North Carolina, to request a meeting on the following day. "You may have seen from the reviews that a number of controversial issues have developed out of the book," Wilmot explained, "and I should value the opportunity of talking with you about certain aspects of Allied strategy during the War." (Wilmot to Marshall, April 26, 1952, GCMRL/G. C. Marshall Papers [Retirement, General].) Marshall agreed and met with Wilmot on the morning of April 27. Later that day Wilmot wrote again to thank Marshall for spending "so much of your time talking with me" and for speaking "so freely and so frankly. I realize that you were talking 'off the record', but I am nonetheless grateful to you for giving me such valuable background information." (Wilmot to Marshall, April 27, 1952, ibid.)

2. "When I return to New York I shall send you a copy of my book and I hope you enjoy reading it even though you will not agree with all its interpretations or conclusions," Wilmot had written on April 27. "After you have read it, I should be most grateful if you could find the time to send me a note about any points that seem to you to have been mis-stated or mis-interpreted by me," as he planned to make "some corrections for a new edition that is being produced in England in the autumn." (Ibid.) *The Struggle for Europe*, originally published by Collins in London in 1952, was published later the same year in the US by Harper.

3. See pp. 696–98.

4. See pp. 679–80 and 701–4.

5. "I left you this morning with some further particular questions," Wilmot's April 27 letter concluded, "and I should regard it as a great favour if you could send me a short note answering those points that we did not have time to consider. If you find that you can't manage this, I shall of course understand, but I am most anxious to ensure that future editions of my book do not go to press with any mistakes uncorrected." (Ibid.) Wilmot had included two pages of questions with his letter but Marshall responded only to questions posed on the second page, where he had added numerals. Wilmot's unanswered questions concerned Russia's entry into the war against Japan. (Ibid.)

Wilmot's questions are inserted in bracketed *italic* type in the text preceding each of Marshall's replies.

6. ROUNDUP had been the codename for a planned cross-Channel invasion of Europe in the spring of 1943. SLEDGEHAMMER was the codename for a much smaller cross-Channel operation in 1942. Marshall strongly opposed the alternative invasion of North Africa in 1942 on the grounds that it would not relieve any German pressure on the Red Army and that it would make ROUNDUP impossible in 1943, but he was overruled by Roosevelt. For numerous documents regarding this controversy, see *Papers of GCM*, 3.

7. Italian dictator Benito Mussolini had been overthrown after the Anglo-American invasion of Sicily in July of 1943.

8. For the numerous wartime controversies regarding and US opposition to operations in the Balkans and Eastern Mediterranean, see *Papers of GCM*, 3 and 4.

415

To General of the Army Dwight D. Eisenhower — July 12, 1952
Leesburg, Virginia

Dear Eisenhower: Congratulations on your fine victory. Katherine and I have followed your course with intense interest.[1]

As you no doubt realized I have carefully refrained from any communication with you because of a continued effort to keep entirely clear of political affairs or implications. But more than that, I felt because of the vigorous attacks on me by various Republicans any communication with you might be picked up as the basis of some strictures detrimental to your cause.[2]

With my best wishes always, Faithfully yours,

G. C. Marshall

DDEL/Dwight D. Eisenhower Papers (Papers as President, Ann Whitman File, Name Series, Box 21)

1. The previous day Eisenhower had secured the nomination as the Republican candidate for president. (W. H. Lawrence, "Eisenhower Nominated on the First Ballot," *New York Times*, July 12, 1952, p. 1.)

2. "My very deep appreciation for your fine note," Eisenhower responded on July 17. "I venture a guess that if I had suggested, at the time you and I were working so hard back in the early spring of 1942, that one day I would be scratching my head over the political and economic problems of the country, with a view to leading a great political party to victory, you would have had me locked up as a dangerous character." (Eisenhower to Marshall, July 17, 1952, GCMRL/G. C. Marshall Papers [Retirement, General].) "I shall," he continued, "fight as hard as I can with the single limit on my efforts defined by honor, fairness and decency. I am firm in my belief that our government cannot stand the excesses that come about through one party domination for too long a time. Many of our present ills stem from this one single fact. But on top of this I am, of course, in disagreement with the present administration on many vital points of policy. Consequently I am buoyed up by the belief that I am performing a real service and I am doing my duty." (Ibid.)

416

To Tazewell Ellett

July 15, 1952
[Leesburg, Virginia]

Dear Ellett: I have received your letter of July 2 with the request that I accept your proposition to have my measurements taken as a preliminary to a monument.[1]

First, let me explain that I am entirely in agreement with Richard Marshall.[2] I would be much opposed to any thought of having such a measure undertaken during my lifetime. Next, I have no objection to the rather gruesome business of the measurements, but suggest that the matter be delayed until my return from Europe the latter part of October.[3] If you get in touch with me then, we can arrange a mutually convenient date.

I am too busy this month, and will be in California all of August. Then, I leave for Europe about September 5.[4] Faithfully yours,

GCMRL/G. C. Marshall Papers (Retirement, General)

1. Tazewell Ellett III (VMI, 1944), a realtor from Richmond, Virginia, had written to Marshall on July 2 "to confirm our conversation at the Institute during finals in June 1952." He explained that he was chairman of a committee assigned "to investigate ways and means of erecting a Statue of you in front of the 'Marshall' arch of the V.M.I. barracks." (Ellett to Marshall, July 2, 1952, GCMRL/G. C. Marshall Papers [Retirement, General].) See pp. 518–23.

2. Ellett had reported that VMI Superintendent General Richard J. Marshall had written that he had "some misgivings about General Marshall's reaction" to the statue and that

the matter "should receive earnest and careful consideration from the Board of Visitors." (Ibid.)

3. The committee, Ellett had persisted, wanted to be prepared "when the proper time comes" and requested that Marshall agree to be measured "at a time and place most agreeable to you." (Ibid.)

4. See pp. 708–9.

417

TO ANNA M. ROSENBERG

July 21, 1952
[Leesburg, Virginia]

Dear Anna: Thank you very much for your letter of July 8 and for the copies of the exchange of correspondence between you and Eisenhower.

I was very much interested in what he had to say and will discuss the matter with you when I see you next.[1] I hope that will be in the early part of September.

Mrs. Marshall and I will be on the West Coast when you return and will not get back to Leesburg until September 1. We leave again on September 4 for Europe. We will be abroad about six weeks, where I will participate in the dedication of our new World War II Cemetery at Suresnes and conduct an inspection of other American Battle Monuments Commission activities in Western Europe and North Africa.[2]

We will arrive in Washington from the West Coast at 11:45 on September 1, and, if it is convenient, perhaps we can get together for lunch before we leave for the country. ~~If this suggestion is not convenient to you, we will be coming into town in time for lunch on September 4.~~ We will fly to New York that afternoon, since we can take no chance on the weather, because we must be aboard the UNITED STATES by eleven o'clock the following morning.

I have asked George to send this letter to your next port of call. We do hope that you are having a pleasant and interesting trip. However, I suggest that you pace yourself and not do more than body and mind will allow.[3]

Affectionate regards, Faithfully yours,

GCMRL/G. C. Marshall Papers (Retirement, General)

1. Eisenhower had previously offered his support for the concept of UMT, both in relation to the 1951 bill (see pp. 208–9) and the 1952 bill (see *Papers of DDE*, 13: 1028–29). After transmitting his comments on UMT to Lovett during the House floor debate on the 1952 bill, Eisenhower qualified his statement to Anna Rosenberg on March 3, recommending that the Defense Department "avoid any reference to me and my opinions" if his February 28 statement contained anything "incompatible" with the department's plans. As he had not had adequate time to study the bill, he added that he had not included any statements about specific proposals since the possibility existed "that there could be some specific feature of the plan that I would earnestly oppose." (*Papers of DDE*, 13: 1028–29, 1040–42.)

Upon his retirement from the army in June 1952 in the midst of the Republican presidential primary elections (see p. 699n2), Eisenhower reaffirmed at a June 3 Pentagon press conference his support for UMT, but he admitted "that he had never understood how Universal Military Training and the Selective Service system could work concurrently," as the 1952 UMT bill had proposed. ("Eisenhower Retires with Defense Plea; Explains Air Stand," *New York Times*, June 4, 1952, pp. 1, 23.) According to Anna Rosenberg, Eisenhower also warned a reporter in Denver on June 19 "that 'the country has more to fear from universal military training than from a small professional army when it comes to the threat of creating a militaristic state,'" although the editors have been unable to verify a source for this quote. These comments had "somewhat disturbed" Rosenberg, she wrote to Marshall on July 8. Following the June 3 press conference, she had "drafted a letter" to Eisenhower "showing the contradictions between his former stand on UMT and the stand he is now taking," although she did not send the letter until learning of his June 19 comment. "I then sent him the original letter with a covering letter. I thought you might be interested in the answer I received from him today, which is difficult to understand. Evidently college professors have made a deeper impression on General Eisenhower than his life-long associates." (Rosenberg to Marshall, July 8, 1952, GCMRL/G. C. Marshall Papers [Retirement, General].) Rosenberg enclosed copies of both of her letters as well as Eisenhower's response.

"Constantly and always, I have insisted that there is nothing to fear from broadly based military training," Eisenhower responded to Rosenberg on July 1, but as he had previously stated, he did "not see how we can manage—at one and the same time—selective service and any system of universal military training." He also admitted his belief "that in justice to the nation and to the individual we should then adopt some form of universal military *service*." He only offered his support for UMT, "a system of training completely separated from the Army itself, because General Marshall and his civilian supporters convinced me that the pursuit of my own convictions would merely result in the defeat of everything." Eisenhower's "own *recent* contacts with a group of college Presidents and others who have been vitally interested in these matters, have led me to believe that we must review the whole situation in light of our present activities (including a costly and indecisive war), in an attempt to find a plan that will be directly related to our present requirements and will have a broad appeal to the people of the United States. I find that every questioner, these days, has a *different conception* of what we mean by UMT. We have argued the matter so long that the entire American public has become confused about the issues involved." Eisenhower concluded his letter by clarifying that he was responding only to Rosenberg's "short letter of the 25th that encloses a very long one which I can read only at a time when I have a bit more leisure. I shall study it carefully and when I have the opportunity to write again, you will hear from me further." (Eisenhower to Rosenberg, July 1, 1952, ibid. See also *Papers of DDE*, 13: 1269–70.)

2. See pp. 708–9 and 724–25.

3. "I am leaving for Europe and North Africa this week as there are several pressing and disturbing problems, and I will be gone for about three and a half weeks," Rosenberg had confided. (Rosenberg to Marshall, July 8, 1952, ibid.)

418

To General Matthew B. Ridgway — July 25, 1952
[Leesburg, Virginia]

Dear Ridgway: Thank you very much for your letter of July 19, in which you confirm the assignment of Walters as my Aide. He is extremely capable, and I am glad to have him.[1]

I was glad to receive your acceptance of my invitation to make the dedication speech, and your doing so pretty well firms up the program.[2]

Mrs. Marshall will accompany me on this trip, as will Miss Mary Lee, who was to have married Clifton in June.[3] We expect to be in Paris on September 12 and 13 and again before we go to England at the end of our trip. We sail from Southampton on October 10. We would be delighted to have dinner with you and Penny.[4]

We appreciate your hospitable thought of us and clearly understand the situation.[5]

I very much appreciate your offer of help, and particularly the fact that I am free to call upon you if the need arises.[6]

With warmest regards to Penny, the little man, and you, Faithfully yours,

GCMRL/G. C. Marshall Papers (American Battle Monuments Commission)

1. Ridgway had replaced Eisenhower as Supreme Allied Commander, Europe on May 31. On July 14, C. J. George had informed Ridgway of Marshall's travel plans and requested that Lieutenant Colonel Vernon A. Walters serve as Marshall's aide in Europe. (Marshall to Ridgway, telegram, July 14, 1952, GCMRL/G. C. Marshall Papers [American Battle Monuments Commission].) See pp. 707–8. Walters, an accomplished linguist who often translated for President Truman at meetings abroad and had assisted Secretary of State Marshall on numerous occasions, was serving under Ridgway at SHAPE, which Walters had helped establish. (See pp. 234–35) "Please tell the General how grateful and honored I am that he asked for me," Walters wrote to C. J. George on July 29. "You know how I feel about him. There is NOTHING I would rather do." (Walters to George, July 29, 1952, ibid.) See pp. 716–18.

2. Marshall had extended the invitation on July 15, which Ridgway accepted in his July 19 letter. (Marshall to Ridgway, July 15, 1952, and Ridgway to Marshall, July 19, 1952, ibid.)

3. See pp. 695n4 and 697–98.

4. "Please do plan while you are here to save Penny and me at least one evening for dinner and a chat," Ridgway had written on July 19. (Ibid.) See p. 405n2. On August 13, the Marshalls agreed to see the Ridgways on September 12, "which will afford us an opportunity to discuss the dedication ceremony on the following day." (Marshall to Ridgway, August 13, 1952, ibid.) See pp. 724–26 and 728–29.

5. Ridgway had regretted being unable to provide overnight accommodations for the Marshalls because their house, "while appearing large from the outside, has only three bedrooms which, with Matty and the nurse, denies us this great pleasure." (Ridgway to Marshall, July 19, 1952, ibid.)

6. "Please let me know of any possible way in which any of us can be helpful," Ridgway had concluded his July 19 letter. (Ibid.)

419

To William D. Hassett July 26, 1952
Leesburg, Virginia

Dear Hassett: I was sorry to hear of your resignation, though I suppose that was your personal desire to gain a little of peaceful surroundings and rest from many and serious daily demands.[1]

You first came to my personal attention through General Bedell Smith when he was my White House liaison officer, and I have grown through the years to admire and appreciate your qualities more and more.[2]

I hope your health is good so that you can enjoy your opportunities for relaxation.

Didn't you think Adlai Stevenson's two speeches, his "welcome" and his "acceptance" were of a high order of construction and effectiveness?[3]

Good luck to you and good health.[4] Faithfully yours,

GCMarshall

FDRL/Papers of William D. Hassett (General Correspondence); H

1. The *New York Times* had reported on July 16 that William D. Hassett had resigned at age seventy-two as secretary to the president, "ending his long service of blending fact and tact, literary phrase and biblical allusion" in the thousands of letters and other documents he had drafted for Presidents Roosevelt and Truman. ("White House Aide Ends Long Career," *New York Times*, July 16, 1952, p. 11.)

2. From 1939 to 1941, Smith served as one of Marshall's assistant secretaries of the General Staff and then secretary of the General Staff as well as unofficial liaison to the White House. In January 1942 he became secretary of the new Joint Chiefs of Staff and Combined Chiefs of Staff before his appointment as Eisenhower's chief of staff later that year. See *Papers of GCM*, 2: 509–10 and 3: 285, 289.

3. Illinois Governor Adlai Stevenson II had "electrified" the Democratic National Convention in Chicago with his opening day speech on July 21. (James Reston, "Stevenson Speech Sends Him to the Fore," *New York Times*, July 22, 1952, p. 1.) Five days later Stevenson accepted his party's nomination for president. (James Reston, "Governor Accepts," *New York Times*, July 26, 1952, p. 1.) "I share your enthusiasm for Adlai Stevenson," Hassett replied to Marshall on August 7. "He is a rare combination of courage, conscience and conviction with vision and imagination too." (Hassett to Marshall, August 7, 1952, GCMRL/G. C. Marshall Papers [Retirement, General].)

4. "I shall always cherish the memory of my association with you and the friendship which has grown out of it," Hassett assured Marshall. "The lesson of all these White House years is that few things are to be taken seriously and nothing is ever to be taken tragically." (Ibid.)

420

TO LIEUTENANT COLONEL VERNON A. WALTERS — July 31, 1952
[Leesburg, Virginia]

My dear Walters: I am delighted, and so is Mrs. Marshall, that General Ridgway has made it possible for you to be with me during my month abroad.[1] I went over a schedule General North sent me, amended it, and told them to send you a copy. From it, you can gather a general idea of what I plan to do, and for Mrs. Marshall and Miss Lee also.[2]

I will add these additional remarks:

(1) We land at Le Havre on the morning of September 10, and I hope you can arrange transportation for us from there to Caen.

(2) Possibly we will have to remain one or two days (September 14 and 15) in Paris after the dedication, though not necessarily.

(3) I do not want to impose on Ambassadors.[3]

(4) I think we should probably arrange to fly from Epinal to Florence, make a 24-hour stop there, and fly on to Rome.[4]

(5) Whether or not Queen Frederika goes through with her invitation (she was without the knowledge at the time of her writing that I was due in Europe, but she does know it now), I do not know. If so, we should fly from Rome to Athens, and back, preferably, to Naples.[5]

(6) Mrs. Marshall thought it would be nice to spend our spare time on Capri until we must start north. If so, maybe someone at the Embassy might have knowledge of someone who has a small place on Capri that they would rent to me for five or ten days, depending on the time available—maybe longer. Such an arrangement would be preferable to the publicity and intrusions of a hotel over a lengthy period.[6]

(7) I plan to ask General Ridgway for a plane to carry me from Naples to Carthage, Africa, for a two-or three-hour stop there; then north to Cannes for a 24-hour stop while I inspect the Draguignan Cemetery; then north to the vicinity of Cambridge, England, for inspection of that cemetery. From there, we could motor via London to Southampton.[7]

I have in mind starting the ladies off with you from Naples or Rome a day or two in advance of my departure for Carthage, motoring along the Italian coast and Grand Corniche drive to Cannes, meeting me there.[8] We can talk all this over when we reach Italy and know definitely about a possible Athens diversion.

(8) The Battle Monument people should be able to provide a car for me in each locality and all over France. I wish you would see if you can procure an Army car for the entire trip on the Continent and another in England.[9] I have already outlined the plane requirements. I suggest that you get and keep in touch with General North, who is in Paris at the Battle Monument headquarters.

I think this covers most of the details. With your usual resourcefulness, you will meet the others.

With warm regards, Faithfully yours,

GCMRL/G. C. Marshall Papers (American Battle Monuments Commission)

1. See pp. 234–35 and 714–15. C. J. George had written to Walters on July 22 "on a personal and confidential basis," explaining that "Because I have the General's power of attorney, I am well aware of his financial situation, which in no way equals his prominence." George continued, "The General will be operating on a per diem basis, which you know from experience is not adequate, but Mrs. Marshall and Miss Lee will have to pay their way" on the ABMC inspection trip. George wrote to Walters again on August 4 requesting that Walters keep receipts for expenses. (George to Walters, July 22, 1952, and George to Walters, August 4, 1952, GCMRL/G. C. Marshall Papers [American Battle Monuments Commission].)

2. For more on Marshall's itinerary, see pp. 724–28. Marshall had informed North that Katherine Marshall and Mary Lee would "probably not do the cemeteries—except that Mrs. Marshall wants to visit Patton's grave" in the Luxembourg American Cemetery. Luxembourg had been headquarters for Patton's US Third Army during World War II. (North to Marshall, July 21, 1952, and Marshall to North, July 31, 1952, ibid.)

3. "I understand the General's desire not to impose on Ambassadors," Walters wrote to George on August 8, "but I still think there will be a lot of invitations when they hear he is coming, not only from Ambassadors but also from governments and organizations." (Walters to George, August 8, 1952, ibid.)

4. The ABMC cemetery at Epinal is located four miles south of Epinal, Vosges, France, on the west bank of the Moselle River. In Florence, Italy, the cemetery is located seven miles south of the city.

5. "Confidentially," Marshall wrote to North, also on July 31, "it may be that we will go to Athens for a personal-private visit with Queen Frederika and King Paul, which may occupy two or three days, or maybe a week." (Marshall to North, July 31, 1952, ibid.) See pp. 708–9 and next document.

6. Capri is an island in the Tyrrhenian Sea off the Campania region of Italy. US Ambas-

sador to Italy Ellsworth Bunker, Commander in Chief of the NATO Forces in Southern Europe Admiral Robert Bostwick Carney, and "the American Express man formed the informal Board" to secure a villa, Marshall confided to C. J. George on September 24. "It is amusing but effective." (Marshall to George, September 24, 1952, ibid.; H.) See pp. 728–29.

7. "With regard to the aircraft, I have ascertained that if General Marshall is travelling on Dept. of Defense orders there will be no difficulty in making a plush C-54 of General Ridgway's available to him," Walters informed George. (Walters to George, August 8, 1952, ibid.) The North Africa Cemetery is near the site of the ancient city of Carthage, Tunisia. Rhone Cemetery is in the city of Draguignan, France, 28 miles west of Cannes. The American military cemetery three miles west of Cambridge, England, is 130 miles from the port of Southampton.

8. The Grande Corniche is a famous coastal road on the French Riviera.

9. "A comfortable car and driver will be made available by General Ridgway for the duration," Walters told George on August 8. "This is over and above the car General North already has." (Walters to George, August 8, 1952, ibid.)

421

To Queen Frederica of the Hellenes — August 1, 1952
Leesburg, Virginia

Your Majesty: I was tremendously interested in your detailed account of the visit to Turkey. While the press have very favourable comments it's too bad they could not have had the full flavor of your letter.[1] I have been waiting Acheson's return to have a talk with him and orient myself on the State Department reactions but his immediate departure for Hawaii has made that impossible at this moment.[2]

You were most kind and generous to give me the benefits of your personal description and reaction to a venture of such great importance to the world at this time. I am deeply appreciative.

We leave early to-morrow morning for Santa Barbara, California for the full month of August, visiting the mother and fiancée of Mrs. Marshall's remaining son who died in May.[3] Then we sail from New York on the S.S. "United States" for Havre, France on Sept 5th. I preside at the dedication of the U.S. War Memorials in the military cemeteries abroad, which is scheduled to take place at Suresnes, France on Sept. 13th. After that I turn to inspecting construction of memorials of the U.S. cemeteries in Western Europe and at Carthage, Africa. We sail for Rome from Southampton, England on October 10.[4] Miss Lee (a great granddaughter of General Robert E. Lee) the young lady I referred to above is going with us.

The heat here has been terrific, almost without precedent and I hope cool Santa Barbara will give us a rest and act as a restorative.

I hope General Ridgway will visit you in Athens. He is a fine fellow and a tremendous fighter. He has been with me a good deal since the days he was a captain in my regiment in China, 18 years ago.[5]

I was much relieved at the outcome of the Republican and Democratic Convention in Chicago. Both candidates are especially fine men. I know them intimately as both have served me, Eisenhower of course with army and Stevenson when I headed the U.S. delegation to the United Nations.[6] We could not have found men of higher integrity, selfless spirit of sincere and broader knowledge of the world to-day. It will be, I suppose, an unusually hard campaign and just now there does not seem to be a marked favourite.

I was very glad to read your comments on the existing state of harmonious public opinion in Greece.[7] Remember what I once told you about your qualities when I had the temerity to speak with . . . frankness to a Queen? I have been proven right time and again since that conversation.

With warmest regards from Mrs. Marshall and me to you and His Majesty, and our love to the children.

With great respect, Faithfully yours,

G. C. Marshall

Lilika S. Papanicolaou, *Frederica, Queen of the Hellenes: Mission of a Modern Queen*, 426–27

1. See p. 709n7. "Greek-Turkish friendship has been put on a very personal basis," Frederica had written to Marshall on June 26. "Every day during our visit brought us closer together with the Turks. The public was quite touching, and the reception we got in Ankara and especially in Constantinople was beyond every description. We were surprised and delighted. You must remember that for 500 years, since the fall of Constantinople, no Greek King has ever entered into this town." (Papanicolaou, *Frederica*, 423.)

2. Acheson was meeting in Honolulu at the beginning of August with the foreign ministers of Australia and New Zealand. ("Acheson Trip Confirmed," *New York Times*, July 1, 1952, p. 6.)

3. See pp. 695n4 and 696–98.

4. See pp. 724–28.

5. See *Papers of GCM*, 1: 391n1.

6. See pp. 711–12, 715–16, and *Papers of GCM*, 6: 266.

7. "Our homecoming was also very satisfactory. We found that our people, completely overcome by the hospitality shown to us by the Turks, showed an enthusiastic and completely united approval of our decision to have gone on this Mission," Frederica had continued in her June 26 letter. "The Country is once again completely united in their approval of the King and Queen." (Papanicolaou, *Frederica*, 425.)

422

To Mrs. Henry H. Arnold — August 22, 1952
Santa Barbara, California

Dear Bee: I noted in the newspaper the other day that you have made a gift to the United States of Arnold's personal papers and that they have been presented to the Library of Congress. It was very good of you to make his writings available to the public.[1]

Seeing this item in the paper and being in California these past few weeks have brought you very much to mind, and it occurs to me that you will be interested in the outcome of a meeting of the Board of Trustees of the National Geographic Society several months ago.

While attending the meeting, I was struck with the thought of the Blythe effigies, which Arnold had told me about and pointed out from the air during the course of one of our inspection trips to the Southwest. I explained to the Board how impressed I was by these effigies and expressed wonderment about their origin. The Board felt that this unusual and interesting phenomenon should be publicized and almost immediately dispatched an expedition to the scene. It was headed by Dr. Frank M. Setzler, Head Curator of the Department of Anthropology [*Archaeology*] of the National Museum, who wrote an article which you will note from the enclosure was prefaced by a short foreword by me.[2]

I am sure that Arnold had mentioned these figures to you, and I am glad that what he pointed out to me years ago resulted in this article, in which I hope you will be interested. Katherine and I are having a most pleasant vacation here at Santa Barbara. We have certainly been fortunate, as the weather has been ideal.[3] We start back home on the eve of Labor Day, but will be there only three days, since we leave on September 5 for Europe, not returning home until October 15.[4]

It has been some time since we have heard from you, and I hope that you are well.[5]

With our warmest regards, Affectionately,

GCMRL/G. C. Marshall Papers (Retirement, General)

1. The *Washington Post* had reported the bequest on August 19. ("Gen. Arnold's Papers Presented to Library," *Washington Post*, August 19, 1952, p. 10.) See p. 47.

2. The meeting had taken place on December 20, 1950. Melville Bell Grosvenor, senior assistant editor of *National Geographic* magazine, had sent a draft of Setzler's article to Marshall on April 1, 1952, and requested that Marshall, as the "father of this project," write an introduction. (Grosvenor to Marshall, April 1, 1952, GCMRL/G. C. Marshall Papers [Retirement, General].) "I do not know whether or not this meets your request," Marshall wrote in an April 17 letter accompanying his draft introduction. "Have your man chop it up in any way that seems advisable." (Marshall to Grosvenor, April 17, 1952, ibid.) Marshall approved a slightly revised version of this draft on May 26; it appeared with Setzler's article, "Seeking the Secret of the Giants: A Flying Archaeologist Attacks the Mystery of Strange Figures, Visible as a Whole only from the Air, Outlined on Desert Mesas," in the September 1952 issue of *National Geographic*. (Marshall to Grosvenor, May 26, 1952, ibid.)

In his draft introduction, Marshall described the 1943 flight during which Arnold had told him "that one of his young pilots had described some curious figures" he had seen from the air, consisting of outlines of a man and of animals "carved in the rocky soil near the lower Rio Grande." Marshall and Arnold changed course to examine the figures and "circled them for a few minutes. They were as accurately described" in Setzler's article. What "interested me especially," Marshall noted, was the fact that these figures were visible only from the air, not from the ground. (Marshall to Grosvenor, April 17, 1952, ibid.)

3. "We had a smooth trip," Marshall had informed C. J. George on August 4. "Weather delightfully cool, very comfortably housed, surroundings lovely, completely relaxed. Mrs. M. already improving." (Marshall to George, August 4, 1952, ibid.; H.)

4. See pp. 708–9 and 724–28.

5. "It was such a pleasant surprise, today, to receive your letter and the copy of the September National Geographic Magazine," Bee Arnold responded. "The article and your introduction were most interesting for, during our tour at March Field, the effigies were a source of constant speculation and I was happy to see such a fascinating subject brought to light." (Arnold to Marshall, August 27, 1952, ibid.)

423

TO PAUL G. HOFFMAN

August 28, 1952
Santa Barbara, California

Dear Hoffman: Thanks for your letter of the 26th with the enclosures and thanks most emphatically for your generously strong statement regarding me personally.[1] I seem to be actively in the midst of this presidential campaign.[2]

Governor [Earl] Warren stopped by to see me the other day and expressed his regrets and apologies for the campaign of invective and misrepresentation directed against me. He also told me some of the convention business.

We leave Sunday night by air. Sail September 5th. In returning we sail from Southampton October 9th.[3] Our warmest regards and sympathy to Mrs. Hoffman, as for you I am always,[4] Faithfully yours,

G.C. Marshall

HSTL/Papers of Paul G. Hoffman; H

1. "The deposition I made in the McCarthy-Benton suit seems to have stirred up quite a bit of turmoil," Hoffman had written to Marshall in Santa Barbara on August 26. (Hoffman to Marshall, August 26, 1952, HSTL/Papers of Paul G. Hoffman.) The *Washington Post* had reported on August 20 that McCarthy was suing Benton for $2 million for libel and slander. See pp. 555–56 and 653. "'I consider those charges fantastically false,'" Hoffman said under oath, adding that "McCarthy's charge that 'the Marshall Plan made mincemeat of the Truman-Forrestal doctrine' to help free nations oppose communism has no basis in fact but 'flies squarely in the face of the evidence.'" (Murrey Marder, "Hoffman Calls McCarthy's Charges False, *Washington Post*, August 20, 1952, pp. 1, 9.)

2. Hoffman had been cochairman of the Citizens Committee for Eisenhower until the nomination; Hoffman then returned as president of the Ford Foundation. (Ibid.) "You may or may not have read the full account of the press conference held by General Eisenhower," Hoffman had written to Marshall. "It seems to me that he made emphatically clear (1) that he would not support any candidate whom he considered unjust, unfair and dishonorable; and (2) that he considered you a great man and a great patriot." (Hoffman to Marshall, August 26, 1952, HSTL/Papers of Paul G. Hoffman.) "'George Marshall is one of the patriots of this country, and anyone who has lived with him, has worked with him as I have, knows that he is a man of real selflessness,'" the *New York Times* quoted Eisenhower from his August 22 press conference in Denver, Colorado. "'I have no patience with any one who can find in his record of service for this country anything to criticize.'" (W. H. Lawrence, "Eisenhower to Back M'Carthy If Named but Assails Tactics," *New York Times*, August 23, 1952, p. 1.) See pp. 852–55.

3. See pp. 708 and 724–28.

4. "It was a great joy to see you and Mrs. Marshall and to meet Mrs. Lee and Miss Lee," Hoffman, who lived in Pasadena, about a hundred miles from Santa Barbara, had written. "We hope you are continuing to enjoy your stay in California." (Hoffman to Marshall, August 26, 1952, HSTL/Papers of Paul G. Hoffman.)

424

TO GENERAL OF THE ARMY DWIGHT D. EISENHOWER

August 30, 1952
Santa Barbara, California

Dear Eisenhower: I am concerned to have you know that I made no such comment as indicated in the attached clipping.[1]

G.C. Marshall

DDEL/Dwight D. Eisenhower Papers (White House Central Files, President's Personal File, 182, Box 935)

1. "Gen. Marshall Lauds Defense by 'My Boys'" was the headline on the clipping from an unidentified newspaper. The article, with a dateline of Santa Barbara, August 29, United Press, said that Marshall "was touched that his 'boys,'" Eisenhower and Democratic presidential candidate Stevenson, "defended him against the attacks of Sen. Joseph R. McCarthy of Wisconsin." ("Gen. Marshall Lauds Defense by 'My Boys'," unidentified clipping, DDEL/Dwight D. Eisenhower Papers [White House Central Files, President's Personal File, 182, Box 935].) At the bottom of Marshall's note, there is an annotation: "DDE has seen." (Marshall to Eisenhower, August 30, 1952, ibid.)

A similar article appeared the same day in the *New York Times*, and *Time* magazine repeated the story in its September 8 issue, supposedly quoting Marshall: "They are both my boys. I sent General Eisenhower to Europe. Governor Stevenson, with me while I was Secretary of State, gave valuable assistance on both the United Nations and our program for economic aid to Europe. My father was a Republican and my mother a Democrat, and my Army service has been so demanding that I have not had time to do much voting or take sides politically." ("Tributes Stir Marshall," *New York Times*, August 29, 1952, p. 10; *Time*, September 8, 1952, p. 53.) See pp. 738–39 and Pogue, *Statesman*, 496–97.

On September 3, Marshall wrote to Truman that he wanted the president "to know that the statement attributed to me about 'My boys' (Eisenhower and Stevenson) had no foundation. I gave no interviews. This was built out of a whole cloth." (Marshall to Truman, September 3, 1952, GCMRL/G. C. Marshall Collection [Truman]; H.)

425

To Brigadier General Thomas North — September 2, 1952[1]
Radio. — Santa Barbara, California

Reference your letters, memorandum, and cablegrams, with regard to invitation to speak from American Club of Paris, please express my regrets.[2]

As to matter of decorations by French government, I am querying Defense Department on this: however, I want it understood that I am not to receive any.[3]

Reference your letter of August 22 to George regarding official and social functions. We might accept a *few* official invitations, but social with old friends only. We can decide on the ground.[4] I approve your proposed program, except that I feel there are too many speeches listed.[5]

With respect to veteran organization and congressional participation, it was wholly impracticable to make any arrangements along the line you suggested; to wit: the designation of one each from both groups because of individuals' geographical locations and some departures from the continent. I believe you are in a better position to make appropriate arrangements.[6]

I received an invitation from Handy to visit Heidelburg and am wiring him that it is highly improbable that I will be able to include it in my itinerary; however, we can discuss this after my arrival.[7]

I have no objections to the disbursement of five hundred dollars to the Paris post of the American Legion for the purpose of assisting financially in the proposed reception.[8]

GCMRL/G. C. Marshall Papers (American Battle Monuments Commission)

1. The Marshalls were in transit from Santa Barbara to Leesburg on September 2. Most of the responses in this radio, sent by C. J. George, had been noted by Marshall on the original documents, probably while in Santa Barbara.

2. See pp. 724–28. General North had radioed Colonel Shaw on August 29 that the club wanted Marshall "to address it on any subject of his choosing and on any date convenient to him." (North to Shaw, radio, August 29, 1952, GCMRL/G. C. Marshall Papers [American Battle Monuments Commission].)

3. In his communication with Shaw on August 29, North had mentioned that "a suggestion has been made that the visiting commissioners" should receive decorations from the French government. North indicated that his "own policy has been to discourage award of foreign decorations" to ABMC personnel but that he "would appreciate chairman's reaction to this proposal." (Ibid.) On September 3, Marshall again cabled North to confirm that "your policy of discouraging such awards is concurred in. I think it best that we not be involved." (Marshall to North, September 3, 1952, ibid.)

4. North had queried George about whether "Mrs. Marshall (and the General) are likely to accept invitations for (a) official (b) social functions while in Europe" because he wondered "whether they will be in mourning." (North to George, August 22, 1952, ibid.) See pp. 697–98.

5. "Arrangements for the dedication ceremony are shaping up," North had written in a detailed memorandum on August 22, which included a tentative program suggesting that a welcome by US Ambassador to France James Clement Dunn, five addresses, a congressional greeting, and two benedictions would follow Marshall's introductory remarks. (North to Marshall, memorandum, August 22, 1952, ibid.) Dunn would represent President Truman and Secretary of State Acheson, whom Marshall had invited on July 28. (Marshall to Acheson, July 28, 1952, ibid.) At General North's suggestion, Marshall had also written to Major General James L. Bennett, chief of chaplains of the Department of the Army, to request "appropriate dedicatory language." Marshall mentioned that "chaplains of the three Faiths from our forces in Europe will participate" in the dedication. (Marshall to Bennett, July 28, 1952, ibid.)

6. North was also concerned that "the number of speakers would become excessive," particularly because "Mr. Keats and General Markey feel that each of the five veterans' organizations representatives who are to be the Commission's guests should make a two-minute address." Instead, North recommended that the veterans "elect one of their number to make a short address (5 minutes) for all of them. This will also justify a suggestion that the four members of the Congress elect a single speaker." (North to Marshall, memorandum, August 22, 1952, ibid.) In his September 3 cable to North, Marshall indicated that "It has been suggested that members representing veterans organizations and Congress be introduced individually on the platform and that they not be scheduled for any speech. I think this is an excellent idea and suggest that you plan the program along this line." (Marshall to North, cable, September 3, 1952, ibid.)

7. See pp. 145–46n2. "We greatly appreciate your invitation," Marshall told General Handy, but explained that "the schedule which is planned is fairly firm and I question the practicability of deviating from it." (Marshall to Handy, telegram, September 2, 1952, ibid.)

8. Marshall had previously indicated to North that the ABMC would not host a reception following the dedication. North responded that "this is appropriate, of course, in view of the solemn nature of the ceremony," but he suggested that the American Legion might hold a reception and asked whether the commission could contribute five hundred dollars to the event. (North to Marshall, memorandum, August 22, ibid.)

426

Article for *Oregon Journal*[1]

September 4, 1952
[Leesburg, Virginia]

Dear Mr. Eyre: Your letter of August 27 was awaiting me upon my return to Leesburg from a month's vacation at Santa Barbara.[2]

As you indicated, Mrs. Marshall and I do have very warm memories of our residence in the Northwest. Consequently, I am glad to send you the enclosed random thoughts, which you may or may not wish to use for the Fiftieth Anniversary of the OREGON JOURNAL.[3]

I should like to congratulate your paper on its achievement of so long a period of public service and acceptance.[4] Faithfully yours,

GCMRL/G. C. Marshall Papers (Retirement, General)

1. "I know that both you and Mrs. Marshall have a warm spot in your hearts for the Oregon Country," *Oregon Journal* Managing Editor David W. Eyre had written on August 27, explaining that the newspaper was planning a golden jubilee edition. "Would you be so good as to put a few of these remembrances and impressions down in print for a Journal article?" (Eyre to Marshall, August 27, 1952, GCMRL/G. C. Marshall Papers [Retirement, General].)

2. See pp. 708–9.

3. Noting the "pleasure and delight Mrs. Marshall and I found in that marvelously beautiful country and the charm and generous hospitality of its people," Marshall described his activities during the two-year period from 1936 to 1938 that he had been at Vancouver Barracks. (See Pogue, *Education*, 300–316, and *Papers of GCM*, 1: 513–607.) These included command of not only "troops at Fort Lewis and as far east as Missoula, Montana," but also "15,000 Civilian Conservation Corps young men and veterans scattered in camps" throughout the Pacific Northwest. "Bi-weekly inspection trips took us over that country time and time again" and enabled the Marshalls to meet numerous people and visit "wonderful fishing streams. These trips have remained a delightful memory." Marshall also noted that Brigadier General Charles H. Martin (USMA, 1887), then governor of Oregon, and his wife were "our close friends," and numerous others in Portland and Vancouver had "remained our intimate friends through the succeeding years. Altogether, we experienced one of our most delightful periods of Army service," one that the Marshalls looked back on "with additional warmth" given the "long years of fearful strain and struggle with a world in turmoil which has not yet subsided." Indeed, their time in the Northwest "appealed to us as a pleasant dream in comparison with the troubled days that followed. The best I can say today," he concluded, "is that we would love to live those two years over again, each day as it was, each of our friends as they were." (Article for *Oregon Journal*, September 4, 1952, ibid.)

4. Eyre wrote again on September 24 to thank Marshall for his "warm and delightful account" of his years in the Pacific Northwest. (Eyre to Marshall, September 24, 1952, ibid.)

LETTERS were sent above Marshall's name on September 4 to the presidents of American television networks informing them about the September 13 dedication of the memorial at Suresnes Cemetery. The message encouraged them to provide "adequate coverage for the benefit of both television and radio audiences of the United States. I believe that you can provide a great public service through such a presentation to the American people, especially those who have lost loved ones through war." (Marshall to McConnell, September 4, 1952, GCMRL/G. C. Marshall Papers [American Battle Monuments Commission].) "American, Columbia, and National Broadcasting Companies have acknowledged your letter," George cabled Marshall in Paris on September 12. "Their local people probably will be in contact with North's office." (George to Marshall, telegram, September 12, 1952, ibid.)

The Marshalls and Mary Lee (see p. 695n4) sailed from New York on the SS *United States* on September 5. Marshall's transportation expenses were covered by his ABMC travel budget, but Katherine Marshall and Miss Lee were guests of General John M. Franklin (see p. 174n2), who had written to Marshall on July 22 to extend "the courtesy of the Line" to them. (Franklin to Marshall, July 22, 1952, ibid.) See p. 717n1. "We had a delightful trip," Marshall reported to C. J. George on September 14. "Most agreeable people, luxurious accommodations and fair weather. Mrs. M. won a Bingo prize of $\$175^{00}$ and I won one of $\$230^{00}$ but had to divide it with another winner—the first time in my life I ever had any such luck." (Marshall to George, September 14, 1952, ibid.; H.)

After landing at Le Havre on September 10, where they were met by North and Walters, Marshall followed an itinerary that had been proposed by North on July 21 while Mrs. Marshall and Miss Lee went immediately to Paris with Walters. Marshall and North visited two cemeteries that day, including the Saint-Laurent Cemetery overlooking Omaha Beach and the English Channel at Normandy. The following day they left Caen and arrived in Paris by noon. (Ibid.; North to Marshall, July 21, 1952, ibid.)

Marshall met with French President Auriol the morning of September 12, then lunched with the Ridgways. That afternoon the Marshalls entertained fifteen guests for "drinks and tea," including US Ambassador to Luxembourg Perle Reid Mesta; Mildred and Robert Woods Bliss; Jacques Adelbert de Pineton, Comte de Chambrun since he had served as General Pershing's French aide-de-camp during World War I (see *Papers of GCM,* 1: 163n1 and 614n1), and his wife, Clara Eleanor Longworth; General North and his wife, the former Ann Ryan; and Frank McCarthy. The Marshalls, Mary Lee, and Frank McCarthy dined at the American embassy that evening. The next day, Foreign Minister Schuman hosted a lunch prior to the dedication for the Marshalls and their guests at the Ministry of Foreign Affairs, on the Quai d'Orsay. (Marshall to George, September 14, 1952, ibid.; H.)

Marshall had sent a memorandum assuring Secretary Acheson on August 1 that Marshall's remarks at Suresnes would be "in strict harmony with our International Policies." He requested that Acheson have "someone in your shop give me a series of paragraphs (not in speech form)" and also "any cautions you may have in mind." (Marshall to Acheson, memorandum, August 1, 1952, ibid.; H.) Undersecretary of State David K. E. Bruce responded with two pages of suggestions. "It might be useful to make references to the cooperative relations which are developing: (a) between France and the United States; and (b) throughout the Atlantic community," Bruce advised. "Stress should be laid on the fact that the mutual defense effort now underway is designed to avoid new wars," he urged.

"Specific references to Germany or other aggressor nations should be avoided. It may be useful to state in positive terms that the American military effort was directed against tyranny in general rather than particular nations," he counseled. "While a dedication ceremony is clearly inappropriate as a sounding board for obvious anti-Communist propaganda, this occasion offers an opportunity to rebuke the Commies for their current 'Americans, go home' campaign." (Bruce to Marshall, August 13, 1952, and Suggestions for General Marshall's statement at dedication of Suresnes Cemetery, n.d., ibid.) Marshall wrote back to thank Bruce for his suggestions. "I found them most helpful in the preparation of my talk." (Marshall to Bruce, August 25, 1952, ibid.) ★

427

Remarks at the Dedication of the Memorial in the Suresnes Cemetery[1]

September 13, 1952
Suresnes, France

My thoughts to-day turn toward recollections of the first memorial service to be held in France in an American military cemetery. The ceremony took place at Romagne on the 30th day of May, 1919, in the hastily prepared plot located in the center of the Meuse-Argonne battlefield. General Pershing presided.[2]

The war was very fresh in our minds that day. The ground still showed fresh scars of the battle. Our living soldiers were daily sailing home in large numbers. Every thought in our minds beyond the sad memories of the day centered on a return to America, to life in a peaceful world, a lasting peace for us and our descendants. That is what we had fought for, had crossed the Atlantic and come to France for.

Yet, on that very ground we were to resume the conflict. As a matter of fact one of our divisions returned here to occupy its exact sector of 26 years previously with the identical supporting division again on its left flank in its same old sector of long ago—a truly remarkable and, I think, significant coincidence. And the young lieutenant of the first mentioned division was now Corps Commander of the two. Later he was to lose his life leading our troops in far off Korea.[3]

What is it all about? Why these terrible repetitions? Living men of this generation, I fear, will never quite find the complete answer.

We are surrounded here by those who paid the price of our mistakes or misconceptions. They paid the full price and this must never be forgotten. Therefore, this ceremony to honor them to-day. To bow in our thanks to them. To show that their fateful contribution is not forgotten and that we are determined that their sacrifice will finally lead to genuine bonds of good will and good faith on this earth. Bonds that will bond us, all together, in a common cause, a common life in peaceful understanding where sovereign nations sink national differences in a fundamental, dominating resolution to live in peaceful concord.

There has been real progress in the last few years toward that end. There have been tremendous strides toward the spiritual unification of Europe. The men who lie buried here in some other world beyond our conception may be aware of the efforts we are making to promote peace and understanding. But I hope they are deaf to the propaganda demands that we living Americans go home and leave Europe to the mercy of a ruthless aggression. The dead cannot go home. They paid too great a price. And we will not go home until our friends here feel that our presence is no longer essential to their security, when we can leave a land free of terrors, a land where the dignity of the individual is supreme, where a feeling of good faith dominates life.[4]

GCMRL/G. C. Marshall Papers (American Battle Monuments Commission)

1. See pp. 707–8. The European edition of the *New York Herald Tribune* reported that a thousand people attended the dedication of the memorial to American dead at Suresnes. The new memorial, which cost five hundred thousand dollars, consisted of two wings with an interior sculpture added to the original memorial chapel, dedicated in 1923 to World War I dead by then ABMC Chairman General Pershing. (Marshall Peck, "Marshall: U.S. Will Not 'Go Home' until Freedom Abroad Is Secure," *New York Herald Tribune*, September 15, 1952, pp. 1, 3.)

After an invocation by army chaplain J. B. Murphy, Marshall presented Ambassador Dunn, who introduced representatives from Belgium, France, Italy, Luxembourg, the Netherlands, the Philippines, and the United Kingdom as well as the American Legion, AMVETS, American War Mothers, the Disabled American Veterans, the Veterans of Foreign Wars, and the World Veterans Federation. See p. 723n6. Brief addresses from President Truman and French President Auriol were read, followed by Marshall's introductory remarks. (Ibid.) Truman's comments were in the form of a letter to Dunn that George had drafted and Marshall then edited and sent to the president. (George draft of Truman to Dunn, revised by Marshall, August 22, 1952; George to Marshall, memorandum, August 25, 1952; and Marshall to Truman, August 27, 1952, GCMRL/G. C. Marshall Papers [American Battle Monuments Commission].)

2. "The 2,500 soldier dead at Romagne were honored by the attendance of a battalion of infantry, a battery of artillery and a regimental band," the *New York Times* reported on May 31, 1919. ("Our Soldier Dead Honored in France," *New York Times*, May 31, 1919, p. 3.) Pershing spoke at Beaumont Cemetery and declared the event "was probably the last time that Americans would assemble in detachments on the soil of France to render honors to American soldiers who had died fighting for freedom." ("Pershing Bids Adieu to Our Heroic Dead," *New York Times*, May 31, 1919, p. 15.) See *Papers of GCM*, 1: 190.

3. Marshall is referring to General Walton Walker, who had led a machine-gun battalion during World War I at St. Mihiel and the Argonne, then commanded XX Corps of Patton's Third Army in World War II. He died in Korea on December 23, 1950. See pp. 171n1 and 308–9.

4. Addresses by Marshal Alphonse Juin, General Ridgway, and French Premier Antoine Pinay followed Marshall's remarks.

THE DEDICATION, Marshall assured C. J. George just before leaving Paris, "went off very well." The next day the Marshalls and Mary Lee had lunch with Frank McCarthy, tea with the Ridgways, and dinner with the de Chambruns. (Marshall to George, September 14 [*15*], 1952, GCMRL/G. C. Marshall Papers [American Battle Monuments Commission]; H.)

Monday, September 15, his final day in Paris, Marshall devoted to presenting Medals of Freedom to twelve French and Belgian superintendents of ABMC cemeteries who had maintained the facilities during World War II "frequently at the risk of their liberty," General North had explained in a letter to Marshall on July

22. (North to Marshall, July 22, 1952, ibid.) North reported to George on October 1 that one of the superintendents was "so seriously ill that the General went to her apartment for a private ceremony—all of which is highly conducive to morale." (North to George, October 1, 1952, ibid.) After presenting the medals, Marshall had lunch with Marshal Juin, attended a reception at the American embassy, and dined with family friend Ann Robertson. See p. 677n5.

Marshall traveled with General North from Paris by air to inspect World War II cemeteries in the Netherlands, France, and Luxembourg. See p. 718n7. By September 24, the Marshalls and Mary Lee had visited Venice, where they "had a delightful stay," Pisa, and Florence, and arrived in Rome, where Marshall made "a round of official calls and lunch at the Foreign Office." He updated George on their plans and reported that "Walters has been perfect and invaluable." (Marshall to George, September 14 [*15*] and 24, 1952, ibid.; H.) From Rome, the Marshalls and Lee went to Anzio, where Allen Brown, Katherine Marshall's son who was killed by a German sniper on May 29, 1944, was buried. (See *Papers of GCM*, 4: 468 and 6: 601.) After Anzio, they planned to spend a week on Capri, where Frank McCarthy would leave them, at a villa owned by Alberto Albertini, "a rich industrialist, and incidentally Lord of the town Council," Marshall explained to George. (Marshall to George, September 24, 1952, ibid.; H.) See pp. 731–32. ★

428

TO MRS. JOHN B. WILSON

October 4, 1952
Naples, Italy

My dear Rose: After 8 days on Capri we came over here today preparatory to flying to Carthage, Africa and Nice, France to-morrow.[1] Your letter of Sept. 20*th* reached me here, via Major George at the Pentagon. We often use the expression "shocked" at such a time, but I am truly shocked terribly at your tragic news of Tom. You did not say what was the trouble so I assume it was heart. It is too hard to realize that the little boy I knew so well at 2400—16*th* Street, punted football with and took sled rides with, has beaten me to the end. With a wife and a fine family of children its hard to explain such workings of providence. Give Susie my affectionate sympathy. She had a fine man who I always admired, especially during the tough days in the depression.[2]

We have been traveling fast except for our rest on Capri. A villa and 6 servants were placed at our disposal and we had a truly charming time—Katherine, Mary Lee and my temporary European A.D.C. [aide-de-camp] Colonel Walters (speaks 7 languages.) Ridgway has loaned me his Constellation for all my flights, which makes European distances melt away. Flew from Nancy, eastern France, to Venice in 1¼ hrs![3]

We reach Niece [*Nice*], France to-morrow evening. Spend ~~Tuesday~~ Monday there (I inspecting a new World War II cemetery) and fly on to Cambridge, England Tuesday.[4] London that night. Lunch with Anthony Eden and dinner with Churchill Wednesday. We sail Thursday on the SS "United States" Thursday from

Southampton October 9th. Go from the ship straight to the airport in New York and fly to Leesburg. Move down to Pinehurst November 1st. Mollie and her family are there in the house she bought. Jim is on sick leave but soon goes to temporary, limited duty and then to the Far East or Germany in the Spring.

With my love and sympathy, Affectionately,

GCM

GCMRL/J. Page Wilson Collection; H

1. See the previous editorial note. Upon his return to the United States, Marshall wrote to Mr. and Mrs. H. J. Hayden that the cemetery at Carthage "has a beautiful location, looking out over the Mediterranean." He added that at their request, he had placed flowers at and photographed the grave of their son, Captain H. J. Hayden III, who had died on May 31, 1943, and was buried at the cemetery. (Marshall to Haydens, October 17, 1952, GCMRL/G. C. Marshall Papers [Retirement, General].)

2. See p. 146n1. "Unfortunately, this note carries tragic news," Wilson had written on September 20, notifying her godfather that her forty-five-year-old brother, Thomas Walker Page III, "died very suddenly after only one day's illness, on September 5." Page, a mining engineer, was survived by his wife, Susan, and three children: Celeste, Virginia, and Tommy. (Wilson to Marshall, September 20, 1952, GCMRL/G. C. Marshall Papers [Retirement, General] and Wilson, *Remembered*, 191.)

3. See pp. 716–17 and 718n7. Marshall reported to C. J. George on October 4 that their stay on Capri "was altogether delightful, lovely villa, skilled servants, beautiful scenery, etc. Had lunch with the famous English vaudeville star Gracie Fields at her beautiful place and she lunched with us yesterday." William and Edna Pawley had arrived in Naples on the airplane the Marshalls had been using, and they would "fly with us to Carthage and Nice" the next day. (Wilson to Marshall, September 20, 1952, ibid., and Wilson, *Remembered*, 191.)

4. Marshall had "no engagements in Nice," he wrote to C. J. George from Naples, although he suspected Katherine Marshall and Mary Lee "will motor along the Riviera with the Pawleys and Walters, play and lunch at Monte Carlo," while he inspected the Nice cemetery. (Ibid.) See pp. 731–32.

Madge Pendleton had requested that Marshall have his picture taken when he visited her brother Robert L. Shedden's grave at Cambridge Cemetery. General North had informed C. J. George on October 1 that "Mrs. Marshall has already asked me to get flowers, and a photo." (George to North, September 22, 1952, and North to George, October 1, 1952, ibid.)

429

To General Matthew B. Ridgway

October 12, 1952
at sea

Dear Ridgway: I wrote you a hurried note from London to express my thanks for all you did for Mrs. Marshall and me but I am going to do it again, more leisurely, to be certain that you are aware fully of my appreciation. The combination of cars, plane and Walters made our trip delightfully comfortable, one that we can always look back on with many choice memories.[1] Katherine stood the rather fast travel very well. I was fearful for her because she had not been at all well and under a great and sorrowful strain—and this recovery largely thanks to you.

Walters made everything smooth for us and added a great deal by his company. The fellow is really unique. He is really cursed by his unusual knowledge of languages, and Europe and Latin America, because his other conspicuous abilities are apt to be ignored. He would be an excellent staff officer in many capacities far beyond that of aide and interpreter.[2]

We had a beautiful sailing, a few rolls but not unpleasant. I am going from the dock direct to the plane and fly into Leesburg. Katherine's grandson, whose father was killed in the Alban Hills north of Anzio on the first rush towards Rome, developed polio three weeks ago. Fortunately the diagnosis was immediate and the treatment prompt so he is now home, with no muscular contractions, after two weeks in the hospital.[3]

We plan to leave Leesburg for Pinehurst N.C. October 31st or thereabouts for the winter. I will shoot for a week on Jim Bruce's island near Savannah, and for ten days with Baruch in So. Carolina during the Xmas season.[4] Otherwise no other plans other than horseback riding and watching famous golfers.[5]

With my love to Penny and you,[6] Affectionately,

G.C.Marshall

P. S. Maybe you saw Katherine' picture. She made the front page in a London, a Paris and a Rome paper riding a donkey—Michaelangelo, in Capri.[7]

USAMHI/Matthew B. Ridgway Collection (Series 2: Correspondence, Subseries 1: Official Correspondence); H

1. See pp. 714–15, 716–18,and 727–28. C. J. George advised General North on October 14 that he had met the Marshalls when their ship docked in New York. "They had a most pleasant trip and were most enthusiastic about their entire journey. They enjoyed themselves immensely." (George to North, October 14, 1952, GCMRL/G. C. Marshall Papers [American Battle Monuments Commission].) See next document.

2. "I agree with you on Walters and shall be alert to expand his sphere," Ridgway responded on October 19. (Ridgway to Marshall, October 19, 1952, GCMRL/G. C. Marshall Papers [Retirement, General].)

3. C. J. George had radioed Marshall on September 24 that Madge Pendleton's son Tupper had been hospitalized "with slight touch of polio. There is no, repeat no, paralysis and child should be home in two weeks. It is a minor case. No temperature and no definite ill effects." George sent another message on September 30 that Tupper had been released from the hospital and would return to school the following week. Marshall instructed George on October 4 to avoid making any arrangements for him and Mrs. Marshall in New York following their arrival, because "Katherine wants to hurry back to see Madge and Tupper and does not feel like undertaking a delay in N.Y. We will want to proceed direct from the dock to the plane." (George to Marshall, radio, September 24 and 30, 1952; Marshall to George, October 4, 1952, GCMRL/G. C. Marshall Papers [American Battle Monuments Commission].)

4. See pp. 669n1 and 743–44.

5. See photo #22.

6. "You were characteristically generous in writing first on the eve of leaving England, then again on arriving home," Ridgway responded. "Your description of plans for the weeks ahead sounds ideal." (Ridgway to Marshall, October 19, 1952, GCMRL/G. C. Marshall Papers [Retirement, General].)

7. The photograph had appeared in the *New York Herald Tribune* on October 5, 1952. "We saw through Walters' eyes the picture of Michaelangelo and had a good laugh," Ridgway added in his own postscript. (Ibid.)

430

To Anna M. Rosenberg

October 15, 1952
Washington, DC

Dear Anna: I have just this moment returned to the office, and on top of a stack of mail which was awaiting me I found your note of October 6 and the enclosure regarding the exemption from draft registration of students enrolled in military colleges. I read it very carefully and believe it fills the requirement.[1]

We have had a most excellent trip, and I was very much interested and encouraged by what I saw at our military cemeteries. Much of the work has been completed, although there are many problems which still have to be worked out. I thought the dedication of the memorial at Suresnes Cemetery went off very well, and I was delighted to see so many of our people in attendance.[2]

While I went about my inspecting, Mrs. Marshall and Mary Lee (she was betrothed to Clifton, Mrs. Marshall's son), accompanied by Colonel Walters, an officer on Ridgway's staff, went on a sightseeing tour. We joined up for our stay with Mrs. Mesta at Luxembourg and then went down to Venice, where we had a very pleasant time. We then went to Florence and Rome and on to Anzio, where we visited the grave of Mrs. Marshall's son, Allen. Then, through the kindness of an Italian industrialist, we occupied his villa on the Isle of Capri for ten days. We had lunch on two occasions with the famous English comedienne, Gracie Fields. She is a most delightful person and has a beautiful villa on the Isle. We then moved over to Nice and, while Mrs. Marshall, Mary, and Walters motored along the Riviera and visited at Monte Carlo, I went to Carthage and inspected the cemetery there. We arrived in London on the 7th and had lunch with Anthony Eden on the 8th and dinner with Churchill that evening. It was all very pleasant and, to add to the occasion, Mrs. Marshall celebrated her birthday. We boarded the liner at 9:00 a. m. on the 9th and moved to Havre to pick up more passengers, and had a very delightful voyage.[3]

Naturally, we are glad to be home and will leave for Leesburg in a few minutes, going by McLean, Virginia, so that Mrs. Marshall can see her grandson, Tupper Brown, who had an attack of polio while we were away. Fortunately, it was a very mild case and, although I have not seen him yet, I understand that he is getting along splendidly.[4]

It was very good of you to arrange for a dinner in honor of Mrs. Marshall and me and I will look forward to seeing you that evening, since I am not sure when I will be back in the building again.[5]

With affectionate regards from us both, Faithfully yours,

GCMRL/G. C. Marshall Papers (Retirement, General)

1. "At long last we have worked out a policy regarding the exemption from draft registration of students enrolled in military colleges," Rosenberg had informed Marshall, and enclosed a copy of "Provisions of the UMT&S Act as Amended, Relating to Military Colleges." (Rosenberg to Marshall, October 6, 1952, GCMRL/G. C. Marshall Papers [Retirement, General].) The provisions defined "military colleges" as those "colleges or universities which confer baccalaureate or graduate degrees; at which the average age of

the students at the time of graduation is not less than 21 years; which require all students to pursue military training throughout the undergraduate course and require all members of the ROTC to be habitually in uniform; which constantly maintain military discipline; which have as objectives the development of the student by means of military training and the regulation of his conduct in accordance with disciplinary principles." (Ibid.)

2. See pp. 726–29.

3. See pp. 724–26 and 727–29. "Everything was made so luxuriously comfortable for us that it was quite an enjoyable experience," Marshall wrote to thank General Franklin on January 9. "I tried to get something in the public ear regarding the [United States] Line at the time of the landing in New York, but the interest, I think, was in other things." (Marshall to Franklin, January 9, 1953, ibid.) See p. 739n1.

4. See previous document, n3.

5. George had radioed Marshall in London on October 7 that "Mrs. Rosenberg proposes dinner in Mrs. Marshall's and your honor October twenty-two, probably Alibi Club." (George to Marshall, October 7, 1952, ibid.)

431

To Jerry K. Nicholson[1]

October 20, 1952
[Leesburg, Virginia?]

Following statement released by me to press this afternoon: Leonard Nicholson's death came to me as very sad news.[2] I have the precious memories of four years of our intimate association as roommates at school, during which we never had a difference. I also have the memories of our many contacts through the following years. In a word, he was a very fine man—clean, honest, and of the highest integrity. He left a fine example of a good citizen.[3]

G. C. Marshall

GCMRL/G. C. Marshall Papers (Retirement, General)

1. Throughout 1951, Marshall and Leonard Nicholson had corresponded extensively on the issue of "the Mississippi River–Gulf Outlet and Mobile to New Orleans Intercoastal Waterway." (GCMRL/G. C. Marshall Papers [Secretary of Defense, Number Indexed, M200-4-36].) In 1952, however, their correspondence shifted to Nicholson's deteriorating health, and Nicholson's adopted son, Jerry, reported to Marshall on August 28 that his father was "extremely ill" and that his passing was "only a question of time." (Marshall to Leonard Nicholson, May 21, 1952, and Jerry Nicholson to Marshall, August 28, 1952, GCMRL/G. C. Marshall Papers [Retirement, General].)

2. Leonard K. Nicholson died in New Orleans on October 19. ("Leonard K. Nicholson Dies, Times Picayune Publisher," *Charleston Gazette*, October 20, 1952, p. 4.)

3. Jerry Nicholson thanked Marshall on October 28 for the "wonderful press release." He was "very happy to tell you that Dad passed very peacefully and was in no pain since he had the strokes right after the Labor Day holidays." (Nicholson to Marshall, October 28, 1952, GCMRL/G. C. Marshall Papers [Retirement, General].)

Another friend of Marshall, Hayden Bartlett Harris, a generous philanthropist and neighbor of the Marshalls in Leesburg who had retired as vice president of the Harris Trust and Savings Bank in Chicago in 1939, had died on October 5, 1951. Marshall had visited with Harris twice in the weeks prior to his death, first while on vacation on Cape Cod (see pp. 603–4), and then in September 1951 while Harris was a patient at a New York hospital. Following Marshall's visit in the hospital, Harris's wife, Lina, thanked Marshall for making "the great effort to come here & give Hayden those moments of happiness. You have so completely become his hero whom he idolizes, that holding your hand meant more to him than I am able to express." (Lina Harris to Marshall, September 22, 1951, GCMRL/G. C.

Marshall Papers [Secretary of Defense, Number Indexed, M200-6-5]; "Hayden B. Harris, 66, Was Chicago Banker," *New York Times*, October 6, 1951, p. 14.)

Harris's son Huntington, also a philanthropist and a neighbor of the Marshalls in Leesburg, wrote to Marshall on November 22, 1952, to request his opinion of Hayden Harris's health "prior to his death" in an attempt to reduce a potentially large tax burden on his father's estate. In his December 4 reply, Marshall recalled his recent visits with Harris. On Cape Cod, Harris "seemed to me to be in good shape—well enough to play golf, drive his car, and follow other normal pursuits." Prior to Harris's hospitalization and Marshall's September 1951 visit, Marshall "had no indication from him verbally, nor could I gather from his appearance and actions, that he was experiencing any physical difficulties. Frankly, I was surprised when I heard of his illness." Huntington Harris thanked Marshall on December 6 for his response. (Huntington Harris to Marshall, November 22 and December 6, 1952, and Marshall to Huntington Harris, December 4, 1952, GCMRL/G. C. Marshall Papers [Retirement, General].)

432

To Mrs. Theodore Roosevelt[1]

October 30, 1952
Washington, DC

My dear Mrs. Roosevelt: I want you to know that I visited Roosevelt's grave overlooking the Normandy Beachhead.[2] I landed at Le Havre at nine that morning and motored directly to the American Cemetery near St. Michel, intending to go to St. Laurent on the Beachhead the next day. However, I found that I would have the time for that inspection that afternoon late, and, therefore, arrived without any flowers, which I had intended to place on his grave. I am sorry.[3]

The memorial structure is about two-thirds on the way to completion. The marble crosses are almost all in—they are placed as rapidly as they are received from the quarries in Italy. It has been quite a job there, because a twelve foot pile has to be sunk for each two crosses; however, that is finished and the top-soil and watering system are in place.

We are exerting some pressure to see if the wreckage of the vessels, especially those which form the artificial harbor, should be left as they are. Many of them have been sold for the metal that was in them. We think it would be much more impressive to allow them to remain in place.

With affectionate regards,[4] Faithfully yours,

GCMRL/G. C. Marshall Papers (Retirement, General)

1. Eleanor Butler Alexander-Roosevelt had married Theodore Roosevelt Jr., son of the former president, in 1910.

2. See p. 347 and *Papers of GCM*, 4: 522.

3. See pp. 724–26.

4. "It was more than kind of you to write me about your visit to my husband's grave," Roosevelt responded on November 7. (Roosevelt to Marshall, November 7, 1952, GCMRL/G. C. Marshall Papers [Retirement, General].) See pp. 759–60.

433

To General J. Lawton Collins

October 30, 1952
Washington, DC

Dear Collins: I attempted to see you this morning, but found that you were at Aberdeen. Therefore, I got in touch with General William Kean with regard to promotions. To my regret, I found that his Board had finished its work, that he was leaving this afternoon, and that there would not be another meeting for twelve months.[1]

My concern is this: General Thomas North, the active, daily director of the American Battle Monuments Commission, retires in April, unless promoted. He has been a Brigadier since the war and has been in active charge of the Commission's concerns for twenty-five years.[2]

At the present time, of the new cemeteries, only five in Europe are half-way to completion of the memorials for which we have had the money. We now have available funds for starting the construction on six or seven more of the memorials. Those now under construction will not be completed before between the summer of 1953 and the winter of 1954. Those about to be undertaken with the new funds available—some $5 million—cannot be completed for about two years from the time of the letting of the contracts.

We are suffering from the effect of the Congressional restriction on numbers, which, when passed, limited us to some 400-odd employees from Manila to Africa. This forced the discharge of many tried men in connection with the engineering and the cemetery work generally, and, following the revocation of this restriction, we are under great difficulties to refill the vacancies because of the fact that all the men with such talent—engineering and otherwise—who can speak the language of the region, have been hired by the Air Force and similar activities in connection with NATO. The result is that we are very much under-staffed, particularly on the technical side. For example, General North has no deputy; and some of our cemeteries have only a Superintendent, without an assistant. General North, working on an eight-hour day, five-day week basis, is confronted with the necessity for being on duty Saturdays and Sundays and working late hours virtually every day.

The amount of work is tremendous, and the contracts are exceedingly difficult to carry out in a satisfactory manner. There are constructions in granites and marble, memorial statuaries, bronzes, mosaics, and matters of that kind, not to mention the straight proposition of seeing that all the cemeteries are in the proper condition as to soil, landscaping, watering systems, reservoirs, pumping plants, etc.

I am fearful of the dilemma we will find ourselves in if we have to replace a man of General North's ability at this particular time. We would have to have a man of sound engineering knowledge and able to speak the language; and it would take him about a half-year to come to know all the various considerations which have to be taken into account.

This, to me, is a very serious matter, and I was distressed to find that I had acted too late in this particular case, unless you can arrange a Special Board—I understand that six members will meet the legal requirements—and pass on this case in time to avoid North's forced retirement.

I am of the opinion that most of those concerned with such personnel matters are quite unaware of the extent of this project and its importance. Then, we constantly find ourselves in difficulty in getting appropriate replacements, because the men must have a certain, special knowledge, must be able to speak the language, and must be suited to be in contact with the public which visits these cemeteries.

Incidentally, I found that at Henri-Chapelle in Holland the weekend visitors numbered about 2,000 and the daily visitors 200 or 300. As these structures reach completion, this will increase very much, because they are going to be works of art and the various touring bus systems, etc., will touch at all of them. We can't afford to make miscues with the relatives of the deceased, which would involve all sorts of political recriminations and pressures.

Please think this over, and I will get in touch with you the first time I come up from Pinehurst, which, in all probability, will be the first week in December.[3]

GCMRL/G. C. Marshall Papers (Retirement, General)

1. Lieutenant General William B. Kean had assumed command of US Fifth Army in Chicago, Illinois, in July 1952. He had served as president of the board that had met on October 15 to recommend the names of fifty officers for recess appointments as permanent or temporary general officers. ("Army General Officers," *Army–Navy–Air Force Register*, July 26 and November 15, 1952, p. 1.)

2. North's association with the ABMC had begun in 1924, when he had become the officer in charge of the Paris office. He had served on Marshall's staff during World War II, and President Truman had appointed him to the position of ABMC secretary on April 18, 1946. (Thomas North obituary, *Washington Post*, June 28, 1990, p. B10.) See *Papers of GCM*, 5: 343n2.

Marshall had written to Frank Pace on October 29, 1951, to recommend that North "be promoted to the permanent rank of Brigadier General and that special consideration be given for his promotion to temporary Major General." Marshall recognized that the board determining promotions "will not consider this latter aspect," but he added that North had "been performing . . . in an outstanding manner for years" and that the ABMC members "urged me to recommend General North's promotion." (Marshall to Pace, October 29, 1951, GCMRL/G. C. Marshall Papers [Secretary of Defense, Chronological, Secretaries, Carlson].)

3. "I am happy to inform you that it will be possible to continue General North in his current assignment, even though the law requires he be retired next year," Collins responded on November 5, noting that the Officer Personnel Act of 1947 made sixty "the mandatory age of retirement for permanent colonels and general officers." Collins proposed, however, "to retain General North on his present assignment by recalling him to active duty the same day that he is placed on the Retired List." (Collins to Marshall, November 5, 1952, GCMRL/G. C. Marshall Papers [Retirement, General].) George informed Marshall that "the matter has been taken up with General North, and he is most agreeable" to Collins's suggestion. On December 5, Marshall wrote again to Collins to thank him and commented that North probably "suffers the misfortune of those who get detached from the regular run of things, however important and excellent the service may be." (Marshall to Collins, December 5, 1952, ibid.) See pp. 784–85 and 951.

434

TO HENRY CABOT LODGE JR. November 6, 1952
Pinehurst, North Carolina

Dear Lodge: I am terribly sorry that the electorate failed you in your state. They made a great error for you were among the most conspicuous statesmen in public office.[1] I anticipated great things for you and maybe in the curious workings of fate this mishap may be a turn for greater things.

Personally, I want to see you Secretary of State preferably. If not, then Secretary of Defense.[2] Some one tells me you came out against any Cabinet position. I hope not. If ever the Country needed a man it needs you![3] Faithfully yours,

GCMarshall

GCMRL/G. C. Marshall Collection (Lodge); H

1. Democratic Representative John F. Kennedy had defeated incumbent Republican Senator Henry Cabot Lodge Jr. of Massachusetts the previous day. ("Lodge a 'Casualty' in Massachusetts," *New York Times*, November 6, 1952, p. 25.) See pp. 617–18 and 621–23.

2. Eisenhower had won 55 percent of the record-breaking popular vote on November 4. ("Eisenhower Wins in a Record Vote," *New York Times*, November 5, 1952, p. 1.) Marshall wrote to the president-elect on November 7 to congratulate him on the "immensity" of his victory and promised to pray "for you in the choice of those to be near you. That choice, more than anything else will determine the problem of the years and the record of history." (Marshall to Eisenhower, November 7, 1952, GCMRL/G. C. Marshall Papers [Retirement, General]; H.) Eisenhower responded that he was "counting heavily upon the help of the finest and most dedicated men and women in our country." (Eisenhower to Marshall, November 10, 1952, ibid.)

Marshall wrote the same day to Adlai Stevenson to offer his sympathy and opined that the Illinois governor's speeches "reached a new high in statesmanship. You deserved far better of the electorate and you will be recognized increasingly as a truly great American." (Marshall to Stevenson, November 7, 1952, ibid.; H.) "Nothing has touched me so profoundly as your thoughtful and flattering note," Stevenson responded on November 20. "I have no regrets, except the disappointment of my friends and supporters, and your letter alone would be sufficient reward for what I did and hoped to do better." (Stevenson to Marshall, November 20, 1952, ibid.)

3. "I cannot tell you how much I prize your letter," Lodge responded on November 14. "My admiration of you goes back many years and for you to consider me worthy of occupying the high offices which you mention will always be a life-long gratification to me." (Lodge to Marshall, November 14, 1952, GCMRL/G. C. Marshall Collection [Lodge].) President-elect Eisenhower nominated Lodge to head the US mission to the United Nations later in November. ("Service to State a Lodge Tradition," *New York Times*, November 30, 1952, p. 63.)

435

TO HARRY S. TRUMAN November 6, 1952
Pinehurst, North Carolina

My dear Mr. President: I want you to know and to feel most sincerely that I am deeply sympathetic with you in the results of the campaign.

For you I will always have the deepest of gratitude, and, I think, of understanding more possibly than any other man. Always you supported me to the full.

Always in International and National Defense matters you took the courageous stand; and for that I am sure history will mark your record clearly as having met the great World problems of the past eight years with initiative, courage and wisdom. I hope your health has not suffered from the severity of the campaign.

With my love to Margaret and my affectionate regards to Mrs. Truman and you personally,[1]

With great respect, Faithfully yours,

GCMarshall

GCMRL/G. C. Marshall Papers (Retirement, General)

1. See previous document, n2. "I did not receive a single letter that I appreciated as much as I do yours," the president replied. "I shall always treasure it and will hand it on to Margaret when the time comes." Truman added his hope that "it won't be too many weeks before I can do as I please to *some extent*." (Truman to Marshall, November 10, 1952, GCMRL/G. C. Marshall Collection [Truman].) See p. 748n2.

436

Statement for the Armistice Day Newspaper Supplement[1]

November 9, 1952
[Pinehurst, North Carolina]

To one who has been deeply involved in the direction of the fighting during the last war, a visit to the cemeteries of our soldier dead abroad makes a profound impression. These men died fighting our battle. They are lost to the joys or sorrows of our living. They do not see the beauty of the young life growing up, nor their wives and mothers as the years pass them into a new maturity. Those men gave all, and they lie buried thousands of miles from home, sometimes in very lonely places, but always, if we do our duty, in very lovely surroundings.

My feelings always turned to what we should do, or could do, to prevent a repetition of the great tragedy that led to their end. It is futile to be merely against war or to demand peace. We must suppress our emotions and try realistically to appraise the problem, and then insist, in a democratic manner, on the necessary action or policy. Action or lack of action as dominated by the emotions is seldom wise. We have repeated the same mistakes time after time. We are doing it again, I fear, by permitting a small minority to dictate our military policy for the long future.[2]

GCMRL/G. C. Marshall Papers (Retirement, General)

1. Clarke Beach of the Associated Press had requested a statement from Marshall in October for an article planned for the commemoration of Armistice Day. (Statement by Marshall, November 9, 1952, GCMRL/G. C. Marshall Papers [Retirement, General].)

2. Beach had written to Marshall on October 20 to thank him for the statement but suggested that readers might be confused without a specific reference to universal military training. (Beach to Marshall, October 20, 1952, ibid.) Marshall responded the following day and requested that the following be added to his statement: "I have in mind, of course, our failure to adopt a program of Universal Military Training. If we do not maintain an enduring posture of military preparedness, some nations are likely to take advantage of us again, as they have twice in the past. I believe that such a training system offers us the

only practical means of keeping our military strength intact without straining our economic resources to the breaking point." (Marshall to Beach, October 21, 1952, ibid.) See pp. 552–53, 558–59, and 679–80.

437

To Brigadier General Marshall S. Carter — November 10, 1952
Pinehurst, North Carolina

My dear Carter: Your lovely one called up on the telephone the day we left Leesburg and said goodbye. You, I think, were at West Point on a sad mission.[1] So this note is to you personally to wish you well on your new duty.[2]

I am very glad you have drawn this assignment for I think it should be most helpful in furthering your career. And you deserve the best.

You are aware of my deep appreciation of the unusually efficient services you have always rendered, particularly during my last job. I will always be grateful for your loyalty and for the exceptional nature of your contribution. We have had a long association through many difficulties and you have never failed me. And you have usually provided plenty of amusement!

With love to all of you, Affectionately,

G.C.Marshall

GCMRL/Marshall S. Carter Papers (Central Files, Selected Correspondence); H

1. Carter may have attended the funeral of Bishop John B. Walthour of Atlanta, who had died on October 29 and was buried at the US Military Academy, where he was the Episcopal chaplain from July 1941 to June 1947. ("Walthour Funeral at West Point Today," *New York Times*, November 2, 1952, p. 89.)

2. Carter became deputy commanding general of the US Army in Alaska at Fort Richardson in November 1952.

438

Proposed Letter to William Fierstein[1] — [before November 12, 1952]
Pinehurst, North Carolina

I have received many queries similar to yours, more of criticism than question, however. It would not be practicable for me to reply to all of them, but I will give you a brief answer to yours.

During the first ten years of my service, I was either stationed in the Philippines or west of the Mississippi, and there was no absentee ballot in force. However, at that early date, I came to the conclusion that it would be better if professional army officers did not vote. Their job was to carry out the directives of the appropriate officials of the administration, and it seemed to me it was advisable for them to keep clear of political implications. Later on, when I reached posts of some national importance, it appeared highly advisable for me to maintain an absolutely neutral position. This was certainly the case during the war years when I had to deal directly with the legislative representatives of both houses of Congress regarding appropriations, proposed laws, etc. There was intense partisan feeling and my neutral position politically gave me a strong platform from which to urge and argue the passage of bills I felt essential to the national defense.

Later on, as Secretary of State, I found myself with tremendous international problems and plans to meet under a Democratic administration and a Republican Congress. I think only my then well-known neutral position politically made it possible to bring forward with hope of success the European Recovery Program and the legislative preliminaries to the North American Treaty Organization with the magnificent senatorial leadership of Arthur Vandenberg.

Again, as Secretary of Defense, I found it very helpful, if not absolutely essential, to meet a great emergency during a very bitter political feud from a commonly accepted neutral position.

In addition, I was then, and have continued to be since, a special advisor to the President and Secretary of Defense in regard to matters concerning national defense.[2]

GCMRL/G. C. Marshall Papers (Retirement, General)

1. Richard Fierstein had written to Marshall on November 5 from Providence, Rhode Island, concerning an Associated Press article that had appeared in his local newspaper on October 14, which stated that Marshall had "never voted, nor do you ever plan to vote." Fierstein explained that he and his friends had "tried to figure out your reason for not voting" and asked Marshall for an explanation. (Fierstein to Marshall, November 5, 1952, GCMRL/G. C. Marshall Papers [Retirement, General].) Variations of the story had been carried by many newspapers. The *New York Times* reported that upon returning from Europe Marshall had said, "I have no comments whatsoever regarding the political campaign," then continued "jovially" that "my father was a Democrat; my mother was a Republican; I'm an Episcopalian. I never voted and I'm not voting this time." ("Marshall Refuses to Talk on Election," *New York Times*, October 15, 1952, p. 28.) Marshall received dozens of letters and telegrams on the subject from around the country; most were critical.

2. Marshall drafted this response to Fierstein's letter and gave a copy to C. J. George to show to Secretary Lovett. "I have in mind possibly sending copies to those who have written me, not in a bitter antagonistic manner, regarding this business," Marshall proposed. "Tell Lovett I have omitted one of my long standing reasons, the end effect of having active military leaders involved in Presidential possibilities, for instance [Major General Winfield] Scott and [General Zachary] Taylor in the Mexican War, [General George] McClelland [*McClellan*] in the Civil War, [Lieutenant General Nelson A.] Miles in the Spanish American War, Leonard Wood in the First World War and MacArthur during World War II and in Japan." (Marshall to George, n.d., ibid.)

George replied on November 12 that he had conferred with Lovett "and his immediate reaction and recommendation, in which I concur, were that nothing could be gained by replying to this letter or any of the letters on this subject. In effect, he thought it might be used publicly, causing divided comment by newspapers. Antagonists would, naturally, broaden the subject, and no good could come from it," George reported. (George to Marshall, memorandum, November 12, 1952, ibid.) Marshall noted "OK," initialed George's next sentence, "He felt strongly that you should not comment in any way," and underlined the word *not*. (Ibid.)

439

MEMORANDUM FOR THE AMERICAN BATTLE MONUMENTS COMMISSION[1]

November 14, 1952
Pinehurst, North Carolina

Between September 10 and October 7 of this year, I inspected all of the World War II American Military Cemeteries in England, Western Europe, and Africa; also several monuments erected by Divisions and the Bastogne memorial.[2] On September 13, I participated in the dedication of the memorial at the Suresnes Cemetery, an exceptionally well-organized and impressive ceremony.[3]

In general, I found the condition of the various cemeteries and the progress of construction satisfactory, considering the limitations due to circumstances beyond the control of this Commission. The various details concerning the progress of construction, contracts, management, etc., will be presented by General North.

I took the liberty of instructing General North to remove the signs forbidding photography, as it seemed best to permit relatives and friends to satisfy their desire for photographs.

It seems desirable to make a renewed effort to make clear to the members of the related Congressional Committees the important reasons for avoiding interruption of scheduled work and crippling restrictions on maintenance, both as to funds and personnel. It might be advisable to address a special letter to this effect to the new Director of the Budget and the new Chairman and members of the related Committees of Congress.

There are several matters that I wish, at this time, to bring to the informal attention of the Commission, later on to be discussed in detail and acted upon as the members see fit:

(a) I think each cemetery Superintendent should be allowed, in effect, a small contingent fund, on which he could draw under certain approved circumstances. I find that these men have been using their own cars and gasoline, and their time after hours, to pick up next of kin or relatives who arrive in the nearest town short of funds or in difficulties as to accommodations. Some Superintendents have even taken into their homes female next of kin who were without funds and actually in want. There are cases of mothers who find themselves in difficulties, and, ignorant of the language and the country, practically stranded. People of financial means can and do take the trip with convenience and security. But at least 75 percent of the wives and parents lack the necessary money and, faced with a wait of indefinite length before the Government makes the necessary provision for the travel, undertake it without sufficient funds.

(b) I think it highly desirable to encourage travel to the various cemeteries, particularly the rather isolated ones. When the memorials are completed, these cemeteries should be interesting points for all local inhabitants and for tourists generally. The memorials will be beautiful works of art in design, construction, statuary, bronzes, and mosaics, which should appeal to all tourists, American as well as others. It is to the advantage of our country to have as many foreigners as possible see this impressive testimony of the sacrifices our men have made in their behalf. Also, I think that relatives of the dead would like to feel that their last resting place is not a dreary, isolated place, however beautiful, but one constantly visited by large numbers of people. I do not think this is at all difficult of arrangement, and we should plan accordingly.

(c) Some arrangement should be made in the case of isolated cemeteries, other than the construction of rest houses, to serve meals, etc., which would take care of relatives arriving without their own motor transportation. Possibly a previously arranged taxi service to the nearest village offering reasonably good accommodations, the cost to be met by the Government, would meet this requirement. The cost for next of kin would be trivial.

GCMRL/G. C. Marshall Papers (American Battle Monuments Commission)

1. C. J. George forwarded this draft memorandum to General North on November 14 with a note that the "General requests your comments, recommendations, and suggested alterations." There is no response from North in the Marshall Papers.

2. Marshall is probably referring to the Mardasson Memorial near Bastogne, in the Belgian province of Luxembourg. The memorial honors the 76,890 Americans killed or wounded in the Battle of the Bulge. The memorial had been dedicated on July 16, 1950.

3. See pp. 626–27.

440

To George Pattullo

December 4, 1952
Washington, DC

Dear George: Katherine and I flew to Washington this morning from Pinehurst to fulfill two commitments. Tonight, we go to the White House for President Truman's farewell dinner to the Cabinet, which will include some former members, such as me.[1]

Upon my desk, I found two cartons of foodstuffs. As usual, Mrs. Pattullo and you are most generous in your thought of us. As I recall telling you some time back, you both are spoiling us with such delicacies, but then you have been doing it for some time.

The second date I have in town is to attend a meeting of the American Battle Monuments Commission tomorrow, after which Katherine and I will fly back to Pinehurst. I am glad to say that we both are enjoying good health, and this retirement business is a delightful experience for me. I have had much pleasure, so far, hunting, fishing, being a member of the gallery at golf tournaments, taking long walks, and, for the most part, just sitting back watching the world go by.

It has been much too long a time since I have heard from you, and I am naturally curious to learn of your goings-on. We should so much like to see you both and, if your travels ever bring you to Washington or the Pinehurst area, or Leesburg during the late spring and summer, I should enjoy very much visiting with you.

Thank you for your thought of us, and Katherine and I send you both our very best wishes for a happy Holiday Season filled with good health and cheer.

With warmest regards, Faithfully yours,

GCMRL/G. C. Marshall Papers (Retirement, General)

1. President Truman hosted the December 4 dinner for present and former members of his cabinet as well as Chief Justice and Mrs. Fred Vinson, Governor Adlai E. Stevenson, "as well as the regular White House aides," recalled Margaret Truman, who also attended. In a biography of her father, she included a note he had made, calling it "a grand affair. I told those present how I appreciated the advice, help and assistance I'd received from all of them and that if I'd had any success as the President of the United States, the greatest office in the history of the world, they had made it possible." (Margaret Truman, *Harry S. Truman* [New York: William Morrow & Company, Inc., 1973], 554.)

441

To Oveta Culp Hobby — December 5, 1952, Washington, DC

Dear Mrs. Hobby: I have waited a bit before sending my congratulations on your selection for a tremendous governmental job. I would have liked to have seen you directly in the Cabinet, but, as a matter of fact, there is more to be done, constructively, where you are going than in most Cabinet positions.[1]

Your record is rapidly becoming the most notable of any other woman in this country, and I am privately and rather smugly proud that I was concerned with its earlier phases.[2]

Good luck to you, and my warm regards to the Governor.[3] Faithfully yours,

GCMRL/G. C. Marshall Papers (Retirement, General)

1. On November 25, President-elect Eisenhower had nominated Hobby to head the Federal Security Agency. ("Mrs. Hobby's Fame Won in War Post," *New York Times*, November 26, 1952, p. 12.) On March 12, 1953, President Eisenhower proposed the creation of the Department of Health, Education, and Welfare and transferring into it the functions of the various units of the Federal Security Agency. Hobby was confirmed as the first secretary of the new department and assumed its leadership on April 11, 1953. ("Senate Group Backs Hobby Nomination," *New York Times*, April 10, 1953, p. 44.)

2. See *Papers of GCM*, 2: 641–42.

3. "I think you must know how much your generous letter meant to me," Hobby replied on December 13. "Because I feel so deeply how much I owe you through the years, and because I am aware that probably I should not have received the present appointment had you not first put your faith in me long ago; I shall attempt always to justify that faith in every future assignment." (Hobby to Marshall, December 13, 1952, GCMRL/G. C. Marshall Papers [Retirement, General].) William P. Hobby, governor of Texas from January 18, 1917, to January 20, 1921, was Oveta Culp Hobby's husband.

442

To John Foster Dulles — December 22, 1952, Pinehurst, North Carolina

My dear Dulles: This note carries both congratulations and Xmas greetings.[1] I waited for the former until you had settled down a little after your Pacific travels. I know you are pleased and Mrs. Dulles must be very happy in your appointment, which seems to have met universal approval.[2]

You will have difficult years and I devoutly hope highly rewarding ones leading to an end of these tragic years of frustration and costly payments. Certainly you of all men are keenly aware of the facts and factors, the individuals and the imponderables. God help you to meet the problems and find the solutions.

Mrs. Marshall and I have been here since October 31 and will be here until May 1. We lead very quiet lives so far as nearby grandchildren permit us.[3] She is not too well, suffers acutely from a lame back and is constantly imprudent, and I am impotent to control her.

Our Xmas greetings and all good wishes for the New Year to Mrs. Dulles and you.[4] Faithfully yours,

G. C. Marshall

GCMRL/G. C. Marshall Papers (Retirement, General)

1. A statement at the bottom of the file copy indicated that this is a transcription of "a note written by GCM's hand." (Marshall to Dulles, December 22, 1952, GCMRL/G. C. Marshall Papers [Retirement, General].)

2. Eisenhower had named John Foster Dulles on November 20 as his choice to succeed Dean Acheson as secretary of state. ("Dulles 'Inherits' Post as Secretary from His Grandfather and Uncle," *New York Times*, November 21, 1952, p. 17.) See pp. 82 and 633. Dulles had rendezvoused on December 8 on Wake Island with Eisenhower after his trip to Korea. Together with other cabinet nominees and advisers, they moved on to Honolulu, Hawaii, where they met for several more days. (*Papers of DDE*, 13: 1446–47.)

3. See p. 39n4.

4. "I cannot tell you how much I appreciate your having taken the trouble to send me this note from your own pen," Dulles replied on January 6. "I remember very proudly my association with you when you were Secretary of State and the confidence with which you honored me." (Dulles to Marshall, January 6, 1953, GCMRL/G. C. Marshall Papers [Retirement, General].) See *Papers of GCM*, 6.

THE MARSHALLS spent five days between Christmas and the end of the year with Bernard Baruch at Hobcaw Barony in South Carolina. (See p. 318n1.) While there, Marshall received orders from the Defense Department signed by Lovett, Rosenberg, and George: "In order to avoid complete extinction of quail in South Carolina and in order to permit Mr. Baruch and General Bradley to enjoy the shooting pleasures at Hobcaw, you are hereby recalled to active duty." (Lovett to Marshall, December 30, 1952, GCMRL/G. C. Marshall Papers [Retirement, General].)

Marshall returned to Pinehurst and birthday greetings from many well-wishers and friends, including President Truman, to whom Marshall boasted that he shot "thirty birds in four days." (Truman to Marshall, December 29, 1952, and Marshall to Truman, January 1, 1953, GCMRL/G. C. Marshall Collection [Truman]; H.) "May your celebration mark the beginning of another year of health, happiness and contentment," President-elect Eisenhower posted from New York City. (Eisenhower to Marshall, December 29, 1952, DDEL/Dwight D. Eisenhower Papers [President's Personal File 182, Box 935].) "Katherine arranged a delightful celebration for me with a group of our friends in and near Pinehurst," Marshall wrote his friends "Flap" and Ruth Adams. "She made the rather uncomfortable business of recognizing another year a very pleasant experience." (Marshall to Adamses, January 14, 1953, GCMRL/G. C. Marshall Papers [Retirement, General].) ★

443

To Robert A. Lovett

January 9, 1953
Washington, DC

Dear Lovett: Enclosed herewith is a letter addressed to you, which was prepared by the Secretary of the American Battle Monuments Commission.[1] The problem he cites has been a particularly difficult one for us, since we have found that time and time again we are asked to release officers of the various Services that have been assigned to the Commission after incomplete periods of duty.

The business of the Commission is quite different from that of any other agency in Government. While it is a small organization in size, it is complete in its operation. It has personnel, construction, architectural, labor recruitment, and language problems, and many other factors which make it unique.

I feel that it is quite important that officers being ordered to duty with the Commission be assigned for the normal length of detail of four years. In this way, after an officer has had his training, we would then receive adequate and valuable service from him. When they are taken away from us after two or three years, our personnel situation is in constant turmoil.

I would appreciate your having your people give real consideration to this request, and I will discuss it with you the next time we can get together.[2] Faithfully yours,

GCMRL/G. C. Marshall Papers (American Battle Monuments Commission)

1. North's letter, over Marshall's signature, referenced Public Law 456, passed by the Seventy-ninth Congress, and Public Law 368, Eightieth Congress. The letter explained the history and mission of the ABMC, then went on to make arguments similar to those Marshall makes in this letter to Lovett. (Marshall to Lovett, January 5, 1953, GCMRL/G. C. Marshall Papers [American Battle Monuments Commission].)

2. Lovett's successor as secretary of defense, Charles Erwin Wilson, the former chief executive officer of General Motors, responded to both letters on February 27, 1953. He acknowledged the importance of continuity in key positions and that very few officers were involved, but he was unwilling to grant Marshall's request on the grounds that "With the reduction in the length of foreign service tours in Korea incident to the rotation program, requirements for officer replacements have increased to such an extent that a drastic decrease in stabilized tours has become necessary." (Wilson to Marshall, February 27, 1953, ibid.)

444

To Frank McCarthy

January 9, 1953
Washington, DC

Dear Frank: I came up to Washington day before yesterday to attend a dinner for Mr. Churchill; another dinner on the same evening of the Trustees of Mr. Truman's proposed Research Library in Missouri. From here, I was to go on today to Columbus, Ohio, to deliver a lecture at Ohio Wesleyan University. However, very foul weather has blocked me at both ends of the flight, and I am leaving in about an hour by train for Pinehurst.[1]

George has told me of your very generous Christmas remembrance, regarding which it remains for Mrs. Marshall to make her selection.[2] I know that she is very much pleased that you not only remember her so generously, but that she can do her own selecting. As a matter of fact, I am glad to have the present come to her in this fashion, because otherwise what generally happens is that the actual gift arrives and in about three hours she has bundled it up and sent it to somebody else. Incidentally, some time back someone sent something to Katherine and she promptly rededicated it to Molly. After the passage of twelve months, Molly sent it on to one of her connections, and that lady received it as a gift she had originally made to Katherine. So, it went around the circuit.

We still have very agreeable recollections of our contact with you in Paris and again on the barge ride out to Capri.[3] Mary Lee stayed on after seeing us off at Southampton and travelled through Spain and Morocco, coming home about ten days ago. I spent my first night here with them at their place "Ravensworth", near Annandale. They both spoke of you.

Mr. Churchill was in great form. He really has done quite a job here: First, in meeting Eisenhower several times in New York at Baruch's; then, coming here and receiving the leaders in Congress for cocktails, seeing the President, and having a select group for dinner at the Embassy. He took off for Jamaica this morning, counting on clear skies over the Caribbean and not the 100 foot ceiling I found awaiting me in Columbus, Ohio.[4]

All good wishes to you in the New Year, and let me know in advance when you are heading homeward so that, if possible, we can arrange for you to see us at Pinehurst. Affectionately,

GCMRL/G. C. Marshall Papers (Retirement, General)

1. Marshall attended "a stag dinner for sixteen" given by Prime Minister Churchill at the British embassy on January 8. ("Truman Plays Farewell, Entertains Churchill and Dinner Guests with Piano Solo," *New York Times*, June 9, 1953, p. 3.)

Marshall wrote to Ridgway on January 8 that he had agreed to speak at Ohio Wesleyan University on January 9 "in payment for something the head of the University did for me while I was head of the Red Cross." (Marshall to Ridgway, January 8, 1951, GCMRL/G. C. Marshall Papers [Retirement, General].) Arthur S. Flemming, president of Ohio Wesleyan since 1948, had held various positions in the Defense Department since February 1951 and had been deputy head of the Office of Defense Mobilization in late 1952. He had served on the US Civil Service Commission in 1939 and on the Commission on the Organization of the Executive Branch of the Government, better known as the Hoover Commission, in 1947. ("Flemming to Stay in Defense Agency," *New York Times*, April 1, 1953, p. 16.) Marshall's talk was rescheduled for early March, but poor weather prevented traveling then as well. Marshall wrote to Arthur Flemming's wife, Bernice, on March 2 that he was "so humiliated over failing twice at the last minute to keep my engagement with your husband that I hardly know how to express myself. This is the first time I recall in my many flights and engagements of this kind that I have ever failed to show up." (Marshall to Bernice Flemming, March 2, 1953, GCMRL/G. C. Marshall Papers [Retirement, General].) On

May 13, at the University of Louisville, Marshall gave a speech almost identical to the one he had prepared for Ohio Wesleyan. See pp. 762–68.

2. McCarthy had written to C. J. George on December 7 asking whether "bottled goods" or "a quantity of the very best *fresh* imported caviar" would be a good holiday gift for the Marshalls. (McCarthy to George, December 7, 1952, GCMRL/G. C. Marshall Papers [Retirement, General].) George wrote to McCarthy on January 22 to explain that the Marshalls' "liquor closet is bulging at the seams as a result of gifts these past three Christmases. He very seldom ever takes an old-fashioned any more, and Mrs. Marshall has given it up. Furthermore, they do very little entertaining." (George to McCarthy, January 22, 1953, ibid.) In thanking Bernard Baruch for his 1950 Christmas gift of bourbon, Marshall had admitted that he took "great liberties" in that period of his life in drinking alcohol, "though I was most conservative during my active Army days." (Marshall to Baruch, February 9, 1951, GCMRL/G. C. Marshall Papers [Secretary of Defense, Number Indexed, M212-2-50].)

3. "It seems only yesterday I was saying goodbye as you left Admiral Carney's boat at Capri," McCarthy had begun his Christmas note to the Marshalls. (McCarthy to Marshalls, December 7, 1952, GCMRL/G. C. Marshall Papers [Retirement, General].) See pp. 727–28.

4. Churchill planned to spend two weeks vacationing on Jamaica. ("Churchill to See President Today," *New York Times*, January 8, 1953, p. 4.)

445

TO DWIGHT D. EISENHOWER

January 21, 1953
Pinehurst, North Carolina

My dear Eisenhower: I did not find an opportunity to speak to you before I left your reviewing box towards the end of the parade yesterday, but I did ask Mrs. Eisenhower to express my very personal thanks for the honor you did me in the seating. I want to repeat that thanks more formally by this note.[1]

That was a great and brave show yesterday and you played your part magnificiently.

My prayers go out for your strength and success.[2] Faithfully yours,

GCMarshall

DDEL/Dwight D. Eisenhower Papers (President's Personal File 182, Box 935); H

1. The *Washington Post* reported that Marshall sat with the "Eisenhower family and friends" in "the simple colonnaded reviewing stand" in front of the White House to view the inaugural parade. ("750,000 on Avenue See Largest Parade," *Washington Post*, January 21, 1953, p. 17.) See Pogue, *Statesman*, 499.

2. "Thank you for your note—I am grateful for the sentiments you express," Eisenhower responded. "For my part, it was a matter of deep personal satisfaction and pleasure that you could be present at the Inaugural ceremonies." (Eisenhower to Marshall, January 26, 1953, GCMRL/G. C. Marshall Papers [Retirement, General].)

446

TO LOUIS MARX

January 21, 1953
Washington, DC

Dear Marx: Your letter of January 12, addressed to Leesburg, reached me after several days' delay at Pinehurst. Actually, it arrived just as I was taking off to come up to Washington for the Inaugural ceremonies.[1] Now that they are over, I am here in my office and will leave in fifteen or twenty minutes for Pinehurst.

I appreciate your telling me of your plan to assemble your three sons and their Godparents at Bradley's some time during the next ten days.[2] As for my participation, I doubt seriously that I will be able to come up. Frankly, in the past several weeks, I have made four trips to Washington, two of which were made under difficult weather conditions.[3] This is about all my strength will allow.

While I have given you my reaction, I think the most important point is that it appears to me to be a very inopportune time for the President. As he has just entered into office, there are many serious and complicated matters which he will have to handle in the next few months. However, if he can spare the time, I am sure it will be a most pleasant little affair.[4]

With warmest regards from us both to Idella, you, and the children. Faithfully yours,

P. S. I don't have the time to wait for this to be typed, so I have asked my secretary to type sign it for me.

GCMRL/G. C. Marshall Papers (Retirement, General)

1. See previous document. Marx was president of the Louis Marx Toy Company.
2. Together with Omar Bradley, Marshall was godfather of Louis Marx's youngest son, Bradley Marshall Marx, born February 6, 1952. (Marx to Marshall, February 6, 1952, and Marshall to Marx, July 9, 1952, GCMRL/G. C. Marshall Papers [Retirement, General].) Marx had included a list of the "'Three Little Generals'" in his January 12, 1953, letter to remind Marshall that Generals Eisenhower and Walter Bedell Smith were the godfathers of his son Spencer Bedell Marx, while Eisenhower and USAF Deputy Chief of Staff for Personnel Lieutenant General Emmett "Rosie" O'Donnell (USMA, 1928) were godfathers of Emmett Dwight Marx. "I have contacted General Eisenhower with the idea of getting together some time after his Inauguration," Marx had written, "just for half an hour, probably at General Bradley's Quarters, so that we can have a photograph taken of the group of godfathers, godmothers and little godchildren." (Marx to Marshall, January 12, 1953, ibid.)
3. See pp. 744–46 and 749.
4. President and Mrs. Eisenhower joined in the occasion at Fort Myer at 4:45 p.m. on April 6. (DDEL/Dwight D. Eisenhower Papers [Papers as President, Presidential Appointment Books].) Marx, who had been an early and generous supporter of Eisenhower's candidacy, was an old friend of the Eisenhowers. General Bradley forwarded a copy of the best of the photographs to Marshall on April 9 and noted that he was "glad that you could come out to visit with the Marx family." (Bradley to Marshall, April 9, 1953, ibid.) See photo #18. Marx's wife, Idella, wrote to Marshall on April 16 to thank him for coming and providing a "tremendous challenge and inspiration" for her sons. (Idella Marx to Marshall, April 16, 1953, ibid.) For more on Marshall's relations with Louis Marx, see pp. 962–63 and 980–82.

447

To the Nobel Committee of the Norwegian Storting[1] — January 31, 1953
Pinehurst, North Carolina

Gentlemen: I have learned that The Honorable Francis Biddle, United States Member of the International Court of Arbitration at The Hague, has proposed to you the award of the Nobel Peace Prize to The Honorable Harry S. Truman, former President of the United States of America.

I enthusiastically endorse Mr. Biddle's nomination.

Having served under Mr. Truman as Chief of Staff of the United States Army, Special Representative of the President of the United States to China, Secretary of State, President of the American National Red Cross, and Secretary of Defense, I know from long experience of his devoted interest in the cause of peace. I think history will rightfully record the tremendous time and energy which he devoted to the welfare and happiness of all peoples.[2] Faithfully yours,

GCMRL/G. C. Marshall Papers (Retirement, General)

1. Francis B. Biddle, former attorney general of the United States from August 1941 to June 1945, had been a member of the Permanent Court of Arbitration at The Hague, Netherlands, since 1951. He had written to Marshall on January 15 explaining that in this latter capacity "I have the privilege of nominating a candidate for the Nobel Peace Award. The day before yesterday I sent a formal nomination," and he was now soliciting letters of endorsement from prominent individuals. "I think a letter from you would carry a great deal of influence with the Committee," Biddle stated, and emphasized that the letter must be sent before February 1. "I saw the President a few days ago and told him I was going to make the nomination," Biddle added. "This pleased him, but of course he doesn't want to take any part in it and hopes it will be handled confidentially." (Biddle to Marshall, January 15, 1953, GCMRL/G. C. Marshall Papers [Retirement, General].) "Not knowing your desire in the matter, alternatives have been prepared for your consideration," C. J. George had written in a memorandum to Marshall on January 30. (George to Marshall, memorandum, January 30, 1953, ibid.)

2. Marshall wrote to Biddle on January 31 that he was "of course, happy to send the Committee my endorsement of your nomination." (Marshall to Biddle, January 31, 1953, ibid.) At the bottom of Biddle's January 15 letter, Marshall had noted, "I mailed letter direct to Oslo." (Biddle to Marshall, January 15, 1953, ibid.) Historian August Schou, director of the Norwegian Nobel Committee from 1946 to 1973, advised Marshall on February 10 that his letter had been received. (Schou to Marshall, February 10, 1953, ibid.)

The week before he sent his endorsement to the Nobel Peace Prize committee, Marshall had sent a handwritten letter to Truman to apologize for missing him and his farewell luncheon at Dean Acheson's home on Inauguration Day, January 20, and to congratulate the now former president on "the splendid demonstration given you enroute west and later. Already the general press comments and editorials give evidence of a far more appreciative understanding of your truly great contributions to the country and the peace." (Marshall to Truman, January 24, 1953, GCMRL/G. C. Marshall Collection [Truman]; H.) "I don't know when I have received a letter that I appreciated more than I did yours," Truman replied. "One of the things that I appreciate more than anything else that has happened to me in the past is the fact that I have you for a friend." (Truman to Marshall, February 7, 1953, GCMRL/G. C. Marshall Papers [Retirement, General].)

448

To Brigadier General Marshall S. Carter — February 7, 1953
Pinehurst, North Carolina

Dear Carter: We were delighted to receive your letter with the photographs and the bear stories. I wonder whether you wrote the letter or merely gave rise to it by your personal bear conduct.

It is fine that all of you are so pleased with your surroundings and you with your job. You are so much better off there than back here at home, particularly in an office job.[1]

I am well but Katherine is having a slow time with her back, improving, but slowly.

You letter arrived while the Pawleys were here. They came Wednesday and left Friday afternoon enroute to their winter place in Havanna. Bill was thick in the business of advising with appointees seeking confirmation. I think he would like to go to Formosa.[2]

Molly has rented her house—a block and a half from us, for $500 a month until May 1st and moved into a place 4 miles from here towards Southern Pines, that gives her an edge of about $350, and a very nice house too. Katherine is motoring there this morning.

George called up yesterday the first time since Wilson was confirmed.[3] Pawley said George's desk was solid in letters a foot high and two rows deep. I go to Washington the 17th for a meeting with the Chiefs of Staff—my cemetery business, and on to Boston for a school speech on the 18th.[4] Then back to Washington for a meeting with Cutler (new White House assistant—from Boston), about what I do not know. I made him a BG when he was on terminal leave in '45. I had only seen him twice before but was so much impressed with him that I took that action, to his complete surprise.[5]

Our love to you all, Affectionately,

GCM

GCMRL/Marshall S. Carter Papers (Central Files, Selected Correspondence); H

1. See p. 738.
2. William and Edna Pawley had known President Eisenhower since August 1946 when, as US ambassador to Brazil, he hosted two receptions honoring the Eisenhowers in Rio de Janeiro. (*Papers of DDE*, 8: 1232.)
3. Marshall is referring to Secretary of Defense Charles E. Wilson.
4. On February 17, Marshall briefed the Joint Chiefs in their conference room about the American Battle Monuments Commission's aims, progress, and problems, then flew the following day to Milton, Massachusetts, to speak at Milton Academy.
5. Eisenhower had named Boston attorney Robert Cutler as his national security adviser, a newly created position. Marshall had promoted Cutler to brigadier general at the end of World War II when he served in the Legislative and Liaison Division in the War Department. "You will recall from President Eisenhower's speeches, as a candidate," Cutler had written to Marshall on February 5, "his great interest in making the National Security Council as effective an instrument as possible for aiding him in the formulation of policies affecting the nation's security." Cutler would "consider it a great privilege if you will permit me to come over to your office sometime and obtain from you an expression of your views on any of the matters I am studying." (Cutler to Marshall, February 5, 1953, GCMRL/G. C. Marshall Papers [Retirement, General].) Cutler wrote again on February 23 to thank Marshall for "having taken the time to see me at such length" on February 19. "Careful note has been made of the points which you made and which will be helpful to me in my planning relative to the National Security Council." Cutler also noted that he was "returning to you herewith the letter from Lord Ismay dated 3 July 1943 together with the memo and attachments concerning the War Cabinet offices. I have read these papers carefully and find them very interesting material." (Cutler to Marshall, February 23, 1953, ibid.)

449

To Robert A. Lovett — February 8, 1953
Pinehurst, North Carolina

Dear Lovett: Your letter of January 29*th* was typical of you, and your character and principals [*principles*] shows in every line.[1]

I was tremendously interested in your summary and profoundly touched by your references to your service with me. I doubt if any man commanded more devoted loyalty combined with remarkable efficiency than I did in you. We had a good many years close together burdened with crises of world wide proportions. Few men in the world have had such an experience, and its authentic history, so far as we were concerned, is a record of complete cooperation, mutual accord and delightful friendship that I cherish and find in it a source of satisfaction in living.[2]

I note that you are flying south.[3] If you should motor, or Adele alone, please do arrange to stop over with us. It would be a great gratification to see you and have you here.

I am well. Katherine recovers slowly with her back, slowly due to indiscretions in serving others, particularly Molly and her children.

We go down to Jim Bruce's Pickney [*Pinckney*] Island for the last week in February—fly down in a plane of one of his companies.[4]

I am due for a conference with the Chiefs of Staff on February 17, a speech in Milton, Mass. on the 18*th* and a meeting at the White House (purpose unknown) with Cutter [*Cutler*] on the 19*th*.[5] Home to Pinehurst that evening.

Our love to you both, Affectionately,

G.C.M.

Yale/Robert A. Lovett Papers (Box 20, Folder 267); H

1. "I believe most of the goals you set in October 1950 were in general attained," Lovett had written at the start of a letter detailing his "stewardship in office" as Marshall's successor as secretary of defense. (Lovett to Marshall, January 29, 1953, GCMRL/G. C. Marshall Papers [Retirement, General].)

2. "I wanted to make this hasty report to you as my boss," Lovett concluded, "and to say that, to the best of our abilities, we have tried to see that the wise policies you laid down for the Department, and the pioneering work done in the development of the new technique of partial mobilization, have been carried forward. I would not have missed the opportunity of serving with you for worlds, and I count myself very lucky to have been given the chance to work in a cause that I believe in profoundly, surrounded by people for whom I have admiration and affection." (Ibid.)

3. Lovett had mentioned that he and his wife planned to fly to their home in Hobe Sound, Florida, "for a long holiday." (Ibid.)

4. See pp. 754n2.

5. See previous document.

450

To George F. Kennan

February 17, 1953
Washington, DC

My dear Kennan: I have your letter of February 9 and think your proposed reply to Mr. Elliston quite appropriate.[1] However, I think you should state that a definite, written recommendation was made (as I recall) by you from the Planning Section, which related directly to the fundamental policy that should govern ~~the~~ a proposal by this Government along the lines of the European Recovery Program.[2]

As I now remember, I called on Chip Bohlen and you to prepare, independent of each other, a definite recommendation on the subject. Also, I grew restless and dictated one of my own, and that the end result was very much a combination of all three.[3]

As you undoubtedly know, the Governmental Affairs Institute is presently preparing a history of the Economic Cooperation Administration and they, of course, are treating the Marshall Plan in connection with it. I have had and will have conferences with the officers of the project, and I am impressed by their intelligent and apparently thorough approach to the subject. I have every hope that the history will prove to be a valuable documentation of these programs and that it will be useful to people like Elliston, as well as others.[4]

I appreciate very much your gracious comments concerning our association at State. I admired and respected your judgment, and you were of great help to me during what I consider a very difficult period.[5]

I read in the newspaper the other day that you were being proposed as Ambassador to Switzerland, and I think you can do your country a great service in that particular post.[6] I regret that you were not able to continue in your post at Moscow, and I suppose the reasons are evident to all.[7]

With warmest regards and belated congratulations to Mrs. Kennan and you on the birth of your son,[8] Faithfully yours,

GCMRL/G. C. Marshall Papers (Retirement, General)

1. *Washington Post* editorial page editor Herbert Elliston had sent Kennan "a query about the origins of the Marshall Plan." Kennan had sent Marshall a draft of his reply explaining that he "would not like to send this unless it meets with your approval." (Kennan to Marshall, February 9, 1953, GCMRL/G. C. Marshall Papers [Retirement, General].) "When General Marshall made his Harvard speech," Kennan told Elliston, "he had in mind, in addition to his own first-hand impressions of Europe, the views of a number of advisors all of whom—I think—were deeply worried about the situation in Europe and convinced that this Government had to take some sort of action looking toward its improvement, if a dangerous further deterioration were to be averted. In addition to that, the General felt strongly that it was advisable for general reasons that this Government take the initiative at that time in its policies toward Europe and not wait until it was pressed by the course of events into what would appear as a late and defensive reaction." (Kennan draft to Elliston, February 5, 1953, ibid.)

2. "You are right that the first task of the Policy Planning Staff consisted in the study of this problem and in the preparation of the advisory opinions for General Marshall both in advance of the Harvard speech and later in the formulation of this Government's reaction to Mr. Bevin's initiative and in the extension of 'friendly aid' to the Europeans in the

drawing up of the program," Kennan had written in his February 5 draft to Elliston. "The Planning Staff was, however, not the only source of advice to the Secretary of State on these questions and I think that a fair picture of the origins of the plan could be obtained only if the major pertinent documents from the Department's files of that period could be released to scholars and students. I have no means of knowing whether the new administration would be prepared to take this step." (Ibid.)

3. See *Papers of GCM*, 6: 139–41 and 147–50.

4. Marshall had met with economists Harry Bayard Price and Roy E. Foulke on October 30, 1952; he would meet with them again the day after he wrote to Kennan, February 18, 1953, at the Pentagon. See pp. 849–50. In January 1951, President Truman had directed all federal agencies involved in emergency programs to prepare histories of their activities. The Economic Cooperation Administration had commissioned the Governmental Affairs Institute, a private research organization, to produce "an independent, objective history and evaluation of the ECA and the Marshall Plan." (Harry Bayard Price, *The Marshall Plan and Its Meaning* [Ithaca, NY: Cornell University Press, 1955], v.)

5. "When you left Government service I refrained from writing to you because I realized how heavy and burdensome personal correspondence must have been for you at that time, and did not want to add to it," Kennan explained. See p. 629. "Enough time has now gone by, however, so that I may be permitted to say what a great privilege I felt it was to be able to serve under you and how grateful I am to you for the lessons I learned from you during that period." (Kennan to Marshall, February 9, 1953, ibid.)

6. "I am still awaiting some word from the new administration as to what they think I might usefully do in the future and I am inclined to think I had better retire as soon as the necessary arrangements can be made," Kennan had confided to Marshall on February 9. "Whether that will be this year or whether I must serve for another year or two, I do not know." (Ibid.) The same day the *New York Times* had reported that Kennan was "expected to be named as Ambassador to Switzerland." ("Alumni to Hear Kennan," *New York Times*, February 9, 1953, p. 29.)

7. On September 19, 1952, while in Berlin en route to a meeting in London of US diplomats posted in Europe, US Ambassador to the Soviet Union Kennan had told reporters that "his isolation in the Soviet capital today is worse than that he experienced as an interned United States diplomat in Germany after Pearl Harbor." (Jack Raymond, "Kennan Describes Isolation in Soviet," *New York Times*, September 20, 1952, p. 3.) As a result, the USSR had accused Kennan of "slanderous attacks hostile to the Soviet Union in a rude violation of generally recognized norms of international law," declared Kennan *persona non grata*, and refused to readmit him into the country. ("Statements in Kennan Case," *New York Times*, October 4, 1952, p. 3.) For more on Kennan's exclusion from Moscow, see John Lewis Gaddis, *George F. Kennan, An American Life* [New York: Penguin Press, 2011], 465–75.

8. Annelise Sorenson Kennan had given birth to a son, Christopher, in 1949. Their daughter Wendy was born in 1952.

451

To Jim G. Lucas[1] — February 18, 1953, Washington, DC

My dear Lucas: Thanks very much for your letter of January 25 and the copy of the proposed editorial which you submitted to your Editor regarding Anna Rosenberg.[2]

I was extremely interested in what you had to tell me of your goings-on in Korea, and I am particularly glad that our people feel as I do about her.[3]

I was very much amused by your stories. They typify the American soldier perfectly.[4] Faithfully yours,

P. S. Major George, whom you know, walked in just as I was finishing up this letter, and he told me that your article had appeared in the New York World Telegram. I know how happy Mrs. Rosenberg must be at this moment and, as I indicated to you previously, she is certainly entitled to all of the praise we can heap upon her. She has done much for the military services and I think her accomplishments will be recognized a great deal later on, rather than at the present. G.C.M.

GCMRL/G. C. Marshall Papers (Retirement, General)

1. Staff writer for the Scripps-Howard news service Jim G. Lucas had been a combat correspondent with the US Marine Corps during World War II. He would win the 1954 Pulitzer Prize for international reporting for his coverage of the Korean War. Marshall had apparently written to Lucas on January 15; that letter is not in the Marshall Papers.

2. "It must be seen to be believed—the affection which this pert little woman engendered in the hearts of so many fighting men," Lucas had written in the story he "filed through the censor" on January 25, when he wrote to Marshall to thank him for the "suggestion that I write about Mrs. Rosenberg in my column." (Lucas to Marshall, January 25, 1953, GCMRL/G. C. Marshall Papers [Retirement, General].)

3. "Korean GI's now are reconciled to the dismaying idea that Mrs. Rosenberg no longer is back there fighting for them. But for a long time they refused to entertain the idea," Lucas had asserted in his column. "Even when she announced she wanted to quit they were sure something would happen. Anna—and that's what most of them call her—simply wouldn't walk off and leave them," he wrote. "Everything she did and everything she said convinced them she was on their side." (Lucas article, ibid.)

4. "Recently, I picked up a soldier and gave him a ride to his engineering battalion." Lucas related. "I asked him who he had been for in the last election. Stevenson, he said. Why, I asked. 'Because that other guy,' he said, 'if they don't watch him, he'll paint the White House olive drab.'" (Ibid.)

452

TO MRS. JOHN B. WILSON

February 20, 1953
Pinehurst, North Carolina

Dear Rose: As usual I was delighted to receive your letter. Sorry I couldn't accept the Red Cross invitation. I have already declined, as you guessed, some fifteen or twenty.[1] And besides I will be near Savannah at that time, and enroute to Columbus, Ohio.

I got in from Washington—Boston—Washington last night and fly off tomorrow for vicinity of Savannah—then Ohio, and will not be back here before March 3d.[2]

I'm well so far. Katherine has been having a hard time with her back, the harder because of her insistence on doing far too much. She has been cook for two weeks, but help arrives Monday—we hope!

Your description of home and family affairs reads attractively.[3]

When I get back I will try to find time and energy to motor up to see you. One sign of age is my reluctance to motor many miles. Also I find I grow very bored and restless sitting in a plane more than an hour or so. Fortunately Washington is only an hour and a half away.[4] *Most* confidentially, I am to go to the Coronation representing the President.[5] I appreciate the compliment but am bored stiff with the prospect. I much prefer peaceful gardening at Leesburg. I don't mind the sea trip, it is restful and pleasantly diverting.[6]

I saw Tom Morgan in Washington on the 14 of January at the Business Advisory Committee. I flew in late and had to fly out in a hurry.

Much love, Affectionately,

G. C. M.

GCMRL/J. Page Wilson Collection

1. The Durham County chapter of the Red Cross had invited Marshall on February 19 to be the "guest of honor at a reception given for the 1953 Fund Campaign Chairman and key workers." (Barnum to Marshall, February 19, 1953, GCMRL/G. C. Marshall Papers [Retirement, General].) Rose Page Wilson, who lived in Durham, North Carolina, had assured Marshall on February 19 that she had explained to the chapter Marshall's hesitancy to accept such invitations, and she had "pointed out further that I could in no way influence you to come. Naturally, it would be 'just lovely' if you would show up and I'd be *delighted* but I am not presuming to urge you." (Wilson to Marshall, February 19, 1953, ibid.)

2. Marshall had given a talk at Milton Academy in Milton, Massachusetts, on February 18, where he saw his longtime friend Lewis Perry, uncle of the headmaster of the school. (Perry to Marshall, February 5, 1953, ibid.) Marshall planned to spend several days in late February shooting with James Bruce on Pinckney Island, South Carolina, then proceed to Ohio Wesleyan University to again attempt to deliver the talk he had been unable give on January 9. See p. 745n1.

3. "News of my family is not exciting but it is pleasant," Wilson relayed. "We are all well, the baby had a brief bout with the flu but is pink and fat now. Page is the honor student of his class, Thomas is the baddest little boy I know, and John works too hard." (Wilson to Marshall, February 19, 1953, ibid.)

4. Marshall later wrote to John D. Biggers, chairman of the Business Advisory Council in 1953, that he was "a little loath" to take lengthy trips, particularly when Mrs. Marshall could not join him. "I have had so many miles to my credit in travel by now—about twelve hundred thousand by air—that I find myself reluctant to fly about much. The reason does not seem to be physical; though, in a sense, the creeping years definitely affect you. I feel more that it is purely laziness, which I frankly cultivate rather carefully." (Marshall to Biggers, June 26, 1953, ibid.)

5. Princess Elizabeth had become queen of the British Commonwealth at age twenty-five after her father, King George VI, died in his sleep on February 6, 1952. On April 28, Buckingham Palace had announced that "Queen Elizabeth II has set Tuesday, June 2, 1953, as her coronation day." ("June 2, 1953, Coronation Is Set by Queen Elizabeth," *New York Times*, April 29, 1952, p. 19.) On March 6, Eisenhower revealed that Marshall would lead the American delegation to the coronation on June 2 of Queen Elizabeth II. ("Marshall to Coronation," *New York Times*, March 7, 1953, p. 2.) See next document.

6. "General Marshall has asked me to write to you regarding a trip to Europe involving Mrs. Marshall and him," C. J. George wrote to General John M. Franklin (see p. 174n2) on February 20. "He regrets that he cannot tell you the circumstances of his trip at this time." (George to Franklin, February 20, 1953, GCMRL/G. C. Marshall Papers [Retirement, General].) George explained that the Marshalls would leave New York on or about May 23 and return "in the early part of the second week of June. He would appreciate your setting aside for him appropriate accommodations." (Ibid.)

HAVING ABANDONED his plans to travel to Ohio to speak at Ohio Wesleyan University due to weather conditions (see p. 745n1), Marshall arrived in

Washington at 9:00 p.m. on March 1. (Marshall to Bernice Flemming, March 2, 1951, and Marshall to Baruch, March 3, 1953, GCMRL/G. C. Marshall Papers [Retirement, General].) He then spent a busy March 3 in his Pentagon office to hold "a number of appointments." He first met with Secretary of Defense Charles E. Wilson at 9:00 a.m. and then spoke with FBI agents concerning Charles E. Bohlen's nomination to replace Kennan as US ambassador to the USSR. ("Senate Approval Asked for Envoys," *New York Times*, February 28, 1953, p. 7.) See pp. 751–52. He would then attend "a decoration ceremony" at 12:45 p.m. at the White House for General Van Fleet, who had announced his retirement from the army. (Marshall to Baruch, March 3, 1953, GCMRL/G. C. Marshall Papers [Retirement, General].) Marshall's last engagement before returning to Pinehurst was "a small, informal luncheon" in honor of Van Fleet hosted by Eisenhower, who had been a classmate of Van Fleet at West Point. (George to Marshall, February 24, 1953, ibid.)

Marshall returned to Washington on March 20 in order to meet with a blue-ribbon committee formed to recommend improvements to the Defense Department. Headed by Nelson A. Rockefeller, chairman of the President's Advisory Committee on Government Reorganization, this Defense Department committee comprised General Bradley; Carnegie Institution President Vannevar Bush; Pennsylvania State University President Milton S. Eisenhower (the president's brother); Arthur Flemming; Robert Lovett; and David Sarnoff. Marshall, Admiral Nimitz, and first USAF chief of staff General Carl Spaatz were named senior military consultants to the committee. The group had first met on March 2 and had been directed to make its recommendations by April 30. (Secretary Wilson Names Committee to Study Defense Department Organization, February 19, 1953, *President's Advisory Committee on Government Organization*, vol. 2, Washington, DC, series, RG 4, Rockefeller Family Archives, Rockefeller Archive Center, Sleepy Hollow, New York; Richard M. Leighton, *History of the Office of the Secretary of Defense*, vol. 3, *Strategy, Money, and the New Look, 1953–1956* [Washington: Historical Office of the Secretary of Defense, 2001], 21–22; DDEL/Dwight D. Eisenhower Papers [Papers as President, Ann Whitman File, Name Series, Wilson, Charles E. (Secretary of Defense) 1953, Administrative Series, Box 40, Folder 7].) Rockefeller had assured Marshall on March 5 that "Every effort will be made to limit the imposition on your time to a minimum." (Rockefeller to Marshall, March 5, 1953, GCMRL/G. C. Marshall Papers [Retirement, General].) After the committee's meeting on March 21, Marshall planned to return to Pinehurst, where Helen and Mary Lee were staying and "taking the Women's Amateur North and South Golf Tournament." (Marshall to Emerson, March 20, 1953, ibid.)

Marshall reported to Edmund Coles on May 13 that the reorganization committee's meetings had required his frequent travel to Washington. "As a matter of fact, from 9:00 a.m. to 6:00 p.m. on Palm Sunday," March 29, "and again on Easter Sunday," April 5, "I was occupied in this duty, which meant I left Pinehurst on Friday afternoon and did not get back until Tuesday." (Marshall to Coles, May 13, 1953, ibid.) A memorandum to the members of the reorganization committee had confirmed that they would meet Saturday, March 28, through Monday, March 30; Saturday, April 4, through Monday, April 6; and Saturday, April 10, through Monday, April 12. (Memorandum for members of the Committee on Department of Defense Organization, March 23, 1953, *President's Advisory Committee on Government Organization*, vol. 2, Washington, DC, series, RG 4, Rockefeller Family Archives, Rockefeller Archive Center, Sleepy Hollow, New York.) The committee issued its report on April 13. (DDEL/Dwight D. Eisenhower Papers [Records as President, Box 22, March and April 1953].) ★

453

To John Foster Dulles[1] — April 7, 1953, [Washington, DC]

Dear Dulles: The Presidential representatives to the Coronation have accepted an invitation from the English-Speaking Union [ESU] for luncheon on June 5.[2]

This will not be my first experience with the Union, and I know that I will be called upon to say something.[3] I would appreciate your Department recommending to me what I might say and what I should avoid saying.

I would prefer that they not outline a speech, but rather a brief summary of the points which might be made.[4] Faithfully yours,

GCMRL/G. C. Marshall Papers (Retirement, General)

1. Secretary of State Dulles's official letter notifying Marshall of his appointment as President Eisenhower's personal representative to the coronation, dated April 10, confirmed that "The President has also appointed General Omar N. Bradley as the Representative of the United States Military Services, with the rank of Special Ambassador; Governor Earl Warren, of California, and Mrs. Fleur F. Cowles as his Representatives, with the rank of Special Ambassador, to attend these ceremonies." Dulles also noted that C. J. George would accompany the Marshalls. (Dulles to Marshall, April 10, 1953, GCMRL/G. C. Marshall Papers [Retirement, General].) "I am honored to receive this appointment and am prepared to fulfill its requirements," Marshall responded on April 20. (Marshall to Dulles, April 20, 1953, ibid.) Fleur F. Cowles was an American writer whose husband was publisher of *Look* magazine and a friend of the president's brother Milton. See *Papers of DDE*, 11: 1056.

2. ESU President William V. Griffin had written to Marshall on March 27. (Griffin to Marshall, March 27, 1953, ibid.) Director-General Frank O. Darvall followed up with details on April 21, explaining that the event would "be held at the Connaught Rooms, the only large banqueting hall which happens to be available in London that day." (Darvall to Marshall, April 21, 1953, ibid.) The Connaught Rooms, located at 61 Great Queen Street, were named for the Duke of Connaught, grand master of the Freemasons in 1908.

3. See pp. 774–77.

4. "I have no particular suggestions," Dulles responded on April 20, but advised Marshall to "check with Ambassador Aldrich after your arrival" about "particular points" to stress or local issues "to be handled with delicacy." (Dulles to Marshall, April 20, 1953, ibid.) See pp. 774–77. On November 30, 1952, President-elect Eisenhower had designated Winthrop W. Aldrich, chairman of the board of Chase National Bank since 1934 and "an ardent advocate of the Marshall Plan," to be US ambassador to Great Britain. ("Role Played by Aldrich in Aid to Britain," *Washington Post*, December 1, 1952, p. 2.)

454

To Margaret Chase Smith April 29, 1953
[Leesburg, Virginia]

Dear Madam Chairman: Your letter of April 21, addressed to me at Leesburg, reached me after some delay at Pinehurst, North Carolina.[1]

I appreciate your suggestions regarding the program of your Subcommittee in connection with the discussions incident to the report of ammunition shortages and subsequent testimony of various officials of the Department of Defense.[2]

There follows a brief summary of my actions in the fall and winter of 1950:

On September 27th, 1950, shortly after I assumed office as Secretary of Defense, I issued a memorandum to the Secretaries of the Military Departments on the subject of guidance for the preparation of a supplemental budget request for Fiscal Year 1951 and the regular annual budget request for Fiscal Year 1952. This guidance contained a series of assumptions, one of which stated "that combat operations will be concluded by June 30, 1951". This assumption followed recommendations made to me at that time by the Joint Chiefs of Staff. As you may know, this assumption was only one of several included in the guidance. Some of the other assumptions were that provision be made also for full training requirements, for a combat pipeline for Korea equivalent to six months of combat at authorized rates and, more important, for additional funding of war reserves necessary to build up to approved levels, which assumption later was modified to provide for war reserves equivalent to six months of combat consumption for all forces planned to be in combat by the end of the first year of an all-out war.[3] From press accounts which I have read, this last mentioned extremely important assumption appears not to have been brought to the attention of the Subcommittee.

On September 28, 1950, after appropriate clearances had been effected with the Secretary of State, I authorized the Secretary of the Army to use as an advance against forthcoming future appropriations the sum of $1.176 billion of MDAP funds. This authority was granted to the Army to permit them to accelerate procurement of necessary Army type items which they deemed it urgent to get under production. Of this amount, $663 million was specifically allocated for the production of ammunition.

By this time, the Department of the Army had received a Fiscal Year 1951 ammunition appropriation of $30 million on September 6, 1950, and a first supplemental appropriation for ammunition of $374 million on September 27, 1950.[4] The total moneys available to the Department of the Army as of September 28, therefore, were $1.067 billion. With these moneys available to it, the Department of the Army was in a position to enter into contracts for ammunition in this amount.

The Department of Defense in the meantime was preparing a second supplemental appropriation request which contained an item for ammunition in the sum of $1.452 billion. This appropriation was enacted by the Congress January 6, 1951. In order not to delay procurement actions until the actual enactment of the appropriation, we directed the military departments to get along with the administrative work required before contracts can actually be signed. It was our intention to speed up the work required preliminary to the actual signing of contracts so that when the money finally became available there would be little or no delay in signing the contracts themselves.[5]

Thus, as to the $1.452 billion which were to become available on January 6, 1951, Mr. Lovett, then the Deputy Secretary of Defense, on December 4, 1950, issued a memorandum to the Joint Secretaries directing them, in the face of the grave danger with which we were faced in the Pacific, to immediately take all necessary actions that would be required short of the actual signature on contracts for the procurement of major items and other supplies and equipment of critical character prior to formal approval by the Congress and the President of the supplemental appropriations then under consideration.

The enactment of the second supplemental appropriation for ammunition of $1.452 billion on January 6, 1951, increased to a total of $1.9 billion the moneys available to the Army on September 28. (The moneys borrowed from MDAP are not included in this total since they were to be returned out of this appropriation.)

In the meantime, I had appeared before the House Appropriations Subcommittee on December 1, 1950, on the occasion of their consideration of the Second Supplemental Appropriation Bill for 1951. At that time, I stated to the Subcommittee that one of the basic principles which we should follow during the very critical days ahead, once reasonably adequate stocks were on hand, was to place maximum reliance upon the creation of a sound, well integrated, well planned industrial base which would provide for us facilities capable of expanding to maximum production within a relatively short period of time, if the occasion so demanded. I must emphasize the importance of this principle. To my mind, it could spell the difference between survival and disaster. My experiences during World War I and World War II led me to the conclusion that the creation of an adequate expansible industrial base in advance of actual requirements was more important than the hurried accumulation of vast quantities of military materiel. I repeated these thoughts when I appeared before the Senate Appropriations Committee on December 9, 1950.[6]

On January 5 and January 13, 1951, memoranda went forward to the Military Department Secretaries enunciating this principle in greater detail. The Secretaries were told that they should plan their production and utilization of funds in such a manner as to insure the establishment of a production and mobilization base that would permit, if needed, a very rapid expansion to full mobilization.

The immediate implementation of this policy required the accelerated use of available funds. For this reason, Deputy Secretary Lovett appeared before the House Appropriations Armed Services Subcommittee on January 19, 1951, to apprise them of the actions necessary to broaden the industrial base. Speaking for me, he stated, in essence, that it would be necessary to utilize all available funds to finance plant expansion to a larger degree than originally contemplated and that the three Military Departments had been instructed to prepare new procurement schedules to carry out this program. Subsequently, as Mr. Lovett testified, he took detailed actions to implement this policy, and he kept me informed of the progress made.

I want to express my appreciation to you for the opportunity you have given me to submit these comments to your Subcommittee. Faithfully yours,

GCMRL/G. C. Marshall Papers (Retirement, General)

1. Senator Smith had written to Marshall on April 21 to inform him that his name "was mentioned in the Senate Armed Service Ammunition Shortage Subcommittee Hearings in connection with a letter signed by you on September 27, 1950, which announced certain budgetary guidelines to the Department of Defense." Smith realized "that this letter was written within a few days of the date you became Secretary of Defense and that undoubtedly it was based on information and studies of others." (Smith to Marshall, April 21, 1953, GCMRL/G. C. Marshall Papers [Retirement, General].) See p. 168n3. The *New York Times* had reported on April 18 that Major General Elbert L. Ford (USMA, 1917), army chief of ordnance, had testified the previous day to Smith's subcommittee that "ammunition deficiencies in Korea were the inevitable result of having had to create a munitions industry 'from scratch' after the fighting had begun." (Harold B. Hinton, "Arms Chief Asks a Ready Industry," *New York Times*, April 18, 1953, p. 9.) Ford told the subcommittee "he had asked for $2,200,000,000 for ammunition in August, 1950," but that this "request was sent back to him by" Lieutenant General Raymond McLain, then army comptroller, "to be cut in accordance with budget assumptions" by Secretary of Defense Marshall "and his staff. One of the assumptions was that combat operations in Korea would be terminated by June 30, 1951." (Ibid.)

2. "The Department of the Army has indicated to our Committee that these guidelines and assumptions, including the assumption the war would end on June 30, 1951, had an adverse effect on the ammunition program," Smith continued, and she felt that Marshall "should be given the opportunity to present your views to the Committee" either in person or in a letter to be made part of the record of the hearings. (Smith to Marshall, April 21, 1953, GCMRL/G. C. Marshall Papers [Retirement, General].) See p. 300 for an earlier excerpt from Marshall's response to Smith.

3. See p. 169n3.

4. For more on the first supplemental budget request, see Condit, *Test of War*, 223–27.

5. For more on the second supplemental budget request, see ibid., 233–40.

6. See pp. 276–78 and 291–93.

455

To Dwight D. Eisenhower — April 29, 1953 [Leesburg, Virginia]

My dear Mr. President: Replying to your letter of April 27 regarding the American Battle Monuments Commission, and your last paragraph, I would prefer not to be consulted as to the choice of the membership.[1]

I take this position particularly because you are retaining me and releasing all of the others, but Leslie Biffle. Incidentally, he is a good man to keep.[2]

General North tells me he is to see you tomorrow. He can give you a pretty good line on everything.

I think your list is very impressive.[3] Faithfully yours,

GCMRL/G. C. Marshall Papers (American Battle Monuments Commission)

1. Eisenhower had sent Marshall "Just a note to make record of my continuing interest in the American Battle Monuments Commission and to express my deep satisfaction in having it under your capable direction." Eisenhower also wondered whether Marshall "might have some ideas from time to time as to the membership of the Commission or perhaps to some other related matter." (Eisenhower to Marshall, April 2, 1953, GCMRL/G. C. Marshall Papers [American Battle Monuments Commission].) Eisenhower had a longtime interest in the ABMC. In January 1927, he was appointed by General John J. Pershing to serve in the ABMC headquarters in Washington, DC, to write a guide to the World War I battle sites and cemeteries in Europe. Eisenhower, known for his writing ability, completed the work in August. In June 1928, Pershing assigned Eisenhower to serve in the Paris headquarters of the ABMC to collect additional data to revise the guides. He did so in September 1929. Eisenhower was also involved in several staffing decisions related to the commission. (Daniel D. Holt and James W. Leyerzapf, *Eisenhower: The Prewar Diaries and Selected Papers, 1905–1941* [Baltimore: Johns Hopkins University Press, 1998], 59–61, 79–84, 99, 104–5.)

Marshall had submitted his resignation to the president on April 4 and added that he had "suggested to all the members of the Commission that they take similar action." (Marshall to Eisenhower, April 4, 1953, GCMRL/G. C. Marshall Papers [American Battle Monuments Commission].) The president had written to Marshall on April 27 to thank him "for the action you have taken to afford me the opportunity to review the membership of the Commission." In his final paragraph, Eisenhower had commented that because Marshall was chairman, he "might prefer not to become directly involved in the selection of members." (Eisenhower to Marshall, April 27, 1953, ibid.)

2. "We have prepared a tentative slate for the new Commission," Eisenhower had explained. "I have no strong feelings on the new membership except that I would like to see a good World War II representation. I think you will agree with the idea of having a prominent negro veteran included, as well as an additional woman member." (Ibid.) Leslie Biffle, secretary of the US Senate from 1945 to 1947 and 1949 to 1953, had served on the ABMC since 1941. See pp. 618–19.

3. In addition to Marshall, North, and Biffle, Eisenhower proposed to retain retired marine General Alexander A. Vandegrift. Others on the list were retired Admiral Thomas C. Kinkaid; retired Brigadier General Benjamin Oliver Davis Sr., the first black general officer in the US Army; retired General Carl Spaatz (see p. 755); Senator Charles E. Potter (R-MI); Representative John Phillips (R-CA); Mrs. Wendell L. Willkie; and Mrs. Theodore Roosevelt Jr. (See p. 733.) Eisenhower's "tentative slate" also included several individuals who were not named to the commission in 1953. New members of the ABMC were announced on July 9. ("President Fills Battle Monuments Group Vacancies," *Washington Post*, July 10, 1953, p. 2.)

"I am very glad that you accepted the President's invitation to serve on the American Battle Monuments Commission, and I look forward to working with you in this important job. I believe you will find the work of great interest," Marshall wrote to the new members of the commission on July 15. (Marshall to Davis, July 15, 1953, GCMRL/G. C. Marshall Papers [American Battle Monuments Commission].) "I am indeed grateful for this evidence that in the midst of his busy life, the President not only remembers my efforts but gives me this great privilege of future service," General Davis replied. "I am also pleased to be again associated with you." (Davis to Marshall, July 27, 1953, ibid.) Mrs. Roosevelt responded on July 20 that "there is nothing I would rather do" than serve on the ABMC. (Roosevelt to Marshall, July 20, 1953, ibid.)

456

Address at the University of Louisville[1] May 13, 1953
Louisville, Kentucky

I first came to Louisville with General Pershing more than thirty years ago.[2] Later, I came as Chief of Staff of the Army during the hurried period in which we were striving to build up a great force of more than eight millions from the small start of about 175,000.[3] In striving to persuade the Navy to build the famous LST's, the great landing craft we used around the world and that made the landing in Normandy possible, the original mock-up or model was constructed at nearby Fort Knox.

My first interest in Louisville lay in the fact that it was the home of General Basil Duke, one of Morgan's famous cavalry leaders, who took my father prisoner, a boy of sixteen, in the border fighting along the Ohio River. Father was in the home guards fighting off a raid by Morgan's cavalry, who were searching for a nearby ford. In the confused struggle in the border states, my father had three brothers in Lee's army, while at the same time he was a member of a local force loyal to the Union. To add to the complications, I believe Duke was a cousin of my father's and, in the fight I have referred to, my father's home was the citadel for the defending home guards. His younger brother, Pickett Marshall, a boy of fourteen, was bayoneted on the stairway leading up to the second floor of the house.[4]

Like all border struggles, it was a generally nasty business, but a very exciting story for me as a boy.

All this was a civil war, and not over the rivalries of countries or kings or despots. We are engaged today in a vast struggle in which our civilization as we know it and love it is threatened by a political or governmental monster, hydra-headed and utterly ruthless, which respects only strength, force, and relentless determination on the part of other peoples and their governments. This situation, therefore, makes our foreign affairs of overwhelming importance in relation to our political future and our economic and military posture.

Concerning foreign policies, I have invariably tried to make the point that it is important for the American public, and especially the young people in high schools and colleges, to cultivate the habit of searching for the facts in any given case. In doing this, one great trouble today is the veritable deluge of statements, the confusion of arguments drenched with political implications, the bitterness of party prejudice, and statements carefully couched in language that will best appeal to the public. While most of these factors are part and parcel of a democracy like ours, when they apply to world issues, rather than to home affairs, as in the old days, a far more searching, impartial analysis is very essential, the more so in the light of our position of world leadership. My suggestion to young people has been to go after the facts and try to avoid the influence of special and partisan pleadings. I have asked them to believe that the spectacular, the exciting, the super-critical, the hasty advocacy of this or that are seldom the part of wisdom. When we come to world affairs, our sudden emotions, our partisanship, and especially our ignorance of the characteristics and history of the peoples involved are usually bad medicine.

It seems important to remember that we are a very young nation. Yet we have been forced into a position which other nations, like the British, for example, have been many hundreds of years in reaching, and that in close contact with the other nations involved. By contrast, we are not only very young, but we are many thousands of miles distant from the Far East and several thousands of miles distant from the nations of Europe and the Mediterranean. We have so much to learn as a people and a nation and so little time in which to learn it, and yet here we are in a position of world leadership such as no other nation has ever approached since the days of the Roman Empire. We have to act and learn at the same time, which means that the public must learn to judge carefully in these grave matters and not to plunge suddenly into violent acclaim or into bitter criticism.

I referred a moment ago to our youth as a nation. Actually, within my lifetime, the United States has risen to international leadership from a position where we were so unimportant to the world at large that not a single nation accredited an Ambassador to this country. A Minister of Legation was the rank they thought suitable for us. Yet today, whether or not we want it, whether we like it or not, we are actually the acknowledged leaders of the free world.

The first great stride into world affairs came with Dewey's victory in Manila Bay on May 1, 1898.[5] From that moment to this, we have literally shot upward to the top of the political, economic and military world, a progression that has previously required hundreds of years on the part of our predecessors across the Atlantic. So I think it should be apparent to all that an exact knowledge of the facts surrounding a situation or a circumstance is most essential to a wise decision by our citizenship.

We are living in a tremendous age, a period which is more critical, I believe, than any other since the fall of the Roman Empire. Wisdom and cool judgments are necessary in the charting of our course through the storms which threaten.

In this connection, consider the solution of the problems which faced our so-called "forefathers"—the drafting of the Constitution of the United States of America. There are several highly interesting factors concerned with the men that performed this duty. They were far more intimately familiar, I am told, with the classics regarding the philosophy of governments down through the centuries than are our college graduates today. They were widely read in the history of the rise and fall of nations. They understood the fundamental requirements for a sound government based on a knowledge of the past dangers and weaknesses displayed by governments.

We who are citizens of a free government usually have a very limited knowledge of the historical development of liberty. We have a limited appreciation of what our "forefathers" sought, of how their hearts and spirits cried out against oppression—a character of oppression which we have never experienced.

But I think the most interesting factor concerned with these men was the extreme youth of the dynamic leaders. Jefferson drafted the Declaration of Independence when he was just 33 years of age. Madison, Monroe and Hamilton were an average age of 20 in 1776. These men, as I have just remarked, were familiar with the lessons of history as they pertained to governments. They had a sound basis for translating these lessons into principles and rules of conduct for the government of a country dedicated to the freedom of the individual. They were men of great ideas, dynamic, pulsating with the vigor of youth.

Sitting with them was one of the wisest and cleverest men of history—Benjamin Franklin, then in his 80's. And presiding over the discussions was the olympian figure of Washington, then in his early 50's. Through the magic of Washington's personality, his great prestige, and his calm restraint in dealing with both the young and the old, he was unique, I think, in the role of a moderator at one of the greatest meetings in history for the chartering of a truly democratic government.

Democracy to these "forefathers" was not a new formula for peaceful pursuit among mankind. As a system, it was the best that had emerged from dark ages of centuries of struggle. It is not much more than that today, although refined by experience and improved by wider understanding. Yet democracy is a very old idea, and its pursuit is even now a race to be won only by the courageous and the determined.

I wonder how many of you are familiar with these immortal words:

"The administration of our Constitution favors the many and not the few—that is why we are called a democracy. Our laws provide equal justice for all. Socially, advancement is based on ability and merit, without regard to considerations of class or financial status. If a man is able to serve the state, he is not to be held back by the obscurity of his position or condition . . .

"And the freedom we enjoy in our government extends also to ordinary life. Each of us goes about his business without encroachment from the other; nor do we cast jealous eyes at a neighbor for doing as he pleases.

"We place our trust less in a rigid system or a rigid policy than we do in the feelings and the native spirit of our citizens.

"Instead of regarding public discussion as a stumbling block to effective action, we regard it as an indispensable preliminary to any wise action at all."

They were spoken by Pericles 2,453 years ago, 500 years before the birth of Christ.[6] You will find in them little that differs from our concept of democracy today. Unfortunately, Pericles could only be heard within the range of his own voice. There did not exist methods for the rapid or wide distribution of his written words.

Apropos of this discussion of the importance of a knowledge of the facts, I might interest you with an example of how great governmental decisions are reached.

At the present time, the Government is struggling with the problem of the tumultuous situation in the Far East—Korea, China, Indo-China, Malaya. The problem was widely discussed in the recent political campaign. It has been written up from almost every point of view. We have the columnists' and commentators' solutions; the editorial and magazine article solutions. We have the emotional appeal and the pure political appeal.

It is very difficult to decide such a matter publicly. Much has already been said which is bound to be of great help to the Soviet Government, while we, by contrast, know relatively nothing of their thoughts or plans. That puts us at a great disadvantage and places the soldier at the front in an added peril to his already perilous position. Some of our public largely base their reaction on the fact that they have relatives on the dangerous ground. Others are strongly influenced from the tax payers' point of view by the tremendous appropriations that are believed to be necessary to meet the situation. Still others are more strongly influenced by their fear of a great world catastrophe. And, behind the scenes, the Administration, in close contact with the Congress, endeavors to arrive at a wise and sound decision.

Let me give you an example out of our experience in the last war, an example of how critical decisions are arrived at under somewhat similar circumstances:

Probably the most far-reaching and bitterly contested decision of the last war was that for the cross-channel invasion of Normandy and the advance across the lowlands of Northern Europe and the Rhine toward Berlin. On a map, it seemed quite logical to make the great thrust in the manner indicated. But there were those that vigorously advocated the advance against Central Europe from the Mediterranean; others thought the drive should be launched across the Western rather than the northern coast of France. Still others strongly favored the great effort being made first in the Pacific. Added to the complication resulting from these heavy pressures was the extremely critical time factor. To stage a colossal effort like the channel crossing, followed by the drive east across France and the Rhine, required at least a year and a half for the assembly of the forces and materiel in England, and it was always a desperate question as to whether or not we would be able to secure the materiel and the vast amount of shipping in time. For evident reasons of tide and weather, the invasion had to be in the late spring or early summer; otherwise, a delay of another year must intervene, which made the consideration of the time factor dominant for this operation.

There was another factor of great importance and that was the fact that during the necessarily long period of preparation the leaders of State, Mr. Roosevelt and Mr. Churchill in this instance, had to meet the insistent public demand for action. Yet such action, meaning other military efforts here and there, would always threaten to absorb so much of troops, materiel and particularly shipping that the concentration for the main effort might be fatally delayed, for in war, one can never tell how prolonged a particular struggle will be, however careful the planning estimates. In this particular case, the reactions from the Pacific, with its fierce island campaigns and resulting heavy casualties, and the popular appeal of subsidiary operation in the Mediterranean, developed pressure which seriously threatened the concentration in England for the invasion of Normandy.

Ocean shipping became a most critical matter. The turn around to England was the shortest haul and therefore more troops, more equipment and more supplies could be moved in a given time. Shipping to the Mediterranean took longer than to England and took much longer to the Southwest Pacific, and shipping was always in short supply and continued to suffer heavily from submarine attack. Then there was the landing craft, the celebrated LST's. There were more arguments regarding the allotment of these craft than over any other subject, for they were the initial basis of any landing operation.

During one of Mr. Churchill's recent visits, we were discussing the fact that in the famous Cairo Conference in December 1943 more bitter differences of opinion related to the disposal of 27 landing craft, the LST's, than to all the great subjects of the Conference combined.

In the face of these many conflicting pressures, we stood by our conclusion that the fundamental operation to precipitate the end of the war lay in the build-up of the forces and means for invading Normandy.[7]

Now please keep this in mind in the light of the Government's problems today—the public could not be informed of either the details or the reasons. Columnists, commentators, newspapers and magazines could discuss and illuminate to prove that this or that plan would be the best plan, but our procedures had to be completely secret; no explanation or defense could be made. Special pleaders to the White House or the Congress or the press were only a little less numerous than starlings in the summertime. It almost seemed a miracle to me that we survived these difficulties.

It is always important to determine the public state of mind in judging the attitude of the Government, the Congress, or the Administration at the time of decision. Otherwise, in later years there would often appear to be no logical explanation for the Administration's action during a particular period. For example: Shortly before I left the office of Chief of Staff, the popular demand for the rapid demobilization of the armed forces had reached such a peak of power that we were compelled to dissipate all that we had so hurriedly built up and at such tremendous cost, and this in the face of a huge Russian Army. There was not time even to protect or ship home the huge dumps of arms and supplies in the Pacific and, in relatively a few months, they were taken over by the jungle. This demobilization continued its wasteful and dangerous pace until later when I, as Secretary of State, was involved in conference with the Soviets in Moscow and we had but four regiments of active infantry in the entire country. There were not enough men to guard the airstrip at Fairbanks, Alaska, against a possible parachute attack from nearby Siberia, yet I was receiving radio messages from patriotic Americans to "give them Hell", meaning the Soviets.[8]

An educated public opinion is the only method I know of to protect us against the dangerous and wasteful procedures that have been so costly in the past.

In the midst of many complications, we are also in the midst of a world revolution. The benighted people, the little people of the earth, have begun to realize how tragic their situation is, how unfair. The Communists seize this growing revolt as a spring-board for their own purposes. They use it. We have largely ignored it through the years, with all our kindly and generous feelings toward our fellow men. Much of our present trouble springs from this source. We can't buy our way out, though we can help, but we must not spread ourselves thinly over the troubled areas of the world. We, in effect, must put our finger in the dike at one place while we first accomplish great things at another, though each region has its special pleaders in our midst. One great trouble during the war was that the public and much Congressional pressure was to do everything at once, which would have meant doing nothing effectively anywhere and very probably being defeated by an enemy who concentrated.

So you see there is much to learn about each situation, so many facts and factors to be considered. They present a wonderful field for you young people in which to play a great part in the leadership of our country through these difficult years, but you must thoroughly understand what you are talking about and not be swayed by every breeze of criticism or clever proponent of this or that conception. While this is democracy at work, our great public in these days of critical international difficulties should be sufficiently well-informed to meet the problems with wisdom and good American common sense.[9]

GCMRL/G. C. Marshall Papers (Retirement, Speeches, Statements, and Writings)

1. Marshall had agreed previously to participate in the University of Louisville's Distinguished Lecturers Series and had written to President Philip Davidson on February 16 to confirm the date of this evening lecture. (Marshall to Davidson, February 16, 1953, GCMRL/G. C. Marshall Papers [Retirement, Chronological].) He also wanted "an indication of the public nature of my lecture, as well as any publicity to be given to my remarks" because that might "restrict my text to a considerable degree." (Ibid.) On May 11, Marshall sent a message to Sam Gifford, program director at a Louisville radio station, that his remarks would "deal generally with the requirements of intelligent citizenship in coping with world problems" but would be "so informal in character" that he felt strongly they would not be interesting for "radio dissemination." (Marshall to Gifford, May 11, 1953, ibid.)

2. In December 1919, while serving as his aide-de-camp, Marshall accompanied Pershing on a tour of army camps and war plants. See Pogue, *Education*, 210–11.

3. Marshall visited Fort Knox, Kentucky, on April 8 and 9, 1941. See *Papers of GCM*, 2: 469.

4. Confederate troops serving under Brigadier General Basil Wilson Duke took George Catlett Marshall Sr. prisoner in Augusta, Kentucky, in September 1862. See Pogue, *Education*, 6–8. Duke's commanding officer was his brother-in-law, Brigadier General John Hunt Morgan.

5. See p. 107n3.

6. Marshall quoted from Pericles' funeral oration. (Thucydides, *The History of the Peloponnesian War*, trans. Richard Crawley [New York: E. P. Dutton and Company, 1910], 119–28.)

7. See pp. 670–71, *Papers of GCM*, 4: 191–96, and Pogue, *Organizer*, 305–9, 317–18.

8. Marshall attended forty-three meetings of the fourth Council of Foreign Ministers in Moscow, USSR, from March 10 to April 24, 1947. See *Papers of GCM*, 6: 72–110.

9. The next day, after an informal morning meeting with students interested in international affairs, Marshall attended a luncheon and made brief, informal remarks to university trustees and officers as well as prominent businessmen in Louisville. (Spilman to Marshall, May 13, 1953, ibid.)

Two years later President Davidson wrote to Marshall that the Distinguished Lecturers Series had "been so successful that we want to publish the lectures" and asked Marshall "to furnish us with a copy of the evening address you gave." (Davidson to Marshall, February 6, 1955, GCMRL/G. C. Marshall Papers [Retirement, General].) Marshall responded that he had "no objection to the publication of this material in the manner you indicate." (Marshall to Davidson, February 15, 1955, ibid.) The university did not publish the lectures.

457

TO ROBERT T. STEVENS[1]

May 13, 1953
Leesburg, Virginia

Dear Stevens: Thank you for your gracious note of May 6.[2]

I was very glad that you agreed to come to the Virginia Military Institute and make the principal address at the inauguration of the new Superintendent. Your talk was inspiring and most appropriate.[3] I am ever anxious to see the Department of Defense evidence a keen interest in the contributions which the Institute has made throughout its history to the armed services, and your participation in these ceremonies did much to encourage the Institute in its efforts.

I enjoyed seeing Mrs. Stevens and you, and Mrs. Marshall joins me in warm regards to you both.[4] Faithfully yours,

GCMRL/G. C. Marshall Papers (Retirement, General)

1. Secretary of the Army Robert Ten Broeck Stevens served in both World War I and II and attended a special civilian course in 1941 at the Army Command and General Staff College at Fort Leavenworth. In 1945, he became chairman of the board of J. P. Stevens and Co. textile manufacturers. In 1951 and 1952, he was chairman of the Business Advisory Council on which Marshall served.

2. Stevens had been the prime speaker at the installation of Major General William H. Milton Jr. (VMI, 1920) as the eighth superintendent of the Virginia Military Institute on May 2. Three days later he had written to Marshall, whom he had seen at the event, that "As always I was favorably impressed with VMI. No one could possibly visit there without being inspired by the esprit de corps evidenced." (Stevens to Marshall, May 6, 1953, GCMRL/G. C. Marshall Papers [Retirement, General].)

3. The *Washington Post* reported that Stevens had declared, "Failure to provide the career soldier at all ranks with proper compensation," which involved "more than just the pay involved," would mean "having to accept less than the best in our regular services." He considered this "false economy at its worst," which "could well jeopardize the very security of this nation.'" (Matt McDade, "VMI Installs Gen. Milton as 8th Chief," *Washington Post*, May 3, 1953, p. M1.)

4. Mrs. Stevens was the former Dorothy Goodwin Whitney.

458

INTERVIEW WITH EDWARD R. MURROW
May 19, 1953 Leesburg, Virginia

AT THE REQUEST of the English-Speaking Union of the United States, Marshall had agreed to an interview with broadcast journalist Edward R. Murrow. ESU President Griffin (see p. 756n2) had asked Marshall to "say a few words" that would "help inform the American people about the commemorative volume" Marshall was to present to the queen during the coronation festivities "as a permanent record of the names of all donors" to the King George VI Memorial Fund. Dedicated to the queen's father, the fund was created to establish scholarships for British students to go to the United States for part of their education. Griffin explained that "we have in hand nearly $275,000 from close to 5,500 contributors, resident in every state in the Union." The interview was recorded at Dodona Manor on May 19, 1953, to be aired the following Sunday, May 24, on *See It Now*, a Peabody and Emmy Award–winning program on CBS television. (Griffin to Marshall, May 15, 1953, GCMRL/G. C. Marshall Papers [Retirement, General].)

In addition to a brief discussion of the fund, Murrow quizzed Marshall on several other subjects, including why he had not yet written a book. "The compelling reason to me is the fact that it would have to be almost entirely personalities," Marshall replied. "I don't wish to go into that. I was in office as Chief of Staff for six years, through a long series of great events; there were changing views all the time; there were passing opinions and as always happens in a case like that, the one unfavorable comment is blown up and exploited and the whole rest of the reference to the individual which may go through hundreds of pages and be high complimentary at least, and at least filled with approval—would be lost." Marshall offered the example of giving promotions during World War II followed by demotions after. "I had to go through the process of making sixteen hundred general officers. That was very hard. Not the juniors; not the brigadiers, but I was dealing with so many of my friends, my contemporaries, and I was going very strong for young men." He noted that Eisenhower was a lieutenant colonel "when I walked into the scene." Lawton Collins was a captain who became a corps commander; Bradley, who was a major, went on to command millions of men in battle; and "Eisenhower had the greatest collection of arms that the world has ever known under one command. Then the worst of it was—I was held on as Chief of Staff under this long six-year period and it fell to me to demote half of those I had made, so while I had, you might say, sixteen hundred friends, I now began to have eight hundred enemies. So I thought that was just going too far." (Marshall interview with Murrow, May 19, 1953, ibid.; used under license.)

Murrow next asked Marshall to discuss his current feelings about universal military training. "We cannot afford a standing army and Universal Military Training is one way of keeping all the world advised that we have a reserve, an available reserve of manpower and young men in arms that makes it quite—most highly dangerous for anyone to question our course in an arbitrary manner," he responded. "I have seen the army disintegrate several times, and I have always been on the receiving end to accept the disintegration and start to reorganize. I was with General Pershing when it dwindled to a force less than we had before we went into the First World War." Marshall recalled that when he became chief of staff in September 1939 he experienced "the difficulties of getting everybody to understand. They spend too much time in trying to find who is responsible for the last thing and too little time in trying to understand what they should do in the future, if I may make that frank statement." Marshall recalled being questioned "as to who ordered the disintegration" of the army after World War II. "Well, the American people backed, supported by their Congress, ordered the disintegration, and that was the end of it." (Ibid.)

Murrow then commented, "General Marshall, you have had most of the honors and some of the abuse that comes to a man in public life," and asked if he had any advice for younger Americans. Marshall countered with laughter that he was "interested in the way you put that question, the 'most' and the 'some.'" He answered that he had tried "my best to influence young people whenever I came in contact with them in public talks, to do one thing: to make it a practice of searching for the facts and not being overwhelmed with the deluge of statements drenched with political phrases, emotions, the appeals that are made through headlines, through a prejudiced paper, columnist, or legislator or member of the administration." He stressed that "this torrent of statements" was "very confusing, very difficult to understand, and when it comes to international affairs, very critical" so he suggested that "our young people should grow up in the habit of trying to get at the facts, instead of merely traveling on the emotions, and for the time being, though that would be asking a miracle, to refrain from opinions. But if they have the facts, they have a great advantage over their elders, particularly at the dinner table." (Ibid.) ★

THROUGHOUT the spring, the Marshalls and C. J. George made preparations to attend the coronation of Queen Elizabeth II. (See p. 754n5.) On April 3, Assistant Secretary of State Livingston Merchant had informed Marshall that he would "be the guest of Her Majesty's Government from May 30 to June 6" and included "instructions as to the dress to be worn during the ceremony and at social functions during the Coronation period." Merchant assured Marshall that "All normal expenses of the designated members of the Special Mission to the Coronation, including the costs of transportation, will be paid by the Department of State." (Merchant to Marshall, April 3, 1953, GCMRL/G. C. Marshall Papers [Retirement, General].)

Festivities filled Marshall's schedule both before and after the coronation. Some invitations designated only members of the delegation (see p. 756n1) while others included Katherine Marshall and newly promoted Lieutenant Colonel George. (See pp.780–82.) Prior to their departure from New York on May 23, the Marshalls had arranged to spend the night of May 22 with Margaret Emerson. The Marshalls and Emerson had accepted an invitation from Anna Rosenberg to attend "a small informal dinner" with Bernard Baruch, Robert Lovett, "and a few other old friends" that evening. (Rosenberg to Marshall, March 25 and April 20, 1953; George to Rosenberg, March 31, 1953; and Marshall to Rosenberg, April 28, 1953, ibid.) On May 5, Marshall had radioed General Ridgway asking for assistance with transportation from Le Havre—where the *America* was due to dock at 11:00 p.m. on May 29—to London. "I am involved in an official function the evening of the 30th and, as the ship is now scheduled for late afternoon arrival at Southampton, we would be considerably pressed for time," Marshall explained. Ridgway offered a C-47 aircraft and Vernon Walters as an escort to expedite the Marshalls' arrival and departure from Le Havre. (Marshall to Ridgway, May 5, and Ridgway to Marshall, May 7, 1953, ibid.) C. J. George traveled to London ahead of the Marshalls aboard the *United States* and would "have two and one-half days there to take care of the necessary arrangements before our arrival." (Marshall to McCarthy, May 22, 1953, ibid.)

Accommodations in London for the American delegation were provided at the Hotel Grosvenor, where the Marshalls joined the rest of the delegation and General Sir Leslie Hollis, senior assistant secretary in the War Cabinet Office during World War II and commandant general of the Royal Marines from 1949 to 1952, who had been named "Gentleman in Attendance on the United States Delegation," for dinner on May 30. (Spilman to Marshall, March 23, 1953, ibid.) Afterward Marshall visited with his old friend Lady Mary Burghley (see pp. 778 and 779n3), then attended the first formal event, a 10:00 p.m. reception at the National Gallery given by the British government. The following day, the Marshalls went to a garden party given by Lord and Lady Salisbury (see p. 773n2). On June 1, the Marshalls lunched with Lady Nancy Dill at the International Sportsman's Club before Marshall proceeded to the British Broadcasting Corporation (BBC) television studios at Alexandra Palace to broadcast a brief address to the United States. (Aldrich to secretary of state, telegram, April 2, 1953, and schedule of coronation activities for General and Mrs. Marshall, ibid.) ★

459

Television Remarks on Coronation Eve[1]

June 1, 1953
London, England

On the very eve of the great event of tomorrow, all our thoughts turn to the beautiful young Queen and the magnificence of the ceremonies. We are all charmed by her as a woman, and profoundly impressed by the display of character and devotion to service of which she has already given evidence. There have been a multitude of statements by world dignitaries to that effect. I fear, however, that few of us are aware of the profound significance of the Coronation ceremony and, for Americans, its intimate historical relation to our government of the people, by the people, and for the people.

The most important single element in the concept of democracy shared by Great Britain and the other nations of the Commonwealth with us Americans is the cardinal principle of the "consent of the governed". Our Declaration of Independence states that, in order to secure the rights of life, liberty, and the pursuit of happiness, governments are instituted among men, deriving their just powers from the consent of the governed.

This basic principle goes back hundreds of years before our own Declaration of Independence and, indeed before the Magna Carta, to the very dim beginnings of Anglo-Saxon democracy, when their chieftans, and later their kings, were elected. This principle has been violated, but has always re-asserted itself. Two examples will suffice: First, when the Norman kings replaced it for a time with the feudal system; and, later, when the right of the governed to give their consent was denied the American Colonies. "Taxation without representation" was a refusal of this right. Abraham Lincoln expressed this great political philosophy when he spoke at Gettysburg in 1864 of "Government of the people, by the people, and for the people".

And this same undying principle of democracy will be acknowledged tomorrow in the opening ceremony of the Queen's crowning, in what is called the Act of Recognition. The Queen will stand alone by the Coronation chair in full view of all. She will then face the four corners, each in turn, as the Archbishop of Canterbury, accompanied by the Great Officers of State, goes to each of the corners and presents the Queen to the people. He asks them if they are willing to render homage and service to the Queen. The people signify their consent to the crowning by replying, "God save Queen Elizabeth".

And so there is thus preserved the act of consent, symbolic in this modern constitutional monarchy of the acceptance of the Queen by all her peoples and of the enduring quality of the ancient precept, precious alike to Americans and Britons: "the consent of the governed".[2]

GCMRL/G. C. Marshall Papers (Retirement, General)

1. Brigadier General Julius C. Holmes, minister to the US embassy in London, had sent Marshall "a short text which you may find of some use for your short television broadcast to the United States tonight." (Holmes to Marshall, June 1, 1953, GCMRL/G. C. Marshall Papers [Retirement, General].) Holmes had been executive officer to the Joint Chiefs of Staff in 1942.

2. "We are most grateful to you for making time to come to Alexandra Palace on 1st June," wrote George Barnes, director of television broadcasting at the BBC. "Your appearance was, by common consent, the highlight of the programme. I very much hope that you did not find your experience too fatiguing." He added that "The programme seems to have been well received and we should like to think that it contributed to good relations between our two countries." (Barnes to Marshall, June 10, 1953, ibid.)

THE CORONATION took place on June 2 in Westminster Abbey. After he returned home, C. J. George recalled in a letter to Frank McCarthy that "One of the most interesting things was when General Marshall entered and started up the aisle toward his seat. The entire gathering arose and the orchestra played. The General was completely ignorant of the fact that this was an honor being paid him, because as he walked up the aisle he glanced over his shoulder to see if there was some important VIP behind. He did not know until the following morning that it was he who should have taken the bow." (George to McCarthy, June 23, 1953, GCMRL/G. C. Marshall Papers [Retirement, General].) Marshall was also honored by the recognition of Prime Minister Churchill and several senior British officers during the procession in Westminster Abbey. See pp. 778–82 and Pogue, *Statesman*, 500–503.

Governor Earl Warren, once back in California, reported to President Eisenhower that "'General Marshall, as head of our delegation, made a profound impression everywhere. Both in the press and in the public eye he was recognized as the outstanding representative of foreign countries. I am sure he did much to impress everyone with our desire for peace and friendship with the rest of the world. He was most considerate of the other members of the delegation and made it a pleasure for all to serve with him.'" (Eisenhower to Marshall, July 6, 1953, DDEL/Dwight D. Eisenhower Papers [Ann Whitman File, Name Series, Box 21].) "I was tremendously impressed," General Matthews, executive aide to General Bradley during the coronation, wrote to Marshall on June 22, "to see first-hand the great admiration and respect the British people have for you. It touched me deeply to hear so many fine things said about you and your service to our country and our allies at the many social and other events which I attended where you were present." (Matthews to Marshall, June 22, 1952, GCMRL/G. C. Marshall Papers [Retirement, General].)

On June 3, Marshall and the rest of the delegation lunched with American press correspondents in London. (Smith to Marshall, March 20, 1953, ibid.) That evening Marshall was the only American who attended the state banquet at Buckingham Palace, which he later described to Truman as "the most brilliant gathering I have ever seen. The Queen's party of about thirty were seated at an oval table in the center of the hall, surrounded by tables of twelve," and Marshall noted that he was "two chairs removed from the Queen." (Marshall to Truman, September 8, 1953, ibid.)

Later that night, General Marshall joined his wife at a ball given by socialite and former US Ambassador to Luxembourg Perle Mesta. John M. Patterson, the "coronation officer" at the US embassy, later reported in a letter to his friend Frank McCarthy that Marshall "danced until 2:30 or later. He looked wonderfully well." (Patterson to McCarthy, June 12, 1953, GCMRL/Frank McCarthy Collection.) For Marshall's first-hand accounts of these and other activities, see the next document, pp. 777–80, his formal report to President Eisenhower on pp. 780–82, and Pogue, *Statesman*, 500–503. ★

460

TO MRS. JAMES WINN

June 5, 1953 2:00 a.m.
London, England

Dearest Molly: We have just come in from an Embassy dinner and ball we left early.[1] We had lunch at 10 Downing St. with the Churchills and Lord and Lady Salisbury.[2] They did some photographing of Churchill on the doorstep saying goodbye to your mother and me which you will probably see. Tomorrow I go at eleven to Buckingham Palace for a reception by the Queen of the delegates like me.[3] Then we lunch with and I speak to the English-Speaking Union.[4] Your mother dines at the Embassy and I at Churchill's banquet for the Queen.[5] Then we join up and go to a reception at Buckingham Palace. The following day lunch with Jockey Club and then the "Derby."[6] Later a reception for me at the Embassy. Sunday lunch with the Duke and Duchess of Gloucester is family affair.[7] Then we head for 3 days in the country.[8] We come to town for a lunch for me by ten special press men and commentators and dinner for me at House of Lords by a group of Lords and House of Commons men.[9] At 9$^{a.m.}$ next day we leave for South Hampton and sail at noon. New York at 8$^{a.m.}$ June 16th.

Your mother is standing up far better than I anticipated and hugely enjoying herself. She has made a *great* impression, has been the literal queen of several affairs, all gravitating to her, especially royalty. She is feeling better I think than back home at housekeeping. We have a delightful suite looking out on Hyde Park and the Parade route. George is square in the middle of things and enjoying himself tremendously. Our first days including Coronation Day were pretty hectic. I went to a tremendous banquet at Buckingham Palace [for] 250 guests. I sat between the Queen Mother and the Princess Alice, the only Commoner at the table of 30.[10] We paraded in after all the other guests were seated, and out the same way. Edinburg, Gloucester and Beucluch [*Buccleuch*] spent the period after dinner before we joined the ladies talking to me.[11] I had ten minutes with the Queen.

I will tell you all when we get back. We have reams of interesting invitations, seatings, descriptions, etc. Love to you and the children. I am sending you the coronation copies of the London Illustrated News.[12]

GCM

GCMRL/© Marshall-Winn Collection (Retirement, Coronation); H

1. At 8:30 p.m. the Marshalls had attended Ambassador Adrich's white-tie dinner for the American delegation at his residence at 14 Prince's Gate.

2. The Marshalls had lunch with the Churchills and Lord and Lady Salisbury on June 4. Lord Salisbury, Robert Arthur James, Gascoyne-Cecil, was leader of the House of Lords from 1951 to 1957. Lady Salisbury was the former Lady Cicely Gore, daughter of the Earl of Arran.

3. The queen's reception for foreign envoys and deputations took place on June 5.

4. See next document.

5. Prior to their dinner engagements on June 5, the Marshalls attended the archbishop of Canterbury's afternoon garden party at Lambeth Palace.

6. The Epsom Derby, Britain's richest thoroughbred horse race, takes place annually on the Epsom Downs in Surrey. See pp. 778 and 780–82.

7. Queen Elizabeth's uncle, Prince Henry, the Duke of Gloucester, was married to Lady Alice Christabel Montagu Douglas Scott. Her sister Mary was Marshall's friend Lady Mary Burghley. See pp. 3–4 and 779n3.

8. See pp. 777–78.

9. See pp. 781n4 and n6.

10. The Queen Mother was Elizabeth, widow of George VI and mother of Queen Elizabeth II. Princess Alice, Countess of Athlone, was a grandchild of Queen Victoria. From 1940 to 1946, her husband, Alexander Cambridge, the Earl of Athlone, had served as governor general of Canada, where the Athlones had met Marshall during the Quebec Conference in September 1944. See *Papers of GCM*, 4: 581–82.

11. "Churchill got hold of me when we took our leave of the ladies and had me sit with him for quite a long time and had me participate with him in the drinks they put on a small table alongside him," Marshall confided to Truman in a September 8 letter. "Before that, the Duke of Edinburgh and the Duke of Gloucester had talked to me for about twenty minutes after we left the ladies." (Marshall to Truman, September 8, 1953, GCMRL/G. C. Marshall Papers [Retirement, General].) Prince Philip, the Duke of Edinburgh, is Queen Elizabeth II's husband. The Duke of Buccleuch, Lieutenant Colonel Lord William Walter Montagu Douglas Scott, was brother to Lady Mary Burghley and the Duchess of Gloucester.

12. For additional details, see Pogue, *Statesman*, 500–503.

461

REMARKS TO THE ENGLISH-SPEAKING UNION OF THE BRITISH COMMONWEALTH[1]

June 5, 1953
London, England

I was much pleased that the English-Speaking Union invited the members of the American Delegation at the Coronation for luncheon today. This will be the second time that I have met with British representatives of the organization. On the previous occasion, I was in London in the fall of 1947 for one of those completely frustrating and prolonged conferences of the Council of Foreign Ministers. There was much that I would like to have said then in extreme frankness that I could not say publicly, much that is now well understood.[2]

I have attended a number of meetings, or rather dinners, of the English-Speaking Union back in my own country and, to be very frank, I always felt that the membership averaged too many years. There was too much of judgment and wisdom and not enough, I thought, of youthful punch. And I must promptly admit that same criticism has very direct application to me, personally, today.

During the recent war years, I made it my business in almost every public utterance to close with an appeal to the American public to do all in their power to promote a generous understanding between themselves and the British people, to understand the great trials, the suffering, you were undergoing, and the absolute necessity for complete teamwork between us. Out of my experience in the last World War and afterward, and my much more limited experience in 1917 and '18, I have been increasingly impressed with the difficulty the people of different countries have in understanding each other, no matter if they speak the same language and are of much the same racial stock.

There is a phase of this difficulty that is usually overlooked. Since 1066, you have been in a continuous process of fusing your Saxon and Norman blood. We, on the contrary, since the recent birth of our Nation, have been most actively engaged in the process of absorbing vast numbers of people of literally every blood stock in Europe. Our respective reactions, therefore, are bound to differ, and was not our great purpose a common one—the liberty of the individual and his freedom to live his own life and develop his aspirations in his own way—we would probably have moved from one misunderstanding to another and more serious one.

Today, we have reason to reach for closer understanding than at any other period in our history and, providentially, your great Prime Minister understands us on both sides of the Atlantic water, politically and historically, better than any other living person.

I first visited this country some forty years ago. I returned to ride in the great victory parade in 1919, and did not again see England until I flew over to meet with your Chiefs of Staff and, later, your War Cabinet in April 1942.[3] Those visits presented strange contrasts, as you can easily imagine. For example, I entered Westminster Abbey for the first time last Tuesday to witness the magnificent ceremony when your altogether lovely and already great Queen was crowned. On a

Sunday morning fifty years ago, Mrs. Marshall and I had set out from our pension near Queen's Gate to attend a special service at the Abbey to be conducted by a prominent Divine. It was a lovely fall morning and, while waiting for the proper bus, one came along labeled "Hampton Court". We took that bus and abandoned our plan for the Abbey.

What happened that day left a very pleasant recollection. We had already seen the Hampton Court, so we hired a punt and I gained my first experience in punting. I did pretty well, but did collide with another punt which was much more skillfully managed by a Britisher. He and his girl were out for a Sunday outing. Instead of recriminations, which might well have been the case, we joined forces and spent the day together—had lunch and tea together, and, in effect, paved the way for my future relations with the British Chiefs of Staff. And so I never entered Westminster Abbey until last Tuesday.

On my brief visit in 1919, there was a Hyde Park review of the American regiment which had come over from France with General Pershing, and it was my honor to escort the Minister of War, Mr. Churchill. After the review, General Pershing presented him with the American Distinguished Service Medal. It was my privilege to read the citation. I did not again see your Prime Minister until the historic meeting at Argentia, Newfoundland, in August 1941, which I attended as Chief of Staff of the American Army.[4]

While my numerous wartime visits to London were during periods of great war strain, my later visit here as Secretary of State was by far the most difficult, involving as it did the fruitless negotiations of the Council of Foreign Ministers, which had followed a similar futile meeting in Moscow.[5] It was my good fortune at that time to work with your late Minister for Foreign Affairs, the Honorable Ernest Bevin. I deeply lament his passing.[6] I had found him a fine man to work with, and I found him also a most able and dependable associate. He rendered a great service.

Incidentally, I had arrived in London for this meeting I have just referred to two days after the marriage of the then Princess Elizabeth, whose Coronation as Queen we are now celebrating. The day before I left, I had the high honor and great privilege of lunching at Buckingham Palace with the Princess Elizabeth, King George and Queen Elizabeth, the Princess Margaret, and the Duke of Edinburgh. There were no other guests, so I enjoyed a rare opportunity, as well as a great honor.[7]

My contacts with your present Minister of Foreign Affairs have been rather intimate and in many parts of the Western World—Newfoundland, Algiers, Cairo, Teheran, France, Canada, Potsdam, and at home in the United States.[8] I am greatly distressed by the painful illness he is suffering and his inability to participate in the Coronation ceremonies.[9] During the war, I took him on a long trip through the South so that he might see at firsthand what we were doing in raising an army and air force of 8-1/2 million men from a small beginning of 175,000.[10] He was and is a great Englishman; I have cherished his friendship and pray for his recovery.

I would like to return again to the matter of British-American relations. During the World War days, I made frequent appeals for a better, more generous understanding between our two countries. As I have already stated, I constantly endeavored to make clear to the American public the severe trials your Nation was enduring with silent, Spartan courage, the heavy loss of life both in soldiers and civilians you suffered, the destruction of much of Britain then in progress and always threatening. Today, the situation is somewhat reversed. The American forces in Korea, as your Prime Minister has pointed out in Parliament, are suffering the greatest losses, except for the South Koreans, of any United Nations force, and our Nation is called upon to make by far the heaviest expenditures. I feel that your public only partially realizes this and, for some reason—probably a result of clever Soviet propaganda and subtle suggestion—seems to believe that America is in a warlike mood, fraught with the possibility of bringing about a general conflagration. Nothing, I know, could be further from the desire of the American people and their leaders. Our public is intent on seeing that nothing be permitted to lend aid to the Communist Chinese forces in maintaining their fight against us.

Allegations are common that we, meaning my Government, do not pay sufficient attention to the advice of our partners on international questions. In my personal experience, as Secretary of State in periods such as the Berlin blockade, and later as Secretary of Defense during the Korean struggle, I think a maximum of attention was paid to the views of our associates, particularly those of the British Government. It is important, I think, that we constantly remind ourselves that we represent a free association of nations, opposed by a group organized into a bloc and held together by a tyranny of force. Our respective publics and our leaders must constantly keep in mind that almost all of our reactions are treated in an open, democratic manner. On the other hand, all is concealed by our opponents, and we are left merely to guess or suspect as to their motives or intentions.

I have somewhat overworked the word "generous" in my remarks, but I must use it again to express my strong personal conviction that a "generous" understanding between the American people and the people of the British Commonwealth is the most important influence in the world today for the peace we all long and pray for.[11]

GCMRL/G. C. Marshall Papers (Retirement, General)

1. See p. 756. On May 16, Undersecretary of State Walter Bedell Smith had sent Marshall a memorandum concerning his address to the ESU. Smith had confided that "our relations with Great Britain are at a low ebb," and added that "The President is worried about this and so are we all." (Smith to Marshall, May 16, 1953, GCMRL/G. C. Marshall Papers [Retirement, General].) Marshall instructed M. L. Spilman to "Call up General Smith and tell him I *very* much appreciated" his suggestions but "I am hustling off to London and could not find time to write my thanks." (Ibid.) Smith's memorandum is not in the Marshall Papers.

2. Marshall was probably referring to the speech he gave to the Pilgrims Society in London on December 12, 1947. See *Papers of GCM*, 6: 287–91. For more on Marshall's participation in the London Council of Foreign Ministers, see *Papers of GCM*, 6: 269–70, 273–75, 277, 280–84, 293–302.

3. Marshall participated in London's victory parade on July 19, 1919, when the horse he was riding "reared and went over backward. Marshall, falling, broke a small bone in his

hand." (Pogue, *Education*, 199–200.) For the April 1942 meetings, see *Papers of GCM*, 3: 157–65.

4. Marshall is referring here to the Placentia Bay conference among Roosevelt, Churchill, and their advisers that resulted in the Atlantic Charter. See *Papers of GCM*, 2: 586–88.

5. Marshall attended forty-three meetings of the fourth Council of Foreign Ministers in Moscow, USSR, from March 10 to April 24, 1947. See *Papers of GCM*, 6: 72–110.

6. Bevin had died on April 14, 1951.

7. Princess Elizabeth and Prince Philip were married on November 20, 1947. Marshall had arrived in London on November 21, 1947. Princess Margaret was King George VI and Queen Elizabeth's younger daughter, sister of Queen Elizabeth II.

8. Anthony Eden had been secretary of state for foreign affairs during World War II and assumed the office again on October 28, 1951.

9. The *New York Times* had reported that on June 10 Eden had undergone bladder surgery in Boston, "the third surgical treatment for the same ailment for Mr. Eden since April and was intended to heal the bile duct." ("Eden Has Operation at Boston Hospital," *New York Times*, June 11, 1953, p. 3.)

10. Marshall, Eden, and Sir John Dill made an inspection tour of military camps in the southern US in March 1943. See *Papers of GCM*, 3: 602–3.

11. The BBC recorded Marshall's and other speeches given at the luncheon for broadcast on its Home Service from 10:00 to 11:00 p.m. that night and extracts were broadcast overseas that night and the next morning. Frank O. Darvall, director-general of the ESU, wrote to Marshall later that day to express the union's gratitude for Marshall's appearance at the luncheon. "Your tremendous contribution to the cause which we all have in common," Darvall declared, "has made your name the most famous and honoured throughout the entire English-speaking world." (Darvall to Marshall, June 5, 1953, GCMRL/G. C. Marshall Papers [Retirement, General].)

Robert Lovett, who had rejoined Brown Brothers Harriman and Company after leaving office on January 20 (see p. 751), informed Carter on July 13 that according to one of his former London partners, "the Old Man was the hit of the affair, ranking second only to the Queen." Lovett reported that Marshall's "endearing quality of modesty made a big hit and his speech before the English-Speaking Union brought the audience to its feet four times. For the British to risk their bunions in such demonstration is a real tribute. I have no doubt that after the warmth of his greeting he said to Lt. Col. C. J. George something like this: 'George, do you think that speech went all right? I want a frank answer.'" (Lovett to Carter, July 13, 1953, GCMRL/Marshall S. Carter Papers [Central Files, Selected Correspondence].)

THE MARSHALLS attended various social engagements over the next two days. See pp. 772–73. On June 7, they were the guests of the Duke and Duchess of Marlborough at Blenheim Palace in Oxfordshire, then continued on to Cottesbrooke Hall in Northamptonshire, where they visited for two days with Reggie Macdonald-Buchanan and his wife, Catherine. Marshall had met Macdonald-Buchanan when he was Field Marshal Sir John Dill's aide-de-camp from 1940 to 1943 and part of the British Joint Staff Mission in Washington. Macdonald-Buchanan was chairman of James Buchanan & Co. distillers and a breeder of racehorses. "They had a beautiful place," Marshall later reported to Truman, but "most of the portraits in the house were of horses." (Marshall to Truman, September 8, 1953, GCMRL/G. C. Marshall Papers [Retirement, General].) On June 10—their final day in London—Marshall spoke to a select group of American journalists, followed by dinner with twenty-five members of Parliament called the Progress Trust. See p. 781n6. ★

462

To Winston S. Churchill

June 10, 1953
London, England

My dear Mr. Prime Minister: I cannot leave England without making plain to you my deep appreciation of the courtesies you have shown me, and Mrs. Marshall, and the distinctions I am sure you have had accorded me during the Coronation ceremonies and festivities.

I feel that as Representative of President Eisenhower, these honors have been paid me and I shall so report, but I also think many of them have been due to your friendship.

Mrs. Marshall and I much enjoyed the luncheon at 10 Downing Street, and we were delighted to have you bring us forward with you in the Stewards Box at the "Derby".[1] Thank you. Affectionately

GCMRL/G. C. Marshall Papers (Retirement, General)

1. "The Queen, the Duke of Edinburgh and about 500,000 persons were at Epsom to witness what turned out to be the gayest and most brilliant Derby in recent years," the *New York Times* had reported on June 7. "The weather was smiling and sunny and the scene was festive." ("Richards' Mount 5–1, Beats Queen's Aureole in Classic," *New York Times*, June 7, 1953, p. S1.) See next two documents.

The same day, Marshall wrote to General Sir Leslie Hollis to express gratitude for his "efforts and attentiveness" during "a very strenuous program" which made matters "very convenient for me as well as for other members of the delegation." (Marshall to Hollis, June 10, 1953, GCMRL/G. C. Marshall Papers [Retirement, General].) Marshall posted a similar letter to D. A. Greenhill of the Foreign Office, who had assisted Hollis in his escort duties, and General Holmes, to thank him for suggestions "made regarding the television show and your comments on my English-Speaking Union speech." See pp. 770–71 and 774–77. (Marshall to Greenhill, and Marshall to Holmes, June 10, 1953, ibid.)

463

To Frank McCarthy

June 15, 1953
at sea

My dear Frank: We land at 8^{am} to-morrow after a wonderful but very strenuous trip. Your radio greeted us in London and we were very appreciative of your sending it.[1]

Katherine has had a very bad back all winter but got through the schedule in very good shape. It was a magnificent show and the banquets at Buckingham and Lancaster House were very splendid affairs, not to mention receptions, garden parties, etc., etc.[2]

Had dinner one night in the country, returning from a garden party, with Mary Burghley, and had lunch, at which she was the third guest, with her sister and the Duke.[3]

Our great regret was to miss your "Command" movie. It was put on the night of the day we sailed. I have not yet heard the reactions.[4] Saw Mountbatten a number of times.[5] In fact he spoke to me from the Coronation procession in the Abbey, as did [Field Marshal Viscount Alan] Brooke, [British Minister of Defense Viscount Harold of Tunis] Alexander, [Field Marshal Viscount Bernard Law] Montgomery. Churchill turned out of the procession to shake me by the hand.[6] Had lunch with him and Mrs. C. Saw him my last afternoon and he sent us off with a full sized painting which had been hung in the National Gallery(?)[7]

Many inquired about you. We missed you. To-morrow we go straight from the boat to the plane (the Navy plane I used as Sec. of Defense by the way.) Should be in Washington by 11:30 and Leesburg—their standard time—before lunch.

George is with me, a new Lieutenant Colonel. I sent him ahead and brought him back with me.[8]

Katherine joins me in love to you. Affectionately,

GCM

GCMRL/Frank McCarthy Collection (Marshall); H

1. "Television interview excellent," McCarthy had congratulated Marshall. (See pp. 770–71.) "Happy coronation." (McCarthy to Marshall, radio, May 25, 1953, ibid.) Due to a reduction in the number of films made and producers employed by Twentieth Century–Fox, McCarthy had reported to Marshall on May 10 that he had accepted the position of director of public relations for the studio "because I like the studio and its people, and the job itself is pretty well down my alley." (McCarthy to Marshall, May 10, 1953, GCMRL/G. C. Marshall Papers [Retirement, General].)

2. Prime Minister Churchill hosted his dinner for the queen on June 5 at Lancaster House, where the Council of Foreign Ministers had met in November and December 1947. See next document.

3. See p. 773n7. Marshall had also seen Lady Mary Burghley on May 31, when she was a houseguest of Conservative Member of Parliament Henry Channon at Kelvedon Hall, his estate in Essex. That night Channon recorded in his diary: "This evening Fleur Cowles, President Eisenhower's personal representative at the Coronation arrived and brought with her General Marshall and Mrs. M, of Marshall Aid fame, an elderly distinguished grey couple. After admiring my now famous gardens, they asked for whisky but their faces puckered with disgust when they found we had given them Scotch and not Bourbon." Channon found Marshall to be "long-winded but a dear." (Robert Rhodes James, ed., *Chips: The Diaries of Sir Henry Channon* [London: Weidenfield & Nicholson, 1967], 475.)

4. McCarthy had informed Marshall on May 13 that his new movie, released in Britain under the title *Single-Handed* and in the United States as *Sailor of the King*, would have "its world premiere as part of the coronation festivities" in London on June 11. (McCarthy to Marshall, May 13, 1953, GCMRL/G. C. Marshall Papers [Retirement, General].) Marshall replied that they would "have to forgo the pleasure" of seeing the film in London "as we leave Southampton at 1:00 p.m. on June 11 for the trip home, but we will look forward to seeing the American version when it arrives in the Leesburg area." (Marshall to McCarthy, May 22, 1953, ibid.)

5. Admiral Lord Louis Mountbatten had been commander in chief of the Royal Navy's Mediterranean Fleet since June 1952. In his September 8 letter to Truman, Marshall explained that because of their "warm friendship and high regard," Mountbatten had facilitated McCarthy's utilization of the British Mediterranean Fleet to duplicate "Galapagos Island on a small island near Malta." (Marshall to Truman, September 8, 1953, ibid.)

6. See p. 771, the next document, and Pogue, *Statesman*, 500–503.

7. "I send you herewith the picture I mentioned to you and your Wife the other day," Churchill had written to Marshall. "It was painted in January 1951 in the Atlas Mountains at a place called Tinherir" in southeast Morocco. "The river which flows boldly out of the mountains soon comes to its end in the Sahara. It was shown at the Royal Academy last year." (Churchill to Marshall, June 10, 1953, Churchill Archives Centre, Churchill College,

Cambridge, UK/Winston S. Churchill Papers [Public and Political: General, Private and Personal].) Katherine Marshall expressed her gratitude to Churchill on June 28, writing that they had hung the painting at Dodona Manor, where it "added so much to the beauty of our living room and has the place of honor." (Katherine Marshall to Churchill, June 28, 1953, ibid.)

8. "I have just had a letter from General Marshall, written on shipboard, telling me of your promotion," McCarthy wrote to George on June 19. "Naturally, I am delighted with this, since I don't think anybody could have a more rewarding assignment than seeing to the proper handling of his and Mrs. Marshall's affairs and nobody could do it so well as you." (McCarthy to George, June 19, 1953, GCMRL/Frank McCarthy Collection [George].)

464

To Dwight D. Eisenhower — June 16, 1953
[Leesburg, Virginia]

My dear Mr. President: I submit herewith a report of my mission to the Coronation of Queen Elizabeth II.

The ceremonies were magnificent, as you have no doubt seen, and we were treated with every consideration. As Chairman of the Delegation representing the President of the United States, I was accorded seemingly unusual honors or distinctions so far as that appeared possible. In that connection, the Prime Minister turned out of the procession into the Abbey to shake my hand.[1]

The American Press entertained me at a luncheon, where my talk was "off the cuff" and supposedly "off the record".[2]

I was called on for remarks at a luncheon of the English-Speaking Union. A copy of what I said is enclosed.[3]

A group of eight American correspondents had me for lunch and a frank talk (New York Times, U. S. News and World Report, Scripps-Howard Press, and Columbia Broadcasting System).[4]

In all my talks or discussions, I made clear that I was reflecting no government policies whatever, merely my personal views, when I expressed any.

I made a very brief television broadcast to close a long program on the eve of the Coronation. I enclose a copy of my remarks.[5]

Finally, on my last night in London, I dined with a group of twenty-five members of the House of Lords (8) and House of Commons (17) called the Progress Trust. I was told that these men represented the most influential group in the two Houses. The dinner was at the House of Lords. I talked intimately for thirty minutes. They questioned me for about an hour and a half.[6] Individually, *each* man devoted his questions to the Middle East, the Suez Canal, and Egypt. They all regarded that situation as extremely critical and argued the world importance of America's moral support. The following day, on the boat train, Soames, son-in-law and Secretary of the Prime Minister, told me that a basis of agreement has been reached between our two governments.[7]

I had lunched informally with the Prime Minister and sat with him at the "Derby", and I called on him the afternoon before my departure.[8] He asked me to carry to you his warm, I believe he said "affectionate", regards. He made no reference to the Middle East, but he did ask me to express to you his interest in Senator Taft's proposal for a Far Eastern Alliance, which appealed to him.[9]

Our Ambassador, Mr. Aldrich, and his people did everything in their power to facilitate our program. He and Mrs. Aldrich gave us a welcoming reception, a large dinner, and several small dinners for the wives and members of the Delegation who were not engaged in the several banquets for or to the Queen.[10]

The other members of the Delegation will, I suppose, report to you direct. In London, they acted with me in close accord.[11]

I wish to express here more formally my deep appreciation of the honor you paid me in this assignment.[12]

With great respect, Faithfully yours

GCMRL/G. C. Marshall Papers (Retirement, General)

1. See pp. 756n1, 772–73, previous document, and Pogue, *Statesman*, 500–503. The September 1953 *National Geographic* magazine published expansive photographic and verbal coverage of the coronation. Marshall is visible in three photographs "in formal dress standing in first row of choir stalls behind the queen." The caption also noted that "Prime Minister and Lady Churchill appear in the rows behind" Marshall. (H. V. Morton, "In the London of the New Queen," *National Geographic*, September 1953, pp. 291–342; Marshall appears in photographs on 323–24.)

2. Marshall had spoken on June 3 at a lunch "given him by the American Correspondents Association at which he really laced into the responsibilities of a free press in a time of national peril," John Patterson had told Frank McCarthy. "He didn't name any names, but he didn't leave much doubt as to what he was talking about. I was sitting near [Hearst Newspapers Editor-in-Chief] Bill and Bootsie [Alma Virginia Walker] Hearst [Jr]. Their expressions were somewhat sour but I hope it did 'em good. He got a standing ovation." (Patterson to McCarthy, June 12, 1953, GCMRL/Frank McCarthy Collection.)

3. See pp. 774–77.

4. Raymond Daniell, chief correspondent of the *New York Times* in London, had written to C. J. George on June 4 that he had arranged "a small luncheon" for June 10 at the Connaught Hotel near the US embassy. "Besides myself, the other guests will be R. H. Shackford of Scripps-Howard Newspapers; Charles Kline of U.S. News and World Report; Howard Smith of Columbia Broadcasting System and E. C. Daniel, Jr., of the New York Times. There will be no other guests and I personally will vouch for each of these. The General can speak with complete freedom and absolute security." (Daniell to George, June 4, 1953, GCMRL/G. C. Marshall Papers [Retirement, General].) For more on E. C. Daniel Jr., see p. 965n4.

5. See pp. 770–71.

6. Sir Guy Lloyd, a Scottish Unionist Party member of Parliament, had initially written on May 8 inviting Marshall to a "special private dinner" while Marshall was in England. Lloyd was chairman of the Progress Trust, whose members were "all either Members of Parliament or Peers, mostly the former" and the organization was "of the highest standing and repute, of which more than twenty ex-Members are now Ministers of the Crown in Her Majesty's Government." (Lloyd to Marshall, May 8, 1953, GCMRL/G. C. Marshall Papers [Retirement, General].)

"I talked for about forty minutes, but could not discuss foreign policy, because I had not been briefed." Marshall reported in more depth to President Truman in a September 8 letter, "and I was only too glad to keep clear of it—so I devoted myself to explaining attitudes in this country in comparison with those in Great Britain, because of the character of our population and theirs, and our tremendous countryside with its different reactions in comparison with their small country and homogeneous population. I went into a great many factors concerned with this, which seemed to surprise them, apparently because they just had not thought it out. Then, I had to agree to be questioned, and every member of the twenty-five questioned me at some length, which carried the dinner on until about 1:00 a. m. Every question related to the same subject—the Suez Canal, which I thought was prophetic." (Marshall to Truman, September 8, 1953, ibid.) On June 12, Lloyd wrote to thank Marshall for "the splendid speech you made, the frank and kindly way in which you answered all our questions, some, I fear, rather embarrassing." (Lloyd to Marshall, June 12, 1953, ibid.) Britain was involved in an ongoing dispute with Egypt over a "multi-billion-dollar" military base maintained by the British in the Suez Canal zone. "The United States position was and is that we agree completely with the British on the necessity of keeping the big Suez base in tip-top working order so that it could be used instantly in case of war or threat of war with the Soviet Union," Chalmers M. Roberts reported in the *Washington Post* on June 26. "The problem has been and remains how to get the British out gracefully and yet be sure that the base will continue to have sufficient technicians to keep it 100 percent useful." (Chalmers M. Roberts, "U. S. Blocked on Egypt by Churchill," *Washington Post*, June 26, 1953, p. 3.)

Marshall had previously attempted to avoid commenting on current events after his retirement. In response to a request from a high-ranking Nationalist Chinese official to provide his opinions or any advice "privately on the Far Eastern situation," Marshall agreed that "the coming year will be a very crucial one for you and the entire Far East," but he declined to express his own views. He knew "nothing of the inside story of negotiations, arrangements, or the situation, as I have kept entirely out of the current since my resignation as Secretary of Defense. I have a hard time making anyone believe this, but it is a literal fact. When one goes out of office, such an office as mine was particularly, leaving a number of men behind me who have been my intimates, more or less my very personal selections, it would only be an embarrassment to them for me to continue to sit on the edge of things, so I keep entirely aloof." (Wang to Marshall, December 10, 1952, and Marshall to Wang, January 8, 1953, GCMRL/G. C. Marshall Papers [Retirement, General].)

7. Christopher Soames was Churchill's parliamentary private secretary as well as a member of Parliament. See p. 671n2.

8. See p. 778 and the previous document.

9. "I think we should have a free hand to form an alliance with the British if we possibly can do so as to how far Eastern affairs should be conducted," Republican Senate Majority Leader Robert A. Taft had opined in a speech in Cincinnati on May 26. (William S. White, "Taft Won't Budge in His Korea Stand," June 6, 1953, *New York Times*, p. 3.)

10. See pp. 772–73 and previous document. Aldrich wrote to Marshall on June 19, "Everyone was so glad to welcome you both again, and your own prestige and popularity added such distinction to the group of representatives of the President!" (Aldrich to Marshall, June 19, 1953, GCMRL/G. C. Marshall Papers [Retirement, General].)

11. See pp. 769–70.

12. "I have read the documents you submitted with great interest." Eisenhower responded on June 17. (Eisenhower to Marshall, June 17, 1953, ibid.) On June 30, Secretary Dulles wrote, "The dignity and understanding with which you fulfilled your mission contributed greatly to the maintenance of those close and friendly relations between the United States, the United Kingdom, and the Commonwealth of Nations which are of such vital importance at this time." (Dulles to Marshall, June 30, 1953, ibid.)

465

TO DWIGHT D. EISENHOWER — June 18, 1953
[Leesburg, Virginia]

Dear Mr. President: Receipt is hereby acknowledged of your directive of May 25, 1953, on the subject of MAKING CLASSIFIED SECURITY INFORMA-

TION AVAILABLE TO FOREIGN NATIONALS.[1] The delay in my acknowledgement has been occasioned by my absence from the United States in service as your representative at the Coronation of Queen Elizabeth II of Great Britain.[2]

I admit to a full understanding of the spirit and letter of your directive. I shall strictly adhere to it, personally, and shall direct the members, officers, and employees of the American Battle Monuments Commission to do the same.[3] Faithfully yours,

GCMRL/G. C. Marshall Papers (American Battle Monuments Commission)

1. Eisenhower had issued an executive order announcing that department and agency heads in the executive branch would be held responsible for insuring that classified security information would be made available to foreign nationals only "on a real need-to-know basis" and "after determination that the furnishing of such information will result in a net advantage to the interests of the United States." The president requested "that the head of each department and agency in the Executive Branch personally acknowledge to me the receipt of this directive." (Eisenhower memorandum, May 25, 1953, GCMRL/G. C. Marshall Papers [American Battle Monuments Commission].)

2. See previous document.

3. Marshall forwarded Eisenhower's directive to General North with instructions to bring it "to the attention of each member, officer, and employee of the American Battle Monuments Commission, in the United States and abroad, with my endorsement and expressed direction that its spirit and letter be adhered to strictly." (Marshall to North, June 18, 1953, ibid.)

466

MEMORANDUM FOR THE ADJUTANT GENERAL

June 24, 1953
Washington, DC

Subject: Efficiency Report on Brigadier General Thomas North, 0 11 879, USA.

Pursuant to the request of The Adjutant General, AGPA-A, dated May 11, 1953, the following letter report is submitted:

a. Period of Report: 1 June 1952–30 April 1953

b. Duties: Secretary of the American Battle Monuments Commission, acting in an executive capacity. His responsibilities are many and varied. Officer's duties encompass all features of a small but complete organization; i.e. management, budget, personnel, field operations, intimate contact with architectural and construction firms. He deals with all agencies of the government, particularly Congress, not only on the budget aspect, but almost all members have a great interest in the Commission's work.

c. General North is an officer of rare ability. He has the primary responsibility for executing all of the work required of the Commission. He has handled his official affairs in an exceptional manner. I consider him to be physically fit, and he is a man of character and integrity, and possesses keen initiative.

d. Officer is a distinct asset to the Service. During the late war years, he occupied positions of great responsibility and, as a result of his training and experience, he represents a real asset to the Army. The construction program of the Commission is, in effect, from Manila, Philippine Islands, to Luxembourg. General North spends considerable of his time in the field supervising this program. He is tireless and imaginative. In all of my service, I consider him one of the most outstanding officers over whom I have had direct supervision.

e. I am unaware of any weakness or defects in this officer's present assignment or any which would adversely affect a totally different assignment.

f. The membership of the American Battle Monuments Commission was delighted with the Department of the Army's action in recalling General North to active duty, and I hope that his current status will not in any way be affected until the completion of the Commission's program.[1]

GCMRL/G. C. Marshall Papers (Retirement, Chronological)

1. See pp. 734–35, 786–87, and 951.

467

To John J. Phillips — July 16, 1953
[Leesburg, Virginia]

Dear Mr. Phillips: I checked with Colonel Shaw yesterday to determine the status of the American Battle Monuments Commission's budget request and was notified that the House had reduced our travel request approximately $14,000, but subsequently the Senate reinstated the original request.

As one of the Conferees on the Independent Offices Appropriation Bill, I hope you will feel free to stress the necessity for the Commission having the entire amount. As you know, the President recently appointed eight new members to the Commission, of which you are one. In this connection, I feel that all or some of the new members should, at the earliest opportunity, visit the installations in Europe so that they will have first-hand knowledge of what has been done and what is planned. I know that with this information they will be better equipped to carry out their new responsibilities.[1]

I have already querried General North, Secretary of the Commission, regarding the possibilities of a meeting. I will let you know of his recommendation, and I will look forward to making your acquaintance.[2]

With best regards, Faithfully yours,

GCMRL/G. C. Marshall Papers (American Battle Monuments Commission)

1. On July 13, C. J. George had received word from Assistant Chief of Staff Major General Robert N. Young that he had directed the adjutant general to retain Colonel Shaw "on active duty until 1 October 1954." (Young to George, July 13, 1953, GCMRL/G. C. Marshall Papers [American Battle Monuments Commission].) Marshall wrote to Young on July 16 to thank him. This assurance, Marshall told Young, "solves an acute personnel problem, particularly since the President has recently nominated eight new members to the Commission" who would "require considerable assistance in the days to come." (Marshall to Young, July 16, 1953, ibid.) See p. 760n3.

North responded to Marshall from Paris on July 20 and concurred that "Each Member should see both the World War I and World War II cemeteries" excluding "the most inaccessible, viz. Gibraltar and Manila, and possibly Brest and Tunis which should be inspected by individual Members designated by the Chairman." (North to Marshall, memorandum, July 20, 1953, ibid.) He estimated a budget of $1,750 per commissioner and "about 21 working and traveling days" and suggested "added time for rest and relaxation." (Ibid.) North noted that "Congress imposes a limit on our travel funds" and warned, "If the cut in our travel funds made by the House is sustained we shall not have enough funds to send any Members abroad, or even carry on adequately our supervision of construction and maintenance." (Ibid.)

2. North recommended that Marshall set a meeting "for some date immediately after 5 October," and proposed that he "come to Washington by air to assist" Marshall "in orienting new members." He also suggested that Marshall "designate two Members to return with me immediately after the meeting to make an inspection," and that Phillips and Senator Potter "be asked to sponsor a request for funds to take the remaining Members who would like to go to Europe—part of them next Spring, part in the Fall," so that their arrival would be within "the capabilities of some of the smaller hotels which we must use." (Ibid.)

On July 27, Marshall notified commissioners that he was calling an ABMC meeting for September 3 and inquired about the possibility of their participation in an inspection trip. (Marshall to Roosevelt, July 27, 1953, ibid.) "I shall be glad to attend the meeting on September 3," Mrs. Theodore Roosevelt replied, "and to go to Europe in September or early October." (Roosevelt to Marshall, July 29, 1953, ibid.) Admiral Kinkaid responded that he "would be delighted to go as my wife and I have wanted to revisit Europe ever since I retired over three years ago." (Kinkaid to Marshall, July 28, 1953, ibid.) See pp. 786–87.

"WE LEAVE for the Adirondacks to spend the month of August, and that should be very pleasant," Marshall disclosed to Reggie MacDonald-Buchanan on July 27 after admitting that since their return from England, "the extreme heat of the past three weeks has been quite a trial." (Marshall to MacDonald-Buchanan, July 27, 1953, GCMRL/G. C. Marshall Papers [Retirement, General].) The Marshalls arrived on August 4 at Raquette Lake in upstate New York "after a most pleasant motor trip from Leesburg," Marshall told Frank McCarthy on August 10. "We are settled in a little cottage alongside the lake and look forward to spending a most pleasant three weeks with Margaret Emerson." (Marshall to McCarthy, August 10, 1953, ibid.) Emerson's first husband, Alfred G. Vanderbilt, had purchased Sagamore "camp" on Raquette Lake in 1901.

On August 11, Marshall sent birthday wishes and money to his godson Page Wilson and expressed regret that he was in a place "where it would be difficult to find you an appropriate present." He also boasted that he was having "very fine" fishing: "my first day—6 large lake trout and a five pound bass that required 25 minutes to land—but since the take has been strictly limited." (Marshall to Wilson, August 11, 1953, GCMRL/J. Page Wilson Collection; H.) A few days later he told Mary Louise Spilman that he had "a 7 lb. whitefish to my credit" when he notified her of their plans to leave Sagamore, spend a night near Tupper Lake, then the "night of the 19th we expect to spend at Lake Placid." (Marshall to Spilman, August 15, 1953, GCMRL/G. C. Marshall Collection [George].)

The Marshalls arrived on August 20 at Topridge, the summer home of Ambassador and Mrs. Joseph E. Davies, located on Upper Saint Regis Lake, where the Marshalls had visited in 1944 and 1945. See *Papers of GCM*, 4: 550 and 5:

302. Davies was a Washington attorney who had been US ambassador to the Soviet Union from 1936 to 1938, as well as having completed numerous special diplomatic missions for both the Roosevelt and Truman administrations; Mrs. Davies was the former Marjorie Merriweather Post. On August 21, Marshall informed Spilman that they would leave Topridge on August 29 and drive back to Leesburg, expecting to arrive on August 31. (Marshall to Spilman, August 21, 1953, ibid.) After Katherine Marshall wrote to thank Mrs. Davies, Marshall on September 8 added his gratitude for the "truly delightful vacation." He reported that Katherine had "improved almost daily" at Topridge, "and to such an extent that, though we motored down in most excessive heat—topping the performance by 106 at Fredericksburg on our last lap—she stood up very well under the extreme discomfort of the trip." In retrospect, "it would have been better to stay by our original plan to fly down, which was a matter of less than three hours." Marshall admitted that he missed "my daily fishing efforts, however penurious I was about delivering the fish; and particularly the activities of the younger group at tennis, and ours at putting. You had a most agreeable lot of guests, which added a great deal to our pleasure." (Marshall to Davies, September 8, 1953, GCMRL/G. C. Marshall Papers [Retirement, General].) ★

468

To General Alfred M. Gruenther[1] — September 3, 1953, Washington, DC

Dear Gruenther: At a meeting of the Battle Monuments Commission today, it was decided that a group of the new members recently appointed by the President should visit Europe and North Africa. Those selected to make the trip are:

Admiral Thomas C. Kinkaid
Brigadier General Benjamin O. Davis
Mrs. Wendell Willkie
Mrs. Theodore Roosevelt

This group will leave New York by water on September 28, arriving at Bremerhaven on October 6, where they will be met by Brigadier General Thomas North. Incidentally, Kinkaid and Davis will be accompanied by their wives.[2] Congressman John Phillips, who is also a newly appointed member, will rendezvous with the party in Paris. He leaves this afternoon by air in connection with Congressional business.

As you know, it takes considerable time to make the circuit and to properly inspect all of the installations. Not only is it time consuming, but at times it is very tiresome. I wonder if it would be possible and convenient for you to arrange military air transportation when necessary? There will only be a few instances when such travel would be required. I also wonder if it would be convenient for you to arrange their return home on one of the scheduled MATS planes.[3] They should be prepared to leave on or about October 27.[4]

I hope that all goes well with you and that you are not suffering too much from the heat.[5] I read the other day of your trip to one of the Scandinavian countries, and I am sure you found the climate there much more to your liking than what you are experiencing there on the Seine.[6]

With warmest regards, Faithfully yours,

GCMRL/G. C. Marshall Papers (Retirement, General)

1. Gruenther had succeeded Ridgway as Supreme Allied Commander, Europe at NATO headquarters outside Paris in July. ("'New' Gruenther Sheds Old Habits," *New York Times*, August 16, 1953, p. 22.)

2. The same day, C. J. George informed the Office of the Secretary of Defense of the travel itinerary and later clarified that "The Commission will pay official expenses of the members" but Kinkaid and Davis would pay their wives' expenses. (George to Riva, September 3, and George to Bergin, September 14, 1953, GCMRL/G. C. Marshall Papers [Retirement, General].)

3. "I shall be delighted to provide air transportation for this group whenever that is necessary," Gruenther replied. "I will have our people work directly" with General North, and Gruenther hoped "to have the pleasure of seeing the group while it is in Paris." (Gruenther to Marshall, September 15, 1953, ibid.)

4. On October 24, North reported to Marshall that "The five Members have arrived in Rome after a strenuous visit." The inspectors, he continued, "so far, have expressed themselves as highly pleased with the opportunity to make the visit and with our arrangements for their travel and housing." He notified Marshall that Kinkaid, Phillips, and Davis would return to Washington by air on October 29 and Roosevelt and Willkie had planned to sail in mid-October. (North to Marshall, October 24, 1953, ibid.)

5. The *New York Times* had reported that high temperatures were "making life in [NATO's] low, prefabricated headquarters uncomfortable." ("'New' Gruenther Sheds Old Habits," *New York Times*, August 16, 1953, p. 22.) The temperature in Washington, DC, on September 3 was ninety-nine degrees. The previous day had been two degrees hotter.

6. Gruenther had left Paris on August 25 "for a week-long tour of Denmark and Norway" to "confer with civil and military leaders." ("Gruenther to Tour Scandinavia," *New York Times*, August 24, 1953, p. 6.)

469

To Mrs. James J. Winn — September 8, 1953, Washington, DC

Dear Molly: Your mother and I came in today for the Wainwright funeral, had lunch at the Pentagon and, while she is doing some shopping, I am finishing up a little business here in the office.[1]

Your mother looks very well, though, of course, she has to be careful about her back. She succeeded in scalding the inside of her right hand yesterday cooking, but it seems to be fairly well recovered today and is painless.

At the funeral, we found ourselves seated with Captain and Mrs. Wainwright. Mrs. Wainwright, Sr., was not there.[2] This was very fortunate, because it permitted your mother to sit down during the ceremony.

Most confidentially, I must tell you that, as you realize fairly well, she is always worrying about your physical health, and was terribly worried when you decided not to come up to Leesburg. I tried to explain to her that it would be very wasteful to try to motor that distance for a five or six day stay, but her reaction was that you had such a hard summer that you were worn down and couldn't make the trip. I claimed you had some diversion in the Smokies, but she said sleeping out in a pup-tent with Jimmy was no vacation, nor cooking meals for him in a cabin.

She would be quite furious with me—rather seriously so—if she knew I were writing you this way, but I am trying to put you a little on guard on what to say, because she reacts so deeply that she finds herself in a continuous state of worry about you and your well-being. Make no reference to this whatsoever—it would probably promote a separation in our family. I find my seemingly logical explanations of things concerning you don't go. I am just registered as unappreciative or uninterested.

I am well, pretty much tanned up, and thoroughly enjoyed the summer. I have just received the keys to a pond and a boat of a Washington man's place near Leesburg with an authority to fish—the pond having been stocked.

The new fencing around the place looks very grand. God knows it should, because my bank account looks very puny. In talking over the matter with Dave Rust at Leesburg, he and some of his friends estimated I could have had the same thing done for $500 ten years ago, instead of $4,000 this year.[3]

Some time this month, possibly about the 20th, I am going to drive out to see Marie and then to Uniontown to attend a dinner in my honor at the dedication of a private dining room at the White Swan Hotel which is being named for me. I am waiting to hear from Marie to set the date. She has taken five days to answer my letter and probably will say she is sorry, but she had an appointment with her hairdresser.[4]

With my love, Affectionately,

GCM

GCMRL/G. C. Marshall Papers (Retirement, General)

1. The funeral for Medal of Honor recipient General Jonathan M. Wainwright (USMA, 1906)—who had died in San Antonio, Texas, on September 2—had taken place at 11:00 a.m. at Arlington National Cemetery. Wainwright commanded US forces in the Philippines between March 12 and the surrender to the Japanese on May 7, 1942, when he became a prisoner of war until August 16, 1945. See *Papers of GCM*, 5: 283, 285, and 290.

In his September 8 letter to Marjorie Davies (see pp. 785–86), Marshall reminisced about his September 10, 1945, flight with actor Walter Huston, the narrator of the "Why We Fight" films commissioned by Marshall during World War II (see p. 32), from the Davies' summer home in upstate New York "to greet Wainwright on his arrival in Washington from his imprisonment." As part of the celebration, Huston had witnessed President Truman present the Medal of Honor to Wainwright, the citation for which Marshall had personally written, "and had a conversation with the President." Marshall and Huston had returned to the Davies' summer home "in time for tea that evening. I do wish I could have seen him there this summer." Huston had died in 1950. (Marshall to Davies, September 8, 1953, GCMRL/G. C. Marshall Papers [Retirement, General].) See also *Papers of GCM*, 5: 290 and 302n1.

2. Jonathan M. Wainwright V was a captain in the naval reserve. (See pp. 923–24.) His wife was the former Elfrida Olsen; his mother, Adele "Kitty" Wainwright, did not attend the funeral at Arlington. ("Gen. Wainwright Laid to Rest in Impressive Arlington Rites," *Washington Post*, September 9, 1953, p. 22.)

3. On July 14, Marshall had written to Molly Winn that he and Mrs. Marshall would have a new "high screening" fence installed around much of the property at Dodona Manor,

"except back of where Jimmy found the blackberries. Pretty expensive—$3,700 plus what we pay locally for clearing the line." (Marshall to Winn, July 14, 1953, GCMRL/© Marshall-Winn Collection [Winn]; H.) Rust was a breeder of thoroughbred race horses and a vestryman at St. James Episcopal Church in Leesburg, which Marshall also attended. ("Landowner David N. Rust, Breeder of Race Horses," *Loudon Times-Mirror*, October 17, 1963, p. A8.)

4. Herman M. Buck, president of the hotel, had written to Marshall on June 15 for permission to dedicate the room in his honor. (Buck to Marshall, June 15, 1953, GCMRL/G. C. Marshall Papers [Retirement, General].) In his next letter, Buck suggested that he would "arrange the opening of the 'General Marshall Room' to coincide with" Marshall's planned visit with his widowed sister, Marie Singer, who lived in nearby Greensburg, Pennsylvania. Buck proposed "a dinner for not more than thirty to 35 persons consisting largely of your Uniontown boyhood friends and a few of our public officials" as well as "a reception for a larger but limited group preceding the dinner." (Buck to Marshall, July 9, 1953, ibid.) Marshall replied that he "would be very glad to participate." (Marshall to Buck, July 16, 1953, ibid.) Marshall pressed his sister on September 8 to confirm the date. "They are waiting to hear from me, and I am waiting to hear from you." (Marshall to Singer, September 8, 1953, ibid.) See pp. 790–91.

470

To General J. Lawton Collins — September 8, 1953, Washington, DC

Dear Collins: I am sorry I was not here—absent in the Adirondacks—to be present at the final ceremonies at the termination of your career as Chief of Staff of the Army. You did a magnificent job and lived up to the very remarkable career that got well underway at Benning. I think, however, your high moment was at the surrender at Cherbourg—at least photographically.[1]

I saw Bradley today at Wainwright's funeral, and he was bragging—an unusual thing for him—of staying in the golf tournament, despite the rain, until they closed the course. He explained to me that he did it for the honor of the Army, without regard for his own feelings.[2]

We spent all of August in the Adirondacks and had a charming summer.[3]

With affectionate regards to Mrs. Collins and you, Faithfully yours,

GCMRL/G. C. Marshall Papers (Retirement, Chronological)

1. Collins was among the future military leaders under Marshall's command at the US Army Infantry School at Fort Benning, Georgia, in 1927. See *Papers of GCM*, 1: 319–21. In June 1944, Collins led the US VII Army Corps in its victorious campaign up the Cherbourg peninsula in France, which resulted in the liberation of the city of Cherbourg. ("Three Veteran U.S. Divisions Won Peninsula," *Washington Post*, June 28, 1944, p. 2.) Photographs of the mayor thanking Collins were widely publicized.

2. See previous document, n1. The *Washington Post* reported that Omar Bradley, who had been playing with Vice President Richard Nixon in the National Celebrities Open golf tournament at the Woodmont Country Club in Rockville, Maryland, "barely beat the rain to the ninth hole and then raced for the clubhouse." ("Celebrities Rained Out, Held Over to Monday," *Washington Post*, September 6, 1953, p. M1.)

3. See pp. 785–86.

471

To Frank McCarthy

October 5, 1953
Leesburg, Virginia

Dear Frank: Thank you for your letter of September 26 and the reviews on your picture. You seem to be getting a good share of complimentary comment, and a profit looks promising.[1]

There has been considerable publicity about the picture THE ROBE and Katherine and I hope to see it.[2]

I hope nothing will come up to interfere with your plans to purchase the house. Is there not any brown or red mink in your area?[3]

The other day we motored up to the mountains to see Marie and, after enjoying a pleasant weekend in that delightful atmosphere, we motored over to Uniontown. We had a very full program. First, there was a luncheon in the mountains near Fort Necessity. That same afternoon, I received the Key of the City from the Mayor and a lifetime membership in the Veterans of Foreign Wars Post, which they so graciously named in my honor. They gathered all the school children in the theatre and I had the opportunity of talking to them for about half an hour. They planned to hold it in the school stadium, but rain forced us indoors.[4] They had a dinner that evening in the new hotel at Uniontown, where I again was paid a compliment when they dedicated the new dining room in my name.[5]

I have been feeling punk since my return. I somehow picked up a virus and Dr. Jackson has been filling me up with aureomycin.[6] At this moment, I feel a little weak, but should soon feel normal again.

We plan to move down to Pinehurst about October 20. When you come East again, please pay us a visit.

I am returning the clippings, as you requested. Faithfully yours,

GCMRL/G. C. Marshall Papers (Retirement, General)

1. See pp. 779n4. "The film has been a great hit in England," McCarthy had reported, which meant "we have to recoup only $500,000 in all the rest of the world." (McCarthy to Marshall, September 26, 1953, GCMRL/G. C. Marshall Papers [Retirement, General].) The Marshalls had attended the premiere of *Sailor of the King* in McCarthy's hometown of Richmond, Virginia, on July 28. Marshall had congratulated McCarthy on August 10 and said he was "delighted to participate in the honors which your townspeople paid you." (Marshall to McCarthy, August 10, 1953, ibid.)

2. *The Robe*, starring Richard Burton and Jean Simmons, was the first film released in Cinemascope format.

3. McCarthy, who was a bachelor, had confided in an August 17 letter that he had "been casting a covetous eye" on a house for sale in Sullivan Canyon, where there was much wildlife. Marshall had responded on September 3 that he hoped there would be "one other bit of animal life due around there—and it must not be a high blonde." In his September 26 letter, McCarthy told Marshall that engineers had discovered problems around the house foundation and teased that "mink is difficult to domesticate. Blonde mink is, of course, out of the question because the Hollywood variety can't be domesticated at all." (McCarthy to Marshall, August 17, 1953, ibid.; Marshall to McCarthy, September 3, 1953, ibid.; and McCarthy to Marshall, September 26, 1953, ibid.)

4. See p. 789n4. After going to Greensburg, Marshall had traveled on September 21 with his wife and sister to Fort Necessity—site of a battle on July 3, 1754, the first in the

French and Indian War—which was undergoing restoration. See pp. 844–47. They then continued on to Uniontown, which he had last visited on September 9, 1939. (See *Papers of GCM*, 2: 54–55.) The *Pittsburgh Post-Gazette* reported that "the key to the city" presented to Marshall had been "made from honey locust wood taken from a tree which formerly stood on the old Marshall homestead," now the location of the Veterans of Foreign Wars Post. Four thousand youngsters heard Marshall speak at the State Theater where he "reminded the students how many great events in the early history of the nation originated in this vicinity." ("Ex-Chief of Staff 'Home,'" *Pittsburgh Post-Gazette*, September 22, 1953.)

5. On September 23, Herman Buck wrote to Marshall to express gratitude and affirm that Uniontown "is tremendously enthusiastic about the two of you." Buck also wrote to C. J. George to thank him for his assistance, and George responded on October 2 that Marshall "thought that everything was well programmed and he was happy to renew old acquaintances and have a good look around the area of his boyhood." (Buck to Marshall and Buck to George, September 23, 1953; George to Buck, October 2, 1953, GCMRL/G. C. Marshall Papers [Retirement, General].)

6. Dr. Jackson may have been Dr. James T. Jackson, who practiced in Leesburg in 1953. Aureomycin is an antibiotic.

472

To Charles E. Wilson

October 9, 1953
Leesburg, Virginia

Dear Wilson: At a meeting of the newly appointed American Battle Monuments Commission on September 3, it was agreed that some recognition be made of Brigadier General Robert G. Woodside's contribution to the work of the Commission covering a period of thirty years.[1]

General Woodside was appointed by President Harding as a member of the original Commission when it was organized in conformity with Public Law 534, 67th Congress, dated March 4, 1923. At the first meeting of the newly organized Commission, Woodside was elected by the members as Vice Chairman. He has given generously of his time and energy without compensation and, during the period of General Pershing's confinement, he assumed the full responsibility of its functions.[2] During this period, he played an important role in the development of our World War I cemeteries.

I know that you are familiar with the Commission's activities and will avoid details. However, I must point out the great contribution that he made to effectively memorialize our war dead interred in beautiful cemeteries abroad. Through his foresight and energy, we were able to, shortly after the termination of World War II, develop a program of cemetery and memorial construction, which is now well on the road to completion. We anticipate that all of the work will be completed in the next two years.

Incidentally, I was appointed a member of the Commission on October 11, 1946, and, after the death of General Pershing, was elected its Chairman, but, because of my various assignments after my period as Chief of Staff, I was unable to devote full time to its work. Consequently, Woodside carried the full load of supervising the Commission's activities.

I know of no other effort which we have made that impresses foreigners as much as our devotion and respect of our war dead and the memorials which have been created in their memory. It leaves such a deep impression on our friends abroad that what has been done for our dead certainly fosters their impression of us as a devoted nation, but, more important, that the sites stand as a permanent monument to those who paid the supreme sacrifice so that others may live in peace.

Woodside is deserving of the highest praise. I request that you consider awarding him "The Medal Of Freedom". It is the least we can do for such a remarkable service to our country.[3] Faithfully yours,

GCMRL/G. C. Marshall Papers (Retirement, General)

1. Woodside, who had retired to Sarasota, Florida, had held various public offices in Pennsylvania and had commanded the state's National Guard during World War II. He was commander in chief of the National Veterans of Foreign Wars five times, and twice headed the Army and Navy Legion of Honor.

2. General Pershing had been a patient at Walter Reed General Hospital in Washington, DC, from May 6, 1941, until his death on July 15, 1948. See *Papers of GCM*, 6: 503–6.

3. Wilson responded on October 30 that he appreciated "the opportunity to recognize the unselfish and devoted service" of General Woodside and approved "awarding to him the Medal of Freedom." (Wilson to Marshall, October 30, 1953, GCMRL/G. C. Marshall Papers [Retirement, General].) President Truman had established the Medal of Freedom on July 6, 1945, to honor civilian service during World War II. He amended criteria for the award on April 3, 1952, so that "without regard to the existence of a state of war or national emergency, the Medal of Freedom may also be awarded . . . for performance of a meritorious act or service in the interests of the security of the United States." Executive Order 10336 stipulated that secretaries of state, defense, and the military services could make nominations. (Executive Order 10336, Amendment of Executive Order 9586 of July 6, 1945, Establishing the Medal of Freedom.)

After General North recommended on January 7, 1954, that General Ridgway be asked to present the medal to Woodside, Marshall suggested "to get the President" to do so "as a favor to me." (North to Marshall, January 7, 1954, GCMRL/G. C. Marshall Papers [American Battle Monuments Commission].) Eisenhower agreed, and Marshall expressed his thanks to the president on January 18 for his "kindness in arranging to take time from your busy day" to make the presentation. Marshall also regretted that he could not attend the ceremony as he did not feel fit to travel from Pinehurst. (Marshall to Eisenhower, January 18, 1954, DDEL/Dwight D. Eisenhower Papers [Papers as President, Ann Whitman File, Name Series, Box 21]; H.) "I am sorry you could not be with us this morning when the Medal of Freedom was presented to General Woodside" at the White House, Eisenhower wrote to Marshall on February 4. "We missed you." (Eisenhower to Marshall, February 4, 1954, GCMRL/G. C. Marshall Papers [American Battle Monuments Commission].)

473

To Major General William F. Dean — October 14, 1953
Leesburg, Virginia

Dear Dean: I have purposely waited until the flood of welcome had somewhat subsided in your case before writing you.[1] Of course, I am delighted with your safe return from a horrible experience, but what I want to say is this:

I feel that the entire country owes you a very special regard for having personally suffered more than any other man for the failures of the period preceding the outbreak of the fighting in Korea. And this, in particular, because of the superb manner in which you met the issue on the ground at the time and suffered for all of the failures of the military, due in the largest measure to the public reactions on Congress.

During the last war, I had somewhat the same feeling regarding the men who were captured on Bataan and Corregidor and other places in the Philippines, particularly those at Bataan.[2] But your case is markedly apart because of the superb manner in which you met the issue on the ground, as I have said.

I wanted you to know that I felt this way about it and, while I did not come again into power in connection with military matters until after your disappearance, I felt a degree of personal responsibility for what had happened.[3]

I know you are happy in the return to your family. I hope your health has not been impaired, and I will continue to feel a lasting indebtedness to you for the sacrifices you had to make and the gallantry with which you made them.[4] Faithfully yours,

GCMRL/G. C. Marshall Papers (Retirement, General)

1. Major General William F. Dean, while commanding the Twenty-fourth Infantry Division, had been captured early in the Korean conflict and held as a prisoner of war near Pyongyang until he was returned to United Nations forces at Panmunjom on September 4, 1953. Marshall wrote to Dean at his home in Berkeley, California.

2. On April 9, 1942, Japanese forces took the Bataan peninsula into which American and Filipino forces had previously withdrawn and sent the approximately seventy-eight thousand soldiers they captured on what became known as the Bataan Death March. Another eleven thousand prisoners were captured when the Japanese took the island of Corregidor in Manila Bay on May 9, 1942. (See also Pogue, *Ordeal*, 259.)

3. While a prisoner of war, Dean had been awarded the Medal of Honor on February 16, 1951. (See p. 471.) The medal citation explained that after facing "a ruthless and determined enemy, highly trained and overwhelmingly superior in numbers," Dean had "remained behind organizing his retreating forces, directing stragglers, and was last seen assisting the wounded to a place of safety." The citation went on to praise Dean's "heroic leadership, courageous and loyal devotion to his men, and his complete disregard for personal safety." (Citation, February 16, 1951, © Congressional Medal of Honor Society.)

4. "Your kind and laudatory letter of 14 October makes me very proud and happy. There is no one from whom I would rather receive a commendation. I only wish that I could make myself believe that I merit all you have said," Dean responded. (Dean to Marshall, October 19, 1953, GCMRL/G. C. Marshall Papers [Retirement, General].)

THE INFLUENZA that had left Marshall "feeling punk" since his return from Uniontown had lingered throughout October. (See p. 790.) "It first started on September 23rd in Leesburg and after having been confined to bed for a week, I was under the impression that I had rid my system of the bug," Marshall explained to Madame Chiang on November 6. "Somehow it stayed with me because shortly after our arrival in Pinehurst on October 20th I had a relapse. For ten days Katherine spent all of her time nursing me, and while there was no fever I had a very aggravating cough." (Marshall to Chiang, November 5, 1953, GCMRL/G. C. Marshall Papers [Retirement, General].) He was still bedridden on October 30 when he received word that the Norwegian Nobel Institute had awarded him the 1953 Peace Prize, no doubt for his work on the European Recovery Program. "I was greatly surprised to hear the announcement. It came about in a very unusual way," Marshall wrote to Thomas A. Morgan, on November 13. "Mrs. Marshall had a telephone call . . . asking for a statement. It seems the award was announced by the Nobel Institute before their telegram, which was addressed to Leesburg, reached me at Pinehurst." (Marshall to Morgan, November 13, 1953, ibid.) The *New York Times* explained that Alfred Nobel, the inventor of dynamite, had stipulated in his will "that the peace prize should go to the candidate 'who has worked the most or best for promoting brotherhood among people, and for the abolition or reduction of the standing armies, and for the establishment and spread of peace congresses,'" and that the 1953 prize would convey more than thirty-three thousand tax-free dollars to Marshall. "In keeping with tradition" the Nobel Institute "gave no explanation" for its selection of Marshall. ("Nobel Prizes to Marshall, Schweitzer," *New York Times*, October 31, 1953, p. 1.) Marshall stated that he could "not find words to express my thanks. This award is a great distinction for which I am deeply grateful. While I have not received official notification, I assume from press dispatches that it is a fact." ("Marshall is Ill of Cold," *New York Times*, October 31, 1953, p. 15.)

The next day, the *New York Times* reported, Marshall "got up from his sickbed to hold a news conference." ("Marshall Talks of his Peace Work," *New York Times*, November 1, 1953, p. 35.) "General Marshall looked rather drawn when he came into the living room from his bedroom but he soon was laughing and joking with photographers," the newspaper described. "He appeared tired and his voice was hoarse but he was in good spirits," and he said that "his greatest contributions to world peace were in speeding United States preparations to fight aggression in 1940 and again in 1950." He recalled that the effort in 1940 "'to persuade the Administration and Congress to get under way with preparations for the inevitable war'" had been "'the hardest thing I ever did.'" Marshall continued, "'Next to that I feel was the struggle in the fall of 1950 to rebuild our forces during the fighting in Korea, trying to do in a month what would normally take a year under great pressure of conflicting opposition in the Congress and in the country as to how this should be done.'" He also mentioned "'the difficulty of keeping one's temper and maintaining one's patience in utterly fruitless negotiations with the Soviet Government.'" (Ibid.)

After receiving news of the severity of Marshall's illness, President Eisenhower arranged for Marshall to be flown on November 1 to Walter Reed Army Hospital, where he would remain for sixteen days. ("Marshall in Hospital," *New York Times*, November 3, 1953, p. 33; "Marshall Going to Oslo," *New York Times*, November 18, 1953, p. 8.) "We had a quiet flight and I slept the latter half," he wrote to Katherine Marshall later that day; "My quarters were all ready for me" at Walter Reed, and "The doctors started in immediately" with tests and medication to quiet his cough. C. J. George stayed with him until 3:30 p.m. and then informed Mrs. Marshall via telephone that her husband was "resting comfortably." (Marshall to Katherine Marshall, November 1, 1953, GCMRL/© Marshall-Winn Collection [Katherine Marshall]; Mace to Marshall, October 30, 1953, GCMRL/G. C. Marshall Papers [Retirement, General].)

There are hundreds of letters of congratulation for the Nobel Prize in the Marshall Papers, although he probably received others that were not catalogued, plus many phone calls. Marshall's responses to most of the letters were very similar. Only those of a more personal nature are included here. Among those not included are letters to Dean Acheson, Eleanor "Bee" Arnold (Mrs. Henry H. "Hap" Arnold), Supreme Court Justice Harold Burton, actress Joan Fontaine, Henry Cabot Lodge Jr., Frank and Frances McCoy, Thomas North, Harold Stassen, Robert T. Stevens, and Thomas J. Watson Jr.

While recuperating, Marshall composed a letter on November 12 to fellow Nobel laureate Winston Churchill, who had been awarded the prize for literature. "I thought, along with the world, that it was wonderfully appropriate," Marshall wrote to him. "You have been prominent in many things in the past twenty-five years, but in nothing more magnificently than in the leadership you have given the world through the medium of your compelling voice." (Marshall to Churchill, November 12, 1953, Churchill Archives Centre, Churchill College, Cambridge, UK/Winston S. Churchill Papers [Public and Political: General, Private and Personal]; H.) ★

474

TO DWIGHT D. EISENHOWER

November 2, 1953
Washington, DC

Dear Mr. President: I am dictating this note as it is rather difficult to write legibly while confined to bed.

Mrs. Marshall conveyed your concern about my health, the offer of your plane and good wishes on the Nobel Award.[1] I am grateful for your interest and am glad to say that I am beginning to feel better. Your Naval Aide was good enough to arrange for one of the fast two-engine aircraft to pick me up at Pinehurst. We arrived at Walter Reed just about lunchtime and the doctors immediately took over.[2] With the care they are giving me I should be on my way home the first of next week.

I have had no official word on the arrangements incident to the presentation, but understand that the ceremony will be held in Stockholm in December.[3] I plan to go by ship and have decided on the Southern route to avoid heavy weather.[4] Needless to say I was very much surprised by the announcement, and in accepting this recognition I do so on behalf of the American people, for it was they who made it possible.

You have been most gracious in your thoughts of me and I am grateful. I hope you will give Mrs. Eisenhower our warmest regards.

With great respect, Faithfully yours,

GCMarshall

GCMRL/G. C. Marshall Papers (Retirement, General)

1. Eisenhower had written on October 30 to express his "sincere congratulations," and acknowledge that while, "at times, I have been completely nonplused in attempting to follow the reasoning of some of the commissions that make awards to individuals in this world—this time, I heartily approve." (Eisenhower to Marshall, October 30, 1953, GCMRL/G. C. Marshall Papers [Retirement, General].) The president was also disappointed Marshall's "slight illness" would "prevent your attendance at the dinner that the Greek King is giving. This distresses me, not only because you apparently are confined to your bed, but because I will be denied the opportunity of having a chat with you." (Ibid.) President and Mrs. Eisenhower had hosted a state dinner at the White House on October 28 for Queen Frederica and King Paul before they embarked on a month-long tour of the United States. Two nights later, the king and queen returned the Eisenhowers' hospitality by giving a dinner at the Greek embassy, which Marshall had been scheduled to attend. ("King Paul, Queen Visit Annapolis," *New York Herald Tribune*, October 31, 1953.)

C. J. George had notified Marshall on September 9 that Queen Frederica had "expressed a desire" to visit with the Marshalls should she and her husband travel to the United States. George had told a counselor at the Greek embassy that the Marshalls hoped the king and queen could visit them in Pinehurst. (George to Marshall, September 9, 1953, GCMRL/G. C. Marshall Papers [Retirement, Chronological].) See pp. 801–2.

2. Eisenhower had initiated Marshall's transport to the hospital on November 1. See *Papers of DDE*, 14: 626n1. "George and I appreciated so much your call and offer of your plane, but this field is too small for it to come in on," Katherine wrote the president in an undated note. "The Navy sent a plane in Sunday." (Katherine Marshall to Eisenhower, n.d., DDEL/Dwight D. Eisenhower Papers [Papers as President, Ann Whitman File, Name Series, Box 21].)

"I came up to Washington yesterday afternoon in hopes that the experts at Walter Reed could clear up this heavy congestion," Marshall confided to Bernard Baruch on November 2. "I have just about worn myself out coughing and have lost some 15 pounds as a result. Last night was the best I have enjoyed in weeks." (Marshall to Baruch, November 2, 1953, GCMRL/G. C. Marshall Papers [Retirement, General].) Marshall complained to Margaret Emerson the same day that he "wanted to stay at home" but his wife "practically insisted so I lost a game but weakening battle. Progress has already been noted, my strength is gradually coming back and the cough has subsided." (Marshall to Emerson, November 2, 1953, ibid.) "Ever since September 23," he admitted to Frank McCarthy on November 3, "I have been fighting a very aggravating case of the flu. Just before leaving for Pinehurst, I thought I had worked it out of my system, but I no sooner got settled down below when it struck again." He had been making "rapid progress" at Walter Reed, however, and "Barring any complications, I should be at home this time next week. I am comfortably situated and there have been so many individuals running in and out with white coats that I mistook the barber for one of the doctors." Three days later, however, he informed McCarthy that he now had "no idea" when the doctors would release him. (Marshall to McCarthy, November 3 and 6, 1953, ibid.)

3. Nobel Prizes for physiology and medicine, physics, chemistry, and literature are presented in Stockholm, Sweden, but the Peace Prize is presented in Oslo, Norway. See pp. 810–16.

4. See p. 799n3.

475

To Gunnar Jahn and August Schou[1]

November 4, 1953
Washington, DC

My dear Mr. Schou: I deeply appreciate your telegram of October 30 in which you notify me that the Nobel Committee of the Norwegian Parliament has awarded me the Nobel Peace Prize for 1953.[2] It is an honor which I gratefully accept on behalf of the American people. The fact that the Committee has singled me out is most heart warming.

I shall look forward to the receipt of your letter and I accept with pleasure the invitation to come to Oslo.[3] I will convey my travel plans as soon as they have been firmed up and, in keeping with the statutes of the Foundation, I will be prepared to give a lecture subsequent to December 10.[4]

I wish you would let those concerned know of my gratitude.

With best regards. Faithfully yours,

GCMRL/G. C. Marshall Papers (Retirement, General)

1. See p. 748n2. Gunnar Jahn was chairman of the Norwegian Nobel Committee from 1941 to 1966.

2. "I have the honor to inform you that the Nobel Committee of the Norwegian Parliament today has awarded to you the Nobel Peace Prize for 1953," Schou had announced. "The prize amounts to 175.292.94 Swedish crowns. Letter follows." (Jahn and Schou to Marshall, telegram, October 30, 1953, GCMRL/G. C. Marshall Papers [Retirement, General].)

3. Jahn and Schou's letter reconfirmed the information in the telegram and mentioned that the prize would be a "medal in gold, on the edge of which will be engraved your name." (Jahn and Schou to Marshall, October 31, 1953, ibid.)

4. "I have also the honor to invite you to come to Oslo and receive the prize on December 10th," Schou's telegram had continued. "According to the statutes of the Nobel Foundation it is incumbent on the prizewinner if possible to give a lecture on his work. Such a lecture can be held in Oslo one of the first days after December 10th." (Jahn and Schou to Marshall, telegram, October 30, 1953, ibid.)

476

To Harry S. Truman — November 4, 1953, Washington, DC

Dear Mr. Truman: I acknowledge with very deep appreciation your telegram of October 31 regarding the Nobel Award.[1] Needless to say, I was surprised when the news first reached me. However, I felt so badly because of this virus I have been carrying around that I could not celebrate the honor. While the recognition is individual in nature, it is, in effect, a tribute to the American people for their unselfish devotion to the welfare of free people everywhere. I hope you will share this distinction with me because it was through your guidance and leadership that the [European] Recovery Plan was made possible.

As I indicated, I have been entertaining in my system an unwelcome guest. It has been with me for five weeks and on Saturday last Katherine, through heavy persuasion, literally forced me into coming up to Walter Reed. I am comfortably situated in the suite that they had arranged for you and which you occupied for a similar ailment.[2] At this particular moment, I am feeling fairly well and, if the progress continues, I should be back in Pinehurst this time next week.

I had prior word from Mr. Edward R. Murrow of the television show last night.[3] I watched it with considerable interest and, as you can well imagine, am deeply appreciative of the honor which you paid me. As usual, you were most generous and kind and, while the years pass into oblivion, I shall never forget your unstinting support in the work which was entrusted me.[4]

I have heard and read of the possibilities of your being signed up on a television network. After watching last night's performance, I think it is a media suited to your talents.

With many thanks again for everything, and with warmest regards to Mrs. Truman, Margaret and you, in which I am joined by Katherine, I am, with great respect, Faithfully yours,

GCMRL/G. C. Marshall Papers (Retirement, General)

1. "They certainly picked the right man," Truman had cabled. "I am just as happy over the award as you are if that is possible." (Truman to Marshall, telegram, October 31, 1953, GCMRL/G. C. Marshall Papers [Retirement, General].)

2. President Truman had been hospitalized at Walter Reed from July 16 to 19, 1952.

3. Truman had been interviewed by Joseph Wershba on *See It Now*. See pp. 767–68. "The nurse on the ward arranged for a TV set and so I was able to see it without leaving my bed," Marshall wrote to Murrow the next day. "Mr. Truman and you were most thoughtful and kind in expressing yourselves on the occasion of the Award. Needless to say, it is a great tribute and I am deeply honored. While it is individual in nature, it truly belongs to all of our people." (Marshall to Murrow, November 5, 1953, ibid.) "Thank you for your gracious letter," Murrow responded. "Please permit me to say I derived deep personal satisfaction from the award to you and from the possibility of using the medium of television to report it at some length." (Murrow to Marshall, November 16, 1953, ibid.)

4. "I think we can look forward to the time when we will have world peace," Truman had told Wershba. "That's what General Marshall has spent the best part of his life working for ever since he was Chief of Staff and I think General Marshall will go down in history as the man of the age." Wershba then asked Truman whether he could find it in his heart "to forgive that little handful of men in public life who attacked General Marshall's personal loyalty and patriotism." Truman replied: "No. That's one of the dirtiest tricks that ever happened. The man who made that attack wasn't fit to shine General Marshall's shoes." (Edward R. Murrow and Fred W. Friendly, *See It Now* [New York: Simon and Schuster, 1955], 197.)

477

To Mrs. John J. Singer — November 6, 1953
Washington, DC

Dear Marie: While I am feeling considerably better at this moment, I still find it very difficult to write in bed and since my throat is no longer giving me any trouble, I find it convenient to dictate.

As you can well imagine I was tremendously surprised when a correspondent of the International News Association called Katherine and asked her for my reaction to the award.[1] It was a little hard to believe at first, because I had no idea that the Institute was even considering me. However, I later found out that the Panel which consisted of five members of the Norwegian Parliament cast a unanimous vote in my favor. Naturally, I felt highly honored and humble. To be the first professional soldier to receive the Peace Award adds luster to its significance.

As you know, I am situated here at Walter Reed Hospital and am most comfortable because I am occupying the President's suite. It is a very delightful arrangement.[2] I have had excellent care and if progress continues, should be home this time next week. I was afraid that Katherine might have worked herself to a frazzle caring for me, but Colonel George tells me that she is in very fine shape. Your post script sounds like you have joined the Chamber of Commerce of Greensburg.[3]

With all my love Affectionately,

GCMRL/G. C. Marshall Papers (Retirement, General)

1. See pp. 793–95. Singer had written her brother that "already three reporters have called me but I told them I knew nothing except what I had heard on the Radio. Is there any honor left for you, for you seem to have had everything. This is just to tell you how delighted and proud I feel." (Singer to Marshall, October 30, 1953, GCMRL/G. C. Marshall Papers [Retirement, General].)

2. See previous document.

3. Marie Singer had suggested that Marshall "should have stayed north in the cold!" (Singer to Marshall, October 30, 1953, ibid.)

On November 11, Marshall wrote his wife that he had also "received a pencil post card of congratulations" from his and Marie's brother, Stuart, and "So I'll have to make a prompt reply or he will be very critical." (Marshall to Katherine Marshall, November 11, 1953, GCMRL/© Marshall-Winn Collection [Katherine Marshall]; H.) Stuart Bradford Marshall (VMI, 1894), an engineering consultant and metallurgist, was for many years president of the Washington, DC, VMI alumni chapter. His "pencil post card" is not in the Marshall Papers. "Thanks for your post card of congratulations," Marshall replied in a handwritten note on November 11. "It was good of you to write." (Marshall to Stuart Marshall, November 11, 1953, GCMRL/Stuart B. Marshall Papers; H.)

Rose Page Wilson had also congratulated Marshall for receiving "the most coveted and distinguished award that can be given." She assured Marshall that "This is no empty compliment, it is an expression of gratitude and honor and I am very proud of you. I have always been proud of you." (Wilson to Marshall, November 2, 1953, ibid.) In his November 6 response, Marshall was "hopeful" that his health would improve enough for him to travel to Oslo. "If I do go," he confided he would depart for Naples on November 28 aboard the Italian Line's SS *Andrea Doria* and fly from Naples to Oslo. He planned to return aboard the *Independence* and arrive in New York on December 22. (Marshall to Wilson, November 6, 1953, ibid.) See pp. 802–4 and 816n1.

478

TO COLONEL JOHN HART CAUGHEY[1] November 6, 1953
Washington, DC

Dear Caughey: I have just received here at Walter Reed your letter of October 31 and taking note of your first paragraph, I'm sure you have heard of the visit by Queen Frederika to the hospital. She paid me a great honor by making a special trip down from New York and we had a most delightful conversation. She stayed for over an hour.[2]

I appreciate what you had to say about the Nobel Peace Prize.[3] It was a great honor and it came as a complete surprise. George is now in the process of making satisfactory arrangements for the trip to Oslo.[4]

It would be very good of you, if you can take the time, to deliver the attached note to Madame Chiang.[5] I hope that you will also convey my best wishes to Dr. Judd.[6]

With many thanks and with warmest regards, Faithfully yours,

GCMRL/G. C. Marshall Papers (Retirement, General)

1. Caughey served as chief of staff on Marshall's mission to China in 1947. See *Papers of GCM*, 5: 408–9. In November 1953, he was serving in the secretary of defense's Office of Foreign Military Assistance.

2. See p. 796n1. "Queen Frederika has stolen the heart of Washington," Caughey had written to Marshall on October 31. "I am sorry that, because of your flu, you were unable to be on hand to assist in greeting and entertaining her—and more particularly, that you have been unable to fulfill your promise to take her through a supermarket." (Caughey to Marshall, October 31, 1953, GCMRL/G. C. Marshall Papers [Retirement, General].) C. J. George had contacted the Greek ambassador on October 29 to explain that Marshall had "suffered a relapse" and would not attend the dinner at the Greek embassy on October 30. (George to Politis, October 29, 1953, ibid.)

"Queen Frederika slipped away" from a reception at the home of Thomas J. Watson Sr. in New York "yesterday and paid an unannounced call" on Marshall in Walter Reed Hospital, the *New York Times* had reported on November 4. ("Queen Slips Away to Visit with Marshall," *New York Times*, November 4, 1953, p. 8.) Undersecretary of State Walter B. Smith had met Queen Frederica at National Airport and escorted her to the hospital. (Dorothy McCardle, "Just Like a Queen in the Story Books, She Came Incognito," *Washington Post*, November 5, 1953, p. 37.)

Watson expressed his regret to Marshall on November 9 that he and Mrs. Marshall could not attend the reception in New York. "Over three hundred people went through the receiving line, whereupon Her Majesty asked Mrs. Watson" for leave to depart the party early so she could attend to "a personal matter." The Watsons "learned the next day that she had flown to Washington to pay her respects to you. She arrived back in New York about midnight to take a 2:00 A.M. train for Boston where Their Majesties had an early morning appointment. We were deeply touched by this evidence of real friendship and appreciation for you." (Watson to Marshall, November 9, 1953, GCMRL/G. C. Marshall Papers [Retirement, General].) Marshall responded on November 20 that Frederica "thought that her trip was a military secret, but, as you know, it is very difficult for a person of her station to move about unobtrusively. She stayed a little over an hour, and we had a delightful talk. I have been following her movements in the newspapers, and she seems to be making a hit everywhere she goes." (Marshall to Watson, November 20, 1953, ibid.)

"I appreciated the great and gracious attention you gave me by your call at the Walter Reed Hospital," Marshall wrote to Frederica on December 20, after he returned from Oslo. "I will never forget it. Its meaning will sweeten my thoughts through the years. No Queen has ever been so gracious and, with your permission, none as lovely." (Marshall draft to Frederica, December 20, 1953, ibid.)

3. "Please accept, sir, from one of the millions who knows and understands what you have stood for and knows how devotedly you have served this country and the interests of all mankind, the most hearty congratulations," Caughey had written. (Caughey to Marshall, October 31, 1953, ibid.)

4. See pp. 802–4.

5. See p. 793.

6. "A study group of the House Foreign Affairs Committee, headed by Dr. [Walter] Judd leaves Washington on 9 Nov. for an Eastern trip," Caughey had explained. See pp. 692–93. Caughey would accompany Judd's group as the Defense Department's representative. He expected to see Madame Chiang and had offered to deliver "some special message" from Marshall. (Ibid.)

COLONEL GEORGE apprised Katherine Marshall of her husband's condition through daily telephone conversations during Marshall's hospitalization. On November 7, Marshall again took up his pen and wrote to her to "apologize for not writing but once I crawled into bed I have remained there without a break and not felt like writing." (Marshall to Katherine Marshall, November 7, 1953, GCMRL/© Marshall-Winn Collection [Katherine Marshall]; H.) "I have been doing pretty well—no coughing spells for 4 days," he continued, "but I woke up at 2 a.m. night before last and coughed for about an hour." He noted that the doctors had prescribed "a hypo of penecillen [*penicillin*]" and "another Xray this afternoon" and assured Mrs. Marshall that "the nurses are very sweet and attentive." (Ibid.)

Marshall also received visits from Helen and Mary Lee, Madge Brown Pendleton, and Generals Ridgway and Harding. (Ibid.) Marshall had "a pleasant chat" with Robert Lovett as well, and reported to Adele Lovett on November 5 that her husband "looks extremely well, which indicates that the pleasant and prosperous obscurity of which he spoke so often seems to be the tonic for good health." (Marshall to Lovett, November 5, 1953, GCMRL/G. C. Marshall Papers [Retirement, General].) Marshall also wrote to Anna Rosenberg on November 5 to thank her for the chrysanthemums she had sent, which added "much color to the room and have been admired by all of my visitors." (Marshall to Rosenberg, November 5, 1953, ibid.)

"Besides your mail I get about 75 pieces a day" Marshall told his wife, and added that "a lot" of mail also went to his Pentagon office. (See p. 696n1.) Marshall revealed that he was signing about a hundred letters a day. (Marshall to Katherine Marshall, November 7, 1953, GCMRL/© Marshall-Winn Collection [Katherine Marshall]; H.)

"The doctor said today that my chest now had entirely cleared," Marshall declared on November 11, and boasted to his wife about all the magazines and Western novels he was reading. He also mentioned that Undersecretary of State Smith "was here after dinner last night and came back today." Like many of their friends, Smith and his wife had sent flowers, but "fortunately," Marshall told his wife, "this is a large room and opens directly onto another so there is room for my floral display." (Marshall to Katherine Marshall, November 11, 1953, ibid.) After he returned home, Marshall wrote to Smith to thank him for "the opportunity to talk things over with you again" because Marshall "realized how little time you had from your oppressing work schedule." (Marshall to Smith, November 20, 1953, DDEL/W. B. Smith Papers [Box 23]; H.)

One sad note Marshall confided to his wife from Walter Reed was that USAF Chief of Staff General Hoyt Vandenberg, who had retired on June 30 after being diagnosed with prostate cancer at age fifty-four, was "dying in the next room." Gladys Rose Vandenberg, his wife, had "been in to see me and is very sad and pathetic." (Marshall to Katherine Marshall, November 7, 1953, GCMRL/© Marshall-Winn Collection [Katherine Marshall]; H.) See pp. 827–28. ★

479

To Robert E. Sherwood — November 10, 1953, Washington, DC

Dear Sherwood: I appreciate your taking the time to write me such a warm and friendly letter on the occasion of the Nobel Award.[1] Needless to say, I was greatly surprised by the action of the Institute and am hopeful of making the trip to Oslo for the presentation ceremony.

I found the Coronation ceremony to be one of the most magnificent things that have come before my eyes. The spiritual procedure and the pageantry were something to behold. I am sorry that we saw so little of each other in London, but the official program kept me on the go constantly.[2]

Since your letter was forwarded to me here by Mrs. Marshall, she read of your good wishes.

Many thanks again for thinking of me in such a gracious way and with best regards.[3] Faithfully yours,

GCMRL/G. C. Marshall Papers (Retirement, General)

1. "I do not presume to congratulate you on this Award, but I should certainly like to congratulate and thank those responsible for it. They have spoken with the voice of history itself," Sherwood had written on November 2. "When I first got into some form of government service in 1940, you were only a vague name to me until Harry Hopkins expressed to me the conviction that George C. Marshall would become one of the truly great names in our American history," Sherwood continued. "Time has proved that never did Harry say anything more prophetic or more accurate." (Sherwood to Marshall, November 2, 1953, GCMRL/G. C. Marshall Papers [Retirement, General].)

2. "Last June I had the honor of being in Westminster Abbey at the Coronation Ceremony," Sherwood had continued. "I was seated where I could see you very clearly; you gave throughout that Ceremony a quiet display of dignity and decency, of substance and strength, and I felt prouder than ever to be your fellow-countryman." (Ibid.) See pp. 771–72 and 880–82.

3. "You have had your detractors," Sherwood had concluded his letter, "but they will go down to ignominy together with others who have slung mud at all of our great men." (Ibid.)

"I HAVE BEEN making good progress and it now looks as though I may be able to start back to Pinehurst this weekend," Marshall wrote to his friend Betty Trippe on Thursday, November 12. "The doctors report that my lungs are clear and I no longer am troubled with a harassing cough." He mentioned that he was hoping for "at least two weeks at Pinehurst before leaving for Oslo on November 28. Katherine will not accompany me as she finds travel difficult." (Marshall to Trippe, November 12, 1953, GCMRL/G. C. Marshall Papers [Retirement, General].) Instead, C. J. George would travel with Marshall to Oslo. The following Monday, November 16, Marshall flew back to Pinehurst. ("Marshall Going to Oslo," *New York Times*, November 18, 1953, p. 8.)

C. J. George informed Marshall on November 20 that "All the necessary arrangements have been made" for their departure on the *Andrea Doria*, which would sail from New York to Naples, Italy, and noted that "the regular fare for your accommodation is $950 each way." (George to Marshall, memorandum, November 20, 1953, ibid.) Marshall had contacted General Gruenther the previous week to request "if practicable, aircraft for flight to Oslo morning of Dec 7." (Marshall to Gruenther, radio, November 14, 1953, DDEL/Alfred M. Gruenther Papers [NATO Series].) Gruenther offered his own plane for the trip to and from Norway. "Trust you will be able to spend at least one day in Paris on your way to or from Oslo," he added. (Gruenther to Marshall, radio, November 15, 1953, GCMRL/G. C. Marshall Papers [Retirement, General].) Marshall agreed to do so, but requested that nothing be scheduled for him in Paris. (Marshall to Gruenther, radio, November 17, 1953, DDEL/Alfred M. Gruenther Papers [NATO Series]; Gruenther to Marshall, November 21, 1953, ibid. [General Correspondence, Box 12].)

Marshall also communicated with US Ambassador to Norway L. Corrin Strong, who cabled on November 19 that he and his wife were "delighted you and Colonel George will be our guests." He advised Marshall that the Nobel Prize presentation ceremony on December 10, where Marshall should be prepared to give a "brief acceptance speech," would take place at 1:00 p.m. and last from sixty to ninety minutes. That evening there would be a white-tie dinner with the Nobel committee where Marshall would be expected to speak for about twenty minutes. Marshall's formal lecture, which was planned to last from fifty to sixty minutes, was scheduled to be delivered at 7:00 p.m. in the auditorium of the University of Oslo on December 11. (Strong to Marshall, telegram, November 19, 1953, ibid.)

Strong requested permission to schedule a press conference and asked "whether Institute or Embassy can receive advance copy of Nobel lecture prior to your arrival." (Ibid.) The following day Strong followed up with a more detailed letter. "I understand that it is the usual procedure for the Nobel Peace Prize winner to give a news conference. The Norwegian press is very friendly toward Americans and I anticipate the interview will be brief and not difficult. One of the pet subjects over here is that of McCarthyism and you just might be asked your opinion on the matter," Strong alerted Marshall. Strong also mentioned that the last president of the League of Nations, Norwegian journalist, author, and prominent statesman Carl Joachim Hambro, who had been a member of the Norwegian Nobel committee since 1940, would give a speech introducing Marshall at the award ceremony. (Strong to Marshall, November 20, 1953, ibid.; "Carl J. Hambro, a Norse Leader during World War II, Dies at 79," *New York Times*, December 16, 1964.) "You may schedule press conference for morning of December 10," Marshall responded. "Since I will write my lecture aboard ship, it is impossible to comply with your request for copy. I have notified the Institute to this effect." (Marshall to Strong, November 24, 1953, GCMRL/G. C. Marshall Papers [Retirement, General].)

Marshall had received a request from the director of the Norwegian Nobel Institute for "the title of the lecture and if possible the manuscript in three copies as soon as possible." (Schou to Marshall, November 11, 1953, ibid.) "As I am now in the process of convalescing from my recent illness, I have not had the opportunity of giving much thought to the content of my lecture," Marshall responded on

November 28. "At this time, I plan to prepare it aboard ship. Consequently, I shall not be in a position to provide you with copies before my arrival at Oslo. I hope this will not inconvenience your arrangements." (Marshall to Schou, November 28, 1953, ibid.) Assistant Secretary of State Carl W. McCardle had sent Undersecretary of State Smith "a memorandum suggesting points General Marshall may wish to make in his address" and indicated that he had discussed its contents with C. J. George. (McCardle to Smith, November 20, 1953, ibid.) On November 25, McCardle had sent an outline of potential speech topics, as well as a "possible informal comment to follow main speech," to George and revealed that Assistant Secretary of State for European Affairs Livingston T. Merchant was "in Pinehurst at the present." (McCardle to George, November 25, 1953, ibid.)

On November 27, Marshall flew from Pinehurst to Newark, New Jersey, on the first leg of his trip. The *New York Times* reported that his plane had arrived at 3:10 p.m. and that he "was driven by military car to an undisclosed hotel." ("Marshall Norway-Bound," *New York Times*, November 28, 1953, p. 16.) "I beat George in by ten minutes," Marshall bragged to his wife. "I have signed the prepared mail and he has gone off with it, and to make some preparations." Marshall also seemed delighted that "Army Secretary Stevens sent me a bundle of westerns!," the novels Marshall most enjoyed reading. See pp. 930–31. (Marshall to Katherine Marshall, November 27, 1953, GCMRL/© Marshall-Winn Collection [Katherine Marshall]; H.)

The next morning, Marshall dashed off another note to tell his wife that he had visited their friend Margaret Emerson in her New York apartment the previous evening. He then left for the ship and an onboard press conference, which was set to begin at 10:30. (Marshall to Katherine Marshall, November 28, 1953, ibid.; H.)

"'I feel so highly honored by this award that it is hard for me to express myself,'" Marshall told the assembled press. The *New York Herald Tribune* reported that Marshall "paid high tribute" to the late Senator Arthur Vandenberg "for his leadership in steering through Congress the program which became known as the Marshall Plan of economic assistance to Europe." Marshall recalled that "'we had the very difficult situation of a Republican Congress and a Democratic administration. Sen. Vandenberg and his bi-partisan approach made it possible for this program to go through, along with the support given by the American people.'" When questioned about the current "status of world peace, Gen. Marshall said, 'That is too complicated for me to attempt to discuss here. The whole struggle for peace involves so many lines of approach that you can't just make one general comment.' He also refused to be drawn out on political questions." ("Marshall, Off for Prize, Gives Credit to Nation," *New York Herald-Tribune*, November 29, 1953, p. 1.) ★

480

TO MRS. GEORGE C. MARSHALL

December 3, 1953
at sea

Dearest, I haven't dressed yet but I have shaved and bathed. The voyage until yesterday has been in mild weather and fairly calm seas. As we cleared the Azores yesterday afternoon we ran into rough waters and things have been knocked about ever since. My suite is luxurious and rather unique. The walls, ceilings, upholstery, even the bath room tiles, tub and basin are in blue and white in the stars and figures of the Zodiac.[1] In addition to the lounge and bed room there is a small dressing room with writing desk where I am now installed. I have gotten along well. George watches over me like an old hen, helps me in dressing and undressing and steadies me in walking about the boat. There is no "Captains table". The ship's officers eat together. George and I have a table with four places and we frequently, almost usually bring a couple to eat with us. Food very good. Wine, etcetera is for me "on the ship".

The winter passenger list "out" (to Europe) is small, about half the full complement. Almost no young people. We have made some interesting friends. Last night, for instance, a Swiss chap older than I am, who seems to be the Chairman of the Board of about every big organization in Europe. A great friend of Bob Lovett's. Had him for dinner—last night.[2] Another interesting friend, a lady of about 42 has a husband in Milan, Italy in a huge company of which this Swiss fellow is the Chairman. She discovered this yesterday so I brought them together at dinner. She is a painter and a sculptress and also a house wife.[3] Almost every one on the boat seems to have heard me talk at one time or another.[4] I am having a terribly hard time getting down to the business of writing my lecture. I cant seem to concentrate.

We touch at Gibralter [*Gibraltar*] to-morrow and I mail this there. I will get off another air mail from Naples.

I had a pretty strenuous press interview—in New York. About 8 large T.V. cameras, 10 small ones and 10 or 12 ordinary cameras. It lasted better than a half hour! I suppose I will have another ordeal at Naples. The Captain met me at the gang plank and stayed with me throughout the performance.[5]

During the movie yesterday a heavy sea ran all the chairs down to one side of the room partially pilling [*piling*] them up there. The racket was terrific. The "grown ups" frightened and the youngest children delighted!

Margaret sent me a variety of candies; the Watsons, who came down to the boat, brought me books, etc. Anna the usual flowers and a very sweet note.[6] There were other things, liquor, books, westerns, magazines, etc. The C. B. S. television man and his wife called and he said he would telephone you when he found the hour ~~of~~ my press conference went on the air. I got word—or at least I think I did—to Mrs. Watson to telephone you of my situation, cabin, etc. I hope she did. I send you a great deal of love, dearest. I miss you in my cabin, at meals and on deck.

I do hope you are well and not concealing some ailment.

GCM

GCMRL/© Marshall-Winn Collection (Katherine Marshall); H

1. Following a news conference in Naples on December 6, the *New York Times* reported that Marshall "found considerable amusement in showing other travelers 'my Zodiac cabin' and explaining 'When I first woke up in here and caught sight of those creatures on the wall, I thought I was losing my mind.'" ("Marshall in Italy on Way to Award," *New York Times*, December 9, 1953.)

2. "At the end of the farewell dinner," the *Times* continued, "Albert C. Nussbaumer, general manager of the Swiss Bank Corporation of Basel, Switzerland, proposed a toast to him for the 'far-seeing policy of aiding the reconstruction of Europe without regard for which countries were friends and which former foes.' The other diners arose and applauded General Marshall, who smiled and gently chided Mr. Nussbaumer for having called attention to him in this manner. Otherwise the general was allowed to go his own way without formalities." (Ibid.)

3. Elizabeth Stetson Barry of New Hope, Pennsylvania, was en route to Milan, Italy, to join her banker husband. (George to Barry, December 18, 1953, GCMRL/G. C. Marshall Papers [Retirement, General].) See photo #19.

4. One passenger who did not recognize Marshall cornered him on the first day at sea and "told him that the entrance of the United States into World War II had been a mistake." Marshall, he reported, "listened thoughtfully." The man was "greatly pleased with the general's considerate reception of his remarks," and concluded that Marshall was "'A real nice man.'" ("Marshall in Italy on Way to Award," *New York Times*, December 9, 1953.)

5. See p. 804 of previous editorial note.

6. The Watsons were probably Mr. and Mrs. Thomas Watson Sr. "In accordance with your instructions, a lovely arrangement of flowers was placed in General Marshall's room prior to his departure for the presentation ceremony," C. J. George wrote to Anna Rosenberg on December 21. "He enjoyed your message and took great delight in telling Ambassador and Mrs. Strong what you had to say." (George to Rosenberg, December 21, 1953, GCMRL/G. C. Marshall Papers [Retirement, General].) Rosenberg's "very sweet note" is not in the Marshall Papers.

THE SEA VOYAGE did not provide the restoration to health Marshall had anticipated. The December 3 letter describing the Atlantic crossing to his wife (see previous document) was mailed as the *Andrea Doria* stopped briefly by Gibraltar "in a rain storm." (Marshall to Katherine Marshall, December 5, 1953, GCMRL/© Marshall-Winn Collection [Katherine Marshall]; H.) When he arrived in Naples at noon on December 6, Marshall met with the Italian press, which "tried to get him, as a former Secretary of State, to comment on the international tension of the day." ("Marshall in Italy on Way to Award," *New York Times*, December 9, 1953.) "The chief personal pride he takes in the world-wide recognition for the Marshall Plan," Marshall told the reporters, "is in the knowledge that he did help to put it through Congress." (Ibid.) He and George then made a four-hour flight to Paris, where he was met by General Gruenther. (See p. 787n1.)

Marshall wrote home again on December 8 to explain his busy time in Paris, including dinner the first night with General J. Lawton Collins, who was the US representative to the Military Committee and the Standing Group of NATO from 1953 to 1954; two other generals; their wives; and the Gruenthers. The next evening it was "just the four of us and we had a movie afterwards." (Marshall to

Katherine Marshall, December 8, 1953, GCMRL/© Marshall-Winn Collection [Katherine Marshall]; H.) Unbeknownst to him, the Gruenthers had turned over their personal suite to Marshall, which he thought was their guest quarters. (Ibid.; Andrew J. Goodpaster, "George Marshall's World, and Ours," *New York Times*, December 11, 2003, p. A43.)

The Nobel address remained unwritten when they arrived in Paris. "I feel that Gen. M— is in trouble re his speech," C. J. George divulged in a brief note to Gruenther on December 7, noting that Marshall "has really done little on it thus far—practically nothing." (George to Gruenther, GCMRL/Andrew J. Goodpaster Papers [SHAPE, Correspondence].) "The first morning a stenographer came in at 9-45," Marshall told his wife. "I grit my teeth and plunged into my lecture. I finished up at 11-30 a.m. She brought me the typed copy at 3 p.m. and I redid a good deal of that." Marshall also received assistance from Gruenther and several officers at SHAPE, including USAF General Lauris Norstad (USMA, 1930), commanding general of the Allied Air Forces in Central Europe; Lieutenant General Cortlandt Van R. Schuyler, Gruenther's chief of staff; USAF Major General Francis L. Ankenbrandt, chief of communications for SHAPE since October 1952; and particularly Colonel Andres J. Goodpaster (USMA, 1939) a special assistant to Schuyler, who had been wounded twice during World War II while leading a combat engineering battalion in North Africa and Italy. He had then served on the War Department General Staff and obtained a doctorate in international relations from Princeton University. Marshall deemed Goodpaster "a brilliant young speech writer." Marshall reviewed their suggestions "and closed the deal. So I dont have to worry any longer." (Marshall to Katherine Marshall, December 8, 1953, GCMRL/© Marshall-Winn Collection [Katherine Marshall]; H; "Andrew J. Goodpaster, 90, Soldier and Scholar, Dies," *New York Times*, May 17, 2005, p. D8.) "I had an interesting one-day job two or three weeks ago," Goodpaster wrote to social sciences professor Colonel George A. Lincoln at West Point on December 30. (See pp. 530–31n2.) "General Marshall passed through here on his way to Oslo and I had the opportunity of assisting him a little with his speech. It was quite an experience to work with the old man again. His mind is as precise and incisive as ever, but he can only sustain close attention for a very short time. He must then relax for a few minutes before he can concentrate again. His stamina has suffered greatly from his illness, but his faculty for going to the heart of a problem is undiminished." (Goodpaster to Lincoln, December 30, 1953, GCMRL/Andrew J. Goodpaster Papers [SHAPE, Correspondence].)

Goodpaster later recalled that he was "serving as an assistant at NATO headquarters, working on policy and strategy issues" when Marshall arrived "with a few central ideas in his head but nothing on paper." (Andrew J. Goodpaster, "George Marshall's World, and Ours," *New York Times*, December 11, 2003, p. A43.) "In the room was a bedridden Marshall, his slate-blue eyes and tight smile unaffected by the cold in his head. He had jotted down a few thoughts on some note cards; we met for 45 minutes and I emerged with a rough outline. I had never seen the general so tired," Goodpaster remembered. "I knew his thinking, however, having worked with him previously, and by our third meeting his health had improved greatly—and his speech was all but finished." (Ibid.) See pp. 816, 817–19, 823–24, and 882–83, as well as Pogue, *Statesman*, 505.

On his final afternoon in Paris, Marshall called on French President Vincent Auriol, then dined with his longtime friends the Comte de Chambrun and his wife, Clara Eleanor Longworth. See p. 725. Marshall and George flew to Oslo the following morning. (Marshall to Katherine Marshall, December 8, 1953, GCMRL/© Marshall-Winn Collection [Katherine Marshall]; H.)

In his letter from Paris, Marshall also informed his wife that he had revised plans for his return to the United States. Instead of sailing back, he had decided to spend three days with Deputy Supreme Commander, Allied Powers General Thomas T. Handy and his wife, Alma, at their home near Heidelberg, Germany, after leaving Oslo. (Ibid.; Handy to Marshall, radio, December 10, 1953, GCMRL/G. C. Marshall Papers [Retirement, General].) See p. 816n1. Marshall would then take advantage of an invitation extended on December 3 by Secretary of Defense Wilson, who would be attending a NATO conference in Paris from December 12 to 16, to join him on his return flight from Paris to Washington. Marshall accepted the offer on December 7 with the comment that he was "now well enough to fly." (Wilson to Marshall, radio, December 3, and Marshall to Wilson, radio, December 7, 1953, ibid.; Marshall to Katherine Marshall, December 8, 1953, GCMRL/© Marshall-Winn Collection [Katherine Marshall]; H.)

Marshall and George arrived in Oslo shortly after noon on December 9. They were met at the airport by Ambassador Strong and members of his embassy staff, as well as Gunnar Jahn, chairman of the Nobel Committee and head of the Bank of Norway; Carl J. Hambro; August Schou; Norwegian Foreign Minister Halvard M. Lange; and Christian Mohr, the Norwegian chief of protocol. (Program of General George C. Marshall for Nobel Peace Prize Award, Oslo, December 9–12, 1953, GCMRL/G. C. Marshall Papers [Retirement, General].) Following lunch at the embassy residence, Schou presented Marshall with the peace prize check for $33,792.55, and the funds were transferred to the Marshalls' bank in Richmond, Virginia. (George to Lovett, December 11, 1953, ibid.)

Ambassador Strong welcomed the Norwegian press at 4:00 p.m. The next day *Arbeiderbladet*, the Labor newspaper, described Marshall's arrival from upstairs in the embassy residence: "he descended carefully, holding on to the railing and did not look up until he had reached the ground." Marshall told the press that he "preferred to avoid political questions." The paper remarked, however, that "a fairly long discussion developed. We had the impression of meeting a wise statesman with a quick and broad intellect—it seemed entirely natural for the man who conceived the great, constructive and simple idea behind the Marshall Plan would be this way." (Summary of Oslo Press Coverage of General Marshall and Nobel Peace Prize Award, December 10, 1953, GCMRL/© Marshall-Winn Collection.) *Nationen*, a Norwegian agrarian publication, reported that "After the General warmed up, it also was clear that he still could handle the press with great ability and vitality. More than once he brought forth laughter, and when he announced with a wave of his hand that something was 'off the record'—which means that the journalists should not take notes—it was meaty and colorful stuff which he served up. His other remarks also did not lack meat, but because he has withdrawn from public life he did not wish to speak about current political matters. In short, it was not some old man who met the press, and it appeared entirely natural that he, in his seventieth year, at the outbreak of war in Korea was called to Washington once more to organize the great democracies' forces." (Ibid.) The press conference was followed by an informal dinner at the residence with Marshall, C. J. George, and Foreign Minister and Mrs. Lange as the only guests.

The next morning Marshall donned his cutaway and went first to the royal palace for an audience with Norwegian King Haakon VII at 11:00 a.m. The award ceremony got under way at 1:00 p.m. in the Oslo University Festival Hall and began with the French ambassador accepting the 1952 Peace Prize on behalf of humanitarian and philanthropist Dr. Albert Schweitzer (see pp. 915–16), who was unable to leave his "hospital in French Equatorial Africa to accept the award in person." ("Nobel Peace Prizes are Awarded in Oslo," *New York Herald Tribune*, Paris edition, December 11, 1953, p. 1.) Carl J. Hambro then delivered an address in Norwegian extolling Marshall. "Nobel's Peace Prize is not given to Marshall for all that he accomplished during the war," Hambro explained. "What he has done after the war to prepare for peace is a corollary to this achievement and it is this great work for the establishment of peace the Nobel Committee has wanted to honour." (Address by C. J. Hambro, December 10, 1953, GCMRL/G. C. Marshall Papers [Retirement, Speeches, Statements, and Writings].)

The proceedings were suddenly interrupted when "young Communist agitators shrilled anti-American invective and scattered propaganda leaflets" from the balcony. Marshall, the *New York Herald Tribune* reported, "stood quietly through the quickly squelched outburst, then received thunderous applause which veteran observers called the greatest ovation ever accorded a Peace Prize winner." ("Reds Heckle Marshall at Nobel Ceremonies," *New York Herald Tribune*, December 11, 1953.) The *New York Times* recounted that Marshall "was coughing" and "had difficulty making himself heard above the applause." Acknowledging the award, he said, "'I accept the honor with profound gratitude, but not for myself but more specifically for the American people, who made it possible to realize the European Recovery Program." ("Reds Protesting Marshall Foiled," *New York Times*, December 11, 1953, p. 8.) See pp. 817–19 and photo #20.

That evening Marshall and George accompanied Ambassador and Mrs. Strong to a white-tie dinner for about eighty guests, including Prime Minister Oscar Torp, at the Grand Hotel. No events were scheduled for the morning of Friday, December 11. At 1:00 p.m. Marshall went to Oslo City Hall to attend "a stag luncheon with about 60 guests, but there will be women present who hold official positions." (Program of General George C. Marshall for Nobel Peace Prize Award, Oslo, December 9–12, 1953, GCMRL/G. C. Marshall Papers [Retirement, General].) At 7:00 p.m. Marshall returned to Oslo University Festival Hall to deliver his Nobel lecture. ★

481

NOBEL PRIZE LECTURE[1]

December 11, 1953
Oslo, Norway

I have been greatly and surprisingly honored in the past twenty-four hours, and in return I have been requested to speak here tonight. While no subject has been suggested, it is quite evident that the Cause of Peace is pre-eminent in your minds.

Discussions without end have been devoted to the subject of peace, and the efforts to obtain a general and lasting peace have been frequent through many years of world history. There has been success temporarily, but all have broken down, and with the most tragic consequences since 1914. What I would like to do is point our attention to some directions in which efforts to attain peace seem promising of success.

I will try to phrase my views or suggestions in the simplest possible terms though I lack the magic and artistry of that great orator whom the Nobel Committee in Stockholm so appropriately honored yesterday.[2] In making my statement I will assume your familiarity with the discussions and efforts of the past eight years and also with something of the conditions which have governed each long continued peace in world history.

I would like to make special mention of the years of the Pax Romana, which endured through almost all the first two centuries of the Christian era. I do so because of a personal incident which made a profound impression on me in the spring of 1919. Arriving late at night in Chaumont, the American Headquarters in France, I sought shelter ~~for the night~~ in the house of a group of friends. I found they were temporarily absent, so I selected an unoccupied room and looked about for a book to read as I waited for sleep to come. The books available were mostly in French or German. Since I was unable to read them with facility, I looked further and finally found an English textbook on the history of Gaul. Casting about for an interesting portion, I landed on a description of the famous Roman Peace. Included in this description was a statement of the dispositions of the Roman troops during this prolonged period, a legion at Cologne, another at Coblenz, a third at Mayence, and the reserve at Trier. Now those happened to be the identical dispositions of our Allied Forces some eighteen hundred years later, with the Peace Commission sitting in Paris and evolving the policy of the League of Nations.[3]

I would not wish to imply that the military deployment I have just described corresponds to the protective NATO deployment of today. The threat of today is quite different, but I do think that this remarkable historical repetition does suggest that we have walked blindly, ignoring the lessons of the past with, in our century, the tragic consequences of two world wars and the Korean struggle as a result.

In my country my military associates frequently tell me that we Americans have learned our lesson. I completely disagree with this ~~assumption~~ contention, and point to the rapid disintegration between 1945 and 1950 of our once vast power for maintaining the peace. As a direct consequence, in my opinion, there resulted the brutal invasion of South Korea, which for a time threatened the complete defeat of our hastily arranged forces in that field. I speak of this with deep feeling because in 1939 and again in the early fall of 1950 it suddenly became my duty, my responsibility, to rebuild our national military strength in the very face of the gravest emergencies.

These opening remarks may lead you to assume that my suggestions for the advancement of world peace will rest largely on military strength. For the moment the maintenance of peace in the present hazardous world situation does depend in very large measure on military power, together with Allied cohesion. But the maintenance of large armies for an indefinite period~~, I think,~~ is not a practical or a promising basis for policy. We must stand together strongly for these present years, that is in this present situation, but we must, I repeat, we must find another solution, and that is what I wish to discuss this evening.

There has been considerable comment over the awarding of the Nobel Peace Prize to a soldier. I am afraid this does not seem as remarkable to me as it quite evidently appears to others. I know a great deal of the horrors and tragedies of war. Today, as Chairman of the American Battle Monuments Commission, it is my duty to supervise the construction and maintenance of military cemeteries in many countries overseas, particularly in Western Europe. The cost of war in human lives is constantly spread before me, written neatly in many ledgers whose columns are gravestones. I am deeply moved to find some means or method of avoiding another calamity of war. Almost daily I hear from the wives, or mothers, or families of the fallen. The tragedy of the aftermath is almost constantly before me.

I share with you an active concern for some practical method for avoiding war. Let me first say that I regard the present highly dangerous situation as a very special one, which naturally dominates our thinking on the subject of peace, but which should not, in my opinion, be made the principal basis for our reasoning towards the manner for securing a condition of long continued peace. A very strong military posture is vitally necessary today. How long it must continue I am not prepared to estimate, but I am sure that it is too narrow a basis on which to build a dependable, long-enduring peace. The guarantee for a long continued peace will depend on other factors in addition to a moderated ~~position of~~ military strength, and no less important. Perhaps the most important single factor will be a spiritual regeneration to develop good will, faith and understanding among nations. Economic factors will undoubtedly play an important part. Agreements to secure a balance of power, however disagreeable they may seem, must likewise be considered. And with all these there must be wisdom and the will to act on that wisdom.

II.

In this brief discussion, I can give only a very limited treatment of these great essentials to peace. However, I would like to select three more specific areas for closer attention.

The *first* relates to the possibilities of better education in the various factors effecting the life of peaceful security, both in terms of its development and of its disruption. Because wisdom in action in our Western democracies rests squarely upon public understanding, I have long believed that our schools have a key role to play. Peace could, I believe, be advanced through careful study of all the factors which have gone into the various incidents now historical that have marked the breakdown of peace in the past. As an initial procedure our schools, at least our colleges but preferably our senior high schools, as we call them, should have courses which not merely instruct our budding citizens in the historical sequence of events of the past, but which treat with almost scientific accuracy the circumstances which have marked the breakdown of peace and have led to the disruption of life and the horrors of war.[4]

There may perhaps have been a "last clear chance" to avoid the tragic conflagrations of our century. In the case of World War II, for example, the challenge may well have come in the early thirties, and passed largely unrecognized until the situation was unlikely to be retrieved. We are familiar with specific events such as the march into the Rhineland or aggression in Ethiopia or Manchuria.[5] Perhaps there was also a last clear chance to begin to build up the strength of the democracies to keep the military situation in equilibrium. There may also have been a last clear chance to penetrate to the spirit of the peoples of the nations threatening the peace, and to find ways of peaceful adjustment in the economic field as well. Certainly, had the outcome of the war, with its devastation and disruption, been foreseen, and had there been an understanding on all sides of the problems that were threatening the peace, I feel sure that many possibilities for accommodation would have been much more thoroughly explored.

It is for this reason that I believe our students must first seek to understand the conditions, as far as possible without national prejudices, which have led to past tragedies and should strive to determine the great fundamentals which must govern a peaceful progression toward a constantly higher level of civilization. There are innumerable instructive lessons out of the past, but all too frequently their presentation is highly colored or distorted in the effort to present a favorable national point of view. In our school histories at home, certainly in years past, those written in the North present a strikingly different picture of our Civil War from those written in the South. In some portions it is hard to realize they are dealing with the same war. Such reactions are all too common in matters of peace and security. But we are told that we live in a highly scientific age. Now the progress of science depends on facts and not on fancies or prejudice. Maybe in this age we can find a way of facing the facts and discounting the distorted records of the past.

I am certain that a solution of the general problem of peace must rest on broad and basic understanding on the part of free peoples. Great single endeavors like a League of Nations, a United Nations, and undertakings of that character, are of great importance and in fact absolutely necessary, but they must be treated as steps toward the desired end.

We must depend in large measure on the impartiality of those who teach. Their approach must be on a scientific basis in order to present the true facts. The scientists, no matter of what nationality, make a common approach to their problems.

For my *second* suggestion, I would like to consider the national attitudes that bear on the great problem of peace. I hope you will not think me amiss if I turn to my own country and certain rather special circumstances found there to illustrate my point. Despite the amazing conquest of the air and its reduction of distances to a matter of hours and not days, or minutes instead of hours, the United States is remote in a general sense from the present turbulent areas of the world. I believe the measure of detachment, limited though it is, has been of help in enabling us on occasion to take an impartial stand on heated international problems.

Also, my country is very specially constituted in terms of population. We have many families of Norwegian ancestry in our population. My country also includes large numbers of former citizens of many of the other countries of Europe, including the present Satellite States. I recall that when the first Polar flight was made by the Russians from Moscow over the top of the world to land on the little airfield of the post I commanded at Vancouver on the Columbia River in the State of Washington, my home was surrounded within a few hours by hundreds and hundreds of Russians, all presumably citizens of the United States.[6] Italians, Turks, Greeks and many, many others who came to our country now constitute an organic portion of our population.

From this fact we have acquired, I think, a feeling and a concern for the problems of other peoples. There is a deep urge to help the oppressed and to give aid to those upon whom great and sudden hardship has fallen.

We, naturally, cannot see a problem in the exact terms as people like yourselves or the Danes, or the Dutch, or the French, for example; people living in the closest contact with each other, yet widely differing in national heritage. I believe there is, however, a readiness to cooperate which is one of the great and hopeful factors of the world of today. While we are not in close contact with the details of problems, neither are we indifferent to them, and we are not involved in your historical tensions and suspicions.

If I am correct in thinking that these factors have given us as a nation some advantage in the quest for peace, then I would suggest that principles of cooperation based on these factors might contribute to a better understanding amongst all nations.

I realize fully that there is another side to this picture. In America we have not suffered the destruction of our homes, our towns and cities. We have not been enslaved for long periods, at the complete mercy of a conqueror. We have enjoyed freedom in its fullest sense. In fact, we have come to think in terms of freedom and the dignity of the individual more or less as a matter of course, and our apparent unconcern until time of acute crisis presents a difficult problem to the citizens of the countries of Western Europe, who have seldom been free from foreign threat to their freedom, their dignity and their security. I think nevertheless that the people of the United States have fully demonstrated their willingness to fight and die in the terrible struggle for the freedom we all prize, to sacrifice their own men in large numbers for this common cause, and to contribute vast sums for the general benefit of the Western countries.

I recognize that there are bound to be misunderstandings under the conditions of wide separation between your countries and mine. But I believe the attitude of cooperation has been thoroughly proven. I also believe that the participation of millions of our young men and women in the struggle in Western Europe, in the closest contact with your people, will bring as its result less of misunderstanding on our side of the Atlantic than perhaps on yours.

In my own case, for example, I spent two and one half years in France during the First World War. Frequently I was quartered in the households of the French peasantry and spent long evenings by the kitchen fires, talking far into the night. I came to know them well, admired them, and in some cases came to love them.[7] Now, how many do you suppose of the present citizens of Western Europe have had a similar look in on the homes of people in the farms and small towns of America. A few may know much of New York, Washington and Chicago, but those great cities do not represent the heart of America.

The *third* area I would like to discuss has to do with the problem of the millions who live under sub-normal conditions and who have now come to a realization that they may aspire to a fair share of the God-given rights of human beings. Their aspirations present a challenge to the more favored nations to lend assistance in bettering the lot of the poorer. This is a special problem in the present crisis, but it is of basic importance to any successful effort toward an enduring peace. The question is not merely one of self-interest arising from the fact that these people present a situation which is a seed bed for either one or the other of two greatly differing ways of life. Ours is democracy, according to our interpretation of the meaning of that word. If we act with wisdom and magnanimity, we can guide these yearnings of the poor to a richer and better life through democracy.

We must present democracy as a force holding within itself the seeds of unlimited progress by the human race. By our actions we should make it clear that such a democracy is a means to a better way of life, together with a better understanding among nations. Tyranny inevitably must retire before the tremendous strength of the gospel of freedom and self-respect for the individual, but we have to recognize that these democratic principles do not flourish on empty stomachs and that people turn to false promises of dictators because they are hopeless and anything promises something better than the miserable existence that they endure. However, material assistance alone is not sufficient. The most important thing for the world today in my opinion is a spiritual regeneration which would re-establish a feeling of good faith among men generally. Discouraged people are in sore need of the inspiration of great principles. Such leadership can be the rallying point against intolerance, against distrust, against that fatal insecurity that leads to war. It is to be hoped that the democratic nations can provide the necessary leadership.

The points I have just discussed are, of course, no more than a very few suggestions in behalf of the cause of peace. I realize that they hold nothing of glittering or early promise, but there can be no substitute for effort in many fields. There must be effort of the spirit—to be magnanimous, to act in friendship, to strive to help rather than to hinder. There must be effort of analysis, to seek out the causes of war and the factors which favor peace, and to study their application to the difficult problems which will beset our international intercourse. There must be material effort—to initiate and sustain those great undertakings, whether military or economic, on which world equilibrium will depend.

If we proceed in this manner, there should develop a dynamic philosophy which knows no restrictions of time or space. In America we have a creed which comes to us from the deep roots of the past. It springs from the convictions of the men and women of many lands who founded the nation and made it great. We share that creed with many of the nations of the Old World and the New with whom we are joined in the cause of peace. We are young in world history, but these ideals of ours we can offer to the world with the certainty that they have the power to inspire and to impel action.

I am not implying in any way that we would attempt to persuade other people to adopt our particular form of government. I refer here specifically to those fundamental values on which our government, like many other democracies, is based. These, I believe, are timeless and have a validity for all mankind. These, I believe, will kindle the imagination and arouse the spirit.

A great proponent of much of what I have just been saying is Dr. Albert Schweitzer, the world humanitarian, who ~~today~~ received the Nobel Peace Award for 1952. I feel it a vast compliment to be associated with him in these awards this year. His life has been utterly different from mine, and we should all be happy that his example among the poor and benighted of the earth should have been recognized by the Peace Award of the Nobel Committee.

I must not further complicate this discussion with the wide variety of specific considerations which will enfold the gradual growth of a sound approach toward some method of securing an enduring peace in the world. I fear, in fact I am rather certain, that due to my inability to express myself with the power and penetration of the great Churchill, I have not made clear the points that assume such prominence and importance in my mind. However, I have done my best, and I hope I have sown some seeds which may bring forth good fruit.

GCMRL/G. C. Marshall Papers (Retirement, Speeches, Statements, and Writings)

1. Marshall's reading copy of his lecture is reproduced here; italicized words were marked by him for emphasis and corrections indicate changes made in his handwriting. The version provided to the press, which differs slightly, was reprinted in its entirety in many newspapers and in the spring 1954 issue of the journal *Social Research*. "Although all Americans who keep abreast of the movement of world ideas have read excerpts from General Marshall's Nobel Prize address," an accompanying editors' note stated, "In spite of General Marshall's modest disclaimer, his address reads as one of the great documents of American intellectual history, the greater because its eloquence clothes itself in straightforward simplicity." (George C. Marshall, "Essentials to Peace," *Social Research* 21, no. 1 [Spring 1954]: 1–10.)

2. Lady Churchill had accepted the Nobel Prize for Literature on her husband's behalf the previous day. See p. 795.

3. Marshall is referring here to the Paris Peace Conference of 1919 that resulted in the Treaty of Versailles and the creation of the League of Nations. At that time Marshall was

aide-de-camp to General Pershing.

4. For additional speeches considering educational themes, see pp. 25–33, 34–37, 57–60, 393–97, 532, and 761–66. See also *Papers of GCM*, 6: 233–34, 288–89, 411, 497–98, and 724–29.

5. On March 7, 1936, German military forces entered the Rhineland in violation of the Treaty of Versailles. For information on the Japanese occupation of Manchuria in 1931 and the Italian occupation of Ethiopia in 1936, see p. 33n6.

6. "Satellite States" was the term used during the cold war to refer to the states of Eastern and Central Europe that had been occupied by the Red Army during World War II and possessed Communist governments loyal to Moscow: Albania, Bulgaria, Czechoslovakia, East Germany, Hungary, Poland, and Rumania. Yugoslavia also possessed a Communist government, but pursued a neutral course during the cold war. On June 20, 1937, three Russian fliers landed at Vancouver Barracks and stayed at the Marshalls' home. See *Papers of GCM*, 1: 545–48.

7. For Marshall's report on his 1948 visit with his World War I landlady in France, see *Papers of GCM*, 6: 588–90.

482

TO COLONEL ANDREW J. GOODPASTER — December 15, 1953
near Heidelberg, Germany[1]

Dear Goodpaster: I want you to know more formally of my appreciation of the very fine assistance you gave me in connection with my Nobel lecture.[2] I felt quite confident, after my departure from here for Oslo, that it was as good as time and energy would allow. While I have not seen too many accounts, those that I have read have been complimentary.[3]

I doubt very seriously that I would have been able to complete the paper without your fine help.

With many thanks again, and with best regards. Faithfully yours,

GCMarshall

GCMRL/G. C. Marshall Papers (Retirement, General)

1. The *New York Times* had mistakenly reported that Marshall had flown from Oslo to Paris immediately after the ceremony. ("Marshall Quits Oslo for Paris," *New York Times*, December 13, 1953, p. 45.) Instead, Marshall and George visited with the Handys near Heidelberg. See p. 808. Marshall wrote to Alma Handy from Paris on December 16 to thank her for their hospitality, which "did much to speed my convalescence." He told her, "We had a pleasant flight to Paris, and I understand that Secretary Wilson is prepared to leave tonight at eleven for the flight home. As it now stands, I should be in Pinehurst by four o'clock, at which time I will unpack my bags and have the high hope of not moving again until we come up to Leesburg in the spring."(Marshall to Handy, December 16, 1953, GCMRL/G. C. Marshall Papers [Retirement, General].) Marshall also left a note of thanks for Mrs. Gruenther for "looking out for my welfare and comforts." Three years later, when he was leaving Paris and retiring from the army, General Gruenther wrote to Marshall that "Mrs. Gruenther and I consider it one of the high points of our tour here that you stopped with us in 1953. You were the perfect guest." (Marshall to Gruenther, December 16, 1953, and Gruenther to Marshall, October 29, 1956, ibid.)

2. See pp. 807–8.

3. "Though it made little impression in this country at the time, Gen. Marshall's Nobel Peace Prize lecture is steadily gaining favorable comment," the *Boston Globe* editorialized on December 22. "General Marshall has set an example of statesmanship in this address

that politicians of all countries would do well to emulate," the *Washington Post* opined on December 16. Marshall's "generous and earnest exposition of American motivations . . . should do much to enhance the good name of this country overseas." ("Marshall Plan II," *Boston Globe*, December 22, 1953; "Marshall on Peace," *Washington Post*, December 16, 1953, p. 12.)

483

TO COLONEL ARTHUR L. LOGAN

December 22, 1953
Pinehurst, North Carolina

Dear Logan: Your letter of November 25 was awaiting me upon my return from Oslo.[1]

I do not recall the incident you mention concerning the fifty reporters.[2] My memory is not especially good. As a matter of fact, I have often wished it were better. Throughout my life I have tried very hard to develop a good memory and whatever success I have achieved in this regard has been the result not of a system, but of concentration. To remember a thing, I find that I must fix it firmly in my mind and pay strict attention to what I see and hear. Unfortunately, even these practices fail me from time to time.

I am sorry that I must ask you not to quote my remarks. Faithfully yours,

GCMRL/G. C. Marshall Papers (Retirement, General)

1. See previous two editorial notes and three documents. "I am writing a book on memory training, one which will help those of us who want to improve our memory enough to make our daily living more efficient," Professor of Air Science and Tactics Colonel Arthur L. Logan had written to Marshall from the University of Virginia on November 25. (Logan to Marshall, November 25, 1953, GCMRL/G. C. Marshall Papers [Retirement, General].)

2. "I have heard that you have an unusual memory, much more keen than most people's. The story is told that while in Washington you asked fifty reporters to give their name and ask one question, and after a short discourse on other subjects, you called each reporter by name and answered his question," Logan continued. "Assuming the story to be true, you either must have a system or have had one in order to train your memory so well." (Ibid.) See Pogue, *Organizer*, 218–19.

484

TO FRANK MCCARTHY

December 25, 1953
Pinehurst, North Carolina

Dear Frank: Your telegram just arrived. Thanks for the greetings.[1] I intended to write to you to-morrow but I'll do so this morning.

Pardon this paper but it is very much easier for me to write on and one of the convalescent remains of this virus flu is a mental inertia that makes writing or rather concentration needed in writing very difficult.[2]

When I went over to Oslo I thought I would do the lecture before the Nobel Institute on the boat enroute, but I reached Naples without a line. I flew to Orly Field and stayed three days with the Gruenthers. The first morning, realizing that I had used up about all my time, I sat up in bed and dictated for an hour and did the business, but it was the hardest doing I have ever attempted. However, strange to say, I apparently did better than on almost any previous effort— Got tremendous distribution; full reprint in hundreds of U. S. papers and abroad.[3]

I was three days with the Gruenthers and three days with the Handys in Heidleberg and a final day with the Gruenthers.[4] I stayed in bed until dinner time each day. Of course I couldn't in Oslo. By the way, the actual business of the Communists would amuse you. Three young men were in the gallery each representing a Communist paper. As the actual award was made to me two threw down leaflets and one started to shout his objects [*objections*?]. He got out just ~~three~~ four— words "I thought this was" when the agricultural attaché of our Embassy klobbered him over the mouth (in George's description) and yanked him back from the rail by his hair. Then the pilot of my plane delivered a one-two knock out and the two Americans evacuated the gent to the first floor and turned him over to the police *when* they showed up. The other two apparently fearing as rough treatment fled down the stairs and jumped into the police wagon uninvited. So the interruption was only momentary. The Norwegians were much embarrassed particularly by the fact that Americans suppressed the demonstration and cleaned out the affair![5]

I flew back with Wilson, returning from his NATO Conference.[6] Had a 70 mile headwind. I landed here after dark and found Katherine waiting on the field. Went straight to be[d] and did not leave the house until yesterday.

I hope you are in good shape physically and in a business way. Katherine has been much better but is pretty down now from Xmas efforts and a cold. Molly and the three children are coming in for Xmas dinner.— I think they all have colds. Jimmy was the senior of the three wise men in the pageant at the church last night. K and I couldn't go see.[7]

With our love Frank and all of our best wishes for your Xmas and the New Year.[8] Affectionately,

G.C.M.

GCMRL/Frank McCarthy Collection (Additions, Box 1); H

1. "Back from almost month in South America just in time send you merry Christmas renewed congratulations and affectionate regards," McCarthy had cabled the Marshalls from Beverly Hills. (McCarthy to Marshalls, telegram, December 25, 1953, GCMRL/G. C. Marshall Papers [Retirement, General].)

2. Marshall's letter was handwritten on lined legal paper.

3. See pp. 808–16, 816n3, and 823–24. "Your Oslo speech was certainly a crowning success," McCarthy replied on December 28. "Although the papers in Los Angeles seldom reprint speeches in full, at least two of them carried the complete text. I thought it was easily one of the two or three best speeches I have known you to make, and the general reaction would seem to indicate that the public did too." (McCarthy to Marshall, December 28, 1953, ibid.)

"I appreciate your remarks on the Oslo speech," Marshall responded to McCarthy on January 8. "I have had quite a large number of complimentary letters, and just the other morning received a letter from a distinguished Swiss banker, whom I met aboard ship, pointing up the possibilities of developing an organization along the lines of UNESCO [the United Nations Educational, Scientific, and Cultural Organization] which would have the responsibility for drafting an educational program affecting all nations. His thought is good, but the matter of implementing the suggestions will have to be done by minds and bodies of a younger vintage." (Marshall to McCarthy, January 8, 1954, ibid.) See 807n2.

4. See pp. 802, 806–7, and 816n1.

5. See p. 809. "Thanks so much for the letter telling me about your visit to Oslo, and most particularly for the inside account of what happened during the award of the Nobel Prize," McCarthy continued. "The press here made the incident sound somewhat more serious than it actually was." (McCarthy to Marshall, December 28, 1953, ibid.)

6. See p. 808.

7. In this and subsequent letters to family and close friends Marshall occasionally refers to his wife by just the letter K.

8. Marshall had written a similar letter the previous day to Truman, who had complimented the Nobel lecture in a December 22 letter to Marshall: "What you said was great for World Peace—right along the line of the Harvard address which won the prize." (Truman to Marshall, December 22, 1953, ibid.)

485

To Lieutenant Colonel C. J. George — December 25, 1953
Pinehurst, North Carolina

Dear George: This carries my annual thanks to you for your good offices in my behalf, your efficient services and your loyal devotion. This year I think I have more to thank you for and I want to be certain that you feel that your services have been appreciated to the full. As a nurse, secretary, aide, and companion, you have been remarkable in your efficiency.

May all good things come to you in the New Year. Affectionately,

GCM

GCMRL/G. C. Marshall Collection (George)

486

To Sir Gyles Isham[1] — January 4, 1954
Pinehurst, North Carolina

Dear Sir Gyles: Through the kindness of Major Reginald Buchanan and Mr. Louis Marx, I received your letter and the medal of Sir Thomas Fairfax. However, I feel that an apology is due you for the delay in my reply.[2]

The package was placed in safe storage by Mr. Marx pending a visit by either my Aide or myself to New York. This we have had no occasion to do. Soon after our return from Oslo, on December 17th, they were persuaded to send the package by registered mail, and for the first time I became aware of your generous gift.

I deeply appreciate the compliment you paid me by presenting such a rare and priceless heirloom. You were most thoughtful in outlining the history of the piece and I was particularly interested in the relationship between the Isham family and Thomas Jefferson.[3]

It was delightful to make your acquaintance and to have the opportunity of seeing the Battlefield of Naseby. I enjoyed our talk and hope that we will meet again.[4]

With my very warm thanks for thinking of me in such a complimentary way and with warmest regards, Faithfully yours,

GCMRL/G. C. Marshall Papers (Retirement, General)

1. Sir Gyles Isham, the twelfth Baronet of Lamport, Northamptonshire, was an actor who had appeared in movies and plays during the 1930s. He served in the King's Royal Rifle Corps during World War II.

2. While the Marshalls vacationed in upstate New York in August 1953 (see pp. 785–86), Marshall had learned from Mary Louise Spilman that Louis Marx had received "a parcel" from Major Reginald MacDonald-Buchanan "containing what they termed 'a priceless medal.'" (Spilman to Marshall, memorandum, August 21, 1953, GCMRL/G. C. Marshall Collection [George].) Sir Thomas Fairfax commanded the parliamentary army in the decisive battle at Naseby on June 14, 1645, during the English Civil War. Isham had offered the medal to Marshall, who had commanded forces "far greater than the twenty-odd thousand men who fought as Naseby," as "a small return for the many kindnesses received from America, and much comradeship in the war." (Isham to Marshall, June 23, 1953, GCMRL/G. C. Marshall Papers [Retirement, General].)

3. Isham explained that only four other Fairfax medals are known to exist. He was "particularly pleased to think that it is going to Virginia" because, he claimed, one of Thomas Jefferson's grandmothers had been an Isham who lived in Henrico County, Virginia. (Ibid.) Mary Isham was actually Thomas Jefferson's great grandmother.

4. "It was a great pleasure to show you the battlefield of Naseby, and I was most interested in your comments," Isham wrote. (Ibid.) Marshall had probably met Isham during his visit with the Macdonald-Buchanans at their home in Northamptonshire in June 1953 after the coronation of Queen Elizabeth II. See p. 777.

CONCERN ABOUT Marshall's health remained high in early 1954. On January 2, he thanked President Eisenhower for birthday greetings and acknowledged that upon his return from Oslo, "I took to my bed again and am still pretty much house bound. The virus business is persistent." (Marshall to Eisenhower, January 2, 1954, DDEL/Dwight D. Eisenhower Papers [Papers as President, Ann Whitman File, Name Series, Box 21]; H.) "I have had to be very careful or I would set up a return to this violent coughing business," Marshall admitted to Rose Page Wilson. "I feel all right but don't dare to take any liberties as this virus business has not yet worn off. I seldom go out and seldom get up before noon. Every one tells me how well I look, but as I have no obligations beyond the house I go along carefully and read too much." (Marshall to Wilson, January 9, 1954, GCMRL/J. Page Wilson Collection; H.) Marshall also complained that he was "having a hell of a time with mail. First about 800 Xmas cards, a third of them with lengthy notes which must be acknowledged; then about 1500 letters and telegrams. The office handles most of them but I have to sign them all. I manage to get off about 7 or 8 long hand letters a day but it is an endless business." (Ibid.)

"General Marshall has not properly convalesced from his attack of virus and, after some insistence, has agreed to check into Walter Reed," C. J. George wrote to Marshall Carter on January 13. "His condition is not alarming, but the weather at Pinehurst has not been conducive to a rapid recovery." (George to Carter, January 13, 1954, GCMRL/G. C. Marshall Papers [Retirement, General].) Marshall made the most of his trip. On the way he stopped in Richmond, Virginia, to attend a meeting of the VMI Board of Visitors. He and Mrs. Marshall then flew on to Washington, DC, where he attended meetings of the Business Advisory Council while she shopped and visited with Helen and Mary Lee. They stayed at Walter Reed Hospital. (Marshall to Miller, January 9, 1954, and Marshall to Armstrong, January 24, 1954, ibid.) On February 3, George wrote again to Carter that Marshall had "had a very thorough check-up and there were no traces of the virus bug. His lungs are clear and the coughing has finally disappeared. I had a long talk with his doctor and they feel that the long siege of flu pulled him down considerably. They were concerned about his heart and the fact that the kidney was not functioning properly. The latter difficulty, however, has been taken care of. As you know, he has an unusual pulse and heartbeat. They had hoped that he would stay with them a little longer in order that they might administer a new medicine. Their approach was a little bad, because it gave the boss the impression they wanted to experiment. I don't believe that there is any cause for concern." (George to Carter, February 13, 1954, ibid.)

After their return to Pinehurst on January 23, Marshall wrote to his childhood friend Catharine Armstrong that he was "still somewhat house bound in largely being careful that I don't start up a relapse," but happy to report that "We flew back yesterday and found our camellias blooming in the snow." (Marshall to Armstrong, January 24, 1954, GCMRL/G. C. Marshall Collection [Armstrong]; H.) ★

487

Memorandum for General Matthew B. Ridgway[1] — January 28, 1954
For the Eyes of General Matthew B. Ridgway Only — Pinehurst, North Carolina

Relative to your message and query of the 27th, I hesitate to advise, as manner of statement depends so very much on what has occurred behind the scenes and on the status of the political reactions or pressures in Congress. The basic principle you state is okay, but the manner of the statement seems questionable.[2]

I think your statement is too lengthy and too complicated. It seems to imply too clearly a preceding fight or struggle in the Pentagon, which would be an invitation to an intense showdown fight on the Hill. If that is what you want, then I guess the statement is okay.

If your desire is otherwise, I think you should state your beliefs in less suggestive form. If the situation develops or has developed in a manner you consider highly dangerous to our defenses, then you have the problem of your manner of carrying the fight to the people, which in effect you would be doing by the character of your proposed statement.

I don't know whether or not you are in the struggle of radically different opinions with the highest authorities, but I am inclined to think, by the very form of your statement, that you are leading with your right.[3]

GCMRL/G. C. Marshall Papers (Retirement, General)

1. Ridgway, US Army chief of staff since August 17, 1953, appeared before the Senate Armed Services Committee on January 28. ("The Proceedings in Washington," *New York Times*, January 29, 1954, p. 9.) On January 18, he had given a speech in Bloomington, Illinois, "hinting at some of his misgivings" about the Eisenhower administration's "political decision . . . to cut military spending by more than $4,000,000,000 as an installment on Republican promises of tax reduction and a balanced budget." ("'Pros' in Pentagon Cool to 'New Look,'" *New York Times*, January 24, 1954, p. 25.) The *New York Times* reported that while "professional soldiers" who had voiced "substantial reservations" about the policy had been "scrupulously careful not to criticize their civilian superiors," Ridgway did obliquely question Defense Department assertions that the cuts would not affect army combat effectiveness. (Ibid.)

2. Ridgway had forwarded to Marshall a draft statement in which he reiterated his oft-stated belief that "the responsibility of the professional military man lies in the professional military field. His over-riding responsibility is to give his honest, objective, professional military advice to those civilians who by our Constitution are his superiors. It is not his responsibility to decide whether the military means which he determines are the minimum essential to accomplish the military task assigned him will cost more than the Nation can afford. He has not been trained for that. It is not, I submit, within his field of responsibility, and if he should seek to so decide, he would seriously impair his greatest value to his Service and his Government. He must be aware, of course, as every senior commander is today, of the major political, economic, financial and social factors which civilian authorities must appraise and equate in reaching their decisions. He must recognize, as every senior commander does today, the imperative necessity of maximum economy and efficiency in the utilization of whatever military means his Government may make available to him. There is no question of this any more than there is any question of the loyalty of these senior officers in carrying out the decisions announced to them by proper civilian authority.

'The point I wish to make here, and I repeat it for emphasis, is that the professional military man has three primary responsibilities:

'First, to give his honest, fearless, objective, professional military opinion of what he needs to do the job the Nation gives him to do.

'Second, if what he is given is less than the minimum he regards as essential, to give his superiors an honest, fearless, objective opinion of the consequences, as he sees them from the military viewpoint, of this shortage, and

'Third, and finally, he has the duty, whatever be the final decision, to do the utmost with whatever he is furnished,'" Ridgway's proposed statement concluded. "I have in mind," he wrote to Marshall, "during course of Congressional hearings which may begin first of next week, adding the following: 'Foregoing has been substantially the same position taken by every recent Chief of Staff.'" (Ridgway to Marshall, January 27, 1954, GCMRL/G. C. Marshall Papers [Retirement, General].) "I would be grateful for any comment of any kind you may care to make," Ridgway concluded. (Ibid.)

3. A note from Mary Louise Spilman at the bottom of this memorandum indicates that it was "dictated over the telephone by General Marshall from Pinehurst, North Carolina, at 3:45 p.m."

488

To Ramon Corazon

February 23, 1954
Pinehurst, North Carolina

Dear Ramon: I am very, very sorry to learn from your letter that you are having a hard time.[1] I have never forgotten your years with me. Mrs. Marshall was very fond of you, as I was.[2]

I will try and see if I can find some manner of helping you.[3] Meanwhile I am sending you a check and my photograph, the latter to identify me and my former close association with you.[4] Faithfully yours,

GCMRL/G. C. Marshall Papers (Retirement, General); H

1. On January 25, Marshall's office had received a letter from Ramon Corazon of Luzon, Philippines. C. J. George forwarded the letter to Marshall because Corazon had expressed "himself in such a way to indicate more than a casual association." Marshall replied that Corazon had been his houseboy from 1913 to 1916 and that he had seen him again in December 1945 while en route to China. "He is a fine fellow. Send him a check for $50.00," Marshall instructed George, "and communicate via Red Cross to see if they can help him." Marshall drafted the letter printed here at the bottom of George's memo. (George to Marshall, February 10, 1954, GCMRL/G. C. Marshall Papers [Retirement, General].)

2. Marshall's first wife, Elizabeth Coles "Lily" Marshall, had accompanied him to the Philippines in August 1913. See Pogue, *Education*, 119.

3. George wrote to American Red Cross Executive Vice President and General Manager James T. Nicholson on March 3 on Corazon's behalf and noted that "The boss asked me to bring this point to your attention." Nicholson responded on March 5 that he would write to the head of the Philippine Red Cross Society to determine whether "some plan could be made for insuring the minimum needs of Mr. Corazon be met." (George to Nicholson, March 3, 1954, and Nicholson to George, March 5, 1954, ibid.)

4. Corazon wrote again to thank Marshall for the photograph and check and requested additional monthly support. George replied that was not possible, prompting Corazon to send another letter, received on May 27, in which he told Marshall that he had not heard from the Red Cross. On this paragraph Marshall noted, "check on this," but there is no further correspondence with the Red Cross regarding Corazon in the Marshall Papers. (Corazon to Marshall, May 27, 1954, ibid.) Corazon continued to petition Marshall for additional assistance throughout 1954 but each time George responded in the negative.

489

To Harry S. Truman

February 25, 1954
Pinehurst, North Carolina

My dear Mr. Truman: I must explain my long delay in writing you a brief on the China affair.[1] The truth is I have been rather down and out since this virus-flu hit me last September. It hasn't yet finally cleared up but I think I am about out of the woods. I would be much worried except that I find much younger men, three down here, who have been having as long drawnout a struggle as I have and longer in several cases.

I had a most difficult time with the Oslo business. I left the Walter Reed and started on the trip. The ocean voyage was rather cold and damp which didn't help matters. It was an eight day affair and I planned to prepare my Oslo so-called lecture enroute. I found it utterly impossible to concentrate and I landed in Naples without a line. I flew up to Gruenthers and there in bed, the next morning I managed to dictate for an hour and a quarter, rather in desperation as my time was running out.[2] That was the lecture. I was very despondent over using it but it turned out I got more of a publicity play than almost any I have done and a few good editorial comments.[3]

I stayed in bed every day in Europe except the two at Oslo and went straight from the plane to bed down here and remained there two weeks and house bound until two weeks ago.

I have gotten my strength back but still find it extremely hard to concentrate.

I about feel up to getting to work on the China business and hope my delay hasn't been embarassing to you, though as I recall you told me you wouldn't have to have it for about a year.[4]

I hope Mrs. Truman and Margaret are both well and are enjoying some recession of public pressures. Katherine is in bed with a cold but has been greatly improved this winter. Our love to all of you.[5] Faithfully yours,

GCMRL/G. C. Marshall Papers (Retirement, General); H

1. Truman was in the process of writing his memoirs. See pp. 833–41, particularly n13.
2. See pp. 806–8 and 817–19.
3. See p. 818n3.
4. "I feel like a heel to have caused you to worry about China and my book," Truman replied in longhand two days later. "What I'd hoped for was your own statement on what happened when you were working with Generalissimo Chiang and Chou-en-Lai on what all of us thought (including Pat Hurley, [Albert C.] Wedemeyer, [Joseph Clark] Grew, et al) was a proper approach to a free China—an approach approved by Stalin, Chiang, Churchill, Attlee, Byrnes and most everyone. But if you do not feel like doing such a statement because of that awful flu or for any other reason it is perfectly all right." (Truman to Marshall, February 27, 1954, GCMRL/G. C. Marshall Papers [Retirement, General].) For more on Marshall's mission to China, see *Papers of GCM*, 5: 371–776, and Larry I. Bland, ed., *George C. Marshall's Mediation Mission to China, December 1945–January 1947* (Lexington, VA: George C. Marshall Foundation, 1998).
5. "Please take good care of yourself," Truman continued. "I want you to live as long or longer than I do because I'm intending to make the Jenners, McCarthys and Knowlands and all the dirty words they've used about you and have a case of political indigestion that would make a first class bellyache feel pleasant." (Ibid.)

490

To Brigadier General Marshall S. Carter — March 9, 1954
Pinehurst, North Carolina

Dear Carter: Thanks for your newsy letter about Alaska, maneuvers and the family.[1] All goes well with us tho I still have to be careful not to precipitate a return of the persistent virus-flu. I would be worried except for the fact that several fellows down here far younger than I am have struggled with it from four to six months. Katherine has about recovered from her lame back and but for occasional colds in in better shape than for several years.

It has been cold down here recently but beautiful clear weather. We can usually sit out on the lawn for hours each day. I am a professional lazy man consuming stacks of Westerns.

Dulles' troubles interest me—now at Caracas, because they merely duplicate mine and I immodestly think that my procedures and public policy statements were less confusing and dangerous than his.[2]

I am due in Washington the 17th and 18th for a BAC meeting and a Battle Monuments Commission meeting. I will only be out one night. The Women's North and South Golf Tournament is on that week and I always get a great deal of pleasure in following that. They play better than the men.

My love to Preot and the children, Affectionately,

GCM

GCMRL/Marshall S. Carter (Selected Correspondence); H

1. "Mild weather is beginning to creep up on us and while we still have our share of snow and a moderate amount of bird shooting, it is time to start working on our fishing tackle," Carter had written on March 5, noting that the temperatures in Alaska hovered "around zero or a little below. We have had very little wind and very dry atmosphere so our outdoor activities have continued unabated." (Carter to Marshall, March 5, 1954, GCMRL/G. C. Marshall Papers [Retirement, General].) He also described maneuvers during the visit of the 123rd Infantry Regiment of the 44th Infantry Division from Fort Lewis, Washington. "The one thing we did prove conclusively is that troops can operate, maneuver, and live in the field at great distances (50–75 miles) from their home base at temperatures below -30°. Up to this point there had always been some doubt about it." (Ibid.)

2. Secretary of State John Foster Dulles was in Caracas, Venezuela, attending the Tenth Inter-American Conference, where he faced considerable difficulty in obtaining Latin American support for an anticommunist resolution aimed at the Guatemalan government headed by Jacobo Arbenz Guzman. The CIA would successfully launch an operation to overthrow Arbenz a few months later. (Stephen G. Rabe, *Eisenhower and Latin America: the Foreign Policy of Anticommunism* [Chapel Hill: University of North Carolina Press, 1988], 49–63.) For more on Marshall's statements regarding Latin America while secretary of state, see *Papers of GCM*, 6: 159, 196–97, 199–201, 203–5, and 426–36.

491

To Richard Arens[1]

March 16, 1954
Pinehurst, North Carolina

Dear Arens: I have just been notified by Senator Robertson that the private bill for the relief of Maria Yutriago [*Intrialgo?*] passed the Senate on March 2.[2]

I very much appreciate all that you did to make it possible.[3] I feel she is entitled to this recognition and I am sure, in due course, that she will take the necessary steps to become a naturalized citizen.

Many thanks again for all of your kindnesses, and with best regards,[4] Faithfully yours,

GCMRL/G. C. Marshall Papers (Retirement, General)

1. Richard Arens was staff director of the Subcommittee on Immigration and Naturalization of the Senate Committee on the Judiciary.

2. Marshall had originally written to Arens on November 18, 1952, requesting a "suspension of deportation" for Maria Yutriago, "who is employed as a member of my household staff." (Marshall to Arens, November 18, 1952, GCMRL/G. C. Marshall Papers [Retirement, General].) "Since Maria's arrival in our household last May, she has proven to Mrs. Marshall and me every attribute which would make her a good citizen," Marshall attested. "I know nothing of her past, but, since coming to our home, she has conducted herself extremely well, and I believe her to be of good moral character." (Ibid.) Arens replied on November 20 that the case had been declined and suggested that Marshall request a private immigration bill from a senator or congressman that "could provide in effect that the subject shall be deemed to be a permanent resident of the United States," and offered "to draft a bill for introduction." Marshall wrote immediately to thank Arens for his offer and added a postscript: "I feel that it is tragic to force this poor woman to return to

Spain. She has been over here seven years and has *studied* hard to prepare for citizenship." (Arens to Marshall, November 20, 1952, and Marshall to Arens, November 20, 1952, ibid.)

On January 2, 1953, Virginia Senator A. Willis Robertson had responded to an inquiry from Marshall that he would "be glad to introduce" a private bill for Miss Yutriago. (Robertson to Marshall, January 2, 1953, ibid.)

3. On July 21, 1953, C. J. George had informed Marshall that the investigating officer had "made a very favorable report to the Senate Judiciary Committee, which will have the final say on the private bill." (George to Marshall, memorandum, July 21, 1953, ibid.)

4. See pp. 921–22.

492

To John White Pendleton — March 19, 1954, Pinehurst, North Carolina

Dear John: We were distressed to receive your Sunday letter and learn of Madge's difficulty.[1] I was provoked with myself because I was in Washington Wednesday afternoon for a meeting of the BAC, and Thursday morning for a meeting of the Battle Monuments Commission and I might have called up and learnt of how things were. Now our information is five days ago. I will set George to work to keep us informed.

Give Madge my love and affection and tell her we are all praying for her.

I flew in last evening at 6-30 p.m. My first plane got its landing gear stuck and I had to turn around at Richmond and go back for another plane.

Katherine is writing. Hastily, GCM

GCMRL/Xerox 2237 (GCM Family, Personal Letters); H

1. Pendleton had written to Katherine Marshall that his wife, the widow of her son Allen Brown, had delivered a premature baby girl by Cesarean section on March 12. "Madge is doing fine," Pendleton had written, but the baby's "lungs were not fully developed, and she is breathing with difficulty." (Pendleton to Marshall, March 14, 1954, GCMRL/G. C. Marshall Papers [Retirement, General].)

On June 17, Pendleton wrote to Marshall that their three children would be baptized together June 25, and asked him to be godfather of the middle child, Hunter, who was named for John Pendleton's father. Their infant daughter was christened Margaret. (Pendleton to Marshall, June 17, 1954, ibid.; "J. W. Pendleton Dies, Oil Firm Executive," *Richmond Times-Dispatch*, April 3, 1971.) Marshall responded on June 21 that he would be "delighted and honored." (Marshall to Pendleton, June 21, 1954, GCMRL/Xerox 2237 [GCM Family, Personal Letters]; H.)

493

To Lieutenant General Lucian K. Truscott Jr.[1] — March 19, 1954, Pinehurst, North Carolina

Dear Truscott: Thank you for your nice letter with its generous comments regarding me, and for the book which has not yet arrived.[2] I will be delighted to have it for several reasons including the interesting review I have read.[3]

It has been a long time since I have been in touch with you. When you were briefly located near Leesburg I counted on seeing much of you but my movements and yours interfered. I do hope to see you when you are on this side again.[4]

We go up to Leesburg about May 1st and probably will be there until next November, except for August.

During the war I always thought of you as one of the most dependable hard fighters no matter what the conditions. You certainly lived up to that estimate. From the start you were a hard bitten fighter.

Good luck and thanks,[5] Faithfully yours,

G.C. Marshall

GCMRL/G. C. Marshall Papers (Retirement, General)

1. After successfully leading the US Fifth Army during World War II, Lieutenant General Lucian K. Truscott Jr. had commanded the US Third Army from October 8, 1945, to April 1946. In 1953, President Eisenhower had approved Truscott's appointment as deputy director for coordination of the CIA.

2. "I cannot tell you how deeply I appreciate the opportunity that you accorded me for service which made the experience which I recounted possible," Truscott had written in a letter on March 11 informing Marshall that he was sending a copy of his new book, *Command Missions*. "You were throughout the war a continuing inspiration to me. I sincerely hope that my narrative will justify some measure of your confidence." (Truscott to Marshall, March 11, 1954, GCMRL/G. C. Marshall Papers [Retirement, General].)

3. Marshall may have been referring to Hanson W. Baldwin's review of Truscott's book in the *New York Times*. (Hanson W. Baldwin, "A Fighting General Speaks Out," *New York Times*, February 9, 1954, p. BR3.)

4. After retiring from the army on September 30, 1947, Truscott and his family had purchased a farm seventeen miles west of Leesburg. Since February 1951 he had been living in Frankfurt as the senior representative of the Central Intelligence Agency in Germany. (Wilson A. Heefner, *Dogface Soldier: The Life of General Lucian K. Truscott, Jr.* [Columbia: University of Missouri Press, 2010], 267–72.)

5. "Rarely do I read any of the war literature, but I found this an intensely interesting exception," Marshall wrote again to Truscott on April 19 after he had read *Command Missions*. (Marshall to Truscott, April 19, 1954, GCMRL/G. C. Marshall Papers [Retirement, General].) "I want you to know that I found it vastly interesting and very informing. I am obliged for the kindly treatment you gave me." (Ibid.) Truscott had recounted numerous encounters with Marshall during the war, and noted "the generous and thoughtful things that always distinguished him in his dealings with his subordinates." (Lieutenant General L. K. Truscott Jr., *Command Missions: A Personal Story* [New York: E. P. Dutton, 1954], 383.)

494

To Mrs. Hoyt Vandenberg

April 8, 1954
Pinehurst, North Carolina

Dear Mrs. Vandenberg: I regretted exceedingly that I could not go up to Washington to pay my last respects to your husband.[1] I was temporarily down with a cold, a mild reaction on my long persistent virus-flu infection.

I send you my deepest sympathy, but to be frank I think the end was a release to him and I know it was a physical release to your nervous system—for I was deeply worried about you.[2]

Time is the only solace or cure for your present sorrow, but you should profit by the thought of the splendid career he left behind and the great service he rendered his country in the finest sense.[3]

We go back to Leesburg May 3d. Maybe I will see you later.

Mrs. Marshall joins me in sympathy and affectionate regards.

GC Marshall

GCMRL/G. C. Marshall Collection (Vandenberg); H

1. General Hoyt Vandenberg had died on April 2. Marshall was listed as an honorary pallbearer at his funeral, which took place on April 5 in the nave of Washington National Cathedral. ("Vandenberg Dies of Cancer at 55; Air Force Chief Retired Last June," *New York Times*, April 3, 1954, pp. 1, 4.)

2. See p. 801.

3. President Truman had extended Vandenberg's term on April 30, 1952, "to permit him to round out thirty years of service in the highest rank he attained." (Ibid.) During World War II Vandenberg was chief of staff of the Twelfth Air Force in North Africa, headed an air mission to Moscow, then returned to the European Theater of Operations. At age forty-nine, he became "the youngest member of the military establishment holding the four-star rank." (Ibid.)

495

To Hanson W. Baldwin

April 15, 1954
Pinehurst, North Carolina

My dear Baldwin: I have received your letter of April 8 with its two questions regarding Mr. Roosevelt and Pearl Harbor.[1]

My embarrassment at present is due to the fact that I have declined to a large number of press inquiries to make a statement beyond saying that I would rest the matter on the record. Despite this, a New York inquiry receiving that reply wrote a lengthy so-called statement of mine, which was without foundation.

A member of the White House press correspondents was sent down here by David Lawrence's magazine to interview me. I made no statement. He was a nice fellow and now, if I meet your request, I will let him down badly.[2] If I could find a way to avoid this embarrassment, I would gladly answer your two questions. My answer would be an emphatic "NO" in both instances. Could you not say that I had answered "NO" emphatically to both questions, and let me go at that?[3]

I am sorry to have been so long in replying to your note.[4] Faithfully yours,

GCMRL/G. C. Marshall Papers (Retirement, General)

1. "As you may know, a new book on Pearl Harbor authored by Rear Admiral [Robert A.] Theobald is about to be published," Baldwin had written, referring to *The Final Secret of Pearl Harbor: The Washington Contribution to the Japanese Attack*. "Admiral Theobald goes so far as to declare flatly that the facts permit no other deduction than to state that the President planned to have Pearl Harbor attacked." (Baldwin to Marshall, April 8, 1954, GCMRL/G. C. Marshall Papers [Retirement, General].) "Admiral Theobald implies that you and Admiral [Harold R.] Stark must have had direct orders from President Roosevelt or some of his subordinates not to alert Pearl Harbor to its dangers." Baldwin then asked whether Marshall ever received "direct or indirect orders or intimations directing you to withhold intelligence information from the commanders in Hawaii or from our commanders in any other areas" and whether he ever gained "any direct or indirect impression that

President Roosevelt or anyone else in the United States government planned deliberately to expose the United States Fleet at Pearl Harbor and our military installations in Hawaii to Japanese attack." (Ibid.)

2. See p. 454n1. In its November 2, 1959, issue (seventeen days after Marshall's death), *U.S. News and World Report* published an article by John P. Sutherland, the news editor in 1954. Sutherland explained that he had met with Marshall three times and claimed that he "took notes, including verbatim quotations, with General Marshall's knowledge and permission. His only stipulation was that his words not be made public during his lifetime." (John P. Sutherland, "The Story Gen. Marshall Told Me," *U.S. News and World Report* 47, no. 18 [November 2, 1959]: 50.) The interviews took place at Pinehurst on March 29, 1954, and April 6, 1955, and at least once in Leesburg. "In all, we spent at least six hours together," Sutherland recalled. (Ibid., 50–51.) Sutherland's article includes quotations from Marshall concerning issues raised in Theobald's book. (Ibid., 51.)

3. On April 12, Admiral Stark had sent to Marshall a copy of a virtually identical letter he had received from Baldwin. "It occurred to me he may have written you a similar letter," Stark wrote. "I'd like to talk to you about it before making a reply" and mentioned that he would telephone Marshall "in a couple of days." (Stark to Marshall, April 12, 1954, ibid.) "In view of your conversation with Admiral Stark this morning," C. J. George wrote to Baldwin on April 15, "I was asked, on behalf of both General Marshall and Admiral Stark, to notify Mr. Sutherland of the U. S. News and World Report that their answer was 'NO' to the question: 'Did President Roosevelt restrain you from sending messages which you otherwise might have sent?'" (George to Baldwin, April 15, 1954, ibid.)

4. "I much appreciate your kind and frank letter," Baldwin replied on April 19. "I tried to follow your suggestions literally and quoted you specifically as you indicated. Indeed, this negative was all I wanted." (Baldwin to Marshall, April 19, 1954, ibid.)

U.S. News and World Report did claim in the "Washington Whispers" column in its February 25, 1955, issue that "Gen. George C. Marshall and the Army are to be blamed—in a history of the Pearl Harbor disaster being written by the Navy—for delay in communications that could have warned of the surprise attack." (*U.S. News and World Report* 38, no. 8 [February 25, 1955]: 6.) Colonel Claire E. Hutchin Jr. informed Marshall that "the Department of Navy Chief of Information has checked with every responsible Naval official who could officially have a hand in writing Navy history and has determined that this report is in error. In other words, it just plain isn't so." He assured Marshall that David Lawrence had been notified. (Hutchin to Marshall, February 23, 1955, GCMRL/G. C. Marshall Papers [Retirement, General].) Marshall assured Hutchin on March 10 that he was "deeply appreciative" for his actions. (Marshall to Hutchin, March 10, 1955, ibid.) For a summary of inquiries into Marshall's role in Pearl Harbor investigations, see Pogue, *Ordeal*, 429–35.

496

PREFACE FOR *FIFTY YEARS IN CHINA* BY JOHN LEIGHTON STUART — April 19, 1954
Pinehurst, North Carolina

It is a great pleasure for me and a compliment to be permitted to write an introduction to the autobiography of Dr. John Leighton Stuart.[1]

I met Dr. Stuart for the first time at Nanking, China, in the late spring, as I recall, of 1946. He was returning from a lengthy visit to the United States recuperating from his years of imprisonment by the Japanese.[2]

We talked over the current situation, and I was so impressed by his reactions that, later on, I proposed to the Department of State that he be appointed Ambassador to China—I was only an Ambassadorial Representative of the President. I took this action because of Dr. Stuart's fifty years' experience in China, and his character, his personality, and his temperament. With Dr. Stuart beside me, I had fifty years of vast experience unprejudiced by personal involvements in Chinese partisanship. On his appointment, I found his advice and leading assistance of invaluable help to me.[3]

I doubt if there is anyone whose understanding of Chinese character, history, and political complications equals that of Dr. Stuart. His high standard of integrity made his opinions all the more important.

I am writing this introduction without having had the opportunity to read the manuscript of his autobiography, but I do not think that is necessary to the purpose of this introduction. It is the man, the character, and the general range of his experience which appealed to me.

GCMRL/G. C. Marshall Papers (Retirement, General)

1. Former president of Yenching University John Leighton Stuart, who had served as US ambassador to China during Marshall's mission to China (see *Papers of GCM*, 5: 620–22), had asked Marshall to write an introduction for his autobiography in March. Marshall responded on March 18 that he would be "very happy" to comply. Stuart thanked Marshall the following day. Stuart wrote again on April 12 that his publishers were "anxious to have the book published on an early date" and requested that Marshall compose his introduction "as soon as convenient." (Marshall to Stuart, March 18, 1954; Stuart to Marshall, March 19, 1954; and Stuart to Marshall, April 12, 1954, GCMRL/G. C. Marshall Papers [Retirement, General].)

2. Marshall met Stuart on May 17, 1946, while they were in Nanking for a conference. See *Papers of GCM*, 5: 587. After the attack on Pearl Harbor, the Japanese placed Stuart under house arrest at Yenching University in the northwestern suburbs of Peking.

3. Marshall wrote to Undersecretary of State Dean Acheson on July 5, 1946, to suggest Stuart's nomination because "he occupies a unique position as the most highly respected foreigner, one whose standards of integrity and actions through the 50 years of his life out here have been a model of the best of the western world." (*Papers of GCM*, 5: 620–22.) Stuart had returned from China in 1949, although he did not formally resign as ambassador until November 28, 1952. He suffered a stroke after his resignation. See p. 945.

497

To Mrs. Harry S. Truman

May 5, 1954
Washington, DC

My dear Mrs. Truman: I just came into the office—the first time since our return from Pinehurst two days ago—and Mrs. Marshall asked me to find out from you whether or not you and Mr. Truman could come down and have lunch with us, or dinner and spend the night (and this, of course, would include breakfast) during your Washington stay.[1]

We are going to try to come up to the Acheson dinner, but beyond that will not attempt to come up to town.[2] Katherine has been having trouble with one eye—not serious, but it affects her comfort, and I have not yet entirely shaken the effects of the virus-flu. So we both avoid engagements which involve any travel.

Please pardon this typewritten letter, but it will get to you promptly, as I understand you are arriving today. Faithfully yours,

GCMRL/G. C. Marshall Papers (Retirement, General)

1. The Trumans had come to Washington to celebrate Mr. Truman's seventieth birthday at events there and in New York to raise funds for the Truman Library.

2. Dean Acheson had invited the Trumans and the Marshalls to dinner at his home on May 10. "Your dinner was quite the most enjoyable event to Mrs. Truman and me, of the whole visit," Truman wrote to Acheson on May 28. "Our conversations with Gen. Marshall gave me a great kick." (Raymond H. Geselbracht and David C. Acheson, eds., *Affection and Trust: The Personal Correspondence of Harry S. Truman and Dean Acheson, 1953–1971* [New York: Alfred A. Knopf, 2010], 52.)

498

To Bill Baker

May 10, 1954
Leesburg, Virginia

My dear Baker: Your letter requesting some statement by me regarding the Battle was addressed to Leesburg. As I was then in Pinehurst, it was forwarded there. Meanwhile, I left Pinehurst to open our home at Leesburg, so your letter was again delayed and forwarded back to Leesburg. It arrived on May 6, and I fear too late for me to meet your request.[1]

I have this to say:

"The Battle of New Market was remarkable for several reasons. It was one of the last desperate efforts of the Confederacy, meaning General Lee, in that theatre to halt the surging Union forces in the final great effort to overwhelm the South.

"It was won by a heterogeneous force, united in spirit, hastily collected by General Breckenridge, who had suddenly been charged with the mission by General Lee, then gripped in a death struggle with Grant's armies. And it included a battalion of boys, Cadets of the Virginia Military Institute, who took a spirited and very effective part in the battle at heavy cost to themselves.[2]

"The gallantry of those boys, their youth and their perfect battlefield discipline, have won historic fame for this contest, rather to the exclusion of the fierce and irresistible fighting of the war worn veterans so hastily called to this field.

"New Market demonstrated to the world the quality of the young men and boys of the South and the character of the Institute from which they came." Faithfully yours,

GCMRL/G. C. Marshall Papers (Retirement, General)

1. Baker, the president of the Battle of New Market Memorial Society, had written to Marshall requesting "a few words" from Marshall to insert into "a souvenir program booklet for our 90th Anniversary" of the Civil War battle. (Baker to Marshall, n.d., GCMRL/G. C. Marshall Papers [Retirement, General].)

2. See p. 522n5.

499

To Admiral Richard E. Byrd

May 13, 1954
Leesburg, Virginia

Dear Byrd: I have been concerned about you ever since our meeting the other day at the National Geographic, and the more concerned when I found you were not able to come to the dinner that night.[1] I am glad you didn't make that effort, but it merely indicated to me the correctness of my estimate.

I am now in my eighth month of virus-flu, and I find I have a number of competitors for time and distance. I tell you now that you can't rush it. It goes through certain stages and so far as I could find out—and I think it was more or less the opinion of Walter Reed Hospital, where I was confined twice—the best cure, certainly in the winter, is Arizona—the dry climate.[2]

The risk in this business is that, when you feel considerably better, you immediately do some things, and then you lose a lot of ground. You have got to be very lazy, very indefinite, altogether worthless, as I am now.[3] You can't beat the game on this thing. I know a number of fellows who have the same trouble, and I have followed their experience rather closely. The poor devils who have a business and have to work command my sympathy, because every effort they make generally sends them back home again.[4]

With affectionate regards and personal concern for your good health, Faithfully yours,

GCMRL/G. C. Marshall Papers (Retirement, General)

1. Marshall had attended a meeting of the Board of Trustees of the National Geographic Society the afternoon of May 5. That evening he attended a dinner honoring Dr. and Mrs. Gilbert Grosvenor at the Chevy Chase Club.

2. See pp. 795–96.

3. "They all tell me that I look very well but under the skin I am not so hot," Marshall had confessed to Frank McCarthy on May 10. (Marshall to McCarthy, GCMRL/Frank McCarthy Papers [Additions, Box 1]; H.)

4. Marshall wrote again to Byrd on June 1 to counsel "extreme patience, especially when you show signs of improvement. The last is where I found trouble." (Marshall to Byrd, June 1, 1954, OSU/Papers of Admiral Richard E. Byrd [Byrd Personal Papers, Sub-Series 3, Marshall, Folder 2207].) Byrd admitted to Marshall on September 10 that he "kept on working" and his condition had deteriorated, so he saw "a famous doctor here in Boston." He reported on September 17 that this doctor quoted Marshall's June 1 advice to Byrd "a number of times," and he joked that "Judging from the doctors' bills, if you should charge me, Dr. Marshall, for your good advice, I would be getting a good size bill from you." (Byrd to Marshall, September 10 and 17, 1954, GCMRL/G. C. Marshall Papers [Retirement, General].) Marshall concluded a September 15 letter to Byrd with a warning: "for goodness sake don't permit your energetic reactions to crowd you into another relapse." (Marshall to Byrd, September 15, 1954, OSU/Papers of Admiral Richard E. Byrd [Byrd Personal Papers, Sub-Series 3, Marshall, Folder 2207].) See p. 971n5.

500

To General Mark W. Clark May 13, 1954
Leesburg, Virginia

Dear Clark: I have just read your note of acknowledgment of our birthday congratulations.[1]

I should have written you a personal note at the time, but involvements in moving from Pinehurst to Leesburg, etc. prevented my doing many personal things. I have wanted to write to tell you how much I have enjoyed reading your last book. I haven't quite finished it yet, but, so far as I have gone, it has intrigued me greatly.[2]

I also want to express our pleasure in having you and Renie as reasonably near neighbors. I know you are going to build a fine place for yourself in the esteem of the Charlestonians, but I find you are also linked rather closely with Charlotte.[3]

With warm regards to you both from Katherine and me,[4] Affectionately yours,

GCMRL/G. C. Marshall Papers (Retirement, General)

1. C. J. George had sent a telegram on the Marshalls' behalf to General Mark W. Clark on his birthday on May 1. "It brought back many memories of my happy association with you in the past," Clark had written. (Clark to Marshall, May 4, 1954, GCMRL/G. C. Marshall Papers [Retirement, General].) During World War II Clark had commanded the Fifth Army and then the Fifteenth Army Group in Europe. As commander in chief of US Occupation Forces in Austria after the war he worked closely with Secretary of State Marshall in Council of Foreign Ministers' meetings in Moscow and London. See *Papers of GCM*, 6.

2. Clark's *From the Danube to the Yalu* had recently been published by Harper.

3. Clark and his wife Maurine "Renie" Doran Clark had moved to Charleston, South Carolina, when he accepted the presidency of The Citadel, the Military College of South Carolina, effective March 1, 1954. The Clarks' link with Charlotte, North Carolina, is unclear.

4. "I deeply appreciate hearing from you and to know that you have read and enjoyed the book," Clark replied. "I hope next fall we can get you and Mrs. Marshall to come down," he continued. "I'd love to have you take a parade and talk to my cadets. They certainly would be proud to have you here." (Clark to Marshall, May 18, 1954, ibid.) On November 26, Marshall tentatively agreed to visit The Citadel on January 21, 1955. He confirmed the date on January 11, but health problems as well as bad weather led him to cancel the trip. (Marshall to Clark, November 26, 1954, and January 11, 1955, ibid.; Marshall to Clark, January 22, 1955, The Citadel Archives and Museum, Charleston, South Carolina; H.)

501

Memorandum for Harry S. Truman on China[1] May 18, 1954
Leesburg, Virginia

The following is a very brief resume of as much of the Chinese situation as I, personally, was intimately familiar with. The difficulty in preparing such a resume is the fact that there is so much of background essential to an understanding (General Hurley's activities, and others of the same nature) that it presents quite a problem as how to prepare a statement without practically getting into a repetition of the China White Paper.[2] While I have sketched below an outline of my initial experience, I find that pages 136 to the middle of 149 of the China White Paper present a clear, chronological statement of the events up to the development of the Manchurian complications. Thereafter, the situation grew so complicated and there were so many related factors that it is exceedingly difficult to treat the affair with any degree of brevity.

When I arrived in China, a few days before Christmas in 1946 [*1945*], a meeting had already been scheduled for January, in which the Communist and other much smaller political parties were to be participants. The meeting was to draw-up the principles to be a basis for drafting a constitution to be considered by the Constitutional Convention scheduled for May 5. The preparatory work leading up to this meeting had been developed largely by General Patrick Hurley, then Ambassador to China, and it came to a head, just prior to my arrival, with the agreement on the actual date for the meeting.

I found that it would be impracticable for me to proceed with my mission to halt the fighting without obtaining a great deal of information, particularly the opinions of people in all walks of life in China and of the various political parties. Therefore, my days were a constant succession of meetings with all manner of people who were then resident at Chunking or came there for the purpose of meeting me. Many of them, particularly women, endeavored to come in secret so their contacts with me would not become public.

These people presented a wide variety of views. The majority of them, other than officials of the Nationalist Government, were bitterly hostile to that Government, particularly the women, though not necessarily friendly to the Communist Party.

Chou En-lai, the representative of the Communists, was then present in Chunking.[3] Just how many of his followers were there, I do not know, but there was not a sizeable number.

It was essential for me to move with all possible expedition, as the meeting of all the political parties had been called by Generallissimo Chiang Kai-Shek for January 10 and he wished to open the meeting with the announcement that the fighting had ceased.

In order to find a basis for terminating the fighting, the Generalissimo appointed a so-called Committee of Three, consisting of myself as Chairman, General Chang Chun representing the Nationalist Government, and Chou En-lai representing the Communist Party.[4] Together, we went over the factors which would be essential to a preliminary agreement. But it was not until the morning of January 10—about one-half hour before the meeting—that we reached a final agreement. This enabled the Generalissimo to make an opening speech of a character appealing to the generous sentiments of all concerned.

Following this period, I in a sense cut myself off from this conference, as it was entirely political and I had been sent to China with instructions to bring the fighting to an end, if that be possible. The agreement reached by the Committee of Three and approved by the Generalissimo had now to be implemented and, for this purpose, I immediately dispatched the Executive Officer of my staff, Colonel Henry A. Byroade, to Peking to organize a headquarters for developing and directing the procedure to bring the fighting to a halt. Utilizing the buildings of the Peking Union Hospital, Colonel Byroade (now Assistant Secretary of State) built up an organization based on the principle of the Committee of Three; that is, an American representative as Chairman of each subdivision and a representative of the Nationalist Government and representative of the Communist Party.[5] Walter H. Robertson, United States Minister to China, was dispatched to Peking to head the organization.[6] There were to be many teams in the field organized in the same manner and provided with radio communication and motor transportation.

The measures followed in bringing at least a temporary halt to the fighting are well-known and are mostly recorded in the China White Paper. I might say in this connection that we found it very difficult in many cases, and usually very important cases, to get at the true facts. The two Chinese members of the teams were not only antagonistic, one to the other, but held to a very strict course of action which would avoid anything prejudicial to their side of the current issue. As a result, it fell more and more to the American representative and Chairman, and at times to me personally, to ferret out the true facts of a case or incident.

For example, we had one situation in Shantung involving coal, a very important issue, where a large number of Nationalist troops were surrounded by a larger number of Communist troops. At the same time, farther to the West, we had almost an exactly similar situation, where a large number of Communist troops were surrounded by a larger number of Chinese Nationalist troops. The Communist representative on the Committee of Three with me was urging me to go personally to settle the western dilemma. The Nationalist representative was opposed to my doing so. On the other hand, the Nationalist representative was pressing me to go to the scene of the difficulty in Shantung, and the Communist member was strongly opposed to that action. This was frequently the case, though not so clearly demarked as in this particular incident.

The information with regard to fighting was very difficult to evaluate because the reports were, as a rule, grossly exaggerated by the side which had suffered the reverse or was charged with the renewal of the fighting, and frequently a light patrol encounter was exaggerated into a large operation. Despite these difficulties, we brought the fighting temporarily to an end.

There now followed a serious dispute over the representation of delegates to the Constitutional Convention scheduled for May 5. This provoked added bitterness both in the field and among the workers behind the scenes politically. The Generalissimo then postponed the meeting of the Constitutional Convention because he stated he could not find a satisfactory basis for the representation of delegates. This was a very serious blow and, from then on, matters proceeded from difficult, to bad, to worse.

During most of the period following January 10, I found the Communist representation and most of their forces in the field to be more responsive to the dictates of the Committee of Three than the Nationalists. It seemed to me the Communists felt that they could win their battle on political grounds more easily than on tactical fighting grounds because they had a more tightly held organization, whereas on the Nationalist side there were many contentious elements. The Communists continued on this line quite definitely, in my opinion, until early in June, after the postponement of the Constitutional Convention. The Nationalist commanders all seemed to be determined to pursue a policy of force.

During this period, and especially later throughout the summer, I was making a strong effort to bring all the small political parties together. These usually represented a rather small number in grand totals, but included a large number of well-informed men. My thought was that, if they could be united under one leader, they would constitute a balance wheel between the Communists and the Nationalists so that, if either broke an agreement, it would find this center group aligned against them. This would not have been too difficult of accomplishment had it not been for the fact that both sides, Nationalist and Communist, endeavored to break down any such grouping by tempting leaders away by choice appointments or otherwise. This continued until the end of my stay in China, but it became quite evident in the Fall that these parties had been broken down to such an extent that I could not hope to make a union among them and, without that, there was little hope of getting any organized setup in China that would lead to an enduring peaceful development.

I received advice from numbers of people in China and elsewhere—Americans, representatives of our press, British, Chinese, and among the latter named certain prominent members of the Government who came to me confidentially and gave me their opinions on the best course to be followed. As the conditions of temporary peace broke down, the agreed arrangements in Manchuria broke with them, and the movement of Communists into that country got underway. The extent of this movement at the start was exaggerated by the Nationalists, in my opinion, but later on there was no question but what large numbers of Communist adherents and troops were filtering into the country.

After the setup for implementing the enforcement of the agreement for bringing the fighting to an end, I next turned to the conference appointed to prepare the basis for the military reorganization. This was again a Committee of Three, though I appeared as an advisor, rather than as the Chairman. Without too much difficulty, an agreement was reached in this matter for the gradual unification of all the military forces in China, which meant in fact the Government and Communist forces. This was formally approved by the Generallissimo and agreed to by Mao Tse tung. Two provisos in this agreement are important to understand:

The first was the fact that the Communists agreed that at the end of eighteen months the Manchurian garrison should consist of fourteen Nationalist Government divisions and *one* Communist division (see page 141 of the China White Paper). The second was the prescribed organization of the country into eight service areas (see Article 3, Section 2, on page 623 of the China White Paper).

The attitude of the Communist regime changed later on, decidedly, in regard to

Manchuria, and the garrison proposed by them was greatly increased with reference to the number of Communist divisions to be located in that region. This action was a direct retaliation of the Communists to what they held were unjustified actions of the Nationalist Government.

The second proviso mentioned was to be the basis for getting the Chinese army out of politics, for breaking down the customary use of military force, which had been wholly unacceptable to a democratic regime.

Following the completion of the military reorganization agreement, I left Chunking with General Chang Chih-chung of the Nationalist Government and General Chou En-lai of the Communist Party on an inspection of the situation in North China and the West to the borders of Mongolia.[7] We endeavored to settle the various military complications which we found during the trip. We paused in Peking to visit the Executive Headquarters established there and endeavored to iron out misunderstandings and various oppositions.

Meanwhile, there had been developing in Manchuria a most serious situation. In the first place, the delay in the Russian withdrawal and their scuttling of all the industrial setups, particularly in the Mukden district, had been a continuing cause of complications. This situation was made the more difficult because of the misunderstanding at Executive Headquarters in Peking that the agreements of the Committee of Three for the implementation of the peace adjustments did not include Manchuria. As early as January 24, 1946, I proposed that Executive Headquarters send a field team to intervene in the fighting which had developed at Yingkow in Manchuria. The Generallissimo was unwilling to agree to this proposal. The Chinese Communist Party gave its approval. Further efforts on my part to establish Executive Headquarters field teams in Manchuria were declined by the Generallissimo. General Chou En-lai personally urged me to visit Mukden, but I did not think this wise at that time. Finally, on March 11, the day of my departure for Washington, the Generallissimo agreed to the entry of field teams from Executive Headquarters, but with such limited powers that the teams would be unable to bring about a cessation of the fighting.

This developing situation in Manchuria became one of the determining factors in breaking down all hope of negotiating a political basis for unity and peace in China.

With the Generallissimo's agreement to the entry of Executive Headquarters field teams into Manchuria, but unfortunately before his limitations on their powers became known, I departed for Washington to apprise the President of the situation and, particularly, to take up the question of the transfer of surplus property and shipping and the problem of loans to China.

In the matter of loans, I had not entered into any detailed discussions with the Generallissimo up to that time. As to the vast accumulations of surplus property in the Pacific, I felt that here was an opportunity to check the inflationary developments in China. This property could be used in many ways to promote trade, to secure for the Government a tremendous cash return, and to provide labor for many engaged in the modification or repair. I felt that the handling of this surplus property afforded a reasonably practical method of combating inflation and I was, therefore, anxious to promote the transfer as quickly as possible.

Another factor was the question of shipping. If China could obtain small coastwise and river shipping in these surplus property transfers, it would provide an effective method of promoting trade relations throughout the river valleys of China. In Washington, agreements were reached which would facilitate the surplus property transfers and guaranteed the provision of coastwise and river shipping for China. My negotiations with the United States Government groups concerned led to an agreement for a loan of $500 million to the Nationalist Government in China. Its conclusion merely lacked the signature of the Generallissimo's representative in Washington—the Chinese Ambassador. The latter came to me with some modifications in the terms of the loan, which the Generallissimo proposed. I informed the Ambassador that I had completed my personal efforts in the matter and, if any changes were to be proposed, they would have to be instituted by the Ambassador. At the same time, I advised him to sign the agreement for the loan immediately. Just what he would have done, I do not know, because on that day the Generallissimo made a speech in China regarding the basis of any political settlement, which caused the Import-Export Bank to withdraw its agreement to the loan.[8]

While I was in Washington, the day after the withdrawal of Russian troops from Changchung, the Communist forces attacked the city and occupied it. From this time forward, there developed a series of incidents provoked in turn by the Chinese Government and by the Communist forces, which led to a complete rupture of the relationships established to terminate hostilities. The recital of these incidents and the discussions related to them would necessarily be a lengthy procedure and virtually a reproduction of the story as recited in the China White Paper. From here on out, the Communists were completely distrustful, in fact rather scornful, of any proposition I made or the Nationalist Government put forward toward finding an adjustment of differences. On the other hand, the Generallissimo, for the Nationalist Government, represented a varying role. At times his attitude was one of sincere endeavor to bring about some reasonable basis of adjustment, but invariably, it seemed to me, behind the scenes, his attitude with his leaders was one provocative of the role of force. Always in my conversations with him I put forward my military opinion that the use of force at that time by the Nationalist Government could not be productive of more success than that of the capture of cities—that the long lines of communication made military operations for the Nationalist Government far more difficult than they were prepared to meet. So long as the Communists confined themselves to attacks on the line of communications and the break down of the influence of the Nationalist Government with the Chinese people, their eventual success seemed to me to be assured.

After my departure from China and appointment as Secretary of State, I encountered the China problem in a somewhat different form than theretofore. It had now become a political issue in this country and the representations were highly colored by purely political motives. One of the most difficult political reactions arose out of the fact that the Nationalist Government of China was not able to procure quickly the military supplies it desired. These delays were charged to our Government. The facts were that our military reserves of modern equipment had been so reduced by allotments to various countries that the War Department could not afford further to diminish them. Even so, a direct purchase was rendered difficult because the money received by the War Department, for example, would have to be turned in to the Treasury and a new appropriation secured, with the possibility of failure. And then there would be the delay in the manufacture of the items, since there was no general market for such supplies. The War Department was loath to enter into the business of these purchases because of their effect on the national defense. Further, the complications in the matter could not well be made plain to the public in the midst of a vigorous political discussion, statements or debate.

In an effort to find some course of action that might be taken to offset the Communist gains in China, General Wedemeyer was sent over to inquire into the situation. It was on my instigation that he was sent to China, but it was his desire, and quite a proper one, that he have a Presidential directive in order that he might have a sound basis for meeting with the officials in China concerned. You are familiar with the issues which arose over his visit.[9]

It has been a great misfortune that throughout this period the Generallissimo has had associated with him individuals who had grown steadily in power from the time of the Generallissimo's march from Canton to the line of the Yangtse. Originally, these were young men, presumably animated with a very fine spirit to free China from the toils and treacheries of the past. But their steady acquisition of great power with virtually no opposition led naturally to a changed attitude until they were opposed to any effort along the line indicated by American policy. Partially discredited in 1946, they steadily regained their power, and found the development of the China political battle in the United States greatly to their advantage.

(Most confidentially, it had been hoped by Ambassador Stuart and me that my statement (page 686 of the China White Paper) following my departure from China, published in Washington on January 7, 1947, would provoke heavy attacks on me by this particular group of men, who seeing me leave the Government service would feel perfectly free to direct their attacks at me without reservation.[10] In this way, we would have had a line-up of the irreconcilables. Unfortunately, however, because, I was told, of some leak at Spartansburg, South Carolina, with relation to the announcement of Secretary of State Byrnes' resignation, it was thought best immediately to publicize my coming appointment as Secretary of State, instead of delaying this for the ten days that I had requested. This announcement was made while my plane was flying homeward over the island of Okinawa.[11] It, of course, resulted immediately in a silence on the part of the irreconcilable group who, in the Chinese manner, retired to their homes sick(?).[12] They did not again appear on the scene until the political fight in the United States on the China question developed. I think that, had the second announcement been delayed the ten days I desired, we would have had a public line-up of the men and their attitude who surrounded the Generallissimo and are now, some of them, associated with him in Formosa.)[13]

GCMRL/G. C. Marshall Papers (Retirement, General)

1. Truman had requested this memorandum from Marshall for use in writing his memoirs. See p. 824n4. "Herewith is an outline of the old China affair," Marshall wrote to Truman on May 18. "It is not much of a paper, but the best I could do at this time." (Marshall to Truman, May 18, 1954, GCMRL/G. C. Marshall Papers [Retirement, General].) This memorandum was published in its entirety but without notes in Bland, *Mediation Mission*, 560–67. For documents relating to Marshall's mission to China, see *Papers of GCM*, 5: 371–776.

2. President Franklin D. Roosevelt sent former Secretary of War Major General Patrick J. Hurley to China in August 1944 as his personal representative to Chiang Kai-shek and appointed Hurley US ambassador to China in November 1944. He left the post at his own request on September 22, 1945, which led Truman to send Marshall to China. Originally issued by the US Department of State as *United States Relations with China, with Special Reference to the Period 1944–1949* (Washington: Department of State, 1949), the China White Paper was republished by Stanford University Press in 1967.

3. For more on Chou En-lai, see p. 13n11 and *Papers of GCM*, 5: 401–2.

4. Chang Chun was governor of Sichuan Province in China from November 15, 1940, to May 14, 1947, and a prominent member of the Kuomintang. See *Papers of GCM*, 5: 411–17.

5. Colonel Henry A. Byroade had been acting director of the US Army's Operations Division's Asiatic Section. He had served in India (1942–43) and China (1943–44) before he joined Marshall's mission to China. (*Papers of GCM*, 5: 377.) Byroade had achieved the rank of brigadier general at age thirty-two in 1946. He resigned from the army in 1952 to become assistant secretary of state for Middle East, South Asia, and Africa.

6. Walter S. Robertson was a banker in Richmond, Virginia, prior to World War II. He became an economic adviser to the State Department, and in April 1945, he was appointed an auxiliary Foreign Service officer and made economic counselor (with the personal rank of minister) to the US embassy in China.

7. General Chang Chih-chung, director of political training for the National Ministries Council, was the director of Nationalist northwestern headquarters from 1945 to 1949 and chairman of the government of Xinjiang province from 1946 to 1947.

8. While in Washington, Marshall urged the Export-Import Bank to extend $500 million credit to the Nationalists and held discussions with the National Advisory Council about making a favorable decision on the matter. See *Papers of GCM*, 5: 516–19, 521, and 6: 30–32, 61, 368–82.

9. For more on Wedemeyer's July 1947 mission to China, see pp. 162, 509, 511–12, and *Papers of GCM*, 6: 170–71, 257; William Stueck, *The Wedemeyer Mission: American Politics and Foreign Policy during the Cold War* (Athens: University of Georgia Press, 1984); and Albert C. Wedemeyer, *Wedemeyer Reports!* (New York: Henry Holt and Co., 1958).

10. For Marshall's full January 7, 1947, statement concerning the "intricate and confused situation" in China, see *Papers of GCM*, 5: 772–76.

11. For Marshall's January 5, 1947, instructions to Marshall Carter concerning release of his statement, see *Papers of GCM*, 5: 770. James F. Byrnes later explained in his autobiography that Truman's December 1946 acceptance of his resignation, which he had submitted to Truman in April, "had been a well-kept secret" until Arthur Krock, Washington bureau chief of the *New York Times*, called Byrnes on January 7 to ask if he had resigned. Byrnes "made several evasive answers" and then informed Truman that the newspaper would likely print a story the next day "speculating on my resignation." He thus suggested that Truman announce his resignation and Marshall's appointment. (James F. Byrnes, *All in One Lifetime* [New York: Harper & Brothers, 1958], 387–88.) Krock did publish such an article the following day, adding that Marshall would succeed Byrnes. (Arthur Krock, "The

President's Tribute," *New York Times*, January 8, 1947, p. 3.) See pp. 859–60.

12. This question mark is in the original version, inserted by Mary Louise Spilman, who transcribed Marshall's draft. "The only formal Government statement" on Marshall's appointment "came from Information Minister Peng Hsueh-pei, who cautiously did not say whether the Government was pleased or displeased." ("Marshall Secret Kept from Staff," *New York Times*, January 9, 1947, p. 3.)

13. "I can't tell you how very much I appreciate your sending me the memorandum on China," Truman responded on May 26. Marshall's "recollection of the situation is exactly in line with my own," Truman added, "but I wanted confirmation of it. As you remember, you and I had many long conversations about it after you returned from China." (Truman to Marshall, May 26, 1954, GCMRL/G. C. Marshall Collection [Truman].) Truman recounted his impressions of Marshall's mission to China in the second volume of his memoirs. (Harry S. Truman, *Memoirs by Harry S. Truman*, vol. 2, *Years of Trial and Hope* [Garden City, NY: Doubleday and Company, Inc. 1956], 66–92.)

502

Statement on John D. Sturgeon's 100th Birthday[1] June 5, 1954
Leesburg, Virginia

My first recollection of Doctor Sturgeon was about 60 years ago when I was a heedless small boy. But I have a clear memory of the Doctor.

My schooling took me away from home at sixteen from early September to July—no vacations. The family usually went to the mountains for the hot months so I saw little of my home town through those years and less later as I went into the army and off immediately to the Philippines.

As a lieutenant on leave, I renewed my acquaintance with Doctor Sturgeon which grew in intimacy with the years, though not through frequent contacts.

My mother admired the Doctor and often spoke of him. He did me a great service in 1906 which I will never forget.[2]

When I saw him last September I was astonished at his apparent well being. He looked well, seemed to feel well and showed far fewer signs of age than most men of seventy.[3]

Several months later I spent an evening with King Haakon of Norway.[4] He is a tall, handsome, alert man of 82. During our conversation he made reference to his age. I did not respond in the usual manner, I think to his surprise, but instead said my views as to age had been greatly altered in the past few months since seeing an old friend, Doctor Sturgeon of Uniontown, Pennsylvania. His Majesty questioned me, "How so?" Thus I told him of the doctor's age, his physical appearance, the few lines in his face, and other lack of the usual signs of many years. The King was greatly interested and talked for quite a bit on the subject of Doctor Sturgeon's state of health and physical appearance. He was quite evidently much interested and possibly taking a new view of his own years.

I am very sorry I can not participate in the Birthday Celebration for Doctor Sturgeon and do him the small compliment of my presence. He represents the best of citizenship, a fine example of service to his fellowmen, a model of integrity and simplicity, and a great doctor of the humanities.

GCMRL/G. C. Marshall Papers (Retirement, General)

1. "On July 12, 1954, Dr. John D. Sturgeon, Sr. will have reached his 100th birthday," Dr. George Tolstoi of the Uniontown Hospital Association had written to Marshall. "Since you know Dr. Sturgeon so well, it would be deeply appreciated if you were to forward to me some of your reminiscences and anecdotes that we may use in our County Medical Journal and newspapers." (Tolstoi to Marshall, June 5, 1954, GCMRL/G. C. Marshall Papers [Retirement, General].)

2. Marshall and his first wife visited Uniontown in 1905 during four months' leave from San Antonio, Texas. (Pogue, *Education*, 89–90.) The editors have not been able to determine the service Dr. Sturgeon provided to Marshall.

3. Marshall had gone to Sturgeon's home during his visit to Uniontown on September 22, 1953. ("Marshall Enjoys First Visit Here in 14 Years," *Uniontown Evening Standard*, September 23, 1953, p. 5.) See p. 790n4.

4. Marshall had met with King Haakon just before accepting the Nobel Peace Prize on December 10, 1953. See p. 809.

503

To Brigadier General Marshall S. Carter — June 25 [*22*], 1954[1]
Leesburg, Virginia

My dear Carter: I enjoyed your newsy letter very much and sent it on to Bob Lovett because I knew he would be intensely interested.

This a.m. came a postal from you sent from Sun Valley where I take it you arrived ahead of Preot and the children.[2]

I envy you there. You are very lucky though you made your luck.

We received invitations today for a White House dinner Friday night for Churchill and Eden.[3] I go. Katherine declines—doesn't feel up to it.

I go in to the Business Advisory Council tomorrow, lunch, afternoon session and dinner—then home late.[4]

I have been doing much garden work, a great deal of watering, particularly on young plants, since we are working into a drought.

I am well with too much blood pressure as a result of my prolonged virus-flu struggle was up to 250. Now about 225. Katherine is suffering again from the effects her last attack of [shingles] on her eyes. But nothing serious. If she didn't overwork she would be all right.

My love to you all— Affectionately,

GCM

GCMRL/Verifax 2037 (Marshall Papers Research File); H

1. The content of this letter indicates that it was written on June 22, although Marshall dated it June 25.

2. Carter had written from Alaska on June 2 that his wife and younger children had already left for their home in Sun Valley, Idaho; he and their daughter Stoney planned to fly there on June 11. (Carter to Marshall, June 2, 1954, GCMRL/Marshall S. Carter Papers [Selected Correspondence].)

3. Marshall planned to attend a dinner for Prime Minister Winston Churchill and Sir Anthony Eden at 8:00 p.m. on June 25. ("Churchill Meets Eisenhower Today, U.S. Doubts Accord," *New York Times*, June 25, 1954, p. 2.) See p. 852.

4. Marshall participated in meetings of the Business Advisory Council on June 23 at the Department of Commerce and the Mayflower Hotel in Washington, DC.

504

To Forrest C. Pogue — June 28, 1954
Leesburg, Virginia

Dear Pogue: Many thanks for your letter of June 11 and for your courtesy in sending me a copy of your book THE SUPREME COMMAND. I have been very much interested in what I have read to date.[1]

During the past several years, I have been asked to reconsider my decision with respect to my participation in the war, and I have answered in each instance that I would not think of undertaking such a task. As you indicated, eighty different volumes will be printed and I think, as a result of this, my participation will be clearly defined.[2]

Confidentially, I have been advised by my doctors to take life leisurely. As you well know, I could not do this if I were to engage in such an effort as you suggest. You have been most gracious in your references to me and I am most appreciative. I hope you will understand my position.[3]

With warmest regards, Faithfully yours,

GCMRL/G. C. Marshall Papers (Retirement, General)

1. "I am completing an official history of THE SUPREME COMMAND IN NORTH-WEST EUROPE, 1944–45, which I have been working on for a number of months for the Department of the Army," military historian Forrest C. Pogue had written to Marshall in 1952. "Although I have gone through many of the papers in the Department of the Army files, the SHAEF files, many of the CCS [Combined Chiefs of Staff] and JCS files, I find there are several questions which only you can answer. This is to ask if you would be willing to grant me an interview sometime at your convenience." (Pogue to Marshall, February 9, 1952, GCMRL/G. C. Marshall Papers [Retirement, General].)

Pogue had written again on May 17, 1954, after presenting President Eisenhower with a copy of *The Supreme Command*, a volume in the official *United States Army in World War II* series, published by the Office of the Chief of Military History in 1954. He expressed his "disappointment" that Marshall "could not be at the White House presentation, since various factors made it impossible for me to interview you while I was writing the book." (Pogue to Marshall, May 17, 1954, ibid.) Pogue thanked Marshall on June 11 for autographing a photograph and assured him that he would "prize it very much." (Pogue to Marshall, June 11, 1954, ibid.)

2. "The war histories we have been writing will show in 80 different volumes the work you performed," Pogue had suggested in his June 11 letter. "But it is important that one volume, bearing the imprint of your papers and your personality, be given to the public in the next few years." (Ibid.) "In writing the volume on General Eisenhower's command in Europe," he continued, "I was given access to your personal correspondence with him, and I was enormously impressed by the close personal interest you took in the choice of commanders, the support of armies, the encouragement of the commanders, and the welfare of the troops. Much of this story is likely to be forgotten in some of the acrimony that has accompanied your fine service since the war." (Ibid.)

"Is there any possible chance that you will reconsider your decision not to write anything relative to the war period?" Pogue inquired. "I realize that you do not want now to undertake the burdensome task of writing a volume or series of articles yourself. But would you consider dictating the answers to certain questions to Mrs. Marshall or to me or to some other person?" he proposed. "It would be absurd for me to suggest that your place in history depends on what you do or do not write. I have every confidence that succeeding years will deal fairly with you. I believe, however, that this generation needs to know what you did for it," he stressed. "There is a danger that the young men just now coming of war age will know only MacArthur and Eisenhower, and not understand that you were the great driving force. I am a great admirer of General Eisenhower, but a study of his papers showed me the great work that you performed." (Ibid.)

3. Forrest C. Pogue became the first director of the George C. Marshall Research Foundation and Marshall's official biographer. See pp. 931–32 and 948–49.

505

REMARKS AT THE CELEBRATION OF THE 200TH ANNIVERSARY OF THE BATTLE AT FORT NECESSITY[1] — July 3, 1954, Fort Necessity, Pennsylvania

Sixty-seven years ago, on a Sunday afternoon, my father took the family on a picnic. We ate our supper on the bank of this stream, probably in this immediate vicinity. He gave us a thrilling description of the battle Washington's small force fought against the French and Indians in this field—Great Meadows, as it was called. I pictured painted redskins behind every tree over there. I clearly recall his showing us the shallow outline of the trench that had been manned by the Colonists.[2]

He told us how Washington passed near this spot a year later, accompanying Braddock's famous Redcoats on their fatal march toward Fort Duquesne; that is, the Pittsburgh of today. He described the near massacre of most of Braddock's command, the retreat, and Braddock's death and burial on the hillside trail a short two miles from here.[3]

That afternoon became a lasting memory. Young though I was, it aroused my deep interest in the history of that period, as it was outlined by great events in this region. Often I was to come in the evening to the site of Braddock's grave in company with my young friends on parties to the nearby mountain house with its chicken and waffle supper as the main event.[4]

The bald knob in the mountain range six miles northwest of here, Dunbar's Camp, where Colonel Dunbar buried the reserve ammunition of Braddock's army and hastily retreated eastward toward Philadelphia, is a familiar sight to many of you.[5] Near its foot is the deep ravine where Washington surprised and almost wiped out Jumonville's small reconnoitering party, firing the opening shot in the war that was to rage in Europe for seven long years.[6] It became a familiar setting for my first trout fishing efforts.

Washington Springs, the site of Washington's meeting with the Half-King; the Washington farm in the fertile valley west of the mountain—all those localities were steeped in early American history, when this was the far frontier, and the struggle between England and France for control of America was a bitter contest.[7]

Hunting the mountain grouse, or pheasant as we called them, made me more and more familiar with these historic surroundings, especially as the birds favored the glades along the Old Braddock Trail. But, very strange to say, practically none of this was touched on in our local schooling. Had it been, I am sure we would have acquired a taste for American history which would have been of great benefit to our opinions as citizens in later years. It would certainly have promoted an early knowledge of the world struggles which, for a time, were centered hereabouts.

Great things had their beginnings here. The man to lead the Colonists in the revolutionary struggle had his start here, an unsuccessful one it must have seemed. His preparation for the long struggle ahead, with its many pitfalls and its awful discouragements, was initiated here.

Few young Americans realize how many powerful nations struggled for a place in this country. The Russians were established as far south as San Francisco Bay. The word "struggled" is hardly applicable to them, because they chose to sell out. New Orleans, with its strategical domination of the entire Mississippi Valley, and Florida, shuttled about between Spain and France, and New England and New York State were in an almost constant state of threat by the British out of Canada.

But there is quite another side to this phase of the development of America. We chose, ourselves, in the war of the Revolution, to make a bid for the control of Canada. Much later on, we fought the Mexicans and took from them much of the southwest and all of California, and we crowded the Indians back all along our frontiers, frequently in violation of their treaty rights. But the start, in effect, was here in the small engagement in this field, with the prodigious results which followed.

So, when we assemble here to celebrate the 200th Anniversary of the Battle of Fort Necessity, we are dealing with the early frontier of this country, the struggle between the French and the British for control; actually the birth of American military power and leadership, a preliminary to the Revolutionary War and our march to the westward.

Since those days, there has been a tremendous shift in power and place, and in tempo. Our most pressing interests today are far remote from the mountains of western Pennsylvania. They concern the Far East, across the Pacific, western Europe, northern Africa, and the Middle East. All of Latin America is much to our interest. But keep in mind one outstanding fact. Nowhere are we grasping for territory. We want peace and, what is far more important, we want a sound basis for an enduring peace.

Turning back again to the historic events of this region and their relation to the future, I think possibly the most telling result which followed the disaster of Braddock's defeat was the initiation of a feeling among the Colonists that they were capable of themselves to fight for independence; that the famous soldiers who then dominated the battlefields of Europe could possibly be discounted. Bunker Hill twenty-two years later confirmed this point of view and awakened a strong determination to fight to a finish, with a Washington to lead them.[8] Of course there was much to learn, mostly of discipline, of stability, of leadership—and the outrageous vagaries of the Continental Congress at times hopelessly confused matters. Only the firm, wise leadership and remarkable personality of Washington saved the situation.

Referring to Washington's leadership in the Revolutionary struggle and his later title as the "Father of his Country", it is very interesting to trace the course of his development to his Revolutionary War status. Here at Fort Necessity, at the ambuscade of Jumonville, he was young, aggressive and fearless—very young as a matter of fact. He goes back to Will's Creek—Cumberland, as we know it—and is given command of a small body of troops to guard the settlers against Indian forays. His forts marked the course of the Shenandoah Valley. He was refused reinforcements for his small command despite frequent massacres of the families of the pioneers; he was denied many necessities to enable him to protect those pioneers. His letters addressed to the Colonial Government at Williamsburg are bitter in recrimination. He was completely outraged by the failure of that Government to support him sufficiently to protect the frontier people against the Indian savagery.[9]

Finally, he resigned and took up his life at Mount Vernon. For years he was not only a leading citizen, the head of a large and valuable plantation, but for fifteen years he was a member of the House of Burgesses at the colonial Capitol of Williamsburg.[10] There, for the first time, he learned something of the difficulties surrounding action by a democratic assembly; he learned the difficulty of obtaining appropriations that involve expenditures for troops. So, when he finds himself at Valley Forge lacking virtually everything for his men—food, clothing, blankets, shoes—when he is beset with the struggle to maintain a dependable army despite short-term enlistments, along with the failure to provide pay, food and clothing, then we find him persistent but patient, determined but respectful, seemingly humble with respect to the governing political body, whatever its action or lack of action may have been. And in that attitude we find the basis for general acceptance of the title of "Father of his Country", bestowed on him by grateful countrymen.[11]

GCMRL/G. C. Marshall Papers (Retirement, Speeches, Statements, and Writings)

1. Reverend William Blake Hindman, chairman of the Fort Necessity Bicentennial Association, had written to Marshall in the spring to invite him to address the group's July 3 event. "With your background and association with Fort Necessity since your boyhood you can give the program a personal touch as no other speaker," Hindman maintained. See p. 790n4. Marshall agreed to do so on April 8 but said that he would "not remain for the banquet." (Hindman to Marshall, n.d., and Marshall to Hindman, April 8, 1954, GCMRL/G. C. Marshall Papers [Retirement, General].) Marshall had also mentioned to Hindman that he might visit with his sister, Marie Singer, while he was in the area, and on May 21, he confirmed to Herman Buck of the White Swan Hotel in Uniontown, Pennsylvania, that he planned to "motor direct from Fort Necessity to Pike Run Country Club, where my sister will be." (Buck to Marshall, May 13, 1954, and Marshall to Buck, May 21, 1954, ibid.)

Marshall's plans apparently changed after writing to Buck; on June 28, he notified the chairman of the Fort Necessity Bicentennial Association that "I intend to arrive at Fort Necessity at 1:45 your time and will go directly to the plane after the ceremony." (Marshall to Hindman, June 28, 1954, ibid.) "I appreciate your invitation for lunch," he explained, "but I will have already had mine before arriving at the Fort." (Ibid.) For Marshall's comments to Forrest C. Pogue on this event, see *Marshall Interviews*, 29–30.

2. "In my day there was just a slight ridge in the field which showed where the entrenchment had been, which my father showed me when I was about seven years old," Marshall recalled. (*Marshall Interviews*, 29.) Lieutenant Colonel George Washington and his troops fortified the British position at the Great Meadows in late May and early June 1754 and

named the circular palisaded stronghold Fort Necessity. They were attacked by combined French and Indian forces on July 3. The battle ended in a truce; the British withdrew on July 4, and the French burned Fort Necessity.

3. Commander in Chief of British forces in North America General Edward Braddock was wounded on July 9, 1755, at the Battle of the Monongahela. Washington, a volunteer aide to Braddock, led the retreating army to a position one mile west of the site of Fort Necessity, where General Braddock died on July 13. Washington officiated the next day at the burial in the trail Braddock's men had cleared.

4. "On this trail, about seven or eight miles from home was the site of Braddock's grave. When they were building the National Road through, they dug up his grave and identified it by the brass buttons and skeleton and other things there, and they reinterred him close by in a very picturesque little plot. I don't think it was over fifty yards square," Marshall reminisced, "but we would go out in that vicinity to picnic. And this little white fence had a flat board on top, and we could sit on the fence, and lots of my early courtship efforts were made sitting on that fence on a moonlight night after one of these picnic suppers in the mountain." (Ibid, 29.)

5. Colonel Thomas Dunbar commanded the rear detachment of Braddock's troops.

6. On May 27, 1754, Washington and thirty-three men under his command as well as some of his Indian allies began the conflict—known in the colonies as the French and Indian War and in Europe as the Seven Years' War—when they surrounded, fired upon, and forced the surrender of a French detachment of approximately thirty-five men, under the command of Ensign Joseph Coulon de Jumonville, who had camped in a ravine near Great Meadows. Some of the French were then massacred by the Indian allies. The dead included de Jumonville as well as approximately a third of his force. This led to the attack on Fort Necessity described in n2 above.

7. Prior to the skirmish at Jumonville Glen, Washington had met with a friendly Seneca chief named Half King. In 1770 Washington purchased "Land at the place called the Great Meadows on both Sides of General Braddocks Road." (W. W. Abbott and Dorothy Twohig, eds., *The Papers of George Washington, Colonial Series*, vol. 8, *June 1767–December 1771* [Charlottesville: University Press of Virginia, 1993], 405–6.) The patent for 234.5 acres was issued on February 28, 1782. (Ibid.)

8. The battle of Bunker Hill took place on June 17, 1775, during the siege of Boston. At the time of the battle George Washington was in New York City, en route to take command of the Continental Army.

9. After Braddock's burial, Washington and his troops retreated to Fort Cumberland, Maryland. As commander in chief of Virginia's western forces, he established headquarters from 1756 to 1758 in Winchester at the head of the Shenandoah Valley.

10. Washington was elected to represent Frederick County, Virginia, in the House of Burgesses in 1758.

11. "I flew over to Fort Necessity near Uniontown this morning—55 minutes. Appeared at the ceremony after it got started. Spoke and left and immediately flew back—50 minutes," Marshall wrote to Molly Winn later in the day. "Was here at 4*15* p.m. Quick business." (Marshall to Winn, July 3, 1954, GCMRL/© Marshall-Winn Collection [Katherine Marshall]; H)

506

TO GENERAL MATTHEW B. RIDGWAY

July 7, 1954
Leesburg, Virginia

Dear Ridgway: Thanks for your telephone offer this morning regarding Baruch's visit here next Friday and Saturday. That was exceedingly thoughtful and I will take advantage of it if anything of that kind promises to come up. As a matter of fact his visit is merely a friendly one long delayed since we couldn't have him at Pinehurst due to my illness. He has often come here and there is nothing else to it. As a matter of fact, confidentially, I studiously keep clear of all official subjects, though he may have a great deal to say.[1]

Thanks also for your nice note after our visit with Penny and you. It was my business to do the writing but I left it to Katherine. She was so pleased to see the lovely setting you had made in her old room, not to mention Penny's hospitality.[2]

The other matter I referred to over the phone was Alexander's visit and his lunching here July 18*th*. It seemed to be indicated that he wanted to see me more or less alone. I doubt this and have put up to him the question as to who he would like me to invite. If, however, the first indication be correct I will guard myself by taking that briefing you offered.[3] With affectionate regards to both of you.

GCMarshall

USAMHI/Matthew B. Ridgway Papers (Marshall); H

1. See pp. 128, 144, and photo #24. Bernard Baruch had written repeatedly in 1954 about visiting the Marshalls. (Baruch to Marshall, April 11 and June 11 and 23, 1954, GCMRL/G. C. Marshall Papers [Retirement, General].)

2. Ridgway had written on May 18 to thank the Marshalls for making "the long trip in to be with us on Saturday afternoon" to attend a garden party on May 15 at their Fort Myer quarters and repeated an invitation "extended with complete sincerity" to stay overnight at any time. (Ridgway to Marshall, May 18, 1954, ibid.) Ridgway wrote again on June 26 after the Marshalls visited "but a few minutes." (Ridgway to Marshall, June 26, 1954, USAMHI/Matthew B. Ridgway Papers [Marshall].)

3. Ridgway had repeated his offer to provide "any briefing you may want at any time on any subject" in his June 26 letter. "If its classified nature should preclude sending it in written form, I shall be glad to send a briefing officer down to meet your convenience." (Ibid.) Alexander was the British minister of defense Earl Harold Alexander of Tunis, who had commanded Allied forces in Burma, North Africa, and Italy during World War II and had served as governor-general of Canada from 1946 to 1952, during which time Marshall had opened the 1951 Canadian National Exhibition (see pp. 607–9). Alexander was invited to lunch at the Marshalls' Leesburg home on July 18, 1954. On July 14, C. J. George sent directions to British Ambassador Sir Roger Makins and informed him that General Sir John Whiteley, chief of the British military mission, and Lady Whiteley would also be guests. (George to Makins, July 14, 1954, GCMRL/G. C. Marshall Papers [Retirement, Chronological].)

507

TO MRS. JAMES J. WINN — July 12, 1954
Leesburg, Virginia

Dear Molly: Thanks for your last letter. K had already decided to make the trip. I told her of your first letter, after she voiced her decision to go.[1]

I'm sure she can find some one who, for a price, will undertake to drive her over to your place each day. She very definitely does not want you to have to do this. Her conception at present is to sleep late, get her breakfast and lunch at the Inn and after a short nap drive over to your place and *back* for dinner with you, at the Inn. I don't think she should leave the Inn or village before about 3 p.m. She is very tired and much in need of a complete rest. Dont let Kitty go into the village and hang on her neck all day. She is not up to it but of course will accept Kitty's desire.

I am sending up with her a small fan for her room if she needs it. Also her special cushion.

I would suggestion [*suggest*]—strictly entré nous—that you do not try to meet her. Let the Sergeant get her settled quietly and then she can rest up and meet you at dinner. Just leave a note of greeting for her.[2]

She really wants to stay 2 weeks but holds forth about me here alone. Make her stay if she finds things comfortable. I am completely *O.K.* and capable of running the house. Keep her off the expense of the servant question and try to get her on more healthy subjects—your health, your over work, etc, etc!![3]

Lots of love Most affectionately,

GCM

GCMRL/© Marshall-Winn Collection (Katherine Marshall); H

1. Marshall had written to his stepdaughter on June 24 after receiving a letter describing her vacation "cottage and surrounding" at a Pennsylvania lake near Binghamton, New York, which he thought "sounded a little grim." Marshall offered that "If it is too much so and you can locate a more pleasurable place in that region take it and I will quietly but gladly meet the expense." He also suggested to his wife that she join the family if Molly Winn "could find a hotel or some one with a comfortable room and breakfast" in the vicinity. Katherine Marshall "said immediately she would love to." (Marshall to Winn, June 24, 1954, GCMRL/© Marshall-Winn Collection [Katherine Marshall]; H; Marshall to Carter, August 24, 1954, GCMRL/Verifax 2037 [Marshall Papers Research File]; H.)

2. Marshall probably is referring to Sergeant William J. Heffner, his orderly, who would drive Katherine Marshall to her destination.

3. "I am so delighted that your Mother seems highly pleased with her vacation," Marshall wrote to Molly Winn on July 19. "You have evidently been extremely thoughtful and she has thoroughly enjoyed herself." (Marshall to Winn, July 19, 1954, GCMRL/© Marshall-Winn Collection [Katherine Marshall].)

508

To Harry B. Price August ?, 1954
Leesburg, Virginia

My dear Price: I have received your manuscript and your letter of August 11. I will look over the former as soon as possible.[1]

After you return from your rest-up, you can take up with Colonel George, my Aide at the Pentagon, the question of an appointment to see me. I seldom go to town, so it will probably have to be at Leesburg.[2] Faithfully yours,

GCMRL/G. C. Marshall Papers (Retirement, General)

1. See p. 752n4. "Since the two very illuminating and helpful talks with you in October 1952 and February 1953, I have completed, in manuscript form, the compressed history and evaluation of ECA and the Marshall Plan operation," Price had written. "I promised that this study would be sent to you in manuscript form for your critical review. If you can take the time to read it, or at least those parts which are of the most interest to you, I shall be most grateful." (Price to Marshall, August 11, 1954, GCMRL/G. C. Marshall Papers [Retirement, General].) On August 24, Marshall drafted a telephone message for

C. J. George to convey to Price: "I am mailing you at General Marshall's direction his comments on the MS on the history of the ECA and the Marshall Plan. He wished me to say that he thought the job had been fairly, clearly and beautifully done. He will probably not be in town for some weeks." (Marshall to George, August 24, 1954, ibid.) Marshall's handwritten comments on the manuscript were:

"Page 2: 'Chief advisor' should read 'advisors' were [then Republican Party Representative] John Foster Dulles, [counselor for the State Department] Benjamin Cohen and [US] Ambassador [to the Soviet Union] W. Bedell Smith." (They ranked about equally in their assistance to me.)

"Pages 3 to 7: Somewhere here I think the factor of possible political reactions that bore on the decisions as to the form of the statement should be referred to. The American people and Congress were aggressively soured on further contributions of money to foreign nations. Reports of mal-administration of generous funds appropriated at the end of the war were rife. The feeling seemed to be that any new proposal for more funds to be appropriated would be ruthlessly repulsed. Therefore, the manner of statement, the first approach, and similar factors had to be most seriously considered. It is easy to propose a great plan, but exceedingly difficult to manage the form and procedure so that it has a fair chance of political survival.

"Page 54: The task of preparing the first draft for a public statement was assigned both to Bohlen and Kennan—to work entirely separately and bring their drafts to me. I meanwhile prepared a draft and, when I had all three, I, in effect, merged them to form the first basis in form of the final draft. [See *Papers of GCM*, 6: 147–50.]

"Page 503: Reference should be made to the strong desire of the principal American representatives then in Europe and England to be permitted to meet the requests of Franks Allied Committee to be given some idea of what our government expected or would possibly approve, and to the fact that I gave positive orders that this should not be done. The first move must be on purely European-English initiation." (Ibid.)

2. "After taking a short vacation," Price explained, "I plan to plunge into the work of revision." (Price to Marshall, August 11, 1954, ibid.) "I appreciate greatly the telephone message and memorandum from you which awaited me on my return from vacation," Price wrote on September 20. (Price to Marshall, September 20, 1954, ibid.) A September 27 note in the file indicates that Price was scheduled to meet with Marshall in Leesburg on October 12 at 11:00 a.m.

"During the past two years, I have had considerable correspondence and discussion with Mr. Harry B. Price," Marshall wrote the following January to a PhD candidate at Tufts' Fletcher School of Law and Diplomacy in Medford, Massachusetts, who had written to Marshall to clarify questions relating to Will Clayton's participation in the development of the Marshall Plan. Marshall emphasized that Price had "gone into the subject very thoroughly." (Pritchard to Marshall, December 12, 1954, and Marshall to Pritchard, January 11, 1955, ibid.) Price's book, *The Marshall Plan and Its Meaning*, was published by Cornell University Press in 1955. See pp. 888–89.

While in Pinehurst on March 27, 1955, Marshall met with Captain George S. Webb, whose master's thesis on the Marshall Plan and Congress had been accepted by Tulane University in December 1953. (Webb to Marshall, March 28, 1955, ibid.) Webb later sent Marshall a carbon copy of his thesis, and Marshall replied on June 16 that Webb had "done a splendid job, and I was much interested to be reminded of various factors and issues that I had forgotten. My only adverse comment" regarding "origin of the Plan" was the emphasis Webb placed on "the statements of a member of the House of Representatives in political discussions. Those points were not concerned at all. As a matter of fact, the deplorable financial situation of England was not a first consideration at all. I conceived the necessity from the viewpoint of the hearts and stomachs of the people of France, Germany and Italy. Those in Holland and Belgium and the Norwegian States were in similar trouble. England was in a great plight. But it was the first—the peoples of the countries I mentioned—that I found being forced into a chaotic, terrible situation." He asked Webb not to quote this response. (Marshall to Webb, June 16, 1955, ibid.)

"THINGS GO ON HERE about the same," Marshall wrote to Marshall Carter on August 24. "I have been going very slowly to recoup from the damage done my heart or circulation by this persistent virus-flu. They tell me I look better than I have for years but I am still very careful." (Marshall to Carter, August 24, 1954, GCMRL/Verifax 2037 [Marshall Papers Research File]; H.)

"Katherine has been much troubled with her left eye, seemingly the returning result of her attack of shingles," Marshall disclosed to Madge and John Pendleton on September 10. (See pp. 42, 62–63, 150.) They had gone to Walter Reed the previous Tuesday for treatment of her eye and his "usual heart examination," as well as dental work, and they would do so again later in September. See next document. (Marshall to Pendletons, September 10, 1954, GCMRL/Xerox 2237 [GCM Family, Personal Letters]; H.)

Gardening remained a favorite pastime. Marshall boasted to the Pendletons that at Dodona Manor they had enjoyed a bountiful "crop of fruit—pears, peaches, tomatoes, and apples, all for the first time." (Ibid.) He told Molly Winn on September 8 that he and Sergeant Heffner had been fertilizing and pruning the fruit trees. (Marshall to Winn, September 8, 1954, GCMRL/© Marshall-Winn Collection [Katherine Marshall]; H.) Winn and her family had spent three weeks with the Marshalls in Leesburg on their way back from their Pennsylvania vacation. See pp. 848–49. "Her three children left their trade marks with us!" he confessed to Robert Lovett on September 12. (Marshall to Lovett, September 12, 1954, Yale/Robert A. Lovett Papers [Box 20, Folder 267]; H.)

Despite his hesitation to travel, Marshall accepted David Rockefeller's invitation to attend the early October installation of John J. McCloy to succeed Marshall as chairman of the board at International House in New York. (Rockefeller to Marshall, June 25, 1954, and Marshall to Rockefeller, June 30, 1954, GCMRL/G. C. Marshall Papers [Retirement, General].) See pp. 145–46. Marshall had known McCloy well during World War II, when he served as assistant secretary of war; he had been chairman of the Chase Manhattan Bank and a trustee of the Rockefeller Foundation since 1953, and in 1954 he became chairman of the Council on Foreign Relations. While in New York, Marshall noted, he would "try to manage as many affairs as have been long waiting for me" there. (Ibid.) Marshall acknowledged to Marshall Carter and Rose Page Wilson that he and his wife were looking forward to their trip, where they would see Bernard Baruch, Margaret Emerson, and Madame Chiang Kai-shek, as well as the David Rockefellers. (Marshall to Carter, August 24, 1954, GCMRL/Verifax 2037 [Marshall Papers Research File]; Marshall to Pendletons, September 10, 1954, GCMRL/Xerox 2237 [GCM Family, Personal Letters]; Marshall to Wilson, September 3, 1954, GCMRL/J. Page Wilson Collection; and Marshall to McCarthy, October 3, 1954, GCMRL/Frank McCarthy Papers [Additions, Box 1]; all H.) Part of the time they planned to stay with the Bruces on Long Island (see next document). "I have arranged for an excellent plane to bring you up from Leesburg or Washington to LaGuardia," James Bruce had written to Marshall on August 26. (Bruce to Marshall, August 26, 1954, GCMRL/G. C. Marshall Papers [Retirement, General].)

"We will do a little quiet fishing," he promised, "and I hope very much that we will be able to get in a pheasant or duck drive. However, in any case, whatever we do won't be any rougher than walking on your lawn at Leesburg." (Ibid.) While there, the Marshalls also visited with Adele and Robert Lovett at their home in Locust Valley on Long Island. "General Marshall seemed to be in fine form, looked tanned and well, and had brought his blood pressure down from over 200 to 150 on the high side," Robert Lovett wrote to Marshall Carter on October 22. "He has succeeded in keeping his weight down, and is in better shape than I've seen him for a long time," (Lovett to Carter, October 22, 1954, GCMRL/Marshall S. Carter Papers [Selected Correspondence].) ★

509

To Frank McCarthy | September 9, 1954
Leesburg, Virginia

Dear Frank: Your long and intensely interesting letter from your resort came this morning.[1] I had previously read your letter to Katherine with its copy of your telegram to the President.[2] First, as to the latter.

I think your telegram was entirely responsible for his statement to the Press. You had stated your proposal in such a manner that a frank response was mandatory, either as actually occurred or by way of refusal. So I'm very appreciative.[3] Of course the break down of McCarthy propitiation loosened up matters as has been evidenced by a number of things. For instance, at the dinner to Churchill and Eden I was placed ahead of all the cabinet except Dulles and the Vice President, and after his toast to Churchill the President toasted me.[4] It's funny and I hold no hard feelings but I think my old assistant on the Hill, General Persons was largely responsible for persuading the president to placate McCarthy.[5] That proved a failure and another course became necessary. The rub of course was that the President could or would ~~loose~~ lose the Senate by [Senator Joseph R.] McCarthy and [Senator William] Jenner out, along with [Senator Robert] Taft to be considered. It's all tough and dirty business.[6]

Another thing. Your fruit of the month has been a long series of delicious or delightful surprises. We are very grateful to you for remembering us so generously.[7] Incidentally, I am still on special occasions drinking your fine whiskey.

Your house plans seem very attractive. I would like to loaf there a few weeks and watch, from a distance, you move through Hollywood's elite set.[8]

We are both well, with reservations. Katherine still has to be careful of her lame back she got when our setter pushed her over a cornice. But the remains of her shingles in the eyes still returns to bother her. Right now she is under treatment as she cannot read and has had headaches. We went together to the Walter Reed Tuesday (first time in town for me in three months) she for her eyes and three fillings and I went for a heart examination and three fillings. We go back the 26th for two days, my semi-annual (10 months this time) physical check up before going south Oct. 15th and K. for further eye treatments.[9]

My case is the result of the virus-flu that hung on for so many months. It sent my blood pressure up to 250, but it is now down to 190-100. Strange to say everyone tells me that I look better than I have for years. Maybe it's the lazy life I lead. But I think I am gradually getting back what I lost by virus-flu disruption.

As you can surmise, we lead a very quiet life. The requests for speaking engagements, statements, etc., pour in but are all declined. The trouble is we can't suppress the telephone requests. And of course the mail and telegrams mount up to fantastic levels over each thing that happens to me in the public eye.[10] George, however, and an excellent secretary handle that very effectively.

You must arrange to really stop over with us whenever you can here or at Pinehurst. We would *literally* love to have you.

We plan to go to N.Y. on Oct. 5, me for Jack McCloy's induction into my old job as President of the International House (I am chairman of the Board, a purely honorary post they put up when I resigned.) I am staying with the David Rockefellers, and K. goes to the Jim Bruce's where I will follow.[11] Then we do five days of seeing friends informally, theaters, etc. My first trip in a long time.

With much love, Affectionately,

GCM

GCMRL/Frank McCarthy Papers (Additions, Box 1); H

1. McCarthy had written to the Marshalls from Rancho Yucca Loma in Victorville, California. (McCarthy to Marshall, September 6, 1954, GCMRL/Frank McCarthy Papers [Additions, Box 1].)

2. On August 5, McCarthy had written to Katherine Marshall because "I know how sensitive General Marshall is to the activities of his friends, so I am sending these messages directly to you with the suggestion that you show them to General Marshall only if you think he would like to see them." (McCarthy to Katherine Marshall, August 5, 1954, ibid.) McCarthy enclosed copies of several telegrams, including one he had sent to President Eisenhower on August 3. "Perhaps no two men in the United States have a more thorough first hand knowledge of General Marshall's selfless contribution to the welfare of the United States than you and I," he had wired the president. "Being proud to share the admiration the gratitude and the affection which I know you feel for this great man I hope you will find it possible through the medium of your press conference tomorrow to strike down and label as false the slanderous attacks leveled against him by Senator McCarthy and Mr. Woodring. In the fourteen years I have known General and Mrs. Marshall they have never asked nor wanted anything but the peaceful and unmolested retirement they deserve. Only through the full application of your unprecedented personal prestige and popularity can we be sure of giving it to them." (Ibid.) See pp. 555–56.

Eisenhower had previously defended Marshall against Senator McCarthy's attacks, but his failure to do so in an October 2, 1952, speech in Milwaukee, Wisconsin, had led to sharp criticism of the then presidential candidate. (See p. 721n2; *Papers of DDE*, 13: 1328–29, 1336–37, 1367–74, and 1421–22). After the 1952 election, the Wisconsin senator had continued his attacks on Marshall. Frank McCarthy's August 3, 1954, request that Eisenhower publicly defend Marshall at his press conference stemmed from the senator's most recent attack on August 2 during which, the *New York Times* reported, he had inserted into the *Congressional Record* a letter from former Secretary of War Harry H. Woodring asserting that Marshall "'would sell out his grandmother for personal advantage; that he would sell his policies, beliefs and standards to maintain his political and military position with the powers that so be.'" ("M'Carthy Quotes Marshall Critic," *New York Times*, August 3, 1954, p. 12.) On the same day, August 2, the Senate sent to a select bipartisan committee a resolution censuring McCarthy that Senator Ralph Flanders (R-VT) had introduced on

July 30.

3. "'[T]here are some things that cause me to be almost emotional,'" the *New York Times* reported that Eisenhower began during an August 4 news conference in response to a question asking for his opinion of the Woodring attack on Marshall. He went on to say that Marshall "'typified all that we call—or that we look for—in what we call an American patriot. I saw many things he did that were proof, to me at least, of his selflessness,'" and cited in this regard Marshall's refusal to let President Roosevelt know how much he wanted a field command during World War II because "'I am here to serve, and not to satisfy personal ambition.'" ("President's Comment on Marshall," *New York Times*, August 5, 1954, p. 6.) "'Now, later on, of course, after the war was over, he went to a different post. What the circumstances were of that post, I know nothing. What were his judgments, what were the things that could have been done that were not done, or should not have been done, I don't know,'" Eisenhower stated. "'But I do know that General Marshall served according to his conceptions of his duty to his chief.'" (Ibid.) "'If you go back through his record, you will find that it was a brilliant record, always serving to the best of his ability,'" the president continued. "'I think it is a sorry reward, at the end of at least fifty years of service to this country to say that he is not a loyal, fine American, and that he served only in order to advance his own ambitions. I can't imagine anyone I have known in my career of whom this is less so than it is in his case. I am sorry if I have made a speech,'" he concluded, "'but that is the way I feel.'" (Ibid.)

The same day Eisenhower had wired a response to Frank McCarthy's telegram: "Confidentially I agree. I hope that my press conference today sufficed." (Eisenhower to McCarthy, August 4, 1954, GCMRL/Frank McCarthy Papers [Additions, Box 1].) McCarthy wired back, "Magnificent is the only word I have for your press conference today. Unfortunately the term is not strong enough to express the full extent of my sentiment and my admiration for what you said and the way you said it." (McCarthy to Eisenhower, telegram, August 4, 1954, ibid.)

"The effect of the President's comment has been electric," McCarthy had written to Katherine Marshall on August 5. "It has provided a stimulus and an occasion for a great many people to express themselves on a subject which has been in their minds and in their hearts for a long time. Every paper in Los Angeles—even the Hearst papers, which are violently pro-McCarthy—ran the story on the first page and carried the President's remarks in full." (Ibid.)

Publicly Marshall refused to comment on the Woodring letter or Eisenhower's comments ("Marshall Has No Comment," *New York Times*, August 4, 1954, p. 6), but in her August 7 reply, Katherine Marshall noted that when she showed McCarthy's August 5 letter to Marshall, "He said—Frank is a 'straight shooter'—There was no way of getting around that wire—No way to hedge—It did the trick. Wires, letters, phone calls are coming in from all over the country. The sheep are following their leader." (Katherine Marshall to McCarthy, August 7, 1954, GCMRL/Frank McCarthy Papers [Additions, Box 1].) "How we wish the credit for this could be given to the one who deserves it," Mrs. Marshall wrote again to McCarthy the next day. "What a service you have done not only for G. but even more for '*The President*.' You gave him the time & place and he grabbed at it. How I wish I could have a talk with you. We are growing old, Frank. Do come and see us as soon and when you can. You have shown great vision. G. is proud of you as always." (Katherine Marshall to McCarthy, August 8, 1954, ibid.; H) See p. 861.

4. See p. 842n3.

5. Brigadier General Wilton B. Persons was head of the Legislative and Liaison Division of the General Staff during World War II. He retired in 1949 with the rank of major general but was recalled as a special assistant to General Eisenhower at SHAPE from 1951 to 1952. He had been a special assistant to the president since 1953.

6. Mid-term congressional elections were scheduled for November 2, 1954.

7. McCarthy's Christmas gift for 1953 had been a membership in the Fruit of the Month Club. (McCarthy to Marshalls, May 22, 1954, ibid.)

8. McCarthy had confided that he had abandoned his "effort to buy a house because I couldn't find anything suitable." Instead, he "paid too much for a beautiful, although

small, lot way up in the Beverly Hills with a spectacular view," and mentioned that his new neighbors would include Hollywood executives and movie stars. (McCarthy to Marshall, September 6, 1954, ibid.)

9. See previous editorial note.

10. "From North, South, East & West the mail is huge & editorials most interesting," Katherine Marshall had told McCarthy on August 8. "We have been deluged with calls & wires & flowers, also clippings." (Katherine Marshall to McCarthy, August 8, 1954, ibid.; H.)

11. See previous editorial note.

510

TO BERNARD M. BARUCH

September 27, 1954
Leesburg, Virginia

Dear Baruch: On September 25, I spent several hours with a Mr. Kerr, who is *the* specialist in amputee training. He had with him a seemingly well-to-do, retired friend, Paul Earl Patersell.[1] To put it exceedingly briefly, he wants help to this end:

He states that surgeons and allied authorities fail to realize that amputees whose legs are off above the knee joint can quickly be trained to activities normal to men in general. Both he and his friend have lost both legs above the knee. He shoots golf in the eighties, played baseball, won lightweight amateur boxing championship, etc., etc.

He trained Lady Halifax's son to walk in five days and he pursues a normal life now.[2]

Kerr met you once when you were watching a demonstration. He tells me the military do a fair job at this business of rehabilitation. He acts, at times, as a supervisor for them. He was employed by Ross McIntyre and the Army Surgeon General during the war years.[3]

He tells me the problem is not directly related to military amputees, and they only constitute a very small percentage of the whole—I think five percent. The larger trouble is among those over fifty-five years—and there are fifteen to twenty thousand of these annually—who feel that the best they can possibly hope for is a slow, short walk with one or two canes. Worse still, according to Kerr, the doctors feel the same way about it. He wants to change their attitude. In effect, it is a matter of rehabilitation. That is why I thought of you.[4] He apparently does not want money. He wants recognition of the possibilities toward leading a normal life. What he needs is expert advice as to how to go about establishing the proven fact that a double amputee, above the knees, has not lost the possibility of living the life of a normal being.

Kerr talks to the convention of the American Medical Association in Atlantic City in November. Unfortunately, he talks last, and he is so absorbed in his subject and experiences that he over-plays and confuses his presentations.

If you are interested in this phase of rehabilitation and would care to see him, his address is:

Charles Macdonald Kerr[5]
Executive Director
The Institute for Amputee Rehabilitation
41 Union Street
Lodi, New Jersey[6]

Katherine and I go up to New York on October 5 and return home on the 9th. She stays with the Jim Bruces. I spend my first night with the David Rockefellers (attending a meeting of the International House Board to install Jack McCloy as President), and then go to the Bruces.[7] I will see you. Faithfully yours,

GCMRL/G. C. Marshall Papers (Retirement, General)

1. The mother of Donald Kerr, executive director of the National Institute for Amputee Rehabilitation in Lodi, New Jersey, had written to Marshall on August 27 informing him that she was a distant relative and requested that he meet with her son. C. J. George replied to her that Marshall "seldom sees anyone except intimate friends at Leesburg; otherwise, he would have no privacy whatever there, but, as he will probably not be at the office any weekend before he leaves for North Carolina, he is willing to arrange for a visit with your son." (George to Mrs. Charles M. Kerr, September 8, 1954, GCMRL/G. C. Marshall Papers [Retirement, General].) Paul E. Patersell was treasurer of the National Institute for Amputee Rehabilitation.

2. Richard Frederick Wood (later Baron Holderness) lost both legs during World War II while serving in the King's Royal Rifle Corps. He was the youngest son of E. F. L. Wood, First Earl of Halifax, who was British ambassador to the United States between 1940 and 1946, and Lady Dorothy Evelyn Augusta Onlsow.

3. Vice Admiral Ross T. McIntire, MD, was surgeon general of the US Navy and President Franklin Roosevelt's personal physician. Army surgeons general during World War II were Major General James C. Magee (June 1, 1939, to May 31, 1943) and Major General Norman T. Kirk (June 1, 1943, to May 31, 1947).

4. Baruch helped establish the New York University Bellevue Medical Center Institution of Rehabilitation and Physical Medicine in 1950. (Margaret L. Coit, *Mr. Baruch* [Boston: Houghton Mifflin Company], 661.)

5. Charles Macdonald Kerr III was known professionally as Donald Kerr.

6. Baruch responded that he would "make some inquiries" among his "people" before contacting Kerr. (Baruch to Marshall, September 30, 1954, GCMRL/G. C. Marshall Papers [Retirement, General].)

Kerr thanked Marshall on October 13 for his helpful suggestions "to reorganize my thinking in this work" and revised his "talks to rehabilitation groups" accordingly. Kerr also asked Marshall for a statement from Marshall or Baruch for the cover of "a comprehensive manual concerning rehabilitation of the amputee" that he and a colleague had just completed. (Kerr to Marshall, October 13, 1954, ibid.) Marshall replied that he thought "it would be much more appropriate for Mr. Baruch to do so because of his strong interest and experience in this field" and suggested that Kerr mail a draft to Baruch. (Marshall to Kerr, November 2, 1954, ibid.)

7. See pp. 851–52.

511

To the First Twelve Marshall Scholars[1] — October 5, 1954
[Leesburg, Virginia]

This note carries my greetings and best wishes to the first group holding Marshall Scholarships to arrive in the United Kingdom. I congratulate the members of the group on winning this great opportunity, and I express again my deep appreciation of the action of the British authorities in making it possible.

A close accord between our two countries is essential to the good of mankind in this turbulent world of today, and that is not possible without an intimate understanding of each other.

These scholarships point the way to the continuation and growth of the understanding which found its necessity in the terrible struggle of the war years.

GCMarshall

GCMRL/G. C. Marshall Papers (Retirement, General)

1. The Marshall Aid Commemoration Act, which had been introduced in Parliament by Sir Roger Makins, had become law on July 30, 1953. This act funded twelve annual Marshall Scholarships for Americans to study at British universities. By the time of the act's implementation, Makins was the British ambassador in Washington, where he was responsible for organizing the Marshall Scholarships program. Marshall remained strictly neutral in the selection of the scholarship recipients, clarifying to the VMI superintendent that he "had a very frank understanding with the British Ambassador that I would stand clear of any personal action in these matters." (Marshall to Milton, October 27, 1953, GCMRL/G. C. Marshall Papers [Retirement, General].)

Chargé d'Affaires at the US embassy in London W. Walton Butterworth had written to Marshall on September 15 that "The first twelve Marshall Scholars in this program are arriving in the United Kingdom next month from the United States. Anthony Eden is giving a reception for them on October 5 and has asked Ambassador Aldrich to extend a word of welcome to them." He explained that "the Foreign Office has suggested that it would be most appropriate if he could read a message from you." (Butterworth to Marshall, September 15, 1954, GCMRL/G. C. Marshall Papers [Retirement, General].) With his letter, Butterworth had sent a draft version composed by Brad Connors, the embassy public affairs officer. "I was pleased to receive your letter, whatever the reason for it," Marshall responded on September 25, when he sent Butterworth this salutation for the first Marshall scholars. (Marshall to Butterworth, September 25, 1954, ibid.) "I am glad to draft a message for the scholarship welcome. Tell Brad Connors that I know his was better, but it had too polished and diplomatic a touch to reveal me." (Ibid.)

"WE LEAVE HERE Saturday afternoon for Pinehurst and six months residence," Marshall disclosed to Admiral Richard E. Byrd on October 15. "I will do little or nothing, as I find rest and leisurely movement conducive to good health. My virus has finally disappeared, but Mrs. Marshall is still troubled with her right eye and right arm." He added that he expected "to see some good golf in the months to come and will probably do some riding. Beyond that, only frequent occupancy of a chaise lounge and a book." (Marshall to Byrd, October 15, 1954, OSU/Papers of Admiral Richard E. Byrd [Byrd Personal Papers, Sub-Series 3, Marshall, Folder 2206].) See photo #22.

Marshall found himself with surprising new responsibilities for the winter of 1954–55. When Molly Winn and her daughters went to live in Japan while Colonel Winn was stationed in Korea, the Marshalls took charge of James Winn Jr., who stayed behind for orthodontic adjustments to his teeth. An addition to Liscombe Lodge's glassed-in porch was built "to accommodate Jimmy, who for the time being occupies the guest room," Marshall explained to Madge Pendleton on October 31, the day the Winns departed. (Marshall to Pendleton, October 31, 1954, GCMRL/G. C. Marshall Papers [Retirement, General]; Marshall to McCarthy, April 6, 1955, GCMRL/Frank McCarthy Papers [Additions, Box 1]; H.) See pp. 864 and 866.

Improvements to Marshall's health continued. "Colonel George has phoned me several times stating that you desired a note from me to have with you during the winter at Pinehurst," Colonel Thomas W. Mattingly, chief of cardiology at Walter Reed Army Hospital, had written to Marshall on October 21. (Mattingly to Marshall, October 21, 1954, GCMRL/G. C. Marshall Papers [Retirement, General].) "When you were seen on 7 September 1954, and again during the latter part of September, I considered your condition to have improved over that of last spring. You have maintained your weight in the 180's and the edema of your legs was absent on the last examination. On 7 September your blood pressure was 190/100, and during the time you were quietly in bed in the hospital, it was as low as 150/100. . . . Your lungs were clearer than I have seen them for a year. Although you still have atrial fibrillation, your pulse rate has remained slow. . . . Your kidney function continues to be adequate." (Ibid.) Mattingly recommended that Marshall "maintain your low sodium diet" and "increase your physical activity during the fall when the weather is cooler, walking a longer distance in the morning and evening, and perhaps taking short horseback rides." The doctor "strongly recommended" that Marshall "make arrangements for a periodic follow-up by a physician in or near Pinehurst while you are away from the Washington-Virginia area." (Ibid.)

"I am at last over ten months of virus-flu," Marshall wrote to Frank Pace Jr. on November 15. "They tell me I look better than for years—a profit I suppose for breaking all records at being lazy. But I have to go slowly until my heart fully recovers, which it apparently has done." (Marshall to Pace, November 15, 1954, ibid.) ★

512

To Dwight D. Eisenhower — October 30, 1954
Pinehurst, North Carolina

Dear Mr. President: I appreciated very much your note regarding Eden. He was more than gracious in his reference to me.[1]

I also greatly appreciated your generous defense of me reference Woodring's indictment.[2] The winds blow pro and con with remarkable contrasts. The latter have not yet invaded my privacy down here. Faithfully yours,

GCMarshall

DDEL/Dwight D. Eisenhower Papers (Records as President, President's Personal File 182, Box 935); H

1. "I have just heard of the splendid tribute paid you by Sir Anthony Eden on a television program last evening," Eisenhower had written, referring to the British foreign secretary's appearance on Edward R. Murrow's *See It Now* on October 26. "Certainly it is a

heartwarming indication of the high esteem in which you are held by the British people." (Eisenhower to Marshall, October 27, 1954, GCMRL/G. C. Marshall Papers [Retirement, General].)

Murrow had alerted Marshall about the program, wiring that "Anthony Eden is saying a few words about you and which I think you will not find displeasing." (Murrow to Marshall, telegram, October 26, 1954, ibid.) On the program, Howard K. Smith asked Eden, "who is the most impressive figure you've met during your career?" (Murrow, *See It Now*, 197.) "Your General George Marshall," Eden replied. "I remember in war how it was he, after all, who chose General Eisenhower, as he then was, for the command on which so much depended, and so many times in our strategy, he gave wise guidance and advice. And then, since the war, Marshall aid was what saved Western Europe." (Ibid.) "I remember Mr. Churchill . . . asking me what I thought of Marshall . . . I said I thought he was like a modern edition of Robert E. Lee. I still think that's not very wide of the mark." (Ibid.)

2. See pp. 555–56 and 852–55.

513

DRAFT OF LETTER TO CONSTANTINE BROWN[1]

November 17, 1954
Pinehurst, North Carolina

My dear Brown: I have just read the attached extract from an article by you in a local North Carolina paper. I recall that a somewhat similar statement was made by you several years ago.[2]

The facts, so far as they concern me were these: In June 1946, General Eisenhower, then Chief of Staff of our Army, arrived in Nanking, China, on a general inspection tour of Army troops. He brought me an oral message from President Truman asking me to accept the appointment as Secretary of State on July 1, next. As I understood it, the message was handled orally in order that no one other than General Eisenhower and I would have any knowledge of the matter.[3]

I asked General Eisenhower to inform the President that I could not accept on the basis of a July 1 appointment, as I was involved in critical negotiations and that, if they were brought to a successful conclusion (they were not), it would be late September at the earliest before I could properly leave China. If the President still desired to go ahead with the matter for an appointment as of July 1, I suggested that he nominate me on that date, get my nomination confirmed by the Senate, and then I would not accept until late September. Otherwise, I must respectfully decline.

I personally arranged a four-word code with General Eisenhower to be utilized in informing me of the President's decision. The code word came back indicating that my proposal for September was accepted. My recollection of this code transmission is a little vague, though I know the President did not press me to accept the appointment for July 1.

Nothing further happened, and I was not nominated. I made no inquiries and, as the Fall of the year came without action, I assumed that the matter had been dropped.

In late December, when I proposed my recall from China, a message came from the State Department, I think, that the President approved my return, and it stated that he considered it important for me to be in Washington January 10. I cabled the President that it would be extremely difficult for me to reach Washington by January 10 and, besides, I had a severe cold; further, if he desired to discuss the same matter as in the last June, that my attitude remained unchanged.[4]

I received authority to come home at a later date and arrived in Washington January 21, 1947, and was immediately sworn in as Secretary of State that morning.

I received no written or cabled mention of my possible appointment as Secretary of State until January 1947. The first mention was by word of mouth in June 1946.

I would prefer to have this treated off the record as merely between us. I only send you this communication in the hope that you will refrain from any further reference to the matter of the circumstances of my appointment. Faithfully yours,

GCMRL/G. C. Marshall Papers (Retirement, General)

1. American journalist Constantine Brown had covered World War I for the *London Times* and was foreign affairs editor for the *Washington Evening Star* before he began, in 1942, to write a column syndicated by the Bell-McClure organization. Marshall sent this handwritten letter, marked draft, to C. J. George to have typed and read to Lovett for his reaction. The editors have been unable to determine if the letter was ever sent.

2. Marshall enclosed part of Brown's November 15, 1954, column in which Brown asserted that "on March 5, 1946, this writer found out that President Truman had cabled General George C. Marshall, who at that time was on a special mission in China, offering him the position of Secretary of State then held by James Byrnes. The reliability of the information's source was such that this reporter wrote the story without any ifs or buts. An avalanche of denials landed on his shoulders. President Truman, who was on a trip to Missouri, denied it to the White House reporters on his train. On his return to Washington he issued an even more vehement denial at his press conference. Secretary Byrnes also issued a strong denial—and justly so, since he did not yet suspect he was being eased out." (Constantine Brown, ". . . Trivial Remark Grew," unknown newspaper, November 15, 1954.) See pp. 840n11.

3. Eisenhower's role in communications between Truman and Marshall is explained in *Papers of GCM*, 5: 546–47.

4. This top secret radio communication with Marshall S. Carter occurred on January 4, 1947, when Marshall explained from Nanking, China, that to arrive in Washington by January 10 would "impose too much of fatigue for my years." See *Papers of GCM*, 5: 768–69.

514

To Dwight D. Eisenhower

December 8, 1954
Washington, DC

Dear Mr. President: I arrived in Washington just prior to noon today to attend the Business Advisory Council meetings, a meeting of the American Battle Monuments Commission tomorrow, and the AMVETS banquet on Friday evening.[1] I will be on my way back to Pinehurst on Saturday morning.

North came over to brief me on the agenda for tomorrow's meeting and brought up the fact that Governor Foss of North Dakota submitted his resignation as a member of the Commission.[2] During the discussion, North mentioned the hope that someone with a broad background in public relations would be a welcome member of the Commission. The name of Ben McKelway, Editor of the Evening Star, was mentioned. I pass this along for your information.[3]

While I have no complaints on the state of my health, Mrs. Marshall has been experiencing great difficulty in the past several months with a case of shingles in the right eye and right arm. This has been a very painful experience for her, but, in recent days, she has shown progress, although it is very slow.

With warmest regards to Mrs. Eisenhower and you, and with great respect, Faithfully yours,

GCMRL/G. C. Marshall Papers (American Battle Monuments Commission)

1. Marshall had accepted Ridgway's invitation to stay at Fort Myer while attending these events in Washington. (Ridgway to Marshall, November 29, 1954, and Marshall to Ridgway, November 30, 1954, USAMHI/Matthew B. Ridgway Papers [Marshall].) AMVETS National Commander Rufus H. Wilson, who received a Purple Heart for injuries sustained in the Battle of Saipan during World War II, had written to Marshall on November 5 to inform him that the organization would present him with an award at its tenth anniversary celebration. (Wilson to Marshall, November 5, 1954, GCMRL/G. C. Marshall Papers [Retirement, General].) Presidents Eisenhower and Truman sent letters of congratulation to Marshall at the December 10 AMVETS banquet, where Foreign Operations Administrator Harold E. Stassen was the principal speaker. "With tears in his eyes," Marshall "gave a ten-minute off-the-cuff address during which he appealed to all Americans to do everything possible to maintain the morale of service men overseas." ("Marshall Lauded for Service to U.S.," *New York Times*, December 11, 1954, p. 7.) "I am just as sorry as I can be that I can't be with you for the honor you are paying General Marshall," Truman had written to Wilson. "I think as highly of General Marshall as one man can think of another. He was the great man of the Second World War; he was a great Secretary of State; he was a great Secretary of Defense, and was one of the greatest Ambassadors that I had in my Presidential family." (Ibid.) Marshall wrote to thank Truman on December 18 and admitted that he was embarrassed that Truman had been "put on the spot as it were by those officials. However that may be, you did me great honor." (Marshall to Truman, December 18, 1954, GCMRL/G. C. Marshall Collection [Truman].)

On February 15, 1955, Marshall wrote to Secretary of Commerce Sinclair Weeks to acknowledge Marshall's new status as "a Graduate Member" of the Business Advisory Council, which required him "to attend but one meeting a year to keep me in good standing." (Marshall to Weeks, February 15, 1955, GCMRL/G. C. Marshall Papers [Retirement, Chronological].)

2. Former marine "flying ace" and Medal of Honor winner Joseph J. Foss had resigned from the American Battle Monuments Commission to become governor of South Dakota on January 4, 1955.

3. In a November 30 memorandum, C. J. George told Marshall that while discussing Governor-elect Foss's resignation with General North, "he invited an opinion from me on a likely successor. I told him that, in view of the fact that he was interested in one who had public relations experience, it might be well to consider Mr. Ben McKelway." (George to Marshall, November 30, 1954, GCMRL/G. C. Marshall Papers [Retirement, Chronological].) See pp. 332–33.

515

TO JOHN C. HAGAN JR.[1]

December 22, 1954
Pinehurst, North Carolina

My Hagan: I appreciate your letter of November 19 advising me that the Department of State, the Department of Defense, and the National Archives will, by Presidential directive, cooperate in providing to The George C. Marshall Research Foundation, Inc., such documentary material relating to my career in public office as may legally be made available. I am glad to learn that the Commonwealth of Virginia will provide land in Lexington for the construction of a building to house the collection of documents.[2]

In accordance with your request, I will turn over to the Foundation those documents in my personal possession which may legally and appropriately be made a part of the collection being assembled by the Foundation.[3] It is my understanding that transfer will not be effected until such time as Federal authorities agree that facilities established by the Foundation are sufficient for safeguarding the documents.[4]

I am honored by the action of the Board of Directors and hope you will let them know my appreciation.[5]

With best regards,[6] Faithfully yours,

GCMRL/G. C. Marshall Papers (Retirement, Chronological)

1. John Campbell Hagan Jr. (VMI, 1921), cofounder and president of a Richmond, Virginia, investment banking firm, was named president of the VMI Board of Visitors in 1953. Marshall had resigned from the Board of Visitors earlier in 1954. (George to Ebeling, December 23, 1954, GCMRL/G. C. Marshall Papers [Retirement, General].)

2. The "Presidential directive" was a memorandum from President Truman dated January 17, 1953, to the secretaries of state and defense and the head of the General Services Administration advising them that "The Board of Visitors of the Virginia Military Institute has arranged for the organization of the George C. Marshall Research Foundation, Inc. [GCMRF], as a non-profit Virginia corporation. The purpose of the Foundation will be to collect and receive papers and records with other historical objects and documents, and to provide a suitable building to house them at VMI. To assist in effectuating this, the General Assembly of Virginia has enacted legislation authorizing VMI to deed land to the Foundation." (Memorandum for the Secretary of State et al., January 17, 1953, GCMRL/Frank McCarthy Papers [Additions, Box 3].) "This building will be a library and museum and will be open to the public," Truman clarified. (Ibid.)

"The establishment of the Foundation has been a matter of great interest to me," Truman continued, "and I have consulted with VMI officials about it over a period of more than a year. In connection with these conferences, I have agreed that the United States Government would in so far as practicable make available to the Foundation documentary material relating to the activities of General Marshall as a soldier, as Secretary of State, and as Secretary of Defense. A committee composed of representatives of the White House, the Departments of State and Defense and the National Archives, has given considerable study to the procedures by which the Government can assist the Foundation in obtaining the documentary material it will want." (Ibid.)

The committee had been established as a result of a meeting on February 19, 1952, during which Truman "left no doubt in our minds that he was determined to have some kind of research foundation established for General Marshall." ("Meeting with President Truman Regarding Establishment of a Foundation for General George C. Marshall," February 19, 1952, NA/RG 59 [Central Decimal File, 114.2/2–1952].) A detailed committee report dated April 1, 1952, identified the location and extent of relevant documents in the files of the Departments of State, Defense, Army, and Navy as well as the National Archives, the Franklin D. Roosevelt Library, and Marshall's Pentagon office. It recommended that as a first step "a program for the selection of pertinent material" be created and that for this purpose a library director be appointed and assured of cooperation by the National Historical Publications Commission. ("George C. Marshall Memorial" and attachment, April 1, 1952, ibid.).

3. Truman related that "The VMI library is equipped to receive and maintain such material on a temporary basis pending construction of the Research Center building." (Memorandum for the Secretary of State et al., January 17, 1953, GCMRL/Frank McCarthy Papers [Additions, Box 3].) "We find that although you have indicated generous cooperation in our talks, we have nothing in writing to supplement these conversations," Hagan had written to Marshall. "We would appreciate it tremendously if you would write a letter to me, as President of the Foundation, stating your intent to give this organization certain papers which you are willing to have included in the collection." (Hagan to Marshall, November 19, 1954, ibid.)

4. "Many of the pertinent Government records will remain classified or will be withheld from the public for a number of years," Truman had explained in his 1953 charge. "I am requesting each of you to bring this memorandum to the attention of your successors in office as a matter of urgency. I feel confident that they will wish to support the efforts that have commenced to provide suitable recognition to one of the greatest Americans of our age." (Memorandum for the Secretary of State et al., January 17, 1953, ibid.) On November 23, Hagan wrote to J. Clifford Miller, president of Miller Manufacturing Company, Incorporated, in Richmond, Virginia, and also a former president of the VMI Board of Visitors who was vice president of the GCMRF board, that he had inquired through Senator Harry Byrd's office about President Eisenhower's feelings concerning Truman's directive. "I have a letter back from Senator Byrd's office stating that General Persons contacted the President and that he was in full agreement with Truman's action concerning the disposition of General Marshall's papers." (Hagan to Miller, November 23, 1954, GCMRL/GCMRF Records [General Correspondence 1951–62].) Hagan also noted that "I have been in touch with Colonel C. J. George, Aide to General Marshall, to enlighten him on various events that have taken place in the Foundation and keep him fully informed." (Ibid.) George had been involved with the foundation since its earliest stages. "The President has asked [White House Press Secretary] Joe Short to organize a small committee to consider the whole matter," Clayton Fritchey wrote to Marshall Carter on February 19, 1952, asking that he attend a meeting in the cabinet room on February 19 at 3:00 p.m. "I think the President and Joe now realize that this undertaking is much more extensive and complicated than they at first realized." (Fritchey to Carter, February 9, 1952, GCMRL/Marshall S. Carter Collection [Department of Defense, Box 14].) Carter responded that his "present activities are such that I would find it impossible to serve on the committee (unless, of course, directed so to do)." Instead, he "strongly" recommended "Maj. C. J. George who has been for the past 5 years and is now Gen. Marshall's alter ego, special assistant, personal assistant, deputy and part-time masseur." (Carter to Fritchey, February 13, 1952, ibid.)

5. The board, which included the superintendent of VMI, had named Frank McCarthy a director at its November 18 meeting in Richmond. "Your close personal relation and friendship with General Marshall, together with your unquestioned competence in the field of public relations will do much to make our plans come to a successful conclusion," General Milton wrote to McCarthy the next day. (Milton to McCarthy, November 19, 1954, GCMRL/Frank McCarthy Papers [Additions, Box 3].) After meeting with Milton and other members of the board, McCarthy and Hagan "put together the necessary papers and framed a letter which we thought General Marshall might write to the Board." McCarthy had planned to deliver these in person to Marshall in Pinehurst but weather conditions made that impossible so, upon returning to California, he sent the documents and draft letter to Marshall. (McCarthy to Milton, November 30, 1954, ibid.)

6. "I am most appreciative of receiving your letter and I am sure that I can speak for the Board of Directors," Hagan responded to Marshall on December 27. "Knowing your feeling in connection with this project, I assure you I will do everything within my ability to proceed with dignity and discrimination, which is characteristic of you," (Hagan to Marshall, December 27, 1954, GCMRL/GCMRF Records [General Correspondence 1951–62].) See pp. 897–99 and 902–3.

516

To Mrs. John B. Wilson

December 22, 1954
Pinehurst, North Carolina

Dear Rose: You beat me to it with your Xmas note. I had your name down on a list on a pad for long hand notes. Our cards go out from Washington. Quite a problem. We only send out 300 now and it used to be 2000. We used to receive about 5000 and now about 1000. So much for statistics!

I was amused at the facial disability of your flock. We have one. Molly's Jimmy is with us for the winter. She is in Tokyo with the two girls. He is 13 and a handful. He has all my early failings.[1]

Katherine has had Shingles in her right eye, arm and hand for nine weeks. Extremely painful. I'm so sorry to read what you said about Tom Morgan's health. He is a very likable and fine fellow. Glad John is so outstanding. He was my bet from the start.[2] With my love and deep affection,

GCM

GCMRL/J. Page Wilson Collection; H

1. See p. 857. On December 26, Marshall told his childhood friend Catharine Armstrong that he was Jimmy Winn's "coach in English and spelling. Do you remember at Miss Thompson's when you headed the line and I was the anchor man!" (Marshall to Armstrong, December 26, 1954, GCMRL/G. C. Marshall Papers [Retirement, General].) At some military schools, the anchorman refers to the person at the bottom of the class. See pp. 868–69.
2. John and Rose Wilson had married in June 1937.

517

To General Matthew B. Ridgway

January 11, 1955
Pinehurst, North Carolina

Dear Ridgway: At the meeting of the Commission on December 9, 1954, the report on North was discussed in a most comprehensive way.[1] It was finally decided that in all but one of the sustained allegations it was not necessarily the fault of the individual, but rather personnel and fiscal ceilings, lack of a law to authorize Stateside leave, budgetary restrictions on overtime pay, difficulties in obtaining qualified personnel, and finally that construction and tourist traffic require the maximum of service during the warm season.

The propriety of issuing change of station orders was discussed. This practice will not be repeated.

I am convinced that this unpleasant experience was brought about as a result of gratuitous and factless criticism by disgruntled employees.

It is the opinion of this Commission that North is not to be condemned for his actions, but complimented on an outstanding performance of duty under difficult circumstances.[2]

With warmest regards, Faithfully yours,

GCMRL/G. C. Marshall Papers (American Battle Monuments Commission)

1. On June 23, Ridgway had sent to Marshall "a letter forwarded to me on 19 May 1954 from the Department of the Air Force." Ridgway explained that during the course of an investigation into "alleged irregularity on the part of an Air Force officer on duty with the American Battle Monuments Commission, Paris, France, two persons made allegations pertaining to Brigadier General Thomas North." (Ridgway to Marshall, June 23, 1954, GCMRL/G. C. Marshall Papers [American Battle Monuments Commission].) Marshall replied that the ABMC "does not have an investigative unit, and in order that this matter may be processed expeditiously and thoroughly, I would appreciate your having the Department of the Army initiate an appropriate investigation to determine the validity of the allegations." (Marshall to Ridgway, June 23, 1954, ibid.) On October 22, Ridgway had forwarded the "conclusions approved by the Inspector General" and reminded Marshall that "Department of the Army policy prohibits the transmission of these conclusions outside the Department of the Army." Marshall acknowledged Ridgway's letter on October 27 and thanked him for his "comprehensive report." (Ridgway to Marshall, October 22, and Marshall to Ridgway, October 27, 1954, ibid.)

Marshall met with North on December 8 to discuss the charges. On December 6, George had prepared a memorandum for Marshall detailing "that 5 of the 23 allegations directed against General North were sustained," including exercising "poor judgment in hiring personnel"; applying "unfair leave policies" and overtime policies; not delegating "appropriate authority to his subordinates" and creating "CONFIDENTIAL files that contained instructions and policies contrary to those publicly announced"; and demonstrating favoritism "among officers and civilians." (George to Marshall, memorandum, December 6, 1954, ibid.)

"I think the allegation you should discuss in detail with him is the matter of the permanent change of station orders and the fact that on two occasions he moved his vehicles to Paris and then disposed of them prior to his departure for home," George advised. "While it must be admitted that General North works constantly while in Europe and takes little or no time for recreation, I think this is a question of propriety." (Ibid.) "It is my opinion that General North is in need of a deputy," George continued. "He is almost 61 years of age and I believe that the pressure of work and travel is beginning to show." (Ibid.)

2. North saw a copy of Marshall's January 11 letter to Ridgway and thanked him on March 2 for his confidence and support in light of the investigation. (North to Marshall, March 2, 1955, ibid.) North clarified however that, by his recollection, one element of the investigation, "'the propriety of issuing permanent change of station orders,'" had been "discussed between ourselves, not in the executive session of the Commission." (Ibid.) North added that "the Adjutant General of the Army confirms my understanding that in the Army when an absence of more than five months is contemplated permanent change of station orders are issued—as I issued them. My contemplated absence was for six months." (Ibid.) Marshall wrote "*noted* G.C.M" at the bottom of North's letter.

518

To Queen Frederica of the Hellenes[1] — January 13, 1955, Pinehurst, North Carolina

Your Majesty: I have wanted to send you and The King my very personal Christmas greetings and, especially, I wanted to thank you for the very lovely

Christmas card, but, to put it very frankly, I thought it better to delay until the anti-American disturbance had somewhat subsided. You wrote me the intimate details of the Cyprus situation, so I was not at all surprised by the reaction which followed our United Nations position.[2]

I am well, but poor Mrs. Marshall is having a prolonged struggle with shingles in her right eye, arm and hand—now an affliction of three months duration. She is slowly recovering, but had decided "ups and downs".

Mrs. Marshall's married daughter left for Japan in early November with her two daughters—6 and 11. She left her 13 year old boy with us for the winter, and I am seriously engaged in coaching him in spelling and English. As I am a famous illiterate in spelling, I am "some" teacher, but he is so bad that I am the proverbial "one-eyed man in the Kingdom of the blind".[3]

I was much interested in what you told me of your proposed cruise with the relations you only saw at funerals—and with the resulting magazine and press reports. Apparently it was a great success.[4]

We are at Pinehurst for the winter and early spring. We return to Leesburg May 1st, as usual.

I sincerely trust that your reported operations were successful and not too painful.[5] Please believe that I had you frequently in mind.

Please make my respects to his majesty and believe me with admiration and, I dare say, affectionate regards, Faithfully yours,

GCMRL/G. C. Marshall Papers (Retirement, General); H

1. Marshall's draft letter, printed here, differs slightly from the typed version that was sent to Queen Frederica. In particular, Marshall made a note to secretary Mary Louise Spilman that he wanted to handwrite the salutation and closing paragraph. (Marshall to Frederica, January 13, 1955, GCMRL/G. C. Marshall Papers [Retirement, General].)

2. The CIA had forwarded to Marshall the queen's most recent letter, dated August 19, 1954, which "was received through our channels with the request that it be forwarded to you." (Fuller to Marshall, September 7, 1954, ibid.) In that letter Frederica had described "our own difficulties with our old friend and ally, the English," over Cyprus, which at that time was still a British colony. "The Cyprus question has become very acute," she told Marshall, referring to an independence movement then gaining momentum and recent British blunders as well as "tactless" statements by British Foreign Secretary Anthony Eden the previous year to the Greek prime minister that had become public. As a result, "During this last year feelings have been rising in Cyprus and Greece, until now they have reached boiling point. There has never been a question of the British losing any bases in Cyprus. We don't want them to leave like Egypt and other countries do. As a matter of fact they can have as many bases as they like on the mainland and on any of our islands. All the Cypriots want is to unite with Greece as have the Ionian Islands Crete and the Dodecanese. It is natural that they refuse to remain 'colonials' considering they are Europeans and Greece such a proven and friendly ally of England." (Papanicolaou, *Frederica*, 432–33.) On December 19, 1954, the *New York Times* reported that "the demonstrations, which began earlier this week in Athens and Salonika and spread to Cyprus, started after the United States had supported the United Nations in a British move to cut off consideration of self-determination for Cyprus." ("Troops Take over City," *New York Times*, December 19, 1954, p. 2.)

3. See pp. 857 and 864. Marshall paraphrased a sixteenth-century proverb by Desiderius Erasmus: "In the land of the blind, the one-eyed man is king."

4. "We are off to Naples to collect about a hundred members of our very large European family for a sightseeing cruise around the Greek islands," Frederica had told Marshall in

her August letter. "My husband and I thought of this idea because we meet Family only at funerals and after all one can't laugh at funerals." (Papanicolaou, *Frederica*, 435.)

5. The *New York Times* reported on November 1 that Frederica had "the first of two ear operations today. A communiqué said the surgery had proceeded normally and she was feeling well. A second operation will be performed in three months. She is suffering from a growth of spongy bone that has caused increasing deafness." ("Frederika Has Ear Operation," *New York Times*, November 2, 1954, p. 2.) See p. 876n2 and n4.

519

TO ALAN BULLOCK

January 18, 1955
Pinehurst, North Carolina

Dear Bullock: In response to the questions you included with your letter of December 30, 1954, the following are my comments on them by number.[1] Should you determine that you wish to quote me, I ask that you first clear it with me:

1) [Marshall Plan. *How far was the initiative taken by Bevin after your Harvard speech in June 1947 and the proposals subsequently put forward by him together with the French discussed with the U.S. Government in advance? Did Bevin anticipate the Russian Refusal?*][2]

   Not more than seven or eight people—all of the State Department—and the President knew anything whatever of the proposed Harvard speech in June 1947, certainly not Mr. Bevin. His actions were on his own initiative entirely.[3]

2) [N.A.T.O. *When was the idea of N.A.T.O. first conceived? How far did the initiative come from Bevin? Am I right in believing that, at the time the Brussels Pact was being negotiated, Bevin already hoped that it would be possible to supplement this with a North Atlantic Agreement?*]

   So far as I can recall, the NATO idea was first considered at the time of first consideration of the Vandenberg Resolution.[4] As to Mr. Bevin's preliminary hopes for a North Atlantic Agreement, I do not know, or do not recall.

3) [Relations with the U.S.S.R. *Bevin's critics have maintained that he missed some (unspecified) opportunity to reach a settlement with the U.S.S.R. Looking back on Bevin's conduct of the negotiations, especially in the Moscow and London conferences, do you feel there is any substance at all to this criticism? Did Bevin ever express the view that President Truman's announcement about Greece might have affected the chances of agreement in Moscow?*][5]

   No substance. Mr. Truman's announcement about Greece was a political necessity made necessary by Bevin's notification, just prior to the Moscow meeting, that the British must withdraw their troops from Greece.[6]

4) [Palestine. *Bevin himself seems to have believed that he could have put through a settlement in Palestine, if the U.S. Government had not been under such heavy pressure from the Zionists that it found it impossible to support him.[7] In your view was this just wishful thinking or was there some substance in his belief?*]

   I don't know or recall.

5) [Bevin as Foreign Secretary. *As a man of working class origins and a trade union leader, Bevin brought an unusual experience to the office of Foreign Secretary. Did this show itself in any particular characteristics of his conduct of foreign affairs?*]

Only that he was realistic, practical and far-sighted. I had great admiration for Bevin and trusted him to the full.[8] Faithfully yours,

GCMRL/G. C. Marshall Papers (Retirement, General); H

1. British historian and Hitler biographer Allan Bullock had written on November 5 that he was the authorized biographer of Ernest Bevin, had been given access to papers in the Foreign Office, and was now "getting in touch with those who were associated" with Bevin "during his career." (Bullock to Marshall, November 5, 1954, GCMRL/G. C. Marshall Papers [Retirement, General].) Marshall replied ten days later that he "was warmly disposed toward Bevin and admired his strong common sense and his courageous attitude in most difficult days." Marshall would be "glad to attempt answers" to any of Bullock's questions, "though whether or not I will agree to direct quotes will depend on the questions." (Marshall to Bullock, November 15, 1954, ibid.) Bullock responded on November 22 that he would pose "one or two questions by letter" and assured Marshall that he would "not dream of using anything you say without your express permission." (Bullock to Marshall, November 22, 1954, ibid.) He had sent a list of questions to Marshall on December 30. (Bullock to Marshall, December 30, 1954, ibid.) Bullock's questions are inserted in bracketed *italic* type in the text preceding each of Marshall's replies. The initial paragraph apparently was drafted by M. L. Spilman; Marshall's responses were handwritten.

2. Bevin contacted French Foreign Minister Georges Bidault on June 6, 1947, the same day Marshall gave the address at Harvard University that initially proposed what came to be known as the Marshall Plan. On June 18, Bevin and Bidault invited Soviet Foreign Minister Vyacheslav Molotov to meet with them in Paris. Molotov did so on June 27, but on July 3, he refused to participate in a positive response to Marshall's offer. See *Papers of GCM*, 6: 175, 220–21.

3. For more on the circumstances leading to Marshall's speech at Harvard, see *Papers of GCM*, 6: 139–42.

4. See p. 384n2.

5. For more on the circumstances preceding Truman's March 12, 1947, address regarding the deteriorating political and economic situation in Greece and Turkey, which became known as the Truman Doctrine, see *Papers of GCM*, 6: 50–51, 55–58, and 67–68. The speech took place while Marshall was in Moscow with Bevin attending a meeting of the Council of Foreign Ministers.

6. Marshall and Bevin discussed funding and the timing of the withdrawal of the British military mission in Greece at a March 22, 1947, meeting. See *Papers of GCM*, 6: 82.

7. Bullock may have been referring here to Bevin's April 1948 proposal that Bullock later described in the third volume of his biography of Bevin, *Ernest Bevin: Foreign Secretary, 1945–1951* (New York: W. W. Norton & Co., 1983), 562–64.

8. "I am most grateful to you for the trouble you have taken in answering my questions," Bullock replied on January 27. "I hope it may still be possible for me to get over to the United States and perhaps see you before I am through with the life of Bevin. In the meantime, I assure you I shall make no direct use of the information you give except with your permission. (Bullock to Marshall, January 27, 1955, GCMRL/G. C. Marshall Papers [Retirement, General].)

MOURNING became a recurrent theme in Marshall's correspondence as his contemporaries passed away more frequently. His brother-in-law, Brigadier General Tristam Tupper, had died at his home in Miles, Virginia, on December

30, 1954. The funeral took place on January 3 in the chapel at Fort Myer, Virginia, and the Marshalls "flew home after lunch, and my time was so short that I had no time for calls," Marshall told Ridgway on January 10. (Marshall to Ridgway, January 10, 1955, GCMRL/G. C. Marshall Papers [Retirement, General].) Lieutenant General Raymond S. McLain had also died in December 1954. (See pp. 558–59n3.) Marshall later wrote that McLain was among the "finest natural battle leaders of our last World War army. Modest in every respect. Inspired in a battle crisis." (Marshall handwritten note, n.d, on George to Marshall, August 3, 1955, ibid.) In February, Marshall attended the funeral of Brehon B. Somervell at the Fort Myer chapel but explained to Mrs. Somervell on February 17 that he dared "not go into the cemetery because of a slight cold and lack of overshoes." (Marshall to Somervell, February 17, 1955, ibid.)

Perhaps the keenest loss was Marshall's longtime friend Frank R. McCoy, who had died on June 4, 1954, after a long illness. ("Gen. McCoy Dies; Served 9 Presidents," *Washington Post*, June 5, 1954, p. 22.) "Thank you for coming to see me the other day," Frances McCoy wrote to Marshall the day after the funeral. "You put great courage into me—for I must confess to feeling only half alive if that." (McCoy to Marshall, June 9, 1954, GCMRL/G. C. Marshall Papers [Retirement, General].) "I want to send you a line of sympathy on the loss of your friend," she continued. "He loved you very dearly, rejoiced in your brilliant accomplishments & took pride in your selflessness & honor." (Ibid.) See next document and pp. 942–43. ★

520

To Major General William S. Biddle[1] — January 24, 1955
Pinehurst, North Carolina

Dear Biddle: I submit the following regarding General McCoy and I hope it will serve your purpose. I am filled with admiration in my memories of the man, but lack the facility to translate that admiration into good English:

"I find it difficult to translate into cold English the depth or quality of my admiration for General McCoy. I first saw him—but did not meet him—enroute to Fort Riley from Fort Leavenworth on the dingy little local train. He sat reading in a rocking chair in the baggage car. I was envious.

"The beginning of our intimacy occurred in June 1917 enroute to France on the S.S. Tenedoes [*Tenadores*] with the headquarters of the 1st Division in the first US convoy of the war with Germany.[2] Thereafter, we were frequently in close touch, particularly at Fort Benning, Georgia, while he was Department Commander stationed in Atlanta.[3]

"But it was not until I became Chief of Staff of the Army and, later, Secretary of State that I saw him in vital roles of national and international importance. Previously, he had risen to National prominence for his great role in Nicaragua, his membership on the Lyton [*Lytton*] Commission to the Far East, and other special missions for the President or the State Department.[4]

"During the tumultuous period of early preparation for World War II and during that war, we came in close personal contact while he served in highly important roles as President of the Military Commission that tried and convicted the Nazi crew of prospective saboteurs who were landed by submarine off Long Island.[5] He was a member of the commission headed by Justice [Owen Josephus] Roberts that investigated the Pearl Harbor tragedy.[6] He headed a commission to survey our procurement program in the light of possible reductions. And, finally, he was made the first Chairman of the Far East Commission on February 26, 1946, and continued in that role until his retirement on November 30, 1949.[7]

"The importance of these various roles was indicative of the complete trust and regard reposed in him by those in high authority, President Roosevelt, Secretary of War Stimson, and the Chief of Staff. Few men of my knowledge over many years of service have commanded so completely the respect, trust and admiration of all who knew him. Among these admiring friends were officials in the Caribbean, Mexico, the Philippines, Japan, England, France, and many other countries.

"As a friend and companion, he displayed qualities of charm and affection, cultivation, breadth of vision, and wide experience rare among men. From the early days of Theodore Roosevelt, General Leonard Wood and Elihu Root, he had been in close touch with the great of America. He commanded not only their respect, but their devotion. Presidents consulted him frequently and utilized his services—Taft, Coolidge, Hoover and Franklin Roosevelt.[8]

"General McCoy was beloved of many men, and he gave them a perfect example of a splendid American, without conceit, unselfish to the extreme, and courageous in principle." Faithfully yours,

GCMRL/G. C. Marshall Papers (Retirement, General)

1. "Mrs. McCoy has done me the great honor of asking that I write the memorial article on the General, to appear in ASSEMBLY," the USMA alumni magazine, Major General William S. Biddle (USMA, 1923), commander of First Armored Division Headquarters at Fort Hood, Texas, had written to Marshall on September 27, 1954. The editor of *Assembly* had instructed Biddle to request a personal tribute from close friends for "a short, informal memoir on Frank McCoy as they knew him." (Biddle to Marshall, September 27, 1954, GCMRL/G. C. Marshall Papers [Retirement, General].) Marshall replied on October 11 that he would "gladly do what I can to help you out, though I may be a little tardy in doing so." (Marshall to Biddle, October 11, 1954, ibid.) See also pp. 935–36.

2. See *Papers of GCM*, 1: 109. For more on Marshall's early association with McCoy, see Pogue, *Education*, 288–89.

3. See *Papers of GCM*, 1: 341–42, 344.

4. Following World War I General Frank McCoy held a number of military and diplomatic assignments in Armenia, the Philippine Islands, and Japan. In 1929 McCoy served as President Calvin Coolidge's personal representative supervising Nicaragua's first peaceful transition of government; then he headed a commission investigating a dispute between Paraguay and Bolivia. As a member of the international Lytton Commission, he spent six weeks in Manchuria in the spring of 1932 attempting to calm growing hostilities between Japan and China, but the commission's report triggered Japan's withdrawal from the League of Nations. The commission was named for its head, Victor Alexander George Robert Bulwer-Lytton, who had been acting viceroy of India in 1926.

5. On June 12, 1942, a German submarine dropped four Nazi spies at Amagansett, New York, on Long Island, where they were discovered. A massive manhunt resulted, but their arrest came after two of the men turned themselves in to the FBI and revealed the additional presence of four others who had landed safely in Florida. McCoy presided over the

military tribunal that convicted the eight men in Operation Pastorius of attempting to blow up strategic American economic targets.

6. McCoy had served on the first Roberts Commission. See pp. 245–47.

7. Details regarding the dates of McCoy's chairmanship of the Far East Commission to determine the fate of postwar Japan were provided by M. L. Spilman. Marshall had left a blank on his handwritten draft.

8. Frank McCoy was an aide to General Leonard Wood during the Spanish-American War and to President Theodore Roosevelt in 1906. After Wood was named army chief of staff by President William Howard Taft in 1910, Wood appointed McCoy a member of the General Staff, which had been organized during the Theodore Roosevelt administration under the tenure of Secretary of War Elihu Root. During World War I McCoy commanded the 165th Infantry of the Forty-second Division and later a brigade of the Thirty-second Division.

521

Letter regarding James Lo[1] February 1, 1955
Pinehurst, North Carolina

To Whom It May Concern James Hung-Ching Lo first came to my attention in 1946 when he was placed in charge of my official residence and office—servants, quarters and mess—by the Chinese National Government. He was employed and paid by that Government, and all the officers of my staff were under his household management.

In all these duties he was exceedingly efficient. He fled from China before the Communist take-over and landed in Hong Kong. His parents and their family had to remain in China and are believed to have been killed.[2]

I assisted in bringing Lo to Washington to attend the Methodist Missionary School in Takoma Park. He had a partial scholarship and it was necessary for him to work very hard to support himself. I then helped him to secure a scholarship at American University, which he was unable to continue because of the hours of work necessary to support himself. He is now working in New York City.[3]

I have kept in touch with him throughout this period. He is a very fine fellow, of high integrity, dependable and hard-working. He will have no trouble in supporting himself.

I urgently recommend favorable action to adjust his immigration status under Section 6 of the Refugee Relief Act of 1953.

GCMRL/G. C. Marshall Papers (Retirement, General)

1. See pp. 704–5. Marshall had sent C. J. George the name of an immigration official on October 4, 1954, with a note that "A combination of Scotch, Burbon, confidential reminiscences, etc. and an emotional account of Mr. Lo's predicament caused him to offer to fix up Lo's status permanently" under article six of the Refugee Relief Act of 1953, signed into law by President Eisenhower on August 7, 1953. (Marshall to George, October 4, 1954, GCMRL/G. C. Marshall Papers [Retirement, General]; H.) George wrote to the US Immigration and Naturalization Service on October 11 and explained that had Lo "remained in China, there would have been a price on his head because of his service" to Marshall. (George to Junghans, October 11, 1954, ibid.)

2. "Since I destroyed when I left home most of the identification and documents showing my relationships with the organizations of the Nationalist Government, which directed my service to the American military personnel, I shall very much appreciate it if you would kindly write for me such a letter indicating my service to them and to you and strongly

expressing that I shall physically be injured by the Communist government and eventually lose my life if I return to China now," Lo had written to Marshall on January 18. (Lo to Marshall, June 7, 1954, ibid.)

3. "I have been accepted into New York University," Lo had written on October 2, and explained that he would be taking evening classes in accounting. (Lo to Katherine Marshall, October 2, 1954, ibid.)

"I AM WELL, though not very ambitious; and Katherine is still struggling with painful shingles in her arm and hand. She has had a long battle of it, and it is telling on her," Marshall wrote to Baruch from Washington on February 17. He had gone to Walter Reed for a check-up, he told Baruch, and "was having a hearing aid checked because my deafness has grown to the point where I will have to begin wearing it pretty continuously." See p. 922 (Marshall to Baruch, February 17, 1955, GCMRL/G. C. Marshall Papers [Retirement, General].)

"We are leading a very quiet life," Marshall summarized. (Ibid.) The same day he reported to Madame Chiang that "at Pinehurst, we have had the coldest weather in fifty years. I think we have been out to meals only twice since October." (Marshall to Madame Chiang, February 17, 1955, ibid.) He was hoping to go hunting "from the 20th to the 27th," Marshall told Madame Chiang, "but I doubt that I shall do much running around. Of course, we will motor behind the dogs and only get out when they point. I have promised to confine myself to not more than two or three hours a day, but I need something to stir me out of the lazy routine I have fallen into." (Ibid.) On February 10, Marshall had received a telegram from James Bruce indicating that General Lucius Clay's plane would stop at Fort Bragg, North Carolina, to pick up Marshall at 11:30 a.m. and deliver him to Pinckney Island. (Bruce to Marshall, telegram, February 10, 1955, ibid.) See p. 669n1. While Marshall was wary about overexerting himself while hunting, he anticipated the spring planting season. ★

522

TO THE W. ATLEE BURPEE COMPANY[1]

March 9, 1955
Pinehurst, North Carolina

4174	Spry Dwarf Double French Marigolds	2 packets	$ .30
3263	Burpee Primrose Tall African Marigolds	1 packet	$ .25
4153	Glitters Flowered Marigolds	1 packet	$ .25
4313	Burbank Zinnias	1 packet	$ .25
4314	Super Giant Zinnias	1 packet	$ .25
3367	Creamy Crinkles California Poppy	1 packet	$ .25
4193	Mixed Tall Large Phlox	2 packets	$ .30
4743	Giant Double Nasturtiums	6 packets	$ .75
4052	Mixed Candytuft	2 packets	$ .20
6136	Early Hybrid Tomatoes	1 packet	$ .50
6042	Salad Bowl Lettuce	1 packet	$ .25
5026	Early Simpson Lettuce	2 packets	$ .30

5043	Crimson Globe Radishes	1 packet	$ .15
6172	Stringless Wax Bush Beans	1 packet	$ .15

GCMRL/G. C. Marshall Papers (Retirement, Chronological)

1. This typewritten list, which is considerably less ambitious than Marshall's February 1949 Burpee order (see *Papers of GCM*, 6: 664–66), included instructions that the seed packets be mailed to Marshall at Liscombe Lodge in Pinehurst.

523

To Philip L. Graham — March 26, 1955
Pinehurst, North Carolina

My dear Graham: I have hesitated over answering your letter of March 14 because I would like very much to oblige you and the Post, but my best judgment dictates my regrets.[1] If it was a mere interview without camera business, I might accept, but my health is not up to the protracted business of the other.

As a favor to my old Secretary of the General Staff, Colonel Frank McCarthy, I gave two entire days to interviews and photographs for an anniversary article similar to your proposal.[2]

Now the "Fund For The Republic", Doctor Hutchins directing, is soliciting quite a bit of my time.[3]

In addition, there are two other requests involving talks and pictures.

I am not well—making a slow recovery from prolonged virus-flu attacks last year and this year. So I have to be very careful.

I'm sorry, but I don't feel up to these various programs. Faithfully yours,

GCMRL/G. C. Marshall Papers (Retirement, General); H

1. "On Sunday, May 8, The Washington Post is planning to present a special television program recognizing the Tenth Anniversary of VE [Victory in Europe]-Day, on our television station, WTOP," Graham had apprised Marshall on March 14. (Graham to Marshall, March 14, 1955, GCMRL/G. C. Marshall Papers [Retirement, General].) "We are especially anxious to have an interview with you, and we can make this as painless for you as possible by sending our people to Leesburg—promising at the same time not to disrupt Mrs. Marshall's housekeeping. Or, if you would prefer, we can do it in our studios here in Washington." (Ibid.)

2. William Arthur, managing editor of *LOOK* magazine, had contacted McCarthy about a "story celebrating the tenth anniversary of V-E Day." McCarthy wrote to Marshall on December 29, 1954, to explain that "The story would be completely personal and would make no reference whatever to politics or controversy of any sort. There would be a good many pictures, but little text." (McCarthy to Marshall, December 29, 1954, ibid.) On January 28, C. J. George confided to Arthur that Marshall's "health is far from perfect, so I imagine that activities will be pretty much indoors and around the house." (George to Arthur, January 28, 1955, GCMRL/G. C. Marshall Papers [Retirement, Chronological].) George notified Marshall on January 31 that Arthur and a photographer would be in Pinehurst on February 3 and 4. (George to Marshall, January 31, 1955, ibid.) "The Magnificent American," which included photos of Marshall grocery shopping and retrieving mail from the post office with Jimmy Winn, appeared in the May 17, 1955, issue of *LOOK* magazine.

3. Robert Maynard Hutchins, president of the Fund for the Republic (a nonprofit educational institution chartered in 1952 under the Ford Foundation) and the former chancellor of the University of Chicago, had written to Marshall on September 23, 1954, to propose that Marshall participate in "a series of television films tentatively entitled 'Great Contemporaries.'" Marshall declined for health reasons, but Hutchins wrote again on December

3 to explain that producer Jack H. Skirball had retained a writer to dramatize Marshall's story, which would "take almost none of your time." (Hutchins to Marshall, September 23 and December 3, 1954, GCMRL/G. C. Marshall Papers [Retirement, General].) Marshall replied on December 22 that "on the basis of what will now be required of me, I accept," and suggested that future meetings take place in Leesburg after his return on May 1. (Marshall to Hutchins, December 22, 1954, ibid.) See pp. 893–95.

KATHERINE MARSHALL'S sister, Allene Tupper Lacy, had returned to Leesburg after her husband, Sterling Byrd Lacy, who suffered from angina, died on March 7 in Daytona Beach, where they had been for a month. ("Sterling Byrd Lacy," *Washington Post*, March 8, 1955, p. 28.) The Marshalls went to Leesburg for Lacy's funeral after just having been to Washington at the end of December for the funeral of Mrs. Lacy's and Mrs. Marshall's brother. See p. 868. (Marshall to McCarthy, April 6, 1955, GCMRL/Frank McCarthy Papers [Additions, Box 1]; H.) Then, on April 1, Marshall wrote to Ruth Adams that "Allene suffered a stroke three days ago," was paralyzed on one side, and remained unconscious. "Katherine left immediately for Leesburg," where she was staying with the Fletchers, their Leesburg neighbors, he reported. (Marshall to Adams, April 1, 1955, GCMRL/G. C. Marshall Collection [Adams]; H.)

"Allene was very bad yesterday," Colonel Robert H. Fletcher (USMA, 1908) disclosed to Marshall on April 4. "This morning her breathing is much easier and she is actually moving her hitherto paralyzed arm and leg a little." (Fletcher to Marshall, April 4, 1955, GCMRL/G. C. Marshall Papers [Retirement, General].) "Katherine is much cheered," he continued, and assured Marshall that his wife "seems in quite good health and between Colonel George, who is a marvel, and the doctors, the Hospital, and her friends," Marshall should "rest assured that she is being taken good care of." (Ibid.) Marshall wrote to Madge Pendleton on April 7 that his wife "finally decided to return here as there was no telling how long Allene would continue in this condition. She arrives here tomorrow." (Marshall to Pendleton, GCMRL/Xerox 2237 [GCM Family, Personal Letters]; H.)

On April 25, C. J. George wrote to Molly Winn in Japan that he was "quite discouraged" about her aunt's condition. "While she has been out of the oxygen tent for several days and seemingly conscious, her eyes are blank and her memory nil. She doesn't even know her closest friend," George confided. (George to Winn, April 25, 1955, ibid.) "In my conversations with your mother, I have given her the picture as I see it. She is optimistic, and I think we should keep her in that frame of mind. You can well-imagine the worry she has experienced so far this year, so I request that in your letters to her you avoid saying anything which might add to her already heavy problems." (Ibid.)

Katherine Marshall became devoted to caring for her sister, who was "still helpless" on July 9 when Marshall wrote to Madge Pendleton that Lacy had "been carried into the house here twice for a brief visit" but there was "no special improvement." Her mind was "fairly clear at times, then completely confused." (Marshall to Pendleton, July 9, 1955, GCMRL/Xerox 2237 (GCM Family, Personal Letters); H.) See pp. 897, 899n4, 901, 912, 979–80, and 986. ★

524

To Robert E. Sherwood April 2, 1955
Pinehurst, North Carolina

Dear Sherwood: Thanks for your letter regarding European impressions, and particularly those northeast of Trieste. When I see you, I will tell you of a curious and rather amusing incident with reference to the Liubljana Gap.[1]

I hope you are correct in your estimate as to the Jugoslavian [Yugoslavian] reactions for the immediate future.[2]

Mrs. Marshall and I have been living quietly in our winter home here at Pinehurst. We return to Leesburg, Virginia, about May 1*st*.

With warm regards, Faithfully yours,

GCMRL/G. C. Marshall Papers (Retirement, General)

1. Sherwood had written to Marshall on March 21 about his first visit to Yugoslavia. "I want to tell you that I encountered deep respect for you in that part of the world; it was respect and I might even say reverence based on more reasons than one. The gratitude for the farseeing Marshall Plan is obvious but, even more than that (and I was talking with officials of the Government), was the admiration for the Grand Strategy which they believe (correctly, I told them) was largely directed by you. Having heard and read through the years endless speculations as the desirability of such channels for invasion as the Liubljana Gap, I was particularly interested to hear the Jugoslavs express vehement conviction that, if the so-called 'soft underbelly' strategy had been followed, the war in Europe would have been greatly prolonged, perhaps into 1947." (Sherwood to Marshall, March 21, 1955, GCMRL/G. C. Marshall Papers [Retirement, General].) Marshall had strongly opposed British proposals during World War II for a movement through the Ljubljana Gap and for other Mediterranean operations, an area that according to Churchill was the "soft underbelly" of the Axis Powers.

2. "I came away from there with the conviction that they will never consent to be a Soviet satellite, that their deepest sympathies and highest aspirations are with the free world." (Ibid.)

525

Tribute to Winston Churchill[1] April 5, 1955
Pinehurst, North Carolina

A great, a very great man has retired from a long and powerful part in World Leadership. The most remarkable career of modern times has reached its active conclusion.[2] I was with him during many critical moments. ~~and days~~ Always he was towering in his strenth [strength] and courage. I am thankful that his voice can still be heard in his beloved House of Commons.[3]

GCMRL/G. C. Marshall Papers (Retirement, General); H

1. "Telephoned to British BBC at request, April 5 1:30 P.M." is written in Marshall's hand at the top of this handwritten statement.

2. Winston Churchill resigned as prime minister on April 5, 1955, at the age of eighty.

3. Churchill remained in Parliament until 1964. Marshall apparently also sent a letter to him. "I am sorry that I have not found an opportunity to answer the letter with which you honoured me last month," Churchill wrote on June 25. "I deeply value all that you say. Our wartime comradeship is one of my most cherished memories of those tremendous days."

(Churchill to Marshall, June 25, 1955, GCMRL/G. C. Marshall Papers [Retirement, General].) Churchill closed the letter "Yours with enduring regard." (Ibid.)

526

To Queen Frederica of the Hellenes[1]

April 13, 1955
Pinehurst, North Carolina

Your Majesty: Your delightful letter gave us great pleasure and not a little amusement. It was very, very good of you to give me so much of your time and effort.[2]

Also I am very deeply indebted to His Majesty and you for your kindness to my friend—Mary (I have forgotten her married name). You were not only most gracious but you went far out of your way to give them extreme pleasure. Mary's letter to me was ecstatic and judging from the other ship's mail I have received the entire passenger list was enthused and charmed—with your action.[3]

Politics and war recriminations fill the air here. Its the way of democracy but it does grow tiresome.

Pinehurst, while the great U.S. golf center (there are four 18 hole courses at the club three blocks from our ~~place~~ cottage) is really a secluded place, but the long distance phone ~~from New York and Washington~~ disturbs our calm many times a day—five times from New York this morning, and five times from Washington.

I am giving you a lot of trivialities when there is so much I would like to talk over with you.

I was relieved to learn of the success of your ear operation. You are too young to have to endure such things.[4] Apparently His Majesty enjoys sturdy good health. That is a blessing for Greece.

Again with my admiration and affection F. Yr.

GCMRL/G. C. Marshall Papers (Retirement, General); H

1. Marshall's pencil draft, printed here, has instructions at the top that it should be typed and filed. (Marshall to Frederica, April 13, 1955, GCMRL/G. C. Marshall Papers [Retirement, General].)

2. "I have been in and out of the hospital these last three months," Frederica had written on March 14. See p. 867n5. The queen admitted that she had "played a rather nasty trick" on her surgeon by telling him "something had gone wrong." With the surgeon's "eyes popping out of his head with concern," the queen "exposed an enormous false ear that I had stuck on. You should have seen the momentary horror in the poor man's face until he collapsed with laughter." (Papanicolaou, *Frederica*, 438.)

3. C. J. George had informed Mary Palmer Rockwell, daughter of General John McAuley Palmer, on February 16 that Marshall had written personal notes to the US ambassador to Greece and Queen Frederica about Rockwell's desire to meet the queen while Rockwell and her husband were on "a Mediterranean Cruise." (Rockwell to Marshall, January 28, 1955, and George to Rockwell, February 16, 1955, GCMRL/G. C. Marshall Papers [Retirement, General]; Marshall to Cannon, February 17, 1955, and Marshall to Frederica, [probably February 15, 1955], ibid; H.)

The Rockwells visited the Greek royal family at their estate north of Athens. (Rockwell to Marshall, March 3, 1955, ibid.) Frederica reported that she "found them very charming," and assured Marshall that he should "not hesitate to recommend any of your friends that may be visiting Greece." (Papanicolaou, *Frederica*, 439.)

4. The queen had written in detail about her two "famous Fenestration" operations. "The result is remarkable," she had written to Marshall. "I suffered hardly at all." (Ibid., 438.)

527

TO CHARLES E. WILSON May 6, 1955
Leesburg, Virginia[1]

Dear Mr. Secretary: I have read the proposed legislation outlining the National Reserve Plan, which you submitted to the Congress for consideration.[2]

My views on the subject of an adequate civilian reserve component have been expressed many times since the end of World War II.[3] I included in my final biennial report to the Secretary of War a recommendation that a plan be formulated to forever eliminate the pressing manpower problems we faced at the start of that conflict.[4] As you know, I made a similar effort while I was Secretary of Defense.[5] The National Reserve Plan does provide six months of training for non-veterans in substantial numbers to meet real requirements and should do much to improve our reserves for readiness in this age.

The position of our reserve forces of all our Services will be sound if we set up machinery which will permit an orderly mobilization of an effective reserve force in a minimum period following any international crisis and resulting in a national emergency for the United States and its allies.

The matter of a reserve force in being has been delayed too long. The wars of tomorrow will not permit a return to the old system of mobilization.

As you know, I feel strongly on the subject and would lend you every support if my health permitted. My hopes have not been diminished, and with an understanding Congress I feel the President's proposal will be enacted. The recent action of the House of Representatives is an encouraging move in that direction.[6]

With best regards, Faithfully yours,

GCMRL/G. C. Marshall Papers (Retirement, General)

1. Marshall also wrote to President Truman on May 6 and mentioned he and his wife had arrived "yesterday afternoon from Pinehurst and are struggling to get settled for the summer and early fall." (Marshall to Truman, GCMRL/G. C. Marshall Collection [Truman]; H.)

2. Implementation of universal military training had not received congressional discussion since the failure to pass the necessary legislation in March 1952. (See pp. 551–53.) Extensive discussions on this topic in the context of reforming reserve policies began within the Eisenhower administration in early 1953. The administration's final proposals, known as the National Reserve Plan, were presented to the press in December 1954 by Secretary Wilson and submitted by Congress by Eisenhower in January 1955. The envisioned program continued many of the current reserve policies, but it included two enlistment options with varying active duty and reserve requirements for men under the age of nineteen who had not been drafted. The bill also clarified training and service obligations for the ready and standby reserve categories. (Leighton, *Strategy, Money, and the New Look*, 399–412; "Wilson Proposes a Reserve of 5,000,000 Trained Men," *New York Times*, December 18, 1954, p. 1; "Eisenhower Urges Military Training of All Fit Youths," *New York Times*, January 14, 1955, pp. 1, 6.)

3. See, for example, *Papers of GCM*, 5: 229–31, 355, and 360.

4. See *General Marshall's Report: The Winning of the War in Europe and the Pacific: Biennial Report of the Chief of Staff of the United States Army, July 1, 1943 to June 30, 1945, to the Secretary of War* (New York: Simon and Schuster, 1945), 117–23. See also p. 178n4.

5. See pp. 325–29, 338–47, 369–71, 409–13, 423–26. 481–84, 551–53. and 558–59.

6. The House Armed Services Committee had passed its own version of the bill on April 27. For more on congressional action on this plan and the provisions of the enacted law, see Leighton, *Strategy, Money, and the New Look*, 412–22, and James M. Gerhardt, *The Draft and Public Policy: Issues in Military Manpower Procurement, 1945–1970* (Columbus: Ohio State University Press, 1971), 198–206.

528

To Virginius Dabney — May 12, 1955
Leesburg, Virginia

My dear Dabney: Thanks for your letter.[1] The points you mention have been brought up countless times over the past ten years.[2]

As to the war period: First, I made three biennial reports—very complete and, I think, very accurate.[3] The last was completed within a few weeks of the close of hostilities and had a circulation of over a million—200 thousand in England alone. This had never been done before in frequency, volume or distribution. For more than a year the last report was, in effect, all the English public had to go on. I did a great deal of this work while flying the oceans or in this country.[4]

While Secretary of State, I made quite comprehensive statements over the radio (and printed) after each great conference, written usually partially at the actual conference table while translations were going on and largely while flying home.[5]

Secondly, the report desired of me now must be largely personal, affecting many individuals—interesting from a news point of view, but hardly helpful. Most of the period I would have to touch on would be from the fall of 1939 to December 1941. Once we were into the war, things were not so difficult.

So many of the incidents of a personal nature have been given a purely political caste without regard to facts well known to the members of Congress concerned. The Pearl Harbor incident, for example—as to where I was and the political purpose to embroil President Roosevelt—after my first day's testimony in the hearings, I checked up carefully and found that I spent that evening in Mrs. Marshall's bedroom, she being ill at the time. This I stated publicly several times, but this was overwhelmed by political assaults for purely political purposes.[6]

Practically anything I wrote now would be brought immediately into the coming political campaign, perverted or otherwise.

I have almost no personal war or other governmental records, as I did not write personally to commanders, in order to avoid confusing the formal *directive* with my personal discussions.[7] Eisenhower, for example, wrote to me frequently and at length, and his letters were very helpful, but I did not write to him. He understood why.[8]

I have testified for as much as a week at a time to committees or joint committees of Congress. All that is in the record and was mulled over in the press at the time.

What is wanted is the personal contacts and reactions. This, I will not do. And I insist that, unless the details of the official dealings are fully stated, then the book, historically, is more harmful than helpful.

There is another factor involved. Though you may praise a man's record over years, one adverse item will be seized upon to an extent that, for the masses, literally blackens the whole. And yet that adverse item may be most important historically, showing the difficulties in preparing for war in a democracy.

This last would seem to be an argument for my writing my personal memoirs. Yet, what I have done was accurate reporting on the war years, and very promptly—more promptly than has any one of my predecessors.

I trust you to hold all this as confidential. I know you will have many answers or rebuttals in mind, but this will have to suffice for me.[9] Faithfully yours,

GCMRL/G. C. Marshall Papers (Retirement, General)

1. *Richmond Times-Dispatch* editor Virginius Dabney had written to Marshall on May 7 and enclosed an editorial he had published that day with an appeal to Marshall concerning "the importance of your handing on to posterity the invaluable knowledge that is yours, and yours alone." (Dabney to Marshall, May 7, 1955, GCMRL/G. C. Marshall Papers [Retirement, General].) In his editorial, Dabney suggested that if Marshall was "unwilling to write full-length memoirs," he should "at the very least prepare a comprehensive memorandum or statement" that would be released "when all the participants in the great drama of World War II and its aftermath are gone." ("General Marshall's Duty to Posterity," *Richmond Times-Dispatch*, May 7, 1955.)

2. See pp. 161, 648–49, 843–44, and *Papers of GCM*, 6: 638, 661, 663, and 743. See also pp. 896–97, 916–17, and 931–32.

3. See *Biennial Report of the Chief of Staff of the United States Army, July 1, 1939, to June 30, 1941, to the Secretary of War* (Washington: GPO, 1941); *Biennial Report of the Chief of Staff of the United States Army, July 1, 1941, to June 30, 1943, to the Secretary of War* (Washington: GPO, 1943); and *Biennial Report of the Chief of Staff of the United States Army, July 1, 1943, to June 30, 1945, to the Secretary of War* (Washington: GPO, 1945).

4. Simon and Schuster, Inc. published *General Marshall's Report: The Winning of the War in Europe and the Pacific: Biennial Report of the Chief of Staff of the United States Army, July 1, 1943 to June 30, 1945, to the Secretary of War* in October 1945. "Mr. Simon has demonstrated an unusual willingness to cooperate in the distribution of your report," Captain James Shepley had informed Marshall after visiting the publisher. (See p. 84n3.) "He has read the manuscript and believes that it conceivably may sell a million or even more copies." (Shepley to Marshall, August 25, 1945, GCMRL/G. C. Marshall Papers [Pentagon Office, General].) The paperback edition sold for one dollar and the cloth for two dollars and fifty cents.

5. See *Papers of GCM*, 6: 77–79, 113–21, 204–5, and 297–302.

6. See Pogue, *Ordeal*, 429–35.

7. On May 21, 1942, Marshall sent a memorandum to Frank McCarthy explaining his policy of not "keeping a memorandum of momentous daily happenings." (Marshall to McCarthy, memorandum, May 21, 1942, GCMRL/Frank McCarthy Papers [US Army, 1941–45].) See *Papers of GCM*, 3: 207–8.

8. "I have followed a practice of almost never writing to a theater commander, to the extent that some of them have been offended because I have not given answers to their frequent communications," Marshall explained to Brigadier General John McAuley Palmer in 1944. (Marshall to Palmer, July 19, 1944, GCMRL/G. C. Marshall Papers [Pentagon Office, Selected].) "The reason for this has been the wish to avoid any misunderstandings as to what was required. Their instructions are prepared by me and edited in the Operations Division, or the reverse, and are usually transmitted by radio." (Ibid.) See *Papers of GCM*, 4: 239–41, and Joseph Patrick Hobbs, *Dear General: Eisenhower's Wartime Letters to Marshall* (Baltimore: Johns Hopkins Press, 1971).

9. Dabney responded on May 16 that he appreciated "the care with which" Marshall had written regarding Dabney's "editorial suggestion." While he wished "it were possible for us to publish" Marshall's May 12 letter or a similar statement of his position, he would "of course regard your communication as confidential." Dabney to Marshall, May 16, 1955, GCMRL/G. C. Marshall Papers [Retirement, General].) Dabney wanted "particularly . . . to get before the public the fact that you were with Mrs. Marshall the night before Pearl Harbor. Although you have testified to this, it doesn't seem to have penetrated the consciousness of the public." (Ibid.)

529

TO JOHN FOSTER DULLES

May 16, 1955
Leesburg, Virginia

Dear Dulles— Your very thoughtful and generous message reference the Austrian settlement came through promptly yesterday.[1]

Thank you for remembering me as you did.

I am sincerely glad the Austrian stalemate has been at last settled. The Soviets took the "profitable" time in making this possible.[2] Anyway it has been done and I hope the poor Austrian people get clear promptly and without complications and resulting pressures.

Again, thank you. Faithfully yours—

Princeton/Papers of John Foster Dulles; H

1. "As I signed the Austrian state treaty a few minutes ago I thought gratefully of your contribution notably at the Moscow conference of 1947," Dulles had cabled Marshall. (Dulles to Marshall, telegram, May 15, 1955, GCMRL/G. C. Marshall Papers [Retirement, General].) Dulles, as representative of the Republican Party, had attended the Moscow conference of the Council of Foreign Ministers with Secretary of State Marshall. See *Papers of GCM*, 6: 73, 92, 104–5, 108–10, 119–20.

The treaty Dulles had signed along with the foreign ministers of Britain, France, the Soviet Union, and Austria ended the Allied occupation of Austria and reestablished it as an independent state.

2. The Soviets received in return for their agreement to end the occupation an Austrian pledge to remain neutral in the cold war.

530

PRESS RELEASE[1]

May 18, 1955
Washington, DC

GENERAL MARSHALL CALLS FOR CONVENTION
TO EXPLORE ATLANTIC UNION[2]

The following statement, made by General George C. Marshall, former Secretary of State and of Defense, to Clarence Streit, member of the Board of Governors of the Atlantic Union Committee and author of *Union Now*, was given out today in Washington by the latter:

"A few days before the death of Justice Owen J. Roberts, I accepted his invitation of May 5 to become a member of the Council of the Atlantic Union Committee which he has headed since its foundation in 1949.[3] In accepting I wrote him on May 12:

"'I am honored to be counted among those who support the unity of free nations.'[4]

"Justice Roberts' services to defense as well as to the judiciary were manifold, but perhaps the finest thing he did was the sacrifice he made in resigning from the Supreme Court to devote himself to the cause of Atlantic Union.[5]

"The subject today is vitally important and the period fateful. All probably agree to the importance of Atlantic unity but few act.

"Recently a resolution calling for action was introduced in Congress by a distinguished bipartisan group from both Houses. It proposes that delegates from the United States and other NATO democracies meet in a Convention 'to explore and report to what extent their peoples might further unite within the framework of the United Nations, and agree to form, federally or otherwise, a defense, economic and political union.' This prudent proposal, which commits us only to exploration, deserves support.[6]

"Thinking back on the development of our own Federal Union—on the doubts and difficulties which preceded the final union of the colonies, on the remarkable advance in freedom, invention, production and living standards which followed on the solution of the early difficulties, and on the high degree to which the States have continued to maintain their individual personality and institutions—Americans should have a sympathetic understanding of this effort to overcome the limitations of national barriers in the approach to a solution for common problems.

"What I said when I addressed the Conference of Governors on July 14, 1947, I would repeat today: 'There is no blinking the fact that this country now stands at a turning point in its relations to its traditional friends among the nations of the Old World.'[7]

"Either it must finish the task of assisting these countries to adjust themselves politically to the changed demands of a new age, or it must reconcile itself to seeing them move in directions which are consistent neither with their own traditions nor with those of this country. Whatever course is adopted will affect the lives and fortunes of people in every State of the Union."[8]

—End Marshall Statement—

GCMRL/G. C. Marshall Papers (Retirement, General)

1. Marshall, "along with 214 other distinguished leaders from nine NATO countries," according to former US ambassador to Norway Lithgow Osborne, had previously signed a "*Declaration of Atlantic Unity*." (Osborne to Marshall, December 30, 1954, GCMRL/G. C. Marshall Papers [Retirement, General].) The *New York Times* had reported on October 4, 1954, that this document called for, in part, increased coordination of "political, trade and defense policies" and the reduction of tariffs and trade restrictions among NATO member nations as well as the creation of "an advisory Atlantic Assembly." ("169 Notables Ask Widening of NATO," *New York Times*, October 4, 1954, p. 5.) Osborne had asked Marshall on December 30, 1954, for a "brief comment or statement on the *Declaration*" to be published in a pamphlet that would include "the text of the *Declaration* and the complete list of signers together with comments on it from the top NATO and civil and military officials."

Marshall handwrote his comment in a note to C. J. George: "All probably agree to the vital importance of Atlantic Unity but few act. This Declaration today is all important and the period fateful." He instructed George to address this comment "to Osborne and sign my name." (Osborne to Marshall, December 30, 1954; Marshall to George, n.d.; and Marshall to Osborne, January 4, 1955, GCMRL/G. C. Marshall Papers [Retirement, General].)

2. Marshall had met with and given this statement to former *New York Times* foreign correspondent and current editor of *Freedom & Union, Magazine of the Democratic World* Clarence K. Streit in Marshall's Pentagon office on May 17. (Streit to Marshall, May 18, 1955, ibid.)

3. Former Associate Supreme Court Justice Owen J. Roberts, who had written to Marshall on May 5, had died of a heart attack on May 17. (Roberts to Marshall, May 5, 1955, ibid.; "Owen Roberts Dies; Former Justice, 80," *New York Times*, May 18, 1955, p. 1.)

4. The full sentence in Marshall's May 12 response to Roberts was, "I regret that I shall not be able to actively participate in the work of the Council, but I am honored to be counted among those who support the unity of free nations." (Marshall to Roberts, May 12, 1955, GCMRL/G. C. Marshall Papers [Retirement, General].)

5. When Roberts, who had resigned from the court on July 31, 1945, was elected to a fifth term as president of the Atlantic Council Committee in 1953, he declared that "he intended to 'work as long as I live, or until we accomplish Atlantic Union, whichever comes first.'" ("Roberts is Re-elected," *New York Times*, November 22, 1953, p. 49.)

6. The *New York Times* had reported in February that "A bipartisan group in Congress urged President Eisenhower today to invite the North Atlantic Treaty Organization powers to a conference looking toward formation of a tighter Atlantic union." ("Congressmen Ask for Tighter NATO," *New York Times*, February 10, 1955, p. 7.)

7. See *Papers of GCM*, 6: 172–76.

8. Streit concluded his May 18 letter to Marshall with his "profound appreciation of your statement yesterday," which he thought would "long warm the hearts of millions all around the Atlantic, and elsewhere." While he hoped "it will not cause you the trouble you foresaw," Streit was "confident" that any negative reaction would fade quickly, and "the honor it will bring you will grow in History." (Streit to Marshall, May 18, 1955, GCMRL/G. C. Marshall Papers [Retirement, General].)

Marshall received letters praising and criticizing his affiliation with the Atlantic Council Committee. (See, for example, Matthews to Marshall, May 19, 1955, and Robinson to Marshall, May 23, 1955, ibid.) He confessed to Thomas L. Robinson, president-publisher of the *Charlotte* [*NC*] *News*, that "Justice Roberts had approached me several times" to join the council while he was still in public service, "and I had always declined." Now, despite C. J. George's opposition due to Marshall's health, he accepted Roberts's request because of the justice's "devoted and, in truth, sacrificial service in the cause of the Atlantic Union." (Marshall to Robinson, June 1, 1955, ibid.)

531

TO WILLIAM M. SPENCER

May 25, 1955
Leesburg, Virginia

Dear Spencer: Thank you for your newsy letter of May 17. George was simply functioning under long-standing procedure in not inconveniencing others when the principal was not available. He was able to work out a most excellent arrangement with General Gay's headquarters. As a matter of fact, Jimmy was given a tour of the Museum of Science and Industry, took in the motion picture "Strategic Air Command", and had a pleasant dinner before leaving on the City of San Francisco [train].[1]

Bradley's position as Chairman of the Committee on Veterans' Affairs will bring him to town several times a year, so our paths will no doubt cross.[2]

Mrs. Marshall has had a very tough winter and spring. Tris' death in December and Stirling Lacy's in March and Allene's two-month illness have taken their toll.[3]

As for Goodpaster, I first met him in Paris in December of 1953 when I was enroute to Oslo for the Nobel Peace Prize. At that particular time, I was both physically and mentally inert and could not develop enough energy to write my speech. However, I knew it had to be done, so just two days before the ceremony I dictated for two and one-half hours without leaving by bed. After I had edited it, I turned it over to Goodpaster to arrange in a more chronological fashion. He did a good job.[4] George tells me that he graduated No. 2 in his class at West Point and is considered one of the bright young men in the Army. This, of course, is evidenced by his appointment as Staff Secretary at the White House. He is an engineer and, after returning from Paris, he had a short tour in San Francisco and, when Pete Carroll died, the President ordered him in as his successor.[5]

When you get to town, I suggest that you give me a ring.[6]

With warmest regards, Faithfully yours,

GCMRL/G. C. Marshall Papers (Retirement, General)

1. Spencer had written to Marshall to explain that because he had been in California, he had not been available to meet Marshall's stepgrandson as he traveled through Chicago, where Spencer lived. (Spencer to Marshall, May 17, 1955, GCMRL/G. C. Marshall Papers [Retirement, General].) C. J. George had begun making arrangements in April for Jimmy Winn to join his family in Japan. (George to Boling, April 16, 1955, ibid.) See pp. 857–58. Molly Winn had written to George on April 12 that friends would "be glad to put Jimmy up and see him on the ship in San Francisco." George assured her on April 25 that he would "see that he gets off in good fashion." (Winn to George, April 12, and George to Winn, April 25, 1955, ibid.) George notified Winn on May 17 that her son had departed from Washington on May 12 via Pennsylvania Railroad and that US Fifth Army commander Lieutenant General Hobart R. Gay had arranged an escort who "entertained" Winn "for twelve hours" in Chicago and put him aboard the train to San Francisco. "He had a pleasant and exciting trip cross-country," George reported to Molly Winn. "I have kept your mother fully informed of his movements and, as you can well imagine, she is gratified that he is on the high seas and on his way to you." (George to Winn, May 17, 1955, ibid.)

2. While in Pasadena, California, Spencer had encountered General and Mrs. Omar N. Bradley, who had been chairman of the President's Commission on Veterans' Pensions since January 14, 1955. "They are delightful people and I was immensely impressed with the General," Spencer commented. "He is indeed a great man." (Spencer to Marshall, May 17, 1955, ibid.)

3. See pp. 868 and 874.

4. "Do you happen to know an Army man named Andy Goodpaster who is now, I believe, an assistant to the President?" Spencer had inquired. (Spencer to Marshall, May 17, 1955, ibid.) See 807 and 817–18.

5. President Eisenhower had named Andrew J. Goodpaster staff secretary and defense liaison officer following the death of General Paul "Pete" Thomas Carroll on September 17, 1954. Carroll had been chief of the Correspondence Section in the Office of the Chief of Staff of General Eisenhower following World War II and military assistant to Eisenhower at SHAPE.

6. Spencer had mentioned that he might be in Washington on May 27. "If so, I would love nothing better than to drop out and drink an Old-Fashioned with you." (Ibid.) See p. 899n1.

532

To Truman Smith

May 28, 1955
Leesburg, Virginia

Dear Smith: Your letter of yesterday and the Report reached me at noon today.[1] As you take off by air Thursday I write immediately and read the suggested chapters of the Report.[2] The last is intensely interesting and I think in style, arrangement and English excellent. I have no other comments.

The State Department's apparent with-holding of your first Report and Ambassador Kennedys cable is not understandable.[3] Elegant language, form and protocol always seem more important than simple facts.

Then another thing which, quite properly, you do not touch on, was the bitter resentment and the serious attacks on you because you recited the facts of the German build up of military power. All these things are an inevitable part of democracy and the consequent political reactions.[4]

I'm glad you are going over. Give my best wishes to von Shell [*Schell*] and his Lady. I would like to have seen him when I was traveling in Germany but in my positions it did not seem wise.[5]

With our best to Mrs. Smith and you. Faithfully yours,

GCMarshall

I am mailing the Report back to you.

GCMRL/Verifax 1117 (Marshall Papers Research File); H

1. Smith, who had returned to Washington from his Berlin assignment after being diagnosed with diabetes in 1939 (see p. 188n3), had served during World War II as an analyst on German military affairs and adviser to Marshall. On May 27, Smith had sent Marshall a draft of his 163-page draft report titled "Air Intelligence Activities, Office of the Military Attaché, American Embassy, Berlin, Germany, August 1935–April 1939, with Special Reference to the Services of Colonel Charles A. Lindbergh, Air Corps (Res.)" with a request that Marshall "examine those portions of my 'Record' in which you have in the past expressed concrete interest or such in which I have quoted you." Smith added that he decided to write "this little narrative" in part as a result of Marshall's numerous requests for him to do so in 1945 and 1946 as well as in 1952 when they saw each other in Cuernavaca, Mexico (see pp. 678–79). (Smith to Marshall, May 27, 1955, GCMRL/G. C. Marshall Papers [Retirement, General].)

2. Smith confided that he was leaving for Germany on June 2 because "old friends in the War Department" had requested that he meet with his "still considerable friends in the German Army," who might be "good contacts for the new group of American officers who are to handle in the future German-American military relations." (Ibid.) Specifically, Smith had requested that Marshall review the sections of his report on "The Inception of Colonel Charles Lindbergh's First Visit to Berlin, July 22–August 2, 1936"; "The General Air Estimate of November 1, 1937"; "Estimate of Lindbergh's Services to the Office of the Military Attaché, Berlin, July 1936–January 1939"; and "Success and Failures of the American Air Intelligence in Germany, August 1935–April 1939." (Ibid. and GCMRL/Verifax 1118 [Marshall Papers Research File].)

Smith predicted that this report would be classified, although he could not "see any legitimate reason" for such action. He planned to place one copy each with the army and air force historical sections and a third in the Lindbergh collection of documents at Yale for use "by legitimate scholars, and future Lindbergh biographers." (Ibid.) Smith's report was eventually published in Robert Hessen, ed., *Berlin Alert: The Memoirs and Reports of Truman Smith* (Stanford, CA: Hoover Institution Press, Stanford University, 1984), 75–166.

3. Marshall is referring not only to Smith's report but also to a cable sent to the State Department on September 22, 1938, by US Ambassador to Great Britain Joseph P. Kennedy in which he summarized a conversation with and a memorandum from Lindbergh warning that "Without doubt the German air fleet is now stronger than that of any other country in the world." (Ibid., 154 and 156.) Kennedy concluded his cable as Lindbergh had his memo: "Germany has such a preponderance of war planes that she can bomb any city in Europe with comparatively little resistance. England and France are far too weak in the air to protect themselves." (Ibid., 155 and 157.) In his 1955 report, Smith indicated that he had found no evidence in State or War Department files that the cable was ever shown to the War Department or, "as Kennedy requested, to the president." (Ibid., 157.)

4. Smith recounted in a 1964 memoir (reprinted in Hessen's book), that after France fell into German hands in June 1940, he had been subjected to "vicious and widespread" attacks in the press accusing him of "being pro-German and anti-American." Smith learned later that Marshall was instrumental in having these attacks cease. (Ibid., 33–36.) On June 30, 1955, Smith sent Marshall a long account of his travels in Germany. "I am so glad," he closed his letter, "that you approved my action in not mentioning my '39, '40 difficulties. After all—personal trials are good for one's soul. I do not regret anything that happened to me. Those years only deepened my loyalty to the US Army (and of course) to you as well." (Smith to Marshall, June 30, 1955, GCMRL/G. C. Marshall Papers [Retirement, General].)

5. In his May 27, 1955, letter Smith mentioned that he planned to see General Adolf von Schell, commander of Germany's Twenty-fifth Panzer Division in 1943, whom both Smith and Marshall had first met when Captain von Schell participated in an advanced officer training from July 1, 1930, to June 30, 1931, while Marshall was assistant commandant and Smith taught military history at the Infantry School at Fort Benning, Georgia. (See *Papers of GCM*, 1: 320, 484, 490, 552, 670.) Smith reported that von Schell "feels that you, and you only were responsible for his release from a British prison in 1946." (Smith to Marshall, May 27, 1955, ibid.) While secretary of state, Marshall had informed Smith on May 26, 1947, that he had forwarded a letter from Smith regarding von Schell's case to the Office of Military Government in Berlin and that he had personally "turned over" a previous letter on the matter to the officials when he stopped in Berlin en route to Moscow in March 1947. (Marshall to Smith, May 26, 1947, GCMRL/G. C. Marshall Papers [Secretary of State, General].) In addition, Marshall Carter, then Marshall's special assistant in the State Department, had asked an official in the Allied Control Council for Germany in an April 18, 1947, memorandum "if there is anything we can do to help" von Schell while emphasizing that there was "no pressure of any kind from the Secretary." (Carter to Draper, memorandum, April 18, 1947, ibid.) After Marshall's death in 1959, von Schell told Smith that Marshall had sent him a personal letter indicating "He had informed the British that he had known me for a long time and he would vouch for me unless there was a concrete case proved against me." ("General Marshall Saves a German General," [1959], GCMRL/Verifax 807 [Marshall Papers Research File].) See p. 920n4.

533

TO ROBERT A. LOVETT

June 16, 1955
Washington, DC

Dear Lovett: I just received your note this morning. It was handed to me as I got in a car at Leesburg, and I am dictating the reply just prior to going over to the luncheon you referred to.[1] I understand perfectly and would have been embarrassed to have you make the trip here in my honor.[2] It was enough of a task for me to motor 37 miles into Washington, where I seldom expose myself to the press.

Speaking of your insecticides, etc., you might be amused by a reaction to mine this morning. As I left, I was looking at our little marigolds, which we cover with pots at night to protect them against the blackbirds which usually are, and now are, rampant. Last year at this time, I came up to the White House—the first time in a long period—and of course was surrounded by the press. I told them that the conversation between the President and myself was for the President to release and not for me. So some fellow came in and said, "What are the prospects for war?". Avoiding the monotony of saying, "No comment", I said the only war I was concerned in was against the blackbirds destroying our marigolds.[3]

I don't know how many letters we got, and I think there was a telegram or two. Both Katherine and I were violently attacked for our injustice to the blackbirds, and I was sent several remedies. So, this time I will have nothing to say on the subject.

I long to see you and Adele and hear your amusing comments. If you do come here, I certainly want to see you at Dodona and give you a restful sleep in our ancient guest room, which sometimes leaks.[4]

With my love to both of you, Affectionately,

P.S. Katherine is not particularly well and is under a heavy strain going to the hospital twice a day to see her sister, who is paralyzed on one side and, at times, very foggy mentally. Today, Katherine is motoring to Richmond with the ashes of Allene's husband, Sterling Lacy, to have them interred in the Tupper lot in Hollywood Cemetery.[5] At the same time, I am going to this luncheon in my honor. Rather a peculiar situation.

I guess that most of the luncheon guests are absent on this bomb trial. The President and several thousand others motored by Leesburg yesterday.[6]

G. C. M.

GCMRL/G. C. Marshall Papers (Retirement, General)

1. Paul G. Hoffman and William C. Foster, who had both left government at the end of the Truman administration, hosted a luncheon at the Mayflower Hotel on June 16 "at which the first copy of 'The Marshall Plan and its Meaning' by Harry Bayard Price will be presented to General George Catlett Marshall." (Invitation, June 16, 1955, GCMRL/G. C. Marshall Papers [Retirement, General].) See pp. 849–50 and 888–90.

2. "The mantle of true greatness which fits you so naturally has, I think been acquired by what you are, and will always be, as well as by what you have accomplished, and it needs no embellishment by anyone," Lovett had written and apologized for not attending because of a prior commitment. (Lovett to Marshall, June 10, 1955, ibid.).

3. The *New York Times* had reported on June 5, 1954, that "General of the Army George C. Marshall, whose big worry just ten years ago was the Normandy invasion, said today that his big problem now is represented by the blackbirds who are 'eating all my marigolds.'" ("Birds Giving Marshall New Invasion Worry," *New York Times*, June 5, 1954, p. 5.) Marshall had attended a June 4, 1954, White House ceremony where the Dutch ambassador "expressed the Netherlands' gratitude by presenting to President Eisenhower a 212-page leather-bound volume entitled 'Road to Recovery'" to mark the end of its participation in the Marshall Plan. ("Dutch Thank U.S. for Aid, Present Book to President," ibid.)

4. Lovett had indicated that he hoped to fly from New York to visit the Marshalls in Leesburg soon to "make sure that you are behaving properly now that the gardening season is in full swing" and mentioned that he continued "to fight a losing battle with bone meal, insecticides," and other products "for the primary position in our household" in his own

gardening efforts. (Lovett to Marshall, June 10, 1955, ibid.) On July 18, Lovett wrote again after a visit with the Marshalls, when he found them "both looking so well in spite of the heat." (Lovett to Marshall, July 18, 1955, ibid.)

5. See p. 874. Hollywood Cemetery overlooks the James River in Richmond, Virginia.

6. The *New York Times* had reported that on June 15 the US would conduct "the first nation-wide Civil Defense test based on an assumed hydrogen bomb attack in which millions of Americans would be killed." During the exercise, the president and at least fifteen thousand "officials and key employees will flee Washington." ("U.S. H-Bomb Alert Today," *New York Times*, June 15, 1955, p. 1.)

534

GIST OF REMARKS FOR A CBS PROGRAM ON THE TENTH ANNIVERSARY OF THE UNITED NATIONS[1] — June 16, 1955, Washington, DC

Question: Do you think membership in the United Nations has served the best interests of the United States?

Answer: Yes, I think membership in the United Nations has served the best interests of the United States.

In the first place, though the Charter undoubtedly has weaknesses which we all deplore, nevertheless, a material change in that Charter in the climate of the present day would, I think, be impossible with the 60-odd nations concerned.

The historic organization was created ten years ago at the close of the modern world's most terrible war. The thoughts of all men were then concentrated on a search for some method or means to divorce war forever from our civilization.[2]

Today, there is a strong, active desire for peace, but some nations now threaten war to obtain their desire, and other nations, like ours, have been forced to arm to maintain the peace.

Under the present United Nations Charter, that organization has saved the world, on occasions, from the tragedy of war. It constitutes a forum where men can state their beliefs before the world and the purposes of their countries. It is a great world safety valve, and no machine which contains explosive power is secure without a safety valve.

Those who deplore the power of the veto and the demoralizing effect it has already had are many, but a cure does not seem practical of accomplishment. Millions demand that the right of veto be stricken from the Charter, but I, personally, do not see a way to manage that at the present time. Some form of restricted use of the veto seems indicated and maybe possible of arrangement. But the great organization must go on.

The very fact that the world's leaders hasten to San Francisco for the 10th anniversary of the birth of the Charter is evidence of its great vitality.[3] The fact that some nations press for membership is another evidence of that vitality.

Here at home, people have had, and in fact are now having, acute feelings over Constitutional issues. The slow, the gradual amendment of our Constitution has been a matter of 166 years. The Charter of the United Nations has been in effect for less than 10. Give it time. Great things, great world changes are not accomplished overnight.

GCMRL/G. C. Marshall Papers (Retirement, Categorical)

1. These remarks were typed from Marshall's handwritten notes. Marshall recorded his comments outside the Pentagon on June 16, possibly for *The American Week*, a half-hour broadcast entirely devoted on June 19, 1955, to the tenth anniversary of the UN. ("Today's TV Programs," *Washington Post*, June 19, 1955, p. J4.)

Senate Foreign Relations Committee chairman Walter F. George (D-GA), whom Marshall had known since at least 1940, had previously asked Marshall to review several documents produced by a special subcommittee which George chaired "in anticipation of an international conference to review the Charter of the United Nations sometime after 1955." He requested that Marshall "discuss in public hearing with us your views and ideas with respect to this matter," particularly Marshall's "comments on the strengths and weaknesses of the United Nations and what changes, if any, in the United Nations system you believe would redound to the benefit of the American people and the cause of peace." (George to Marshall, March 2, 1955, GCMRL/G. C. Marshall Papers [Retirement, General].) Marshall declined this request due to his health and his unfamiliarity with the functioning of the UN since his resignations as secretaries of state and defense. (Marshall to George, March 15, 1955, ibid.)

2. The initial meeting of the United Nations (more formally known as the United Nations Conference on International Organization) was held in San Francisco between April 25 and June 26, 1945.

3. President Eisenhower was scheduled to give the opening address on June 20 at the tenth anniversary meeting of the United Nations in San Francisco, followed on succeeding days by addresses by British Foreign Secretary Harold Macmillan, Soviet Foreign Minister Vyacheslav Molotov, French Foreign Minister Antoine Pinay, and Secretary of State John Foster Dulles. ("Broad Coverage Set for U.N. Fete," New York Times, June 16, 1955, p. 63.)

535

To Paul G. Hoffman

June 23, 1955
Washington, DC

Dear Hoffman: I greatly appreciated the very gracious treatment received at the Marshall Plan luncheon the other day.[1] Your courtesies and expressions were more than any man could hope to receive.[2]

I have been troubled this past week by the manner in which I spoke of your successful administration of the program.[3] Secondary comments are like a correction in the newspaper, relegated to the last page. My feelings then and now are more easily defined as a "case of acute humiliation". Had I known remarks were expected and had Stassen's appearance been on schedule, my tongue would have been prepared to say what was in my mind and heart.[4] You are entitled to, and have, my apology for slipping up. The credit you deserve for a job "well done" is so great it is difficult to express in words, but I know you are aware of my feelings.

I am writing Foster a similar letter.[5]

With many thanks again, and my affectionate regards to Mrs. Hoffman and you,[6] Faithfully yours,

GCMRL/G. C. Marshall Papers (Retirement, General)

1. See p. 886n1. The *New York Times* reported that Presidents Eisenhower and Truman, Dean Acheson, and New York Governor W. Averell Harriman sent Marshall letters of congratulations, which were read at the event. ("Leaders Pay Tribute to Marshall for European Recovery Program," *New York Times*, June 17, 1955, p. 3.) "Through a long lifetime devoted to the good of his country," the president had written, Marshall "has given much to the maintenance of our national security, the preservation of freedom, and the establishment of a just peace in the world. He has demonstrated his greatness as a soldier, as a statesman, as an American citizen dedicated in his country's service." (Eisenhower to Foster, June 15, 1955, DDEL/Dwight D. Eisenhower Papers [Papers as President, President's Personal File 182, Box 935].) "It is personally gratifying to know of your meeting in recognition of his many achievements and particularly of his contribution to free world strength through the Marshall Plan." (Ibid.) Marshall thanked the president on June 22 for his "contribution to the honors which were paid me the other day. . . . As usual, you were most generous and gracious in your expressions of me, and I am duly appreciative." (Marshall to Eisenhower, June 22, 1955, GCMRL/G. C. Marshall Papers [Retirement, General].)

2. The *New York Times* recounted that at the luncheon, "Mr. Hoffman described General Marshall as the most selfless man he had ever known." ("Leaders Pay Tribute to Marshall for European Recovery Program," *New York Times*, June 17, 1955, p. 3.) Hoffman had returned to South Bend, Indiana, as chairman of the board of Studebaker Corporation in 1953.

3. The *Times* reported that "Marshall, still trim and soldierly at 74, came out of retirement long enough today to reminisce about the beginnings of the Marshall Plan." (Ibid.) "Addressing a small audience of officials and newsmen who had been active in Washington when the European Recovery Plan was in operation, General Marshall emphasized that the main thing in all Government activity was not to conceive great plans but to devise effective ways of carrying them through." (Ibid.) "His purpose was not to claim credit for the success of the economic plan that bears his name but to pass the credit on to many former associates." (Ibid.)

4. Harold E. Stassen, representing Eisenhower, made formal remarks to the audience. Since 1953, Stassen had been in charge of American foreign aid programs as director of the Foreign Operations Administration, and in 1955 Eisenhower named him special assistant to the president for disarmament matters, with cabinet rank. ("Harold E. Stassen, Who Sought G.O.P. Nomination for President 9 Times, Dies at 93," *New York Times*, March 5, 2001, p. B6.) "The Marshall Plan for European Recovery has given every evidence of being the right answer at the right time," Stassen told Marshall at the luncheon. "Perhaps you, General Marshall, were the only man to make that answer—the man most qualified by experience and practice and heart." (Address of the Honorable Harold E. Stassen at Luncheon Honoring George C. Marshall on the Occasion of the Release of the Book "The Marshall Plan and Its Meaning," June 16, 1955, GCMRL/G. C. Marshall Papers [Retirement, General].) Stassen asserted that "The immediate objectives of the Marshall Plan were attained more quickly and more surely than many people expected. And we have seen the emergence of a concept new in our history, a possibility of applying the lessons of partnership not just to winning a war or recovering from a war but, even more important for the future, to winning the utmost and ultimate victory of lasting peace." (Ibid.)

5. See p. 76n1. Marshall sent an identical letter to luncheon co-host former deputy secretary of defense William C. Foster, who had been president of the Manufacturing Chemists Association Inc. since 1953. (Marshall to Foster, June 23, 1955, GCMRL/G. C. Marshall Papers [Retirement, General].)

6. Hoffman was married to the former Dorothy Brown. He thanked Marshall on July 1 for his "warm and gracious note," although he admitted that he "was surprised" by Marshall's apology. "As hosts at that luncheon, Bill Foster and I felt somewhat embarrassed by the flattering statements you made about the manner in which we administered the Marshall Plan. If you had said any more, it would have been just too much." (Hoffman to Marshall, July 1, 1955, ibid.) "I do appreciate your kind words," Foster assured Marshall. "I understood the thought and thank you for it. It is a matter of great pride to me to have had your full confidence in some of our mutual endeavors." (Foster to Marshall, June 24, 1955, ibid.)

On July 22, Marshall wrote to Dean Acheson, who had been at a reunion at Yale at the time of the luncheon, to thank him for his "very gracious letter," which had been read at the luncheon. (Marshall to Acheson, July 22, 1955, ibid.; H.) "It is sober historical fact that nothing like the Marshall Plan in grandeur of conception and magnitude of effect has ever occurred in the peacetime relations of independent states," Acheson wrote. "All of us who served under you in any part of this work will never forget the creativeness of those days and the inspiration of your leadership." (Acheson to Marshall, June 14, 1955, ibid.)

536

To Mrs. M. C. Long[1]

June 23, 1955
Washington, DC

Dear Mrs. Long: I have delayed in replying to your letter and request of January 21 because of temporary ill health—virus flu. Also, I have been much puzzled as to just how to approach the subject.[2]

Alanbrooke and I were thrown into intimate contact on many critical occasions from December 1941 to the more or less final settlements at Potsdam in 1945. Always, I found him a great gentleman and a more or less inflexible British military leader.

I counted him as a friend and still do, probably more so now than during the trying war years. He has been a guest in my home at Leesburg, Virginia (while he was a Director of the Hudson's Bay Company).[3]

On the friendly side, I was most impressed by him as a guest of mine when I was entertaining the British Chiefs of Staff with Lord Wavell and his subordinate Chiefs at the restored, ancient Colonial Capital Village at Williamsburg, Virginia.[4] Some swam (the Sea Lord Dudley Pound), some occupied themselves in photography (Lord Wavell), but Alanbrooke, with his field glasses, devoted his time to a study of the Virginia birds in that locality. His persistence and his pleasure in the task were very appealing.[5]

We had been having a very hard time in Washington reaching agreements, but the weekend in Williamsburg with no business discussions cleared the air entirely.[6]

Alanbrooke and I occupied the leading car from the airport over the twenty miles to Williamsburg.[7] At one point, I stopped our car and ushered Brooke out. As the others gathered with us, I announced that they were engaged in a peaceful, and I hoped pleasurable visit. I did not want them to pass by the historic spot that marked the virtual close of our American Revolutionary War—Yorktown—the site of Cornwallis' surrender to General Washington. There was much laughter, but I was somewhat humbled to find one or two who had no recollection of that event.[8] The tremendous happenings on the Continent of Europe had absorbed their memory, along with the record of Cornwallis' services in India.[9]

In summary, I would say that Field Marshal Lord Alanbrooke rendered a tremendous service to his Country by his actions and his wisdom as Chairman of the British Section of the Combined Chiefs of Staff. He was determined in his position, and yet amenable to negotiation. He was generous in his judgments and delightful in his friendship. He worked from a wide experience, particularly in France in the opening phases of the Second World War. He had a hard schooling in the Battles of the Somme in earlier years and had suffered the sudden shock of the highly modernized Nazi Army. This, for a year or more in our earlier negotiations, made it difficult for him to meet our theory and battle inexperience with his practical and rather desperate experience. All of this washed away as the war developed, and we came more and more into mutual understanding.[10]

But the great point was that I felt a complete confidence in his sincerity, his integrity, and his willingness to negotiate toward a solution. Those factors were of vital importance in the waging of a war where two great allies were striving to act in concert.[11] Faithfully yours,

GCMRL/G. C. Marshall Papers (Retirement, General)

1. Marian C. Long had been appointed by the Royal Regiment of Artillery to gather and organize material for a biography of Lord Alanbrooke to be written by British historian Sir Arthur Bryant. (Arthur Bryant, *The Turn of the Tide: A History of the War Years Based on the Diaries of Field-Marshal Lord Alanbrooke, Chief of the Imperial General Staff* [Garden City, NY: Doubleday and Company, Inc., 1957], vii; Arthur Bryant, *Triumph in the West: A History of the War Years Based . . .* [Garden City, NY: Doubleday and Company, Inc., 1959.]) In her January 21 letter to Marshall, Long had explained that she "used to be on Admiral Mountbatten's staff during the war." (Long to Marshall, January 21, 1955, GCMRL/G. C. Marshall Papers [Retirement, General].) Lord Alan Brooke, wartime chairman of the British Chiefs of Staff, became Baron Alanbrooke, of Brookeborough in 1945, and Viscount Alanbrooke in 1946.

2. "I am taking the liberty of writing to you on the advice of Sir Anthony Eden," Long wrote. (Ibid.) "What I seek are intimate pictures of the Field Marshal both at work and at play, which will as it were clothe the bare bones of history, and illustrate the man." (Ibid.) She claimed that the biography would not be published in Alanbrooke's lifetime "but we are collecting material now while people's memories are still green, so as to get an accurate picture of the man in addition to the soldier, as seen by his American and British Colleagues." (Ibid.)

3. Lord Alanbrooke became a director of the Hudson Bay Company in 1948.

4. This trip to Williamsburg took place on May 15 and 16, 1943. Less than a week later, commander in chief of the Eastern Army Field Marshal Sir Archibald P. Wavell was named viscount of Cyreniaca and Winchester, and viceroy of India during the Third Washington Conference (TRIDENT) held from May 12 to 25.

5. On February 26, 1954, Lord Alanbrooke wrote to Marshall to thank him for sending a book about photographing birds. "You could not possibly have sent me anything that would have given me greater pleasure." (Alanbrooke to Marshall, February 26, 1954, ibid.) "I treasure it all the more as being a link with those days when we worked together during the last war." (Ibid.) Admiral of the Fleet Sir Dudley Pound was first sea lord of the British Navy. Other guests at Williamsburg in May 1943 were Air Chief Marshal Sir Charles Portal, chief of the British air staff; Admiral Sir James Somerville, commander in chief of the Eastern Fleet; and Lieutenant General Sir Hastings Ismay. See also Pogue, *Organizer*, 202–3.

6. This and the paragraph above from "I was most impressed" are quoted in a footnote on pp. 506–7 of *The Turn of the Tide*.

7. Frank McCarthy's memorandum to Marshall outlining plans for the trip proposed a flight from Washington to Langley Air Force Base in Hampton, Virginia, followed by a drive to Williamsburg on the Colonial Parkway, "which parallels the York River and is particularly beautiful at this time of year." (McCarthy for the Chief of Staff, memorandum, May 13, 1943, GCMRL/Frank McCarthy Collection [Williamsburg Trip].) The official report of the weekend indicated that Marshall and Lord Wavell rode in one car and Chief

of the Imperial General Staff General Sir Alan Brooke rode in a different car with Air Chief Marshal Portal. (Gerald Horton Bath, "A Report on the Visit of the British High Command to Colonial Williamsburg, May 15th and 16th, 1943," ibid., p. 25.)

8. Major General Charles, Earl of Cornwallis surrendered to George Washington at Yorktown on October 19, 1781, ending the American War for Independence from Great Britain. The driver of Admiral Somerville and General Ismay's car reported that they asked "many questions" on the approach to Yorktown where, the driver mentioned, "'the British didn't do so well,' to which General Ismay replied, 'Ah yes. Let's see, what was the name of that chap who did so badly here?'" (Ibid., p. 30.)

9. Cornwallis had led troops in the Seven Years' War in Europe prior to the American Revolution, and after was named governor-general and commander in chief of India, in 1786.

10. This paragraph, from "determined in his position," is quoted in on pp. 290–91 of *The Turn of the Tide*. "'There was a great charm and dignity about Marshall,' Brooke wrote, 'which could not fail to appeal to one; a big man and a very great gentleman who inspired trust but did not impress me by the ability of his brain.'" Bryant noted that Brooke "continued to be critical of Marshall's strategic outlook," and Marshall felt the same about Brooke's. "The two soldiers met as the protagonists of contending points of view each rooted in his country's military past." (Bryant, *Turn of the Tide*, 290.)

11. "I had heard from Lord Alanbrooke how much he had enjoyed his visit with you to Williamsburg, and he told me how that visit had been a god-send after the strain you had all been under," Long wrote to Marshall in reply. (Long to Marshall, July 8, 1955, GCMRL/G. C. Marshall Papers [Retirement, General].) "Your summary was intensely interesting for it confirms the opinions I have collected to date, and is the more valuable in that it comes from you, an ally, who can judge more dispassionately than one of his own countrymen," she observed. (Ibid.)

Alanbrooke wrote to Marshall on October 14, 1956, to request permission to publish two quotations from this letter. Marshall responded on October 29 that he had "no objection whatever to it being printed. The question really is: Do you object? It was all devoted to you." (Alanbrooke to Marshall, October 14, 1956, and Marshall to Alanbrooke, October 29, 1956, ibid.) See pp. 982–83.

"LAZY AND generally good for nothing," was Marshall's description of himself to Madge Pendleton on July 9. "June was delightful," he reported, but he complained that "July has been fierce, above ninety almost daily" and "rabbits have eaten up most of our garden." On August 1, he told her, they would leave for "Eagles Mere in northern Pennsylvania where we have taken a cottage." (Marshall to Pendleton, July 9, 1955, GCMRL/Xerox 2237 [GCM Family, Personal Letters]; H.)

Joe Hussey, a golf pro at Pinehurst, had suggested Eagles Mere to the Marshalls as a place to escape the summer heat in Leesburg. C. J. George had arranged their rental of Twin Wicks cottage in Eagles Mere Park where, George was confident, the Marshalls would "have a pleasant month." (George to Marshall, memorandum, May 18, 1955, GCMRL/G. C. Marshall Collection [George].) Sergeant Heffner drove them to Eagles Mere on an "exceptionally hot" day, General Marshall reported to C. J. George on August 2. Their "maid seems quite satisfactory," and the four-bedroom cottage was "large" with a verandah and "lots of comfortable furniture." Even in the mountains, however, the weather was "too hot to go out on the Lake or do much of anything outdoors unless you are young and vigorous," but two days later he told Heffner that the evenings were cool and requested that he send a jacket. (Marshall to George, August 2, 1955, GCMRL/G. C. Marshall

Papers [Retirement, General]; GCMRL/William J. Heffner Collection [Correspondence]; both H.) See photo #25.

"I am well now and go down on the beach to watch Gen. M. go in" the lake, Katherine Marshall wrote to Heffner on August 10, and she mentioned that James and Ellen Bruce would spend a long weekend at the nearby Forest Inn. (Katherine Marshall to Heffner, August 10, 1955, ibid; H.) Admiral and Mrs. Harold Stark, who had a summer residence on Lake Carey in Tunkhannock, Pennsylvania, about an hour away from Eagles Mere, also visited with the Marshalls, for lunch on August 24. (Katherine Marshall to Heffner, August 25, 1955, ibid.; H.)

Marshall was clearly excited to accept the invitation of Little League Baseball President Peter J. McGovern to attend the Little League World Series in Williamsport, Pennsylvania. (McGovern to Marshall, August 9, 1955, GCMRL/G. C. Marshall Papers [Retirement, General].) He wrote to Heffner on August 25 and announced that he was "going to the 'Little Base Ball' game ending their annual world series!" (Marshall to Heffner, August 25, 1955, GCMRL/William J. Heffner Collection [Correspondence]; H.) The *New York Times* reported that the Marshalls attended the final game of the Little League World Series on August 26, which "was played before a packed park of 10,000 fans." ("Jersey Nine Bows in Title Final, 4–3," *New York Times*, August 27, 1955, p. 10.)

In October, when Marshall wrote to his goddaughter, he recalled Eagles Mere as the place "we enjoyed more than any locale visited in a long while." (Marshall to Wilson, October 7, 1955, GCMRL/J. Page Wilson Collection.) Indeed, the village became a focus in the Marshalls' plans for the future. See pp. 895, 906, and 907–8. ★

537

To Lieutenant Colonel C. J. George[1] August 8, 1955
Eagles Mere, Pennsylvania

Colonel George— I have hurriedly gone over this and have some questions to ask and comments to make.

In the first place, what is my part? Do I have to appear in part of this. It would be most distasteful in view of the highly complimentary account of me throughout. In fact in reading I grew a little sick of myself.[2]

Cantigny: It seems to me this is far too much talk of me and by me.[3]

Pages 44-45. General Pershing talks of open warfare and an American push thru towards Berlin. He refers to the German, as well as the French and British armies as in a trench warfare stalemate. The later implication then carrys thru to the Meuse-Argonne as being our break out. As a matter for fact the great, very great German offensive of Mch. 21 to April 3*d* was a break out into open warfare; in a way the only one of the war unless we count the German break thru to Chateau Thiery [*Thierry*] and the Marne in the first week in June 1918.[4]

Meuse-Argonne: The initial plan for the Meuse-Argonne was drawn up by *other* officers. I had *no* part in it. I was busy with the St. Mihiel and the *concentration* of *troops for* the Meuse-Argonne. I did not become chief of operations of the First Army until October 10th or 12th. I merely helped before that.[5]

These are hurried notes with no records of any kind available. But to avoid long delays in the preparation of the script I give them off hand. *That must be* emphasized to Skirball.

GCM

See additional notes to be inserted in above

Mrs. Marshall's Comments

Too long. Too much detail in build up. Too much discussion with General Pershing—not sufficient climax

She suggests it *start* with discussion of three officers with General Pershing at Walter Reed.

Then a quick build up from the VMI days to first decision at Quebec, avoiding so much of present details.

Then debate over my staying in Washington or going in command.

Then final decision at Cairo following my reply to Roosevelts question "In your opinion where would you render the most important service to your country" and my reply "Mr. President I cannot evaluate my own services. You'll have to make the decision. I will do cheerfully whatever you decide" He replied "I could not rest easy with you out of Washington.[6]

Finally my long hand message to be radioed to Eisenhower telling him of his selection to command.[7]

GCMRL/G. C. Marshall Papers (Retirement, General); H

1. "You will recall accepting Dr. Robert Hutchins' invitation to participate in the program, 'The Great Contemporaries,'" C. J. George had written to Marshall on August 3. (George to Marshall, memorandum, August 3, 1955, GCMRL/G. C. Marshall Papers [Retirement, General].) See p. 873n3. Skirball had met in Washington with George, who had provided background material for the scriptwriter, and by July 14, George had received a first draft of the script, which he promised to read and send "to the General for his perusal." (Skirball to George, June 22, 1955, ibid.; George to Skirball, July 14, 1955, GCMRL/G. C. Marshall Papers [Retirement, Chronological].) The following are Marshall's notes concerning the first draft of the script for the dramatization of elements of Marshall's life, as well as comments by Katherine Marshall on its dramatic sequencing, all in Marshall's handwriting.

2. In an August 11 letter to Skirball that conveyed the Marshalls' observations on the script, George mentioned that "in view of the highly complimentary account of his activities, it would be distasteful to [Marshall] if he had to appear in the film." (George to Skirball, August 11, 1955, GCMRL/G. C. Marshall Papers [Retirement, General].)

3. For more on the Battle of Cantigny, see *Papers of GCM*, 1: 136–39, 142–43, and Marshall, *Memoirs*, 87–99.

4. For Marshall documents relating to March through early June 1918, see *Papers of GCM*, 1: 136–41.

5. Marshall detailed his activities relating to the Meuse-Argonne offensive in Marshall, *Memoirs*, 138–74.

6. Marshall related this conversation in February 1947 to Robert Sherwood as Sherwood researched his Pulitzer Prize–winning *Roosevelt and Hopkins: An Intimate History*. See *Papers of GCM*, 6: 54. Marshall recounted a more detailed version in *Marshall Interviews*, 343–44.

7. "I have noted the criticisms and suggestions and wish you would express to both General and Mrs. Marshall our sincere thanks for their splendid cooperation," Skirball responded to George's August 11 letter. (Skirball to George, August 22, 1955, ibid.) Marshall sent further comments on a later draft of the script in November. "You write Skirball that the treatment is satisfactory to me except as to the Meuse-Argonne battle," Marshall wrote. "I was not involved in the preliminary planning as I was more or less responsible for the operational conduct of the St. Mihiel battle *then* in progress. I was withdrawn from my connections with the St. Mihiel during its final phase to move the troops to the Meuse-Argonne front. A night movement of some 3 or 500,000 I think. When that was completed I joined the First Army G-3 staff without formal assignment, but on October 10th I was made chief of operations of that army and so continued until its final phase. I was made Chief of Staff of the Army Corps, tho I remained in my post as Chief of Operations until after armistice day." (Marshall to George, November 14, 1955, ibid.) George returned the script to Skirball on November 15 with Marshall's clarifications. On January 23, 1956, Skirball's secretary responded with an apology for the delay and indicated that a revised script would be forthcoming. There is no additional correspondence on this subject in the Marshall Papers, and the editors have not been able to determine if the program was ever produced.

538

To Mrs. John B. Wilson

September 12, 1955
Leesburg, Virginia

Dear Rose— I have a faint recollection of writing to you after I received Page's letter of thanks. Maybe not, so here goes an~~d~~ acknowledgement of your sweet letter of a few days ago.[1]

I was amused at his deliberation about expending his ten dollars.[2] I was not so wise. I was crazy for a clock (imitation) with a cuckoo on or in it. When I finally raised the 1^{00} I bought it despite the protests of Mother. I grew tired of it in one day and I have never forgotten that lesson.

I am well. Just had a four day checkup in the Walter Reed which they claimed proved that the disintergrating [*disintegrating*] process at [*had*?] subsided and I was better off than two years ago, Maybe!

Katherine went with me and had a similar workout.[3] She is much better off than a year ago. Shingles has been her trouble. First ten months and recently a four month siege—eye, arm and hand, the last the most painful.

We leave for Pinehurst about October 20th and are thinking of selling Leesburg place—too big, servants too hard to find for a six months period. In that case we will take a house at Eagles Mere, Penna for the entire summer and early fall, leaving Pinehurst about June 1*st*.[4]

I feel more vigorous now as my virus-flu wears off and perhaps I can drive up to see you and your family.[5]

We may go out to Honolulu, Samoa, New Zeleand, Australia and home via Japan and Honolulu next February. We have the invitation to join the Board of Directors of Pan American. Every year we have declined such trips. Possibly this year we will accept—but I doubt it.[6]

My love to you Rosie, Affectionately,

G.C.M.

GCMRL/J. Page Wilson Collection; H

1. Wilson had sent Marshall a chatty letter about her family, reporting that "our home is a mad house" thanks to all of her children's different interests and personalities. (Rose Wilson to Marshall, September 6, 1955, GCMRL/G. C. Marshall Papers [Retirement, General].)

2. Marshall had written to his godson from Eagles Mere, "May you have more of these birthdays than I have had and each better than the other." (Marshall to Page Wilson, August 26, 1955, GCMRL/J. Page Wilson Collection; H.) "Ten dollars is a lot of money for me," Page wrote after receiving his birthday money from Marshall. "I may get a good baseball glove." (Page Wilson to Marshall, August 29, 1955, ibid.) In her September 6 letter, Rose Wilson had described Page's trip to a sporting goods store, where "He looked at everything, tried out everything, and finally came out with his $10 still in his pocket. He said, 'I can't just blow in $10, I have to think about it more.'" Instead, he "came home and oiled up his old baseball mitt," Wilson wrote. "He's going to wait until he has a desperate need for something special." (Rose Wilson to Marshall, September 6, 1955, ibid.)

3. See next document.

4. See pp. 892–93, 906, and 907–8.

5. Instead, the family visited the Marshalls in Pinehurst in early November, which Rose Wilson recalled in her memoir, *General Marshall Remembered*. (Wilson, *Remembered*, 374–79.) She wrote a few days later that she hoped the Marshalls had "recovered from the onslaught," adding that the children "had a wonderful time" and that seeing the Marshalls "is always one of my greatest pleasures." (Wilson to Marshall, November 14, 1955, GCMRL/G. C. Marshall Papers [Retirement, General].) Page and Thomas Wilson also wrote to thank their hosts and report on their Halloween adventures, which prompted Marshall to reply, "We too had a busy 'Trick or Treat' night. Some 45 young people called on us and left us bankrupt." (Marshall to Page and Thomas Wilson, November 7, 1955, GCMRL/J. Page Wilson Collection; H.)

6. Marshall served on the board of Pan American World Airways in 1949–50 and remained friendly with its president, Juan Trippe. See p. 4n3 and 173n3. In 1954, Marshall had written to Trippe to thank him for his "generous South American proposal" but Marshall had not accepted. (Marshall to Trippe, December 24, 1954, GCMRL/G. C. Marshall Papers [Retirement, General].)

539

To Colonel Edward R. Bowditch — September 16, 1955
[Leesburg, Virginia]

Dear Peter: Katherine and I read your very interesting letter written on Labor Day, and we were especially glad to hear that your lady is making good progress.[1]

I enjoyed your reminiscing because it brings back one of the richest phases of my life.[2] Seriously, I have never given any thought to writing of my association with General Pershing.[3] As a matter of fact, during the past ten years I have received every pressure from many quarters to write my own memoirs. This, I will not do.[4]

Speaking of McCoy, Katherine and I spent five days at Walter Reed having our autumn check, which we do every year before moving down to Pinehurst.[5] On the eve of our departure from the hospital, we had Frances over for dinner, together with a young Lieutenant Colonel named [Vernon] Walters who served me well as a remarkable linguist on many of my overseas trips.[6] Frances is in excellent health and very happy with her work in the Government.

My doctors have advised against any strenuous exercise, so my garden efforts have been very meager.

With our thanks again for your fine letter, and with warmest regards to you both. Faithfully yours,

GCMRL/G. C. Marshall Papers (Retirement, General)

1. Marshall's longtime friend had written that his wife, Agnes, had been "improving in health every day" since they had arrived in San Mateo, California, on July 26. (Bowditch to Marshall, September 5, 1955, GCMRL/G. C. Marshall Papers [Retirement, General].)

2. "Do you remember that inspection or 'look see' trip we took," Bowditch recalled, and cited several anecdotes from an inspection of army installations with General Pershing and others during the winter of 1919–20. "Memories. Oh why did I ever resign from the regular service?" Bowditch wondered. (Ibid.) See *Papers of GCM*, 1: 194.

3. "Have you ever considered writing your reminiscences of General Pershing?" Bowditch had asked. "They would be interesting to all. How I wish you would write your story. From a historical point of view they'd be valuable." (Ibid.) Marshall had, in fact, written a manuscript about his experiences with Pershing during World War I and also kept a diary covering his travels in Europe with Pershing in 1919. They were published together in 1976 as *Memoirs of My Services in the World War 1917–18*. Marshall told his stepdaughter Molly Brown in 1940 that "he had written it while stationed in Washington just after the First World War. He had wanted to put his impressions of that war down on paper while they were still fresh in his mind." Katherine Marshall believed her husband had directed that the manuscript be destroyed but Winn discovered it years after Marshall's death in the attic of the Marshalls' Leesburg home. (Marshall, *Memoirs*, viii.)

4. See pp. 647–48, 648–49, 845–46, and *Papers of GCM*, 6: 638, 661, 663, and 743. See also pp. 878–80, 896–97, 916–17, 931–32, and 947–48.

5. "Lord how I miss Frank McCoy," Bowditch wrote. (Ibid.)

6. See pp. 234–35 and 716–18.

540

To Frank McCarthy

September 20, 1955
Leesburg, Virginia

Dear Frank: Some luscious peaches just arrived from Oregon—thanks to you.

This note, aside from mention of the peaches, is merely to tell you that I have decided to go along with the proposals from Hagan and you regarding my memoirs. I have George working up a draft of my agreement and after I work over it I will advise you accordingly.[1]

My idea is to have the agreement in a single brief form, rather than the present letterwise discursive manner. Also I have not quite decided how to word the portion dealing with release dates. I have in mind the possibility of so arranging the stuff that most of it can be published at a not too distant date in easily readable form. Certain specifically personal phrases can be omitted with only a check reference for them as a sort of supplementary pamphlet.[2]

In this way maybe the VMI can get some financial benefit at an early date.[3] We'll see.

Allene leaves for Warm Springs, Georgia on Monday. Harry DeButts has placed a private (or work) car at her disposal for the trip to Atlanta. An ambulance must do the remainder of the journey.[4]

Katherine and I had a fine month of August in the mountains at Eagles Mere Penna—we'll certainly go back next year, and for longer.[5] Affectionately,

GCM

Remember me to [Darryl F.] Zanuck.

GCMRL/Frank McCarthy Papers (Additions, Box 3); H

1. See pp. 862–64. Marshall Foundation President John C. Hagan Jr. had written to McCarthy on March 31 that he and VMI Superintendent Milton "had a very cordial, interesting meeting with the President," on March 30. (Hagan to McCarthy, March 21, 1955, GCMRL/Frank McCarthy Papers [Additions, Box 3].) "The President said that he would take up with his Cabinet on Friday the idea of trying to expedite the declassification of a lot of papers." (Ibid.) "Arrangements are being made by the Department of State, the Department of Defense, and the National Archives to cooperate fully with VMI and the Foundation subject to applicable provisions of the law," Eisenhower assured Hagan in an April 1 letter. "It is the policy of this Administration to remove security classification from government documents of historical importance at the earliest possible time consistent with the national interest. I am confident that a continuing flow of documents can thus be made available to the Foundation for reproduction." (Eisenhower to Hagan, April 1, 1955, GCMRL/G. C. Marshall Papers [Retirement, General].)

McCarthy and Hagan visited the Marshalls in Leesburg on June 18. (Hagan to Marshall, June 20, 1955, ibid.) "It did me good to see you both looking so well," McCarthy wrote to them on June 23. (McCarthy to Marshall, June 23, 1955, ibid.) "I have asked for additional details and guarantees on the research project which we discussed, since I should not wish to have it on my conscience that I had urged you to do anything which might become a nuisance later on." (Ibid.) On July 15, Hagan sent draft letters from McCarthy and him to C. J. George for comment. "In my opinion, the most important element at this time is the selection of a project director," George responded. (George to Hagan, July 18, 1955, ibid.) See p. 953n2. "As papers of great significance are made available to the project director," he advised, Marshall could "dictate his comments on a tape recording machine. In this way, I think you could maintain a continuity of papers and, most importantly, finish up the General's participation in a relatively short time. You could then have competent help transcribe his comments as footnotes and the tape placed in safe deposit and retained until the statute of time had expired." (Ibid.) See next document. George also recommended that the project director proceed "on a chronological basis, presenting those papers having great significance to the General with the suggestion that he add a footnote. This would give him the opportunity of concentrating on a single issue without any possible deviation. My thought there is that in general conversation it seems to be the normal tendency to sort of roam around the issue at point. . . . Once you get his mind on the subject, there is a natural enthusiasm applied to the work." (Ibid.)

McCarthy's July 27 letter to Hagan reflected George's suggestions, and noted that "General Marshall can set his own date for the release of whatever information he gives the director in his interviews." (McCarthy to Hagan, July 27, 1955, ibid.) McCarthy emphasized that the project director's meetings with Marshall "could be held at any time of day suitable to General Marshall, and it would be clearly understood that there would be no social obligation of any type." (Ibid.) McCarthy's letter also discussed the likelihood of a one-hundred-thousand-dollar grant to the Marshall Foundation "if General Marshall decides he wishes to go ahead." (Ibid.) See p. 917n1. McCarthy's letter was enclosed with one from Hagan, who further explained that "If this sum is made available so that we could start the actual accumulation of various historical data, etc. I will immediately start proceedings on the raising of funds for the building and the endowment for the maintenance and operation of the building." (Hagan to Marshall, August 1, 1955, ibid.)

"I read the attached letters which you received from Jack Hagan," C. J. George wrote to Marshall at Eagles Mere on August 16. "If the Marshall Research Foundation is to be what so many people hope it to be, I feel that your participation is necessary. For the past three years, many men have devoted a lot of their time and energy and have created a plan which is now in the stage of implementation. The fact that one foundation is prepared to contribute $100,000 as an initial sum is, to me, a strong indication of the intention to make the foundation one of the finest of its kind." (George to Marshall, August 16, 1955, GCMRL/G. C. Marshall Papers [Retirement, Chronological].)

2. See pp. 902–3.

3. The Virginia Military Institute Foundation was the base for early fundraising efforts for the Marshall Foundation.

4. See p. 874. Marshall had written to Harry A. deButts (VMI, 1916), president of the Southern Railway System, on September 16 explaining that Mrs. Lacy and her private nurse would require special transportation to Atlanta on September 27. (Marshall to deButts, September 16, 1955, GCMRL/G. C. Marshall Papers [Retirement, Chronological].) Fred Botts, director of admissions at the Warm Springs Foundation, wrote to C. J. George the following day to report that "when meeting Mrs. Lacy at the door she smiled and said she had a pleasant trip." (Botts to George, September 28, 1955, GCMRL/G. C. Marshall Papers [Retirement, General].) See p. 901.

5. See pp. 892–93.

541

To Colonel William M. Spencer

September 28, 1955
Leesburg, Virginia

Dear Spencer: Mrs. Marshall and I were very glad to hear from you and, particularly, to know that you both had a very interesting visit to Europe. Your expressions of Bohlen merely confirmed my opinion of him. As you know, he served with me at State during my tenure, giving an exceptional performance. When I next write him, I will tell him what you said.[1]

From what I can gather, speedy progress is being made on the terms of reference for the Marshall Foundation. I have been told that, if the thing is to be a success, it will take a little more than minor participation on my part.[2] I now have a dictaphone, but your suggestion on the tape recorder appeals to me because it would be a more convenient way of doing the job.[3]

We are both feeling very well and have recently received an encouraging report from General Heaton at Walter Reed.[4] We spent five days there in the early part of this month receiving our autumn check before our move to Pinehurst.

I am making very good use of the chair and, for some reason, it is so clearly identified as being mine that even our guests pass it up.

With our warmest regards to you both, Faithfully yours,

GCMRL/G. C. Marshall Papers (Retirement, General)

1. Spencer had written to Marshall on May 17 that he and his wife, the former Gertrude White, were planning to travel to Russia in late August and early September and had "even applied for a visa to Moscow, foolish as that may seem." (Spencer to Marshall, May 17, 1955, GCMRL/G. C. Marshall Papers [Retirement, General].) Spencer had written again to Marshall on July 26 to say how much he enjoyed "being with you and Mrs. Marshall the other evening" and to update his travel itinerary. (Spencer to Marshall, July 26, 1955, ibid.) "I will, of course, check in at the Embassy anyway, as the State Department has so requested, but it is always nice to have a friend at court if we should get into trou-

ble—which I do not anticipate." (Ibid.) On August 8, Marshall wrote to Charles E. "Chip" Bohlen, who had been US ambassador to the Soviet Union since April 20, 1953, to inform him of the Spencers' upcoming ten-day visit to Russia, "dividing the time between Moscow and Leningrad. They have no favors to ask of you; Spencer merely wanted to be known at the Embassy in case they got into trouble or needed assistance." (Marshall to Bohlen, August 8, 1955, ibid.) Spencer notified Marshall on September 13 "that we are back from a most interesting trip to Russia and Germany. Mr. Bohlen was kind enough to invite us for luncheon." (Spencer to Marshall, September 13, 1955, ibid.) "He is tops in every respect, and this country is fortunate indeed to have him as our representative in Russia." (Ibid.)

Marshall also wrote on September 28 to thank Bohlen for his hospitality to the Spencers: "They were deeply appreciative, and he was quite enthusiastic about you." (Marshall to Bohlen, September 28, 1955, ibid.; H.)

2. See pp. 862–64, previous document, and 902–3.

3. Spencer had offered to give Marshall a tape recorder, which C. J. George had already determined would be helpful as Marshall coordinated with the as-yet undetermined director of the George C. Marshall Foundation. (See previous document n1.) "I am sending off today to Pinehurst a Bell & Howell tape recorder," Spencer wrote on October 7. "Once you get the hang of the thing, you can sit back and relax and talk into the microphone at your leisure." (Spencer to Marshall, September 13, 1955, and October 7, 1955, ibid.) Marshall wrote to thank him on December 24, having "inadvertently mislaid" Spencer's letter. "I appreciate your gift of the tape recorder and, since I now have the theory of its operation, I will give it a practice run when I next dictate." (Marshall to Spencer, December 24, ibid.) See pp. 967–68.

4. Major General Leonard D. Heaton, a surgeon, had been commanding general at Walter Reed Army Medical Center since April 1, 1953.

542

To Major General Arthur R. Wilson — October 7, 1955, Leesburg, Virginia

Dear Wilson— I had clean forgotten my part in the maneuvers you described in such detail regarding the Truman Committee. Some portions, I still do not recall. Too much was evidently happening.[1]

Your write as though you were no longer engaged in traveling abroad, and had settled down.[2]

Give my best to your wife, and believe me always,[3] Faithfully yours,

GCMRL/G. C. Marshall Papers (Retirement, General); H

1. Wilson had written to Marshall on September 22 and enclosed a copy of a five-page letter he had sent to West Virginia Senator Harley M. Kilgore concerning a recent interview in which the senator discussed the origin of the Senate Special Investigating Committee, popularly known as the Truman Committee, on which Kilgore and Wilson had served. (Wilson to Marshall, September 22, 1955, GCMRL/G. C. Marshall Papers [Retirement, General].) In his letter, Wilson recalled that while working for Marshall in January 1941, he had suggested "'we try to get the President to appoint a committee to investigate the war as the war goes on, while the actors are still alive and the records are available.'" (Wilson to Kilgore, September 16, 1955, ibid.) Marshall agreed and Wilson planted the idea with his friend and President Roosevelt's adviser Harry Hopkins. Wilson proposed Senator Harry S. Truman as chairman of this committee. because he "had always been active in the military since World War I, was presently a colonel in the Reserve and was a profound student of Military History and especially familiar with investigations following the Civil War, Spanish American War, and World War I." (Ibid.)

2. Marshall and Wilson, who owned the Mount Ida olive grove near Oroville, California, had maintained sporadic communication since World War II. On November 3, 1953, Wilson had written that he had "spent weeks in Egypt, Greece and since May have been to every country in Europe" studying the culture of growing olives and noted that everywhere he traveled he saw "the great benefits of 'the Marshall Plan.'" (Wilson to Marshall, November 3, 1953, ibid.)

3. Ellen Kormann Arends was Wilson's wife. (Arthur Wilson, "Ex-general, Dead," *New York Times*, August 12, 1956, p. 85.)

AS 1955 PROGRESSED, Marshall continued to reach out to longtime friends but often found his efforts frustrated. The Marshalls had encountered Lorenzo Gasser at Walter Reed during their semiannual checkups, and on September 12, Marshall wrote that he had been "very glad" to see Gasser because he "seldom" got "to town. As a matter of fact, I avoid it because it always involves me in a number of engagements with people I would rather not have to trouble with." Nevertheless, he had several friends who lived in the same Washington apartment building as Gasser, and Marshall wondered whether "some day" he "could drive into town and, if agreeable to you, make your suite my headquarters while I undertook these brief calls." (Marshall to Gasser, September 12, 1955, GCMRL/G. C. Marshall Papers [Retirement, General].)

M. L. Spilman had notified Marshall on May 2 that "General and Mrs. John McAuley Palmer both are now residing here permanently." (Spilman to Marshall, May 2, 1955, GCMRL/G. C. Marshall Papers [Retirement, Chronological].) Spilman had learned the news from Anne Peek, "who was a neighbor of yours many years ago at Leavenworth." (Ibid.) Peek had reported that the Palmers were "in very poor health, but are able to get around a bit. She says that General Palmer is perpetually grateful for your birthday remembrances and any communications he gets from you." (Ibid.) "I will be delighted to see you; your plan will work," Gasser assured Marshall on September 16. (Gasser to Marshall, September 16, 1955, GCMRL/G. C. Marshall Papers [Retirement, General].) There is no evidence that the visits occurred before John McAuley Palmer died on October 26 and Gasser on October 29. See pp. 906–7. Marshall later wrote to Gasser's brother that when he recently saw his friend of "many years," Lorenzo Gasser had "appeared at that time to be feeling well and, of course, his death came as a shock." (Marshall to Earl Gasser, November 14, 1955, ibid.)

Marshall's plans may have been disrupted by the news from the Warm Springs Foundation that it could not treat Allene Lacy's paralysis. (See p. 899n4.) On October 7, Marshall wrote to Rose Page Wilson that he and his wife were "rushing to Pinehurst early next week to superintend her arrival at a convalescent home there." (Marshall to Wilson, October 7, 1955, GCMRL/J. Page Wilson Collection.) They were in Pinehurst on October 11 in time to meet her train. See p. 914. ★

543

To John C. Hagan Jr.

October 20, 1955
Washington, DC[1]

Dear Hagan: In your letter of August 1, enclosing a letter from Frank McCarthy dated July 27, you requested my concurrence in your plans for the George C. Marshall Foundation.[2] As I mentioned to you in subsequent conversations, I will be very glad to cooperate with the Foundation, subject to the following understanding:

1) That the selection of the project director will be the responsibility of the Board of Directors of the Foundation without reference to me for comment or concurrence.

2) That the selection and processing of the papers which are made available to the Foundation will be the responsibility of the project director and his staff working under the guidance of the Board of Directors and in accordance with the rules of procedures established as a result of the President's memorandum of April 1, 1955.[3]

3) That title to my personal papers will pass to the Foundation upon my death.

4) That additional information will be provided by means of recorded answers to specific questions prepared by the project director, or by direct discussion with the project director, or otherwise.[4]

5) That any statement or comment by me regarding personalities or events of a personal nature will be made available to the public only with my written consent or, subsequent to my death, with the approval of the Board of Directors of the Foundation.

6) That any funds accruing to the Foundation from commercial publication or project connected with material relating to me will remain with the Foundation.[5] Faithfully yours,

GCMRL/Frank McCarthy Papers (Additions, Box 3)

1. This letter was typed on Marshall's Pentagon stationery but on October 11 the Marshalls had moved to Pinehurst. See previous editorial note and pp. 910–11.

2. See pp. 897–99.

3. See p. 898n1.

4. See pp. 898n1, 899–900, 960–61, and 967–68.

5. A handwritten note to Hagan attached to a rubber-stamped copy of this letter in the Marshall Foundation 1955 correspondence file says "We are leaving for Pinehurst Tuesday for the winter. If par. 6 is not in the exact terms you would like let me know. *GCM*" (GCMRL/GCMRF Archives [General Correspondence 1951–62, Box 1].) Hagan replied on October 21 that "These conditions are acceptable to me as President of the Foundation and I am confident that this will be concurred in by the Board." (Hagan to Marshall, October 21, 1955, GCMRL/G. C. Marshall Papers [Retirement, General].) "I am confident that I am expressing the feeling of the entire Board of Directors of the George C. Marshall Foundation for your magnanimous contribution to this project." (Ibid.)

On October 28, M. L. Spilman forwarded a copy of Marshall's letter to Frank McCarthy at Marshall's request. "I think General Marshall's letter is excellent, but we must remember that his first qualification places a tremendous responsibility upon us," McCarthy wrote to Hagan on November 22. "The entire success or failure of this project will depend upon selecting the man who is to conduct interviews with General Marshall." (McCarthy to Hagan, November 22, 1955, GCMRL/Frank McCarthy Papers [Additions, Box 3].) "I would like to ask the special privilege of meeting and talking to the candidates before a selection is made. My reason for this is that I have had the opportunity to know and understand General Marshall better than almost anybody around him," McCarthy continued. "Since the General will not himself even make a comment on the prospective director, I think we must exercise extraordinary care in his selection." (Ibid.) See p. 953n2.

544

STATEMENT FOR *COLLIER'S* MAGAZINE[1]

October 26, 1955
Pinehurst, North Carolina

There was some comment when the Nobel Peace Prize for 1953 was awarded to me, a soldier. Many people saw in this a serious inconsistency. To me, it did not appear remarkable for a soldier to be regarded as a worker for peace. They know much better than others what war is really like; and I, as Chairman of the American Battle Monuments Commission, have a constant reminder of its aftermath. One of my duties is to supervise American military cemeteries overseas where Americans have lost their lives in battle. The cost of war is constantly spread before me in huge ledgers whose columns are gravestones.

No one can accurately foresee the future, but one vast fact about another world war appears clear to me. It is this: even the victorious power will stand or totter amidst its own ruins with little or no strength left to rehabilitate itself or to assist its neighbors. It will be an empty triumph of inheriting the responsibility for a shattered world.

It is my hope to protect our future against the agonies and miseries of war. We should concentrate now, with earnestness comparable to our zeal in time of war, on finding peaceful solutions to the world's critical problems. Peace must be more than a negative condition that is merely the absence of armed hostilities.

The present period in some respects is even more critical than the recent war years. Problems are different, but no less vital to the national security than those when the fighting was fiercely active. But we no longer display the intensity, the unity of purpose that marked our war efforts. Because immediate peril is not plainly visible many of our people have become indifferent to the dangers to our security. Yet our attitude and our actions as we face international problems will largely determine our future. The attitude of the spectator is not enough. Spectators of life are not those who will fight to retain their liberties.

There is no shortage of people who deplore, but there always has been a shortage in the number who will do something. "Man is born to act," said the late Mr. Justice Holmes. "To act is to affirm the worth of an end, and to affirm the worth of an end is to create an ideal." The attitude of the mere spectator—and I say this with all earnestness—is the culminating frustration of man's nature.[2]

There are many ways in which peace can be promoted. For the moment, the maintenance of peace in a very hazardous world must depend to a large degree on military power, together with Allied cohesion. But the maintenance of large military forces for an indefinite period is not a promising basis for policy. I regard the present dangerous situation as a special one, which naturally dominates our thinking. However, it should not be made the basis for our reasoning toward a condition promising a long continued peace. A strong military posture is necessary today. How long it will continue so I am not prepared to estimate, but I am sure it should not govern our long-term effort toward a peaceful world.

The great fundamental in our search for durable peace lies in the educational world. The schools have a key part to play in this quest. There should be a searching study of the factors that have gone into the breakdown of peace in the past. Our schools, and I do not mean our colleges only, but more especially our high schools, should have courses to instruct young people in the sequence of events and circumstances which have marked the oncoming of war. Students should learn, so far as possible without national prejudices, what has led to past tragedies for mankind.[3] I am certain that a solution of the general problem of peace must rest on an unprejudiced and basic understanding on the part of free peoples.

We now need, and must have, the deepest and nearest approach possible to a scientific study of what has caused the wars of the past, and what steps or conditions or attitudes might have averted at least some of them.

Closely related to deep study by millions of individuals into the reasons why peace so often has been shattered, is the attitude of nations toward one another. If we educate enough of our individuals in the fundamentals of peace and security, frictions and irritations between countries will rapidly diminish. When millions of men and women the world over realize, from their studies, that war is not a necessary activity for survival in this modern world, we will be on the road toward its abandonment.

A third course of action for development of lasting peace is intelligent concern for the people who live under sub-normal conditions. Democracy must be presented to them as a force holding within itself the seeds of unlimited progress for them, and for all mankind. Remember always that democratic principles, good-will among men and nations, do not thrive on hunger, ignorance or disease.

The only good that can be said of war is that it may have been the lesser of two great evils. It is better than appeasement of aggression because appeasement encourages the very aggression it seeks to prevent. And it is better than submission to tyranny and oppression because, without freedom and respect for human dignity, life would not be worth living.

Unless faced with these two terrible alternatives, we should concentrate resolutely on finding peaceful solutions for world problems. They must be practical and not emotional. We should support to the full every existing instrument for building a more stable world. So long as there is a forum such as the United Nations for open discussion of international disputes, the United States should be a participant. So long as there remains a conference table around which nations can gather, the United States should be the first to attend and the last to retire.

There are no limits to the blessings of peace and progressive civilization. It is not impossible for us to attain both. I have suggested a few areas for close attention. Underlying achievements in these areas, and giving vitality to our efforts in them, is a great but intangible essential which I cannot describe better than to call it spiritual regeneration. This is a condition that must come, if we are to maintain peace, from within our hearts as individuals and as nations. Sympathetic understanding, patience, tolerance of differences, generosity will mark the relations of man to man and nation to nation if a spiritual regeneration dominates the world.

GCMRL/G. C. Marshall Papers (Retirement, Speeches, Statements, and Writings)

1. Journalist Theodore H. White initially had contacted Marshall on June 22 and recalled their meeting in 1948 prior to White's departure for Europe as a correspondent. "You said then, that the Russians would never negotiate seriously with us so long as they thought our civilization was in decay and theirs firm; therefore, we had to have the Marshall Plan to firm up Western Europe and force the Russians to take us seriously and, if we were resolute, some day we might force the Russians to bargain realistically." (White to Marshall, June 22, 1955, GCMRL/G. C. Marshall Papers [Retirement, General].) "Now," White suggested, "the strategy conceived in 1947 is finally paying off." (Ibid.) This was probably a reference to the "thaw" in cold war relations that had accompanied the July 1955 Geneva Summit Conference. White explained that he was now a contributing editor of *Collier's* magazine, which was planning "to publish a series of conversation pieces with those people in American life whose thinking probes the frontiers of our problems." (Ibid.) "There are few people in the world whose opinion counts on the strategic choices that lie ahead. Yours, pre-eminently, is an opinion that the country needs." (Ibid.) Marshall made a note to C. J. George at the top of the letter: "Tell him not now—but I'll let him know a little later." (Ibid.)

On October 4, *Collier's* Associate Editor Theodore Strauss wrote that the magazine planned a Christmas issue with a central theme of peace and was requesting brief essays from several Nobel Peace Prize winners for an honorarium of one thousand dollars. On October 13, James C. Derieux, the magazine's senior editor in its Washington office, sent C. J. George a draft of "the kind of statement Collier's would like signed by General Marshall. It is made up of selections from the several speeches you showed me. Words have been changed only for the purpose of organizing the General's paragraphs as he had written them from time to time." (Derieux to George, October 13, 1955, ibid.) George sent a draft to Marshall on October 19, which Marshall edited heavily in his own hand. A clean, typed version was given to Derieux on October 26. "Peace Must Be Waged," by General George C. Marshall, appeared in the December 23, 1955, issue of *Collier's* magazine.

2. US Supreme Court Justice Oliver Wendell Holmes, 1902–32, included the following in his June 28, 1911, speech delivered at the fiftieth anniversary of his Harvard University graduation: "Man is born a predestined idealist, for he is born to act. To act is to affirm the worth of an end, and to persist in affirming the worth of an end is to make an ideal." (*Speeches by Oliver Wendell Holmes* [Boston: Little, Brown, 1934], 96–97.) Marshall quoted the same passage in a speech given at Princeton University on February 22, 1947. See *Papers of GCM*, 6: 47–50.

3. "I have always been deeply interested in history and feel that, today, the subject is not being covered adequately in our schools," Marshall had written in 1953 to a couple who were "trying to find a way to make the world and its problems vitally important" to their two young sons. Marshall advised them that "There is a serious failure to tie up cause with effect. A date is usually of little importance, but the future effect of the occurrence marked by that date is the important consideration." (Housers to Marshall, February 22, 1953, and Marshall to Housers, April 29, 1953, GCMRL/G. C. Marshall Papers [Retirement, General].)

545

To General Charles D. Herron — November 7, 1955
Pinehurst, North Carolina

Dear Herron: Many thanks for your letter of October 27 and my letter of ancient vintage in which I make a postscript comment on Slappey. I will make mention of the letter to him at Christmastime, but I think you should decide on the disposition of my letter to you.[1]

It was a source of regret to me not to be able to come up for Palmer's interment, but I find it mandatory to preserve my health, which is seemingly good at the moment.[2] Long trips are arduous and it takes me several days to recuperate. I wrote Maude a letter and, in addition, had my Aide call Mary.[3] Gasser's passing certainly came as a surprise, because we exchanged letters a few weeks ago and he made no mention of his health.[4]

The decision to sell the Leesburg place wasn't an easy one to make, but it became evident that it was too much house for just the two of us, and the domestic situation made the problem more acute.[5] We will spend most of the year at Pinehurst and are hoping for long summers at Eagles Mere, Pennsylvania.[6] While this may lessen the chances of our getting together, I will keep in touch with you on my infrequent visits to the city.

Katherine joins me in affectionate regards to Louise and you. Faithfully yours,

GCMRL/G. C. Marshall Papers (Retirement, General)

1. "I came across the enclosed a few days ago in sorting out some old papers and thought of sending it on to the Slappeys, but it occurred to me that you might want to send it to them yourself," Herron had written in a postscript to his letter. (Herron to Marshall, October 27, 1955, GCMRL/G. C. Marshall Papers [Retirement, General].) Marshall apparently returned the "letter of ancient vintage" to Herron. Marshall had known Eugene N. Slappey since at least 1934, when both were instructors with the Illinois National Guard. (Slappey to Marshall, May 14, 1934, GCMRL/G. C. Marshall Papers [Illinois National Guard].) By the 1950s, Slappey and his wife, Katherine, lived in Leesburg, Virginia. (Katherine Slappey to Marshall, August 26, 1956, GCMRL/G. C. Marshall Papers [Retirement, General].)

2. See pp. 176 and 354–55. General John McAuley Palmer's funeral took place in the chapel at Fort Myer on October 27. "He was buried near General Pershing and the day was the most perfect of October days," Herron reported. (Herron to Marshall, October 27, 1955, ibid.) Palmer, Herron continued, "was a faultless character and he was an outstandingly useful officer." (Ibid.)

3. Maude was General Palmer's widow and Mary Palmer Rockwell, his daughter.

4. See p. 901. "Some ten days before his death I went to see" Gasser, Herron wrote to Marshall on November 13, "in his apartment and we had a very pleasant talk, in the course of which he showed me your letter, which pleased him very much. He said that he had answered it, but you had not yet replied." In his October 27 letter, Herron mentioned that Gasser "was not well enough to come" to Palmer's funeral. (Herron to Marshall, October 27, 1955, ibid.) On November 13, Herron wrote "more of the passing of that staunch friend and gallant soldier 'Cap' Gasser." (Herron to Marshall, November 13, 1955, ibid.) "As you know, Gasser got pneumonia in England when he went over during the war and never was the same afterwards, as it recurred several times later, each time leaving his heart and lungs weaker. About a year ago he had a severe heart attack and last spring they discovered that he had TB," Herron continued, and detailed his interactions with Gasser during his final

days. "He was a man of enormous courage and complete integrity and I mourn him, as I know you do!" Herron concluded. (Ibid.)

5. See pp. 907–8 and 943n5.

6. See pp. 892–93.

546

To General Walter Bedell Smith — November 9, 1955, Pinehurst, North Carolina

Dear Smith— I appreciated your note but was disturbed by you reference to your state of health. Its no use advising or cautioning you, I know too well, and you are happier and more content when fully occupied, regardless of ailments. But please do be careful and not bring down the house on your head.[1]

Mrs. Marshall's sister has had another stroke, slight but devestating none the less. The strain on Katherine is too severe and she is wearing down. I, as usual, am worthless with circumstances and unable to curb Katherine's efforts.[2]

The weather here has been perfect. My love and affection to Norry.[3] As ever—

GCMarshall

Don't answer.

DDEL/Walter Bedell Smith Papers; H

1. Walter Bedell Smith had left government service after thirty-seven years on October 1, 1954, from his position as undersecretary of state and entered private industry as vice president of American Machine and Foundry Company. On August 24, while the Marshalls were vacationing in Eagles Mere (see pp. 892–93), C. J. George wrote to a friend in New York that he was "surprised to learn that General Smith had taken ill and that surgery was necessary." (George to McGlincy, August 24, 1955, GCMRL/G. C. Marshall Papers [Retirement, General].) As soon as he returned to Leesburg, Marshall wrote to Smith that he hoped "all goes well and that you are an obedient patient—which I very much doubt." (Marshall to Smith, September 1, 1955, ibid.) Marshall wrote again on October 15 to say he was "much distressed to miss you two the other day" after the Smiths had driven to Leesburg "on the off chance that we might find you at home," Smith replied on November 7. "I am a good deal less than fit, but I have so much to do that I can't seem to stop." (Marshall to Smith, October 15, 1955, DDEL/Walter Bedell Smith Papers; Smith to Marshall, November 7, 1955, GCMRL/G. C. Marshall Papers [Retirement, General]; both H.)

2. See pp. 874, 899n4, and 901.

3. Nory was Mary Eleanor Smith's nickname.

547

To Thomas J. Watson — November 12, 1955, Pinehurst, North Carolina

Dear Tom: I have purposely delayed answering your interesting letter until we received the package you mentioned. It arrived Wednesday morning, and Katherine and I are delighted with this lovely remembrance of our Silver Anniversary from Jeannette and you. Many, many thanks for your gracious thought of us. It is truly beautiful.[1]

We were very glad to have the news of your activities and to be reassured that you both are in fine fettle.[2]

We had a delightful month at Eagles Mere, Pennsylvania, this summer and enjoyed it so much that we are seriously considering spending the torrid months there in the future. We have decided that the Leesburg place is more than the two of us need, so it will be up for sale when we return there in the spring. We plan to spend most of each year here and then go North for the few really hot months.[3]

The one dark cloud on our horizon has been the serious illness of Katherine's sister following a stroke in the early spring. She is now in a nursing home near here, where she has recently suffered another stroke and is steadily sinking.[4] Katherine feels her duty to such an extent that I fear her attendance on Allene is producing a serious physical and emotional strain upon her, but there seems to be no solution to the problem.

I am well—but lazy. It seems that to be lazy is the only way I can stay well.

Katherine joins me in sending you both our thanks, again—and our warm and good wishes. Faithfully yours,

GCMRL/G. C. Marshall Papers (Retirement, General)

1. "Jeanette and I saw in the newspaper the other day a nice picture of both of you taken in your garden at the time of your silver wedding anniversary," Watson had written on October 27. (Watson to Marshalls, October 27, 1955, GCMRL/G. C. Marshall Papers [Retirement, General].) He also mentioned that they were sending "a little gift as a remembrance of this occasion and as a token of our friendship for both of you." (Ibid.)

2. Watson reported that he and his wife had spent the summer in New Canaan, Connecticut, and Vermont. (Ibid.)

3. See pp. 895–96. "Dodona Manor, historic Colonial home of Gen. and Mrs. George C. Marshall, is being offered for sale," the *Washington Evening Star* had reported on October 19. ("Marshall to Sell Dodona Manor," *Evening Star*, October 19, 1955, p. D-8.) The next day the *Washington Post* noted the "asking price of $75,000." ("Marshall Plans Sale of Home," *Washington Post*, October 20, 1955, p. 59.) See pp. 909–10 and 947n5.

4. See pp. 901 and 910–11.

548

FOREWORD FOR *SOLDIER: THE MEMOIRS OF MATTHEW B. RIDGWAY*[1]

November 19, 1955
Pinehurst, North Carolina

I first knew General Ridgway as a young Captain in China, and later at the celebrated Infantry School at Fort Benning, Georgia, where I came to know him intimately.[2] I found him on the General Staff of the Army when I was sent to Washington in 1938.[3]

As the designated Chief of Staff in May 1939, he was a member of my staff on a military mission to Brazil.[4]

As our preparations to meet the threat of war progressed, he became the commander of the celebrated 82nd Airborne Division, which he led to fame in the invasion of France and in the desperate fighting of the Battle of the Bulge.[5]

General Ridgway has firmly established himself in history as a great battle leader. The advance of his Army Corps to the Baltic in the last phase of the war in Europe was sensational to those fully informed of the rapidly moving events of that day. His campaign in Korea will be rated as a classic of personal leadership. As Supreme Commander of the North Atlantic Treaty Organization in Europe, he did a splendid job. And he culminated his military career as Chief of Staff of the Army.[6]

I have not read his manuscript, but I am confident of the integrity of his account.[7]

GCMRL/G. C. Marshall Papers (Retirement, General)

1. Ridgway, who had retired as army chief of staff in June 1955, had written to Marshall on November 7 that he was "polishing up some memoirs which were worked up between retirement and taking over my new post" as chairman of the board of trustees at the Mellon Institute of Industrial Research in Pittsburgh. He asked Marshall to write a foreword for the book. (Ridgway to Marshall, November 7, 1955, GCMRL/G. C. Marshall Papers [Retirement, General].) Marshall was "complimented" by the request, he replied on November 19, and if the draft "is not to your taste," he encouraged Ridgway to "recommend alterations" or "abandon the idea altogether." (Marshall to Ridgway, November 19, 1955, ibid.)

2. Ridgway had commanded a company of the Fifteenth Infantry in Tientsin, China, from July 25, 1925, to May 1, 1926. He had been a student at the Infantry School during the 1929–30 academic year.

3. Ridgway's memoirs state that in 1937 he "reported to the Presidio of San Francisco as G-3 [operations] for the Fourth Army." (Matthew B. Ridgway, *Soldier: The Memoirs of Matthew B. Ridgway* [New York: Harper & Brothers, 1956], 46.) His next assignment was "to report to the War Plans Division in Washington" in the summer of 1939. (Ibid., 47.)

4. Marshall and his staff embarked for a goodwill tour to Brazil on May 10 and returned on June 20, 1939. See Ridgway, *Soldier*, 47–48, and *Papers of GCM*, 1: 715–20.

5. At Ridgway's suggestion, Marshall revised this paragraph in order to clarify that Major General James M. Gavin (USMA, 1929) was in command of the Eighty-second Airborne Division during the Battle of the Bulge. (Ridgway to Marshall, November 28, 1955, GCMRL/G. C. Marshall Papers [Retirement, General].) Marshall made a note at the bottom of the letter: "Done and mailed." (Ibid.)

6. See pp. 309n1, 715n1, and 822n1.

7. "I am deeply honored that you should honor my request and write a foreword for the memoirs I plan to publish," Ridgway replied on November 25. (Ridgway to Marshall, November 25, 1955, ibid.) "No military man since George Washington has, I think, made such a contribution to our nation or had such an enduring impact on the Officer Corps of our military establishment as you. Certainly, of those with whom I was privileged to serve, no one so profoundly influenced my thinking and service as you, my wonderful father, and General Frank McCoy." (Ibid.)

549

To Mrs. John White Pendleton — December 9, 1955
Pinehurst, North Carolina

Dear Madge: I was both amused and delighted with your notice of election as Secretary of the Ladies Auxiliary. Amused because of your reaction to me.[1] That is really fine and I know John must be proud of your success, which of course means much to him in his work. I can still picture his father passing the plate in church during my cadet days.[2]

Congratulations.

Katherine is off at the Convalescent Home where she goes each morning.[3] We are flying up to Washington and the Walter Reed ~~of~~ the 14*th* for three days largely on Katherine's account though I will come in for a check up.

Molly and the family arrive this afternoon. K. has worked herself to death getting their house in order but she labors under a complete lack of knowledge of their plans, whether they will be here a few days or a month, etc. I know they saw you, at least their post cards indicated that intention.[4]

I do hope you have a delightful family Xmas. K., incidentally, has not even be able to get started on her Xmas packages, selection of presents, etc.

My love to you Madge, and the family. Affectionately,

GCM

Fine that Tupper is doing so well.[5]

GCMRL/Xerox 2237 (GCM Family, Personal Letters); H

1. "I can't wait another minute to write to you of my major social triumph down here," Madge Pendleton had written on December 6 to Marshall from Tuscaloosa, Alabama, where John White Pendleton had become assistant to the president of the University of Alabama. "I have just been made secretary of the Ladies Auxiliary of the Episcopal Church, one of its four officials!!! In Washington, the equivalent would be appointment to the Cabinet. Not bad, do you think, having been here just over a year, having the few attributes with which you accredit me and a Yankee to boot?" (Pendleton to Marshall, December 6, 1955, GCMRL/G. C. Marshall Papers [Retirement, General].)

2. See p. 43n1.

3. See next document.

4. "I have just written to Mrs. Winn asking them all to come over here for the day while Molly and family are there," Pendleton added in a postscript. It will be such fun for us and I certainly hope they can manage it." (Ibid.) Colonel James Winn's mother, Ellene Winn, lived in Birmingham, Alabama.

5. Madge's son—who was also Katherine Marshall's grandson—Tupper Brown was a student at Lawrenceville School just outside Princeton, New Jersey.

550

To Queen Frederica of the Hellenes — December 13, 1955[1]
Pinehurst, North Carolina

Your Majesty: I was surprised and much ~~flattered~~ complimented to receive your lengthy personal discussion of the situation in Greece, Syracuse [*Cyprus*] and Turkey and the serious reactions resulting. I was also much distressed to learn of the reactions of the Greek people with regard to the United States, though probably the Turkish reactions are of much more serious consequence. You were very good to have written to me, and I deeply appreciate your doing so.[2]

Since receiving your letter, I have been scratching my head trying to decide just how I can be of help without violating your confidence, and also without inflaming Dulles who you tell me has not been too friendly on his part.[3] You may be sure that point of view here officially will receive my earnest consideration.

Mrs. Marshall and I came south early this year, and suddenly, because of her sister's serious ~~state~~ condition. She, the sister, suffered several strokes last March.

We got her accepted at the famous Warm Springs Sanatorium in Georgia that Mr. Roosevelt built. When they there found they could do nothing for her, we had to vacate her room in a week and had her moved to a convalescent home here, and had to hurry south to meet her train.[4] The strain of spending most of her mornings daily at the hospital, or home, has been very exhausting for Mrs. Marshall. Incidentally, she is there now as I am writing.

We had an unusually hot summer but escaped to a cottage in the Pennsylvania mountains in August.[5]

Mrs. Marshall's daughter with her Army Colonel husband and three children are due here today, returning he from Korea and all of them from Japan.[6] Much excitement, of course.

I, as usual, am lazy and good for nothing, declining about two invitations a day to speak somewhere in the U.S. or write or make statements. Each foreign complication sets my telephone ringing by the press.

I pray that you and your family will have a happy Christmas, and I always pray a little for you personally, for my affectionate admiration is constant.

With my most respectful regards to His Majesty, and with great respect, Faithfully yours,

GCMRL/G. C. Marshall Papers (Retirement, General); H

1. Marshall's handwritten draft of this letter, transcribed here, was dated December 13. The version reproduced in Papanicolaou, *Frederica*, 445–46, is dated December 16, which is the date of the typed version sent to Queen Frederica.

2. "Cyprus dominates today the heart, the soul and the brain of every Greek," Frederica had written to Marshall on October 13 in a long letter about the ongoing political crisis over Cyprus. (Papanicolaou, *Frederica*, 440–41.) See p. 866n2. "The Greek people feel (and I tell you this quite honestly, as I have always been honest in the expression of my feelings to you) that America, the country to whom we looked as giving moral leadership to the world, has for God knows what material and political reasons betrayed her own ideals." (Ibid., 441.) "The United States decision to vote against inclusion of Greece's appeal to place the Cyprus issue on the United Nations agenda stunned Athens tonight," the *New York Times* had reported on September 22. ("Greece is Stunned," *New York Times*, September 22, 1955, p. 8.) On October 10, the newspaper related that "according to reports to the State Department, in Greece a considerable sector of public opinion holds the United States partly responsible for the sequence of events that led to the anti-Greek rioting in Turkey on Sept. 6." ("Washington Eyes Uneasy Mid-East," *New York Times*, October 10, 1955, p. 2.) Frederica informed Marshall that "the Turkish riots in Constantinople and Smyrna" resulted in the destruction of more than sixty Greek churches. (Papanicolaou, *Frederica*, 441.)

3. "What put still more oil into the fire was a message coming from Mr. [John Foster] Dulles that was addressed to the Greek and Turkish Governments alike, urging both to quickly make up and kiss each other, as otherwise American dollars would have gone to waste, or words to this effect dressed in more diplomatic language." (Ibid.)

New York Times columnist C. L. Sulzberger noted on September 24, that "The Greeks felt as if, having been beaten up in an unprovoked fight, they were being hauled into the same dock as the bully who assaulted them." (C. L. Sulzberger, "Foreign Affairs," *New York Times*, September 24, 1955, p. 18.) "Mr. Dulles' words had the effect of gasoline poured on fire," Sulzberger echoed Frederica. (Ibid.)

4. See pp. 874–75 and 901.

5. See pp. 892–93.

6. See pp. 857–58.

551

To Mrs. Egbert Armstrong — December 25, 1955, Pinehurst, North Carolina

Dear Catherine. I was delighted to receive the note on your Xmas card. It gave me your address and put me in touch with you again. I had been wondering what your correct address might be.

Mrs. Marshall's daughter with her Colonel husband and three children (7-12-14) just arrived from Japan so we have been having a lively Xmas. You may have noticed the picture of one Louis Marx on the cover of Time Magazine a week ago—a big toy manufactor [manufacturer]. He sent us, as usual about 100 toys, large and small and I have been busy distributing them.[1] Some were very handsome and elaborate. Our colored couple have 2 children, our laundress and cleaner has 12, Molly's garbage man has 9 and her yard man 8, so we had a good beginning.[2]

I had Mrs. Marshall up at the Walter Reed Hospital in Washington last week for a check up. I took one also. She has been "run down" looking after her older sister who suffered a paralysizing [paralyzing] stroke last March and another recently. She is in a Convalescent Home here, fortunately a very fine one.[3]

I am much as usual, lazy and restraining myself from much activity. They all tell me I look better than I have for years—but it is largely from the neck up.

If I get to Richmond, which I used to do quite frequently, I will certainly call on you. With the season's greetings and affection [affectionate] regards—

GCMarshall

GCMRL/G. C. Marshall Collection (Armstrong); H

1. For several years Marx had shipped packages of toys to Marshall for distribution to children in Pinehurst. *Time* had featured Marx on the cover of its December 12, 1955, issue, accompanied by an extensive article. See pp. 746–47 and 962–63.
2. Julia and Ray Floyd were the Marshalls' servants in Pinehurst. See photo #21.
3. See pp. 874 and 901.

552

To Dwight D. Eisenhower — December 30, 1955, Pinehurst, North Carolina

My dear Mr. President— I greatly appreciated your generous and thoughtful birth day greetings which found me in reasonably good shape.[1]

I won't comment on your health with all the World, the Press and the Commentators doing so.[2]

I saw that very sweet and gentle daughter-in-law of yours at the Walter Reed, and sent her a note of congratulations on her Xmas gift.[3]

Thanks again for you message, Faithfully yours,

GCMarshall

DDEL/Dwight D. Eisenhower Papers (Papers as President, Ann Whitman File, Name Series, Box 21); H

1. "This year it is a deeply felt privilege to send congratulations on another yearly milestone in your brilliant career of service to our country," the president had wired from Key West, Florida, on December 30. (Eisenhower to Marshall, December 30, 1955, DDEL/Dwight D. Eisenhower Papers [Papers as President, Ann Whitman File, Name Series, Box 21].) The *New York Times* reported on its front page that Marshall would be spending his seventy-fifth birthday reading messages "pouring into" his Pinehurst home "from all over the world, from heads of state and from men who were buck privates under his command." ("World Leaders Laud Marshall, 75," *New York Times*, December 31, 1955, p. 1.) The article explained that Marshall's birthday plans included "a luncheon to be given by James Bruce, a former Ambassador to Argentina. Tomorrow night other friends will give a dinner. General Marshall was keenly disappointed that bad weather has delayed a visit by Bernard Baruch, financier." (Ibid.)

On January 6, Marshall informed Walter Bedell Smith, who had joined Joseph Davies in calling Marshall on his birthday, that "there were three cameramen working in the cottage" at Pinehurst in addition to "thirty guests, including lively children" when they had called. (Marshall to Smith, January 6, 1951, GCMRL/G. C. Marshall Papers [Retirement, Chronological].) Katherine Marshall acknowledged to M. L. Spilman on January 14, "This house was a 'madhouse' for a week." (Marshall to Spilman, January 14, 1956, GCMRL/Katherine Marshall Correspondence Collection.) See photo #21.

2. President Eisenhower had suffered a coronary thrombosis on September 24 in Denver, Colorado. He had recuperated on his farm in Gettysburg, Pennsylvania, following his release from the hospital in November, then celebrated Christmas at the White House with his family before going to Key West from December 28 until January 8.

3. Barbara Jean Thompson Eisenhower, wife of the Eisenhowers' son Major John Eisenhower, had given birth to her fourth child, Mary Jean, on December 21 at Walter Reed. ("President Plans to Resume Talks with Press Soon," *New York Times*, December 22, 1955, p. 1.)

553

To Major General Marshall S. Carter — January 10, 1956
Pinehurst, North Carolina

Dear Carter: First I owe you thanks for an interesting letter with the report on the Carter family and the picture of your beautiful and talented wife.[1]

I am also indebted to you and the Command for the telegram of birthday greetings and good wishes to Mrs. Marshall and me.

I was glad to learn that the two children will come to Virginia for their schooling. VMI, while not successful in signing you up, will eventually have a Carter on the roster.[2]

With our affectionate regards to the family and every good wish for the New Year, Faithfully yours,

G C Marshall

P.S. Delighted with the news of your promotion. I had hoped it wouldn't have taken this long.[3] Incidentally a major general's wife doesn't cook. She just presides—and how![4]

GCMRL/Marshall Carter Collection (Marshall Correspondence)

1. Carter had sent a picture of his wife and their Labrador puppy as "evidence of success" hunting near their new "huge quarters" at Fort Sheridan, Illinois, near Chicago, where he was commanding officer of the Fifth Army Antiaircraft Region. (Carter to Marshall, December 16, 1955, GCMRL/G. C. Marshall Papers [Retirement, General]; H.)

2. "Stoney, (my 17 yr. daughter) has applied for admission to Mary Washington College (of The Univ. of Va.) for next September," Carter reported. "And my 15 yr. old son, Marshall, plans on entering the Institute in 1958—both are rebels I guess—born in Virginia anyway." (Ibid.)

3. Carter had received word in late December of his promotion to major general.

4. This final, handwritten comment, was in response to Carter's account that his wife, "Préot remains chained to the kitchen stove but seems resigned to her fate—the quality and quantity of her productions remain at their amazing high level." (Ibid.) "Préot got a wonderful laugh out of your remark," Carter replied on February 27, "but I also sensed a hollow ring to it. I think the only way she ever expects to get out of the kitchen is after we get the three children successfully married off or self-employed. I think she is right too!" (Carter to Marshall, February 27, 1956, GCMRL/Marshall Carter Collection [Marshall Correspondence].)

554

To Frank McCarthy — January 11, 1956
Pinehurst, North Carolina

Dear Frank: When your letter of December 30 reached me, Mrs. Marshall suggested that we postpone an immediate reply and talk about the prospects of our coming to the Coast. The invitation which you extended in behalf of Mr. Engel was most enticing because it also would permit us the opportunity of meeting old friends and enjoying some relaxation.[1] However, when we got down to the root of the matter, Mrs. Lacy's condition is such that it is impossible to predict day-to-day occurrences. Mrs. Marshall has given so much of her time to her sister that she is pretty well worn out. Besides, both of us have reached the point where we no longer find long trips pleasant.

Mr. deMille paid me a high compliment and I am only sorry it is not possible to participate in the tribute which the Guild plans to pay him. I hope you will find the opportunity to tell him of my deep appreciation for his having me in mind.[2]

We had a very pleasant Christmas and a quiet, but stimulating birthday. Many thanks for your telegram, as Mrs. Marshall and I were very glad to have some word from you.

With many thanks again to Mr. deMille, Mr. Engel and you,[3] Faithfully yours,
GC Marshall

GCMRL/G. C. Marshall Papers (Retirement, General)

1. "Each year the [Screen Producers] Guild gives its Milestone Award to a man who has made a great contribution to the progress of motion pictures," McCarthy had written to Marshall on December 30. (McCarthy to Marshall, December 30, 1955, GCMRL/Frank McCarthy Collection [Additions, Box 1].) On January 22, a dinner to honor movie director and producer Cecil B. deMille would take place in Beverly Hills, California. McCarthy extended an invitation to the Marshalls on behalf of Samuel G. Engel, president of the guild. "Your only obligation would be to attend the dinner and make a little talk," McCarthy explained.

2. "When asked what national figure he would like to have invited, he named you," McCarthy explained. (Ibid.) When McCarthy received Marshall's regrets, he wrote to C. J. George that Marshall included a note expressing the desire to write "something which can be read" at the event, which would host "one thousand dinner guests, including every top actor, actress, and creator in town." (McCarthy to George, January 14, 1955, ibid.)

3. "While not present for the tribute being paid you tonight, I should like to join in the congratulations on your great contribution to the motion picture industry and the pleasure you have provided people everywhere, including myself," Marshall wired deMille on January 19, to be read at the dinner. "Your thought of me is reassuring, complimentary, and deeply appreciated." (Marshall to Engel, January 19, 1956, GCMRL/G. C. Marshall Papers [Retirement, Chronological].) "Sam Engel has just called me and read the telegram he received from you," McCarthy notified Marshall on January 20. "It is perfect for the occasion, and it will be greatly appreciated by deMille and by all others who hear it or read it." (McCarthy to Marshall, GCMRL/Frank McCarthy Collection [Additions, Box 1].) "Although we have received about 50 messages from people prominent in various fields, only two will be read at the dinner, yours and the President's." (Ibid.)

555

To Albert Schweitzer[1] — January 16, 1956, Pinehurst, North Carolina

Dear Dr. Schweitzer: I was delighted to receive your letter of December 16, carefully translated by Dr. Ross.[2] While in due time I would have been able to read your longhand effort, he facilitated your message. My French has suffered badly since World War I.

I feel highly complimented by your gracious expressions and the thought which encouraged you to write me such a fine letter.[3]

Word came to me of the Nobel Award when I was confined to bed with a severe case of virus-flu. Unfortunately, it continued with me during the voyage and while waiting in Paris for the flight to Oslo. I had hoped that the trip via the southern route would provide the sun and possibly the cure; however, the weather was bad and no progress was realized. Incidentally, I wrote my talk just three days before it was given.[4]

As a soldier being honored with a peace award and being associated with you, a distinguished doctor and humanitarian, this was one of the greatest honors that has been paid me.[5]

I do agree that, should a trip to Europe develop, I will be in touch with you. Perhaps there is time remaining to afford me the great pleasure of meeting you.

Mrs. Marshall is most appreciative of your message.[6]

With many thanks again for your remembering my birthday, and with high regard and respect,[7] Faithfully yours,

GCMRL/G. C. Marshall Papers (Retirement, General)

1. In November 1954, Marshall had been asked for a statement to accompany a photographic essay in *Life* magazine. (Stoddard to Marshall, November 9, 1954, GCMRL/G. C. Marshall Papers [Retirement, General].) "LIFE's graphic illustration of Doctor Schweitzer, the man, and the character of his contribution to his fellow man in Africa is a testimony to the grandeur of his beneficent work. I, myself, felt especially honored to receive the Nobel

Peace Award in his company, though not in his actual presence," Marshall wrote. "The world, these days, sorely needs the example offered by the life of Doctor Schweitzer." (Statement for *Life* magazine, November [19], 1954, ibid.)

2. Emory Ross, treasurer of the Albert Schweitzer Fellowship of New York City, had translated and forwarded the letter written by Schweitzer as he returned from Europe to Lambarene in French Equatorial Africa, where he directed a hospital. The Southern Pines, North Carolina, *Pilot* reprinted Ross's translation of Schweitzer's letter in its entirety on January 12, 1956. ("Dr. Schweitzer Ponders Problem of Peace in Greeting to Gen. Marshall," [*Southern Pines, NC*] *Pilot*, January 12, 1956, p. 1.)

3. Schweitzer admired Marshall's "clearsightedness and your courage" because "after having done your duty during the war, you put yourself at the service of peace" and "approached the realities with a spirit of idealism that was rational and poised." As a result, Marshall had gained Schweitzer's "profound sympathy." (Ibid.)

4. See pp. 807–8. Schweitzer noted that his "joy was double" to have received the Nobel Prize at the same time as Marshall. "We both of us know how little we have been able to do for the coming of peace," he confided. "In working out my talk for Oslo on the problem of peace I was as if crushed by this sentiment." (Ibid.)

5. Because their "two names have been put forward together" Schweitzer believed he and Marshall were "united in the humility of appreciation of our role in the service of peace, to which we are vowed, each one in his place, each one with his means." (Ibid.)

6. "I beg you to present my respects to Mrs. Marshall," Schweitzer closed his letter and added a postscript suggested that perhaps they might rendezvous in Europe sometime in the future. (Ibid.)

7. Emory Ross responded on January 26 that he had forwarded Marshall's letter to Dr. Schweitzer and closed "with warm appreciation of the influence of Mrs. Marshall and yourself in so many ways on our generation." (Ross to Marshall, January 26, 1956, GCMRL/G. C. Marshall Papers [Retirement, General].)

556

TO MRS. JOHN WHITE PENDLETON — January 16, 1956
Pinehurst, North Carolina

Dear Madge: Relative to your New Yorker friend Kahn, in a literal sense I am not writing my memoirs. The VMI foundation really does it, hires the editor, searches the records, etc. I only agree to fill in the blind spots, and that at my entire convenience. They manage all, hire, supervise, etc. The Rockefeller Foundation (this is confidential) supplies the needed funds. I stipulate that I am not to be worried by decisions—choice of editor, etc.[1]

Isn't this the fellow that wrote a profile of me and had ping pong as my principal diversion—Chief of Staff of the Army and ping pong!?[2]

We are gradually cleaning up the holiday and birthday fuss. Three secretaries and my aide have been and still are working on the flood in Washington.[3]

Allene seems much better mentally though not physically, is trying to write some stories— Katherine is resting up some but not enough. I am, as usual, lazy and generally good for nothing.

One Hudson Strode sent me his life of Jefferson Davis. He now seems to be trying to start up a correspondence. He knows and admires you and John. What sort of a chap is he?[4]

Molly and her crew seem to have settled down pleasantly at Fort Ritchie. She has a beautiful house, built as a summer home for the Governor of Maryland on the *once* National Guard reservation.[5]

My love to you all. Affectionately,

GCM

GCMRL/Xerox 2237 (GCM Family, Personal Letters); H

1. See 905–6. On November 16, 1955, Jack Hagan had written to Frank McCarthy that Carlisle Humelsine, Marshall's World War II assistant and later a deputy undersecretary of state who had been executive vice president of Colonial Williamsburg, Virginia, since 1953, was having conversations with John D. Rockefeller Jr. about supporting the planned biography of General Marshall. (Hagan to McCarthy, November 16, 1955, GCMRL/Frank McCarthy Collection [Additions, Box 3].) "Everything O.K. for $100,000.00. This definite," Hagan wired McCarthy on December 19. "Will probably have lunch with him tomorrow to get details on how news release will be made." (Hagan to McCarthy, December 19, 1955, ibid.) Hagan wrote to Rockefeller on December 30 that historians at the State and Defense Departments and the archivist of the United States "estimate that the cost of documenting [Marshall's] papers, including an outstanding historian with a proper staff to catalogue, microfilm and develop questions for General Marshall's interpretation, will cost approximately $150,000. It is with this latter phase of the work of the Foundation that I hope you will be interested, knowing of your interest in education and your great philanthropic work to preserve history." (Hagan to Rockefeller, December 30, 1955, ibid.)

2. Madge Pendleton's "*New Yorker* friend Kahn" may have been E. J. Kahn Jr., who was a staff writer for the *New Yorker* magazine from 1937 to 1994. Marshall may have confused Kahn with A. J. Liebling, who had written a profile of Marshall for the October 26, 1940, issue of the *New Yorker*, in which he reported that Army Chief of Staff Marshall "was known to neighbors" at Katherine Marshall's Fire Island, New York, cottage "as a ping-pong expert, a good bridge player without being fanatical about it, and an unimpressive swimmer." (A. J. Liebling, "Profiles, Chief of Staff," *New Yorker*, October 26, 1940, p. 35.) Liebling was a staff writer for the *New Yorker* from 1935 to 1963.

3. See photo #21. Articles about Marshall's seventy-fifth birthday had appeared in newspapers across the United States, which generated hundreds of letters from well-wishing friends and admirers. Marshall personally responded to very few but each letter received a response from his office. See next document.

4. A professor of creative writing at the University of Alabama, Hudson Strode had written to Marshall on January 13 to explain that "Because of a longtime admiration for your qualities and accomplishments, last week I took the liberty of sending you an inscribed copy of my recent biography of Jefferson Davis." (Strode to Marshall, January 13, 1956, GCMRL/G. C. Marshall Papers [Retirement, General].) Strode mentioned that he was "very fond of Madge and John Pendleton, and it is a delight to have them in Tuscaloosa. Such couples turn up only too rarely." (Ibid.)

5. See p. 930n5.

557

To Major General Edwin Forrest Harding — January 19, 1956
Pinehurst, North Carolina

Dear Harding: I will be much interested in seeing and reading the article you mention.[1]

As to the question of engaging an historian, etc., I have nothing to do with that (by express stipulation). The Foundation acts without disturbing me. I am not *writing* my memoirs. I only fill in the blank spots in the records.[2]

We had a fine Christmas with the family all here and some New York and Washington guests staying at the hotel, but virtually living at our house.

The birthday tumult pretty much upset things—hundreds of telegrams, constant telephone messages, a great number of letters, and cards without number.[3]

Give my love to Eleanor. Faithfully yours,

GCMRL/G. C. Marshall Papers (Retirement, General); H

1. See pp. 417–18. Harding had written at length to Marshall on January 10 about *Victory in Papua* by Samuel Milner, which had not yet been published, in the official *United States Army in World War II* series. "I was and am personally interested in having you read the book since it establishes the fact that Harding and his battered and depleted cohorts were in there fighting all the way and doing about as well as could be expected with what they had. I have had misgivings that you might have thought, or even be thinking, that I didn't keep pushing," Harding admitted, referring to his experiences commanding the Thirty-second Infantry Division in the Battle of Buna-Gona in New Guinea. (Harding to Marshall, January 10, 1956, GCMRL/G. C. Marshall Papers [Retirement, General].)

Marshall had previously been asked to comment on other volumes in the ongoing *United States Army in World War II* series and had done so (see pp. 147–48 and *Papers of GCM*, 6: 687–93), but early in his retirement he replied to General Ward that he had "no comment to make" on the two chapters from what would become in 1953 *The Fall of the Philippines* by Louis Morton. "The statements and interpretations appear to be correct, in my opinion," he added, but "I have no access to records down here." (Marshall to Ward, December 4, 1951, GCMRL/G. C. Marshall Papers [Secretary of Defense, Selected].) He also offered no comment on the manuscript for *Stilwell's Mission to China* by Charles F. Romanus and Riley Sunderland, which was also published in 1953. (Ward to Marshall, April 4, 1952, GCMRL/G. C. Marshall Papers [Retirement, General].)

2. See pp. 902–3. Harding wrote that he had "long felt that what you, and only you, know concerning the great historical events in which you played a leading part just had to get in the record somehow." (Harding to Marshall, January 10, 1956, ibid.) Apparently Milner, an historian with the Air Transport Command of the Army Air Forces in World War II, had written to Harding in October declaring his interest in working on Marshall's biography. (Ibid.)

3. See previous document, p. 913n1 and photo #21.

"I HAVE BEEN at Walter Reed since last Thursday, but am hopeful of getting away this Friday," Marshall wrote to Frank McCarthy on February 2, 1956. He described "a rash which circled my waist" for several weeks that "the doctors at Pinehurst were unable to cure." More important, he acknowledged that "A second problem was the inability to focus my right eye, which was caused by the rupture of a vein in my head. It appears that both problems have been resolved." (Marshall to McCarthy, February 2, 1956, GCMRL/Frank McCarthy Papers [Additions, Box 1].)

Marshall told McCarthy that he looked forward to returning to Pinehurst, where he could "enjoy the lazy life I have now become accustomed to," but on March 18 he admitted to Marshall Carter that he "brought back a mild case of intestinal flu from my Walter Reed trip and gave it to Katherine!!" (Ibid.; Marshall to Carter, March 18, 1956, GCMRL/Marshall Carter Collection [Marshall Correspondence].) "I had a tough trip home," Marshall wrote to C. J. George on February 7. He explained that his plane had landed at Raleigh, North Carolina, rather than Fort Bragg because of heavy fog. "Katherine and Heffner met me at 5:45" but they did not arrive in Pinehurst until 8:00 p.m. in a downpour. (Marshall to George, February 7, 1956, GCMRL/G. C. Marshall Collection [George]; H.)

Marshall's hearing also continued to deteriorate. See p. 872. C. J. George confided to Carter on March 8 that "there is at least a sixty percent deficiency in his left ear and fifty percent in the right. Some months ago, I talked him into being fitted for a hearing aid, which he only uses for the movies and television. I would imagine that if he does not curtail the shipment of batteries, he will have to vacate his room." (George to Carter, March 8, 1956, GCMRL/G. C. Marshall Papers [Retirement, Chronological].) ★

558

To Ellene Winn — February 13, 1956, Pinehurst, North Carolina

Dear Ellene— Thanks a lot for sending me your tale of the princess and the witch. You did a grand job and I have no suggestions to make—only compliments to send. You are going to be a fine writer.[1]

I am sending you back the manuscript for your own records, as it is your first effort and therefore will be an important incident in the history of your life. Keep it carefully.

We were glad to learn that you were giving Bones exercise in the woods behind your house. That is good and will keep him in fine health.[2] Affectionately,

GCMRL/G. C. Marshall Papers (Retirement, General); H

1. "I have written a story to be published," Marshall's stepgranddaughter had written to him on February 6. "If you see anything wrong with it please send it back and I will correct it and return it to you." (Winn to Marshall, February 6, 1956, GCMRL/G. C. Marshall Papers [Retirement, General].)

2. Bones was the Marshalls' dog.

559

To Colonel Truman Smith — February 20, 1956, Pinehurst, North Carolina

Dear Smith: Thanks very much for your gracious letter—and for the book. I know you would want me to be honest in the matter—Reeder sent me the book sometime ago. I read it with great interest. It was very well done. I wrote and told him so.[1]

It brought up the same reaction in me it did in you.[2]

I knew an old Lieutenant Colonel who was a "trooper" in the charge described. Also, my fifty-eight year old teamster "Nate Cox" in 1905 was the son of the man whose horses were run off by the Mexicans. Either Nate or his brother rode in on the expedition.

I mapped 2,000 square miles along the Rio Grande with Nate and a pack train of thirty-six mules under an old packer of sixty years.[3]

My best to you and Mrs. Smith. Faithfully yours,

P.S. I had a nice letter from von Shell (also a Christmas card this year), but no acknowledgement of a photograph I sent him. I guess it got lost.[4]

G. C. M.

GCMRL/G. C. Marshall Papers (Retirement, General); H

1. Smith had sent a copy of Colonel Russell P. "Red" Reeder Jr.'s *The MacKenzie Raid* to Marshall as a belated birthday gift along with a long letter explaining how much he had enjoyed the book. (Smith to Marshall, February 5, 1956, GCMRL/G. C. Marshall Papers [Retirement, General].) While the Marshalls were vacationing in Eagles Mere, Pennsylvania, in August 1955 (see pp. 892–93), C. J. George had written to Reeder (USMA, 1926) on Marshall's behalf to thank the author, promising that "in the cool of the evening I will sit down and read your treatment of the military history of 1873. Knowing of your fine ability as a soldier and fighter should make the book very interesting." (Marshall to Reeder, August 8, 1955, ibid.) Marshall probably first met Reeder at Fort Benning, where he was a student officer in 1932–33. He served as a member of Marshall's General Staff during World War II and wrote a report titled "Fighting on Guadalcanal" for which Marshall wrote a foreword and ordered one million copies printed and distributed to troops. Reeder commanded the Twelfth Infantry Regiment of the Fourth Infantry Division when it landed on Omaha Beach on June 6, 1944. After the war Reeder established a leadership course at West Point and, in 1954, began writing novels, military history, and biographies for young readers. ("Russell Reeder, 95, Leader in Invasion on D-Day, Dies," *New York Times*, March 1, 1998, p. 35.)

2. *The MacKenzie Raid* "was 'escapism' to be sure," Smith opined, yet "It seemed to me that it was one of the best tales of the old Regular army I had ever read." (Smith to Marshall, February 5, 1956, ibid.) The book is a novelized account of the US cavalry's 1873 raid into Mexico, led by Colonel Ranald S. MacKenzie (USMA, 1862), against Kickapoo Indians who had been marauding the frontier of Texas.

3. In an undated reminiscence, Marshall recalled his 1905 mapping expedition from Fort Clark, Texas, which "supplied me with an escort wagon and a four-line mule team driven by Nate Cox of Bracketsville [*Brackettville*, Texas], whose father brought Nate when he was 6 years old through Dead Man's Pass, near Shumla, Texas, then to Silver Lake. His earliest recollection was watching his father stand in the doorway of the cabin with a rifle to keep off a band of Comanches, his mother loading the rifle." (GCMRL/G. C. Marshall Collection [1905 Mapping Expedition].) In 1957 Marshall recalled the mapping project as "the hardest service I ever had in the army." (*Marshall Interviews*, 144.) "This required, in a sense, more leadership on my part than almost anything else, because it was all hard going and at times rather dangerous going. I remember one stretch there, the old packer and myself were without water for eighteen hours and had to travel pretty nearly fifty miles. This was an endurance contest of the first class." (Ibid., 145.) For more on Marshall's 1905 assignment, see Pogue, *Education*, 86–89 and *Papers of GCM*, 1: 28–34.

4. See pp. 885n3, 884n1, and 885n5. German General Adolf von Schell had written on August 27, 1955, to thank Marshall "by all my heart for all you have done for me in the past, especially in those days when you saved me from being turned over to the Poles by the English." (Schell to Marshall, August 27, 1955, ibid.) He wrote again on September 19 to thank Marshall "for those two wonderful pictures you have sent me." He would frame and place them on his desk to remind him "of you and all the other good friends whom I formed in Benning and the American army as well." (Schell to Marshall, September 19, 1955, ibid.) After Smith informed von Schell that Marshall did not recall receiving this letter, von Schell wrote again "by the hand of Truman Smith" to ensure that his "heartiest thanks" for the photographs would reach Marshall. (Schell to Marshall, May 5, 1956, ibid.)

560

To Emanuel Celler[1] February 21, 1956
Pinehurst, North Carolina

Dear Mr. Chairman: I have just been notified by Congressman Devereux that the Private Bill S. 1682, which was introduced in the Senate by the Honorable Willis A. Robertson and passed on July 28, 1955, was not favorably considered by a Subcommittee on the Judiciary.[2]

This news is very discouraging to Mrs. Marshall and me, because we felt all along that Maria Intriago Martinez was such a worthy person that she would soon enjoy the maximum of her wishes—permanent residency.

I have been told that the reasons for the Subcommittee's action were that Maria's case did not fall within the provisions of hardship.[3] This is so, because Maria has consistently squeezed her budget tightly so that when the day arrived for retirement she would be completely independent. I am sure the record will disclose that she has invested considerable of her money in War Bonds, has paid her income taxes when due, has been a consistent contributor to the Red Cross Blood Bank, and has shown natural attributes of character and integrity.

It would be a shame if this woman would have to leave the Country after she has proved so clearly a great desire of becoming a resident and citizen of our Country. I know you will give every consideration to this request, and I am hopeful that your Committee will react favorably.[4] Faithfully yours,

GCMRL/G. C. Marshall Papers (Retirement, General)

1. Congressman Emanuel Celler (D-NY) was chairman of the Committee on the Judiciary of the House of Representatives.

2. See pp. 825–26. On July 26, 1955, Senator Robertson had written to advise Marshall that "yesterday the Senate passed the bill which I introduced for the relief of Maria Intriago Martinez." (Robertson to Marshall, July 26, 1955, GCMRL/G. C. Marshall Papers [Retirement, General].) Brigadier General James P. S. Devereux, who had been awarded the Navy Cross for leading the defense of the American outpost on Wake Island during the Japanese siege from December 7 to 22, 1941, before being taken prisoner of war, was a Republican member of Congress from Maryland. On July 12, 1955, he had written to Marshall that he had introduced a bill "in behalf of Maria" before the House Judiciary Committee; he wrote again two weeks later that "this bill cannot be considered during this session of Congress but at least Miss Martinez will be allowed to remain in this country until August 1, 1956." (Devereux to Marshall, July 12 and July 25, 1955, ibid.)

3. "I am indeed sorry to have to relay such discouraging news and to advise that there is nothing further which can be done," Devereux wrote to Marshall on February 23. (Devereux to Marshall, February 23, 1956, ibid.) "Unfavorable action was based on the fact that the Committee did not feel Maria's case fell within the provisions of hardship despite all the evidence submitted in her behalf," Devereux explained. (Ibid.)

4. "Your letter of February 21 was delivered by hand to my office yesterday, and it was immediately brought to my attention," Celler responded on February 22. (Celler to Marshall, February 22, 1956, ibid.) "After a discussion it has been agreed that although the case represents certain appealing aspects, it still does not possess sufficient equities for setting aside the general law and enacting private legislation in behalf of a person who is not a refugee, not threatened with deportation to a country practicing persecution on political, racial, or religious grounds, not related to United States citizens, and not having anyone depending on her for support. I might add that it is our well established policy to

act favorably on private immigration bills only when they cover cases where at least one of the above summarized factors is present." (Ibid.)

561

To Harry S. Truman — March 3, 1956
Pinehurst, North Carolina

My dear Mr. Truman I have waited until your "Life" series was completed before writing.[1]

Thank you very, very much for the generous and flattering manner in which you dealt with me in your descriptions involving my work with you.[2] I found I had forgotten much that you recited and naturally I was deeply interested.

All that you wrote was intensely interesting and remarkably effective. It must have been a tremenduous task.[3]

Katherine and I had not had a good winter but we are O.K. now. Only she has a daily duty with her sister that pretty much takes it out of her each day. But it can't be helped.

I was up at the Walter Reed recently for eight days and had a successful trip if that ever can be said of hospital experiences.[4]

I hope Mrs. Truman and you are well—and Margaret. Katherine asked me to tell Mrs. Truman very often she thinks of her. She is firm in the opinion that Mrs. Truman was the most gracious and best balanced lady she had ever seen in the White House.

With affectionate regards to both of you.[5] Faithfully yours,

GCMarshall

GCMRL/G. C. Marshall Collection (Truman); H

1. Extensive excerpts from Truman's memoirs, published in two volumes in 1955 and 1956 by Doubleday, had appeared in *Life* magazine between September 1955 and February 1956. See p. 841n13.
2. Truman praised Marshall many times throughout both volumes of the memoirs.
3. "Getting that book together was about the most awful task that ever faced me," Truman responded on March 14. (Truman to Marshall, March 14, 1956, GCMRL/G. C. Marshall Papers [Retirement, General].) "More than a million and a half words were dictated, written and transcribed. Then came the cut to 1/3. Now the boys who write reviews seem to know more than I could find out when I was doing the job and with all the documents before me! But it is down in black and white, as my mother would say, and that is what I wanted." (Ibid.)
4. See pp. 918–19.
5. "Never have I received a letter more appreciated than yours of Mar. 3rd about my much talked about book," Truman replied. "If you are pleased with it, I am very happy." (Ibid.)

562

To Sinclair Weeks

March 7, 1956
Pinehurst, North Carolina

My dear Mr. Secretary: I am told that the position of Superintendent of the United States Merchant Marine Academy, under your jurisdiction, is soon to become vacant.

I take the liberty of suggesting for your consideration the name of Jonathan M. Wainwright, 5th, for appointment to this post.[1]

Enclosed is a summary of his service in the Merchant Marine covering a period of twenty-five years—eighteen years of sea duty, and including the Distinguished Service Medal for hazardous conduct during the landing operation on the beach at Salerno, Italy.[2]

Since my withdrawal from Governmental posts, I have made no recommendations of individuals. There is a special reason for this exception.

I have always felt that the Government and the people owed a special debt of reparation to General Wainwright [IV] and his associates for the tragic dilemma into which they were precipitated by the utter unpreparedness of this Country on its entry into the war with Japan. Within the powers of my positions in the Government, I did a little, and at General Wainwright's funeral I told this then young man he should call on me if I ever was in a position to be of assistance.[3]

Therefore this recommendation, which I think the records show is fully deserved.[4] Faithfully yours,

GCMRL/G. C. Marshall Papers (Retirement, General)

1. Wainwright, the son of Medal of Honor recipient General Jonathan M. Wainwright IV, had written to Marshall on February 28 to thank him for "the privilege of conferring with you." (Wainwright to Marshall, February 28, 1956, GCMRL/G. C. Marshall Papers [Retirement, General].) With his letter, Wainwright included a request to be considered for appointment as superintendent of the Merchant Marine Academy at Kings Point, New York. "The present Superintendent is in over service category and the Maritime Administrator is presently planning a change in command and is seeking a candidate for the assignment," Wainwright indicated. "My service experience and background qualifies me for the position." (Ibid.)

2. The December 23, 1943, citation accompanying the Merchant Marine Distinguished Service Medal noted that Wainwright's "unfaltering courage, indomitable determination, and expert seamanship in accomplishing his missions under unusually trying circumstances were in keeping with the finest traditions of the United States Merchant Marine." (Wainwright citation, December 23, 1943, ibid.)

3. See p. 788n2.

4. Secretary of Commerce Weeks responded on March 16 that "no current vacancy exists in this post, and none is anticipated in the immediate future." (Weeks to Marshall, March 16, 1956, ibid.) The misunderstanding "stems from the fact that the present Superintendent, Rear Admiral Gordon McLintock, U. S. Maritime Service, was, upon his reappointment some four years ago advised by Admiral [Edward Lull] Cochrane, who was then Maritime Administrator, that his term of appointment would expire March 31, 1956"; however, the administrator had recently advised McLintock that his appointment would be continued "until further notice." (Ibid.) Weeks acknowledged that Wainwright's "unusual background of training and experience, coupled with his distinguished service in the U. S. Merchant Marine, makes him fully deserving of the confidence you have expressed in his

character and abilities. Under these circumstances, you may be sure that we shall be glad to see that he is given appropriate consideration whenever it becomes necessary for us to make an appointment to this post." (Ibid.) In a brief note, Marshall asked C. J. George to forward Weeks's letter to Wainwright "on a confidential basis." (Marshall to George, n.d., ibid.) Wainwright retuned the letter on March 30 and informed George that he had received a letter with the same information from Clarence G. Morse, who had been maritime administrator since 1955. (Wainwright to George, March 30, 1956, ibid.)

563

To Queen Frederica of the Hellenes[1] March 8, 1956
Pinehurst, North Carolina

Your Majesty: I just received your letter of February 29 an hour ago. The delay was due to the fact that it was addressed to Leesburg, Virginia, and we are at our winter home, a cottage at Pinehurst, North Carolina.

This letter of mine is not an answer to yours—merely an acknowledgement. My reply will go later, as soon as I can go over the situation here, mainly political, with some care.

First though, we are vastly complimented and charmed by your suggestion. You have done us a great honor.[2]

Second, for reasons that I will explain we cannot go North and open our Leesburg home before late in April. Mrs. Marshall's older sister is in the hospital here half paralyzed and critically ill. She has been so for months, and Mrs. Marshall cannot leave here. We are trying to arrange to move her North as soon as it warms up somewhat.

Now, as to the important factors: I must, for your sake, be very frank and I will first have to go about finding out whether my premonitions are sound. I will do so with great secrecy, entirely outside of the Administration.

The situation is that I have so completely withdrawn from any governmental contacts and political manifestations that the entire basis of my information is the press or radio.

Important groups of the Republican Party are extremely hostile to me in the pre-election endeavor to tear down everything the Democratic Administration did, and are now attacking foreign relief or assistance. Also, in the South, some Democrats are attacking foreign relief—in fact, undercutting their representatives in Congress who are committed to such a course. You may not be aware of the fact that I have been more viciously attacked than any other public figure in this generation.[3]

In view of these conditions, I fear that my assistance in the manner suggested would concentrate a bitter and hostile press attack. I am only guessing at this and will quickly inform myself through an expert or two at this business—close friends of mine in Washington. Then, I will write you immediately of my opinion as to the result desired.

This is an embarrassing letter to write, as you will understand. The one person in this world who we would most love to have in our home suggest it—and that person, a great Queen, and her Country facing a desperate crisis.[4] With great respect and admiration,

G. C. Marshall

P.S. I hope my fears are unfounded. Believe me, Your Majesty, I will seek the wisdom to advise you to the best interests of your Country and you personally.[5]

GCMRL/G. C. Marshall Papers (Retirement, General); H

1. At the top of his handwritten draft of this letter, Marshall scrawled, "I sent this long hand. Type for Smith to see." Smith was probably Walter Bedell Smith.

2. "We have just passed the most difficult time since my husband's coming to the throne," Frederica had confided to Marshall on February 29. (Papanicolaou, *Frederica*, 447.) She wrote urgently requesting "a courageous action now on behalf of America towards Greece" particularly in terms of military materiel. (Ibid., 448.) "My husband and I feel so strongly that America must now come full out in support of Greece that we think it might be helpful if I went to the States privately in order to meet the right people and talk to them privately and unofficially." She wondered whether the Marshalls could invite her to stay with them at Dodona Manor and help her to meet there with those who "would be responsible for giving military, naval and any financial aid to Greece?" (Ibid.) Frederica acknowledged that she was "taking tremendous advantage of our friendship." (Ibid., 449.)

3. See pp. 555–56, 721–22, 852–55, and 858–59. Attacks on Marshall, particularly relating to foreign aid, had continued. On February 4, 1956, the *Washington Post* had reported that while in New York for a Democratic fundraising dinner, former President Truman had berated "the Republican Administration in his speech for making a 'shambles of bipartisanship in foreign policy.'" ("Truman Snubs Nixon for 'Traitor' Charge," *Washington Post*, February 4, 1956, p. 2.) "'The Republicans had made political capital of charges of treason against the Democratic Party,'" Truman continued, and noted that "'They even called Gen. George C. Marshall and me traitors, and if we're traitors, the country is in a hell of a fix.'" (Ibid.)

4. "America must win in Greece again now or else there is fear Greece may be lost forever," Frederica had warned. (Papanicolaou, *Frederica*, 449.) "The West will lose a very strong position and thus the gates will be opened to swamp the already rather shaky position in the Middle East." (Ibid.)

5. See next document.

564

To Queen Frederica of the Hellenes — March 20, 1956[1]
Pinehurst, North Carolina

Your Majesty: After many delays, due to the temporary absence from Washington of the individuals I most trusted as to secrecy as well as expert knowledge on the subject concerned, I am now in a position to make a formal reply to your letter.[2]

First, there is a complete unanimity in the feeling that it would be very unwise for you to come over to influence the decision regarding U. S. contributions to Greece in materiel and funds. It could not be done secretly, as you apparently thought possible, and the hostile reaction would be immediate and probably bitter.[3]

Strange to state, if you were less of a person, had less charm and beauty, the opposition would be less to your efforts.

This morning's papers on the Congressional reactions to the President's proposals on foreign aid are plainly indicative of what I have just written.[4]

My advisors are the most fully informed men outside the State Department and Congress. They were "my men" at one time and I could trust them completely.

In my investigation of the situation I have already been able to do some positive good to influence the allotment of materiel, and especially as to the policy which tends to regulate such dealings. I think that I have awakened a strong feeling that the political situation in Greece must be strongly supported against the Communist thrust. The pre-election build-up is heavily involved.

How the financial allotment will go will first depend initially on the Congressional decision as to the President's proposal of this morning for foreign aid.

I find that there are several other countries bringing the heaviest pressure on our government. I have sought to intrude the feeling that what this Country has already invested in Greece or done for her must not be canceled by some small "across the board" ruling concerning allotments of materiel to various countries.

As to me personally, I must admit that there was also unanimity regarding my feelings that I personally would stir up a storm of political opposition by the virulent group in the opposition. They count all the billions my policies have already cost the American tax payer and, in this pre-election demagogic scramble, they want no more of my influence or interference.[5] I feel I have already been able to do some good behind the scenes and I hope I can do more.

In all of this I have been completely frank and I trust to your goodness to understand me. All of this has been very difficult for me to write, but it is directed by my heart as well as my head.[6] With increased admiration and devotion,

G. C. Marshall

P.S. I hope my fears are unfounded. Believe me, Your Majesty, I will seek the wisdom to advise you to the best interests of your Country and you personally.

GCMRL/G. C. Marshall Papers (Retirement, General)

1. Marshall's longhand draft of this letter in the Marshall Papers is undated but the published version in Papanicolaou's *Frederica, Queen of the Hellenes: Mission of a Modern Queen* is dated March 20, 1956.

2. See previous document, n2. On March 8, C. J. George had mentioned to Marshall Carter that "a touch of flu has slowed me down, but only temporarily." (George to Carter, March 8, 1956, GCMRL/G. C. Marshall Papers [Retirement, General].)

3. See previous document, n3.

4. President Eisenhower delivered a major message on foreign policy before Congress on March 19, 1956, in which he requested $4.9 billion. The *New York Times* reported that he asked for $3 billion for military aid, compared to about $4 billion the previous year. ("Eisenhower Maps New Aid Strategy," *New York Times*, March 18, 1956, p. 9.) On March 21, the *Washington Post* reported that "Acting Secretary of State Herbert Hoover Jr. yesterday met a surprisingly gentle reception from Congress as he opened the Administration's case for a $4.9 billion foreign aid program." ("Hoover Calms Opposition to 10-Year Aid," *Washington Post*, March 21, 1956, p. 2.) Marshall received the *Washington Post* daily with his mail. (Marshall to Elmore, January 23, 1956, GCMRL/G. C. Marshall Papers [Retirement, General].)

5. Marshall is referring to expenditures relating to the European Recovery Program.

6. "Thank you very much for your two letters," Frederica responded on March 29. "I appreciate deeply the thought and effort you put into finding the right decision, which I

consider absolutely correct and wise. I thank you especially for the frankness in which you write because that is what I feel friends are there for, especially friends in whom one has absolute confidence." (Papanicolaou, *Frederica*, 452.)

565

TO JOHN WHITE PENDLETON

March 23, 1956
Pinehurst, North Carolina

Dear John: We both were delighted to receive your fine, newsy letter. Thank you for troubling to write in such detail.[1]

As to Saudi Arabia, I am reluctant to advise.[2] As I see it—

The problem of a disturbed Middle East has to be considered.

The isolation in a somewhat barren country is a problem, but you will probably have an interesting group.

The thought of advance assignment after some years to a United States or British post is a consideration, without which I wouldn't want the job.

I suppose with their own planes your family might get flights to Europe from time to time.

Do you get clear on taxes?

Tupper seems to have landed on his feet at Lawrenceville.[3] Madge must be very proud of him.

The V.M.I. finals engagement was, or is, surrounded with "ifs" by me. I may not get there after all.[4]

We are both well. Allene unchanged, though stronger.

Molly was due Monday for a short visit, but the snow and sleet stopped her. Will try to come later.

My love to both of you. Affectionately,

GCMRL/G. C. Marshall Papers (Retirement, General)

1. Pendleton had written on March 18 with news of his family. He acknowledged that he had been "unusually busy with all the trouble here lately" at the University of Alabama, where race riots had taken place after a black graduate student enrolled. "Feelings have been running high, and I'm afraid the world at large has a very one-sided picture. . . . It's hard to see what the solution will be—time, I suppose." (Pendleton to Marshall, March 18, 1956, GCMRL/G. C. Marshall Papers [Retirement, General].)

2. Pendleton mentioned "the possibility of our going to Saudi Arabia with the Arabian American Oil Company." They had been weighing the offer and would "be most grateful" if Marshall could provide his opinion. (Ibid.) See p. 949.

3. See p. 910n5. Pendleton had reported that his stepson, Tupper Brown, "is doing well at Lawrenceville. We talked to him over the telephone the other night, and he seemed very happy indeed." (Ibid.)

4. See pp. 934 and 938–42. Pendleton, who was a VMI alumnus, had seen in the *Rockbridge County News* that Marshall was scheduled to speak at VMI on June 12. "If I am in this country, I shall certainly make an effort to go." (Ibid.)

566

To Rear Admiral Samuel E. Morison[1] March 27, 1956
Pinehurst, North Carolina

Dear Morison: I have no clear recollection of the remark quoted by Slessor. A southern port was a necessity. Eisenhower's "right" demanded an aggressive front. I recall that the gasoline for half of Patton's troops came through from the south.[2]

The editorial in LIFE appeared shortly after the landing, as I now recall.[3]

Mrs. Marshall appreciated your messages. Faithfully yours,

GCMRL/G. C. Marshall Papers (Retirement, General)

1. Historian Samuel Eliot Morison had recently retired from Harvard University, where he taught for forty years. During World War II, President Roosevelt commissioned Morison to write a multivolume history of US naval operations from an insider's perspective. "I should very much like to have a talk with you about the strategy for Operations OVERLORD and DRAGOON, as I am working on the volume of my naval history that covers the liberation of France," he had written to Marshall on February 17. (Morison to Marshall, February 17, 1956, GCMRL/G. C. Marshall Papers [Retirement, General].) Marshall replied on February 25 that he would be "glad to see you at my home" in Pinehurst. (Marshall to Morison, February 25, 1956, ibid.) Morison sent a note of thanks on March 8 for the Marshalls' "kind & hospitable reception of me and to you for answering my questions and giving me such interesting data on the war and after." (Morison to Marshall, March 8, 1956, ibid.) C. J. George wrote to another military historian who, on March 13, had requested a meeting with Marshall that "he recently devoted four afternoons to interviews in his home, and they have proved too exhausting. The number of requests he receives is so great that he is not up to the task." (George to Higgins, March 26, 1956, ibid.)

2. Morison wrote to Marshall on March 16 that he had recently seen Sir John Slessor, who had recalled a conversation between Marshall and "'Jumbo' Wilson at Caserta in late June 1944. He quoted you substantially as saying 'We have about 50 new divisions building up in the U.S. and we owe it to the American people to use them as an argument for *Dragoon* rather than an eastern operation.' He said he was sure you meant that with all these divisions ready to throw into the European theatre, we must have a big port like Marseilles. Do you remember the incident?" (Morison to Marshall, March 16, 1956, ibid.) Marshal Sir John Slessor was deputy air commander in chief Mediterranean Allied Air Forces in mid-June 1944, when General Marshall met with Field Marshal Sir Henry "Jumbo" Maitland Wilson in Caserta, Italy, to discuss the invasion of southern France, originally code-named ANVIL, and later renamed DRAGOON. For more on these meetings, see *Papers of GCM*, 4: 405–8. In 1950, Slessor succeeded Lord Tedder as chief of the British air staff. He retired in 1952.

3. "In your talk with me you mentioned an editorial in *Life* Magazine about Torch operation which you commended as being excellent," Morison had written, and explained that his assistant had not found the item. (Ibid.) Marshall had probably referred to the commentary in the November 23, 1942, issue of *Life* that considered the Allies' invasion of North Africa within the context of recent history, and noted how Depression-weary Americans were eager "to be Americans again—to do things in a big, imaginative way, to act with an efficiency that left observers breathless." ("Action is What We All Needed and Action Is What We All Got," *Life*, November 23, 1942, p. 44.) "Here was the American war machine in action at last, in full view of all the world, well-timed, well-concealed, effective, and geared to the British in so practical a manner that the two nations were to all intents and purposes acting as one." (Ibid.)

567

MEMORANDUM FOR LIEUTENANT COLONEL C. J. GEORGE March 27, 1956
Pinehurst, North Carolina

The following is merely a repetition or confirmation of instructions I gave to you some years ago.

In the event of my death *I wish*:

a The services to be conducted in the Fort Myer chapel.

b. To be buried in my lot in Arlington Cemetery. (a new headstone will be necessary to include Katherine's name)

c The services in the cemetery to be private.

d The selection of the pall bearers to be left to you, except to include you, Sergeant Powder, Sergeant Heffner, Bedell Smith if he is in town, the following *if convenient* to them: Lovett, Jim Bruce, Frank M^c^Carthy.[1] No long list

GC Marshall

GCMRL/William J. Heffner Collection; H

1. Master Sergeant James W. Powder was Marshall's chief orderly during World War II.

568

TO FRANK MCCARTHY April 5, 1956
Pinehurst, North Carolina

Dear Frank— I am wondering if Daryl Zanuck's change of station has effected you materially? I do hope not unless favorably.[1]

We think of you often and your monthly fruit offering makes a frequent decided impression.[2]

Katherine has at last gotten fairly well over her shingles and back injury. Allene's daily requirements keeps her, K, down a little, but not as much as I feared. Allene's condition is unchanged though she grows stronger.

We were talking today with regret at how Virginia Stettinius had dropped out of our lives. As we don't get to Richmond we have no contacts.

I am well, but careful as usual.

We plan to go to Leesburg about May 1st. Heffner goes up a few days ahead to open the house. Our fine colored couple her[e] plan to go with us, which, if they do, will be a blessing.[3] We want to go to the Penna. mountains in August but can't make definite plans.[4]

Molly is happy in her lovely house at Fort Ritchie near Hagerstown, Penna, though it has been very cold, being in the mountains. It is the caretaking garrison for the underground headquarters for the Administration and the Chiefs of Staff.[5]

Pinehurst is lovely with the dogwood in full bloom.

Give my regards to Zanuck. Affectionately

GCMRL/Frank McCarthy Collection (Additions, Box 1); H

1. "Darryl F. Zanuck's decision to relinquish his post as vice president in charge of pro-

duction for Twentieth Century-Fox and go into independent production with the company is the result, in part, of the fact that high taxes are eating up most of his $260,000-a-year salary," the *New York Times* had reported on February 12. ("Hollywood Levies," *New York Times*, February 12, 1956, p. X5.) McCarthy responded on April 28 that it was "difficult to say" how "Zanuck's change of status may eventually affect me." (McCarthy to Marshall, April 28, 1956, GCMRL/G. C. Marshall Papers [Retirement, General].) He mentioned that he had been offered a partnership in a public relations firm but would "rather remain at 20th Century-Fox." (Ibid.)

2. See p. 854n7.

3. See p. 912n2.

4. See pp. 892–93, 906, and 907–8. Following their stay in Eagles Mere, Pennsylvania, in August 1955, newspapers had published stories about the Marshalls' plans to spend future summers there. When they received word that Twin Wicks cottage, which they had rented the previous summer, was available in August, Marshall had informed C. J. George that they were "so involved" with Mrs. Lacy's care and the "possible sale of Dodona etc. that we are unable to make an early reservation." (Laing to Spilman, March 28, 1956, GCMRL/G. C. Marshall Papers [Retirement, General].)

The Marshalls had received numerous offers for assistance in purchasing property in Eagles Mere. "Mrs. Marshall and I are very fond of the place and have hopes of buying a cottage," Marshall had written to William B. Forney Jr., director of Graphic Fashions in Philadelphia, Pennsylvania, on January 23, 1956. "We have several letters on the availability of houses, but we will wait until late Spring before deciding." (Marshall to Forney, January 23, 1956, ibid.) On January 26, Marshall received a long letter from Henry M. Gross, who informed him about several properties that might be available. "You are quite correct in your assumption that we need easy accessibility to the community's services," Marshall responded, "but that *privacy is paramount* in importance." (Marshall to Gross, January 31, 1956, ibid.) On February 3, Katherine Marshall also wrote to Gross that "We are looking forward with a great deal of pleasure to spending this summer at Eagles Mere." (Katherine Marshall to Gross, February 3, 1956, ibid.) On July 6, Marshall received word about another cottage but C. J. George responded on Marshall's behalf that "for a number of reasons we have been unable to come to a decision. However, it appears that we have to exclude a visit to the mountains at this time." (George to Kirk, July 30, 1956, ibid.)

5. Fort Ritchie and Hagerstown are located in Maryland near the Pennsylvania border.

569

To Bennett Foster

April 9, 1956
Pinehurst, North Carolina

My dear Foster: Copies of both TURN LOOSE YOUR WOLF and THE KID FROM DODGE CITY have arrived and been already read and much enjoyed. Thank you very much.[1]

I get a pleasant relaxation from "Westerns" if they are printed in plain type, particularly because I have been over much of the country depicted on horseback in my earlier Army days—mapping, maneuvers, marches, etc. I have been over much of southwestern Texas and along the Rio Grande (I mapped 2,000 square miles there on horseback in 1905, and did part of my "fill-in" sketching in Roy Bean's famous old cabin at Langtry), Arizona, New Mexico, Utah, Wyoming, along the Columbia River, the Blue Mountains in Oregon, etc.[2]

Carl Brandt informed me of your letter to him of March 9 and I am most appreciative of your gracious remarks of me.[3]

My thanks again for your thoughtfulness in sending the books.[4] Faithfully yours,

GCMRL/G. C. Marshall Papers (Retirement, General)

1. Bennett Foster was a writer of Western novels who lived in Albuquerque, New Mexico. On March 9 he had written to his New York literary agent Carl Brandt and recommended his book *Turn Loose Your Wolf* be sent to Marshall on Foster's account. "I believe it is as good a one as I ever wrote," and allowed, "it would be a small mark of my respect and admiration for the General." (Foster to Brandt, March 9, 1956, GCMRL/G. C. Marshall Papers [Retirement, General].) "The only other book I have in print is a reprint . . . under the title THE KID FROM DODGE CITY." (Ibid.)

2. See pp. 919–20. For more on Marshall's 1905 mapping assignment, see *Papers of GCM*, 1: 28–34, and Pogue, *Education*, 86–89. Roy Bean was a saloonkeeper in Langtry, Texas, who served as a justice of the peace off and on from 1882 to 1896 and billed himself as the "law west of the Pecos." He died in 1903. His exploits were dramatized in several Western films and books and inspired a television series that aired during the 1955–56 season.

3. Brandt had written to Marshall on March 13 and enclosed Foster's letter to Brandt in which he recalled having met Marshall in San Antonio, Texas, during World War II and praised him as "a great man." (Brandt to Marshall, March 13, 1956, ibid.)

4. "My kind of writer," Foster responded to Marshall on April 16, "serves no very useful purpose unless he entertains and it is nice to know you enjoyed the books." (Foster to Marshall, April 16, 1956, ibid.)

570

To Forrest C. Pogue

April 18, 1956
Pinehurst, North Carolina

Dear Pogue: Thank you for your letter of April 2 with the information that you have arranged to have mailed to me a copy of the book THE MEANING OF YALTA. I will read it with interest.[1]

I have not in any way altered my original decision with regard to my memoirs.[2] As a matter of fact, I am not writing my memoirs. The processing and possible release of any papers will be done by the Marshall Research Foundation, to a large extent without reference to me. I but agreed to fill in the portions the records do not cover.

I appreciate having your opinion of my attitude regarding unfavorable remarks made of me, as well as your comments regarding the Nobel ceremony. Frankly, I did not learn the exact details of what occurred until after the ceremony was over.[3]

With many thanks for having me in mind, and with warm regards,[4] Faithfully yours,

GCMRL/G. C. Marshall Papers (Retirement, General)

1. See pp. 843–44. Pogue was a contributor to *The Meaning of Yalta: Big Three Diplomacy and the New Balance of Power* (Baton Rouge: Louisiana State University Press, 1956), a volume edited by John L. Snell that made use of the extensive Yalta Conference documents published in 1955 by the State Department in a special volume of *FRUS* subtitled *The Conferences at Malta and Yalta, 1945*. In his April 2 letter to Marshall, Pogue had noted that his contribution to *The Meaning of Yalta* "is based on the published docu-

ments, but reflects the viewpoint towards your work and that of President Roosevelt which I gained in writing the official history of THE SUPREME COMMAND, which was sent you two years ago." (Pogue to Marshall, April 2, 1956, GCMRL/G. C. Marshall Papers [Retirement, General].)

2. "I was pleased to hear a short time ago that you had reversed your previous decision not to write on the war and had agreed to write something which would be published later," Pogue continued. "It was that which I was urging in my letter to you in 1954. I think it most important that the next generation have your story." (Ibid.) See pp. 843–44. For more on Marshall's refusal to write his memoirs, see *Papers of GCM*, 6: 638, 661, 663, and 743. See also pp. 161, 647–48, 648–49, 878–80, and 896–97.

3. "I have spoken often to friends of the Nobel Prize ceremony which I attended at Oslo when you received the award," Pogue wrote, and complimented Marshall's "calm bearing in the face of the Communist shouts when you stood to speak." (Ibid.) See p. 809. "It has also been a wonderful thing to see the way you have taken the false and malicious attacks on your policies. I am sure that the truth will win, but it is good to know that you have agreed to set down explanations which you alone can give." (Ibid.)

4. On April 25, C. J. George wrote to J. Clifford Miller, vice president of the Marshall Foundation, to recommend that Forrest Pogue be considered as foundation director. "I would like to suggest that in connection with my mentioning Pogue's name you write to his former chief, Major General Orlando Ward, who lives at Grand Lake, Colorado. He was head of the Historical Division during the period of Pogue's service there." (George to Miller, April 25, 1956, ibid.) See pp. 952–53.

571

To Tom Humphrey — April 24, 1956
Pinehurst, North Carolina

My dear Humphrey: I fear I cannot help you much on your write-up of Vancouver Barracks.[1] All I know is, or was, in my head. It wasn't much to begin with and has shrunk or evaporated considerably.

While I read a great deal of Vancouver history (all of which is available to you), much of my information came from Governor Martin who had reported there from West Point, spent many years on the post, married there, and finally returned to the political life of Oregon.[2]

One thing I recall as a remarkable coincidence: We officers gave him a dinner on the 50th anniversary (I think) of his reporting for duty there. The original commanding officer's quarters had, in my time, been converted into a club. Governor Martin was seated at the head of the table with me. Actually, and quite unintentionally, his chair marked the identical spot in his recollection where he had stood in reporting to Colonel Anderson fifty years earlier, very scared and humble in much travel-worn civilian clothes, his baggage carrying his uniforms having been temporarily lost. The Colonel refused to accept his report and sent him back to Portland to find his uniform.

The Russian affair is covered in detail in Mrs. Marshall's book TOGETHER or ANNALS OF AN ARMY WIFE.[3]

I was told General Nelson Miles built the present commanding officer's quarters, but before they were completed had to leave for the Geronimo Campaign in Arizona.[4]

At the moment, I don't think of anything that would be pertinent to your proposed article that you wouldn't already have. I don't know whether or not General Kearney served there.[5]

I recall Martin saying that for many years Vancouver Barracks was the center of civilization for a radius of 1,000 miles. When I was there, it was a back bay in general affairs.

I'm sorry I can't give you anything of value.[6] Faithfully yours,

GCMRL/G. C. Marshall Papers (Retirement, General)

1. "Revisiting Vancouver barracks the other day, in the process of developing material for a series of articles I am preparing," *Oregon Journal* Editor-at-Large Tom Humphrey had written to Marshall on April 12, "reminded me of the days when you were commandant and of several interesting events in which you figured prior to the war." (Humphrey to Marshall, April 12, 1956, GCMRL/G. C. Marshall Papers [Retirement, General].) Humphrey was preparing "a profile of the Vancouver community from the old Hudson's Bay fur trading post days to today." (Ibid.) "Remembering your interest in and knowledge of Northwest history and your sentimental interest in Vancouver Barracks, I'm wondering whether you could give me a hand to the extent of some personal observations about Fort Vancouver, its place in military history and about some of the officers who later were stationed at the Barracks." (Ibid.)

2. See p. 724. Vancouver Barracks was then Lieutenant Martin's first assignment after graduating from West Point in 1887. He married Louise J. Hughes, in Portland, Oregon, in 1897. Martin retired from the military in 1927 and returned to Portland. He represented Oregon in the House of Representatives from 1931 to 1935 and served one term as governor from 1935 to 1939.

3. "I remember particularly the arrival of the Russian fliers (that certainly was a tricky one to handle)," Humphrey reminded Marshall. (Ibid.) The Marshalls had entertained three Russian fliers who landed unexpectedly at Vancouver Barracks on June 20, 1937. See *Papers of GCM*, 1: 545–47, 549, 551; Pogue, *Education*, 306–7; and Marshall, *Together*, 25–28.

4. Nelson A. Miles had volunteered for the Union Army in 1861 and had been promoted to the brevet rank of brigadier general by the end of the Civil War. He received the Medal of Honor in 1892 for his actions during the 1863 Battle of Chancellorsville. Miles led many of the army's campaigns against American Indians following the Civil War before he assumed command of the Department of the Columbia, with headquarters at Vancouver Barracks, on August 2, 1881, with the permanent rank of brigadier general. In 1886 Miles commanded the campaign against Apache leader Geronimo and his warriors, and in 1895 he was named commanding general of the US Army, the senior officer in the army at the time. While in this position, he led the Puerto Rico campaign during the Spanish-American War as well as the military government established on the island following the war. He was promoted to lieutenant general in 1900 and retired in 1903.

5. Humphrey listed several prominent military officers associated with Vancouver Barracks and ended by asking Marshall "Was Kearney there too?" (Humphrey to Marshall, April 12, 1956, GCMRL/G. C. Marshall Papers [Retirement, General].) Humphrey probably referred to Brigadier General Stephen W. Kearny, who led forces that conquered California in the Mexican-American War.

6. "I discovered when I tried to purchase a copy of Mrs. Marshall's book that it is out of print," Humphrey told Marshall when he wrote on June 19 to thank him for his response. (Humphrey to Marshall, June 19, 1956, ibid.)

572

To Major General William H. Milton Jr. April 24, 1956
Pinehurst, North Carolina

Dear Milton: Many thanks for your note of April 16 and for the copy of the Resolution passed by the Board of Visitors on April 13. I am both pleased and gratified at these gracious expressions. Please accept for yourself and express to the Board my thanks.[1]

I, too, am looking forward to attending Finals, but I must caution you not to count too heavily on my being present, because my energy is an erratic factor which may desert me at the last moment and prevent my making the trip.[2]

With best wishes, Faithfully yours,

GCMRL/G. C. Marshall Papers (Retirement, General)

1. The VMI Board of Visitors had gone "on record" at its April 13 meeting with a "testimonial of its confidence and trust in the loyalty and integrity" of the Marshall Foundation Board of Directors and "its implicit confidence and trust in its affairs to carry on the same to a successful termination." (VMI Board of Visitors resolution, April 13, 1956, GCMRL/G. C. Marshall Papers [Retirement, General].) The Board of Visitors also pledged "its hearty cooperation to the George C. Marshall Research Foundation in all things deemed advisable to successfully carry out its most laudable undertakings." (Ibid.)

2. Milton closed his cover letter "With best regards of all of us at the Institute, who are looking forward with much anticipation to your being here at Finals, and with my own warm personal regards." (Milton to Marshall, April 16, 1956, ibid.) See pp. 938–42.

573

To Charles E. Wilson May 7, 1956
Leesburg, Virginia

Dear Mr. Secretary: Thank you very much for your letter of April 25 and enclosures regarding the organization of the Department of Defense. Up to now, I have hastily checked through the pamphlets, but I will give them a closer reading in the week to come.[1]

I appreciate your asking me to join the Committee for luncheon and a meeting on May 23. Barring any unforeseen complications, I will be there.[2] Faithfully yours,

GCMRL/G. C. Marshall Papers (Retirement, General)

1. "It is almost three years since the Rockefeller Committee on the Organization of the Department of Defense turned in its report," Secretary of Defense Wilson had written to Marshall on April 25. See pp. 755–56. "Since that time we have made a very serious effort to implement its recommendations and, in addition, have made a number of organizational and operational changes that we feel are in consonance with those recommendations." (Wilson to Marshall, April 26, 1956, GCMRL/G. C. Marshall Papers [Retirement, General].) Wilson enclosed information from an advisory committee on fiscal organization and procedures as well as the Hoover Commission's conclusions on business organization in the Department of Defense. (Ibid.)

2. "I hope you will be able to join with all the members of the Rockefeller Committee

for a luncheon here in the Pentagon at 12:30 on May 23rd and that we will have a chance for several hours of discussion on these matters following luncheon," Wilson urged. (Ibid.) On May 1, Nelson Rockefeller also wrote to Marshall and urged him to attend the luncheon. (Rockefeller to Marshall, May 1, 1956, ibid.)

574

STATEMENT FOR THE GENERAL FRANK MCCOY MEMORIAL[1] May 23, 1956
Leesburg, Virginia

Among the many friends I have had in my military service—the men I have grown to admire, the men for whom I developed a deep affection—none quite reached the position of General McCoy. He had qualities so fine and so rare as almost to be unique in the exact meaning of the word.

His standards of honor and the integrity of his every action were clearly apparent to the most casual acquaintance. He was generous to a fault in every phase of his career. To know him intimately was a rare and genuine privilege.

I did not know General McCoy during his younger Army years. I knew he had a fine record at West Point and was catcher of the Cadet ball team. I knew he was wounded at San Juan in 1898 and later became one of General Leonard Wood's most trusted assistants in Cuba and the Philippines. He was a Presidential Aide and intimate companion of Theodore Roosevelt.

I came to know him on our entry into the First World War. His career in France was outstanding, both as a GHQ staff officer and as a fighting regimental and brigade commander.

Later he was called upon by Presidents—I am using the plural—to perform missions of critical and international importance, notably the pacification and reorganization of Nicaragua and the Lytton Commission to China. He was, in effect, a leading man in the State Department.

During the last war we came into close association on a number of issues. Always General McCoy was selfless, calm, sane and wholly dependable.

Altogether his varied career as an Army Officer furnishes a model, a wonderful example for the young officers who choose to make that a career. Unfortunately he moved about so quietly, so modestly that few who did not come in personal contact with him are aware of his record.[2]

His death created a great void in my life, because his friendship was one of my most cherished possessions. I am delighted that his home town people have concluded to pay him this high honor. I had hoped to be present so that I might more adequately and abundantly convey my real feelings for General McCoy, but I am sure that General Groninger, in his reading of this brief message, has expressed quite fully my impression of a great American.

I should not close without mention that through a great part of his service General McCoy greatly profited by an ideal wife and helpmate. She was all things that a woman should be to the man she chooses for life partnership.[3]

GCMRL/G. C. Marshall Papers (Retirement, General)

1. This statement was read by Major General Homer Groninger (USMA, 1908) on June 4, 1956, at the unveiling of a memorial honoring General Frank McCoy in Lewistown, Pennsylvania. Groninger, who was commanding general of the port of Brooklyn during World War II, had retired to Port Royal, Pennsylvania, seventeen miles from Lewistown, where the McCoy memorial was to be dedicated.

2. For another tribute to General McCoy by Marshall, see pp. 869–71.

3. See p. 942.

575

To Gladys Marion Brooks[1] May 23, 1956
Leesburg, Virginia

My dear Gladys: Both Mrs. Marshall and I were delighted at your winning a National Merit Scholarship and being accepted by Swarthmore College. Your mother should be very happy.[2]

I have complete confidence in your ability to make a fine record there. I hope that from time to time you will send me a note telling me how well you are doing, because I would be much interested.[3] Faithfully yours,

GCMRL/G. C. Marshall Papers (Retirement, General)

1. Gladys Brooks's mother had worked as a housekeeper at Eagles Mere, Pennsylvania, in 1955, where she met Marshall and asked him to provide a recommendation for her daughter's college applications. See pp. 895–96. On August 30, 1955, Brooks sent Marshall a three-page summary of her "scholastic attainments" in high school, which Marshall asked M. L. Spilman to "type in third person, correcting spelling if necessary, or sentence structure." (Brooks to Marshall, August 30, 1955, GCMRL/G. C. Marshall Papers [Retirement, General].) On January 10, 1956, Swarthmore College informed Marshall that Brooks had given his name as a reference on a scholarship application. (Keeny to Marshall, January 10, 1956, ibid.)

2. "I believe my mother has sent you a newspaper clipping about my winning a National Merit Scholarship," Brooks had written to Marshall on May 17, and told him that she had been accepted by Swarthmore, which was "the fulfillment of all my dreams." (Brooks to Marshall, May 17, 1956, ibid.) She expressed her "deep gratitude for your part in bringing about these opportunities, and I promise to do everything in my power to justify your trust in me." (Ibid.)

3. Marshall and Brooks corresponded again during her freshman year. (See Marshall to Brooks, December 31, 1956, and Brooks to Marshall, February 4, 1957, ibid.) Gladys Brooks Block went on to earn a PhD from the Johns Hopkins School of Public Health and become a professor at the University of California at Berkeley.

576

To William Arthur[1] June 6, 1956
Leesburg, Virginia

Dear Mr. Arthur: During the period July 16–30 this Commission will dedicate six World War II Cemeteries in Europe.[2] The program has been arranged as follows:

July 16—Cambridge, England[3]
July 19—St. Laurent, France
July 20—St. James, France
July 23—Epinal, France
July 26—Draguignan, France
July 30—Anzio, Italy[4]

The [American Battle Monuments] Commission has been most fortunate in obtaining acceptances of invitations from a number of distinguished Americans and foreign nationals.[5] Incidentally, the three Service Secretaries will participate in the dedicatory programs.[6]

As you might well know, the American Government has expended millions of dollars in creating beautiful Cemeteries and Memorials to perpetuate the memory of those who gave their all.[7] I think it only fitting that the whole of our People know what is being done. I would like to request you to consider the prospects of running an appropriate article and, as they often say that pictures speak more clearly, I think if our People could see the visual results of our Government's effort they would most certainly appreciate what has been done.[8] Faithfully yours,

GCMRL/G. C. Marshall Papers (American Battle Monuments Commission)

1. Arthur was the managing editor of *LOOK* magazine. See p. 873.
2. The American Battle Monuments Commission had issued a press release on April 9 announcing the dedication ceremonies. (ABMC press release, April 9, 1956, GCMRL/G. C. Marshall Papers [American Battle Monuments Commission].) "Civilian and military officials . . . will be invited to attend the ceremonies." (Ibid.)
3. "Our dedication ceremony at Cambridge went off splendidly, without a hitch," General Thomas North wrote to Marshall on July 18. "Even the prolonged rains which we have been having ceased during the ceremony and resumed immediately afterwards." (North to Marshall, July 18, 1956, ibid.)
4. In a September 25 memorandum ABMC Vice Chairman Admiral Thomas C. Kinkaid reported to Marshall that "audiences numbered from 1,200 to 2,000, of whom perhaps 10 to 15 per cent were Americans." (Kinkaid to Marshall, memorandum, September 25, 1956, ibid.) See p. 956.
5. Major General William J. Donovan, who was head of Office of Strategic Services in World War II, participated in all of the ceremonies as President Eisenhower's representative. (Ibid.) Veterans of Foreign Wars, the American Legion, Disabled American Veterans, American War Mothers, and AMVETS also sent representatives to each event and "a total of 23 veterans of the three Services, decorated with the Medal of Honor, Distinguished Service Cross, or Navy Cross attended the ceremonies also as special guests of the Commission. A minimum of four such veterans were present at each ceremony; on some occasions eight attended." (Ibid.) Commissioners Kinkaid, Leslie L. Biffle, General Alexander A. Vandegrift, Mrs. Theodore Roosevelt, Brigadier General Benjamin O. Davis, General Carl Spaatz, and Senator Charles E. Potter represented the ABMC. (Ibid.)
6. "I was particularly delighted to receive word from Colonel George that the Secretaries of the Army, Navy and Air Force had accepted the invitation to participate in this Commission's dedicatory programs in Europe," Marshall had written to Secretary of Defense Wilson on May 23. "I know that their presence and participation will add considerably to the occasions." (Marshall to Wilson, May 23, 1956, ibid.)
7. "In each cemetery a memorial has been erected which contains a small chapel, an engraved list of those who have no known graves or who were lost or buried at sea, and large maps outlining the achievements of American forces in these regions." (ABMC press release, April 9, 1956, ibid.)

8. An identical letter was sent to the editor of the *Saturday Evening Post* but "they felt their article of several months ago was all that they could do at this time." (George to North, June 14, 1956, ibid.) William Arthur replied to Marshall that he was "pleased that you wrote to LOOK in connection with this project" and proposed that the magazine would feature the six cemeteries in its regular "LOOK Applauds" feature in an issue that would be published "around Armistice Day." (Arthur to Marshall, June 8, 1956, ibid.) One photograph appeared in the November 13, 1956, issue of *LOOK* magazine.

On December 3, Marshall sent President Eisenhower "an album of photographs, press reports, and other documents" concerning the dedication cereomies and encouraged him "to read Admiral Kinkaid's memorandum to me, because he provides a very comprehensive report on the dedicatory program." (Marshall to Eisenhower, December 3, 1956, ibid.) Marshall had written to Kinkaid on September 28 that he regretted "that it was not possible for me to make the trip, and I was glad when you agreed to act in my stead." (Marshall to Kinkaid, September 28, 1956, ibid.)

577

Remarks to the Graduates of the Virginia Military Institute

June 12, 1956
Lexington, Virginia

When you have reached my age you feel rather free to make highly personal comments—which is my excuse for doing so right now. I have not participated in any public gatherings for almost two years. I had a ten-month bout with virus flu and that wasn't included in the curriculum here, and I haven't fully recovered. But when I was told by General Milton that a committee of the first class had expressed a personal desire to have me participate in their final ceremony of their cadet careers, I accepted immediately. I stipulated, however that I wouldn't talk more than five minutes, which, of course, is a rather difficult thing because when you have to say very little, you have to say something![1]

And the other day I finally got around to it and I wrote out a little sketch of what I might say in five minutes, and then in following my usual custom, I read it to Mrs. Marshall—this is advice to you who have not yet married! When I got through—she's always very frank; she's interested in my career, my reputation—so I asked her, "How about it?" She said, "It's terrible." So I said, "That's my opening speech. I'll just throw this aside and I'll talk about what appeals to me in the spirit of the moment." So what I'm saying is off the cuff, as it were.

Under similar circumstances I was reminded last night that I had talked here sixteen years ago and that I was moved up to the very commencement of the program because we had just learned of the fall of Paris to the Germans and President Roosevelt had sent word down here for me to return immediately. So I made my speech and left for Washington.[2]

That seems a long time ago and there were terrible years to follow, particularly for the young graduates that I addressed that day and for their contemporaries throughout the country.

At the present time we have a peace, but it's a nervous peace. That's what we all strive for, peace, but we are under a tension with a very large part of the population of the world. The daily grist—in the papers, the commentators, columnists, the radio, TV, oratory in Congress—relates to this. And we have many critical situations which are always dangerous because nobody can tell to what they might lead. So it occurred to me that probably the best I could do would be to make some reference to you to the state of the world into which you are entering in active citizenship.

I might say in the first place that it is extraordinarily hard to evaluate these various critical situations, and one of the great weaknesses in the situation for us is that so few of our people and few of our leaders are intimately familiar with the exact conditions. Most of our people don't understand the traditions, the deep feelings, the habits of life, the aspirations of other peoples. It is in such great contrast to our own life. We are impatient and want things to happen very, very quickly. And we are dealing with nations whose histories go back hundreds and hundreds and hundreds of years. And they feel very deeply about this and that we are wholly unaware of it. And we can offend bitterly and be totally unconscious of doing so. We have fixed opinions about a thing and are woefully ignorant of what the background is. It all makes for a very complex situation and of course it is further complicated, it seems rather paradoxical, by the fact that the news from here from all over the United States circulates all over the world in virtually a few minutes.

I remember once when I was Secretary of State and we were dealing with great difficulty in Congress with what was to be the European Recovery Program, the so-called Marshall Plan, and one of the members of the Cabinet got one sentence into something he said. He didn't mean it in the way it was taken, but the next morning my desk was just covered with reports from all our ambassadors giving me the headlines in all the various European papers. They had turned on us *en bloc* in antagonism to what this man had said without any comprehension that he had in any way irritated them.

We are the richest country in the world. That is a great danger, as well as a great satisfaction, to our citizenship because the whole world in a sense is a little suspicious and jealous of such great riches. The generosity is not thoroughly understood. That shouldn't prevent it. It's like our wealthy men and all. You don't have that reaction abroad. It's a sporting proposition. They build up great wealth and then they get rid of it. The great foundations that you see illustrated here almost every day, notably recently the Ford Foundation—that doesn't occur in the same sense abroad. They just think that we are dollar marks but we are just exactly the opposite.

We are the most generous people under the heavens, but the great difficulty is for our people to understand, for you young men to understand, the situation where countries are jammed up against each other, where they speak different languages, where they have jealousies that go back two or three hundred years. All of them try to get together despite all these differences that are almost ineradicable. But you have to deal with it.

And in the usual thing, we being a democracy, it is complicated by what is said and what is printed. Now I talk to you, young men, about this because you are just entering into your active citizenship. You have better trained minds, far above the average. You also have a sense of discipline, respect for authority, things of that sort, integrity which is often referred to, which is of vast importance in the body politic. So I think I will risk advising you to go very carefully in making up your mind about these various things. Don't be wedded to one pleasant voice, don't be wedded to one attractive way of writing things, maybe some columnist, but try to search out for what seems to be the fact. And if you have time look into the racial history of the people involved and get some idea as to what it's all about from that point of view. Then you are in a position to express an opinion. You can't very well avoid it because it is a daily topic of conversation, the grist of the papers, all the news that comes to you. That's the big item along with several other local ones, but it's one of the big items in our daily life.

It is certainly very critical in a sense, these foreign complications. They're the most difficult things of all to compose. I recall once hearing the conference of governors out in Salt Lake City.[3] I got in for the discussion. I was to make a talk that night and I flew out and just heard the end of the thing. They had been discussing all day long the unification of state and federal tax affairs where one intruded on the other. And, of course, taxes intrude on everything political and also on your own pocketbook—you haven't got one yet but you will have one pretty soon. And they said at the end of it, two or three of them in succession, when it was hopeless to take this up in just one day, that you couldn't possibly find any adequate recommendations on such short consideration. Well, at that time we had a group headed by an English chairman representing the countries of Western Europe trying to make a proposal to us for what eventually was the European Recovery Program. I declined to let our people suggest anything. It had to come entirely from the other side. And they had been at it for about two weeks. Members of Congress were very impatient because they didn't settle this in two weeks. It involved sovereign rights; it involved everything about their citizenship. You couldn't have gotten anything that would have more deeply affected the whole life of all of those countries. And our people thought two weeks was too long. These governors, that all spoke the same language, had been talking about this all the time and had a whole day to discuss it, thought it couldn't possibly be settled in that time. It was going to take a long time to do it. But over here, with all these conflicting languages and traditions, feelings, it was supposed to be settled in two weeks.

There is a lack of comprehension of what it is abroad, what the countries are like, the whole set-up politically, the human particularly, and you have to know something about that, not the tourist reaction but the main reaction. I sometimes think that maybe the tourist reaction is a little harmful because it is so hasty. You don't draw all your conclusions at the Bois de Boulogne and the Cafe de la Paix.[4] It doesn't come out that way.

The effort to get at the facts is the important thing. And if you will permit me I will counsel you to try to do that. It's not so difficult as it might seem.

We all know there are some newspapers that print the facts and not just one political side or another political side, always with ulterior motives. There are certain columnists that are well known for the fact that they deal with the facts and not with the prejudices. So if you take a careful resume of the whole thing and don't be devoted to one voice or one method of writing, you begin to get something which approaches the facts. It's very difficult but it's very important. You have to remember that in our country, take it geographically, the Wyoming cowboy and a Wall Street broker are miles apart, a Northwest lumberman and a Georgia cotton grower, they don't speak the same language at all, in a sense, yet they are all Americans and they are all patriotic. We have that all over our country because we are very widely spread, and that is one of the complications. England is a very cohesive, small country and they have Welshmen, of course, and Yorkshiremen and all that, but they have a common bond that is very close and very understanding. But here you have the Rocky Mountain states, the Deep South, this, that and the other all over, and there's a different language up in Boston, New York, down in Savannah, out in San Francisco—and a brand new one coming out of Los Angeles with the movement of the new settlers into that region.

So it's a very disturbed world. It's a very critical world. And if you will permit the suggestion from me—and I know of my own feelings as a young man listening to the commencement day orations that I always got sore when they began advising me—my best advice that I could give you in the present day is, Don't be a deep feeler and a poor thinker. I'll repeat that again, Don't be a deep feeler and a poor thinker.[5]

I am very grateful for the invitation to come down. I'm very glad to see you all and it's very stimulating for me to be here in assemblies like this again and I thank you very much.[6]

GCMRL/G. C. Marshall Papers (Retirement, General)

1. "Many members of the Corps of Cadets have expressed a great desire to have you visit the Institute and talk to them," General Milton had written to Marshall on February 29. Despite some hesitation to make such a request, Milton invited Marshall to speak at VMI's graduation ceremony on June 12 and to attend "festivities surrounding Finals" beginning on June 9. (Milton to Marshall, February 29, 1956, GCMRL/G. C. Marshall Papers [Retirement, General].) Marshall accepted on March 5 with several conditions. He requested that Milton "make the real address and I finish with a mere five-minute speech"; that he would not be required "to participate in any receptions or hand-shaking affairs"; that these "restrictions" not be publicized to prevent any embarrassment; and that he would not arrive on post "until the evening before" graduation. "I am sorry to be so demanding, but it's the only basis on which I can accept." (Marshall to Milton, March 5, 1956, ibid.) Milton was "delighted" with Marshall's acceptance and assured Marshall on March 9 that "the conditions that you make are most acceptable to us and fully understandable." (Milton to Marshall, March 9, 1956, ibid.) See p. 934.

On June 4, C. J. George had confirmed to the VMI commandant that Marshall would "arrive by air at Lexington around 2:30" on Monday afternoon, June 11. (George to Kerlin, June 4, 1956, ibid.)

2. For excerpts from Marshall's June 12, 1940, commencement speech at VMI, see *Papers of GCM*, 2: 244–45n1.

3. Marshall had addressed the National Governors' Conference in Salt Lake City, Utah, on July 14, 1947. See *Papers of GCM*, 6: 172–76.

4. The Bois de Boulogne is a public park in Paris, and the Café de la Paix is a restaurant in Le Grand Hotel in Paris.

5. See p. 960.
6. "I very much enjoyed my visit to the Institute and the brief participation in the graduation exercises," Marshall wrote to General Milton on June 19. "I feel that I slipped out unnoticed, and I had a convenient ride back to my quarters in the State Police car. I believe that this visit was the most relaxed one that I have ever had, and the interest you showed in me is very much appreciated. I hope you will let Mrs. Milton know of my thanks for her many courtesies and for providing me a protective corner on her porch." (Marshall to Milton, June 19, 1956, ibid.)

578

TO MRS. FRANK MCCOY — June 20, 1956
Leesburg, Virginia

Dear Francis, Your sweet note was greatly appreciated, and I was so glad to learn that the affair went off so beautifully.[1]

Sorry as I was not to be there I quickly learned at the V.M.I. finals that it had been a wise decision.

The VMI affair was my only engagement I can think of in the past two years. While it was only a forty five minute flight and was cool weather I found that I could not do much. I went to no parades or receptions, stayed in my rooms most of the time and made but a five minute talk. I left the ceremony immediately I finished talking and went to bed. While I was only there 24 hours and did almost nothing it pretty well tired me out.[2]

Katherine is pretty well but worries too constantly about Allene and seems to spend her time writing to her and the nurse and searching Allene's trunks and bags for this and that.[3]

We are getting our place in order but I have not made notable progress with the flowers. Our Colored man who came up from Pinehurst with us—and [h]is wife and two young children, has done a small garden.[4]

Some viewers are coming to see the house to-morrow. We put it back on the market ten days ago.[5] It seems very sad to think of leaving, but unless we have a guarantee of good servants it is too much for Katherine We do have an excellent couple now, the ones we had all winter—but you never can tell. Affectionately,

GCM

GCMRL/G. C. Marshall Collection (Frances McCoy); H

1. "The Mifflin County Historical Society is planning a Memorial for General Frank McCoy on Monday, June 4, 1956, the anniversary of his death, at which time his widow will present the Society his numerous commissions and mementos," Senator Edward Martin had written to Marshall on January 27. (Martin to Marshall, January 27, 1956, GCMRL/G. C. Marshall Papers [Retirement, General].) See pp. 869–71. "You being a very close friend of General McCoy and one of Pennsylvania's most outstanding sons of all times, we feel it would be appropriate if you could be present on this occasion." (Ibid.) Marshall responded on February 20 that he would "very much" like to attend but that he could not commit so far in advance. (Marshall to Martin, February 20, 1956, ibid.; H.) Reverend Henry A. Riddle of Lewistown, Pennsylvania, chairman of the historical society's McCoy Memorial, had also written to invite Marshall to speak at the event. (Riddle to Marshall, January 26, 1956, ibid.) See pp. 935–36.

"I was very much touched, pleased & honored by your charming message to the Lewistown meeting which Gen. Groninger read—we missed you—but knew you were with us in spirit & feeling," Frances McCoy had written to Marshall on June 11. "I kept thinking how much Frank would have been overcome by it and how he could have enjoyed telling the people how he felt about *you*." (McCoy to Marshall, June 11, 1956, GCMRL/G. C. Marshall Papers [Retirement, General].)

2. See previous document.

3. On May 23, Katherine Marshall had written to Mrs. Jefferson Caffery that Allene Lacy "wished to remain in the Pinehurst Convalescent Home" when the Marshalls returned to Leesburg for the summer. (Katherine Marshall to Caffery, May 23, 1956, ibid.) Mrs. Marshall had known Mrs. Caffery when Jefferson Caffery was US ambassador to France from 1944 to 1949. See *Papers of GCM*, 6: 560–61.

4. See p. 912n2.

5. See pp. 906–7 and 907–8. The Marshalls signed a contract on June 6 listing Dodona manor for seventy-five thousand dollars with the George Mason Green Company of Arlington, Virginia, "exclusively and irrevocably until the 31st day of October 1956." (Dodona Manor contract, June 6, 1956, GCMRL/© Marshall-Winn Collection [Household files, Dodona Manor].)

NEWS OF THE DEATH on June 25 of Fleet Admiral Ernest J. King at the naval hospital in Portsmouth, New Hampshire, "shocked" Marshall. ("Eisenhower Pays Tribute to Admiral; Former Comrades Also Praise Career," *New York Times*, June 26, 1956, p. 28.) Vice Admiral James L. Holloway Jr. (USNA, 1919), chief of Naval Personnel, wired Marshall the following day to request that he "act as honorary pall bearer at funeral service to be held in Washington National Cathedral at 1300 hours on the 29th of June. Burial will be in the Naval Academy Cemetery at Annapolis the same date." (Holloway to Marshall, telegram, June 26, 1956, GCMRL/G. C. Marshall Papers [Retirement, General].)

M. L. Spilman advised Holloway that Marshall would attend the service "in civilian dress." (Spilman to Marshall, June 27, 1956, ibid.) She assured Marshall that he could go directly to the cathedral rather than assemble two hours earlier with the other honorary pallbearers at the Army-Navy Club. (Ibid.) At the end of her instructions, Spilman added "a personal comment: I was sorry to learn that you plan to attend these services. I fully appreciate why you want to and feel you should pay your final respects to Admiral King. But the heat in Washington is and has been so intense that I fear you may subject yourself to more than just discomfort by making the trip. I feel that Washington is no place to be right now unless the need is quite urgent." (Ibid.) Marshall attended the funeral at the cathedral but it is not clear whether he joined in the burial ceremony. ("Tribute Is Paid to Admiral King," *New York Times*, June 30, 1950, p. 17.)

More distressing was the loss of "one of my closest friends," Major General Walter S. Grant, who had died on March 4 at Walter Reed Hospital, where he had been confined for several years with Parkinson's disease. Marshall wrote the next day to Grant's widow that he "admired and respected his character above most men I have known." (Grant to Marshall, telegram, and Marshall to Grant, March 5, 1956, GCMRL/G. C. Marshall Papers [Retirement, General].) Marshall had known Grant since they served together in France in World War I. (See Marshall, *Memoirs*, 207.)

Another sad note came with word of the death of Thomas J. Watson Sr., who died on June 19 after a brief illness. ("Thomas J. Watson Sr. Is Dead; I.B.M. Board Chairman Was 82," *New York Times*, June 20, 1956, p. 1.) Watson was one of the very few men he met late in life whom Marshall addressed by first name. (See p. 22.) Watson's final letter to Marshall, dated February 24, 1956, conveyed their reciprocal affection: "The increasing years bring increasing appreciation of friendships such as yours, and I want you to know that I was deeply touched by your remembrance," he wrote, referring to Marshall's birthday greeting on February 17. (Watson to Marshall, February 24, 1956, GCMRL/G. C. Marshall Papers [Retirement, General].) Marshall, who was "laid up" at the time of Watson's death, handwrote his widow a note on July 24, acknowledging that he admired Watson "greatly as did thousands of others who knew him. His accomplishments were truly magnificent, but most of all I admired his family life as a husband and a father." (Marshall to Watson, July 24, 1956, ibid.; H.)

Marshall also learned that Ralph C. Kennedy, a fellow Uniontown native, died in June. "We were very old friends," he wrote their mutual friend, philanthropist and fellow VMI Board of Visitors member Jay Winston Johns; Marshall added that he would miss Kennedy's "engaging, though infrequent, letters." (Johns to Marshall, June 22, 1956, ibid.; Marshall to Johns, July 5, 1956, CWM/Jay W. Johns Papers.) In 1954, Kennedy had forwarded a photograph taken during Marshall's September 1953 trip to Uniontown. See p. 794n4. The picture showed Marshall with a youngster whose father "had taken his son to the hotel and got you to pose with him because the boy, too, has a December 31st birthday." (Kennedy to Marshall, July 27, 1954, GCMRL/G. C. Marshall Papers [Retirement, General].) Marshall made a note at the bottom of Kennedy's letter that he was "only too glad to oblige. Nice looking boy but I look like hell." (Ibid.)

Earlier in the year Marshall had received a report about Edmund Coles (brother of his first wife, Lily Coles Marshall), who had suffered a stroke the previous May. Coles had fallen several times, had pneumonia and a severe rash resulting from an allergic reaction to penicillin, and possessed virtually no memory but his wife assured Marshall that Coles "*never* complains." Marshall responded to Sadie Coles on June 27 that he was "relieved for you that Edmund is still able to move about with assistance and is in such a warm frame of mind." (Coles to Marshall, February 20, and Marshall to Coles, June 27, 1956, ibid.)

Marshall continued to advise his contemporaries about the dangers of attempting to rush recovery from illness such as he had experienced in 1953–54 (see pp. 793–95 and 832). "I had a ten-month case of virus-flu that just about ruined me," he wrote on July 17 to Wendell Hammond, who had trained under Marshall at the CCC camp at Fort Douglas, Utah, in 1916. Marshall emphasized that "only time and patience seemed to be the cures," and warned, "You may feel temporarily better, but, if you resume any activity, you pay a heavy price in returns." (Marshall to Hammond, July 17, 1956, ibid.; H.) Hammond had been sending the Marshalls annual shipments of cherries from his property in Bountiful, Utah, since at least 1949. (Hammond to Marshall, June 27, 1949, ibid.) "Now we come to the time when usually I send you a box of cherries," Hammond had written earlier in July but "for several weeks I have been ill and at home, perhaps due to overwork and an attack of the flu" and mentioned that he was "taking one of the new wonder drugs which aid such a condition." In response, Marshall cautioned Hammond that "The doctors seem to know little about this virus business, except if you take the so-called miracle drugs within the first 36 hours, you may beat the attack, but after your system once gets saturated with the germ, whatever it is, then it's a prolonged ordeal." (Hammond to Marshall, July 10, 1956, and Marshall to Hammond, July 17, 1956, ibid.)

Good news came on July 18 when Marshall learned that his friend John Leighton Stuart (see pp. 829–30) was "improving steadily" after a setback, according to Philip Fugh, who was Stuart's personal assistant when he was president of Yenching University and US ambassador to China. "We hope that he will be back to his old self again in the course of a few weeks." (Fugh to Marshall, July 18, 1956, ibid.) Marshall had visited Stuart in September 1955 and afterward wrote to C. J. George that he found Stuart "completely paralyzed, hands and legs, but looking surprisingly well in the face." (Marshall to George, September 12, 1955, ibid.) Stuart wrote to Marshall on April 20 to commemorate the tenth anniversary of their first meeting in Nanking. He assured Marshall that he was "very contented" and grateful for "the devotedly vigilant care of Philip and his family." (Stuart to Marshall, April 20, 1956, ibid.) Marshall responded to Fugh's July 18 letter that he was "very happy" to receive the "good news," and admitted that in June he also had been "somewhat under the weather." Marshall suggested that "If I get to the point of driving into Washington again, I will try and arrange to call on Doctor Stuart." (Marshall to Fugh, July 30, 1956, ibid.) ★

579

To the Adjutant General[1]

July 1, 1956
Leesburg, Virginia

I would repeat my comments on his last two efficiency reports.[2] And add: He performs duty in a superior manner more appropriate to the grade of brigadier general. He strikes all levels of his duties with equal energy and efficiency. He is exceptionally efficiency [efficient] in all matters which I have had to do concerning foreign relations.[3]

GCMRL/G. C. Marshall Collection (C. J. George); H

1. The following are Marshall's handwritten notes on a form "worksheet for efficiency report" for C. J. George.

2. On June 16, 1954, Marshall had deemed George "A most exceptional (superior) officer" in his annual evaluation. Marshall also noted that his aide's "efficiency covers a wide range in international meetings at home and abroad, relationships with our Embassies in Europe and So. America and with foreign officials of *all* ranks, United Nations organization, wide and intimate acquaintance with officials and distinguished civilians in this country, exceptional organizer and executive, gets along smoothly with everyone or organization, performs all duties from the most formal to the most personal and even humble

in this same fine spirit. (Marshall to adjutant general, note, June 16, 1954, GCMRL/G. C. Marshall Collection [George].)

3. On July 12, Marshall also signed off on C. J. George's "suggested rating" for General Thomas North's efficiency report, which read in part: "General North continues to perform his duties in an exceptional manner. He is an indefatigable individual of high character and integrity." (George to Marshall, July 12, 1956, GCMRL/G. C. Marshall Papers [Retirement, General].) "I know that every member of the [American Battle Monuments] Commission shares my opinion and confidence in General North." (Ibid.) See pp. 734–35, 783–84, and 951.

580

TO F. WARREN PERSHING

July 2, 1956
Leesburg, Virginia

My dear Warren: Your letter of June 21 has been received.[1]

The Congress has authorized the American Battle Monuments Commission to recommend a site and type, and ascertain the cost of an appropriate memorial to your Father—all of which are to be presented to the Congress for approval. The site preferred by the A. B. M. C. is the rectangle on Pennsylvania Avenue between 14th and 15th Streets. The Commission had an architect draw-up what the Commission approved as an appropriate memorial. But the Fine Arts Commission, informally, has declined to approve the memorial *for that site*. They would approve it for another site, perhaps in the region between the First and Second Division memorials. The Fine Arts Commission and the A. B. M. C. both are anxious to have the Pennsylvania Avenue rectangle site for the memorial, and we believe we can secure the approval of the Fine Arts Commission if we can have an appropriate memorial designed which would include a large fountain. As soon as we receive an official statement on our proposal from the Fine Arts Commission, the A. B. M. C. can proceed further.[2]

As to the inscription, I will give it some careful thinking before answering your question.[3]

I'm glad to hear of the health and prosperity of your family. Give my best to your wife.[4]

With warm regards,[5] Faithfully yours,

GCMRL/G. C. Marshall Papers (Retirement, General)

1. "I noticed in the paper some time ago that Congress had authorized a memorial to my Father," New York stockbroker F. Warren Pershing, only son of General John J. Pershing, had written to Marshall. If this was under Marshall's purview as chairman of the ABMC, Pershing "would be interested in knowing what your thoughts are." (Pershing to Marshall, June 21, 1956, GCMRL/G. C. Marshall Papers [Retirement, General].) General Pershing had preceded Marshall as chairman of the ABMC.

2. The ABMC had officially presented the plans for its proposed memorial to General Pershing at Pennsylvania Avenue and Fourteenth Street to the Washington, DC, Fine Arts Commission on June 12. While the Fine Arts Commission "complimented" the design and presentation, it did not accept the ABMC proposal. John Harbeson, a consulting architect to the ABMC, opined that the Fine Arts Commission, "perhaps at the urging of the" National Capital Planning Commission, "feels that this site should be used for a big foun-

tain because of its relation to the view down Pennsylvania Avenue toward Treasury and the White House. If ABMC would consider a fountain as suitable for [the] Pershing Memorial, they would be glad to approve." (Harbeson to North, June 15, 1956, GCMRL/G. C. Marshall Papers [American Battle Monuments Commission].) Colonel Shaw, officer in charge of the ABMC, later clarified that the Fine Arts Commission believed the ABMC design "was too peaceful . . . for the hustle and bustle at that noisy and busy location." He anticipated that the Fine Arts Commission would recommend a memorial "with greater strength and action than what we had proposed." (Shaw to Spilman, ibid.)

Marshall wrote to Harland Bartholomew, a noted urban planner and chairman of the National Capital Planning Commission, on July 17 to explain the background of the ABMC's actions on the proposed memorial. He assured Bartholomew that the ABMC would "once again study the problem" and consider the views of the Fine Arts Commission, including its insistence of "the undesirability of erecting anything resembling a building at this site." He would recommend that the ABMC "appoint an architect for this project," since the new Congress would not convene for "several months." (Marshall to Bartholomew, July 17, 1956, ibid.)

3. Warren Pershing had requested Marshall's thoughts about "an appropriate inscription" for the pedestal of a statue of his father that had been commissioned by the State of Missouri. (Pershing to Marshall, June 21, 1956, GCMRL/G. C. Marshall Papers [Retirement, General].)

4. Warren Pershing had announced that his wife "Muriel and the boys are in good shape and we are moving that part of the family up to Narragansett for the summer over this weekend, and I will begin my weekly commuting." (Ibid.)

5. "I shall look forward to having your ideas of a suitable inscription," Pershing responded on July 9. C. J. George informed Pershing on October 26 that Marshall had reviewed General North's recommended inscriptions for the Missouri statue the previous day. (George to Pershing, October 26, 1956, ibid.)

Pershing Park, featuring a statue of General Pershing and a fountain, opened to the public on May 14, 1981, at Pennsylvania Avenue and Fourteenth Street NW in Washington, DC.

581

To J. H. Berkowitz — July 17, 1956
Leesburg, Virginia

Dear Mr. Berkowitz: I have your letter of July 4, which was prompted by a public statement made by me in connection with my memoirs.[1] I appreciate the compliment implied by your reference to the Adams and Jefferson papers, and your suggestion that mine should receive the same treatment as theirs.[2]

I might tell you that there has been organized a George C. Marshall Research Foundation, which will have the responsibility, with Government cooperation, for being the repository for all of my papers, both official and personal. The Foundation will be so organized that students, teachers, historians, researchers, and others might study actions taken by me.[3]

This should indicate that I am not going to write my memoirs, but simply make my records available to the public.

With my thanks for your good wishes, and with best regards,[4] Faithfully yours,

GCMRL/G. C. Marshall Papers (Retirement, General)

1. On July 1, newspapers throughout the United States had published an Associated Press article by Roger D. Greene, who had interviewed Marshall in Leesburg. "Marshall's mode of living is simple, almost Spartan, compared to the luxury he might enjoy if he had accepted fabulous offers to write his memoirs," Green wrote. "He is one of the few great wartime leaders who has persistently refused to write his own story." (Roger D. Greene, "On WWII Duty: 'I am Here to Serve and Not to Satisfy Personal Ambition,'" *Durham [NC] Morning Herald*, July 1, 1956, p. 3.) "'There are too many people still alive who could be hurt,'" Greene quoted Marshall about why he had consistently rejected offers from publishers. (Ibid.)

2. Research consultant and counselor at law J. H. Berkowitz had written from New York that the Adams and Jefferson Papers had "contributed to our better apprehension of the country's history, thanks to the historians who have been drawing upon them, since it was not vouchsafed to the authors of those 'papers' to perpetuate them in print." He encouraged Marshall to preserve, as Adams and Jefferson had, "the recorded details of events" and publish "for this and future generations the record of your participation in the epochal events in which you had so significant and noble a part, nobly performed." (Berkowitz to Marshall, July 4, 1956, GCMRL/G. C. Marshall Papers [Retirement, General].)

3. See pp. 862–64, 897–99, and 902–3.

4. The Associated Press article also generated an inquiry from Celeste Page Morgan, the sister of Rose Page Wilson, both of whom Marshall had known since they were children. "My autobiography is an old story," Marshall responded to his friend. "I'm afraid I am no good now." (Marshall to Morgan, July 17, 1956, ibid.) He added a note that he hoped Celeste's husband, Tom Morgan, with whom Marshall had served on the Business Advisory Council, "is in good shape." (Ibid.) See p. 673n1.

582

To John C. Hagan Jr. — August 2, 1956, Leesburg, Virginia

Dear Hagan: Thank you very much for your letter of July 23 with the announcement of Dr. Pogue's appointment as Director of the Research Center.[1]

Please assure him that my cooperation in his endeavors will be limited only by my ability and energy.[2]

With warm regards, Faithfully yours,

GCMRL/G. C. Marshall Papers (Retirement, General)

1. "Dr. Pogue is coming to us with very strong recommendation from the Chief Historian of the Defense Department [Rudolph Winnacker], the State Department [George Bernard Noble], Army [Major General Albert C. Smith], as well as Mr. Arthur Minnich, Assistant Secretary of the White House and many others too numerous to mention. This decision has been made by the unanimous vote of the Board," Hagan had notified Marshall. (Hagan to Marshall, July 23, 1956, GCMRL/G. C. Marshall Papers [Retirement, General].) See pp. 843–44. Hagan explained that the board had considered "some 20 odd people" for director of the Marshall Foundation. "I hope we have decided on the right person for we have checked on his security record, and that of his wife as well." (Ibid.) Pogue, a professor of history at his alma mater, Murray State College in Murray, Kentucky, was married to librarian Christine Brown Pogue.

2. Apparently Hagan had met with Marshall the previous year in Eagles Mere (see pp. 892–93) and in his letter he reiterated that if "at any time" working on interviews with Pogue was "not agreeable," Marshall should "advise me. I will see that your work load is lightened." (Ibid.) A press release issued by the Marshall Foundation on July 24 had announced that Pogue would begin his duties on August 15. (George C. Marshall Research

Foundation Press Release, July 24, 1956, ibid.) "I appreciate your efforts in my behalf and hope I can live up to your expectations," Pogue wrote to C. J. George on August 3 after learning that George had been an advocate for his candidacy. (Pogue to George, August 3, 1956, ibid.) See p. 932n4. On September 5, Marshall wrote again to Hagan that George had informed him about a luncheon Hagan arranged to introduce Dr. Pogue to foundation staff. "The time and effort you are putting into this project are tremendous," Marshall acknowledged, "and I continue to be greatly complimented by the interest you and others are showing in it." (Marshall to Hagan, September 5, 1956, ibid.) See pp. 952–53.

583

To Mrs. John White Pendleton — August 9, 1956
Leesburg, Virginia

Dear Madge— I have been a long time writing you since we learned of John's landing in the Middle East, but not of his arrival at his home port.[1]

I hope all goes well with you; that you have no servant difficulty like Marion in Montgomery; and that the children are in shape for the trip.[2]

We have had an unprecedented streak of cool, damp, humid, rainy weather. The farmers are about ruined, their wheat, corn, alfalfa, tomatoe crops etc, ruined. They haven't been able to put up any hay.[3]

All Leesburg caught cold and K and I each got bad cases of bronchitis. We finally went to the Walter Reed for a week.[4] Better now, but the sun came out only yesterday and the house is still damp.

Molly [Winn] got tired and blew in yesterday with Ellene. Left this afternoon. Looks well and Ellene cute.

I have practically not been off the place but I'm going out to a men's dinner tonight.

Katherine sends her best—with me, to you and John. Affectionately,

GCM

GCMRL/Xerox 2237 (GCM Family, Personal Letters); H

1. John White Pendleton had taken a position with ARAMCO Saudi Arabian Oil Company in Dhahran, Saudi Arabia.

2. Marion Tupper, widow of Katherine Marshall's brother, General Tristam Tupper, had moved to Montgomery, Alabama, where she worked for the Alabama State Crippled Children's Service. (Tupper to George, May 21, 1955, GCMRL/G. C. Marshall Papers [Retirement, General].)

3. "The Washington area was drenched by 5.88 inches of rain last month, making it the wettest July since 1945," the *Washington Post* had reported on August 1. "More than half the total rainfall fell between July 20 and 27," and temperatures were also considerably cooler than normal for July. ("Rain Brought Wettest July Since '45," *Washington Post*, August 1, 1956, p. 26.)

4. On July 31, C. J. George had written to Frank McCarthy that "both General and Mrs. Marshall are occupying comfortable rooms in Ward B at the Walter Reed Hospital. Fortunately, their illness is not serious, though uncomfortable. They both have a touch of bronchitis, or, to an old Pennsylvania Dutchman like me, a summer cold." (George to McCarthy, July 31, 1956, GCMRL/Frank McCarthy Collection [Additions, Box 1].)

FRANK McCarthy had visited the Marshalls at Dodona Manor in July (see photo #23) while he attended the Strategic Intelligence School in Washington, DC. (McCarthy to George, August 9, 1956, GCMRL/G. C. Marshall Papers [Retirement, General].) "I do not think you can know what your all-too short-visit did for us both," Katherine Marshall wrote to McCarthy on July 18, adding that her husband "keeps referring to this and that—and it will remain with us for many a day." (Katherine Marshall to McCarthy, July 18, 1956, GCMRL/Frank McCarthy Collection [Additions, Box 1]; H.) Marshall wrote to McCarthy on August 11 about their illnesses (see previous document) and admitted that it was fortunate that "we did not go up in the Penna mountains for we would have frozen or gone moldy. The weather up there was wretched." (Marshall to McCarthy, August 11, 1956, ibid.; H.)

"I travel very little these days," Marshall admitted on September 12 to his childhood friend Catharine Armstrong. "We were here at Leesburg all summer and it was cool and generally delightful, though too much rain. We couldn't go farther away on account of Mrs. Marshall's sister who suffered a stroke and was quite helpless. We couldn't bring her up from the very fine convalescent home at Pinehurst," he explained, but they were able to "keep in close touch from here." (Marshall to Armstrong, September 12, 1956, GCMRL/G. C. Marshall Collection [Armstrong]; H.) See pp. 874, 899n4, 901, and 910–11. He wrote a newsy letter to Allene Lacy on August 20, telling her that he and Katherine Marshall had gone to Washington recently "to shop" and visit with Leesburg neighbors "the Dave Rusts. He looks badly, seriously so. She is well and chirpy as usual." (Marshall to Lacy, August 20, 1956, GCMRL/G. C. Marshall Papers [Retirement, General].) While in the city, Marshall also paid "his final respects" to Colonel James Kimbrough, chief of urology at Walter Reed Hospital, who died on August 19. (George to Pifer, August 28, 1956, ibid.) Marshall mentioned to his sister-in-law that they had installed "an air-conditioner in the library, but never had to turn it on until a few days ago, and only for a short time." He told her that the reason he was writing in place of his wife was because her "eye is troubling her again—a return of her shingles ailment, so she writes with difficulty. I am attempting to fill in for her." He closed by joking that he was "no good as usual, but improving in worthlessness." (Marshall to Lacy, August 20, 1956, ibid.) ★

584

TO AUGUST HECKSCHER

August 10, 1956
Leesburg, Virginia

Dear Mr. Heckscher: I have your letter of July 31 and greatly appreciate the action of the Board of Directors of The Woodrow Wilson Foundation in nominating me for the 1956 award.[1]

While I am highly complimented by the action of the Board in paying me such a high tribute, I feel that it is necessary for me to withdraw because of my inability to attend the dinner.[2]

With my thanks again for thinking of me in this way, and with warmest regards,[3] Faithfully yours,

GCMRL/G. C. Marshall Papers (Retirement, General)

1. "It has seemed to the Trustees that your life-long service to the United States is in keeping with the ideals of character which Woodrow Wilson emphasized in his teaching and by his example," August Heckscher, president of the Woodrow Wilson Foundation, had written to Marshall. "They have felt also that in launching the Marshall Plan you gave a fresh expression to the ideals of internationalism for which Wilson fought." (Heckscher to Marshall, July 31, 1956, GCMRL/G. C. Marshall Papers [Retirement, General].)

2. Heckscher also explained that the award, "made from time to time to an individual who has rendered meritorious service to democracy, public welfare, or peace through justice," would be presented at a dinner in New York City on December 27, the eve of Woodrow Wilson's one hundredth birthday. (Ibid.)

3. Heckscher assured Marshall on August 15 that the Woodrow Wilson Foundation "would be glad to make the presentation in any way that would be acceptable to you, perhaps in a very simple way at Leesburg." (Heckscher to Marshall, August 15, 1956, ibid.) Marshall replied on August 28 that "under these circumstances I am honored to accept." (Marshall to Heckscher, August 28, 1956, ibid.) See pp. 954–55 and 957.

585

To Brigadier General Thomas North | August 28, 1956
Leesburg, Virginia

Dear North: Before you get back into other business, I want you to know of my very warm appreciation for the outstanding job you did in arranging the numerous details of the dedicatory programs. I have had indirect word that each of the programs was conducted in a dignified and most efficient manner. This was very fine news to receive and, since you bore the brunt of the whole affair, the majority of the compliments are yours. I am sure that every member of the Commission would second the endorsement of the fine job you did.[1]

I should have liked to have been present, but, as you know, it would have been an impossible task for me to undertake.

It is difficult for me to understand the reason behind the action on your promotion. I regret that such a thing happened, because you are certainly worthy of the recognition.[2]

With my thanks again, and with best wishes, Faithfully yours,

GCMRL/G. C. Marshall Papers (American Battle Monuments Commission)

1. See pp. 936–38. "All of the dedications are now over and I am happy to say that all were completely successful and most impressive," North had reported to Marshall on August 6. (North to Marshall, August 6, 1956, GCMRL/G. C. Marshall Papers [American Battle Monuments Commission].)

2. "You may have learned that Sen. Potter's bill concerning the Commission was enacted, except that the House struck out the authorization for my promotion," North added in a handwritten postscript to his letter. (Ibid.) Senator Charles E. Potter was a member of the ABMC. See pp. 734–35, 783–84, and 945–46.

586

TO MRS. JOHN B. WILSON

September 21, 1956
Leesburg, Virginia

My dear Rose Some time in mid-August I sent Page a Birthday note and his annual ten bucks. As he has always been meticulous with his thanks I fear something has gone wrong. Hence this note.[1]

I have not done very well this summer but am improving. Katherine is in better shape, thank goodness. I do hope all goes well with you.[2]

I went to town the first time in three months yesterday for the Business Advisory Council. Stayed only part of the session—no dinner. I did not see Tom Morgan. Maybe he's not a member now or was not well.[3]

With love, Affectionately

GCM

GCMRL/J. Page Wilson Collection; H

1. Page Wilson had written to thank Marshall for "the money and the card" on August 21, and expressed the hope that the Marshalls were "over the flew [*flu*] all right." (Page Wilson to Marshall, August 21, 1956, GCMRL/G. C. Marshall Papers [Retirement, General].) He also mentioned that he might see Marshall during his Christmas vacation because he hoped to "go up to Pinehurst to play in a golf tourney." (Ibid.) Rose Wilson responded on September 24 that Page had "bought himself an eight iron to match his golf clubs" with the money Marshall had sent and boasted that her son was a "runner-up in the championship for boys through eleven yrs old in North & South Carolina." (Rose Wilson to Marshall, September 24, 1956, ibid.)

2. "I do not like the news that you were not well this Summer," Marshall's goddaughter concluded her newsy letter. "I would love to come to see you. I think I'd better come alone; after that big dose of my kids you got the last time, I think you'd rather wait until they were older when I bring them again," and suggested that she would "drive down for lunch or tea or something." (Ibid.) See p. 899n5.

3. Marshall had attended the BAC meeting on September 20. (George to McCarthy, September 25, 1956, GCMRL/G. C. Marshall Papers [Retirement, Chronological].) Wilson reported that her brother-in-law "is said to be getting along exceptionally well" according to her sister, Celeste, but their mother had confided that Tom Morgan "has aged tremendously." (Rose Wilson to Marshall, September 24, 1956, GCMRL/G. C. Marshall Papers [Retirement, General].)

587

TO MISS EUGENIA D. LEJEUNE

September 21 [*19*], 1956[1]
Leesburg, Virginia

Dear Miss Lejeune: I have your note of September 15, in which you express an interest in obtaining the position of Librarian-Archivist with the Marshall Foundation.[2] Incidentally, Mr. John C. Hagan, President of the Foundation, and Dr. Pogue visited with me yesterday morning.[3] I told them of your interest, and I feel confident that Mr. Hagan will write you shortly.

I remember your Father very well and also the occasion of my visit to Norfolk. He was a highly regarded man whose name is legendary in the Marine Corps, and his work at V. M. I. is well-known.[4]

I appreciate the interest you expressed in becoming a member of the Foundation, but since I have no official connection the response to your request will come from its President.[5]

With best regards, Faithfully yours,

GCMRL/G. C. Marshall Papers (Retirement, General)

1. This letter, drafted by C. J. George, is stamped September 21; however, Katherine Marshall wrote to Frank McCarthy that Marshall's "Biographer with Mr. Hagan & Col. George were here on Tuesday," September 18, which implies this letter was actually written on September 19, 1956. (Katherine Marshall to McCarthy, September 22, 1956, GCMRL/Frank McCarthy Collection [Additions].)

2. Eugenia Lejeune, a major in the marine corps and a librarian at the Armed Forces Staff College Library in Norfolk, Virginia, had written on September 15 that it would be "an honor to be associated with your life's history and works" through employment at the Marshall Foundation. She assured him that she and her late father, Lieutenant General John A. Lejeune, commandant of the US Marine Corps from 1920 to 1929 and superintendent of VMI from 1929 to 1937, admired Marshall, and she felt she "could materially contribute to the success of the Foundation with my military background and training, plus the happy combination of my fourteen years' library and archival experience." (Lejeune to Marshall, September 15, 1956, GCMRL/G. C. Marshall Papers [Retirement, General].)

3. Forrest Pogue thanked Marshall on September 21 for the visit and for his comments on "the 1939–41 period," which "illuminated the difficulties of those years and threw new light on the problems you faced then." He added that some of Marshall's "little asides . . . were valuable reminders of obstacles to military preparations which many people have forgotten or which they never knew. I think military and political leaders—and taxpayers—can profit immensely from this type of information which you alone know." (Pogue to Marshall, September 21, 1956, ibid.) Pogue also thanked Marshall for granting him use of Marshall's Pentagon office when he was in Washington to conduct research and interviews, and mentioned that C. J. George would "arrange interviews for me with former associates of yours who may be visiting the Pentagon." (Ibid.)

4. "I recall vividly your visit to us here in Norfolk when you addressed the VMI Club and Father's remarks about you at that time," Lejeune had noted. (Lejeune to Marshall, September 15, 1956, ibid.) Marshall spoke to VMI alumni in Norfolk on September 16, 1939. (Jacob to Marshall, September 7, 1939, GCMRL/G. C. Marshall Papers [Pentagon, Selected].)

5. Pogue informed Marshall on June 13, 1957, that the foundation had hired Lejeune as of July 1. "For approximately a year she will do research in the Army records for 1939–45. This work will be done in Alexandria [Virginia] where the records for this period have been stored." (Pogue to Marshall, June 13, 1957, GCMRL/G. C. Marshall Papers [Retirement, General].)

588

TO ROBERT A. LOVETT

October 11, 1956
Leesburg, Virginia

Dear Bob— We were delighted and greatly surprised to receive the portable T.V. set. You and Adele were so kind to make the long trip down here, then your gifts and now the T.V. Thank you very much.[1]

We shall take it to Pinehurst.

It is quite cold now and we are running both the furnaces and open fires.

The time is drawing very near to leave for our winter home—November 1st.

Our gardens have been demolished, or winterized. Fortunately we got hold of a lot of manure to straighten up things.

We go into the hospital for a check up before leaving, then fly down.[2]

With my thanks again, Affectionately,

GCM

Yale/Robert A. Lovett Papers (Box 20, Folder 267); H

1. Lovett had returned as a partner of Brown Bothers, Harriman & Co. in New York after leaving the Defense Department in 1953; he had been a director of Union Pacific since 1926. ("R. A. Lovett, Ex-chief of Defense Who Pressed Buildup in 50's Dies," *New York Times*, May 8, 1986, p. B24.) On September 30, the day before an appearance before the Interstate Commerce Committee on October 1 concerning the Union Pacific Railroad Company's business, Lovett and his wife had traveled to Leesburg to see the Marshalls "and were delighted to find you both looking so well and chipper." (Lovett to Marshall, September 17 and October 4, 1956, GCMRL/G. C. Marshall Papers [Retirement, General].) "I noticed that you are a television fan," Lovett continued, so he had shipped a small set "in the hope that you may find it convenient to have in your bedroom if you want to see the morning newscast, or if you want to watch the shows in some other room in the house. These little 14″ portable sets have just been perfected," he explained, and hoped that Marshall "may get some pleasure from it and be reminded of our affectionate regards." (Ibid.)

Marshall wrote to Lovett again five days later to congratulate him on becoming president of the Union Pacific. "I'm *so* glad to see you finally honored as you should have been long since. And I am humiliated that I have been so long in congratulating you. One does not become President of a great trans-continental railroad every day," Marshall stressed, and added that Lovett's "record of public service and private performance is above and beyond most Americans." (Marshall to Lovett, October 16, 1954, Yale/Robert A. Lovett Papers [Box 20, Folder 267]; H.) Lovett quickly clarified that "In reporting to Mrs. Marshall on the Lovett family happenings, Adele says she got her titles a little mixed," and explained that he was chairman of the executive committee of the Union Pacific, "a post which delights me because my father held it for many years. The President is the 'operating' man, and is in Omaha, while the Executive Committee is domiciled here in New York and is charged with general policy and, specifically, with all financial matters." (Lovett to Marshall, October 22, 1956, GCMRL/G. C. Marshall Papers [Retirement, General].) Judge Robert Scott Lovett was chairman of the board of directors of the Union Pacific System of railroads from 1909 until his death in 1932.

2. C. J. George had suggested that prior to their departure for Pinehurst the Marshalls have their semiannual check-ups at Walter Reed, just after the presentation of the Woodrow Wilson Award in Marshall's Pentagon office on October 25. (George to Marshall, October 10, 1956, ibid.) See next document and p. 962.

589

To General Alfred M. Gruenther — October 25, 1956
Washington, DC

Dear Gruenther: Many thanks for your cabled congratulations on my selection to receive the Woodrow Wilson Foundation Award. The presentation has just been made in my office.[1] You were kind to remark on it.[2]

I know you must be very busy as your time to leave SHAPE approaches. I imagine, too, that your feelings are mixed as your retirement from the Army nears. You are better off than some, for not only do you have a career of fine achievement behind you, but you have also youth and the prospect of worthwhile achievement ahead. It will seem strange not having you in Paris, but I am sure that the organization you leave behind will continue in the same commendable fashion.[3]

I again would like to add my thanks for the many courtesies and kindnesses which I have received from Mrs. Gruenther and you. Your attentiveness to me during the winter of 1953 will long be remembered.[4] It has been a source of regret to Mrs. Marshall and me that we could never get together on some of your trips home. Perhaps the future will permit such an opportunity.

With our warmest regards to Mrs. Gruenther and you,[5] Faithfully yours,

GCMRL/G. C. Marshall Papers (Retirement, General)

1. See pp. 950–51. The *New York Times* reported that Marshall received the award "at an informal gathering in his Pentagon office." Former Secretary of State Dean Acheson and Woodrow Wilson's widow also attended the ceremony. ("Marshall Gets Wilson Citation," *New York Times*, October 26, 1956, p. 3.)

2. Gruenther's brief congratulatory cable had arrived in Marshall's Pentagon office on October 22. (Gruenther to Marshall, cable, October 22, 1956, GCMRL/G. C. Marshall Papers [Retirement, General].)

3. Gruenther was scheduled to leave his post as supreme commander of the Allied Powers in Europe on November 21 and retire from the military on December 31. (Gruenther to Marshall, October 29, 1956, ibid.)

4. The Gruenthers were Marshall's hosts in Paris en route to Oslo to receive the Nobel Peace Prize in December 1953. See pp. 803, 806–7, and 816n1.

5. "How very thoughtful of you to give such a generous estimate of my military career," Gruenther replied on October 29. "You are quite right when you speculate that my feelings are mixed. SHAPE has been a vital part of my life for almost six years now, and I shall leave a large part of my heart behind when I finally fly away," he confessed. (Ibid.) "Mrs. Gruenther and I consider it one of the high points of our tour here that you stopped with us in 1953," he added. "You were the perfect guest." (Ibid.)

Marshall wrote again to Gruenther on November 15 to congratulate him for accepting the presidency of the American Red Cross, effective January 1, 1957. "It is a great organization and I know its fine work will continue and progress under your capable leadership," Marshall affirmed. (Marshall to Gruenther, November 15, 1956, GCMRL/G. C. Marshall Papers [Retirement, Chronological].)

590

TO ARTHUR HOLLY COMPTON[1] October 25, 1956
Washington, DC

Dear Doctor: Yesterday, I received the autographed copy of your book, for which I am very grateful. Previously, the publishers had sent me the book, which I read immediately.[2]

It was intensely interesting to me, particularly as there was so much of it with which I was not familiar.

I marvel at the numerous understandings which had to be reached among so many people of different nationalities. Possibly science provides a common denominator for such men as are involved in your story, but from my own experiences it is most remarkable to me that you men were able to do as you did.

I have never forgotten my brief visit to Mrs. Compton and you. While I lunged so suddenly into the tide of affairs in Japan and Korea after leaving you, I did not forget and have not forgotten the very pleasant hours I spent with you.[3]

With warm regards to you both, Faithfully yours,

GCMRL/G. C. Marshall Papers (Retirement, General)

1. Compton had written to Marshall the previous year that he was writing *Atomic Quest, A Personal Narrative*, "which is concerned among other things with the decision to use the bomb against Japan." He sent a draft of a chapter about May 1945 meetings of the Interim Committee, a group that had been assembled by then Secretary of War Henry L. Stimson to advise President Truman on issues relating to nuclear energy. Compton had quoted "an opinion as I recall it expressed by you. Also I quote from a conversation between ourselves when you spoke at Washington University's commencement some years ago." (See pp. 541, 546–47.) "It will be of very considerable help if you will corroborate or correct my recollections and if you will comment on the appropriateness, relative to security, that these views of yours should be made public." (Compton to Marshall, August 27, 1955, GCMRL/G. C. Marshall Papers [Retirement, General].) Compton mentioned that the manuscript would be reviewed by the Atomic Energy Commission for clearance before publication. (Ibid.) Compton wrote again on September 21 to thank Marshall for "taking time to review the section of the manuscript I sent you, and I am pleased to know that your recollection of the meeting of the Interim Committee is in accord with mine." (Compton to Marshall, September 21, 1955, ibid.)

2. The publicity manager at the Oxford University Press had sent a prepublication copy of the book to Marshall on September 18. "We should be happy to have your comments on it," he wrote. (Boardman to Marshall, September 18, 1956, ibid.) "I have known the writer a good many years," Marshall responded. "I read the book with considerable interest; however, I have no comment for publication." (Marshall to Boardman, September 28, 1956, ibid.)

3. Compton was married to the former Betty Charity McCloskey. Immediately after his June 6, 1951, address at Washington University, Marshall had departed for his secret trip to Japan and Korea. (See pp. 541, 546–47.) "One of my prized memories is that of walking with you under the trees back of the Chancellor's residence at Washington University, as we were discussing these matters," Compton handwrote at the bottom of his August 27, 1955, letter. (Compton to Marshall, August 27, 1955, ibid.)

In *Atomic Quest* Compton asserted that during the May 31, 1945, meeting of the Interim Committee, Marshall had at first argued against using the bomb "at least if its existence could be kept secret. Such use, he said, would show our hand. We would be in a stronger position with regard to future military action if we did not show the power we held." Even though he was thus noting "a real military objection to any demonstration of the bomb," Compton continued, "he seemed to accept the view that its use was nevertheless important. This I verified in subsequent discussions. He was fully convinced at this time that the bomb should be used. This was primarily to bring the war quickly to a close and thereby to save lives. He never believed that the Japanese would surrender solely as a result of further naval operations and conventional air attacks." (Arthur Holly Compton, *Atomic Quest, A Personal Narrative* [New York: Oxford University Press, 1956], 237–38.) The similar but somewhat different version in Compton's draft can be found with his August 27, 1955, letter to Marshall cited in n1 above.

591

To T. Townsend Brown

October 25, 1956
Washington, DC

Dear Mr. Brown: I received your communication on the subject of unidentified flying objects and your committee's interest in undertaking an investigation in the hope of securing authoritative information.[1]

I do not feel free to comment on the question posed, but not because of a lack of interest. My mail brings me numerous demands of one nature or another, and I lack the energy to take the time and thought necessary for constructive or affirmative replies.

I hope you will understand. Faithfully yours,

GCMRL/G. C. Marshall Papers (Retirement, General)

1. T. Townsend Brown, the executive vice chairman of the National Investigations Committee on Aerial Phenomena, based in Washington, DC, was an American inventor who studied unusual electrical effects. He had written to Marshall about "a subject of inevitable concern in every major phase of human welfare" and sought Marshall's support for the creation of a civilian committee to investigate aerial phenomena. (Brown to Marshall, October 18, 1956, GCMRL/G. C. Marshall Papers [Retirement, General].) At the bottom of his letter, Brown noted that their "mutual neighbors in Leesburg felt that you especially would be interested." (Ibid.)

592

To Dwight D. Eisenhower — October 27, 1956
Leesburg, Virginia

Dear Mr. President: I greatly appreciated the telegram you sent me regarding the Woodrow Wilson Award. Your gracious and exceedingly generous expressions will remain in my memory.[1]

I found the arrangements for the presentation of the Award most convenient, since I planned to come to town at this time for my semi-annual checkup at Walter Reed prior to leaving for Pinehurst on November 1.[2]

Mrs. Marshall sends her thanks with me to Mrs. Eisenhower for her warm expressions.

I was especially touched by your pausing in the midst of the strain of this campaign to remember me.[3]

With great respect, Faithfully yours,

GCMRL/G. C. Marshall Papers (Retirement, General)

1. See pp. 950–51. The award, Eisenhower had written, "gives me another opportunity to reaffirm the admiration, respect and esteem that I have always held for you. In 1948 I tried to express my feelings, thinking of you mainly as an outstanding war leader. But I could well have added what I then felt and feel now, that though I have met all or most of the so-called prominent and great in the world, you head my list of those who, I believe, deserve the most from their country and from the free world, and who have provided the rest of us with an exemplary standard of service." (Eisenhower to Marshall, October 25, 1956, GCMRL/G. C. Marshall Papers [Retirement, General].) On November 18, 1948, Eisenhower had sent Marshall one of the first copies of *Crusade in Europe*, published in 1948, with a letter stating that he would "ever be deeply grateful to you for wise leadership, friendly advice, and warm support during a great national crisis." (*Papers of DDE*, 10: 311–12; Dwight D. Eisenhower, *Crusade in Europe* (Garden City, NY: Doubleday, 1948.)

2. See p. 954n1.

3. President Eisenhower was campaigning for reelection. See p. 961.

593

To Elmo Roper November 6, 1956
Pinehurst, North Carolina[1]

Dear Roper: I received your letter of the 24th together with the manuscript of your proposed chapters regarding me.[2] I have nothing to say regarding the manuscript other than that you treated me very generously—and two comments regarding my service as Chief of Staff.

There are two things connected with that service which I think have a very important bearing on my conduct of the business. One is the fact that by an Executive [*military*] Order of the President I was made directly responsible to him for training, organization, operations, and strategy.[3] That left to the Secretary of War the general supervision of mobilization, which I, of course, was greatly concerned with. But in these other matters my responsibility within the War Department was complete, and I held it directly to the President.

I may say that this was really quite a blow to Mr. Stimson, but he took it in a very fine manner, and I, on my part, tried to include him, as it were, in these matters so far as practicable.[4]

I was particularly concerned with the affairs of the Chiefs of Staff and the Combined Chiefs of Staff. Here, it was a little difficult for me to include him because that, in a sense, required the agreement of the Navy representative, Admiral King, and the British. But I managed to keep him reasonably well-informed.[5]

The other item which had a great bearing on my conduct of affairs as the Chief of Staff was the fact that I travelled hundreds of thousands of miles to keep in constant touch with the mobilization and training of the troops and the conduct of their operations all over the world. I forget what my total mileage was at the end of the war, but I know that while I was Secretary of State it was added up and found to be 1,400,000 miles.

Early in the mobilization, I used to average about 60,000 miles within the Continental United States, I think, a year. I started to say "a month," but that doesn't sound reasonable. Anyway, it was 60,000. And, as part of this, Congress, without my request, gave me first $25 million and later $100 million which I could spend as I saw fit without making any report. This enabled me to take action wherever I might happen to be when something came up that needed immediate attention, rather than the long, painful course of getting it estimated to Washington and then several months in getting it through Congress.

As a matter of fact, the history of this fund was quite interesting. It really became a revolving fund and most of it was returned to me. The largest portion that was expended without return was that I sent to Australia in the endeavor to get supplies to MacArthur on Corregidor.

I didn't intend to go into so much detail, but it may be of some interest to you.

I am returning the manuscript.[6] Faithfully yours,

GCMRL/G. C. Marshall Papers (Retirement, General)

1. "The Marshalls left last evening by rail for Pinehurst," C. J. George had informed

Marshall Carter on November 2. (George to Carter, November 2, 1956, GCMRL/G. C. Marshall Papers [Retirement, Chronological].)

2. Pollster Elmo Roper had explained to Marshall that he was writing a book of profiles of ten American leaders during 1935 to 1955. "I shall try to be as factual as I know how in describing simply how the people looked at these men over the years, put into the context with what was going on at the time." (Roper to Marshall, October 24, 1956, GCMRL/G. C. Marshall Papers [Retirement, General].) Roper also planned to include "any personal impressions I might have gained from knowing the man myself." (Ibid.) "I should like very much to tell the story of your relations with the present Administration as you told me," Roper added, "but I have guarded that secret closely and shall continue to do so unless you should happen to feel that the time has come for me to put in a paragraph about it." (Ibid.)

3. President Franklin D. Roosevelt issued an executive order on July 5, 1939—effective July 1, 1939—which directed members of the Joint Army-Navy Board on which Marshall and his navy counterpart sat to report directly to him rather than the service secretaries.

4. Harry H. Woodring was secretary of war when Roosevelt issued the order. Henry L. Stimson replaced Woodring on July 10, 1940. (Mark S. Watson, *Chief of Staff: Prewar Plans and Preparations*, in *United States Army in World War II* [Washington: GPO, 1950], 5–7, 310–11.) For more on later developments with Woodring, see pp. 852–55 and 858–59. For more on Marshall's reminiscences about his relationship with Stimson, see *Marshall Interviews*, 315–16.

5. For more on Marshall's reminiscences about his relationship with Admiral Ernest J. King, see *Marshall Interviews*, 434–36.

6. On January 15, 1958, Roper sent Marshall an advance copy of *You and Your Leaders, Their Actions and Your Reactions, 1936–1956*, which would be released by William Morrow and Company on April 1. (Roper to Marshall, January 15, 1958, GCMRL/G. C. Marshall Papers [Retirement, General].) Marshall thanked him on February 10, noting that he read the book "with great interest." (Marshall to Roper, February 10, 1958, ibid.)

594

To Ellen Hagen Ture Nerman[1] — November 15, 1956
Radio. — [Washington, DC]

My Government has clearly and forcefully stated its position with regard to Hungary. As an active member of the United States Government I agree in the action taken but feel it would be inappropriate for me to take individual action on the basis of my Nobel association.[2]

GENERAL GEORGE C. MARSHALL

GCMRL/G. C. Marshall Papers (Retirement, General)

1. Ellen Hagen Ture Nerman, a member of the Swedish Committee of the Congress For Cultural Freedom, had wired Marshall on November 10 to ask for his support of a letter to Soviet Premier Nikita Khrushchev to condemn and protest the Soviet crushing of the Hungarian uprising that had begun on October 23. Nerman's committee had sent the same appeal to twenty-eight other Nobel Prize recipients, and asked Marshall "to cable us your adhesion." (Nerman to Marshall, telegram, November 10, 1956, GCMRL/G. C. Marshall Papers [Retirement, General].)

2. Marshall also sent this reply to another Nobel laureate who had asked him to endorse the letter, and he declined participation in a new organization that was forming in response to the Soviet invasion. (Muller to Marshall, telegram, November 13, 1956; George to Muller, November 15, 1956; Liebman to Marshall, November 14, 1956; Marshall to Liebman, December 3, 1956, ibid.)

595

To John C. Hagan Jr. November 17, 1956
Pinehurst, North Carolina

Dear Hagan: Thanks for your letter of November 9 and for The Cadet. I appreciate your sending it to me, and both Mrs. Marshall and I found it of interest. Incidentally, she was the one who coined the phrase, "Don't be a deep feeler and a shallow thinker."[1]

They did a good job on Forrest Pogue. He has been spending several afternoons with me going over some papers. We seem to have hit on a good arrangement. At least I find this way of doing it less tiresome.[2]

We appreciate your open invitation to drop by the farm, but I hold little prospect of going North. If I have to, it will be for a brief period only. However, I am glad to have the map in case we find an opportunity to pay you a visit.[3]

With our warmest regards to Mrs. Hagan and you, Faithfully yours,

GCMRL/G. C. Marshall Papers (Retirement, General)

1. Hagan had sent Marshall a copy of the September 24 issue of the VMI student newspaper that mentioned Marshall's "inspiring talk to the graduating class" on June 12 in which he had offered Katherine Marshall's advice. See pp. 938–42. ("'Don't Be a Deep Feeler . . . ,'" *VMI Cadet*, September 24, 1956, p. 2.)

2. Pogue had visited Marshall for lunch in Leesburg on September 28. "The afternoon interview was most helpful and gave me a good start," Pogue wrote on October 1, and added that he was "delighted at your suggestion for further interviews." (Pogue to Marshall, October 1, 1956, GCMRL/G. C. Marshall Papers [Retirement, General].) Pogue wrote on October 18 that he had been ill and hoped to be well enough for another visit the following week. He thought that "it might help prepare for the next interview, if I sent along questions which I have prepared on some of Matloff's early chapters." Pogue was referring to Maurice Matloff, chief of the Strategic Plans Section of the Office of the Chief of Military History, who, with fellow military historian Edwin M. Snell, had produced *Strategic Planning for Coalition Warfare 1941–1942* in the *United States Army in World War II* series in 1953. "In some cases where it seemed to me that Matloff's conclusions were sweeping or where he seemed to be guessing, I have merely asked 'Does this seem adequate' or 'does this seem fair.' Since this is an official volume, I should like to see the account accurate there." (Pogue to Marshall, October 18, 1956, ibid.)

On November 1, Spilman had sent Marshall "the two sets of notes made on your two conferences with Dr. Pogue. I do this without Dr. Pogue's knowledge—as a protection for you and to relieve myself of a considerable sense of responsibility in your behalf." (Spilman to Marshall, November 1, 1956, GCMRL/G. C. Marshall Papers [Retirement, Chronological].) "I have the feeling that these notes *may* some day be made available for public inspection or perhaps be quoted in a future publication of the Marshall Research Foundation." She particularly referenced notes "on your conference of October 29 that you, in no instance, specified that any remarks were to be 'off the record.'" (Ibid.) She pointed out if Marshall were "to edit or delete from the notes, I would be in an embarrassing position with Dr. Pogue. In that event, therefore, I would like your permission to tell Dr. Pogue that you instructed me to submit these notes to you for editing." (Ibid.) "Notes on Comment by General George C. Marshall at a Conference with Dr. Forrest C. Pogue at Leesburg, Virginia, on October 5, 1956," which cover a wide range of subjects on World War II, are in the chronological files of the George C. Marshall Research Library. (Ibid.) There are no notes for an October 29 meeting in this file.

"Dr. Pogue will arrive in Southern Pines at approximately 8:00 a.m. on Tuesday, November 13," C. J. George had informed Marshall on November 7. "I have shipped out via Railway Express the recording machine. I suggest that [Sergeant William J.] Heffner uncrate it and have it ready when Dr. Pogue arrives." (George to Marshall, November 7, 1956, GCMRL/G. C. Marshall Papers [Retirement, General].) "George's biographer Dr. Pogue has been at the Hotel for two weeks," Katherine Marshall wrote to her friend Ellen Bruce on November 27. "He comes three days a week and asks George questions—and G. answers into the Dictaphone—So they will have a record in his voice. He left yesterday." (Katherine Marshall to Bruce, November 27, 1956, GCMRL/Katherine Marshall Papers.) See pp. 967–68.

3. Hagan had invited the Marshalls to visit him at his farm when they returned to Leesburg from Pinehurst. (Hagan to Marshall, November 9, 1956, GCMRL/G. C. Marshall Papers [Retirement, General].)

596

TO DWIGHT D. EISENHOWER — November 18, 1956
Pinehurst, North Carolina

My dear Mr. President: I have, as usual, waited for the flood to subside before adding my congratulations on your tremenduous victory. As you well know you have received an unprecedented vote of approval, affection and encouragement in a turbulent World.[1]

I pray that the great effort of the campaign did not too heavily wear down your strength.

Judging from the TV Mrs. Eisenhower seemed to gain strength and health as you went along. She must be very proud.[2] With great respect,

GCMarshall

DDEL/Dwight D. Eisenhower Papers (Papers as President, Ann Whitman File, Name Series, Box 21); H

1. Eisenhower won forty-one states in the November 6 election, garnering 457 electoral votes to Adlai Stevenson's 73.

2. "I am more than grateful for your longhand note of felicitations on my re-election," Eisenhower responded on November 23. "Actually, I found the campaign this year fairly easy—at least by comparison with the '52 effort. I tried to make most of the trips one-day affairs, which, while temporarily exhausting, did give me time both to catch my breath and to keep up with the necessary official business." (Eisenhower to Marshall, November 23, 1956, GCMRL/G. C. Marshall Papers [Retirement, General].) The Hungarian uprising (see p. 959) as well as a crisis in Suez involving Great Britain, France, Israel, and Egypt, had occupied much of the president's time and energy between August and November. For more on Eisenhower's impressions of the 1956 campaign and simultaneous world events, see Dwight D. Eisenhower, *Waging Peace* (Garden City, NY: Doubleday & Company, Inc., 1965), 3–19 and 31–90.

597

TO MRS. JOHN B. WILSON — December 17, 1956
Washington, DC

Dear Rose: I flew up from Pinehurst after lunch today and stopped at the office for an hour and am taking the opportunity of dictating a number of notes with

Christmas reactions. I haven't heard from you yet, but I assume I will, so am sending you now my love and affectionate greetings.[1]

I will only be here about two days for this meeting and for a little check-up at Walter Reed.[2] I am in a curious position. So many people say I look better than I have for years and yet, as a matter of fact, I have great difficulty in walking—that is, my sense of balance seems to have vanished with I don't know what, my hearing or something of that sort.[3]

When the spring opens up maybe you will feel inclined to make that threatened visit, though I won't be able to accompany you around the golf course. I can watch you from a distance, but that's all.

I do hope all goes well with John and your children—and of course with you.

With my love and affectionate greetings, Faithfully yours,

GCMRL/J. Page Wilson Collection

1. Marshall's goddaughter responded on January 7 with news about her "most strenuous" Christmas due to attending social engagements and assembling complex toys for her children. (Wilson to Marshall, January 7, 1957, GCMRL/G. C. Marshall Papers [Retirement, General].)

2. The same day Marshall wrote to Frances McCoy that Mrs. Marshall had not accompanied him on this trip to Washington to attend a meeting of the American Battle Monuments Commission, "the first I have attended for a long time. And then I am going directly to the Walter Reed to see the dentist and to have a small check-up." (Marshall to McCoy, December 17, 1956, ibid.) Marshall had also made arrangements to see Helen and Mary Lee the evening of December 17. (George to Marshall, November 28, 1956, GCMRL/G. C. Marshall Papers [Retirement, Chronological].)

3. Marshall also confided to his longtime friend Colonel Edward R. "Peter" Bowditch, "there are a great many things about me that are failing, notably my hearing and, I must admit, my sense of balance. I have been told many times that I was off balance, but now I can understand it." (Marshall to Bowditch, December 17, 1956, GCMRL/G. C. Marshall Papers [Retirement, General].)

598

To Louis Marx[1]

December 17, 1956
Washington, DC

Dear Marx: I received the notices of your having entered subscriptions for me to Fortune Magazine and the National Geographic. Thank you so much. You certainly are good about these things. I have never known anybody of wealth who did so much in delightful things for other people as you do.

The major portion of your toys are being distributed now for the children of Pinehurst, but I take particular pleasure, and my orderly Sergeant also does, in a recent widow whose husband died of lingering cancer and who earns a very modest income in a little 10¢ store (though it is hard to find anything for a dime in it these days), and who was left with five children, the oldest one being ten. So the Sergeant and I took particular pains in arranging her Christmas from you. Another we do from you is our occasional maid of all work, who is the mother of thirteen. She never celebrated Christmas until you barged into our neighborhood, because they couldn't buy Christmas gifts. Katherine objected to my giving them the White House to build. She said they wouldn't know what it was. Well, I took exception and they have got it, or will have it.[2]

With affectionate regards to you and Idella, Faithfully yours,

GCMRL/G. C. Marshall Papers (Retirement, General)

1. See pp. 746–47.
2. Marx had written to the Marshalls on December 10 that he was having "an assortment of toys" shipped from "our various factories" in Pennsylvania, West Virginia, and New Jersey. (Marx to Marshalls, December 10, 1956, GCMRL/G. C. Marshall Papers [Retirement, General].) Marshall noted on Marx's letter that the "wonderful collection" had "arrived in excellent shape." (Ibid.)

599

To General and Mrs. Matthew B. Ridgway — December 17, 1956
Washington, DC

Dear Ridgways: We received your lovely card and particularly appreciated the note. I hope you will pardon a dictated acknowledgement. The truth is that I seem to have gotten beyond longhand performance.

Katherine and I are getting along pretty well considering the years, but we could do better. The joke of it is—if there is any joke about it—that I was rather resentful of hearing her on the telephone answering inquiries about me and giving the impression that she has to look after me. But the truth of the matter is that now she does.

Another humiliating fact is that I used to make fun of my mother through her 70's and into her 80's about the valise she had full of medicines, and I called her by a medical term, Madame Blank—and now, by glory, I have as many as she had.[1]

It was very good to hear from you. Affectionately,

GCMRL/G. C. Marshall Papers (Retirement, General)

1. Ridgway replied on December 27 with birthday wishes "of admiration and affection." (Ridgway to Marshall, December 27, 1956, GCMRL/G. C. Marshall Papers [Retirement, General].) "And may the medicine cabinets gather thick cobwebs in 1957," he added. (Ibid.)

600

To Dwight D. Eisenhower — December 19, 1956
Washington, DC

My dear Mr. President: Heaton gave me your gracious message a few minutes ago, and I was not only pleased to receive it, but much more pleased to find out how well you were doing.[1]

As I am in your suite until tomorrow, I think it is about time that I thanked you for your consideration in always placing it at my disposal. This is deeply appreciated.

With the Season's Greetings to Mrs. Eisenhower and to you, and with the hope that all goes well with you physically and politically—and with your family,[2] Faithfully yours,

GCMRL/G. C. Marshall Papers (Retirement, General)

1. General Heaton had successfully operated on the president for ileitis in June 1956.

2. Eisenhower asked the Marshalls to be his "personal guests" at his second inauguration on January 21, and he invited Marshall to attend a reception for judicial and military officials scheduled for February 7. Marshall declined both invitations. (Eisenhower to Marshall, December 22, 1956, GCMRL/William Heffner Collection; Eisenhower to Marshall, January 16 and 28, 1957, GCMRL/G. C. Marshall Papers [Retirement, General].)

Marshall also dictated a letter to Queen Frederica on December 19, which was "about as much as I can manage these days." He admitted that his hospital room at Walter Reed "has never looked the same since" she visited in 1953. (See p. 801n2.) He added that he and Mrs. Marshall "have had a rather difficult summer and fall. The principal difficulty is 'years' I am not up to much of anything these days. They say I look better than I have for a long time, but my limitations are more numerous." He also apologized for his inability to "tell you very much because I move about so little and do so little that I am completely out of the world, as it were. And I know for you and His Majesty there is constant tribulation." (Marshall to Frederica, December 19, 1956, ibid.)

601

To General Walter Krueger[1]

January 4, 1957
Pinehurst, North Carolina

Dear Krueger: I was very much pleased to receive your birthday telegram. You were good to think of me.[2]

Just the other day my mind went back to 30th Infantry days in 1903 to one night you took me into your mess in Manila. I think it was the first time I met you. I had come up from southern Mindoro.[3]

With affectionate regards, Faithfully yours,

GCMRL/G. C. Marshall Papers (Retirement, General); H

1. General Walter Krueger commanded the Sixth Army in the Pacific in World War II. For Marshall's assessment on his long-term impressions of Krueger, see *Papers of GCM*, 2: 473–74.

2. Krueger had sent Marshall "Best wishes and warm regards for a happy birthday and many more of them." (Krueger to Marshall, telegram, December 31, 1956, GCMRL/G. C. Marshall Papers [Retirement, General].)

3. In a 1957 interview with Forrest Pogue, Krueger recalled "young Marshall as a green second lieutenant who reported for duty in a fresh uniform and with evident distaste for his new surroundings." (Pogue, *Education*, 82–83.) Major General R. W. Stephens, chief of military history for the Department of the Army, had sent to Marshall on November 9 for comment a draft of the first four chapters of *Triumph in the Philippines*, a volume to be published in the *United States Army in World War II* series, which perhaps sparked Marshall's renewed thoughts of his time in the Philippines.

602

TO HARRY S. TRUMAN

January 14, 1957
Pinehurst, North Carolina[1]

Dear Mr. Truman: I greatly appreciated your telegram of birthday greetings. It was very thoughtful of you to remember my day. For some reason or another, they seem to be arriving much more rapidly.[2]

Mrs. Marshall and I were distressed to read of Mrs. Truman's accident. We hope she is not too uncomfortable and in good time will be back on her feet again.[3]

We haven't read anything of Margaret lately, so we suppose she is playing the role of a dutiful housewife.[4]

With many thanks again, and with our warmest regards to you both,[5] Faithfully yours,

GCMarshall

GCMRL/G. C. Marshall Papers (Retirement, General)

1. This letter was typed on Marshall's Washington, DC, office stationery but Marshall had dictated it from Pinehurst.

2. Truman's birthday message had arrived on January 1. (Truman to Marshall, telegram, January 1, 1957, GCMRL/G. C. Marshall Papers [Retirement, General].) President Eisenhower had sent "birthday felicitations" on December 29. "I rather suspect that you—along with a lot of us—would just as soon these dates be forgotten, but it gives me the greatest enjoyment to send my very best wishes to you," Eisenhower had written. (Eisenhower to Marshall, December 29, 1956, DDEL/Dwight D. Eisenhower Papers [Papers as President, President's Personal File 182, Box 935].)

3. "Mrs. Bess Truman," the *New York Times* had reported on January 4, "fractured her left ankle in a fall at their home." ("Mrs. Truman Hurt," *New York Times*, January 4, 1957, p. 18.)

4. Margaret Truman had married Elbert Clifton Daniel Jr., an assistant foreign news editor for the *New York Times*, on April 21, 1956. "The idea of getting married in a week seems as though it must be happening to someone else," Margaret Truman had written to the Marshalls in April. "He is very nice, very handsome, very intelligent with great integrity and 'you can't hardly find them no more.' I do hope he will have the opportunity of meeting you someday soon." (Margaret Truman to Marshalls, April 19, 1956, GCMRL/G. C. Marshall Papers [Retirement, General].) By January 1957, she was pregnant with her first child. "A son was born to Mr. and Mrs. Clifton Daniel," the *New York Times* reported on June 5, 1957. ("Truman's Daughter Has 6½-Pound Boy," *New York Times*, June 5, 1957, p. 1.)

The *New York Times* had reported in 1956 that "Margaret Truman has been signed to a new one-year television contract by the National Broadcasting Company," effective September 1. ("Miss Truman Gets New TV Contract," *New York Times*, July 21, 1956, p. 47.)

5. "Mrs. Truman is getting along all right," Truman responded on January 28. "Her left foot is in a cast that reaches half-way to her knee, and she spends a great deal of her time bemoaning the fact that she has to wear it." (Truman to Marshall, January 28, 1957, GCMRL/G. C. Marshall Papers [Retirement, General].)

603

To Robert A. Lovett — January 22, 1957
Pinehurst, North Carolina

Dear Lovett: I very much appreciated receiving your multiple purpose letter of January 7. Many thanks for the birthday greetings from Adele and you, and our thanks for your New Year greetings and news of your current activities.[1]

I know you bankers are having quite a problem figuring out what the future offers and, since you are inexperienced as a crystal gazer, much thought will have to be given to every degree of business pulse, whether up or down.

I appreciated your reaction to the new Mid-East doctrine and was amused, in part, with Acheson's remarks.[2] I think he is apt to get a check from Readers' Digest when they quote his expression, as they so often do with others who make significant one-sentence remarks. I, personally, have not become aware of the prospects of inflation or deflation in the past several years, except to wonder what my barber will charge me on my next visit.

So far this year, the weather has been good to us. We have had our share of rain and wind, but nothing of a nature requiring a long stay indoors. I am feeling as well as can be expected, but occasionally I find myself having difficulty with balance. Many have told me that the problem is the inner ear, but the people at Walter Reed who checked me over recently do not share that opinion. Actually, they found nothing wrong with me except that age has its way of taking advantage of one's physical capabilities. Mrs. Marshall, I am happy to say, is the stronger of the two and, except for a bout with fatigue shortly after the Christmas Holiday, she has been well. I might say that she put together 65 packages and, as usual, refused any assistance.

You seem to have a good living arrangement to avoid the hazards of weather, and I suppose you both are looking forward with great relish to your planned trip to Florida.[3]

With our thanks to Adele and you for your good wishes and affection, which we so gladly return, Faithfully yours,

GCMRL/G. C. Marshall Papers (Retirement, General)

1. "We send you our love and best congratulations on your steady climb toward par—the goal of all bond traders," Lovett teased Marshall about passing his seventy-sixth birthday. "It seems to me significant that, while Government bonds are going steadily down and are now at a new low, you keep moving up which proves, in the bond dealers' lingo, that the Marshalls of 1957 have better intrinsic value and offer a better yield than Governments. No one in their right mind has ever had any doubt about this, but it is nice to have this neat statistical proof." (Lovett to Marshall, January 7, 1957, GCMRL/G. C. Marshall Papers [Retirement, General].)

2. In what became known as the "Eisenhower Doctrine," President Eisenhower had on January 5 requested Congressional authorization to commit US forces "to secure and protect the territorial integrity and political independence" of nations in the Middle East who requested such aid "against overt armed aggression from any nation controlled by international communism." (See Dwight D. Eisenhower, *Public Papers of the Presidents: Dwight D. Eisenhower, 1957* [Washington: GPO, 1958], 6–16.) "With the announcement of the so-called Eisenhower doctrine," Lovett had written to Marshall, "the business com-

munity is trying to figure out the prospects for 1957 with some rather amusing political byplay. Most of the commentators have pointed out that there is nothing new in the concept of negotiating from strength, except that it has not been tried for the last three years—and even a normally self-restrained Dean Acheson was quoted, in today's press, as having said that it had been described to him as a program 'To fight an enemy that's not going to attack with forces that don't exist, to carry out a policy you haven't decided upon yet.'" (Lovett to Marshall, January 7, 1957, ibid.)

3. "We spend most of the week in town and go out to Locust Valley for Saturday and Sunday, and thereby escape some of the discomfort and hazards of travels on the icy roads around here at this season. We expect to fly down to Hobe Sound for the month of March for our holiday, and I may have to go to the West Coast on business a couple of times before then." (Lovett to Marshall, January 7, 1957, ibid.) The Lovetts owned a "small cottage, not very comfortable, but two story" in Locust Valley on Long Island, New York. (Robert A. Lovett interview with Forrest C. Pogue, August 28, 1973, p. 22, GCMRL/Oral Histories.) They also owned a home at Hobe Sound, Florida.

"I WAS IMPRESSED with the degree to which General Marshall has aged during the last six months," Frank McCarthy, after a brief trip to Pinehurst, confided in a letter to Jack Hagan on January 25. "Although his morale is fine and he has every comfort, I felt he was less vigorous than I have ever seen him before." To the Marshalls, McCarthy wrote that he enjoyed visiting their "warm and comfortable and delightful house," and added that it gave him "and your many other friends" satisfaction " to picture you in such a pleasant atmosphere and to know that you are surrounded by such faithful people." (McCarthy to Hagan, January 25, 1957, and McCarthy to Marshalls, January 30, 1957, GCMRL/G. C. Marshall Papers [Retirement, General].) Marshall wrote on February 2 to convey "special thanks for making the long trip down from New York" to McCarthy and told him the effort was "greatly appreciated." (Marshall to McCarthy, February 2, 1957, GCMRL/Frank McCarthy Papers [Additions, Box 1]; H.)

In January, Marshall was busy recording his recollections for Forrest Pogue on the tape recorder given to him by William Spencer. See pp. 899–900 and 960–61. "When I first wrote you my thanks, the contraption was still a mystery to me," Marshall admitted to Spencer on January 30. "However, now that the Marshall Research Foundation has become a functioning organization and is energetically amassing a record of my life and career, I find myself continually subjected to the chore of personally answering in detail the thousands of questions its Director poses in an effort to fill the gaps in the official written records of my activities. His interviews with me were a burden and inconvenience to us both. But now we have come to the happy solution of his writing the questions out and sending them to me and, when I am in the mood and find it convenient, I record the answers on your machine and send the finished tape to him. The machine is so simple to operate and so remarkably sensitive that I find it a joy to use." (Marshall to Spencer, January 30, 1957, GCMRL/G. C. Marshall Papers [Retirement, Chronological].)

In his letter to Hagan, McCarthy reported that "General Marshall seems greatly interested in the project, but I don't think he had any conception of the volume of work to be done when he gave us his agreement. He didn't complain about this, but he did mention two or three times during the day that 'this is going to take years, and years, and years.'" McCarthy opined that "the personal interviews" should be kept "to an absolute minimum" and recommended "pushing the questions to him for tape recorded replies as fast as possible." McCarthy assured Hagan that Marshall's "memory is phenomenal, but at the same time he is subject to periods of lethargy which could affect the quality of his replies." (McCarthy to Hagan, January 25, 1957, GCMRL/G. C. Marshall Papers [Retirement, General].) On February 19, C. J. George wrote to Hagan that he was "more than pleased with the progress that is being made. It would do your heart a world of good if you could sit in our office here and listen to the tapes that General Marshall has been recording. Pogue just ran one off and the elapsed time was two hours. The General's voice was as strong at the finish as it was at the beginning." (George to Hagan, February 19, 1957, ibid.)

Still, Marshall acknowledged to his old friend Bill Pawley on February 5 that he was "not up to travel and visiting yet. My trouble is fading somewhat but not sufficiently for me to do much. I feel well. They tell me I look well, but I am troubled by lack of balance when I walk." Pawley had invited the Marshalls to visit him and his wife in Miami, Florida, as they had in 1949. See *Papers of GCM*, 6: 674–75. Pawley proposed to fly the Marshalls in a private DC-3 direct from Pinehurst, which Marshall considered "very generous." (Marshall to Pawley, February 5, 1957, GCMRL/William D. Pawley Collection; H; Pawley to Marshall, February 1, 1957, GCMRL/G. C. Marshall Papers [Retirement, General].) "Much as I tried to encourage both of them to take advantage of the hospitality you so generously offered, I lost the battle of words," C. J. George wrote to Pawley on February 6. "I, personally, am sorry, because I think it would have done them both a world of good." (George to Pawley, February 6, 1957, ibid.)

Change continued in the Marshall family circle. At the end of January, Marshall wrote to his cousin Elizabeth Bradford Harbeson that his brother Stuart had "passed away on last November 11 of hypertensive heart disease." He also noted that his sister Marie was "fine and has just recently celebrated her eightieth birthday. I hear from her rather regularly and find that she is busy with her bridge playing, luncheons and dinners." He also mentioned that Allene Lacy was "still helpless in a nursing home near Pinehurst." (Marshall to Harbeson, January 31, 1957, ibid.) Marie Singer wrote to Marshall to express condolences on the December 29, 1956, death of his former brother-in-law, Edmund Coles, "but he was old enough to go, as I am," she declared. (Singer to Marshall, n.d., ibid.; H.) See p. 944. Marshall responded on January 22 to thank his sister for "the beautiful basket of fruit. My departure for Walter Reed and absence until the day before Christmas must be accepted as my practical apology." (Marshall to Singer, January 22, 1957, ibid.) ★

604

To Melville Bell Grosvenor[1] February 5, 1957
Pinehurst, North Carolina

Dear Grosvenor: Thank you for your letter introducing Mr. Fisher and your son, Gilbert.[2] I enjoyed their visit and think it went very satisfactorily. Their work on the American Battle Monuments Commission article is in fine shape, and I am sure it will be very impressive to the public—especially the many persons whose loved ones are interred in these cemeteries so far from home.[3]

Mrs. Marshall and I will be delighted to see Mrs. Grosvenor and you on March 17. Just give us a call when you arrive at the village.[4]

With best wishes, Faithfully yours,

P. S. Warmest congratulations on your election to the offices of President and Editor of the Society.[5]

GCMRL/G. C. Marshall Papers (Retirement, General)

1. Melville Bell Grosvenor was the son of National Geographic Society founder Gilbert Grosvenor. He succeeded John Oliver LaGorce as president and editor at the January 8, 1957, meeting of the Board of Trustees.

2. Grosvenor had written to Marshall on January 26 to announce that his son Gilbert and Allan C. Fisher, both members of the *National Geographic* magazine staff, would be coming to Pinehurst to show Marshall the "first drafts of the proposed articles" as well as "the dummies of the twenty-one pages of color plates covering the American Battle Monuments scheduled for the June issue of the Magazine." (Grosvenor to Marshall, January 26, 1957, GCMRL/G. C. Marshall Papers [Retirement, General].) Grosvenor explained the issue would lead with an introductory article by Marshall as chairman of the ABMC. (Ibid.)

3. Marshall reported to Grosvenor on February 26 that Fisher's article was "admirable," and he offered "no suggestions" for revisions. (Marshall to Grosvenor, February 26, 1957, ibid.) Grosvenor thanked Marshall on March 7 for reviewing the thirty-eight–page ABMC article "proof so carefully." He thought it was going to be a unique and "extraordinarily popular contribution to the Magazine." (Grosvenor to Marshall, March 7, 1957, ibid.)

4. Grosvenor had mentioned that he and his wife hoped to pass through Pinehurst on their way to Florida. (Grosvenor to Marshall, January 26, 1957, ibid.)

5. "I appreciated very much your congratulations," Grosvenor replied on February 14, although he regretted that Marshall was not "present on that—to me—momentous occasion!" (Grosvenor to Marshall, February 14, 1957, ibid.)

At Marshall's request, Grosvenor agreed on March 13 to provide approximately five thousand reprints of the article to the ABMC. (Grosvenor to Marshall, March 13, 1957, ibid.) Marshall approved a cover letter drafted by General North to be included with the reprints, which would be sent to "public libraries, Members of Congress, etc." (North to George, June 4, 1957, GCMRL/G. C. Marshall Papers [American Battle Monuments Commission].) The letter stated the ABMC's hope that the reader find the article "of interest and also that it may bring to the attention of more of the American people just what their Government is doing to honor the memory of those who served the armed forces during the war." (Cover letter for *National Geographic* article reprint, May 30, 1957, ibid.)

"The War Memorials article is beautifully done," Marshall wrote the editor after receiving advance copies of the June issue. He and the entire ABMC were "tremendously pleased and grateful for the Society's generous cooperation" in publicizing the ABMC's "achievements" and were confident the public would have "great" interest in the subject. (Marshall to Grosvenor, May 21, 1957, ibid.) Marshall received numerous letters that praised the article, including correspondence from veterans of both world wars. (Giles to Marshall, May 27, 1957, and Hawkes to Marshall, June 25, 1957, GCMRL/G. C. Marshall Papers

[American Battle Monuments Commission].) He commented to John Oliver La Gorce that the response to the article was "extraordinary," although he was "embarrassed by the compliments I have received for something your gifted editor wrote. It seems to have made a deep impression on the public." (Marshall to La Gorce, June 17, 1957, GCMRL/G. C. Marshall Papers [Retirement, General].) Marshall expressed similar sentiments to Allan Fisher, who responded that Marshall had "underestimated your own contribution to the article." Marshall's "desire to reassure families, your wish that more people visit the cemeteries, the episode of the Gold Star mother at Epinal—these thoughts and others supplied the framework and coloration of the story. You gave generously of your time and imbued me with your own deep convictions on the subject." (Marshall to Fisher, June 25, 1957, and Fisher to Marshall, June 26, 1957, ibid.)

605

To Mrs. John B. Wilson — February 9, 1957, Pinehurst, North Carolina

My dear Rose I am going to inflict on you one of my limping long-hand letters.

For some queer reason I write with great difficulty. My hand is unusually steady—and I have no difficulty in mental composition, but I can not write.

I can dictate fast and accurately—did 32 letters in one hour of dictation while I was at the Walter Reed the other day, but no long hand.[1]

Your reply was such a lengthy newsy letter that I thought it merited a written reply, which is the best I can do down here.[2]

I have been quite well this winter, no colds or other afflictions. Katherine the same. She has a hard time with her ordinary duties and spending considerable time with her paralyzed sister at the Convalescent Home.[3]

It has been miserably rainy and cold for weeks. I am in hopes that the weather will finally clear for spring. I have no Washington engagements, declined an invitation to the Inauguration, and had stayed strictly at home. Read all morning, breakfast at 8-30 but do not get up until noon.

I liked your proposal to come down alone and stay with us. We will try and arrange a date later.[4]

With love, Affectionately,

GCM

GCMRL/J. Page Wilson Collection; H

1. Marshall's most recent stay at Walter Reed Army Medical Center was from December 17 to 24, 1956, when he dictated letters, particularly holiday greetings, to many close friends, including Lady Mary Burghley, Catharine Armstrong, Frances McCoy, and John Leighton Stuart.

2. See p. 962n1. Wilson had reported on Christmas activities and had given Marshall an update on various family members in her January 7 letter. (Wilson to Marshall, January 7, 1957, GCMRL/G. C. Marshall Papers [Retirement, General].) She also related that her son Page, who was also Marshall's godson, "has started dancing school and loves it. This is a great surprise. He even goes to dances." (Ibid.)

3. See pp. 874, 899n4, and 912.

4. In her memoir, Wilson commented that in the winter of 1956–57 "Colonel Marshall and I talked on the phone from time to time, as usual," which may explain the source of this suggestion. (Wilson, *Remembered*, 382.)

606

To Rear Admiral Samuel E. Morison[1] March 19, 1957
Pinehurst, North Carolina

Dear Morison: I have your letter of March 7.[2]

I recall some bicycle talk, but thought it was by President Roosevelt, and maybe not about the Ruhr.[3]

I do not recall threatening to resign. Don't believe it.[4]

We all argued very strongly, and as I recall, the United States group were close together.

I am terribly saddened at Byrd's passing. The world's loss is immense.[5] Faithfully yours,

GCMRL/G. C. Marshall Papers (Retirement, General)

1. See p. 928.

2. "May I ask you to give me the benefit of your recollections on one small matter" relating to the book he was writing about the invasion of France and Germany in World War II, Morison had written to Marshall. (Morison to Marshall, March 7, 1957, GCMRL/G. C. Marshall Papers [Retirement, General].) Morison questioned Fleet Admiral Ernest J. King's account in his autobiography of discussions among the Combined Chiefs of Staff "at the Malta Conference of 30 January–3 February 1945," when "the C.C.S. was deadlocked between [Field Marshal Bernard Law] Montgomery's plan to cross the Rhine at only one or two places, and Eisenhower's to cross at several places at once." (Ibid.)

3. In his book, King had described his and Marshall's meeting with President Franklin D. Roosevelt onboard the cruiser *Quincy* at Malta on February 2, 1945. "When Marshall and King insisted upon the soundness of Eisenhower's idea the president asked for a map. After examining it, he recalled that he had made a bicycle tour through the very area involved, and as he knew the terrain, he understood Eisenhower's basic idea at once, and approved of it." (Ernest J. King and Walter Muir Whitehill, *Fleet Admiral King, A Naval Record* [New York: W. W. Norton & Company Inc., 1952], 585–86.) Morison questioned this account, stating that it "Sounds a little fishy, King pronouncing on ground-force strategy when you and Bedell Smith were present." (Morison to Marshall, March 7, 1957, GCMRL/G. C. Marshall Papers [Retirement, General].)

4. Morison also doubted what he incorrectly understood to be Robert Sherwood's version of the events during the disagreement, that Marshall "threatened, if the Monty plan were approved, to be asked to be relieved." (Ibid.) In *Roosevelt and Hopkins: An Intimate History*, Sherwood actually wrote, "The arguments reached such a point that Marshall, ordinarily one of the most restrained and soft-spoken of men, announced that if the British plan were approved by the Prime Minister and President he would recommend to Eisenhower that he had no choice but to ask to be relieved of his command." (Sherwood, *Roosevelt and Hopkins*, 848.) Morison concluded his letter by asking Marshall whether he remembered "King taking the lead in the argument, or merely pointing out one factor—the encirclement of the Ruhr—which made the Eisenhower plan more acceptable; and whether Sherwood represents your attitude correctly, and whether F.D.R. did intervene." (Morison to Marshall, March 7, 1957, GCMRL/G. C. Marshall Papers [Retirement, General].) Morison also contacted Bedell Smith for his recollection of events. "I doubt very much if Sherwood is correct in saying that General Marshall threatened or asked to be relieved," Smith concluded an April 26 letter to Morison, which he shared with Marshall. "During all of the time I have known [Marshall] and served under him he has never, even by implication, used as a threat the inference of his personal relief to support an argument which might have gone against him." (Smith to Morison, April 26, 1957, ibid.)

5. "Rear Admiral Richard E. Byrd, U.S.N., retired, the first man to fly over the North and South Poles, died in his sleep," the *New York Times* had reported on March 12. ("Admi-

ral Byrd Dies at 68; Made 5 Polar Expeditions," *New York Times*, March 12, 1957, p. 1.) The next day Marshall sent a telegram to Byrd's widow. "My deepest sympathy goes to you. I have lost a generous friend who did much for me in difficult times. He was a great man." (Marshall to Byrd, telegram, March 13, 1957, GCMRL/G. C. Marshall Papers [Retirement, General]. See also Marshall to Byrd, May 1, 1957, GCMRL/G. C. Marshall Papers [Retirement, Chronological].)

607

To Frank McCarthy

April 3, 1957
Pinehurst, North Carolina

Dear Frank: I have just had word from General Milton of your gift to V. M. I. and particularly the Marshall Arch. I am deeply grateful to you for this generous and gracious thought of me. Only you would think of such a thing.[1]

Katherine and I have been getting along in good fashion. It is quite remarkable to me, with all she has to contend with, that her health has not suffered. Frankly, she seems to improve from day to day. As for myself, at times I feel inert, but there is enough going on to keep me fairly occupied, and I suppose that is the best medicine possible.[2]

Incidentally, I took in the North-South Women's Amateur Championship Tournament and the results were very pleasing. A young lady by the name of Barbara McIntire, representing the Mid-Pines Club at Pinehurst, took top honors. I followed the play very leisurely in an electric cart.[3]

I hope you are getting along well—and please be sure to stop in on us whenever you are East. Your last visit was stimulating.[4] Faithfully yours,

GCMRL/G. C. Marshall Papers (Retirement, General)

1. "It has been a long time since I was in Lexington, but on my last visit I noticed there was no appropriate lighting in the Marshall Arch," McCarthy responded on April 13 about his idea to illuminate the arch at the Virginia Military Institute that had been dedicated to Marshall on May 15, 1951. See pp. 518–23. (McCarthy to Marshall, April 13, 1957, GCMRL/G. C. Marshall Papers [Retirement, General].)

2. C. J. George reported to Marie Singer after a March 22 visit to Pinehurst that her brother was "looking especially well" and in "fine spirits," while Mrs. Marshall "appears and feels much better than she has in many years. I doubt she has any complaint, except for the distress of her sister's illness." (George to Singer, March 26, 1957, ibid.) George also wrote to Adlai E. Stevenson with news about the Marshalls and mentioned that "while paralyzed," Allene Tupper Lacy "is still constitutionally strong and mentally alert." (George to Stevenson, March 29, 1957, ibid.)

3. "Barbara McIntire of Toledo, Ohio, leading from the third hole, won the North and South women's amateur golf tournament," the *New York Times* had reported on March 26. ("Barbara M'Intire Takes Golf Final," *New York Times*, March 26, 1957, p. 39.)

4. See pp. 967–68. "It is good to know that you are occupied," McCarthy noted in his April 13 letter. "I saw Forrest Pogue in Washington about a month ago and he was delighted with the results which you are achieving. So are we all." (McCarthy to Marshall, April 13, 1957, ibid.)

608

TO GENERAL MAXWELL D. TAYLOR

April 4, 1957
Pinehurst, North Carolina

Dear Taylor: I should like to acknowledge with appreciation the approval of my appraisal of Miss Mary Louise Spilman's performance of duty.

She has been for me a most competent assistant, and I feel that she is most certainly entitled to a promotion, in lieu of a cash award which I understand may accompany the "Outstanding" rating. Miss Spilman has been most valuable; she has great initiative and has independently taken action on many matters of importance. I have never had occasion to differ from her judgment.

I should like to point out that Miss Spilman's grade classification was designated as GS-10 at the time she became my secretary early in 1952. For these past five years, she has been a great asset to this office and I find her help invaluable.

I strongly endorse the promotion of Miss Spilman to the next highest grade.[1] Faithfully yours,

GCMRL/G. C. Marshall Papers (Retirement, Chronological)

1. "Thank you for your note of April 17 advising me of the approval of my recommendation for Miss Spilman's promotion," Marshall wrote to Taylor on April 23. "I appreciate your consideration of the matter and assure you that both she and I are very much pleased." (Marshall to Taylor, April 23, 1957, GCMRL/G. C. Marshall Papers [Retirement, Chronological].)

SHORTLY BEFORE the Marshalls made the transition from Pinehurst to Leesburg on May 3, Katherine Marshall had confided in her friend Ellen Bruce that "G. is very frail & seldom goes out even for a drive now." (Katherine Marshall to Bruce, April 26, 1957, GCMRL/Katherine Marshall Correspondence.) Marshall's sister wrote to Colonel George that she "had not had a line from them for weeks," and wondered "What is the matter with George, do you know? I have never been able to find out!" (Singer to George, April 3, 1957, GCMRL/G. C. Marshall Papers [Retirement, General].) On May 6, General and Mrs. Marshall moved into Walter Reed Army Hospital for semiannual check-ups, and while his wife was completing her appointments Marshall dictated to Mary Louise Spilman more than two dozen letters. His correspondents included former President Truman (see next document), family members, and longtime friends. He told Madge Pendleton that Katherine Marshall had been down with "an attack of intestinal flu, which struck everybody at Pinehurst" but overall, she enjoyed "the best winter she has had for years." He reported that they left his sister-in-law, Allene Lacy, "about the same. She is right cheerful and seems to be in good shape physically. In fact, she is better rested up than any of us, and she seemed quite content at Katherine's departure from Pinehurst." See p. 874. He wrote to Lacy to apologize for not seeing her before they left Pinehurst, "but I find that I am not up to visiting around and I had to conserve all my energy for the trip." (Marshall to Pendleton and Marshall to Lacy, May 10, 1957, ibid.)

"I have had a pretty sorry winter," he confessed to Queen Frederica. (Marshall to Frederica, May 10, 1957, ibid.) He disclosed to Madame Chiang Kai-shek that over the winter Katherine Marshall had "a great deal to do in nursing me as a matter of fact, and I have had to place a great deal of dependence on her." (Marshall to Madame Chiang, May 10, 1957, ibid.) "My trouble seems to be largely this lack of balance I suffer from and a lack of appetite so that I am losing weight, which I shouldn't do," he confided to Bernard Baruch. "I enjoy my breakfast hugely, but then I just cannot eat the other meals." (Marshall to Baruch, May 10, 1957, ibid.) "The lack of balance only affects me in a forward way," he explained to Bill Pawley. "After I walk a little bit, I feel like I am going to fall on my nose." He also mentioned to Pawley that "Bedell Smith is in the next room to me having a bad time with his eyes as he had a hemorrhage." (Marshall to Pawley, May 10, 1957, ibid.) Marshall also wrote to Anna Rosenberg the same day with a further description of "poor old Smith, who is having a long bout with patience, as he has to lie quiet in bed with his head sandbagged into place while this business of his eye heals up. He had his operation last Thursday. I have talked to him quite a bit, but it is an effort to talk to me because I have gotten pretty deaf and he can't raise his voice. So we are not much help to each other." (Marshall to Rosenberg, May 10, 1957, ibid.) "I enjoyed so much chatting with you," Smith wrote to Marshall on May 24 from the Massachusetts Eye and Ear Infirmary, where he had undergone further surgery, "and I hope we can do it again soon but in a more pleasant surrounding." (Smith to Marshall, May 24, 1957, ibid.)

"I haven't done anything for Pogue for some weeks," he admitted to Jack Hagan, but promised that after he "got rested up a little at Leesburg, I will go to work again. Fortunately I find that dictating does not tire me particularly." (Marshall to Hagan, May 10, 1957, ibid.) Marshall also corresponded with Catharine Armstrong, Sir Anthony Eden, Robert Lovett, William M. Spencer, Rose Page Wilson, Generals Mark Clark and Matthew Ridgway, and others while he was at Walter Reed. ★

609

To Harry S. Truman — May 8, 1957
Washington, DC

Dear Mr. Truman: Mrs. Marshall and I came up from Pinehurst three or four days ago and have moved into the hospital for our semi-annual check-up.

I appreciated very much your letter to me—particularly the postscript—expressing your regret that I could not appear at the dedication of your Library.[1] The truth of the matter is that I have been suffering all this winter from a peculiar ailment, which consists largely of a lack of balance. For example, I can't write longhand. I get about half a line done and then I fade out, and yet my hands are not at all tremulous. I can dictate by the hour and it doesn't seem to tire me much, so I have no trouble with that.

As I have no secretary at Pinehurst, I am very much limited in my writing.

Most of it is done for me up here in my Washington office. Otherwise, you would hear from me more frequently and at greater length.

As I have said, I came into the hospital here two days ago for a semi-annual check-up, and so far they find me quite perfect, except that they can't help me at all.

I just learned by accident a moment ago that this is your birthday, so this letter is a birthday greeting. Please give my love to Mrs. Truman, and I know Mrs. Marshall would want to join me in this and in congratulations on your birthday. She is in the hospital with me having her semi-annual check-up, which tires her out quite a bit, but she has been better off this winter than for several years.

If everything proceeds in a normal way, we will be at Leesburg until we go South again the first of next November. If it becomes very warm, we may go up to the mountains, but it is so much more comfortable at Leesburg that we hang on there until we are driven out by the heat.

With affectionate regards and my devotions,[2] Faithfully yours,

GCMRL/G. C. Marshall Papers (Retirement, General)

1. On April 15, Marshall had sent a letter of regret to Basil O'Connor, president and chairman of the Truman Library's executive committee, concerning the dedication of the Truman Library. (Marshall to O'Connor, April 15, 1957, GCMRL/G. C. Marshall Papers [Retirement, General].) "This is a very sad disappointment," Truman had written in his April 29 letter. "I had hoped that you, more than anyone else, could be here, but the one thing that concerns me more than the dedication of the library is your continued good health." (Truman to Marshall, April 29, 1957, ibid.) The handwritten postscript urged Marshall to "Please take good care of yourself and Mrs. Marshall. Hope to see you both in the not too far distant future. HST" (Ibid.) Truman wrote again on June 21 after the dedication that "the darned thing has turned out so much better than I ever had any idea that it would, that I am really overwhelmed. You know that's hard to do to me." (Truman to Marshall, June 21, 1957, ibid.) "You know from experience how a corporal in National Guard Field Artillery in 1906—by accident became C in C [commander-in-chief]. Thanks to you and men like you he was not a complete failure," Truman concluded his letter. (Ibid.)

2. Truman responded on May 23 and mentioned that he "had a fine interview the other day with Mr. Pogue, who told me that he is making good progress in his work. Please remember that any papers or information I have that might be of interest to you are available for any use you wish to make of them." (Truman to Marshall, May 23, 1957, ibid.)

610

To Frank McCarthy May 10, 1957
Washington, DC

Dear Frank: I checked-up on your promotion prospects and I believe the action will come in June. If it doesn't, I'm going to raise a little bit of Hell.[1]

Katherine and I came into the Walter Reed on the 6th, but we expect to go back to Leesburg in a day or two. She seems to be in good shape and very much relieved to find that her eyes are 20-20 and in good condition. She had suffered considerably with her eyes as a result of the shingles, but that seems to be wearing off now.

They find me all right too, except that I have a lack of appetite and a lack of balance. Affectionately,

GCM

GCMRL/Frank McCarthy Papers (Additions, Box 1)

1. McCarthy had remained in the active reserves since leaving the army after World War II. (See p. 950.) After returning from his visit with the Marshalls in Pinehurst (see p. 972n2), C. J. George had discussed the issue of McCarthy's promotion at the Pentagon and informed Marshall that he had "been advised that Frank's recommendation will be considered by the Board when they convene in the first part of June and, from all indications, it appears that his promotion is a foregone conclusion." (George to Marshall, memorandum, March 27, 1957, GCMRL/G. C. Marshall Papers [Retirement, Chronological].) He assured Marshall that "Your attitude in this matter has been made known to General [Maxwell] Taylor. (Ibid.) "You have been nominated for promotion to Brigadier General. Congratulations and affectionate regards," Marshall wired McCarthy on July 12. (Marshall to McCarthy, telegram, July 12, 1957, GCMRL/Frank McCarthy Papers [Additions, Box 1].) "The Secretary of the Army passed through Los Angeles ten days ago and pinned the star on my shoulder," McCarthy wrote to Marshall on September 3. (McCarthy to Marshall, September 3, 1957, ibid.)

611

Remarks upon Receiving an Award from the Organization for European Economic Cooperation[1] — June 5, 1957, Washington, DC

It is with very real humility that I come here today to receive your expressions of appreciation for the attitude of the people of this Country toward all of Western Europe in their tragic dilemma at the close of the Second World War. That attitude was helpful to a degree without precedent, I believe, in history.

It was my good fortune to be in the position to give expression to this rather typical American reaction, which came from the very heart of its people. And, in a way, it has set an example for the succeeding years, though the corrosion of ten years ago still persists to trouble the world and poison the course of history.

I accept this medal with deep humility as a profound tribute to my countrymen.[2]

GCMRL/G. C. Marshall Papers (Retirement, General); H

1. "In a ceremony at Blair-Lee House" across from the White House, the *New York Times* reported on June 6, General Marshall "was honored on the tenth anniversary of the address that outlined the Marshall Plan for assisting war-torn Europe." ("Marshall Is Honored on 10th Anniversary of Aid Plan," *New York Times*, June 6, 1957, p. 1.) See *Papers of GCM*, 6: 147–50. President Eisenhower briefly attended the ceremony and gave Marshall a letter declaring that at the time Marshall gave his speech at Harvard University on June 5, 1947, "The fate of all Western Civilization hung in the balance, and there were many to whom disaster seemed inevitable. That this tragedy was averted is due in large measure to the bold and imaginative undertaking which you proposed and which rightfully bears your name." (Eisenhower to Marshall, June 3, 1957, GCMRL/G. C. Marshall Papers [Retirement, General].)

2. The silver medal, given by the Organization for the European Economic Cooperation, and presented by the British ambassador, bore the inscription "Salus Europae: Pax terra marique parta," which translates as "The Salvation of Europe: Peace by land and sea." ("Marshall Is Honored on 10th Anniversary of Aid Plan," *New York Times*, June 6, 1957, pp. 1, 6.)

612

TO MISS BERTHA R. SKINKER June 11, 1957
Leesburg, Virginia

My dear Miss Skinker: I appreciated your letter referring to Lily Coles, who was later Elizabeth Coles Marshall.[1] She died in 1927 in Washington after twenty-five years of, to me, charming and delightful married life.[2]

The cemeteries in Europe were not damaged and are maintained in beautiful condition.[3]

I am glad you found my article of interest.[4] Faithfully yours,

GCMRL/G. C. Marshall Papers (Retirement, General)

1. Bertha R. Skinker of La Jolla, California, had introduced herself as a close childhood friend of Marshall's first wife, Elizabeth "Lily" Coles. Skinker had "lost sight of her completely" after Coles had moved "back to Lexington." She had heard that Coles "had married a captain in the Army," and while Skinker knew "nothing further" about the marriage, she "did eventually hear more of the captain." (Skinker to Marshall, May 29, 1957, GCMRL/G. C. Marshall Papers [Retirement, General].)

2. For more on Marshall's first marriage, see Pogue, *Education*.

3. Skinker had inquired if "Romagne and the other 1918 cemeteries still stand" or if they had been damaged during World War II. Her brother had been killed on the first day of the battle of the Argonne, although his body had been returned to the US due to their father's belief that the Germans would "invade France again" and "take special pleasure in destroying the United States cemeteries" there. (Ibid.)

4. See pp. 969–70.

613

TO REAR ADMIRAL SAMUEL E. MORISON June 11, 1957
Leesburg, Virginia

Dear Morison: Thanks for the Times clippings re Alanbrooke's diary. You were thoughtful to send them and very vigorous in your comments.[1]

The N. Y. Times had a good review.[2]

So goes it! It's as bad as Gettysburg.[3] Faithfully yours,

GCMRL/G. C. Marshall Papers (Retirement, General); H

1. See p. 891n1. "I thought you might be interested in the English clippings covering my two lectures here on U.S. contributions to the strategy of World War II," Morison had written to Marshall from Oxford, England, on May 18. "They are, in a way, an answer to the Alanbrooke diaries, which have created a furor here." (Morison to Marshall, May 18, 1957, GCMRL/G. C. Marshall Papers [Retirement, General].) Alanbrooke's diaries were also very critical of Marshall. The *London Times* reported that in his lectures, Morison "attacked the Alanbrooke diaries as being indiscreet and answered a number of points raised in them." ("Anglo-American Wartime 'Strategic Mistake,'" *Times* [London], May 17, 1957.)

2. On February 17, the *New York Times* had published a brief summary of *The Turn of the Tide*, and Morison wrote a highly critical review of the book for the May 19 issue of the newspaper. ("Briton Analyzes President at War," *New York Times*, February 17, 1957, p. 3; Samuel Eliot Morison, "The British General Kept a Diary," *New York Times*, May 19, 1957, pp. BR1, 28.)

3. Marshall had thanked Viscount Alanbrooke on March 13 for sending an inscribed copy of *The Turn of the Tide*. "I shall read the book with much interest," Marshall wrote. (Marshall to Alanbrooke, March 13, 1957, GCMRL/G. C. Marshall Papers [Retirement, General].) *Washington Post* publisher Philip L. Graham wrote to Katherine Marshall on June 20 that he was infuriated after reading the book, so he wrote to Viscount Brendan Bracken, who had served as Britain's minister of information from 1941 to 1945. Graham forwarded a copy of Bracken's response to Katherine Marshall to ensure she would have an opportunity to read the letter before showing it to General Marshall. (Graham to Katherine Marshall, June 20, 1957, ibid.) Bracken's letter to Graham rejected Alanbrooke's claims and praised Marshall's rare "moral distinction," character, humility, intellect, and pervasive influence on President Roosevelt, which was his "biggest contribution to the war effort." (Bracken to Graham, June 12, 1957, ibid.)

On June 24, Katherine Marshall drafted a response to Graham that included a message to him from General Marshall: "To evaluate Brooke's biography you have to keep in mind *when* it was written—it was taken from notes in his diary at a time when there was dissension between the British and American Chiefs of Staff as to the conduct of the war. Brooke at that time was a very bitter and disappointed man. I feel that if he had written an *autobiography after the war* the tone would have been very different." (Katherine Marshall to Graham, June 24, 1957, ibid.) Katherine Marshall's own assessment of Alanbrooke was "not as generous," though. Noting that Alanbrooke had visited the Marshalls on several occasions during the war and had autographed "one of the first copies" of his book for Marshall the previous Christmas, she commented that "the British are not noted for their tact nor intuition. This has been illustrated lately at Gettysburg . . . and will long be remembered." (Ibid.) Field Marshal Bernard Law Montgomery had toured the American Civil War battlefield at Gettysburg, Pennsylvania, with President Eisenhower on May 12. Two days later the *New York Times* reported they had sparked controversy when "They agreed that both General [Robert E.] Lee and his opponent, Gen. George G. Meade, should have been dismissed, the Southerner for having ordered the ill-fated Pickett's Charge that resulted in a Confederate defeat, and the Union leader for not having followed up on his advantage." (Allen Drury, "South Opens Fire on Montgomery," *New York Times*, May 14, 1957, p. 36.) Montgomery was surprised but "undaunted by the outcries his remarks had touched off among Southerners." (Ibid.)

614

To Mrs. Anna M. Rosenberg — July 25, 1957, Leesburg, Virginia

Dear Anna: Thanks for your note about the Sunday Star article.[1] You always do the nice thing.

The Lovetts had dinner or lunch with us a few weeks ago.[2] It was fine to see them, and they both look well.

I am pretty much house-bound, but I get around on the place a little.[3] It has been much too hot to go out recently. This entire area is suffering greatly from lack of rain. Any crops that are not already harvested will never be. It is a very bad year for the farmers.

Thanks again for writing. Affectionately,

GCMRL/G. C. Marshall Papers (Retirement, General)

1. Rosenberg had written to Marshall about an article, published July 7, by *Washington Star* editor James Birchfield, who lived near Leesburg. (James Birchfield, "A Neighborly Call on Gen. Marshall," *Sunday Star Magazine*, July 7, 1957, p. 12.) "Reading it and see-

ing your pictures gave me a very warm feeling," Rosenberg told Marshall. (Rosenberg to Marshall, July 17, 1957, GCMRL/G. C. Marshall Papers [Retirement, General].)

2. C. J. George had sent Marshall a memorandum on June 12 concerning plans for a luncheon with the Lovetts at Dodona Manor on June 14. (George to Marshall, memorandum, June 12, 1957, GCMRL/G. C. Marshall Papers [Retirement, Chronological].)

3. Marshall drafted his response by hand at the bottom of Rosenberg's letter. The following sentences were added by M. L. Spilman to the typed version mailed to Rosenberg.

On July 25, Marshall also wrote to Lawrence H. Whiting, president of several companies in Chicago—including the American Furniture Mart—and a longtime friend of William M. Spencer, who had visited Marshall on June 16. (Spencer to Marshall, June 17, 1957, GCMRL/G. C. Marshall Papers [Retirement, General].) Marshall wrote to thank Whiting for the "lovely summer furniture" he had shipped to Dodona Manor; however, "a heavy flight of pestiferous insects" made "sitting outdoors uncomfortable. But we are using it to full advantage indoors or on our terrace." He encouraged Whiting to telephone ahead when he was in the area because "the servants turn" away "a constant flow of curious people who claim at the door to be intimate friends of mine." (Marshall to Whiting, July 25, 1957, ibid.)

615

To Mrs. John White Pendleton — August 14, 1957
Leesburg, Virginia

Dear Madge: Katherine and I received your long, interesting, and most welcome letter. We were especially delighted to know that all goes well with you and the family. It appears that you are getting a theoretical and practical education in far-off Saudi Arabia.[1]

Incidentally, George tells me that King Saud made quite an impression when he visited the Pentagon.[2] I suppose the manner of dress and the colorful attendants had much to do with this reaction.

I am sorry that the book on Indians took so long to reach you, but I'm glad that you were in quick receipt of the National Geographic article on our overseas cemeteries. I think the Society did a masterful job, and I hope that many millions of our people get to see it.[3]

Your resume of Tupper's activities was most interesting, and we hope that if you make any snapshots of the family you will include us in the distribution.

Allene had a very strong urge to move north, and some several weeks ago she came up by train with her nurse and is now comfortably situated in a nursing home at Williamsport, Maryland. It is a short distance from Hagerstown, and not too many miles from Molly. She makes frequent visits, and Katherine has been up several times. It is a few hours from Leesburg, through a very picturesque countryside.[4]

Physically, I have been holding my own and have no particular complaint, except that I lost considerable weight and now find it difficult to put it back on. For some little time, I was not eating very well, but am doing much better at the moment.[5]

Katherine, I think, has done very well this fall, spring and summer, but on occasion she had the same old trouble with her eyes.

I have never had lamb in the desert. Perhaps the atmosphere and style of eating makes it more attractive.

With love to you all, Affectionately,

GCMRL/Xerox 2237 (GCM Family, Personal Letters)

1. Madge Pendleton and their children had joined her husband in Dhahran, Saudi Arabia, where John Pendleton had taken a position with ARAMCO Saudi Arabian Oil Company. See p. 927n2.

2. The Saudi Arabian king had lunch with Secretary of Defense Wilson on February 1 at the Pentagon. (Russell Baker, "Dulles Is Optimistic on Talks with Saud," *New York Times*, February 2, 1957, p. 3.)

3. See pp. 969–70.

4. C. J. George had notified Sergeant Heffner on June 17 that arrangements had been made to transport Allene Tupper Lacy by rail from the nursing home in Pinehurst, North Carolina, to one in Williamsport. (George to Heffner, June 17, 1957, GCMRL/G. C. Marshall Papers [Retirement, Chronological].) "I go up to Williamsport, Md. Sanatorium every two weeks to see my sister," Katherine Marshall had written to her friend Ellen Bruce on August 3. "This is my only trip off the place." (Katherine Marshall to Bruce, August 3, 1957, GCMRL/Katherine Marshall Correspondence.) See p. 986.

5. Mrs. Marshall also confided to Mrs. Bruce that the doctor "comes down from Walter Reed to give George his injections so we have not had to take that trip up to Washington." (Ibid.) On August 16, C. J. George advised Heffner that Colonel Francis W. Pruitt, chief of the medical service at Walter Reed Army Hospital, recommended that Marshall increase his "dosage of Diamox," a medication to treat dizziness and glaucoma, "to two tablets a day." The doctor also reminded George and Heffner to "be very conscious of the fact that General Marshall is on a low salt diet." (George to Heffner, August 16, 1957, GCMRL/G. C. Marshall Papers [Retirement, Chronological].)

616

To Westbrook Pegler[1]

August 14, 1957
Leesburg, Virginia

Dear Pegler: Replying to your letter of June 18 from Tucson:[2]

I bought the stock mentioned—ten shares for One Hundred Dollars. After a short period—about a year I think—it began to pay yearly dividends. The purchase was in 1945 I think. It has paid very large dividends, but they have decreased a little the last few years.[3]

Your letter, by implication, reflects on Marx and expresses surprise that I should have had contact with him. I regret this attitude or implication because I value Marx as a good friend and have had numerous occasions to receive evidence of his character.[4]

The following I trust to your eye with the understanding that it will be treated as purely confidential. I feel that I owe it to Marx as evidence of the nature of our relations.

When I became Deputy Chief of Staff in the fall of 1938, General [Henry H.] Arnold showed me a lot of toys Marx had sent for distribution to our Air Corps children—he seemed very enthusiastic about the Air Corps. I was told he had been sending them for several years. I did not meet Marx until Arnold took me to a Joe Louis prize fight in New York, where we were his guests for the evening, returning to Washington that night.[5] I did not see him again for quite a long time.

Meanwhile, the following incident developed:

The German Army had just completed its overwhelming action in conquering France, in which low-flying airplanes played a demoralizing part. We had a few planes and it would be a long time before others would commence to pour off the lines in true quantity production fashion. The ground officers were appealing for planes to train with them. The public was pressing and the Air Corps resisting, since they had only a very limited number of planes for their own training. Pressures were great, feelings ran high, and the tension was growing.

After one particular dramatic description of the effect of the German planes on the ground troops and fleeing multitudes in the demoralized retreat in France, General Arnold came into my office (Chief of Staff) and suggested that we work up some air-ground training. As that was what I had been trying to promote for sometime, I welcomed his suggestion.

Bedell Smith—a Lieutenant Colonel or Colonel—was present at the time. He made a very sarcastic comment to the general effect that "it was about time," etc.

When Arnold left, I called Smith back and told him that I would attend to the correction or reprimand of the high ranking Generals, and that was not the function of a Lieutenant Colonel staff officer. He apologized and left the room. The remainder of the affair I learned later from Arnold.

Smith had gone directly to Arnold's office, reported what I had said to him, and sincerely apologized. Arnold, in his always friendly manner, had patted Smith on the back and told him not to mind—that he, Arnold, understood. Then he went further. He told Smith to take the afternoon off and go with him to shoot some pheasants. Smith, being a keen hunter, joyfully accepted and they went over to Maryland on some leased ground good for pheasants, and there met Marx, who controlled the plot.

That was Smith's introduction to Marx, whom I had yet to meet personally. The two became shooting associates for a time, Marx controlling several plots of ground, one near Manassas, his wife's home.

I tell you all these details because I have the highest opinion of Smith officially and personally and I like Marx.

The lovely wife from Manassas gave rise to the only request Marx ever made of me. She developed cancer, and penicillin had just been produced. The Army controlled the limited supply. When Mrs. Marx was near death he appealed to me to release enough for a trial treatment of her. It failed.[6] Faithfully yours[7]

GCMRL/G. C. Marshall Papers (Retirement, Chronological)

1. In late 1952 newspaper columnist Westbrook Pegler asked Marshall if information he had received about Marshall being employed as a director for a company owned by Louis Marx and paid $10,000 annually was true. Marshall responded that "I have never had any position with his company, never been a director, never been asked to be a director, never rendered any services." (Pegler to Marshall, November 28, 1952, and Marshall to Pegler, December 4, 1952, Herbert Hoover Presidential Library/James Westbrook Pegler Papers [Louis Marx].) Pegler reminded Marshall of this correspondence in a June 18, 1957, letter

stating that "Bedell Smith told me that you, he and Eisenhower" as well as two other generals "all had received from Marx stock in a company which he organized as a subsidiary of his toy company," and asking if this was correct as well as why they "ever came to put yourselves into such association with such a man" and why Marx had been permitted to live at Eisenhower's headquarters during and after World War II. When Marshall did not reply Pegler asked him again on July 24. (Pegler to Marshall, November 28, 1952, and July 24, 1957, ibid.)

2. C. J. George had advised Marshall on August 1 not to send this detailed reply on the grounds that some of the details were not relevant or necessary and that "the least said in a matter of this kind is best." Consequently he drafted an alternative reply, but Marshall declined to use it. (George to Marshall, August 1, 1957, GCMRL/G. C. Marshall Papers [Retirement, Chronological].) George's alternative reply is not in the Marshall Papers, but the version of Marshall's response transcribed here is in the Pegler Papers with Marshall's signature and handwritten explanation at the end that his "long delay" in responding "has been due to my illness." (Marshall to Pegler, August 14, 1957, Herbert Hoover Presidential Library/James Westbrook Pegler Papers [Louis Marx].)

3. On July 2, 1946, Louis Marx had written to Marshall instructing him "to send $100.00 made out to—The Charmore Company" and on August 29—when Marshall was in China—Marx mailed the stock certificates to Marshall's Pentagon office. (Marx to Marshall, July 2, and August 29, 1946, GCMRL/G. C. Marshall Papers [Pentagon Office, Selected].) In 1950, Marx informed Marshall that the dividend check for his Charmore stock was "the same rate as last year," which was "$150 per share." (Marx to Marshall, February 13, 1950, ibid.) For more on this transaction, see Pogue, *Statesman*, 494–95.

4. For more on Marshall's relations with Louis Marx, see pp. 746–47 and 962–63.

5. "I want you to know how much I appreciated your fine hospitality the other night," Marshall wrote to Marx after the June 18, 1941, prize fight between Joe Louis and Billy Conn at the Polo Grounds in New York City. (Marshall to Marx, June 23, 1941, GCMRL/G. C. Marshall Papers [Pentagon Office, Selected].) "We got back to Washington in the morning so had plenty of time to get ready for the next day's pressures." (Ibid.)

6. Marx wrote to Marshall on January 31, 1944, that his wife René had cancer that had metastasized and appealed to Marshall to inquire about the efficacy of penicillin as a treatment. (Marx to Marshall, January 31, 1944, ibid.) Marshall responded that "our leading medical man informs me that penicillin has proven ineffective and therefore is not employed in such cases," but after another plea from Marx he explained how Mrs. Marx's doctor might be able to obtain the drug. (Marshall to Marx, telegrams, February 1, 1944, and March 15, 1944, ibid.) Marx obtained the drug, but Mrs. Marx died soon thereafter and Marshall wired his condolences on April 26, 1944. (Marshall to Marx, March 25, 1944, and Marshall to Marx, telegram, April 26, 1944, ibid.).

7. "Many thanks for your note of August 14," Pegler replied. "I am sorry to hear of your illness," he continued, while noting that Marshall had not addressed his question about Marx's presence at Eisenhower's headquarters and asked that he do so when he could. "My opinion of Marx is not the same as yours," Pegler continued, followed by a series of specific questions about the episode. (Pegler to Marshall, August 27, 1957, GCMRL/G. C. Marshall Papers [Retirement, General].) There is no Marshall reply in either the Marshall or the Pegler Papers.

617

TO MRS. JOHN B. WILSON

September 23, 1957
Leesburg, Virginia

Dear Rose: Thank you very much for your newsy letter of September 3. I was delighted to hear from you and to learn something of the family. However, I am concerned about your worries over your Mother's health and that of Tom Morgan.

It seems that your sister has her hands full, and I hope that she bears up under the pressures.[1]

It was very thoughtful of your husband to send me a recording of the Commencement speech by Barbara Ward. As you suggested, I will write to Justice Reardon and thank him for his efforts in arranging it.[2]

I have had two letters from Page, which I enjoyed very much. It is always good to hear from him, and I am delighted that he is making such good progress.[3]

I have not been feeling very well. I have considerable difficulty with my balance and suffer from an almost total lack of energy. I stay close to home and participate in very few activities.[4]

Katherine is in better shape, although she is having some trouble with her back. Mostly, she is doing too much for me. In addition, her sister is now in a convalescent home at Williamsport, Maryland, and she makes frequent trips to visit her there.[5]

We plan to make the move back to Carolina around November 1.

With warm and good wishes to all of you,   Affectionately,

GCMRL/J. Page Wilson Collection

1. Rose Page Wilson had confided to Marshall that her mother suffered "from severe arthritic pains in her head and neck which sap all her energy," and her brother-in-law, Tom Morgan, had undergone surgery that "left him weaker than he was before." Her sister, Celeste Page Morgan, "rushes from one to the other with little time for anything else." (Wilson to Marshall, September 3, 1957, GCMRL/G. C. Marshall Papers [Retirement, General].)

2. The Wilsons had traveled to Boston, Massachusetts, to attend festivities for John Wilson's twenty-fifth class reunion at Harvard University. British economist and author Barbara Ward, who had just completed her first term as a visiting professor at Harvard, gave the commencement speech, which celebrated the tenth anniversary of Marshall's "big Marshall Plan speech," according to Wilson. "I was so impressed by her suitable tributes to you that I made arrangements to get the tape for you." (Ibid.) She explained that Paul Reardon, the chief justice of the Massachusetts Superior Court and one of John Wilson's classmates, had agreed to forward the recording to Marshall. (Ibid.) Marshall wrote to Reardon on October 15 to thank him. (Marshall to Reardon, October 15, 1957, ibid.)

3. Page Wilson had written on August 19 that he "was very happy and honored" to receive a birthday telegram from his godfather. (Wilson to Marshall, August 19, 1957, ibid.) His mother reported that his "academic record so far has been better than average and his athletic ability is far better than average." (Wilson to Marshall, September 3, 1947, ibid.)

4. Marshall wrote Secretary of the Army Wilber M. Brucker the same day to apologize for missing a luncheon given by Defense Secretary Wilson on September 17 because he "did not feel equal to the trip" to the Pentagon for the event. (Marshall to Brucker, September 23, 1957, GCMRL/G. C. Marshall Papers [Retirement, Chronological].)

5. See pp. 979–80 and 986.

MARSHALL'S CONDITION did not improve in the remaining months of 1957. C. J. George wrote to Marshall Carter on September 23 that he had "motored down to Leesburg" the previous week "to learn first-hand how General and Mrs. Marshall were getting along." Marshall, he continued, "is very frail, weighing only about 150 pounds. His equilibrium is poor and, from my observation, he is bored to death." (George to Carter, September 23, 1957, GCMRL/G. C. Marshall Papers [Retirement, General].) The next day Colonel George confided to Queen Frederica that Marshall had not been well "for quite a long time, and he has been unable to write longhand for some several months. He finds it difficult to dictate." (George to Frederica, September 24, 1957, ibid.) "He is unable to do more than walk with a cane or with Mrs. Marshall's help around his place in a very limited way" but, George assured the queen, Marshall "suffers no painful ailments of any kind. It is merely a lack of strength, a lack of appetite, and too great a loss of weight." (Ibid.) Frank McCarthy visited the Marshalls in Leesburg on October 11 and later wrote to say he was "happy to find both of you comfortable and well." (Marshall to Brucker, November 1, 1957, ibid.; McCarthy to Marshall, November 13, 1957, ibid.) On October 15, Colonel George wrote to Margaret Emerson to bring her up to date on the Marshalls' situation and mentioned that they were at Walter Reed "undergoing some tests. The doctors are concentrating on the General to determine what they can do to increase his energy and appetite." George also disclosed that the Marshalls planned to fly to Pinehurst on November 1. (George to Emerson, October 15, 1957, ibid.) Katherine Marshall wrote to President Eisenhower from Walter Reed to say how much her husband "appreciated the lovely red and white carnations which came with such a kind note," and reconfirmed that Marshall was "very frail." (Katherine Marshall to Eisenhower, October 15, 1957, DDEL/Dwight D. Eisenhower Papers [Papers as President, President's Personal File 182, Box 935].) Unlike the energetic torrent of correspondence accomplished during his hospital stay in May 1957 (see pp. 978–81), Marshall did not dictate a single letter while in Walter Reed in October of the same year.

Queen Frederica's brother, Prince Paul of Hanover, visited the Marshalls in Pinehurst on Thanksgiving Day. (George to Frederica, December 9, 1957, GCMRL/G. C. Marshall Papers [Retirement, Chronological].) See pp. 987–88. On December 2, C. J. George wrote to former ambassador Lewis W. Douglas that Marshall "has no specific complaint, but lacks energy and the ability to personally take care of his correspondence." (George to Douglas, December 2, 1957, ibid.) "I usually telephone General Marshall around noon on Mondays and, when I talked to him last, his voice seemed somewhat stronger and he reported that he was feeling somewhat better," George wrote to Elizabeth Barry on December 9. "I only hope that this is an indication of a return to normal health." (George to Barry, December 9, 1957, GCMRL/G. C. Marshall Papers [Retirement, General].) ★

618

TO HARRY S. TRUMAN

December 23, 1957
Pinehurst, North Carolina

My dear Mr. Truman I did not want to type a letter to you and I may not be able to complete one in longhand—but I'll try.

Katherine is well but pretty hard worked keeping house and looking after or nursing me. I am about the same—possibly a little better off than last year—Less of unbalancing.

I want [*walk*] about 6 blocks a day—but some one with me. In other words I am a poor specimen of a man.

They tell me I look well, but I am very thin. You knew me at 200 lbs. I now weigh 150.

I hope Mrs. Truman and you are both well. Margaret seems to be blooming. What a wonderful thing it is for Margaret to have that fine baby and a fine husband.[1]

The weather is lovely here. We have been sitting on the lawn to day.

I just heard a few minutes ago from Jack McCloy. Earlier in the day from Bob Lovett—two of my old faithfuls.

I saw Margaret the other night. She is really a fine actress—so natural.

My Xmas greetings to Mrs. Truman and you—and a Happy deserving New Years. Mrs. Truman continues to be Katherine's Washington favorite. She would send love but she is asleep.[2] Affectionately,

GCMarshall

GCMRL/G. C. Marshall Collection (Truman); H

1. See p. 965. Frank McCarthy and Margaret Truman Daniel had sent a note to the Marshalls in late November when she joined a dinner party at McCarthy's home in Hollywood, where she was "doing some TV shows." (McCarthy to Marshall, November 29, 1957, GCMRL/G. C. Marshall Papers [Retirement, General].) "Frank has the most magnificent house I've ever seen!" Daniel enthused. "I wish you could see my baby. I miss him and his father so much but I'm leaving for home this weekend." (Ibid.)

2. "You'll never know how highly appreciated your letter of Dec. 23 is," Truman responded on January 7. "I sincerely hope your health will improve and that it will be my privilege to see you and Mrs. Marshall before many moons roll around." (Truman to Marshall, January 7, 1958, ibid.)

MARY LOUISE SPILMAN arrived in Pinehurst on January 10 to assist General and Mrs. Marshall with their correspondence. Over two days they responded to dozens of holiday, birthday, and other greetings. Marshall sent a brief note to Bedell Smith to say that "It was very, very good of you to go to the trouble of telephoning me, and I want you to know that I appreciate it very much." (Marshall to Smith, January 11, 1958, GCMRL/G. C. Marshall Papers [Retirement, General].) He assured his friend Lady Mary Burghley that "It is always a treat for me to hear from you," and chided Mrs. David Rockefeller because her Christmas card had not included a photograph of her children. "I always thought you had one of the most charming young families I have ever seen. It has been a joy to me to see them as they grow up," he acknowledged. (Marshall to Burghley and Marshall to Rockefeller, January 11, 1958, ibid.) To Catharine Armstrong, his childhood friend from Uniontown, he admitted, "You and I are about the only ones of the old crowd of our early teens that still survive. I think actually we are the only ones, though I am inclined to think you do a better job of surviving than I am doing." (Marshall to Armstrong, January 14, 1958, ibid.) ★

619

To Mrs. Robert Ernest Dismukes Sr.[1] January 10, 1958
Pinehurst, North Carolina

Dear Lenora: I am answering your note of December 29 to Katherine, which contained birthday greetings to me.

She is well, but rather tired, having recently returned from Allene's funeral in Richmond. Allene died of a stroke on January 2. Molly and Jim were there and also Allene's relatives in Richmond. Although long expected, it was quite a blow to Katherine, and the trip tired her out greatly.[2]

I am not of much help these days. I have no suffering of any kind, but I am getting pretty old, and I am confined to the house except for about a half-mile or a mile of walking every day.[3]

With our affectionate regards, Affectionately,

GCMRL/G. C. Marshall Papers (Retirement, General)

1. Lenora Dismukes and her husband were among Marshall's friends from Columbus, Georgia, to whom he sent an announcement of his marriage to Katherine Tupper Brown on October 15, 1930. (List for Marshall-Brown wedding announcements, GCMRL/© Marshall-Winn Collection [Fort Benning].) Robert E. Dismukes owned an insurance firm in Columbus and was chairman of the board of the local hospital center. (Dismukes to Marshall, January 20, 1958, GCMRL/G. C. Marshall Papers [Retirement, General].)

2. Allene Tupper Lacy died at the Williamsport Sanitarium in Williamsport, Maryland, and was buried in Hollywood Cemetery in Richmond, Virginia, on January 4. Marshall wrote to John C. Hagan on January 11 to express appreciation for his help to Katherine Marshall while she was in Richmond. "Mrs. Hagan and you made things as easy for her as they could have been made and she is immensely grateful, and I am even more so for your kindness." (Marshall to Hagan, January 11, 1958, GCMRL/G. C. Marshall Papers [Retirement, Chronological].)

3. A few days later Marshall wrote to Madame Chiang Kai-shek that his wife had "to devote a great deal of her time to nursing me, and I feel rather humiliated to be failing in my duty to her to this extent." (Marshall to Madame Chiang, January 14, 1958, GCMRL/G. C. Marshall Papers [Retirement, General].)

620

To Winston S. Churchill January 10, 1958
Pinehurst, North Carolina

My dear Sir Winston: Your Christmas card, after several forwardings, has reached us here at our winter home in North Carolina. It was a highly valued greeting.[1]

Mrs. Marshall and I are here for the winter. She is well, but I am not doing quite as well, I believe, as you are, though I have several years' advantage of you.

It is very pleasing for me to be remembered by you, for I am always pleased with a retouch of our earlier associations.

I don't know anyone with whom I had more arguments than with you, and I don't know anyone whom I admire more. Your later writings shame me with your fascinating literary products.[2]

With affectionate regards to Lady Churchill and you,[3] Faithfully yours,

GCMRL/G. C. Marshall Papers (Retirement, General)

1. Churchill's Christmas cards to the Marshalls featured reproductions of his paintings. (Churchill to Marshall, n.d., GCMRL/G. C. Marshall Papers [Retirement, Separated Materials, Christmas Cards].)

2. From 1956 through 1958 Churchill produced four volumes of *A History of the English-Speaking Peoples*. (Winston S. Churchill, *A History of the English-Speaking Peoples* [London: Cassell, 1956–58].)

3. "It was a great pleasure to hear from you," Churchill responded. "I am so glad you have found pleasure and interest in the books that I have written." (Churchill to Marshall, January 31, 1958, GCMRL/G. C. Marshall Papers [Retirement, General].)

621

To Queen Frederica of the Hellenes — January 11, 1958
Pinehurst, North Carolina

Your Majesty: My secretary arrived from Washington, so I take this opportunity to dictate a note to you and the King. I asked Colonel George to write you a note of what had happened here, but I will tell you nevertheless.[1]

We found your brother most attractive, and we were sorry he could only remain for a single meal. I was much flattered that he made the tedious trip down here—this is not an easy place to get to—to see me and for that, of course, I have you to thank.[2]

I have been better off here than I was at Leesburg. We left there on November 1 and will remain here until May 1. I am now able to get in one-half mile to a mile of walking a day, which is just that much more than I was able to do when I was up in Virginia. While Pinehurst can grow pretty cold at times, nevertheless it has a fairly agreeable winter climate. I have not been able to sit out on the lawn as much as usual, but I have had several meals there and a few drinks.

I never see your photograph—I am now referring to that on your Christmas card—without recalling the first time I saw you standing by the fire in your little sitting room at Claridges.[3] That made an unforgettable impression on me, but not so much as your resume of what was the matter with Europe and what would have to be done to correct it. I only got so far in the battle, but we seem to have lost a good bit of ground, although I am not at all familiar with the circumstances today.

For a while, they tried to keep me in touch, but I more or less declined that because they would expect me to have a well-advised opinion in keeping with my past experience, which is not at all the case. People are always questioning me on the subject of Europe and the Middle East and will never believe me when I assure them that I know no more than I see in the paper or hear on the television, and Mrs. Marshall is better informed that way than I am.

Judging from your card, your oldest girl is an exact replica of you as you must have been as a younger woman.[4] The youngest lady is charming looking. She counters her father's serious aspect.

With New Year greetings to both of you, and always my most affectionate regards, Faithfully yours,

GCMRL/G. C. Marshall Papers (Retirement, General)

1. C. J. George had written to Frederica on September 24 to say that Marshall had hoped "he could handle this very personally, but he feels that word to you has been too long delayed." George gave a description of Marshall's infirmities and explained that "he is loath to confess that he is reduced in physical activity." (George to Frederica, September 24, 1957, GCMRL/G. C. Marshall Papers [Retirement, General].) See p. 984.

2. George had reported to Frederica on December 9 about Prince Paul's lunch visit with the Marshalls on Thanksgiving Day. (George to Frederica, December 9, 1957, ibid.)

3. "Do you remember when you came to see me the first time in London? I was very upset," Frederica had recalled when she wrote to Marshall in October. See *Papers of GCM*, 6: 353–54. "Well, many years have passed since then and we met only once or twice since then, yet I feel as if we have known each other all our life." (Frederica to Marshall, October 28, 1957, ibid.) Mary C. Carrolou had written to Colonel George on December 16 "upon the express wish of H.M. the Queen in order to get information about General Marshall" and to confirm that he had received her letter. (Carrolou to George, December 16, 1957, ibid.) "Please advise Her Majesty that General Marshall did see her letter, and the delay has been occasioned by his desire to write a personal note," George had responded. (George to Carrolou, December 27, 1957, ibid.)

4. At the close of her October letter, the queen had mentioned that she hoped "to come to the States some time in Spring with my eldest daughter [Sophia]. We shall then meet again." (Frederica to Marshall, October 28, 1957, ibid.)

NEIL H. McELROY, secretary of defense since October 9, 1957, wrote to Marshall on January 29 requesting Marshall's advice regarding "another study of the Defense organization." (McElroy to Marshall, January 29, 1958, GCMRL/G. C. Marshall Papers [Retirement, General].) Marshall agreed to meet with Charles A. Coolidge, special assistant to McElroy on organizational matters, and on March 7, Coolidge and Colonel George flew to Pinehurst. George later reported to Robert Lovett that they "had what proved to be a most interesting three hours with General Marshall." (George to Lovett, March 12, 1958, GCMRL/G. C. Marshall Papers [Retirement, Chronological].) "We had a delightful lunch, after which we got down to the business of discussing the proposed re-organization of the Defense Department. At the outset of the conversation the General went on record as saying that he was too far removed to make any substantial contribution. However, it later proved that he was most helpful because Mr. Coolidge asked him specific questions," George recounted. "The General made some very keen answers, and it was obvious to me that his response was welcome to Mr. Coolidge." (Ibid.) George related that Marshall "reminisced quite a bit, almost entirely along the lines of the importance of a unified and well-coordinated team. His experiences prior to and during World War II and the contributions of the Joint Chiefs and Combined Chiefs were pointed out. I believe that the General made specific comment on at least ten points, ranging from the single Chief concept to the promotion techniques of 3- and 4-star ranks." (Ibid.) ★

622

To Mrs. Egbert Armstrong [April 1, 1958]
Pinehurst, North Carolina

My dear Cathremine[1] Thank you very much for your sweet note and especially for the photograph and old print evidently taken at the Blisses.[2] I am so glad to have the photograph of you. I know you have some of me of the last ten years.[3]

I would like to write you long hand but it's too difficult and disreputable. Tho I do believe I will send you this "as is".

I am pretty poorly off these days and I don't grow better with time.

Our occasional notes are a great pleasure to me.[4] My very affectionate regards.

GCM

GCMRL/G. C. Marshall Collection (Armstrong); H

1. Marshall scrawled this undated note on a yellow legal pad and misspelled the name of his longtime friend, Catharine Lindsey Armstrong. (Marshall to Armstrong, n.d., GCMRL/G. C. Marshall Collection [Armstrong].)

2. "If one of your young friends received an Eastman Kodak [camera] for Christmas, have them take a snapshot of you. I would like so much to have one," Marshall had written to Armstrong on January 14. (Marshall to Armstrong, January 14, 1958, ibid.) The Blisses may have been the adult children of George Catlett Marshall Sr.'s partner, Arthur Weir Bliss, in the coal and coke business in Uniontown, Pennsylvania. See Pogue, *Education*, 10–12, and 20–21.

3. Marshall wrote to Armstrong again in June to thank her for the same pictures. (Marshall to Armstrong, June 1, 1958, ibid.; H.) "Blessed be forgetfulness when I receive a *second* note of thanks from you for the old photographs!" Armstrong replied on June 21. (Armstrong to Marshall, June 21, 1958, GCMRL/G. C. Marshall Papers [Retirement, General].)

4. "We had a rough air trip up this spring and poor weather here, but the garden is blooming and shrubs sprouting," Marshall told Armstrong in his June letter, and admitted that he missed "gardening more than anything else. I like dirt and growing things and there is lots of both here." (Marshall to Armstrong, June 1, 1958, GCMRL/G. C. Marshall Collection [Armstrong].) "Katherine is well but too worn down looking after me which of course she denies." (Ibid.)

THE WINTER OF 1958 was extraordinarily difficult, with memorable snowfalls in Washington and "weeks of cold, rainy weather," Katherine Marshall reported to Ellen Bruce on April 1. "Last week we were at Fort Bragg, George in the hospital there both Srg. Heffner and I with him. He is home now & up and about the house." (Katherine Marshall to Bruce, April 1, 1958, GCMRL/Katherine Marshall Correspondence.) The Marshalls flew back to Washington on April 30 and Mrs. Marshall wrote to C. J. George three days later that she "was certainly glad to see you at the air-port for all the way up I was very frightened about Gen. M. and his weak condition to start the trip." (Katherine Marshall to George, May 3, 1958, ibid.) George told William Spencer that "while frail," General Marshall was "in high spirits and looking forward to the coming of warm weather with a great degree of enthusiasm." (George to Spencer, May 2, 1958, GCMRL/G. C.

Marshall Papers [Retirement, General].)

General and Mrs. Marshall checked into Walter Reed for their semiannual checkups on May 11. Ten days later Colonel George wrote to Mrs. Marshall, who was visiting her daughter, that General Marshall "admits to feeling fairly good. His color is good; his step a little stronger; and his appetite is ravenous. The nurses report that he has been 'eating like a little pig,' and he did away with a super-duper banana split." (George to Katherine Marshall, May 22, 1958, GCMRL/G. C. Marshall Papers [Retirement, Chronological].) Marshall returned to Leesburg on May 24. Nine days later C. J. George wrote to Marshall Carter that Katherine Marshall "reports that, while General Marshall continues to eat well, he has no taste for exercise. He spends practically all of the day in his room—which of course means in bed—and I am fearful that, unless he changes, he will become so weak that exercise in any form will be almost impossible." (George to Carter, June 2, 1958, ibid.) ★

623

To Colonel John L. Ames Jr. May 15, 1958
Washington, DC

Dear Ames: I appreciate tremendously the thought of me in connection with the First Division dinner. Recalling the vital and lively dinners of the past, I feel the more gratified at greetings from the "old timers" and more recent ones too, now that I am so poor a hand these days.[1]

I appreciate the advance information regarding the dinner for this time next year; however, I doubt my ability to attend, since the years have a way of curtailing all desirable activity. I am no longer active and must take things very easy.[2]

With warm regards, Faithfully yours,

GCMRL/G. C. Marshall Papers (Retirement, General)

1. Marshall handwrote these sentiments at the bottom of a letter from Colonel Ames, who had written to Marshall on April 30 extending "warmest greetings to a comrade we hold in greatest affection," from the "old-timers" of the Officers of the First Division organization, which had recently held its thirty-ninth annual dinner. John L. Ames Jr. served in the 28th Infantry, First Division during World War I and was recalled to active duty during World War II, when he served on General Omar Bradley's staff. He retired from the military in 1955.

2. This paragraph was drafted by C. J. George at Marshall's request.

624

To Nunnally Johnson July 1, 1958
Leesburg, Virginia

Dear Mr. Johnson: Through the kindness of Frank McCarthy, I received the map which you had received from the widow of Field Marshal [Erwin] Rommel. It is an interesting piece of paper and makes a most welcome addition to the Foundation Library. Dr. Forrest Pogue, the Staff Director of the Foundation, will have the map examined by an expert so that an appropriate synopsis may be written to take its place alongside the map.[1]

It was very thoughtful of you to turn it over to me, but what I especially appreciate is the fact that you wanted the map to be a part of my collection.[2]

With many thanks for your personal message, and with warm regards, Faithfully yours,

GCMRL/G. C. Marshall Papers (Retirement, General)

1. As he prepared to write and produce *The Desert Fox: The Story of Rommel*, American filmmaker Nunnally Hunter Johnson had visited Lucia Rommel, the field marshal's widow. See p. 365n3. "As a souvenir of the call," Frank McCarthy had explained to Marshall on June 3, "Frau Rommel gave Mr. Johnson one of the sketches that her husband drew when he was planning the battle of El Alamein. Mr. Johnson told me he would like to give the sketch to a worthwhile military museum." (McCarthy to Marshall, June 3, 1958, GCMRL/G. C. Marshall Papers [Retirement, General].) After McCarthy told Johnson about plans for the Marshall Museum, Johnson agreed to make the gift and wrote to McCarthy that "'Maybe an expert on the North African campaign could recognize what the map means, but it's no use asking me.'" (Ibid.)

2. On September 28, C. J. George informed William M. Spencer, who had recently met in Chicago with Marshall Foundation President John C. Hagan, that Alonzo Gentry, the architect selected to design the Marshall museum and library in Lexington, Virginia, had visited with the Marshalls in June, but that Forrest Pogue's most recent meeting with Marshall had occurred on November 24, 1956. (George to Spencer, September 29, 1958, ibid.) "As a matter of fact," George assured Spencer, "every effort is being made to avoid seeing General Marshall" on issues relating to the Marshall Foundation. (Ibid.) "I do not know what the prospects are of getting further interviews with General Marshall," Pogue wrote to Hagan on September 10. "Colonel George has broached the subject to him several times, but nothing has come of it." (Pogue to Hagan, September 10, 1958, GCMRL/GCMRF Archives [General Correspondence 1951–62, Box 1].) See *Marshall Interviews*, 11.

625

To Dwight D. Eisenhower — August 14, 1958
Washington, DC

Dear Mr. President: I greatly appreciated your note of August 8 and the fine arrangement of flowers.[1]

I arrived here Monday a week ago to have corrected some trivial matters, such as a cyst and hair follicle in the left eye and some dental work. These were taken care of expeditiously and I had hoped to be on my way back to Leesburg when, through my own stupidity, I fell and cracked a rib. It was very troublesome for the first few days, but I am now vastly improved. For some time, it was a question of my appetite and a loss of weight; however, I am eating extremely well and my chart indicates a gain of eight pounds since my arrival. This is hard for me to believe, but they say figures never lie.

I am comfortably situated in your fine suite and, again, you have my deepest thanks for this gracious gesture on your part.[2] As usual, I am receiving the best attention, which of course is typical of Heaton and his people.

Both Mrs. Marshall and I appreciate the greetings from Mrs. Eisenhower and you and, in turn, we send our thanks and warm regards.[3]

With great respect, Faithfully yours,

GCMarshall

DDEL/Dwight D. Eisenhower Papers (Papers as President, President's Personal File 182, Box 935)

1. President Eisenhower's note extended "affectionate regard" and the hope that Marshall would "soon be able to leave Walter Reed." (Eisenhower to Marshall, August 8, 1958, GCMRL/G. C. Marshall Papers [Retirement, General].)

2. Marshall had also occupied the president's suite in May when he was in Walter Reed receiving "excellent treatment." (Marshall to Eisenhower, May 16, 1958, ibid.)

3. Marshall remained in Walter Reed for three weeks and was discharged on August 23. Marshall "Pat" Carter and Robert Lovett had joined Marshall for lunch one day and left "pretty much concerned with General Marshall's condition," according to a letter from C. J. George to Lovett. "It is a rather strange thing," George explained, "because one day he will be quite cheerful, bright, and lucid, and the next day, the complete opposite." (George to Lovett, August 11, 1958, GCMRL/G. C. Marshall Papers [Retirement, Chronological].) "I think Pat [Carter] was more shocked than I since he had not seen the General in some time," Lovett responded. "While the Old Man was feeble, he still seemed to me to be cheerful and eager, and that is really what counts in this case." (Lovett to George, August 13, 1958, GCMRL/G. C. Marshall Papers [Retirement, General].) After he returned to Colorado Springs, General Carter wrote to Lovett that he "felt incoherent and completely demoralized as a result of General Marshall's apparent condition. I had not seen him for almost 9 months and while I had anticipated some degradation in his physical condition, I thought I detected a degree of faltering in his mental processes that I had never before experienced." Carter told Lovett that he received regular reports from Colonel George that Marshall "does not eat at all well at Leesburg and that he has practically nothing to inspire him mentally or physically." (Carter to Lovett, September 8, 1958, GCMRL/Marshall S. Carter Collection [Box 19, Folder 20].) "I went through the same inner turmoil a few months ago," Lovett replied to Carter, "when I went down to see him at Leesburg." (Lovett to Carter, September 16, 1958, GCMRL/Marshall S. Carter Collection [Box 9, Folder 1].) "Maybe a campaign to get visitors there would help but on some occasions I am told it does actual harm in that the effort exhausts him. This is not true in the hospital, where he can stay in bed and feels none of the responsibilities of a host." (Ibid.)

Toward the end of Marshall's hospital stay, Mrs. Marshall visited Molly and Jim Winn at Fort Ritchie. Marshall told his friend Helen Lee that his wife's "stay was most restful and relaxing." Marshall declared that when she returned, Mrs. Marshall "looked simply wonderful" and surmised that "the absence of household duties and the responsibility of looking after me were the major reason for her appearance." (Marshall to Lee, August 21, 1958, GCMRL/G. C. Marshall Papers [Retirement, General].) During her absence, C. J. George kept Katherine Marshall apprised of her husband's progress. "Each afternoon the physiotherapist puts him through a series of leg exercises," George reported, and assured her that Marshall "had been eating substantial meals ever since he arrived." (George to Katherine Marshall, memorandum, August 14, 1958, GCMRL/G. C. Marshall Papers [Retirement, Chronological].)

AS GENERAL MARSHALL neared the end of his August hospitalization, C. J. George wrote a memorandum for the record concerning recommendations made by Brigadier General Thomas W. Mattingly, chief of medicine at Walter Reed, who thought "it would be extremely wise to have an attendant attached to General Marshall while in residence at Leesburg." Mattingly, George wrote, "indicated that it was unlikely that General Marshall would get over his problem of equilibrium and that there was always the prospect of his falling." (George memorandum, August 21, 1958, GCMRL/G. C. Marshall Papers [Retirement, Chronological].) Colonel George called Katherine Marshall on August 21 to convey Mattingly's advice. "While she indicated her appreciation of their concern, she stated that she felt such an arrangement would not be practicable," George noted. Mrs. Marshall had, she told him, "provided a bedroom for the General on the first floor adjacent to lavatory facilities; that a buzzer arrangement exists between the General's room and Sergeant Heffner's room; that she, herself, is in almost constant attendance on General Marshall; and that Sergeant Heffner is practically always available." (Ibid.) "I received the definite impression that Mrs. Marshall was not disposed toward such an arrangement," George concluded." (Ibid.)

After Marshall's return to Dodona Manor on August 23, Katherine Marshall confided to Ellen Bruce that "the shock of the fall—also all the injections and medication they gave him have weakened him greatly— He insisted on coming home—but is really a hospital case." Her husband, she wrote, was "seldom out of bed" but she felt he was "happier here than any place and as long as possible—I want to keep him out of the Hospital." (Katherine Marshall to Bruce, August 26, 1958, GCMRL/Katherine Marshall Correspondence.) By September 8, Mrs. Marshall wrote to Colonel George that she had "gotten in a male nurse from the hospital here on an 8 hour shift 3 pm. to 11 pm. to relieve me or Srg H. He came yesterday & if this does not work out—I shall have to close up here & bring Gen. M. back to Walter Reed & will go to the hostess house myself until I can make other arrangements." (Katherine Marshall to George, September 8, 1958, ibid.)

In his September 16 letter to Marshall Carter about Marshall's decline, Robert Lovett conceded, "There is no question that his machinery is wearing out." (Lovett to Carter, September 16, 1958, GCMRL/Marshall S. Carter Collection [Box 9, Folder 1].) "I have an uncomfortable hunch that he would really be much better off at Walter Reed with professional care than at Leesburg," but, Lovett cautioned, "I don't know how anyone could make such an offensive suggestion without doing great damage." He hoped that "the doctors would insist on it" and advised that neither Carter, George, nor Lovett "could have any part in it." (Ibid.)

By September 23, Marshall had been readmitted to Walter Reed and arrangements were being coordinated with Fort Bragg to transfer him to Pinehurst. (George to Sink, September 22, 1958, GCMRL/G. C. Marshall Papers [Retirement, Chronological].) Queen Frederica, who planned a trip to the United States in November, had cabled Marshall about a possible visit. "Frankly, I am in poor health and, in all probability, I will be in Pinehurst at that time. I am most anxious that you not tax your energy nor burden your schedule with such a lengthy trip," Marshall replied. "Besides, I am so weak that I am sure you would find me a poor conversationalist. However, should I still be here at Walter Reed, it will be easy to arrange things." (Cable to US Army Military Attache, Athens, October 9, 1958, GCMRL/G. C. Marshall Papers [Retirement, General].)

"It was particularly rewarding to see you enjoying good health and in high spirits," Marshall wrote on October 14 to his sister, Marie Singer, who had recently come to Walter Reed. "As you well know, I envy you your stamina and the great joy you get out of life." (Marshall to Singer, October 14, 1958, ibid.) "I was so relieved and delighted to see how well you looked—I thought you looked better than when I saw you in Leesburg," Singer told Marshall upon her return to Pennsylvania. (Singer to Marshall, October 12, 1958, ibid.) C. J. George notified Mrs. Singer that her brother left Walter Reed on October 16. "He seemed to be feeling fine, and I know he looked forward to joining Mrs. Marshall. As you know, he is very fond of Pinehurst, and I am hopeful that he will have a good winter. (George to Singer, October 17, 1958, GCMRL/G. C. Marshall Papers [Retirement, Chronological].) ★

626

TO HENRY CABOT LODGE JR. October 18, 1958
Pinehurst, North Carolina

Dear Lodge: Miss Spilman told me of your telephone call with the inquiry regarding my health.[1] I will admit that I am not stepping very high, but there does not seem to be anything of a specific nature of which I can complain. I had a fairly long visit at Walter Reed, which gave the doctors an opportunity to conduct a very thorough physical evaluation. In their verbal report to me, they indicated that all the vital signs were good, which led me to conclude that it is all a matter of age.

I left Washington Thursday afternoon and had a most pleasant flight to Pinehurst, where I joined Mrs. Marshall. We look forward to a pleasant stay here.

With my thanks for your interest, and with warmest regards, Faithfully yours,
GCMarshall[2]

GCMRL/G. C. Marshall Papers (Retirement, General)

1. "Ambassador Lodge had telephoned from New York City" after he learned about his most recent hospitalization, Spilman had informed Marshall on October 13. Lodge was "much relieved to know that the rumor of your serious illness was false—and he wishes you a pleasant season in the South." (Spilman to Marshall, memorandum, October 13, 1957, GCMRL/G. C. Marshall Papers [Retirement, General].)

2. This is the last known letter that bears Marshall's signature. All subsequent correspondence sent over General Marshall's name appears to have been drafted by his staff, primarily C. J. George.

Afterword

LISCOMBE LODGE was being "run as a small hospital," Katherine Marshall confided to Ellen Bruce six days after Marshall was flown by air evacuation transport from Walter Reed Army Hospital to Pinehurst. (Katherine Marshall to Bruce, October 22, 1958, GCMRL/Katherine Marshall Correspondence; H.) Queen Frederica visited on October 25 and stayed for an hour, which "cheered George greatly," his wife wrote to Frank McCarthy. (Katherine Marshall to McCarthy, November 3, 1958, GCMRL/Frank McCarthy Collection [Additions, Box 1]; H.) Robert and Adele Lovett paid their respects on Marshall's birthday, December 31. (Lovett to Heaton, May 28, 1959, GCMRL/G. C. Marshall Papers [Retirement, General].)

On January 16, 1959, Marshall suffered the first of two strokes and was immediately taken to Womack General Hospital at Fort Bragg, North Carolina. According to a report from M. L. Spilman, there was "no paralysis." (Spilman to Harbeson, January 16, 1959, GCMRL/G. C. Marshall Papers [Retirement, Chronological].) After two visits to the hospital, C. J. George wrote to Marie Singer on January 29 that Marshall was "sitting up in bed, bright-eyed, cheerful, and conversant." The doctors predicted he would remain at the hospital for "at least six weeks," and Katherine Marshall was staying in "a room just across the hall." (George to Singer, January 29, 1959, ibid.) The second stroke occurred on February 17. "He is desperately ill," Katherine Marshall confessed to Frank McCarthy two days later, as this "last attack" had affected his eyes and throat and "he can neither see nor speak. He is not suffering and this is my one comfort." (Katherine Marshall to McCarthy, February 19, 1959, GCMRL/Frank McCarthy Collection [Additions, Box 1]; H.). On February 24, C. J. George joined the Marshalls at the hospital and reported to M. L. Spilman by telephone on February 26 that Marshall's condition had "stabilized" and that he "awoke bright-eyed and more alert." Spilman noted that he was "making a great effort to speak more and more often—and is succeeding." (Spilman to McCarthy, February 26, 1959, ibid.)

On March 11, Marshall returned to Walter Reed by ambulance after transport from Fort Bragg on an evacuation aircraft. President Eisenhower visited on March 13, as did Molly Winn and Mary Lee. Katherine Marshall moved into a nearby apartment on the hospital grounds. (Katherine Marshall to Bruce, postcard, March 15, 1959, GCMRL/Katherine Marshall Correspondence; H.) C. J. George wrote to Marie Singer on March 24 that "slow progress" was occurring since her brother had sat up in bed one day for five minutes and three days later "spent ten minutes in a wheel chair; and today, he did the same. For the most part, he has been bright and cheerful. Upon occasion, his voice is strong and clear." (George to Singer, March 24, 1959, GCMRL/G. C. Marshall Papers [Retirement, Chronological].)

On April 10, George informed Madge Pendleton that Marshall was "beginning to enjoy visitors," which George considered beneficial because "conversation stimulates him and we feel that having old friends drop by will provide a most useful tonic." (George to Pendleton, April 10, 1959, GCMRL/G. C. Marshall Papers [Retirement, General].) Visitors included "the Maxwell Taylors," who Katherine reported had brought homemade cookies and a cake, a relief "after four months of Army food," as well as Generals Lawton Collins and Harold "Pinky" Bull and Anna Rosenberg. George mentioned to Mrs. Singer that her brother's "vision has not yet improved to the point where he can read" but he was listening to recordings for the blind. (Katherine Marshall to Bruce, postcard, April 11, 1959, GCMRL/Katherine Marshall Correspondence; H; George to Singer, April 17, 1959, GCMRL/G. C. Marshall Papers [Retirement, Chronological].) Eisenhower and Churchill saw Marshall on May 5, "unfortunately," George reported, one of Marshall's "poorer days." (George to Bowditch, May 15, 1959, GCMRL/G. C. Marshall Papers [Retirement, General].) See also Pogue, *Statesman*, 509–11. Katherine Marshall recounted to Ellen Bruce that she had enjoyed "quite a visit" with Mamie Eisenhower and "Even Nixon" had come by "to shake hands." (Katherine Marshall to Bruce, n.d., GCMRL/Katherine Marshall Correspondence; H.) Lovett had visited "about every two weeks" since December, and in late May he wrote to General Heaton to express gratitude for the "superb care and thoughtful attention devoted" to Marshall by the medical personnel at Walter Reed. (Lovett to Heaton, May 28, 1959, GCMRL/G. C. Marshall Papers [Retirement, General].)

"For a while we took General Marshall outside each morning to enjoy an hour or more of the sun," George wrote to a Pinehurst friend on June 18. Katherine Marshall herself became ill with "a heavy cold and congested lungs," George told Bernard Baruch the same day, and mentioned that General Marshall had "slipped somewhat in the past two weeks." George informed another family friend that Marshall was "unusually frail and very weak" and commented that "he does speak, but these instances are becoming more rare." (George to Jones, George to Baruch, and George to Hibbs, all June 18, 1959, ibid.) George admitted to General Ridgway on July 14 that he was "amazed" by Marshall's alertness at certain points; but "then he slips into what is termed 'twilight.'" The same day George divulged to Marshall Carter that Marshall's weight had slipped to 136 pounds, which "should be a clear indication to you of how he looks," but added that occasionally Marshall was "mentally alert and talkative." (George to Ridgway and George to Carter, July 14, 1959, GCMRL/G. C. Marshall Papers [Retirement, Chronological].) On September 2, he informed Lovett that "at times," Marshall "appeared to be slipping away, and 24 hours later he is bright-eyed and making every effort to respond to simple questions." George noted that "All his vital signs are good, and I credit his life to that amazing food pump, devoted attention, and professional care." (George to Lovett, September 2, 1959, ibid.)

Sometime in June Katherine Marshall reviewed plans for Marshall's funeral and added names to the list of those who would be invited to the service at Fort Myer Chapel, where seating capacity was limited but where, C. J. George noted,

General Marshall had expressed a desire for the chapel's "tradition and simplicity." (George memorandum, June 9, 1959, GCMRL/Katherine Marshall Correspondence.) On September 1, Mrs. Marshall moved into an apartment at 1900 Q Street NW, about twenty minutes from the hospital, and told C. J. George that "she had no intention of ever returning to Leesburg to live." Instead, the Winns, who had already moved in, would purchase Dodona Manor. (Katherine Marshall to Bruce, September 3, 1959, ibid.; H; George to Lovett, September 2, 1959, GCMRL/G. C. Marshall Papers [Retirement, Chronological].)

The end came at 6:08 p.m. on October 16, 1959, when General of the Army George C. Marshall died of a "cerebrovascular accident due to hypertension." (Statement of Death, issued October 19, 1959, GCMRL/Xerox 2818 [GCM Family].) General Orders No. 39 announcing Marshall's death was issued on October 17 by Chief of Staff General Lyman L. Lemnitzer. (General Orders No. 39, Headquarters, Department of the Army, Washington, DC, October 17, 1959, GCMRL/G. C. Marshall Collection [Box 3, Folder 2].)

The solemn but reserved service Marshall had requested took place at Fort Myer and Arlington National Cemetery on October 20. (See p. 929 and Pogue, *Statesman*, 511–13.) In a memorial address delivered at VMI the following day, Frank McCarthy noted that "old friends, including cabinet officers, ambassadors, generals, admirals, and associates" from Marshall's "school days, his early service in China and the Philippines, and his retirement at Leesburg," as well as Sergeants Heffner and Powder, were among those invited to attend the graveside ceremony "on a gentle hillside overlooking Washington and the Potomac." (Address by Brigadier General Frank McCarthy, October 21, 1959, GCMRL/Frank McCarthy Collection [Additions].)

The day of the funeral President Truman issued a statement proclaiming Marshall "the greatest general since Robert E. Lee" and "the greatest administrator since Thomas Jefferson." Truman concluded, "I sincerely hope that when it comes my time to cross the great river that General Marshall will place me on his staff so that I may try to do for him what he did for me." (Truman statement, October 20, 1959, GCMRL/G. C. Marshall Collection [Truman].)

General Marshall's legacy endures in the accomplishments of the George C. Marshall Foundation. John C. Hagan Jr., the foundation's first president, died on November 9, 1959, less than a month after Marshall himself. In September 1959, General of the Army Omar N. Bradley had assumed the presidency, while Forrest C. Pogue remained its director; in 1987, Pogue published the fourth and final volume in his biography of Marshall. The publication of this seventh and last volume of *The Papers of George Catlett Marshall* concludes another of the original missions of the foundation. ★

Glossary

Abbreviations, Code Names, and Sources

If an abbreviation or code name is used only within one document, it is explained in brackets in the text or in a footnote.

ABMC = American Battle Monuments Commission
AEC = Atomic Energy Commission
AEF = American Expeditionary Forces
AFB = air force base
ANVIL = code name for the invasion of southern France, summer 1944 (renamed DRAGOON)
AP = Associated Press
ARC = American Red Cross
ASAF = Associated Services for the Armed Forces, Inc.
BAC = Business Advisory Council
BBC = British Broadcasting Corporation
CBS = Columbia Broadcasting System
CCC = Civilian Conservation Corps
CCPB = Civilian Components Policy Board
CCS = Combined Chiefs of Staff
CDU = Christian Democratic Union Party of Germany
CIA = Central Intelligence Agency
CINCFEC = commander-in-chief, Far East Command
CINCUNC = commander in chief, UN Command
CIS = Congressional Information Service
CNO = Chief of Naval Operations
CWM = Manuscripts and Rare Books Department, Swem Library, College of William and Mary
DDEL = Dwight D. Eisenhower Presidential Library, Abilene, Kansas
DOD = Department of Defense
DPRK = Democratic People's Republic of Korea (North Korea)
ECA = Economic Cooperation Administration
ERP = European Recovery Program
ESU = English-Speaking Union
EST = Eastern Standard Time
EXOS = Executive Office of the Secretary
FBI = Federal Bureau of Investigation
FDRL = Franklin D. Roosevelt Library, Hyde Park, NY
FEAF = Far East Air Forces
Finals = annual festivities surrounding commencement at the Virginia Military Institute
FRUS = *Foreign Relations of the United States*
FY = fiscal year
G-1 = personnel
G-2 = intelligence
G-3 = operations
G-4 = logistics
GCM = George C. Marshall
GCMRF = George C. Marshall Research Foundation, Lexington, Virginia
GCMRL = George C. Marshall Research Library, Lexington, Virginia

GPO = Government Printing Office
GS = General Services
H = document handwritten by author
HR = House Resolution
HSTL = Harry S Truman Library, Independence, Missouri
IADB = Inter-American Defense Board
ISAC = International Security Affairs Committee
JCS = Joint Chiefs of Staff
JNPR = Japanese National Police Reserve
JUSMAG = Joint US Military Advisory Group
KAMAG/KMAG = United States Military Advisory Group to the Republic of Korea
MAAG = Military Assistance Advisory Group
MATS = Military Air Transport Service
MDAP = Mutual Defense Assistance Program
MSFE = Senate Committee on Armed Services and Committee on Foreign Relations, *Hearings to Conduct an Inquiry Into the Military Situation in the Far East* (MacArthur Hearings). . . , 82d Cong., 1st sess. (Washington: GPO, 1951).
MTDP = Medium Term Defense Plan
NA = National Archives and Records Administration, Washington, DC, and College Park, MD
NATO = North Atlantic Treaty Organization
NBC = National Broadcasting Company
NCO = non-commissioned officer
NSC = National Security Council
NSRB = National Security Resources Board
OAS = Organization of American States
ODM = Office of Defense Mobilization
OPI = Office of Public Information, OSD
OSD = Office of the Secretary of Defense
OSS = Office of Strategic Services
OSU = Ohio State University, Byrd Polar Research Center Archival Program
OVERLORD = code name for the cross-channel invasion of France
POW = prisoner of war
PRC = People's Republic of China
Princeton = Princeton University Library, Seely G. Mudd Manuscript Library Department of Rare Books and Special Collections
RCA = Radio Corporation of America
RDB = Research and Development Board
RG = Record Group
ROK = Republic of Korea (South Korea)
ROTC = Reserve Officer Training Corps
SACEUR = supreme allied commander, Europe (NATO)
SACLANT = supreme allied commander, Atlantic (NATO)
SACMED = supreme allied commander, Mediterranean (NATO)
SCAP = supreme commander for the allied powers in Japan
SHAEF = Supreme Headquarters, Allied Expeditionary Force
SHAPE= Supreme Headquarters Allied Powers Europe
SPD = Social Democratic Party of Germany
SR = Senate Resolution
UDF = United Defense Fund
UMST/UMTS = universal military service and training
UMT = universal military training
UN = United Nations
USA = United States Army
USAF = United States Air Force

USAMHI = US Army Military History Institute, Carlisle Barracks, Pennsylvania
USMA = US Military Academy, West Point, New York
USN = US Navy
USNA = US Naval Academy, Annapolis, Maryland
USO = United Services Organization
USSR = Union of Soviet Socialist Republics
V-E Day = Victory in Europe Day, May 8, 1945
V-J Day = Victory over Japan Day, September 2, 1945
VFW = Veterans of Foreign Wars
VMI = Virginia Military Institute, Lexington, Virginia
WAC = Women's Army Corps
Yale = Manuscripts and Archives, Sterling Memorial Library, Yale University

Appendix

Published Congressional Testimony of George C. Marshall, 1949–51

Marshall's facility in informing and persuading Congress was an important aspect of his work from 1939 to 1951. Only selected portions of Marshall's published testimony have been reproduced in the Marshall Papers; others have not because they are widely available, the quantity is large, or the transcripts contain significant amounts of non-Marshall material. The following list includes the published proceedings of hearings at which Marshall testified before various congressional committees from October 1949 to July 1951.

The list gives the date Marshall testified, the committee before which he appeared, the title of the publication, and certain locating information. The latter includes (in parentheses) the size of the publication; the pages on which Marshall's testimony appears (e.g., GCM = pp. 597–606); the Congressional Information Service, Inc., accession number to *U.S. Congressional Committee Hearings on Microfiche* (e.g., CIS = [81]H1263-8); and the Superintendent of Documents number (e.g., Y4.Ar5/2:D36). Included in the list is Marshall's statement to the House Committee on Public Works on February 21, 1951, which because of Marshall's illness that day, was read to the committee by John D. Small.

Marshall's appearances before Congress for which testimony was not published are noted in the Marshall chronology in the front of this volume. The editors are aware of three such appearances: November 27, 1950; February 8, 1951; and June 14, 1951.

Additionally, classified portions of Marshall's testimony on May 7–12 and 14, 1951, were excluded from the *Military Situation in the Far East* hearings published that year. His unpublished testimony was declassified and released in 1975. The declassified transcripts are available in the George C. Marshall Research Library (GCMRL/Xerox 1584) and in the National Archives (RG 46, Records of the Senate Foreign Relations Committee).

1949	*81st Congress, 1st Session*
Oct. 21	HOUSE COMMITTEE ON ARMED SERVICES: *The National Defense Program—Unification and Strategy, Hearings. . . .* (v+639 pp.; GCM = pp. 597–606; CIS = [81]H1263-8; Y4.Ar5/2:D36)

1950	*81st Congress, 2d Session*
June 7	HOUSE COMMITTEE ON FOREIGN AFFAIRS: *To Amend the Mutual Defense Assistance Act of 1949, Hearings. . . .* (iii+164 pp.; GCM = pp. 85–108; CIS = [81]H1288-7; Y4.F76/1:As7/2/950)

June 7	SENATE FOREIGN RELATIONS COMMITTEE: *Executive Sessions of the Senate Foreign Relations Committee (Historical Series),* Volume II, *81st Congress, 1st and 2d Sessions, 1949–1950* (Washington: GPO, 1976), "Mutual Defense Assistance Program—Continued." (vi+840 pp.; GCM = pp. 425–35; CIS = [81]SFo-4; Y4.76/2:Ex3/2/v.2)
July 5	SENATE COMMITTEE ON FOREIGN RELATIONS, SUBCOMMITTEE: *Expanded International Information and Education Program, Hearings . . . on S. Res. 243, a Resolution Favoring an Expanded International Information and Education Program by the United States.* (iii+165 pp.; GCM = pp. 21–26; CIS = [81]S945-3; Y4.F76/2:In3/2)
Sept. 19	SENATE COMMITTEE ON ARMED SERVICES: *Nomination of General of the Army George C. Marshall to be Secretary of Defense, Hearing. . . .* (ii+25 pp.; GCM = pp. 1–25; CIS = [81]S959-7; Y4.Ar5/3:M35)
Dec. 1	HOUSE COMMITTEE ON APPROPRIATIONS, SPECIAL SUBCOMMITTEE ON NATIONAL DEFENSE APPROPRIATIONS: *Second Supplemental Appropriation Bill for 1951, Hearings. . . .* (ii+350 pp.; GCM = pp. 15–37; CIS = [81]H1309-3-A; Y4.Ap6/1:Ap6/2/951-3/pt.1)
Dec. 9, 11	SENATE COMMITTEE ON APPROPRIATIONS: *Second Supplemental Appropriation Bill, 1951, Hearings. . . .* (ii+405 pp.; GCM = pp. 1–31, 43–58; CIS = [81]S958-6; Y4.Ap6/2:Ap6/2/951-3)
1951	*82d Congress, 1st Session*
Jan. 10	SENATE COMMITTEE ON ARMED SERVICES, PREPAREDNESS SUBCOMMITTEE: *Universal Military Training and Service Act of 1951, Hearings . . . on S. 1, A Bill to Provide for the Common Defense and Security of the United States and to Permit the More Effective Utilization of Manpower Resources of the United States by Authorizing Universal Military Service and Training. . . .* (xix+1243 pp.; GCM = pp. 25–37; CIS = [82]S960-9; Y4.Ar5/3:M59/6)
Jan. 23, Mar. 1	HOUSE COMMITTEE ON ARMED SERVICES: *Universal Military Training, Hearings . . . on H.R. 1752, A Bill to Provide for the Common Defense and Security of the United States and to Permit the More Effective Utilization of Manpower Resources of the United States by Authorizing Universal Military Service and Training. . . .* (969 pp.; GCM = pp. 8–42, 436–40; CIS = [82]H1453-0.4; Y4.Ar5/2a:951-52/4)
Feb. 15	SENATE COMMITTEE ON FOREIGN RELATIONS AND COMMITTEE ON ARMED SERVICES: *Assignment of Ground Forces of the United States to Duty in the European Area, Hearings . . . on S. Con. Res. 8, . . .* (iv+819 pp.; GCM = pp. 38–75; CIS = [82]S963-7; Y4.F76/2:G91)
Feb. 21	HOUSE COMMITTEE ON PUBLIC WORKS: *St. Lawrence Seaway, Hearings . . . on H.J. Res. 2, H.J. Res. 3, H.J. Res. 4, H.J. Res. 15, H.J. Res. 102, H.J. Res. 122, H.J. Res. 159, and H.R. 2536, Approving the Agreement between the United States and Canada relating to the Development of the Resources of the Great Lakes–St. Lawrence Basin for National Security and Continental Defense of the United States and Canada; Providing for Making the St. Lawrence Seaway Self-Liquidating; . . .* (vi+630 pp.; GCM = p. 62; CIS = [82]H1325-2A; Y4.P96/11.82/2)

May 7–12, May 14	SENATE COMMITTEE ON ARMED SERVICES AND COMMITTEE ON FOREIGN RELATIONS: *Military Situation in the Far East, Hearings . . . to Conduct an Inquiry into the Military Situation in the Far East and the Facts Surrounding the Relief of General of the Army Douglas MacArthur from his Assignments in That Area.* (iii+3691 pp.; GCM = 321–724; CIS = [82]S985-1-A; Y4.Ar5/3:M59/7/pt.1)
May 29	SENATE COMMITTEE ON BANKING AND CURRENCY: *Defense Production Act Amendments of 1951, Hearings . . . on S. 1397, A Bill to Amend the Defense Production Act of 1950 . . . , Part 1.* (vi+1079 pp.; GCM = pp. 787–828; CIS = [82]S969- 0-A); Y4.B22/3:D36/2/pt.1)
June 29, July 2	HOUSE COMMITTEE ON FOREIGN AFFAIRS: *The Mutual Security Program, Hearings . . . on (H.R. 5020 and H.R. 5113). . . .* (xi+1600 pp.; GCM = pp. 81–124; CIS = [82]H1332-4; Y4.F76/1:M98)
July 18	HOUSE COMMITTEE ON APPROPRIATIONS, SUBCOMMITTEE ON DEPARTMENT OF DEFENSE APPROPRIATIONS: *Department of Defense Appropriations for 1952, Hearings . . . Part 1. . . .* (ii+261+iii pp.; GCM = pp. 195–203; CIS = [82]H1334-3-A; Y4.Ap6/1:D36/5/952/pt.1)
July 27	SENATE COMMITTEE ON FOREIGN RELATIONS AND COMMITTEE ON ARMED SERVICES: *Mutual Security Act of 1951, Hearings . . . on S. 1762, A Bill to Promote the Foreign Policy and Provide for the Defense and General Welfare of the United States by Furnishing Assistance to Friendly Nations in the Interest of International Security.* (iv+801 pp.; GCM = pp. 35–68; CIS = [82] S983-4; Y4.F76/2:M98/2)

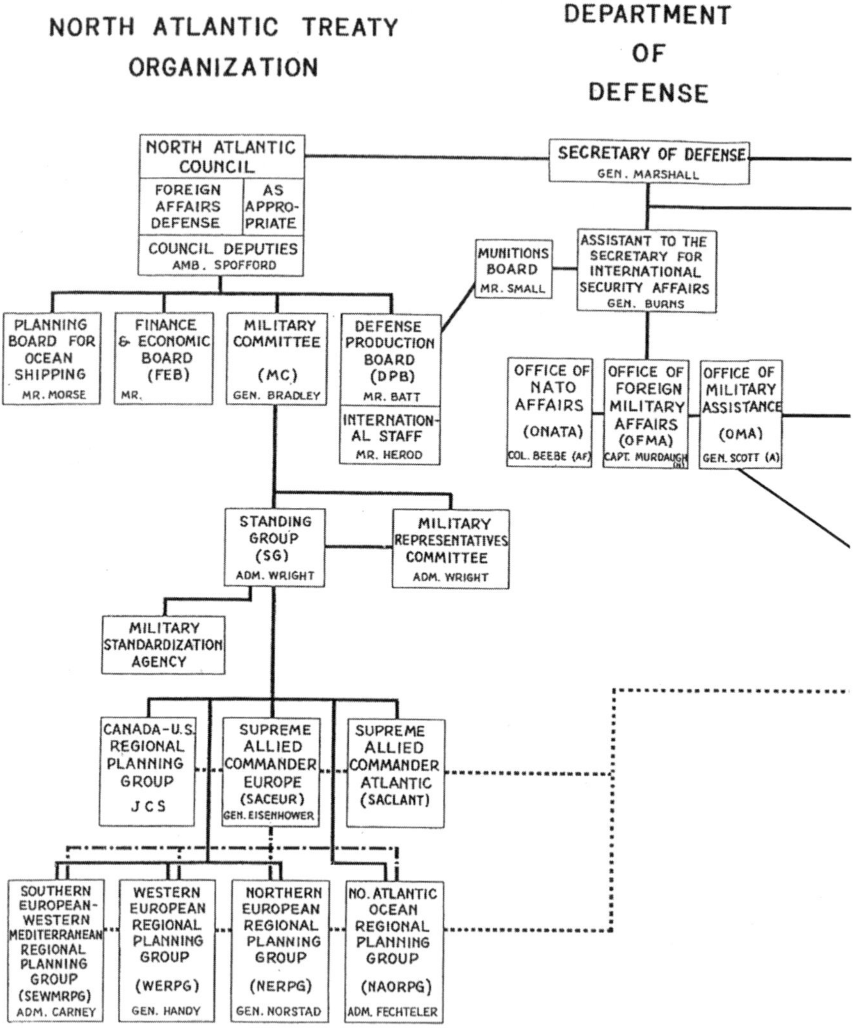

Source: NA/RG 330, CD 091.3 (MDAP, Gen.)

INTERNATIONAL SECURITY AFFAIRS ORGANIZATION

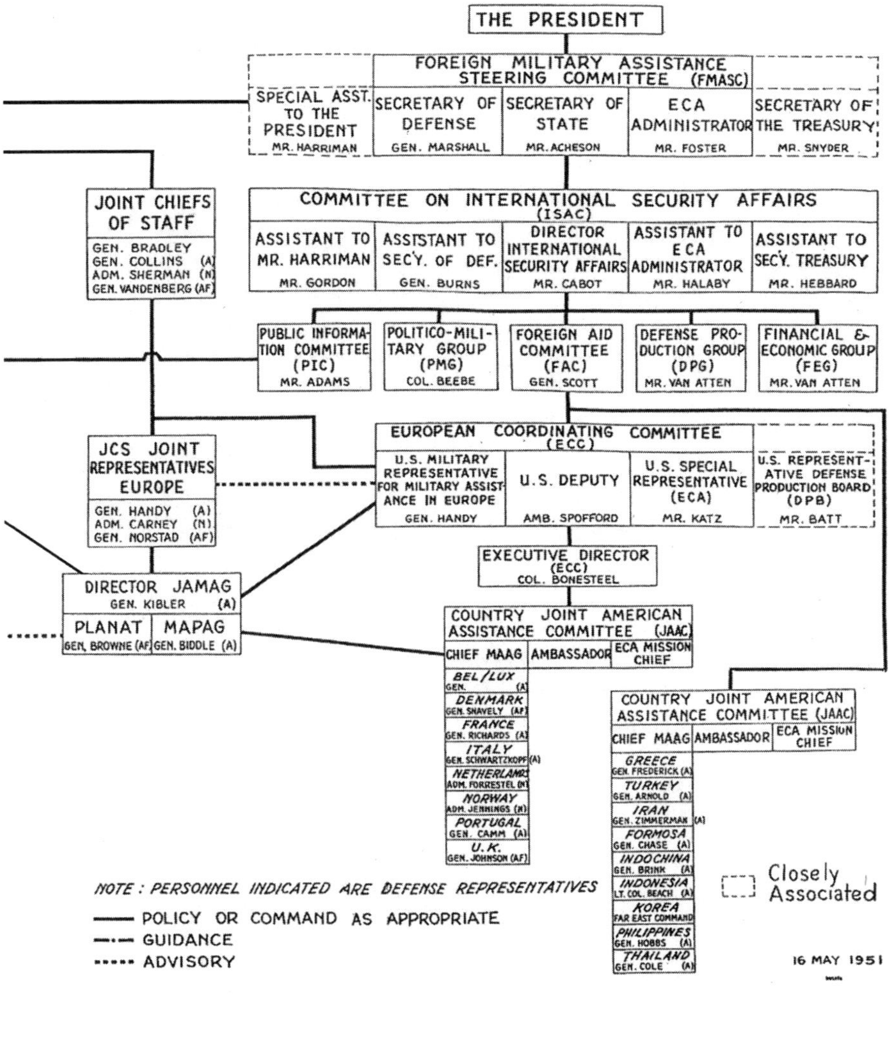

OFFICE OF THE SECRETARY OF DEFENSE

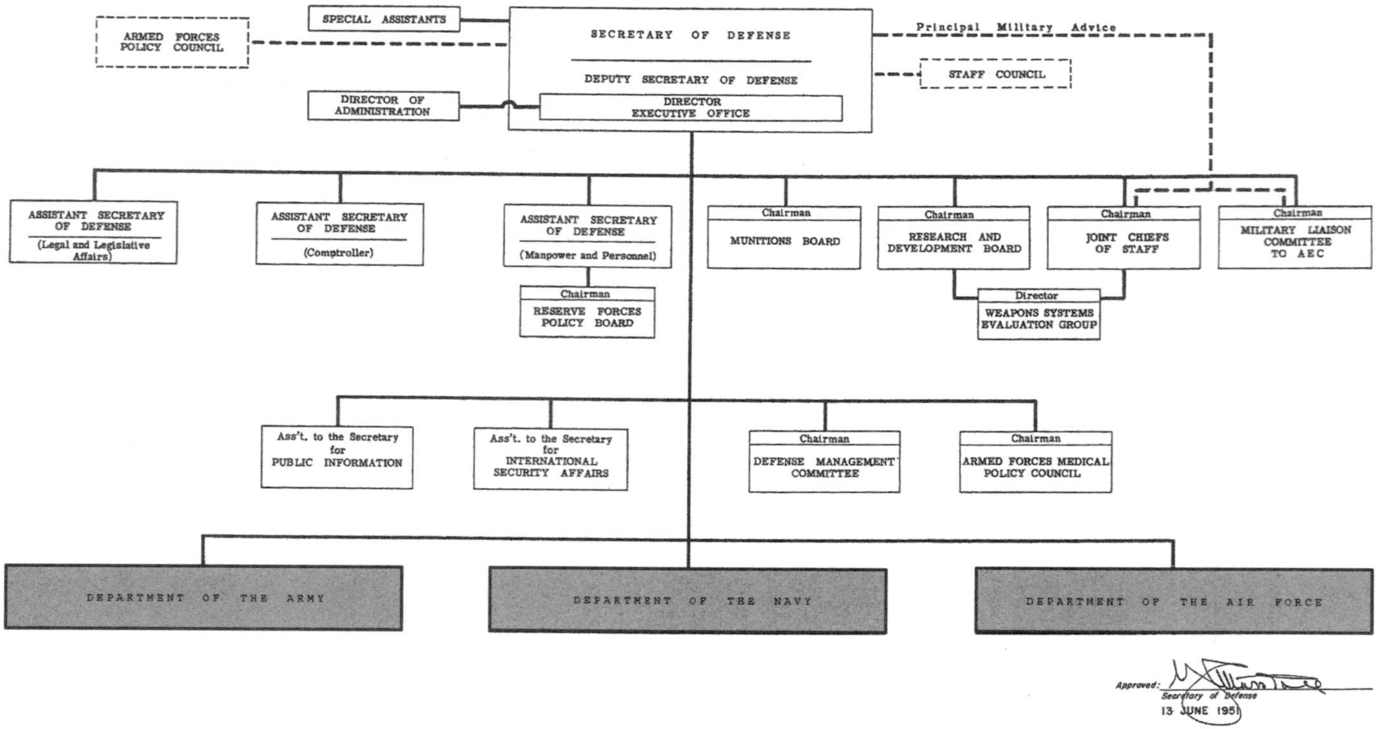

Source: GCMRL/Marshall S. Carter Papers (Department of Defense, Director, Executive Office of the Secretary of Defense, 1951–1970)

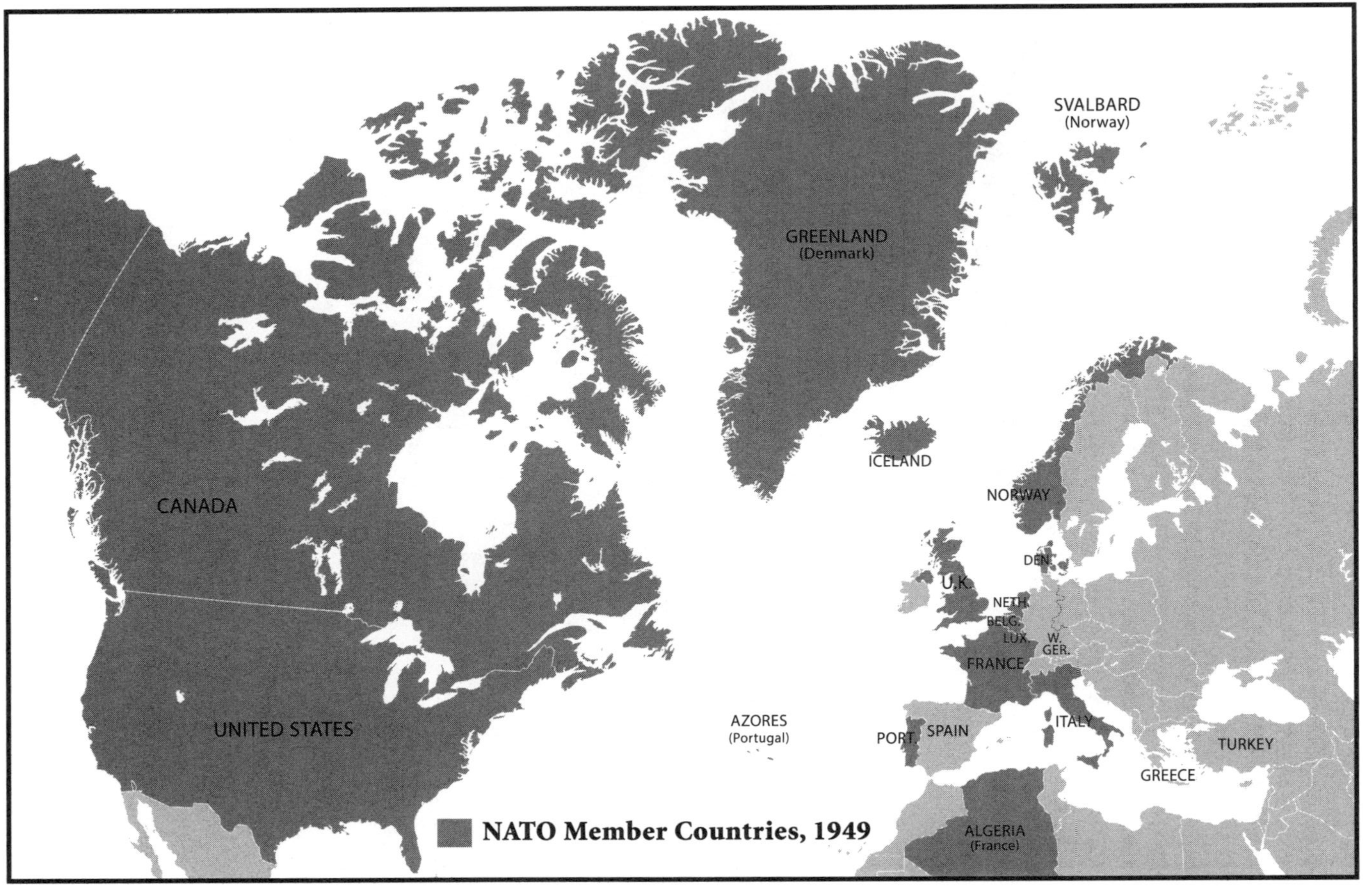

NATO Member Countries, 1949
SVALBARD
(Norway)
GREENLAND
(Denmark)
ICELAND
CANADA
UNITED STATES
AZORES
(Portugal)
NORWAY
DEN.
U.K.
NETH.
BELG.
LUX.
W.
GER.
FRANCE
PORT.
SPAIN
ITALY
GREECE
TURKEY
ALGERIA
(France)

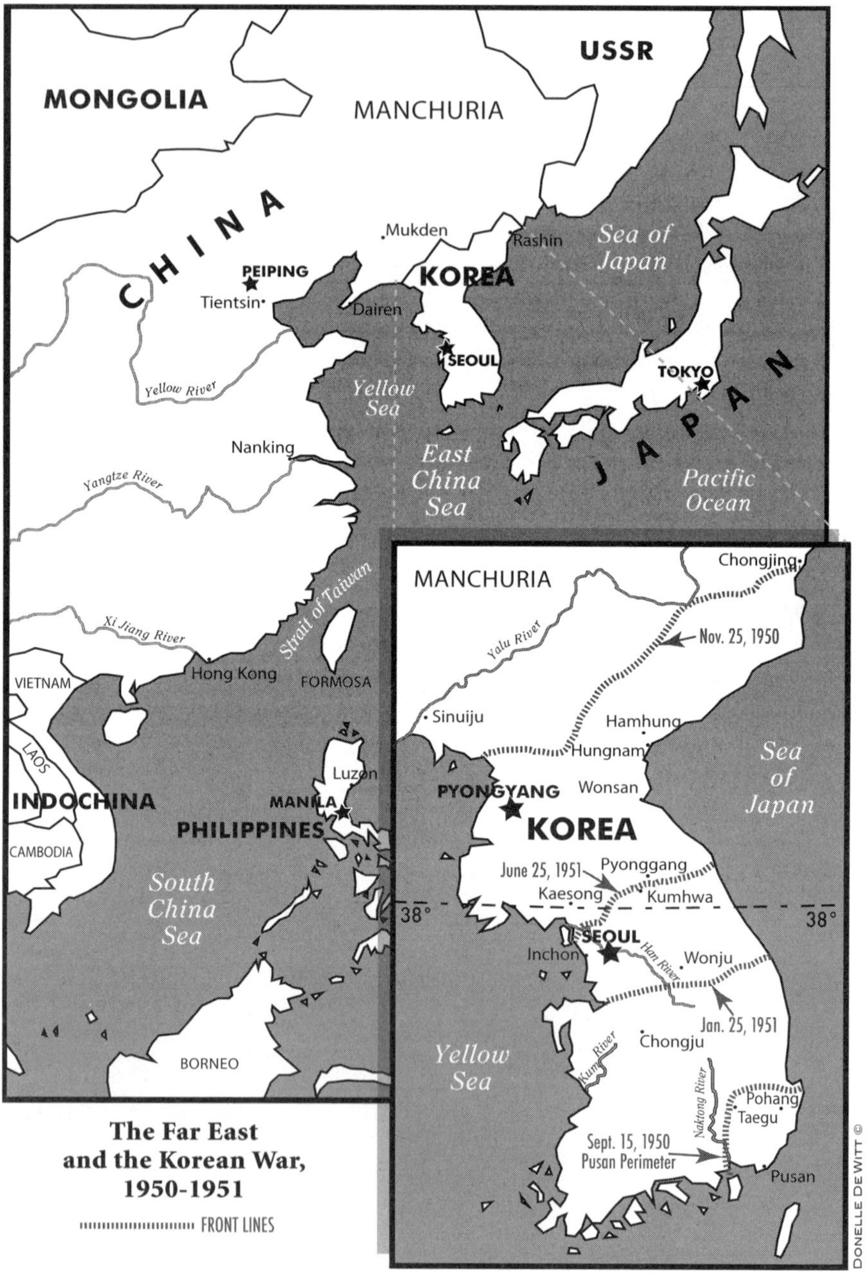

The Far East and the Korean War, 1950-1951

FRONT LINES

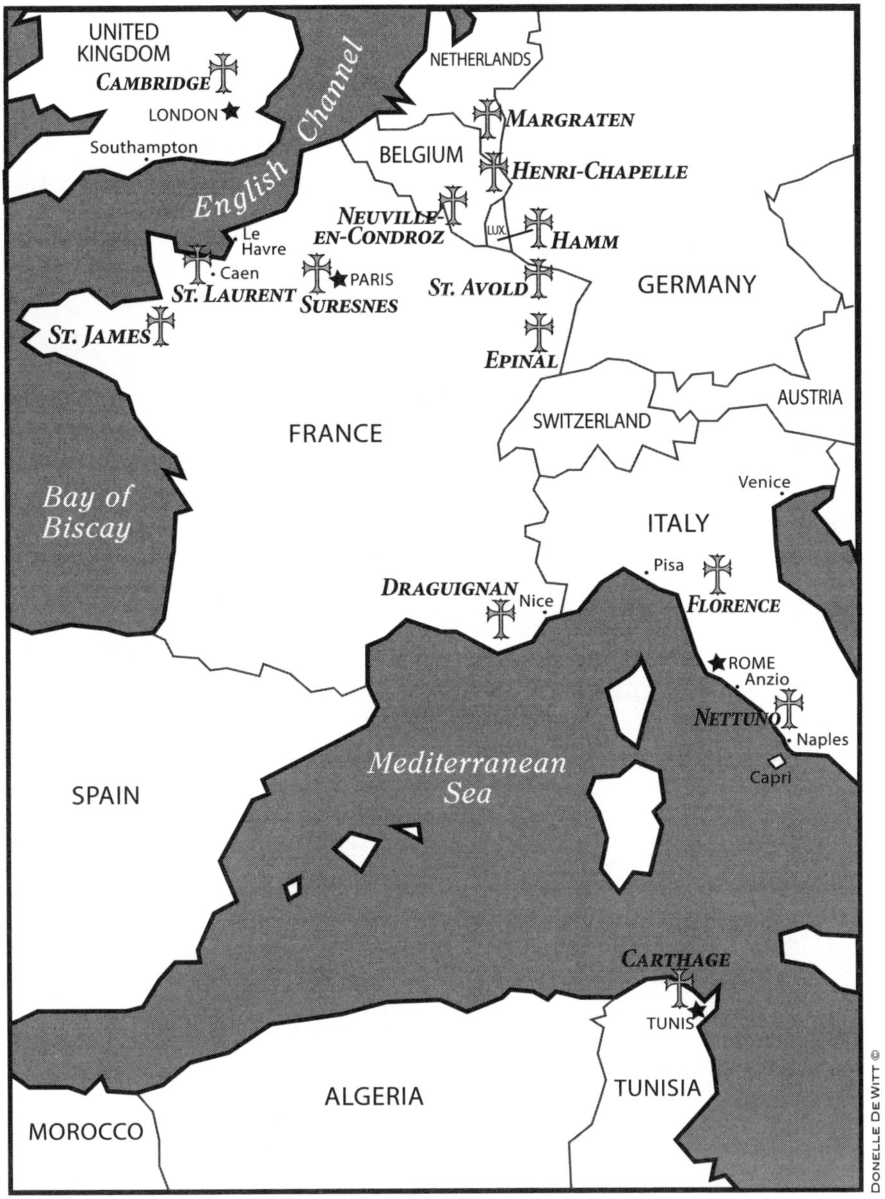

ABMC Cemeteries Visited by Marshall, September 10–October 7, 1952

Index